THIRD EDITION

HIV and the Pathogenesis of AIDS

THIRD EDITION

HIV and the Pathogenesis of AIDS

Jay A. Levy

Department of Medicine, Laboratory for Tumor and
AIDS Virus Research and Cancer Research Institute
University of California, School of Medicine
San Francisco, California

ASM
PRESS

WASHINGTON, D.C.

Address editorial correspondence to ASM Press, 1752 N St. NW,
Washington, DC 20036-2904, USA

Send orders to ASM Press, P.O. Box 605, Herndon, VA 20172, USA
Phone: (800) 546-2416 or (703) 661-1593
Fax: (703) 661-1501
E-mail: books@asmusa.org
Online: estore.asm.org

Library of Congress Cataloging-in-Publication Data

Levy, Jay A.
   HIV and the pathogenesis of AIDS / Jay A. Levy. — 3rd ed.
      p. ; cm.
   Includes bibliographical references and index.
   ISBN-13: 978-1-55581-393-2 (alk. paper)
   ISBN-10: 1-55581-393-3 (alk. paper)
   1. HIV (Viruses) 2. HIV infections—Pathogenesis.   I. Title.
   [DNLM: 1. HIV Infections—etiology.   2. HIV Infections—phys-
iopathology.   3. Acquired Immunodeficiency Syndrome—etiology.
4. Acquired Immunodeficiency Syndrome—physiopathology.
5. HIV. WC 503.3 L668h 2007]

   QR201.A37L48 2007
   616.97′9207—dc22

                                        2006100552

10 9 8 7 6 5 4 3 2 1

Cover: "The Cell #4," painting by George Habergritz. Photo by Keiko Banks.

To Sharon, for her continual support and encouragement.

Contents

Preface

It hardly seems possible that nearly 10 years have passed since the second edition of this book was written. It is fitting to complete this third edition on the 25th anniversary of the recognition of AIDS in the world (1576). It has been quite a task, but also a pleasure, to cover the past decade of scientific articles in many different areas of HIV/AIDS research and to select those that have contributed the most notable new information to the field. Most of the new knowledge has added incrementally to the past information that was established in the first 15 years of research on this major human epidemic and was covered in the second edition. For this reason, several of the early quite definitive original articles in each topic remain cited in the book, but subsequent articles confirming the findings without adding much new information were deleted. They can be found in the first or second editions of this book.

New knowledge in basic and clinical research, as well as epidemiology and social science, has helped improve our understanding of HIV/AIDS and has provided novel approaches in prevention and treatment. The most recent contributions to these fields are cited in each chapter. Features of AIDS pathogenesis, including aspects of the HIV-1 and HIV-2 isolates involved; the cells infected; the consequences of this infection; and the host immune response to HIV are discussed in this book. Moreover, potential approaches for therapy and a vaccine for the prevention of HIV infection and AIDS are considered. Because of the interactions among the various chapters, readers are directed in the text to various sections in the book that cover the topic in greater detail. As an example, R5 and X4 subtypes are introduced very early in the book, before their definition in the text (Chapter 4). The term HIV is used generically to indicate observations with HIV-1 and HIV-2.

The Pioneers in HIV Research cited in the book are individuals who were actively involved in HIV research from the early 1980s (1981-83) and who continued to contribute to the field. Many of them have served as mentors to a large number of currently active HIV/AIDS investigators.

Among the major additions to our knowledge of HIV over the past decade has been the elucidation of intracellular controls of HIV replication that have been identified by genetic studies. APOBEC3G and TRIM5a, which block HIV replication, provide approaches for novel antiviral therapies (Chapter 5). The identification of genetic markers for susceptibility to HIV infection and determinants of the clinical course has been greatly expanded (Chapter 13). Moreover, for therapy, the development of decoys for cell surface proteins, including chemokine coreceptors used for entry, has resulted in an emphasis on entry inhibitors along with virus fusion inhibitors that can serve as new targets for the anti-HIV drug armentarium (Chapter 14).

Clinical trials have clarified to some extent what drugs to use in initiating therapy and take into consideration the potential toxicities of the treatments. In many cases, protease inhibitors are now avoided because of the clinical disorders particularly linked to these drugs. The use of combination therapy with one pill taken once daily has certainly enhanced the adherence of individuals on drug therapy and hopefully will limit development of virus resistance (Chapter 14). In this regard, the timing for the initiation of drug administration in chronically infected people is now better appreciated. The threshold for beginning highly active antiretroviral therapy (HAART) has been raised so that individuals who are healthy but have $CD4^+$ cell counts of >250 cells/ml may not need therapy; viral loads are not as important in the decision for treatment (see Table 14.3). At the same time, the initiation of therapy in primary infection still requires further evaluation. Some results have suggested that treatment prior to seroconversion can be of clinical benefit to the HIV-infected individual (Chapters 4 and 14). Currently, ongoing studies are evaluating if and when one could stop HAART (i.e., structured treatment interruption [STI]) and permit the patient to be treatment-free for a while. STI for chronic infection has thus far not been encouraging, but in patients treated during acute infection, the procedure may be possible (Chapter 14).

Whereas 10 years ago I was surprised that viral latency was not as well researched as it had been in the first 5 years of this epidemic, more recently this topic has received further attention (Chapters 5 and 14). The interest stems from the discovery of residual virus-infected cells that remain in individuals who are on very effective anti-HIV therapy. Not surprising to those working with retroviruses, an agent like HIV, which becomes part of the genetic machinery of the cell, cannot be eliminated with the drugs currently available. Although the present anti-HIV treatments can make progeny viruses noninfectious (protease inhibitors) or not replicative competent (reverse transcriptase inhibitors), they still leave cellular reservoirs of the virus, even at low numbers, that can rebegin the infectious cycle and give rise to resistant strains (Chapter 4). Thus, approaches targeting a variety of cellular reservoirs need to be given continued attention (Chapters 5 and 14).

Also very important over the last 5 years has been the appreciation of the importance of innate immunity both as the first response to HIV (Chapter 9) and for its likely role in preventing infection in exposed seronegative individuals (Chapter 13). This arm of the immune system certainly plays a role, along with adaptive immunity, in maintaining virus control in several untreated healthy individuals infected for more than 25 years. This feature is dramatically illustrated in long-term survivors or long-term nonprogressors (Chapter 13). More knowledge of the immune system has led to further, though not sufficient, attention to immune system-based therapies, particularly using cytokines (e.g., interleukin-2 and interferon α) and dendritic cell approaches (Chapter 14).

Vaccine development has received greater emphasis over the past 10 years but has not yet revealed an approach for effective prevention of HIV transmission (Chapter 15). Completion of the first phase III trials provided important information on various legal, social, and public health issues and procedures that are needed to establish an effective vaccine trial, although they did not show efficacy. Other phase III and phase II trials are in progress, keeping this important topic in the forefront of clinical studies. Nevertheless, it is obvious to most investigators that a vaccine will not be available in the very near future. Thus, education on how to prevent the infection as well as the use of antiretroviral drugs in low-resource countries should help limit transmission (Chapter 3) and reduce the spread of the epidemic.

Other advances since 1997 that have improved our understanding of HIV pathogenesis and treatment include the following:

1. Additional HIV-1 clades have been identified in the M (main) group of HIV-1 (K and L), and clades E and I have now been recognized as recombinant viruses (Chapter 1). In addition, the O (or outlier) clade has been found to have many representatives. The past decade has also revealed a new group (N [non-M, non-O]) that has had very few isolates in human populations; they most resemble the chimpanzee isolate. Thus, HIV as a zoonotic infection has been further emphasized (Chapter 1). Importantly, HIV appears to be continually evolving perhaps with founder viruses entering human populations with specific genetic features and immune responses (Chapters 1, 7, 8, and 13).

2. Several HIV-2 isolates have been found, and more extensive classification of this subtype has been established, with five new groups (notably not clades) recognized (Chapter 1).

3. The increasing incidence of recombinant viruses indicates that dual infection and superinfection can occur (Chapter 4). Recombination brings new types of viruses to human populations. Some of these may carry resistance to anti-HIV immune responses and therapies. For that reason, this ongoing viral process must be considered in curtailing the epidemic.

4. The role of immune activation in HIV pathogenesis has received much more appreciation, particularly in its induction of cell loss by cytokine-induced apoptosis (Chapters 5 and 13).

5. The field of HIV research has helped to redefine subsets of CD4$^+$ and CD8$^+$ T cells which reflect their naïve, or memory, status, whether activated or resting (Chapters 4, 8, and 11). The varying abilities of R5 and X4 viruses to infect subsets of cells have been shown to influence the pathogenic pathway (Chapters 4 and 13). It has become evident that HIV can infect resting T cells through cytokine exposure or the nature of the particular resting cell subset. The virus infects, integrates, and then can become latent in these cells.

6. Novel new functions of viral accessory genes are now highlighted (Chapter 7). The vast number of intracellular activities seems too large to be attributed solely to each of the viral proteins, but these pleiotropic functions are impressive. Targeting these viral gene products or the cellular proteins involved in their function offers new directions for therapy.

7. As noted above, great progress has been made in identifying genetic factors that are associated with the susceptibility of individuals to infection and a clinical course, reflecting either very rapid progression or long-term survival (Chap-

ter 13). These observations give further support to the importance of both innate and adaptive immunity as targets for approaches to control HIV infection.

8. In the field of adaptive immunity, various different functioning subsets of cytotoxic T cells can now be distinguished, which helps to explain why tetramer-positive or HIV-specific CD4$^+$ and CD8$^+$ cells may be detected (e.g., by Elispot or intracellular cytokine production) but may not function as cytotoxic cells (e.g., lack perforin) (Chapters 11 and 13).

9. Some new information has been obtained in our understanding of neutralizing versus enhancing antibodies. Monoclonal antibodies with exquisite epitope selectivity have helped define regions in the viral envelope that can elicit broadly reactive humoral responses. The recognition that the removal of certain regions of the viral envelope (e.g., V2) may increase sensitivity of viruses to neutralization and help in the induction of neutralizing antibodies may provide novel approaches for vaccines (Chapter 10). Nevertheless, some broadly reactive antibodies have been found to cross-react with normal cellular proteins. Thus, how to induce virus-specific antibodies with strong neutralizing activity against a variety of diverse HIV groups and clades remains a challenge.

10. HIV neuropathogenesis has been further explored. Although new observations are limited, there is a greater acceptance of other cell types (e.g., astrocytes or oligodendrocytes) besides macrophages/microglia that can be infected by HIV and contribute to central nervous system disorders (Chapter 8).

11. The field of HIV enteropathy is better appreciated than it was 10 years ago, with the recognition of massive CD4$^+$ cell infection and destruction in the gastrointestinal tract early in infection (Chapters 4 and 8). Infection of other organs such as the kidney and the compartmentalization of viruses in various tissues (e.g. the brain or testes) where they can undergo independent evolution have been noted (Chapters 4 and 8). Thus, having an absence of detectable virus in the blood does not necessarily indicate that there is no infectious virus elsewhere in the body, particularly in the gastrointestinal tract and genital fluids (Chapters 2 and 3).

12. In HIV-related cancers (Chapter 12), greater knowledge has been gained on the viruses associated with the malignancies (e.g., KSHV/HHV8, EBV, HPV) and HAART has reduced the incidence of most of these cancers. Several important steps, from infection to tumor development, remain to be elucidated.

13. Microbicides have been emphasized for prevention of HIV infection (Chapters 2 and 3). The progress in this field has not been dramatic, although clinical trials of diaphragms to block transmission via the cervical canal may provide encouraging results. Currently, it appears that microbicides that cover the vaginal wall and prevent contact with HIV-infected cells and the free virus would be the best approach. In this way, the antiviral compounds will not induce lesions in the vaginal and anal canals that could enhance virus infection.

14. In vaccines, the use of DNA as a vaccine approach has been less encouraging because it does not induce good humoral immunity and induces only limited cellular immunity. Prime/boost approaches continue to show promise, although the use of two different modalities has not been as popular as it was several years ago (Chapter 15).

15. Within the past 3 years, a greater emphasis has been given to the development of an AIDS vaccine through funding from the Bill and Melinda Gates Foundation, the National Institutes of Health, the International Agency for Vac-

Table A Number of HIV-infected persons (2006)[a]

Country	No. of infected persons (millions)
India	6.5
South Africa	5.5
Ethiopia	4.1
Nigeria	3.6
Mozambique	1.8
Kenya	1.7
Zimbabwe	1.7
USA	1.3
Russian Federation	1.0
China	1.0

[a]Estimates based on data available at http://www.unaids.org.

cine Initiative (IAVI), and other international organizations. With this new support, one can hope for advancements and development of an effective vaccine in the very near future. In addition, further attention to the immune system and treatment strategies to harness immune responses against HIV should receive even greater emphasis.

Since 1998, the pandemic of HIV infection has continued to increase, with several additional countries (e.g., India, China, Nigeria, and Russia) experiencing the speed with which this infection can spread (Table A). The factors that are associated with the emergence and spread of the AIDS epidemic remain the same (Table B). Fears of similar large epidemics in countries such as Indonesia are surfacing. Education is the immediate approach available, and a vaccine is a vital necessity. It can be estimated that a new infection takes place in the world every 7 seconds and a death from HIV infection occurs every 10 seconds. In 1996, it was projected that by the year 2000, over 100 million individuals would be infected by HIV-1 or HIV-2 (2794). Because of the introduction of HAART, the number is now estimated to be about 40 million people infected with HIV worldwide (http://www.unaids.org) (Figure A) (Table A), and 22 million persons have died.

In the United States 40,000 new cases were reported in 2005. In 2006, 1 million people in the United States were living with HIV/AIDS (660). In the first edition of this book, 1 in 250 Americans was estimated to be infected by HIV,

Table B Factors conducive to the emergence of the AIDS epidemic

- Migration of carriers into cities – increased interpersonal contacts
- Poverty, prostitution
- International travel
- Sexual behavior
- Intravenous drug use
- Receipt of blood and blood products

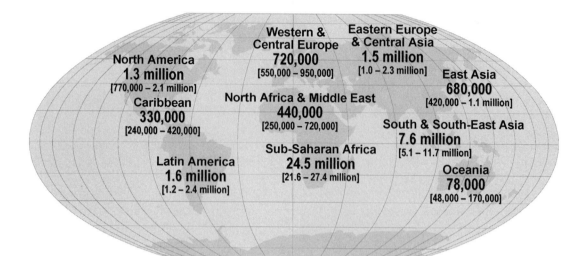

Total: 38.6 (33.4 – 46.0) million

Figure A The global HIV/AIDS epidemic. Estimated number of persons living with HIV infection or AIDS by region at the end of 2005. (Source, http://www.unaids.org; accessed 6/15/2006.)

including 1 in 100 males and 1 in 800 females. That number has not changed appreciably, indicating that either the prediction in 1993 was too high or the rate of new infections has stabilized. Nevertheless, the total number of U.S. cases of HIV infection since AIDS was recognized in 1981 has now reached nearly 2 million. More than 500,000 Americans have died from the disease. It is estimated that 275,000 people in the United States are HIV infected but have not been tested and identified. Until 1996, AIDS in the United States was the leading cause of death among young people, both male and female, between 25 and 44 years of age. Death from AIDS has now decreased because of the success of the antiviral therapies (Chapter 14). However, since 1992, non-Hispanic blacks, Hispanics, and women have accounted for increased proportions of AIDS cases. In 2005, women represented 25% of all U.S. adult cases reported. Currently, less than half of the new AIDS cases in the United States result from transmission by homosexual and bisexual men (45%) (660).

Papers published on HIV and AIDS have increased at a rapid rate. As of December 2006 (2952), a total of about 250,000 articles have been written on this subject since the initial report on AIDS in 1981 (652). The number of papers published on HIV and AIDS peaked at 19,721 in 1996. For this edition, about 5,000 have been cited.

To gain a perspective on the changes in our knowledge of HIV/AIDS and emphasis in research, readers are recommended to read the Prefaces to the first and second editions of this text. Criteria for AIDS as defined by the Centers for Disease Control are found in Appendices I and IV. The well-known relationship of CD4$^+$ cell number to the risk of opportunistic infections and cancer is shown in Appendix V. The research conducted by my co-workers and myself was supported by grants from the National Institutes of Health, the California State

Universitywide Task Force on AIDS, the American Foundation for AIDS Research, the Campbell Foundation, and the James B. Pendleton Charitable Trust. In addition to my gratitude to those who provided helpful suggestions and advice on the initial text in *Microbiological Reviews* and the other editions of this book, I want to thank the following individuals for their assistance with the present edition: Lena Al-Harthi, Marcus Altfeld, Brigitte Autran, Edward Barker, David Blackbourn, Susan Buchbinder, Rick Bushman, Dennis Burton, Michael Busch, Andrew Carr, Mary Carrington, Cecilia Cheng-Mayer, Mario Clerici, Deborah Cohan, Suzanne Crowe, Tony Cunningham, Andrew Davison, Steven Deeks, Lisa Demeter, Josef Eberle, Lawrence Fong, Donald Forthal, Donald Francis, Robert Garry, Stephen Goff, Marie-Lise Gougeon, Carl Grunfeld, Phalguni Gupta, Ashley Haase, Beatrice Hahn, Marc Hellerstein, Walid Heneine, James Hoxie, Shiu-lok Hu, Rachel Kaplan, Paul Klotman, Bette Korber, Donald Kotler, Alan Landay, Nathaniel Landau, Michael Lederman, Alexandra Levine, Paul Luciw, Francine McCutchan, Preston Marx, Susan Moir, Laura Napolitano, Philip Norris, Jorge Oksenberg, Nancy Padian, Joel Palefsky, Tristram Parslow, David Pauza, Matija Peterlin, John Phair, Vicente Planelles, Lynn Pulliam, Jacqueline Reeves, Edward Robinson, Mario Roederer, Robert Seder, Haynes Sheppard, Robert Siliciano, Gregory Spear, Leonidas Stamatatos, Ralph Steinman, Jeffrey Ulmer, Eric Verdin, Robert Winchester, and John Zaunders. I thank Julie Winters and Pamela Lacey for their help in editing and production, Krista Preckel for her assistance, Ann Murai for her excellent help with the manuscript, and particularly Kaylynn Peter for her close attention and overall handling of this book.

I hope this newly revised text will continue to be a helpful resource for researchers, clinicians, health care providers and students, who are all part of the important group dedicated to finding a solution to this devastating epidemic.

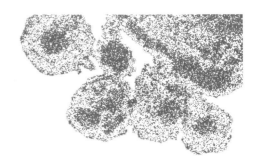

Discovery, Structure, Heterogeneity, and Origins of HIV

1

Discovery of the AIDS Viruses
The HIV Virion
Virus Heterogeneity
Origin of HIV

THE HUMAN IMMUNODEFICIENCY VIRUS (HIV) is a member of the genus *Lentivirus* in the *Retroviridae* family. Retroviruses are so called because their RNA genome is transcribed into a DNA within the cell using the viral enzyme reverse transcriptase (RT). This DNA then enters the nucleus and integrates into the cellular chromosome (see Chapter 3). Retroviruses were first recognized as the cause of leukemias and lymphomas in birds and rodents; these types of viruses form different genera (formerly known as the *Oncovirinae*) of this virus family (827) (see http://www.ncbi.nlm.nih.gov/ICTVdb/index.htm).

Lentiviruses consist of a diverse group of animal viruses (Table 1.1) (827, 1683, 2514). The human counterpart, HIV, was discovered because of its association with the acquired immune deficiency syndrome (AIDS) (1577). This clinical condition is characterized by a marked reduction in CD4$^+$ cells and the development of opportunistic infections and cancers (Tables 1.2 and 1.3). These conditions result from the persistent replication and spread of HIV (see Preface).

Ironically, one of the first viruses identified in nature was a lentivirus, the equine infectious anemia virus, discovered in 1904 (4541). It induces episodic autoimmune hemolytic anemia in horses, with devastating effects on the equine population in many parts of the world, particularly Japan. This agent, although initially demonstrating some characteristics of a retrovirus (2512), was only later identified as an RNA virus containing RT and a member of the lentivirus genus (695). Similarly, lentiviruses of sheep (visna/maedi virus) and goats (caprine arthritis-encephalitis virus) have been known for many years to be associated with a long illness and clinical symptoms not generally characteristic of retrovirus infection (703, 916, 1683, 2514).

Table 1.1 Lentiviruses

Virus	Host infected	Primary cell type infected	Major clinical disorder
Equine infectious anemia virus	Horse	Macrophages	Cyclical infection in the first year, autoimmune hemolytic anemia, sometimes encephalopathy
Visna/maedi virus	Sheep	Macrophages	Encephalopathy/pneumonitis
Caprine arthritis-encephalitis virus	Goat	Macrophages	Immune deficiency, arthritis, encephalopathy
Bovine immune deficiency virus	Cow	Macrophages	Lymphadenopathy, lymphocytosis, central nervous system disease (?)
Feline immunodeficiency virus	Cat	T lymphocytes	Immune deficiency, encephalopathy
Simian immunodeficiency virus	Primate	T lymphocytes	Immune deficiency and encephalopathy
Human immunodeficiency virus	Human	T lymphocytes	Immune deficiency, encephalopathy, and enteropathy

Instead of malignancies, they can cause pathological entities such as autoimmunity, pneumonitis, and brain and joint disorders (Table 1.1 and 1.3).

In this chapter, the discovery of HIV type 1 (HIV-1) and HIV-2, their structural and genetic features, and their classification and proposed origin are discussed.

I. Discovery of the AIDS Viruses

A. HIV-1

If, in hindsight, AIDS researchers had looked for an agent that would cause first an immune disorder in humans and later neurologic syndromes, certainly a lentivirus would have emerged as a prime candidate. Instead, in the early 1980s, the search for the cause of AIDS focused on a variety of viruses,

Table 1.2 Average CD4⁺ cell count at diagnosis of an AIDS-defining condition[a]

Opportunistic infection	CD4⁺ cell count/µl
Non-Hodgkin's lymphoma	240
Primary cerebral lymphoma	<50
Kaposi's sarcoma	220
Pneumocystis jiroveci pneumonia[b]	120
Toxoplasmic encephalitis	98
Cryptococcal meningitis	73
Mycobacterium avium complex infection	<50
Cytomegalovirus retinitis	<50

[a]Reprinted from reference 2824 with permission.
[b]Formerly *P. carinii* (1509).

including retroviruses, but also parvoviruses and herpesviruses, which are known to cause immune deficiency (3283, 3819). Even after HIV was discovered, its classification as a lentivirus took a year (Table 1.3) (754, 1559, 2541, 3649).

The first indication that AIDS could be caused by a retrovirus came in 1983, when Barré-Sinoussi and associates at the Pasteur Institute (272) recovered a virus containing RT activity from the lymph node of a man with persistent generalized lymphadenopathy (PGL). At the time, some physicians suspected that this syndrome was associated with AIDS (12), but there was no conclusive evidence. Since enlarged lymph nodes are observed during several viral infections, many clinicians believed initially that PGL resulted from infection with a known human virus such as Epstein-Barr virus or cytomegalovirus. In addition, the characteristics described for the retrovirus recovered by the Pasteur Institute group (272) included some that were reported for the human T-cell leukemia virus (HTLV) (for a review, see reference 4327). Thus, most investigators believed initially that the lymph node isolate was a member of this already recognized human retrovirus group. This conclusion was influenced by the concomitant publication in the same issue of *Science* that HTLV was isolated from AIDS patients (1421).

The possibility that HTLV was the etiologic agent of AIDS, however, seemed unlikely because of its low-level replication in cells and its close association with the cell membrane (3035, 3547,

Table 1.3 Characteristics common to lentiviruses

Clinical
- Association with a disease with a long incubation period
- Association with immune deficiency
- Involvement of hematopoietic system
- Involvement of the central nervous system
- Association with arthritis and autoimmunity

Biological
- Host species specific
- Exogenous and nononcogenic
- Cytopathic effect in certain infected cells, e.g., syncytia (multinucleated cells)
- Infection of macrophages—usually noncytopathic
- Accumulation of unintegrated circular and linear forms of viral cDNA in infected cells
- Latent or persistent infection in some infected cells
- Morphology of virus particle by electron microscopy: cone-shaped nucleoid

Molecular
- Large genome (≥9 kb)
- Truncated *gag* gene: several processed Gag proteins
- Envelope gene is highly glycosylated
- Polymorphism, particularly in the envelope region
- Novel central open reading frame in the viral genome that separates the *pol* and *env* regions

4327). Since AIDS had been reported for hemophiliacs (653), how could this type of virus be transmitted by cell-free plasma products such as factor VIII? HTLV is rarely found as a free virion in the blood. Moreover, HTLV does not kill lymphocytes; it often immortalizes them into continuous growth (3547, 4327). Thus, the characteristic loss of CD4$^+$ lymphocytes in AIDS patients (1576, 3008, 4246) could not be explained by an HTLV infection (Table 1.4).

Table 1.4 Comparison of HIV and HTLV[a]

Parameter	HIV	HTLV
Retrovirus genus	Lentivirus	HTLV/BLV
Genome size (kb)	9.8	8.5
Core morphology	Cone	Cuboid
Accessory genes	6	2
Infects CD4$^+$ lymphocytes	++	++
Infects CD8$^+$ lymphocytes	−	++
Wide tissue tropism	+	+
Causes syncytium formation	++	+
Cytotoxic	++	−
Transforms cells	−	++[b]
Replicates to high titers	++	−
Mostly cell associated	−	++
Can exist in a latent state	+	+
Associated with immune deficiency	++	+
Associated with neurologic disorders	++	++[c]

[a]Plus signs indicate the relative presence of each characteristic.
[b]T-cell leukemia.
[c]Tropical spastic paresis.

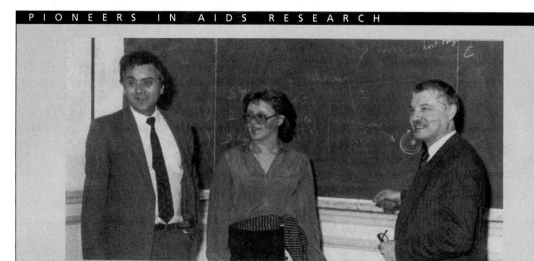

Jean Claude Chermann, Françoise Barré-Sinoussi, and Luc Montagnier (left to right)

Dr. Montagnier (co-founder of the World Foundation for AIDS Research and Prevention and co-director of the Program for International Viral Collaboration, Director of Research at the National Center for Scientific Research [CNRS] of France),

Dr. Chermann (Chief Scientific Director of Urrma Biopharma based in Montreal, Canada, and Research & Development Director of URRMA R&D, Aubagne, France), and Dr. Barré-Sinoussi (Director of the Regulation of Retroviral Infections Unit, Pasteur Institute, Paris) were the first to isolate HIV. The virus was recovered from an individual with lymphadenopathy syndrome. Originally called LAV (lymphadenopathy-associated virus), the virus proved to be the cause of AIDS.

Further studies by Montagnier and coworkers (3059) clarified these questions in relation to the PGL agent. Their results indicated that this human retrovirus, although similar to HTLV in infecting CD4+ lymphocytes, had quite distinct properties. Their virus, later called lymphadenopathy-associated virus (LAV), grew to substantial titer in CD4+ cells and killed them, instead of establishing the cells in continuous culture as is characteristic of HTLV. These observations on LAV provided important evidence supporting the potential etiologic role of a retrovirus in AIDS.

Several other laboratories were also searching for the agent responsible for this immune deficiency syndrome. In early 1984, Gallo and associates reported the characterization of another human retrovirus distinct from HTLV that they called HTLV-III (1420, 3580, 3922, 4009). It was isolated from the peripheral blood mononuclear cells (PBMC) of adult and pediatric AIDS patients. These researchers noted the lymphotropic and cytopathic

properties of the virus and reported that HTLV-III cross-reacted with some proteins of HTLV-I and HTLV-II, particularly the core p24 protein (1420). Thus, they believed it merited inclusion in the HTLV group, even though their newly isolated virus was cytopathic and did not induce an established cell line from infected lymphocytes.

Levy and coworkers (2537) at the same time reported the identification of retroviruses they named the AIDS-associated retroviruses (ARVs). These viruses were recovered from AIDS patients from different known risk groups, as well as from symptomatic and some healthy people. Finding ARV in asymptomatic individuals indicated for the first time a healthy carrier state for the AIDS virus. ARVs showed some cross-reactivity with the French LAV isolate when examined by immunofluorescence techniques (2537). Moreover, they grew substantially in PBMCs, killed CD4+ lymphocytes, and did not immortalize them. Thus, the three newly identified retroviruses had similar characteristics. Most

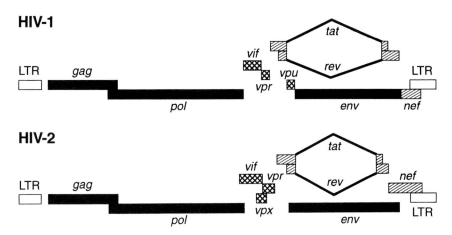

Figure 1.1 Genomic maps of HIV-1 and HIV-2. Note the unique presence of Vpu in HIV-1 and Vpx in HIV-2. Reprinted from reference 2518 with permission. Copyright © 1989, American Medical Association. All rights reserved.

importantly, infection by these viruses, as described in 1984, was not limited to AIDS patients. The viruses were also recovered from healthy individuals as well as those with other clinical conditions, including lymphadenopathy. The last observation supported the conclusion that PGL was part of the disease syndrome.

Within a short time, the three prototype viruses (LAV, HTLV-III, and ARV) were recognized as members of the same group of retroviruses, and their properties identified them as lentiviruses (Table 1.3). Their proteins were all distinct from those of HTLV; their genomes showed only remote similarities to the genome of HTLV, no more than that of chicken retroviruses (3649). Thus, the initial cross-reactivity of HTLV-III with HTLV proved incorrect. The AIDS viruses had many properties distinguishing them from HTLV (Table 1.4). For all these reasons, in 1986 the International Committee on Taxonomy of Viruses recommended giving the AIDS virus its separate name, HIV (826).

In several studies, the HTLV-III isolate was confirmed to be the same virus as the LAV isolate (683, 738, 1665). The Pasteur Institute group had sent LAV to the National Institutes of Health (NIH), where it appears to have contaminated a culture in the NIH laboratory (683, 1705). This occurrence explains the unique molecular similarities between HTLV-III and LAV, in contrast to the sequence diversities observed with ARV-2 (now called HIV-1$_{SF2}$) and other strains (306, 542, 2541, 3156, 3673, 3908,

4651). Ironically, the French agent (LAV) also was a contaminant in culture. At first considered an isolate from one patient (BRU), it was found to originate from a different individual (LAI). The LAI isolate overgrew the BRU virus in a presumed mixed culture (683, 4652). Thus, HIV-1$_{LAI}$ is another name for the LAV/BRU and HTLV-III isolates.

HIV isolates were subsequently recovered from the blood of many patients with AIDS, AIDS-related complex, and neurologic syndromes, as well as from the PBMCs of several clinically healthy individuals (2550, 2551, 3888). Thus, the widespread transmission of this agent was appreciated, and its close association with AIDS and related illnesses strongly supported its role in these diseases. Soon after the discovery of HIV-1, a separate subtype, HIV-2, was identified in West Africa (792). Both HIV subtypes can lead to AIDS, although the pathogenic course of HIV-2 appears to be longer (see below).

It is now known that some HIV-1-infected individuals can remain asymptomatic for up to 28 years and still have virus recoverable from their PBMCs (259, 545, 2520, 2597, 3849) (see Chapter 13). Also noteworthy for these "long-term survivors," or "long-term nonprogressors" (606, 2520, 3416), is the relative stability of the CD4$^+$ cell numbers, which remain in the normal range, in contrast to the reduced CD4$^+$ cells observed with HIV-induced disease (see Chapter 13). The factors in HIV infection that influence this resistance to progression to AIDS are a major topic of this book.

B. HIV-2

1. DISCOVERY AND CHARACTERISTICS

Shortly after the identification of HIV-1, a second AIDS virus was recovered in Portugal from AIDS patients from West Africa, particularly the Cape Verde Islands and Senegal (792). This virus, as determined by cloning and sequence analysis, differed by more than 55% from the previous HIV-1 strains isolated and was antigenically distinct. Thus, it was designated a new type of HIV (792, 826, 1678) (Figure 1.1). Other HIV-2 isolates were subsequently recovered from individuals from Guinea Bissau, The Gambia, and Ivory Coast (52, 638, 1232, 2271, 2338). The genome of HIV-2 is very similar to that of HIV-1 except for the absence of *vpu* and the presence of *vpx*; *vpx* appears to be a duplication of *vpr* (4475).

The major serologic difference between HIV-2 and HIV-1 isolates resides in the envelope glycoproteins (Figure 1.2). Antibodies to HIV-2 will generally cross-react with the Gag and Pol proteins of HIV-1 but might not detect HIV-1 envelope proteins and vice versa (793, 1535). For this reason, blood banks are required to use assays to detect both HIV-1 and HIV-2 proteins (3304) (see Chapters 2 and 4). Sera from some individuals from Africa have reacted with both HIV-1 and HIV-2 proteins, suggesting cross-reactivity or dual infection. In certain cases, infection by both types of virus was documented (1232, 1491, 3456, 3677). No effect of HIV-2 on HIV-1 replication or subsequent survival has been noted (50) (see below).

HIV-2 glycoproteins appear to cross-react serologically with envelope proteins from isolates of simian immunodeficiency virus (SIV) (793) (Figure 1.2), a complex group of primate lentiviruses (29). Since antibodies to SIV and HIV-2 cross-react and their sequences are similar, many investigators believe that HIV-2 was derived from SIV sometime in the near distant past (Section IV.C) (1192, 1845, 2851) (for a review, see reference 3684).

2. EPIDEMIOLOGY OF HIV-2 INFECTION

HIV-2 isolates have been recovered from patients in several parts of Africa, primarily in the western region. They have been detected in individuals in Europe, the United States, and South America (3304, 4717). HIV-2 infections have been increasing rapidly in India (2794) (UNAIDS website [http://www.unaids.org]). In the United States, as

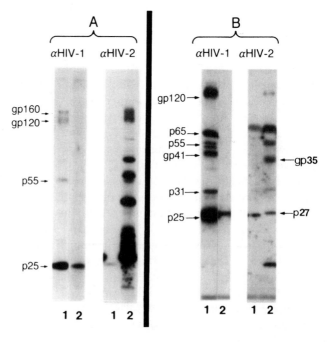

Figure 1.2 Immunoblot analyses showing antibody reactions with HIV-1, HIV-2, and SIV proteins. (A) Serum from an African patient with HIV-1 and HIV-2 infections was tested for reactivity against electrophoretically separated cell lysates containing HIV-1 (lane 1) and SIV$_{mac}$ (lane 2). Note the differential detection of the envelope gp160 and gp120 proteins. (B) Proteins from purified HIV-1 (lane 1) and HIV-2 (lane 2) isolates were reacted with serum from an HIV-1- or HIV-2-infected individual. Reprinted with permission from reference 1231. Copyright 1988 AAAS.

of 2002, about 100 HIV-2-infected individuals had been reported to the Centers for Disease Control and Prevention, of whom about half were of West African origin (659). The spread of HIV-2 throughout the world, therefore, has not been as extensive as that of HIV-1 (see below).

3. PATHOGENESIS

In terms of levels of disease, individuals infected solely by HIV-2 have developed AIDS, but the infected people usually survive longer without disease than those infected with HIV-1 (2091, 4747; for a review, see reference 3684). Moreover, in a study of female commercial sex workers in Senegal, the HIV-2-infected women showed a markedly reduced rate in transmission and in the loss of CD4$^+$ lymphocytes compared to HIV-1-infected women (1111). As with HIV-1 infection, the baseline HIV-2 RNA level can also predict the rate of disease progression (147). Thus, subjects with higher viral loads soon after infection need to be followed with the possibility of initiating antiretroviral therapy (see Chapters 2 and 3).

The reasons for the potential differences in HIV-2 transmissibility and pathology compared to HIV-1 are not clear, but several features offer an explanation (Table 1.5) (983). The epidemiological observations could reflect the low plasma viral load in HIV-2-infected individuals, which can be 100-fold less than in HIV-1-infected subjects (983, 4036, 4152, 4216). Lower levels of HIV-2 than of HIV-1 are found in semen (1575). Moreover, since a large number of circulating virus-infected cells can be found in the infected people, HIV-2 production by infected cells must be low in comparison to that of HIV-1 (388a, 3581).

In support of the decreased replicative ability of HIV-2 (and perhaps, therefore, a reduction in emergence of pathogenic variants) is the observation that the intrapatient nucleotide variability rate in the V3 region of the *env* gene of HIV-2 was 0.6% for healthy HIV-2-infected individuals and 2% for those with clinical AIDS. For HIV-1-infected patients, the V3 sequence heterogeneity can be as high as 6.1% (3914); for a review, see reference 2820. These findings cannot yet be fully explained but could reflect the single NF-κB site in the HIV-2 long terminal repeat (LTR) that influences virus replicative ability (4446) (see Chapter 7).

Another potentially relevant observation with some HIV-2 isolates has been their reduced cytopathic properties in cell culture and lack of modulation of the CD4 antigen on the cell surface (638, 1231, 2271, 2345). The findings could indicate the presence of relatively noncytopathic strains of HIV-2 in certain infected populations (1231).

Other investigations have indicated that there is reduced immune activation (3000, 4216) and T-cell apoptosis (2730, 3000) with HIV-2 infection compared to HIV-1 infection. Moreover, the lower virulence of HIV-2 could reflect a reduced affinity of the envelope gp105 versus gp120 for cell surface receptors (4036). In addition, an increase in β-chemokine production is induced by the HIV-2 envelope that could have an antiviral effect (see Chapter 3). Another explanation has been the down-modulation of the CCR5 receptor, perhaps mediated by CD8$^+$ cell release of β-chemokines (4078).

The delay in pathogenesis might also result from a strong host immune response that limits the replication of HIV-2. For example, autologous

Table 1.5 Features of HIV-2 infection that could explain its less pathogenic nature compared to HIV-1 infection

- Lower viral load in blood and genital fluids (983, 1575, 4152)
- Replication to lower titers in infected cells (3581)
- Reduced cytopathicity (1231, 1736)
- Lack of modulation of CDA protein on the cell surface (1231)
- Reduced immune activation (3000, 4216)
- Decreased T-cell apoptosis (2730, 3000)
- Reduced affinity of the envelope gp105 (vs gp120) for cell surface receptors (4036)
- Increase in β-chemokine production induced by the HIV-2 envelope, with subsequent down-modulation of the CCR5 receptor (4078)
- Autologous neutralizing antibodies found more frequently than with HIV infection (388, 4098)
- HIV-2-specific T helper cells more preserved and functional (1154, 4944)
- Enhanced CD8$^+$ cell noncytotoxic immune response (39)
- CD8$^+$ cells have a more diverse T-cell receptor repertoire (2665)
- Strong CD8$^+$ cell noncytotoxic antiviral response (39)

neutralizing antibodies have been found more frequently in HIV-2-infected than in HIV-1 infected subjects (388, 4098). Moreover, some HIV-2 isolates can enter cells by a CD4-independent mechanism that appears to be more sensitive than HIV-1 to antibody-mediated neutralization (4421). The delayed clinical course in HIV-2 infection could be related as well to effective recognition of viral epitopes by HIV-2 specific T helper cells (4944). This antiviral $CD4^+$ T memory cell response is well preserved and functionally active (1154). In addition, the HIV-2-specific $CD8^+$ T cells in comparison to $CD8^+$ cells from HIV-1-infected subjects have a more diverse T-cell receptor usage, which permits broader recognition of variant epitopes. Also, the $CD8^+$ cells show a strong noncytotoxic anti-HIV response (39) (see Chapter 11). These observations could be an explanation for some presumed cross-protection from HIV-1 infection by a prior HIV-2 infection (1615, 2665, 4462, 4548, 4748). However, these findings have not been consistently obtained (148). Perhaps related are studies showing an inhibition of HIV-1 replication when PBMC are coinfected by HIV-1 and HIV-2. The mechanism is not at virus entry but appears to involve virus assembly and release (1052). These observations on dual infection require further evaluation.

II. The HIV Virion

A. Structure

Viewed by electron microscopy, HIV-1 and HIV-2 have the characteristics of a lentivirus, with a cone-shaped core composed of the viral p24 Gag capsid (CA) protein (Figure 1.3). By convention, the viral protein (p) is designated with a number corresponding to the protein size, ($\times$ 1,000). The virion is about 100 to 120 nm in diameter, with heterogeneous morphological shapes (2359). Infectious viruses contain the envelope and three structural Gag proteins: matrix (MA, p17), CA (p24), and nucleocapsid (NC, p7), (for a review, see reference 1555). MA forms the inner shell in the particle just below the viral membrane, CA forms the conical core enclosing the viral genomic RNA, and NC interacts with viral RNA inside the capsid. These viral proteins are generated by the viral protease (PR) processing the HIV-1 p55 Gag precursor polypro-

tein. The locations of the Gag proteins on the p55 precursor are as follows: p17/p24/p2/p7/p1/p6. The uncleaved Gag p55 has three major domains referred to as membrane targeting (M), interaction (I), and late (L) (1555). M, located within the MA region, is myristoylated and targets the Gag protein to the plasma membrane. I is responsible for Gag monomer interaction and is found within the NC. The L domain, also within the NC, mediates retroviral budding, which involves the p6 region of the Gag polyprotein (1360).

Inside the Gag capsid, or nucleoid, are two usually identical RNA strands with which the viral RNA-dependent DNA polymerase, Pol, also called RT (p66, p51), and the NC proteins (p9 and p6) are closely associated (Table 1.6). As noted above, the inner portion of the viral membrane is surrounded by a myristoylated p17 core protein (MA) that is part of the viral structure (1483, 1484) (Figures 1.3 and 1.4). The assembly of HIV most likely requires protein:nucleic acid interactions at the center of the particle (506). It is known that MA is needed for incorporation of the Env proteins into mature virions (4893).

Closely associated with the core are the Vif and Nef proteins (586, 2631, 3400). Estimates of 7 to 20 molecules of Vif per virion have been made (586). Also found within the virion and most likely outside the core is the viral accessory gene product Vpr (and Vpx for HIV-2) (Figure 1.4) (2682, 4891) (see Chapter 5). The presence of all these viral proteins within the virion particles suggests that they play a role in early events of HIV infection (see Chapter 3). Certain cytoskeletal proteins (e.g., actin, ezrin, emerin, moesin, and coflin), perhaps cleaved by the HIV-1 PR, have also been detected within virions (3358); their role in HIV infection, if any, is unknown (see below). However, emerin appears to be necessary for HIV replication by helping in the interaction of the viral cDNA with chromatin and subsequent integration (1992). Emerin bridges the interface between the inner nuclear envelope and chromatin. Moreover, heat shock protein 70 (hsp70), found within the membrane of HIV-1 cores, helps to maintain the core's structural integrity (1674). Finally, as with other retroviruses (2513), HIV isolates have demonstrated selective incorporation of specific lipid domains from the host cell membrane

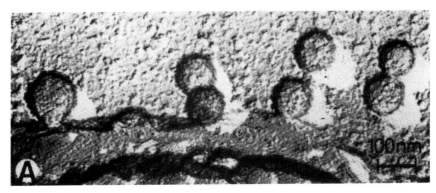

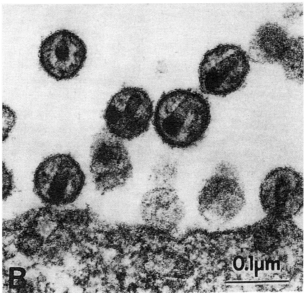

Figure 1.3 (A) Scanning electron micrograph of budding particles, most probably HIV, on the surface of a T lymphocyte. This process can incorporate cell surface proteins onto the surface of the virus and has been considered responsible in part for false-positive reactions in enzyme-linked immunosorbent assay (3941). Antibodies to normal T-cell proteins (e.g., HLA and CD4) could show a positive reaction. Photomicrograph courtesy of H. Gelderblom. (B) Transmission electron micrograph of HIV replicating in a T cell. Photomicrographs provided by R. Munn.

during viral budding (73) (Figure 1.3A). The latter is reflected in the molar ratio of cholesterol to phospholipid (73).

The envelope proteins are derived from a 160-kDa precursor glycoprotein, gp160, which is cleaved inside the cell (most likely by cellular enzymes in the Golgi apparatus) into a gp120 external surface envelope protein and a gp41 transmembrane protein (2904).

The surface of the virus was initially described as having up to 72 knobs containing these envelope glycoproteins (Env) as trimers (676, 1162, 1483, 4710, 4718). However, by the time the virus is released from a cell, only 7 to 14 trimers (Env spikes) appear to be present on the virion surface as detected by electron microscopy (740, 2438, 4953) and most recently by cryoelectron microscopy tomography (4954). These spikes are arranged as tripod-like structures on the virus. The low number of envelope proteins on the surface of a virion reflects a reduction in Env formation within the cell rather than envelope shedding (740). Atomic

Table 1.6 HIV proteins and their functions

Proteins[a]	Designation(s)[b] and size (kDa)	Function
Gag	p24	Capsid (CA), structural protein
	p17	Matrix (MA) protein, myristoylated
	p7	Nucleocapsid (NC) protein; helps in reverse transcription
	p6	Role in budding (L domain)
Polymerase (Pol)	p66, p51	Reverse transcriptase (RT): RNase H—inside core
Protease (PR)	p10	Posttranslational processing of viral proteins
Integrase (IN)	p32	Viral cDNA integration
Envelope (Env)	gp120	Envelope surface (SU)[c] protein
	gp41	Envelope transmembrane (TM)[d] protein
Tat[c]	p14	Transactivation
Rev[c]	p19	Regulation of viral mRNA expression
Nef	p27	Pleiotropic, can increase or decrease virus replication
Vif	p23	Increases virus infectivity and cell-to-cell transmission; helps in proviral DNA synthesis and/or in virion assembly
Vpr	p15	Helps in virus replication; transactivation
Vpu[c, d]	p16	Helps in virus release; disrupts gp160:CD4 complexes
Vpx[e]	p15	Helps in entry and infectivity
Tev[c]	p26	Tat/Rev activities

[a]See Figure 1.3 for location of the viral genes on the HIV genome.
[b]Numbers in designations are sizes, in kilodaltons.
[c]Not found to be associated within the virion.
[d]Only present with HIV-1.
[e]Only encoded by HIV-2. May be a duplication of Vpr.

force microscopy, however, suggests that the envelope proteins on a virion exist as 70 to 100 tufts made up of trimeric gp41 with various numbers of gp120 monomers not in the classic trimeric form (2359). Therefore, the true nature of the envelope structure on an infectious virion has not been resolved.

The envelope proteins are transported to the cell surface, where part of the central and amino-terminal portion of gp41 is expressed on the outside of the virion. The loop segment of gp41 is important for membrane fusion (3431). The central region of this transmembrane protein binds to the external viral gp120 in a noncovalent manner,

Figure 1.4 An HIV virion with the structural and other virion proteins identified. The exact locations of Nef and Vif in association with the core have not been well established. The abbreviated viral protein designations are those recommended (2484).

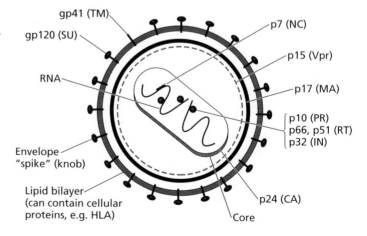

primarily at two hydrophobic regions in the amino and carboxyl termini of gp120 (1799). The long cytoplasmic tail of gp41 appears to be required for HIV-1 envelope glycoprotein incorporation into virions (3173). Some analyses suggest that a knob-and-socket-like structure is involved (4008), and that several envelope regions, including the V1/V2 and the C2 and V3 domains of gp120 (Color Plate 1, following page 78), help stabilize the association (4334, 4768). Recently, the tail-interacting protein of 47 kDa (TIP47) has been shown to interact with the viral envelope and bind MA to form a ternary complex which is important for envelope incorporation during viral assembly (2667a).

The virion gp120 located on the virus surface contains the binding site(s) for the cellular receptor(s) and the major antibody-neutralizing domains. The external portion of gp41 has also been reported to be sensitive to neutralizing antibodies (688, 958) (see Chapter 10). In general, the virion has 60 to 100 times more p24 Gag protein than envelope gp120 (740, 2438, 3090) and 10 to 20 times more p24 than the polymerase molecule (2438).

B. Genomic Organization

The genomic size of HIV is about 10 kb, with open reading frames coding for several viral proteins (Table 1.6 and Figures 1.1 and 1.5) (see also Chapter 7 for further detail on the viral accessory proteins). The primary transcript of HIV is a full-length viral mRNA, which is translated into the Pol and Gag proteins (Figure 1.5). The Pol precursor polyprotein is autocleaved by its PR region into products consisting of the viral enzymes RT, PR, and integrase (IN). By proteolytic cleavage, the Gag precursor p55 gives rise to smaller proteins, including p24, p17, p9, and p6, cited above, as well as p2 and p1. The Gag and Gag-Pol products are synthesized in a ratio of about 20:1 (3347). Splicing events are important in producing many subgenomic mRNAs responsible for the synthesis of other viral proteins. The relative amounts of the unspliced to singly and multiply spliced mRNAs appear to be determined by the *rev* gene, which is itself a product of a multiply spliced mRNA (1266, 4197).

As noted above, the envelope gp120 and gp41 proteins are made from the precursor gp160, which is a singly spliced message from the full-length viral mRNA. Proteolytic cleavage of gp160 is mediated by furin, an endoprotease (1701). Gene products of other spliced mRNAs make up a variety of viral regulatory and accessory proteins that can affect HIV replication in various cell types (Figure 1.5) (see Chapter 7).

One regulatory protein is Tat, a transactivating protein that, along with certain cellular proteins, interacts with an RNA loop structure formed in the 3' portion of the viral LTR called the Tat response element. Tat is a major protein involved in up-regulating HIV replication (for reviews, see references 1620 and 3483).

Another viral regulatory protein, Rev (regulator of viral protein expression), mentioned above, interacts with a *cis*-acting RNA loop structure called the Rev-responsive element, located in the viral envelope mRNA (1266, 4197). This interaction involves cellular proteins and multimers of the Rev protein and permits unspliced mRNA to enter the cytoplasm from the nucleus and give rise to full-length viral proteins needed for progeny production. Tat and Rev are RNA binding proteins that interact with cellular factors for optimal activity.

The viral protein Nef (negative factor) appears to have a variety of potential functions, including cell activation and enhanced infectivity. It interacts with cellular proteins to elicit its function in signal transduction and cell activation (3937). Viruses lacking *nef* usually do not replicate well in PBMC or in vivo (614) (see Chapter 7).

Other accessory HIV viral gene products, Vif (4632), Vpr, and Vpu/Vpx, affect events such as assembly, cell cycling and budding, and infectivity during the production of infectious viruses (Table 1.6) (1620, 3362, 3483). The importance of Vif in countering the intracellular resistance factor APOBEC3G is discussed in Chapter 5. Some studies have suggested that the accessory genes *nef*, *vpr*, and *vpu/vpx* are more important for HIV-1 replication in macrophages than in CD4$^+$ lymphocytes (231).

As described in reviews on the molecular features of these viral gene products (1620, 3362, 3483), the regulation of virus expression involves the interplay of many viral proteins and cellular factors, leading to either high or low production of HIV or even the establishment of

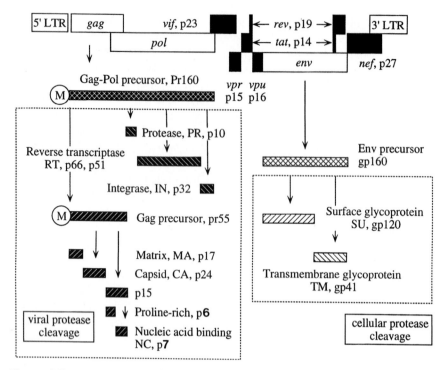

Figure 1.5   Processing of viral proteins. Some HIV-1 proteins, which are translated from 10 distinct viral transcripts, are further processed by viral and cellular proteases. From 46 translated open reading frames, which include Tev (not diagrammed), 16 viral proteins are made. They form the virion structure, direct viral enzymatic activities, and serve regulatory and accessory functions. The Gag-Pol precursor of 160 kDa is processed by the viral (as-partyl) protease into seven proteins, which include four Gag proteins (MA, p17; CA, p24; late domain, p7; and NC, p9), protease (P, p10), reverse transcriptase/RNase (RT, p66, p51), and integrase (IN, p32). The Env precursor (gp160) is processed by a cellular protease into the surface glycoprotein (SU, gp120) and the transmembrane glycoprotein (TM, gp41). Viral regulatory and accessory proteins, which include Tat (p14), Tev (p20), Rev (p19), Nef (p27), Vif (p23), Vpr (p15), and Vpu (p16), are not processed. M, myristoylated. Figure provided by M. Peterlin.

a latent state. For example, production of Rev in the later phases of the viral replicative cycle can down-regulate its own expression as well as that of Tat and Nef. Virus replication would then be limited.

It is noteworthy that HIV codes for three major enzymes that function at different times during the replicative cycle. As expected, they have been prime targets for antiretroviral approaches (see Chapter 14). The RNA-dependent DNA polymerase (with its RNase H function) acts in the early steps of virus replication to form a double-stranded DNA copy (cDNA) of the virus RNA (see Chapter 2 for details on HIV replication). The

IN functions inside the cell nucleus to incorporate the viral cDNA into the host chromosomal DNA. The PR, by processing the Gag and Gag-Pol polyproteins mostly within the budding virion, induces the maturation of the viral particle into an infections virus (1620, 3483).

III. Virus Heterogeneity

A. General Observations

The extensive biologic and serologic heterogeneities of HIV isolates are mirrored in the variable genetic sequences of the viruses (Figure 1.6).

How these diverse strains of HIV arise is not clear, but the viral RT is very error prone and thus appears to give rise readily to changes in the genome (829, 3602, 3753, 4371). The fidelity of this enzyme has been found to be severalfold higher with RNA than with DNA, suggesting that most mutations occur with the DNA template-DNA primer (473). It has been estimated that up to 10 base changes in the HIV genome can occur per replicative cycle (829). Molecular techniques have helped to define the variations in the viral genome associated with HIV heterogeneity (see Chapter 7).

B. Genome Sensitivity to Restriction Enzymes

One of the first differences recognized among HIV-1 isolates was the variation in sensitivity of the cloned, proviral genome to digestion by restriction enzymes. When the restriction enzyme patterns of two prototype isolates, HTLV-III and LAV, were examined, they were found to be virtually identical (62, 1691), but that of the third, ARV-2 (HIV-1$_{SF2}$), showed marked differences (542, 2690). The latter observation became the rule as various isolates were recognized by their different restriction enzyme patterns (2541) (Figure 1.7).

Viruses recovered from one individual appear to conserve several restriction enzyme sites and thus can be identified as coming from the same person (306, 731, 1693). Similarly, HIV-1 isolates from a mother and child, individuals receiving a blood transfusion or clotting factor from the same donor, or two sexual partners could show a close relationship among the viruses by similar restriction enzyme patterns (2238).

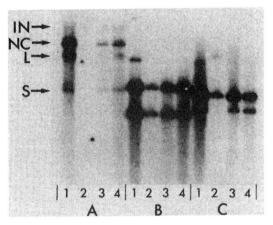

Figure 1.7 Restriction enzyme differences among various HIV isolates. HUT 78 T cells were acutely infected with HIV-1$_{SF2}$ (formerly ARV-2) (lane 1), SF-4 (lane 3), and SF-19 (lane 4). Lane 2 contains a HUT 78 line chronically infected with HIV-1$_{SF2}$. High-molecular-weight DNA was prepared from whole cells and treated with restriction enzymes and blotted as described previously (2541). Panel A contains undigested high-molecular-weight cell DNA. The positions of unintegrated forms of HIV-1 DNA are shown. IN, integrated; NC, nicked circles; L, linear (9.7 kb); S, supercoils. Integrated viral DNA in undigested DNA samples is at the exclusion limit of the agarose gel (greater than 20 kDa). Reprinted from reference 2541 with permission.

Another technique involving DNA heteroduplex analysis on an agarose gel has been used to detect HIV-1 quasispecies diversity when evaluating different genetic regions (Figure 1.8). This approach is a rapid procedure for studying genomic differences among HIV isolates and the evolution of genetic variants over time (1045).

Figure 1.6 Estimated similarities in amino acids for the different HIV-1 gene products. Figure compiled from data analyzing several early HIV-1 isolates worldwide (3185) and provided by C. Kuiken.

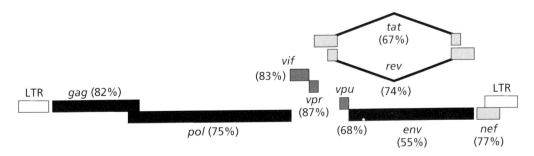

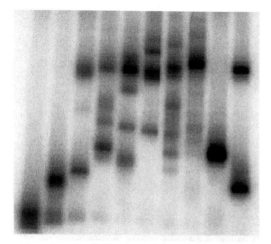

0   1   3   3.5   4   4.5 5.5 6.5 C3.5 C4

Figure 1.8 DNA heteroduplex tracking analysis of HIV envelope gene quasispecies collected over 6.5 years and of derived isolates. The Env V3–V5 region was nested PCR amplified from longitudinally collected PBMC starting at seroconversion (labeled in years starting at year 0) and from two in vitro-amplified cultures (labeled C with year of origin). Time zero PCR product was radiolabeled and reannealed to excess DNA from the same and other samples. Labeled DNA heteroduplexes were separated by nondenaturing polyacrylamide gel electrophoresis and exposed by autoradiography. Analysis shows clearance over time of the earliest time zero variant reflected by the disappearance of the fastest-mobility labeled DNA homoduplex, increasing genetic diversity noted by the large number of DNA heteroduplex bands, and appearance of slow labeled mobility heteroduplexes. The cultured isolates show reduced genetic diversity relative to the uncultured PBMC samples. Provided by E. Delwart.

C. Genetic Sequence Differences

When complete genetic sequence data were available for the initial HIV-1 isolates, it again became evident that HTLV-IIIB and LAV were the same isolate (HIV-1$_{LAI}$), whereas SF2 and subsequently other HIV-1 isolates could be differentiated by their viral genomic sequences (63, 3156, 3673, 3908, 4651). At least 6 to 10% of the total viral genome can differ among isolates from different individuals. Some viruses vary widely in both synonymous sequence changes (mutations that do not affect amino acid representation) and nonsynonymous sequence changes (mutations that affect the amino acid expressed). The greatest

nonsynonymous sequence heterogeneity is observed in the genes of the regulatory and envelope proteins (2846, 2987, 3189); with some isolates, nearly 40% differences in amino acid sequences in certain viral genes can be appreciated (Figure 1.6) (3189) (see also http://hiv-web.lanl.gov/content/index).

D. Groups and Sequence Subtypes (Clades) of HIV-1 and HIV-2

1. HIV-1

The amplification of parts of a viral genome by PCR followed by DNA sequencing has been very helpful in conducting rapid comparisons of different sequences among HIV-1 and HIV-2 isolates (2365, 2673, 2846, 2907, 2909, 3361, 4098), particularly in the envelope region. By amino acid analyses, this procedure has shown extreme envelope diversity as well as certain similarities among viruses. Currently, based on full-length viral genome sequencing, there are three HIV-1 groups called M (main), O (outlier), and N (non M or O). Eight HIV-2 groups have been identified (3684) (see below).

Nine HIV-1 clades (or subtypes) have been recognized within the M group (3460, 3755) and are designated A to D, F to H, J, and K. Some subtypes have been distinguished for group O, but only a few isolates of group N have been identified. No subtypes of the HIV-2 groups have yet been identified (3755). Each HIV-1 M clade differs from the others in amino acid composition by at least 20% in the envelope region and 15% in the Gag region (3755) (see also http://hiv-web.lanl.gov/content/index). The groups show more than a 25% difference in sequences in the envelope and *gag* regions. The clades are approximately equally distant from each other. To be considered part of a clade, the isolate must resemble another member within sequences crossing the entire genome (3460).

The interrelationship of groups and clades has been established by phylogenetic trees which can be drawn either as phenograms along a vertical axis line (Figure 1.9A) or as a radial unrooted tree (Figure 1.9B). In the HIV-1 M group, clade (subtype) A is found primarily in Central Africa, clade B in North America and Europe, clade C in South Africa and India, and clade D in Central Africa. Subtype F

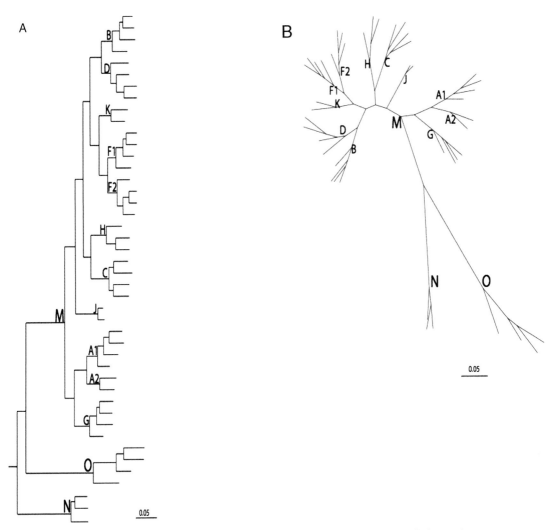

Figure 1.9   Two representations, vertical (A) and radial (B), of the same phylogenetic tree. The distances between the HIV-1, M, N, and O groups, and the M group, are illustrated. At the tip of each branch is a modern sequence, and the phylogeny is an attempt to reconstruct their evolutionary relationships—which viruses are most closely related and how far they have evolved. In the radial tree (B) there is no root, but the branching order is identical to the phenogram (A). The branch length reflects the genetic distance, or the number of mutations that could have occurred between two sequences as they diverged from a shared ancestor. Only the horizontal branch lengths are counted in the phenogram, and the sum of the branch lengths between any two sequences is the same in either representation. This tree was made using the program PAUP and is a neighbor-joining tree. Provided by B. Korber and the Los Alamos HIV Database.

includes a few isolates from Brazil (3591) and all of the viruses thus far characterized from children in Romania (1149). Some investigators now suggest subdividing subtype A into A1 and A2 and clade F into two subclades: F1 (from Brazil, Romania, and Finland) and F2 (from Cameroon and the Democratic Republic of Congo) (1426, 4472). In this regard, the viruses in clade F from Brazil have GPGR in the V3 loop crown, whereas the clade F isolates from Romania have GPGQ (1149). Other sequence subtypes of group M include viruses from Russia (G) (415), Africa and Taiwan (H) (3187), Zaire (clade J) (2424), and Cameroon (clade K) (3795) (Figure 1.9).

Recombinant viruses (discussed in Chapter 4) emerge frequently in human populations where multiple clades cocirculate. In some cases, a recombinant form becomes an epidemiologically important lineage. These are then called circulating recombinant forms (CRFs) and are numbered sequentially with the clades involved cited by letter. When the parental strain is unknown, a U symbol is used. Viruses which are recombinants involving four or more subtypes are called complex and designated *cpx*. Presently there are 16 recognized CRFs (http://hiv-web.lanl.gov) (3460, 3755) derived from the group M HIV isolates.

In this regard, two previously designated HIV-1 clades, E and I, represent recombinants. Subtype E (A and E) has been renamed CRF-01AE, although no full-length subtype E representative has been found (Figure 1.10). It is particularly prevalent in Thailand. The subtype I virus, initially found in Cyprus (2291), is considered a recombinant (114) and is now designated CRF-04cpx since this recombination involves at least four subtypes with about 11 points of recombination (1425, 3755). CRF-02AG dominates the HIV epidemic in some parts of Africa (Figure 1.10).

For a new subtype, clade, or CRF to be named, three representative full-length genomes need to be sequenced from individuals not linked epidemiologically (3755). Globally, clades A through D and the CRF-01AE and CRF-02AG recombinants account for more than 90% of infections worldwide (370) (Figure 1.11). Close to 75% of the new infections occurring in the world are caused by subtypes A, C, and CRF-02AG. Clades C and E are the most prevalent in the world, with C spreading though Central Africa down to South Africa. Clade C is becoming dominant in parts of China, India, and Ethiopia and may represent today up to 50% of all HIV infections worldwide (http://www.unaids.org).

In addition to the M group, other isolates initially found in Cameroon (3187, 3457) are considered outliers and form the O group (see below). They can be distinguished by their genetic sequence, which places them apart from the M group (Figure 1.9). They have also been found at low frequency in other African countries (2849, 3457) (Table 1.7). About 25% of isolates from Cameroon are of the O clade genotype (183). The existence of subtypes of this O group has been suggested by some analyses of variants of the prototype ANT 70 virus (2007, 4848) but not by others (3797). The genetic distances between subtypes of this group are similar to that of group M clades, and therefore a separation of group O viruses into

Figure 1.10 Map along the HIV-1 genome showing the patterns of recombination in the two most common circulating recombinant forms, CRF01 and CRF02. Such recombinants are complex and can be important as major epidemic strains. Provided by B. Korber and C. Calef.

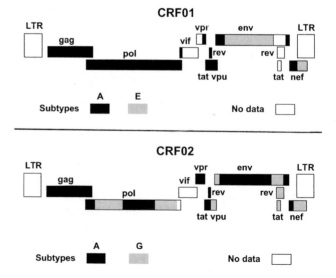

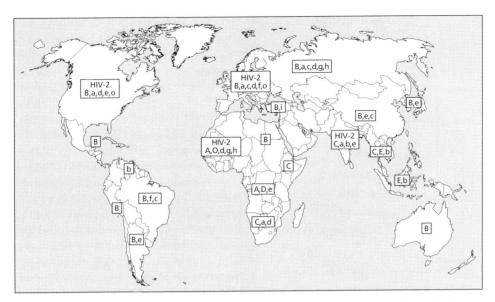

Figure 1.11 HIV-1 is the predominant HIV type distributed throughout the world, but HIV-2, which is less common, has still been found in West Africa and most recently in India at an increasing rate. The distribution of the various subtypes (clades) of the HIV-1 M group is indicated by letters. The HIV-2 groups are not shown separately. Source, UNAIDS, 1996.

five phylogenetic (I to V) classifications (4846) has been proposed.

It is noteworthy that the earliest documented infection by HIV-1 was in three Norwegian people (a couple and their daughter) who died in 1976 after ten years of clinical evidence of HIV infection (2611). The virus present in these individuals was clade O (2046). These results therefore indicate that this recently recognized HIV-1 group existed long before the emergence of the present epidemic.

In addition to the M and O groups is the N group of HIV-1, found in a few HIV infection cases in Cameroon (3460, 4153) (Table 1.7). These viruses appear to show more sequence similarity to SIV (see below). The prototype virus of the N group was recovered in 1995 from a 40-year-old Cameroonian woman with AIDS (4153). By the phylogenetic relationship of structural and regulatory genes, this virus was equidistant from the group M and the SIV$_{cpz}$ viruses (Figure 1.12). The N group of HIV-1 appears to be closer to chimpanzee SIV than either the M or O group of HIV-1. Thus, the evolutionary ancestor of N viruses could have been nonhuman primates. However, in serologic studies in Cameroon, very little prevalence has been found for the group N

HIV-1 viruses. Moreover, very few N group viruses have been identified (2849) (Table 1.7). With the most recent evidence of group N viruses in a husband and wife in Cameroon, the number of group N isolates has reached 10 (4847). The N group of viruses also appears to be a recombinant

Table 1.7 Infection rate of HIV groups and clades[a]

HIV group or subtype	No. of infections (% of total)
HIV-1	
Group M	45,000[b] (99.6)
Group N	10 (0.000013)
Group O	10,000[b] (0.22)
HIV-2	
Group A	50,000[b] (0.11)
Group B	25,000[b] (0.06)
Group C	1 (0.0000002)
Group D	1 (0.0000002)
Group E	1 (0.0000002)
Group F	1 (0.0000002)
Group G	1 (0.0000002)
Group H	1 (0.0000002)

[a]Adapted from reference 2849 with permission.
[b]Estimate.

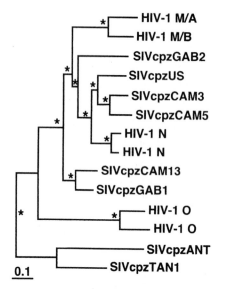

HIV-1 M/A
HIV-1 M/B
SIVcpzGAB2
SIVcpzUS
SIVcpzCAM3
SIVcpzCAM5
HIV-1 N
HIV-1 N
SIVcpzCAM13
SIVcpzGAB1
HIV-1 O
HIV-1 O
SIVcpzANT
SIVcpzTAN1

0.1

Figure 1.12 Evolutionary relationships of SIV$_{cpz}$ and HIV-1 strains based on maximum-likelihood phylogenetic analyses of full-length envelope protein sequences. SIV$_{cpz}$ strains from *P. troglodytes troglodytes* and *P. troglodytes schweinfurthii* are highlighted in red and blue, respectively. Representative strains of HIV-1 groups M, N, and O are included for comparison. Asterisks indicate internal branches with estimated posterior probabilities of 95% or higher. The scale bar denotes 10% replacements per site. Reprinted from reference 4074 with permission.

between an ancestral virus related to the HIV-1 group M and an SIV$_{cpz}$ strain found in Cameroon (892, 1424, 3796, 4073, 4153). It is, therefore, unknown whether this group is emerging in the epidemic or declining (184).

All of the HIV-1 groups and clades identified as well as seven of the CRFs have been found in Africa (2672, 3460), with most clades cocirculating in Central Africa (http://data.unaids.org/Publications/IRC-pub05/HIV-genetic-variability_en.htm). Great diversity has also been reported in Cuba (930) and Latin America (3201, 4424). The distribution of clades in other countries varies but most likely reflects the number of viruses recovered as well as epidemiological spread. For example, in servicemen returning to the United States in the 1990s, viruses from two other M clades (A and D) besides subtype B and the recombinant CRF-01AE were detected (519).

In a recent study of blood donors in the United States, 6 out of 312 infected blood samples showed

one HIV-2 infection and 5 had non-subtype B strains (1043). The extent of virus replication appears to influence the interpatient variation that develops during the spread of virus subtypes through populations in the world (2284). Similarities among clades obtained from various countries could indicate a recent introduction of the virus into these countries. Great diversity would suggest a longer period that these viruses have existed and spread in the population (Figure 1.13).

Also noteworthy has been the genetic characterization of an HIV isolate detected in a 1959 plasma sample from Zaire (3199). It was shown to be an ancestral form related to clades B and D (4956). This information has encouraged the concept that the spread of HIV-1, particularly in Africa, is leading to the establishment of various diverse viruses that can change sufficiently in replication to be characterized as different subtypes. Moreover, the finding suggests that HIV was in human populations a long time before AIDS was recognized (see below).

2. HIV-2

Eight distinct sequence groups of HIV-2 (A to H) have been identified (964a, 3684). Groups A and B are the most commonly identified groups thus far (Table 1.7). HIV-2 group A is generally found in Senegal and Guinea Bissau; group B is found in the Ivory Coast (3460). The others have only one representative. Group G was isolated from a blood sample in the Ivory Coast, and groups C, D, E, and F came from rural areas in Sierra Leone and Liberia (718, 3460). Group D also appears to be closely related to SIV isolates, leading some researchers to conclude that SIV has entered humans on more than one occasion (1427) (see below). The HIV-2 viruses appear to be most related to the SIV$_{smm}$ isolates obtained from sooty mangabeys found in the same areas (719, 964a, 3460) (Figure 1.14). In this regard, the HIV-2 LTR, similar to that of SIV, has only one NF-κB site (4446).

E. Biologic Differences among Viral Groups and Clades

Virus replication differences involving the NC protein have been described for the HIV-1 group M and group O viruses. The O viruses do not appear to be very sensitive to cyclosporine in

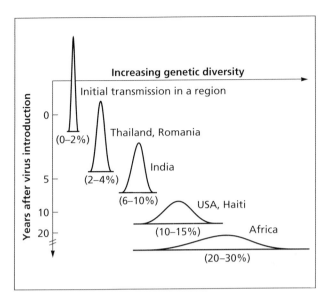

Figure 1.13 Relationship between the degree of genetic diversity of a genotype and the duration of the epidemic in a region. Each curve represents the expected distribution of intrasubtype nucleotide substitution frequencies, expressed as a percentage, among all possible pairs of a typical sample of sequences from a country or area. Examples named reflect the most recently reported genetic divergence. The width of each curve represents the approximate range of these frequencies, and the height represents the relative proportion of pairs with that frequency of substitution. Genetic divergence is believed to increase at a rate of approximately 0.5 to 1% per year. Reprinted from reference 4726 with permission.

culture, suggesting that the interaction of the karyophilin complex with this Gag protein is not required for group O replication (478) (see Chapter 5). The relative effect of the intracellular resistance factor, TRIM5α, on these different clades merits evaluation (see Chapter 5). Moreover, in vitro studies with PBMCs as well as dendritic cells suggest that group M isolates replicate up to 100-fold better than group O or HIV-2 strains (144). The relationship of these findings to the in vivo biologic heterogeneity of HIV-1 isolates is not certain.

In other studies in which clade B and C HIV isolates from group M were added simultaneously to PBMC at similar viral inputs, the subtype C viruses were found to be less fit than the subtype B viruses (229). These results were noted in primary CD4+ T cells and macrophages from different donors but not in human Langerhans cells. The efficiency of host cell entry seemed not to be involved; subtypes B and C could infect and spread equally, but subtype C replicated to a lesser extent. Therefore, this clade could be associated with a slower disease progression (229). However, these in vitro studies do not necessarily reflect the clinical observations with the clades (see also Chapters 7 and 13). They do not explain, for example, the rapid spread of clade C throughout Africa and certainly Asia. A greater function of the clade A and C proteases has beeen noted which could influence the dominance of

these subtypes in Africa (4578). Some studies suggest that clade A virus infection may have a slower disease course (2072, 2092). Other evidence suggests that clade C is present at higher levels in vaginal fluid than are clades A to D (2039). Moreover, recent simian/human immunodeficiency virus (SHIV) studies with rhesus macaques suggest that the clade C virus-derived chimeric viruses, in comparison to the clades C and E SHIVs, replicate best in the interleukin-7 (IL-7)-sensitive gut-associated lymphoid tissues (662) (see Chapter 8).

As with HIV-1, the biologic phenotypes of HIV-2 can be distinguished by their ability to form syncytia and to grow rapidly to high titer or slowly to low titer (53) (see Chapter 4). Many HIV-2 isolates often use a broader range of alternative coreceptors for infection in vitro than do HIV-1 isolates, and some can enter cells by a CD4-independent mechanism (3684, 3686) (see Chapter 3).

It seems apparent that several regions within a virus need to be considered when the final genetic and biologic classification of HIV-1 isolates takes place. Nevertheless, the distribution of virus subtypes according to sequence should focus on the genetic structure of the viral envelope region, which is very important for vaccine development. How the clade classification relates to antigenic subtypes is an important, unresolved area of study (see Chapter 10).

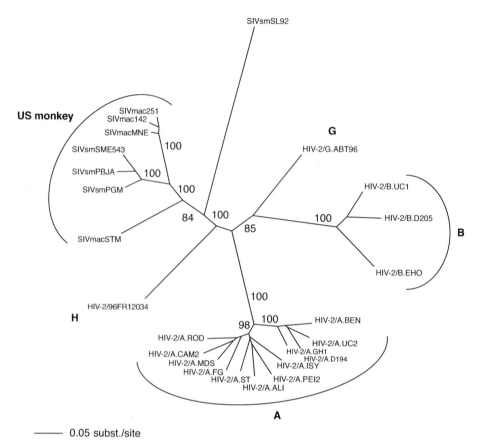

Figure 1.14   Unrooted phylogenetic tree showing the relationship of HIV-2 groups and SIV$_{sm}$ representatives inferred from the complete genome alignment by maximum likelihood. The numbers near the nodes indicate the percentage of bootstrap replicates supporting a clade. Bootstrap values greater than 70% are shown. The scale indicates substitutions per site and refers to the branch lengths. Reprinted from reference 964a with permission.

IV. Origin of HIV

A. Overview

After examining sequence variations among the three HIV-1 groups and the several HIV-1 subtypes or clades, several investigators have proposed that HIV-1 entered the human population from primates as early as 30 to 100 years ago (2282, 2483, 3188, 3189, 3890; for a review, see reference 4073) (see below). Similar analyses, particularly full-length envelope tree analyses, suggested that the founder of the B subtype came to the United States in about 1967 (for reviews, see references 2282 and 3747) and subtype C emerged in Africa in the middle to late 1960s (4463). Still other researchers question the early origin of HIV-1 and

suggest that the virus could have emerged in human populations many years before (1580, 3655, 3890; for a review, see reference 2483). In this regard, some molecular clock analyses suggest that the common ancestor of the group M HIV-1 and SIV$_{cpz}$ lineages could date from the end of the 17th century (3890). Importantly, which HIV-1 group or clade first entered the human population is not yet certain, although group O does appear to have been present very early (2046) (see below).

As noted above, the earliest documented evidence of HIV infection in humans came from an African seropositive serum sample collected in 1959 from the Congo (3199). The sequence of this virus appeared to place it at the ancestral node of clades B and D (4956). It is also noteworthy that the sequences of a virus from blood samples from a Norwegian family infected by HIV in the mid-1960s (1377) were very similar to those of the current circulating group O viruses. The father had traveled to Africa. The findings seem to reflect slow evolutionary properties of the group O viruses (2046). However, other samples taken from many parts of Africa up to the mid-1970s did not show serologic evidence of HIV infection (2547, 3186). Thus, how, where, and when HIV emerged in human populations and existed in various groups and clades (3755) are not clearly evident.

The existence of clades can reflect the extensive heterogeneity of HIV-1 and HIV-2 that results from the high mutation rate from the viral error-prone RT, its rapid replicative ability (24 h), and its extensive progeny production (i.e., 1,000 virions/cell) (829, 3655) (see Chapter 4). Virus recombination (see Chapter 4) can also be a major mechanism for formation of new clades and, as noted above, was responsible for the development of the previously considered clades, E and I (114) (Section III.D). It is feasible that viruses maintained and spreading in one habitat could, after several transmissions and immune selection in different hosts, evolve with sufficient mutations to be classified as a separate clade. The extent of virus replication obviously influences the interpatient variation that develops during the transfer of virus subtypes through populations in the world. As noted above, great diversity would reflect a longer time the virus has been present in the population (Figure 1.13).

It is noteworthy that a study of viral isolates circulating in the Democratic Republic of Congo (formerly Zaire) through the 1980s indicated that up to 37% of the strains already were recombinant viruses. Multiple infections were documented. The results suggested that the HIV epidemic was already well established in Central Africa in the early 1980s (2074). The diversity at that time was more complex than in isolates currently found in other parts of the world. The data question further whether subtypes that are now circulating represent true evolution of HIV M group viruses or recombinant viruses.

It is also curious that the distribution of virus groups and clades worldwide has remained relatively constant (Figure 1.11). For instance, the lack of a large number of people infected with clades other than B in North America raises questions about the singular emergence of certain virus subtypes in other countries. The presence of N and O clades primarily in Cameroon and the dominance of clades in some parts of the world, such as Romania (F) and Russia (G), reflect this occurrence. Whether a virus founder effect can explain these observations is not known.

PIONEERS IN AIDS RESEARCH

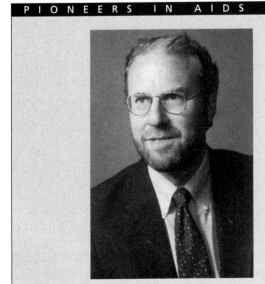

Michael D. Gottlieb
A physician in Los Angeles, Calif., Dr. Gottlieb is credited as being one of the first to describe the clinical syndrome of AIDS.

B. Theories on the Origin of HIV-1

Several explanations for the origin of HIV have been presented. The most common is the transfer of virus from primate reservoirs to humans. Derivation of the nine HIV-1 clades could then have resulted from a founder effect when a virus subtype was introduced by zoonotic infection into a particular human population. Recombinant viruses could have emerged later. Many investigators propose that the M, N, and O HIV-1 groups were introduced into humans by three separate cross-species transmissions of SIV$_{cpz}$ from chimpanzees, particularly the subspecies *Pan troglodytes troglodytes* living in the West Central region of Africa (e.g., Cameroon) (892, 1927, 3455) (for a review, see reference 4074) (Figure 1.12).

Thus far, two different SIV$_{cpz}$ clades have been recognized that appear to be related to HIV-1 groups M and N (2145) (Figure 1.12) (see below). However, no SIV$_{cpz}$ isolate closely resembling group O HIV-1 isolates has yet been found (2145). Comparison of the nucleic acid sequences among SIV and HIV isolates shows similarities of about 80% (Table 1.8). Just recently, SIV infection in wild gorillas was noted, and the virus (SIV$_{gor}$) resembles the HIV-1 group O-like viruses. Thus, the group O virus may have been transmitted to humans from gorillas (4550a).

Evaluation of three HIV group N isolates from Cameroon has suggested a single chimpanzee transfer event (3796). As noted above, the HIV-1 N group isolates have also been considered recombinants since only the *env* region resembles the SIV$_{cpz}$ isolate from a Cameroonian chimpanzee (892). One unifying theory on the origin of HIV-1, which relates to the emergence of all the groups (M, N, and O) in Cameroon, would take into consideration the fact that the chimpanzees whose viruses most resemble HIV-1 have all been found in Cameroon (*P. troglodytes troglodytes*) (see above).

Another chimpanzee virus (SIV$_{cpz}$ANT) has been identified in Tanzania from a different chimpanzee subspecies (*Pan troglodytes schweinfurthii*). Its sequence is further distanced from virus isolates from Gabon and from group O HIV-1 viruses (3455, 4568) (Figure 1.12). It has not been linked to HIV transmission. SIV has not been found in two other chimpanzee subspecies (*Pan troglodytes. verus* and *Pan troglodytes vellerosus*) (4074).

Up until 2005, very few SIV$_{cpz}$ isolates were detected in wild chimpanzees (3235, 3916, 4352). Recently, using fecal samples, a large number of wild chimpanzees in Cameroon from the *P. troglodytes troglodytes* subspecies has been noted to carry SIV$_{cpz}$ (2145). The prevalence of SIV$_{cpz}$Ptt ranged from 4 to 35% depending on animal communities in the Cameroonian forests. These viruses showed a close relationship to HIV-1 groups M and N. Since no chimpanzee counterpart for group O has been found, this virus, evident in the earliest human infection by HIV-1 (1377, 2046), could have already been present in human populations in the past. Alternatively, chimpanzee colonies elsewhere in Cameroon or Africa carry an SIV$_{cpz}$ counterpart of group O viruses. The new findings have led to the conclusion by researchers that the HIV-1 group M most likely came from chimpanzees in southeastern Cameroon and group N from a lineage of SIV$_{cpz}$Ptt in chimpanzees in southcentral Cameroon (2145).

Further support for the theory of HIV-1 originating from chimpanzees comes from the fact that this primate virus (SIV$_{cpz}$) and its ancestral viruses as well as HIV-1 have the *vpu* gene (220, 1556, 4476). Moreover, simian retrovirus infections of people exposed to monkeys have been reported (4802). Evidence now indicates that SIV$_{cpz}$ is a recombinant of ancestral SIVs (220). The 3' region containing the *vpu* gene came from an SIV of the greater spot-nosed monkey (SIV$_{gsn}$) and the 5' region from the red-capped mangabey. Notably, the

Table 1.8 Sequence similarities between SIV and HIV[a]

For HIV-1 vs SIV$_{CPZ}$

HIV-1 group M (HXB2) vs SIV$_{CPZ}$Ptt (MB66)
   Nucleotides: 78.7% (L = 7,029)
   Amino acids: 76.6% (L = 2,343)
HIV-1 group N (YBF30) vs SIV$_{CPZ}$Ptt (EK505)
   Nucleotides: 85.7% (L = 7,056)
   Amino acids: 84.9% (L = 2,352)

For HIV-2 vs SIV$_{SMM}$

HIV-2 group A (ROD) vs SIV$_{SMM}$ (PBj)
   Nucleotides: 79.5% (L = 7,065)
   Amino acids: 81.9% (L = 2,355)

[a]Average percent sequence identity values based on the comparisons of the *gag*, *pol*, and *env* genes. The values that contributed to the averages are weighted according to the sum lengths (L) of the three viral sequences and proteins evaluated (in parentheses). Table provided by B. Hahn, E. Bailes, and P. M. Sharp (see also reference 2145).

habitat of the greater spot-nosed monkey overlaps with that of the *P. troglodytes troglodytes* chimpanzee (220, 4074), the suggested primate source of HIV.

Additional support for the chimpanzee origin of HIV-1 in recent time includes reports from anthropologists who have documented over 100,000 years of human habitation in Central West Africa. Moreover, over 300 years ago slaves were taken to the Americas from the same regions where the SIV-infected sooty mangabeys and chimpanzees lived; therefore, AIDS should have appeared long ago (2849). However HIV is not in the descendants of these African populations. The reason could relate to the relatively low prevalence of SIV_{cpz} in the chimpanzee population (see above) and a lack of the ability to capture these animals in the past (e.g., without guns).

The relation of SIV_{cpz} to the transmission of HIV-1, however, is not clear. The genetic sequences of HIV-1 and SIV_{cpz} can differ by more than 20% (3423) (Table 1.8), and this divergence of the primate and human viruses does not support a recent direct transfer of HIV-1 between humans and chimpanzees. If a transmission took place, the differences suggest that other processes were required for SIV_{cpz} to evolve into HIV (2849). In addition, the closest relatives of SIV are HIV-1 group N and HIV-2 groups C through G (see below). Each of these HIV types has only infected a limited number of humans (Table 1.7), and thus they do not represent viruses of the present epidemic (2849).

Importantly, the zoonosis hypothesis usually implies transmission of a *disease*-causing agent from animals to humans. It suggests that changes in the transferred virus can occur readily within people after a limited amount of interhuman transmission and, thus, cause disease (2849, 3186). There is no evidence that SIV_{cpz} can cause AIDS in humans, and thus other factors need to be considered. Some argue that experimental or accidental transmission of SIVs to different species occurs rarely and without AIDS (130, 1135). Moreover, after 25 years no marked evolution of clade B to a different clade or a different pathogenic potential has been seen. The group O viruses have also not changed substantially over a long period (2046). In contrast, Africa has all the HIV-1 clades (4601, 4602), strongly suggesting that this continent was the first affected by HIV-1 many years ago. A global origin in the Congo for the group M clades has been proposed (3655, 4601,

4956), and Cameroon seems to be the dominant center for groups N and O. One could surmise that the virus over a long period has been evolving in Africa and that the groups and clades were only recognized when AIDS became apparent.

Notably, if SIV_{cpz} is the origin of HIV-1, this virus is nonpathogenic in chimpanzees. Moreover, many SIVs do not grow well in human PBMC (1450), and very little evidence is available for the ability of the recently described SIV_{cpz} isolates, identified only by PCR, to grow in human cells (130). Therefore, what changes had to occur to render SIV_{cpz} pathogenic in humans require further evaluation (for a review, see reference 4074). Conceivably, if this chimpanzee transfer took place, HIV-1 could have been present in the human population for many years before AIDS was recognized (1377). The serologic studies of McCormick and colleagues support this conclusion (3302). When they studied sera collected in 1976 from a small village in the Congo, a 0.76% prevalence of antibodies to HIV-1 was found. Then 10 years later, when the infection raged 10 to 15 miles away, the seroprevalence was the same. Without a change in social and economic structure, the virus remained as a low-level pathogen. Determining the genetic, economic, and social factors that helped to enhance this virus' spread and pathogenicity in the mid-20th century is an important objective (2849). Finally, consideration of lentiviruses from other animal species (Table 1.1) whose origins remain a mystery also suggests that the simian and human viruses could have evolved independently from a progenitor lentivirus that entered the animal kingdom thousands of years ago.

All these findings, while very suggestive of a chimpanzee origin for HIV-1, do not lead to a firm conclusion that the infection of humans took place in the recent past from these nonhuman primates. However, the search for the origin of HIV-1 has permitted appreciation of how living in close proximity to animals will encourage zoonotic infections that can give rise to new agents that can be pathogenic in humans.

C. Origin of HIV-2

A connection between SIV from monkeys and HIV-2 provides the most compelling evidence for a human infection, although it is also not conclusive. SIVs in monkeys originating in West Africa, particularly sooty mangabeys (SIV_{smm}),

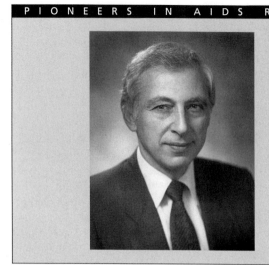

Robert C. Gallo

Director, Institute of Human Virology, University of Maryland. Dr. Gallo was among the first to identify HIV as the cause of AIDS and originally called it HTLV-III.

are genetically related to several of the HIV-2 groups (2820, 3917). Eight known groups of HIV-2 have been identified, but only five have been traced to a likely point of origin in primates. E and F are related to SIV_{smm} in Sierra Leone (718); HIV-2 group D is closely related to a Liberian strain (719, 1428). The most prevalent groups, A and B, are believed to have their geographic origin in sooty mangabeys living in the Tai Forest in the Ivory Coast (3917).

The most common viral ancestors of HIV-2 groups A and B were estimated to have been transmitted from monkeys in the 1940s (2487). Nevertheless, the genomic heterogeneity among SIV and HIV-2 strains, which continues to be appreciated as more viruses are isolated and sequenced, still questions the conclusion that HIV-2 came recently from nonhuman primate lentiviruses (29) (for a review, see reference 3684). In this regard, an SIV antibody study of 11 different primate species showed widely varying prevalence rates and the absence of viral infection in certain primates. Nonetheless, the results, indicating differences in susceptibility of various nonhuman primates to SIV infection, help to elucidate the importance of these animal reservoirs for potential human infection (29). Moreover, a seroepidemiological survey of 10,000 rural villages in northern Sierra Leone showed no evidence of SIV_{smm} transmission (718). However, in other parts of West Africa the conditions may be more favorable for virus transmission (3917). Several years

ago, a laboratory worker was infected by an SIV_{smm} strain (B670) (2174) and remains asymptomatic with persistent infection. Rhesus macaques that usually develop AIDS from SIV_{smm} did not become infected by this virus recovered from the laboratory worker (2174). The future course of this SIV_{hu} infection, which is now clinically silent, could influence the thinking on this issue.

D. Theories on HIV Emergence and the AIDS Epidemic

While the exact time of HIV-1 transmission and emergence in the human population is not conclusive, two recent hypotheses have been proposed to explain the sudden onset and spread of the HIV-1 and HIV-2 epidemics over the past 30 years. One, pioneered by Edward Hooper (1888), posits that chimpanzee kidney cells cultivated in Africa for oral poliovirus vaccines were contaminated with the chimpanzee SIV isolate, SIV_{cpz}. This virus was then passed directly or after recombination with a variety of other chimpanzee virus isolates to poliovirus vaccine recipients in various regions of Africa. The receipt of this human oral attenuated poliovirus vaccine in the 1950s correlates with the outbreaks of HIV-1 in several regions of Africa. However, no evidence of chimpanzee DNA could be found in several vials of the oral poliovirus vaccine (401, 3549). In addition, SIV_{cpz} does not grow well in human kidney cells. The natural anti-HIV substances in the oral cavity (see Chapter 3) would also seem capable of blocking an effective transmission of SIV$_{cpz}$ to humans during the oral vaccination process. Finally, the hypothesis does not explain the emergence of HIV-2.

An alternative view presented by Preston Marx and associates (1135) as well as others (1528) suggests that the use of needle injections following the development of syringes in the past 60 years has permitted the spread of a virus that was most likely present in African populations for many years. They propose that deforestation and increased hunting exposed humans to SIVs that were not commonly encountered. Then, unsafe injections and transfusions in postcolonial Africa enabled the transferred SIVs to adapt through serial passage with perhaps recombination (2849). A strong association has been made in Africa between HIV seropositivity and the receipt of medical injections (2074, 2795). This means of virus transfer could partially explain the emergence of HIV-2, since its resemblance to monkey SIVs would suggest that an occasional transfer and establishment of SIV infection in humans may have occurred and its transmission was enhanced by needle injections. However, the geographic distribution of AIDS cases through Africa does not necessarily correlate with needle use. Another possibility, not fully explored, is that the worldwide immunization against smallpox may have spread the viruses through contaminated injection materials. Again, however, the time frame of these vaccine programs to the emergence of AIDS seems too short to explain the epidemic.

E. Conclusions

SIVs have now been found in more than 35 African primate species (29), and HIV-1 is thought to have been transferred from chimpanzees to humans at least three times to form the HIV-1 lineages M, N, and O (4074) (Figure 1.12). Similarly, the origin of HIV-2 has been related to a transfer from sooty mangabey into human beings on multiple occasions (719). Only a relationship of SIV$_{cpz}$ to groups M and N has been suggested (2145). In support of these theories are the genetic relationships between the human and the nonhuman primate viruses that could indicate multiple transmission events. However, the genetic distances in the phylogenetic tree (Figure 1.12) reflect ancient divergence between the SIVs that are found in different African primates. One sequence of each clade of the M group, representative of the global diversity, is very small when considered in the context of the divergence of all SIVs (B. Korber, personal communication). Conceivably, HIV reflects very selective transmission events.

Nevertheless, none of these theories has been fully substantiated, and thus the outbreaks of HIV-1 and HIV-2 infections in the last century are not conclusively explained. While some believe that the virus could have been transferred from chimpanzees and monkeys in the 1930s through preparing and eating bush meat (1692), it seems surprising that this type of transfer did not take place many years before since bush meat has been a popular diet in many parts of Africa. Perhaps capturing the animals without modern methods (e.g., guns) was more difficult. However, it also seems very possible that HIV has been present in African populations for many hundred of years but until relatively recently never reached an infection threshold sufficient for epidemic spread. Similar to the observations in the Congo by McCormick and colleagues (see below) (3302), HIV-1 may have been in such small numbers of humans that it took a long time for the virus to evolve to be more pathogenic and when pathogenic would not have been recognized because the threshold of infection never reached proportions that would be recognized for AIDS cases. The breakdown of borders, economic stress, political trafficking (2487), prostitution, and most likely needle-injecting devices all increased during the last half of the past century (753). These factors could have favored the spread of HIV-1 and HIV-2 and their various clades into many more human populations. During this time, virus recombinants were also formed.

The emergence of HIV has alerted public health officials and governments worldwide to the constant threat of new infectious agents that can be spread rapidly. Through the present-day means of international communication, newly established international surveillance units are helping to prevent emergence of new epidemics of potential human pathogens (1453). Research on HIV and approaches for its control should provide insights into future microbial challenges to the well-being of human and animal populations.

1. HIV, first identified in 1983, is the causative agent of AIDS. It is a member of the lentivirus genus of retroviruses. The earliest documented case of HIV infection appears to have occurred in 1959, and the epidemic phase became apparent in 1981.

2. AIDS is defined by the reduction in CD4$^+$ cells (less than 200 cells/μl) and the onset of opportunistic infections (particularly *Pneumocystis jiroveci [carinii]* pneumonia) and malignancies (e.g., Kaposi's sarcoma and B-cell lymphomas). Neurologic and gastrointestinal disorders are also commonly found in AIDS patients.

3. The basic pathology in AIDS is a loss of CD4$^+$ lymphocytes and a variety of disorders in immune function.

4. Development of disease results from a lack of control of HIV replication by the host immune system.

5. Two types of HIV exist in the world: HIV-1 and HIV-2. Their genomic structures are similar, but they can be distinguished by sequence, particularly in the envelope glycoprotein.

6. The HIV genome contains two structural proteins (Gag and Env), three enzymes (polymerase, integrase, protease), and six accessory genes that help to regulate virus replication (*tat, vif, vpu, vpr [vpx], nef,* and *rev*).

7. The replicative cycle of HIV involves reverse transcription of the viral RNA into a DNA copy and subsequent integration of the viral genome into the cell chromosome. Thus, the virus-infected cell is an important reservoir for HIV infection in the host.

8. Individual HIV-1 and HIV-2 isolates can be characterized by a variety of biologic, immunologic, and molecular features.

9. Three HIV-1 groups (M, N, and O), nine group M clades (A to D, F to H, J, and K), and five group O clades have been identified based on sequence differences; only rarely have group N viruses been isolated. Five HIV-2 groups have been found.

10. The origins of HIV-1 and HIV-2 are not conclusively known, although many investigators believe that HIV-1 came from chimpanzees (SIV$_{cpz}$), particularly those living in Cameroon. Others posit that HIV-2 was transferred from monkeys to humans within the near distant past. Support for these hypotheses comes from similarities in SIV and HIV genes and the prevalence of SIV in primates living in Africa, where the AIDS epidemic appears to have begun.

11. Another possibility is that the viruses were derived from a progenitor virus that entered the mammalian species thousands of years ago. This concept considers the presence of lentiviruses in several distinct animals (e.g., cat, goat, and horse). Only low-level prevalence of HIV could have been maintained in humans until recently.

12. Spread of HIV and the AIDS epidemic could have taken place by injection devices as well as social and behavioral changes in human populations.

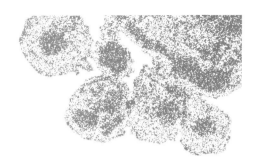

Features of HIV Transmission

2

HIV in Blood

HIV in Genital Fluids

HIV in Milk, Saliva, and Other Body Fluids

HIV Transmission by Blood and Blood Products

Sexual Transmission of HIV

Mother-Child Transmission of HIV

THE TRANSMISSION FREQUENCY OF A VIRUS such as HIV is influenced by the amount of the infectious agent in a body fluid and the extent of contact an individual has with that body fluid. Establishment of infection depends on three points of a classic epidemiological triangle (Figure 2.1): characteristics of the infectious agent (e.g., virulence and infectiousness), host-related factors (susceptibility, contagiousness, and immune response), and environmental factors (social, cultural, and political). The same features can influence disease development.

Epidemiological studies conducted during 1981 and 1982 first indicated that the major routes of transmission of AIDS were intimate sexual contact and contaminated blood (1994). The syndrome was initially described in homosexual and bisexual men and intravenous drug users (1576, 2868, 3008, 4135), but its transmission through heterosexual activity was soon recognized as well (1741). High-risk sexual behavior early in the epidemic caused the rapid increase in HIV transmission (2905). Moreover, it became evident that transfusion recipients and hemophiliacs could contract the illness from blood or blood products (653) and that mothers could transfer the causative agent to newborn infants (99, 3329). These three principal means of transmission—blood, sexual contact, and mother-child—have not changed (3635) and can be explained to a great extent by the relative concentration of HIV in various body fluids (Table 2.1).

The high virus load in blood observed during acute HIV infection or the symptomatic period (Section I) appears to correlate with the greatest risk of HIV transmission (3636). For conclusive evidence, however, relative levels of virus in genital fluid at these times must be considered, but these numbers are still somewhat inconsistent (Section II).

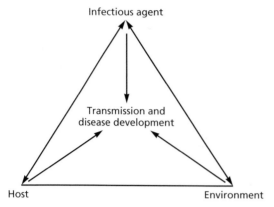

Infectious agent

Transmission and
disease development

Host   Environment

Figure 2.1   Epidemiology of infectious diseases. A variety of host and environmental factors, as well as characteristics of the infectious agent, determine transmission of the agent and induction of disease. Reprinted from reference 3831 with permission. Copyright © 1997 Massachusetts Medical Society. All rights reserved.

It would be most important to know the virus biotype that is first transferred by all the routes of transmission. That information may be obtained through analysis of blood, vaginal secretions, or cervicovaginal biopsy samples as well as samples taken from the rectal canal. It is certain that the mixed virus population in genital fluids will contain a virus that can be preferentially transmitted by sexual activity. During intravenous drug use, such a selection may be less evident but could reflect virus that can more readily infect circulating $CD4^+$ T cells or those cells present in highest number within the lymph node (see below).

In this chapter, the evidence on virus load in various body fluids is reviewed and the findings are considered in relation to virus transmission. The value of anti-HIV antibodies in assessing HIV infection is discussed in Chapter 4.

I. HIV in Blood

Because of the great concern for the reported transmission of AIDS by blood, major efforts were made early in the study of HIV to quantify virus in this body fluid. The results indicated that both free infectious virus and infected cells were present in blood, and HIV-infected cells appeared to be more numerous than infectious virus (Table 2.1). In blood, as well as other body fluids, noninfectious viruses and cells containing defective

viral genomes detected by PCR were found in the largest quantities but did not represent sources of transmission. Currently, HIV-1 clade B dominates virus infection of blood donors in the United States, although 2% of people show infection by other M clades and by HIV-2 (1043) (see Chapter 1 for virus classifications).

A. Infectious Virus

In the early studies of viremia, methods for detecting infectious virus had to be established and optimized. The initial data suggested that free infectious HIV was present in the blood of about 30 to 50% of infected individuals (1244, 2996). However, improved virus detection procedures later showed that most blood samples contain circulating infectious virus whether the HIV-infected individual is asymptomatic or has AIDS

Table 2.1 Isolation of HIV from body fluids[a]

Body fluid	Virus isolation[b]	Estimated quantity of HIV[c]
Cell-free fluid		
Plasma	33/33	1–5,000[b]
Tears	2/5	<1
Ear secretions	1/8	5–10
Saliva	3/55	<1
Sweat	0/2	
Feces	0/2	
Urine	1/5	<1
Cervicovaginal fluid	5/16	<1
Semen	5/15	10–50
Milk	1/5	<1
Cerebrospinal fluid	21/40	10–10,000
Infected cells		
PBMC	89/92	0.001–1
Saliva	4/11	<0.01
Bronchial fluid	3/24	NK
Cervicovaginal fluid	7/16	NK
Semen	11/28	0.01–5

[a]For cell-free fluid, values are infectious particles per milliliter; for infected cells, values are percentages of total cells infected. PBMC, peripheral blood mononuclear cells. NK, not known.

[b]Number of times infectious viruses or infected cells were isolated per number of samples tested.

[c]High levels associated with symptoms and advanced disease.

Table 2.2 Titer of infectious HIV-1 recovered from plasma in relation to CD4+ cell count

No. of CD4+ cell/ml	No. of individuals	Range of HIV titers (TCID*a*/ml)	Mean of HIV titers (TCID/ml)*b*
≥ 500	13	1–500	114
300–499	8	1–500	205
200–299	4	25–500	381
<200	8	25–5,000	1,466

*a*TCID, tissue culture infectious dose.
*b*The trend of finding increased virus titer with lower CD4+ cell counts was statistically significant (Kruskal-Wallis test; data from reference 3396).

Table 2.3 Plasma viremia and clinical stage*a*

Clinical stage	Viremia (virions/ml)
Acute (primary) infection	5×10^6
Asymptomatic	8×10^4
Early symptomatic	35×10^4
AIDS	2.5×10^6

*a*Summary of qualitative competitive PCR data from reference 3528. Representative values are shown. Culturable infectious virus ranged from 100- to 100,000-fold less.

(875, 1853, 3396). The quantity can reach 100 to 1,000 infectious particles (IP) per milliliter of blood (Tables 2.1 and 2.2). Importantly, the level is very low in healthy subjects and often undetectable in people who remain healthy without therapy after 10 years of infection (i.e., long-term survivors) (see Chapter 13) (606, 3416). To quantify optimally the level of free infectious virus in blood, the plasma needs to be tested within 3 h after venipuncture. Otherwise, neutralizing antibodies, complement (4332), and other undefined factors in the plasma (for a review, see reference 4218) reduce the infectivity of HIV (3396). An important procedure for detection of infectious virus in plasma is to allow at least a 24-h incubation with the target cells (3104).

Infectious HIV is readily found during acute infection (i.e., first 7 to 14 days) (790, 947, 2541, 3396), but within weeks the level of this virus detected in the blood is markedly reduced (875, 1221, 1853, 3396, 3502). The reason for this decrease in viremia is linked to an active antiviral immune response (see below and Chapters 9 to 11). Then, as disease develops with its characteristic loss of CD4+ cells, the concentration of infectious HIV in blood rises substantially (Table 2.2), reflecting the increased virus load in PBMC and lymphoid tissues (see Chapter 4) (875, 1181, 1853). Thus, as noted above, the risk of transmission of infectious HIV would seem to be highest in the early stage of infection and during the symptomatic periods (see Section IV).

B. Viral Antigen and RNA Levels

Other procedures for measuring virus can greatly increase the sensitivity for detection of HIV in blood and other body fluids. However, they do not distinguish between infectious and noninfectious virions. These methods include the measurement of viral p24 antigen (1579), directly and after acid dissociation (429), and of HIV RNA by PCR (1879) and quantitative competitive (QC) PCR techniques (2974, 3502). The early QC PCR data supported the observations on high viremia during acute infection and AIDS (Table 2.3).

Very sensitive methods for detecting HIV RNA include reverse transcription-PCR and a procedure based on the attachment of branched oligodeoxyribonucleotides to viral RNA for subsequent signal amplification (4528, 4551) (Figure 2.2). The sensitivity of these procedures is usually better than that of QC PCR. Detection of viral RNA to levels of ~50 copies/ml or lower can be achieved (3648). Most recent viral RNA assays can even detect virus levels as low as 2 RNA molecules/ml (1286, 3395). These molecular approaches are very valuable for measuring the relationship of viremia to the clinical condition and the response to therapy (1854, 4700). They have provided an important advancement in handling clinical approaches to HIV infection (see Chapter 14). In resource-poor countries or areas where viral loads cannot be measured by the above techniques, dried blood samples on filter paper have been useful to detect HIV infection (858).

With these techniques available, two groups of investigators, using antiretroviral drugs to suppress virus replication in vivo, calculated the potential kinetics of virus replication and time for removal of HIV from the peripheral blood (see also Chapter 14). These studies with symptomatic patients suggested that the half-life of HIV in plasma (measured by RNA) is about 6.5 h (1854, 3471, 4700)

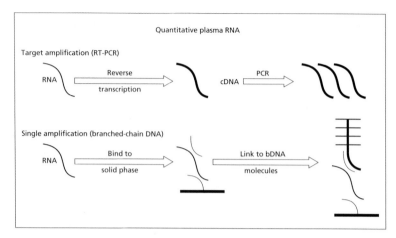

Figure 2.2 Schematic representation of the reverse transcriptase PCR and branched-chain DNA techniques for amplification and quantitation of viral RNA in blood and body fluids. Adapted from reference 1707 with permission.

and that up to 10 billion virus particles could be present in the circulating blood of symptomatic patients (3471). Subsequent studies using plasmapheresis gave estimates of the HIV half-life as 28 to 110 min and that of hepatitis C virus (HCV) as 100 to 182 min (3660). The half-life of HIV is so short that it is estimated that half the entire plasma virus population is replaced in <30 min (3660).

Additional observations on infected individuals in different clinical states indicated that high levels of viremia correlated with progression of disease. Small decreases in plasma viral RNA levels have been reported in women during ovulation, most likely reflecting the effect of certain hormones (e.g., human chorionic gonadotropin) on HIV replication (466, 1616). In long-term survivors, as noted above, free infectious virus and viral RNA are very low or undetectable in the blood (606, 1443, 3416). Thus, the absence of plasma viral RNA has been considered a good prognostic sign (see Chapter 13). This finding sparked interest in beginning antiretroviral therapy in infected individuals at early stages in infection. The objective was to reduce the viral load to undetectable levels (i.e., less than 50 copies of viral RNA/ml of blood) for long periods. The timing for treatment, however, has been controversial and is not yet resolved (see Chapter 14).

The relationship of data on viral RNA levels measured by these molecular procedures to the number of *infectious* particles, the potential source of HIV transmission, is important. It is estimated that up to 100,000 (average, 60,000) more noninfectious virions than free infectious viruses are present in the plasma of seropositive individuals (2438, 3502). These noninfectious viruses would be the majority of virions detected by the quantitative antigen and RNA analyses cited above. Thus, in considering transmission, appreciation of the amount of infectious virus in the blood is obviously necessary. For efficacy of antiretroviral drugs, viral load is the best surrogate marker. Moreover, for prognosis, the extent of viral RNA production, as it reflects the overall clinical state, can be a valuable parameter (2969) (see Chapter 13). Currently, however, levels of CD4$^+$ cells are considered more important than viral load in assessing the need for therapy and the seriousness of the clinical state (see Chapter 14).

C. Virus-Infected Cells

Despite this attention to free virus particles in the blood, their relationship to virus-infected cells remains an important question. In many cases, levels of free virus, even following antiviral therapy, have not consistently shown a correlation to virus in PBMC (2467) or in the lymph node (838) (see Chapter 14). The total number of HIV-infected cells has been estimated to be several hundred billion (1194), a much greater number than the free virions usually found in blood (see above and Chapter 13). Moreover, studies have indicated that one infected cell can produce from 200 to 1,000 particles per day (average 200 infectious viruses) (1089, 2522, 2548). Thus, the total number of infected cells responsible for the high viral RNA level in the blood could represent only a small fraction (10 to 20 million) of cells known to be infected (1194, 2522, 2525). This observation emphasizes a concern about concluding that a block in de novo virus infection by using current antiretroviral drugs will give long-term benefit. Many virus-infected cells remain in the body and can be a continual source of new infectious viruses (2517, 2522, 2525, 3858) (see Chapters 13 and 14).

As with free virus, the number of infected cells is increased with symptomatic disease in association with reduced CD4$^+$ cell counts (Table 2.1). Initially, the number of virus-infected cells detected by in situ hybridization techniques ranged from 1:10,000 to 1:100,000 PBMC (1736). Subsequent studies using PCR procedures increased this number to an average of 1 in 1,000 to 1 in 10,000 PBMCs in healthy individuals and 1:10 PBMCs in AIDS patients (1907, 3990). In studies using in situ PCR hybridization and flow cytometry, 1 in 10 PBMCs were found to be infected in some symptomatic patients (216, 3442). Most of the infected cells (50 to 90%) contained HIV in a latent (unexpressed, or "silent") state (3442) (see Chapter 5). Using a microculture assay, optimal procedures for measuring the number of cells capable of producing virus have been reported (4024). Close to 50% of the virus-infected cells in lymphoid tissue from some infected individuals appear to contain infectious virus (397).

The majority of cells showing HIV infection by these molecular techniques are CD4$^+$ lymphocytes (211, 3442). Not many circulating macrophages are found to be infected (see Chapter 4). The nature of the latent virus in the unproductively infected cells is not well defined; it could be replication defective or in a silent state (646; for a review, see reference 4141) (see Chapters 5 and 14). When the infection is latent and infected cells contain infectious virus, what activates virus production in the cells is an important factor in HIV pathogenesis (see Chapters 5 and 13).

For concerns about transmission and spread of virus in the host, the virus-infected cell becomes more important than infectious virus load in the blood (Table 2.4). The total amount of free infectious virus in asymptomatic individuals can be 100 IP/ml of blood (1853, 3396), whereas the average number of virus-infected cells in these individuals is about 1 in 1,000 PBMC, (211, 510, 1736, 1907, 3611, 3993) (see Chapter 4). Once again, total viral RNA (containing mostly noninfectious virions) will be up to 100,000-fold higher but not a factor in transmitting HIV. With at least 5×10^6 white cells/ml of blood, there can be about 5,000 infected cells/ml of blood in a healthy individual. From this total amount, one can estimate that at least 50% of these cells can release infectious virus (397). Thus, the number of infected cells in blood is at least 25-fold greater than the amount of free infectious virus. In addition, each cell could produce many IP daily (1089, 2548).

During symptomatic infection, especially AIDS, the number of infectious viruses and infected cells is usually much higher (e.g., 1,000 IP/ml; up to 1:10 CD4$^+$ cells/ml) (211, 214, 1907, 2521, 3990) (Tables 2.2 and 2.3). Thus, the chance of transmitting infection, particularly by cells containing HIV, could be even greater (2517, 2521, 2522). Furthermore, even if a latently infected cell was transferred, it could serve as a source of HIV

Table 2.4 HIV pathogenesis: importance of the virus-infected cell[a]

- Present at higher levels in the body (>200 billion cells) than free virus (1–10 billion particles)
- Reservoir for persistent virus production (1,000 particles/day)
- Present at higher levels (5 to 50 times) than free virus in genital fluids and blood
- Remains viable in genital fluids and blood longer than free virus
- Transfers HIV to new cells more effectively than infection by free virus
- Can induce apoptosis by cell-to-cell contact
- Releases viral products that are toxic to the host (e.g., gp120, gp41, and Tat)
- Releases toxic cellular products (e.g., TNF-α and IL-6)

[a]TNF-α, tumor necrosis factor alpha; IL-6, interleukin-6.

transmission after its activation in the new host (2807).

It is noteworthy that HIV-1 RNA and infectious virus can be found bound to erythrocytes, platelets, neutrophils, CD8$^+$ cells, and B lymphocytes without infecting these CD4$^-$ cells (1827, 1995, 2530, 3048, 3330) (Figure 2.3). Virus can be passed to susceptible target cells such as CD4$^+$ T cells. Even in the absence of plasma HIV RNA, HIV, in association with erythrocytes, can be detected as it has been in circulating immune complexes (IC) (3115). Some of this IC virus appears to be neutralized (1076). HIV ICs have also been found on follicular dendritic cells in lymphoid tissue (1783, 4230). The virus bound to these uninfected cells can be more stable and infectious than cell-free virus (3330) (see Chapters 8 and 13). Other uninfected CD4$^-$ cells in the body (e.g., fibroblasts and epithelial cells) could be important transmitters of infectious virus within the host and conceivably in genital fluids (for a review, see reference 2530).

Figure 2.3 Many cell types can bind HIV directly through specific cell surface receptors (e.g., DC-SIGN) or via attachment of HIV immune complexes to cellular receptors (e.g., CD21 and CD35). Infectious virus can then be transferred to various target cells. Reproduced from *The Lancet* (2530), copyright 2002, with permission from Elsevier.

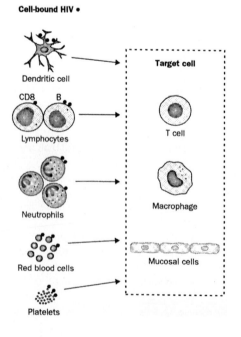

II. HIV in Genital Fluids

A. General Observations

In the case of sexual transmission, the amount of virus in genital fluids is important. Generally, seminal and vaginal fluids have shown the presence of free infectious virus and/or virus-infected cells in 10 to 30% of specimens (112, 1857, 2517, 2521, 4564, 4620, 4800, 4906; for reviews, see reference 877 and 4589) (Figure 2.4). However, the levels of free infectious virus detected in these body fluids (estimated at 1 to 50 IP/ml) have not been reported from a large number of individuals, and the quantity of virus found can vary considerably (2517, 4589) (Table 2.1).

Measurements of viral RNA levels have shown a greater frequency of free virus in these fluids than infected cells, but the risk of transmission will depend on the number of infectious virions (for a review, see reference 877). Moreover, the potential influence of anti-HIV antibodies (3258), anti-HIV cytotoxic T lymphocytes (1922) (CTLs), and innate antiviral factors (3514) in genital fluids on the risk of transmission merits consideration. Biologic and epidemiological factors that can influence virus shedding in the genital tract are listed in Table 2.5 (3143).

B. HIV in Seminal Fluid

1. FREE VIRUS

High viral load in semen has been detected in HIV-1-infected subjects at all stages of the disease and correlates strongly with blood plasma viral load (1671). The relationship of seminal viral load with blood CD4$^+$ T-cell count is controversial. In some studies, a correlation was observed (1671); in others, only a weak association was noted (4586). Longitudinal analysis of subjects who progressed to AIDS showed that the seminal viral load increased markedly in most cases as the disease progressed (1671). Higher efficiency of virus isolation from semen with subjects with lower CD4$^+$ cell numbers further supports these findings (878, 4588). Furthermore, a longitudinal study indicates that in most HIV-1-infected subjects, the virus is shed intermittently in semen, and such intermittent shedding reflects the compartmentalization of HIV-1 between semen and blood (1670).

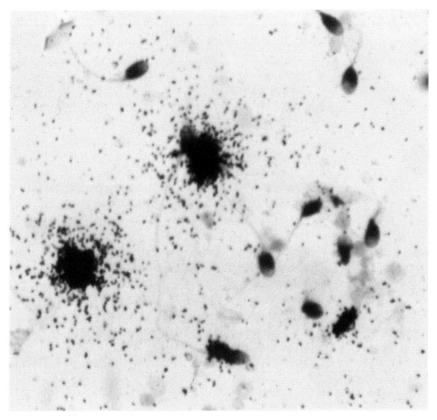

Figure 2.4   HIV-infected cells detected in seminal fluid by in situ hybridization. Magnification, ×40. Reprinted from reference 2517 with permission. Copyright © 1988, American Medical Association. All rights reserved.

As noted above with plasma virus, the largest amount of infectious virus in genital fluids might be expected in the acute phase of infection and during the symptomatic periods (Section I). In this regard, transmission has been found to be increased when the male partners with disease or high viral RNA levels engage in heterosexual or homosexual activity (3351, 3636, 3920). Both syncytium-inducing (SI) X4 and non-syncytium-inducing (NSI) R5 viruses (see Chapter 3 for description of virus phenotypes) can be isolated from semen (4590). The majority of viruses present appear to be of the R5 type (878, 1670, 3422). In some studies, HIV RNA associated with shedding of seminal cells was found in over 80% of seminal plasma specimens, and levels of virus were lower than in plasma. In the presence of genital tract inflammation and sexually transmitted dis-eases, HIV levels are higher in seminal fluid (169, 3515) (Table 2.5) (see below).

Others have reported that the quantity of HIV in semen may not reflect the level of plasma viremia (3515). In this regard, one small group of men (high producers) had RNA levels in seminal plasma comparable to or higher than that detected in blood plasma (4357). They could represent high virus transmitters. Recovery of infectious virus from semen is greatest from men with low CD4$^+$ cell counts (112, 4587). Nevertheless, several studies suggest that the presence of infectious virus recovered primarily from infected cells in seminal fluid does not necessarily correlate with the clinical state (1704, 2329; for a review, see reference 877). Moreover, the level of HIV RNA in semen does not correlate with the frequency of HIV-specific CD8$^+$ cells (4094). These and other

Table 2.5 Factors affecting HIV-1 shedding in the genital tract[a]

Status	Factors in:	
	Females	**Males**
Confirmed correlates[b]	Pregnancy	HIV disease stage
	Oral contraceptives	CD4$^+$ lymphocyte count
	Cervical ectopy	CD8$^+$ lymphocyte count
	Cervicitis	Antiretroviral therapy
		Leukocytospermia
		Gonorrhea
		Urethritis
Potential correlates	HIV disease stage	Plasma viremia
	Phase of the menstrual cycle	Viral phenotype or subtype
	CD4$^+$ lymphocyte count	Vasectomy
	Plasma viremia	Circumcision status
	Viral phenotype or subtype	Nutritional deficiency states
	Antiretroviral therapy	Nongonococcal urethritis
	Injectable contraceptives	Mucosal HIV antibodies
	Nutritional deficiency state	
	Specific cervical or vaginal STD[c]	
	Lactobacillus and H$_2$O$_2$ production	
	Mucosal HIV antibodies	
	Douching or drying agents	

[a]Adapted from reference 3143 with permission.
[b]The confirmed correlates listed are those which have been significantly associated ($p<0.05$) with HIV-1 detection in genital tract fluids in one or more studies.
[c]STD, sexually transmitted disease.

findings (3512) suggest a separate seminal tissue compartment for HIV with the viruses produced by different cells in the male genital tract (4590) (see Chapter 4).

Further support for a seminal compartment for HIV comes from finding that the virus in semen does not always show the same biologic or genetic phenotype as that found in the blood (i.e., R5 versus X4) of the same infected individual (575, 1670, 3422, 3512, 4587, 4958). Moreover, in one study, HIV levels measured weekly for 10 weeks showed no HIV shedding in semen in 28% of subjects, continuous shedding in 28%, and intermediate shedding in 44%. There was no change in blood plasma virus levels during the same time period (1670). Similarly, no correlation of plasma viremia to viral levels (measured by reverse transcription-PCR) in semen or saliva was found when all three body fluids were examined (2643). Apparently, direct infection (2976) or local in-

flammation in these various body compartments can be the important factor in the level of virus present. The reactivation of cytomegalovirus may increase the extent of HIV shedding in semen (4095). Finally, virus has been detected in semen by cell culture or PCR techniques despite antiviral therapy when plasma virus levels were low or undetectable (878, 1220, 1704, 2330, 4587). These findings probably reflect the inability of some drugs to penetrate the blood-testis barrier (253) (see Chapter 14) and emphasize the ability of an infected person to transmit HIV despite low viremia levels.

2. HIV-INFECTED CELLS

The prevalence of virus-infected cells appears to be an important variable in genital fluids (2521, 4619, 4804). In seminal fluid, the number can range from 0.01 to 5% (2517) (Table 2.1; Figure 2.4). Semen from healthy uninfected individuals usually

Harold W. Jaffe

Former Director, Division of AIDS, STD and TB Laboratory Research, National Center for Infectious Diseases, Centers for Disease Control and Prevention. Dr. Jaffe was among the first to pioneer efforts at tracing the epidemiology of AIDS.

has over 1 million white cells/ejaculate (111, 3332, 4803), but levels and subsets of cells can vary widely from day to day in the same person (D. Phillips, personal communication). Nevertheless, the HIV-infected cells (>10^4 cells/ejaculate in some cases) would seem to be a greater source of transmission than free infectious virus. Moreover, if venereal disease is present, many more inflammatory cells, and thus virus-infected cells, would be present in both seminal and vaginal fluids (see Section V). In one study, HIV DNA was found in urethral cells during gonococcal urethritis, and the number of infected cells detected was decreased by antibiotic treatment (3139). Moreover, latently infected cells have been consistently found in semen as well as blood after prolonged antiretroviral therapy (912, 3479). Their potential role in transmission must be appreciated.

3. SOURCE OF VIRUS

The cellular source of HIV-infected cells in seminal fluid is not well defined, and the cells could be from several sites. Some believe that the virus comes from the blood (for a review, see reference 2674). Others conclude that the virus-infected cells come from the testes and the free virus comes from the prostate gland (3422). Others have considered distal genitourinary sources aside from the prostate as a source (876). By culture and in situ PCR hybridization procedures, HIV has been detected in large quantities in the testes of infected

individuals. It has been found in urethral cells (3139), spermatogonia, spermatocytes, and rare spermatids, but not in Sertoli cells (3293) (see Chapter 4). Testicular atrophy can take place in HIV infection and thus limit the detection of virus in this tissue (3293). In some cases, this pathology probably reflects the pathogenic effects of the virus. The presence of HIV in spermatogonia could explain the puzzling finding of HIV DNA in the mid-portion of some spermatozoa, as noted by in situ PCR hybridization (210). Since only the head enters the egg during fertilization, the possible germ line transmission of HIV has no likely relevance. Nevertheless, a glycolipid resembling galactosyl ceramide on the middle portion of the sperm tail (520) could serve as an attachment site for HIV, as it does on some brain and bowel cells (see Chapter 3). In HCV-coinfected men, HCV particles originating from the blood have been found in semen (502).

HIV has been isolated from semen from vasectomized men (113), and after vasectomy, many lymphocytes can be found in the ejaculate (3332). Infectious virus has been recovered as well from pre-ejaculatory fluid from infected men (1952, 3613). In some studies, HIV has not been detected in the epithelia of the prostate, epididymus, seminal vesicles, or penis of men with AIDS by in situ PCR hybridization procedures (3293). In summary, while HIV transfer from blood is possible, the differences in virus isolates suggest that HIV and virus-infected cells in semen can come from the testes, urethra, prostate, and other secretory glands (944, 2449, 3422). Evidently, the initial HIV infection must lead to subsequent virus transfer, most likely from the blood to the genital tract, where selection of specific virus variants that are shed into the semen takes place.

C. HIV in Vaginal Fluid

Vaginal fluid has been found to contain free infectious virus only rarely (1813, 4800); generally, infected cells are detected (1813, 4619, 4620, 4800), but the quantity has not been reported (Table 2.1). Even by PCR analysis, only 28% of infected women showed HIV in cervicovaginal secretions (3258). As with seminal fluid, plasma viremia can (1746, 2307) but does not always correlate directly with the extent of virus shedding in the vaginal canal (1746, 3258, 3671). Moreover, the prevalence of free virus in cervicovaginal secretions does not necessarily reflect the clinical state, antiretroviral therapy, or risk group (1746, 1813, 3671). Nevertheless, anti-HIV therapy has dramatically reduced cervicovaginal HIV RNA levels (929).

Vaginal fluid RNA is higher in women with cervical ectopy, abnormal vaginal discharge, or severe vitamin A deficiency or in those taking oral contraceptive pills (7973 for a review, see reference 3831) (Table 2.5). Viral shedding also may correlate with certain phases of the menstrual cycle (305, 3689), perhaps due to vaginal cytokine levels (49). Some studies suggest that clade C virus infection is associated with increased HIV-1 vaginal shedding (2039). Again, however, the number of subjects with infectious virus studied has been too low to make definitive conclusions on the risks of virus transmission. Importantly, even with highly active antiretroviral therapy (HAART), cell-free virus has been detected in cervicovaginal fluids (3291).

With regard to viral types, several studies have revealed that viruses in cervical secretions can differ genotypically from those found in the peripheral blood (1191, 3500, 3588). These differences become very evident during antiviral therapy (1002). This recognition of tissue-specific variants, as well as differences in plasma and vaginal fluid HIV RNA levels cited above, support the conclusion, noted with seminal fluid, that a separate distribution (or evolution) of viruses can be found in the genital tissues in comparison to the blood. In a recent study, Env RNA sequences from plasma and genital compartments from HIV-infected women during primary infection showed great similarity. In contrast, when these sequences were studied in chronically infected women, the viruses retrieved from the genital epithelia were found to be different than the viruses found in the blood. Moreover, in the chronically infected women, some of the original transmitted virus persisted (763). These observations again indicate how compartmentalization of HIV-1 occurs following acute infection; the initially transmitted virus, most likely in blood, infects the genital tract and can undergo a separate evolution in the different tissues infected (1388).

The source of HIV in vaginal fluid is not known but is probably the secretory glands in the vagina or cervix, white cells in the uterine cavity, and, in some cases, menstrual blood. HIV has been detected in the cervix (3567), where, by in situ PCR hybridization procedures, it is found in monocytes and macrophages (3294) and in the glandular epithelium in the zone of transformation between columnar and squamous cells (3294). The cervix is a more frequent source of virus than the vagina (797; for a review, see reference 3831).

In all these studies on genital fluids, detection of infectious virus was probably limited, since culturing of HIV can be technically difficult. These body fluids can be cytotoxic in cell culture, and survival of virus can depend on the pH and potential antiviral factors present (3311). In this regard, several vaginal fluid cationic polypeptides used together have shown anti-HIV activity (4581). Moreover, a delay in assaying genital or other body fluids probably decreases detection of virus, as noted with plasma samples (3396).

D. Rectal Secretions

Studies to examine anal/rectal virus shedding have shown that inflammation and human papillomavirus infections are associated with the presence of viral RNA and HIV-infected cells (2218). High plasma HIV RNA levels correlated as well with the presence of virus in anal and rectal cells and anal secretions (2218). Viral RNA has also been detected in feces (see Section III.C) (4547) and in diarrhea fluids (4882). Local virus replication in the bowel (see Chapter 8) appeared to be a major mechanism for HIV expression when plasma viral loads were low. In some studies, HIV RNA levels were higher in rectal secretions than in blood plasma or seminal plasma and the virus did not appear to be sensitive to antiviral therapy (4983). Whether this finding reflects the anal canal as a separate compartment for HIV evolution remains to be determined.

III. HIV in Milk, Saliva, and Other Body Fluids

A. Milk

Maternal milk is an important source of infectious HIV that can be transferred to a newborn (1151, 4544, 4962). This transmission is associated with high milk viral loads, a large number of infected breast milk cells, and mastitis (3820, 4042). The probability of transmission by 1 liter of milk

ingested by the newborn can approach that of heterosexual transmission per unprotected sexual act (3724) (Table 2.6). Some studies suggest that colostrum and early breast milk contain primarily infected CD4$^+$ macrophages, which can be a source of macrophage-tropic R5 HIV-1 (3928). This infection, by HIV via maternal milk, can occur not only by secreted viruses but also by HIV transfer via macrophages expressing DC-SIGN (see Chapters 3 and 9) to cells in the gastrointestinal tract even in the presence of acidic gastric fluid (3928).

HIV-1 core antigen has been detected in 24% of milk specimens obtained from women within days after delivery, but not in subsequent samples (3840). In addition, by PCR procedures, virus-infected cells were detected in 58% of milk samples from more than 100 infected African women. Recent studies suggest that breast milk and infected CD4$^+$ T cells produce more infectious virus particles than blood-derived CD4$^+$ T cells (291). The importance of these cells in mother-to-child

Table 2.6 Estimates of risk of HIV transmission and global importance[a]

Type of exposure	Likelihood of infection after a single exposure (%)	Global total (%)
Sexual intercourse	0.0–1.0	70–80
Receptive vaginal	0.01–0.32	60–70
Receptive anal	~1.0	5–10
Insertive anal	0.06	
Insertive vaginal	0.01–0.1	
Injecting drug use	0.5–1.0	5–10
Maternal transmission		
Pregnancy/delivery[b]	12–50	5–10
Breast milk	12[c]	Not quantified
Medical interventions		
Blood transfusions	>90	3–5
Blood products	Not quantified	Not quantified
Organ transplantation	Not quantified	Not quantified
Artificial insemination	Not quantified	Not quantified
Health care work (needlestick, etc.)	0.1–1.0	<0.01

[a]Data obtained from references 1125, 1141, 1767, 3377, and 4761. Table provided by R. Kaplan, L. DeMaria, and N. Padian.
[b]Rate of infection diminished greatly by antiviral therapy during pregnancy and neonatal period (see text).
[c]Risk for continuous breast-feeding, not a single exposure.

transmission must be appreciated. Shedding of free virus in breast milk is intermittent and can differ between the two breasts of an individual woman at a given time (4780). Whether these findings reflect infectious viruses that can be transmitted by milk is the important question. Low CD4$^+$ cell counts and vitamin A deficiency are associated with the highest risk of having virus-infected cells in milk (3227).

Transmission by milk carries the greatest risk early after delivery (3821) and when the mother is infected shortly after birth (e.g., by blood transfusion). In the latter case, the infectious virus content in milk at the time would be high because of a lack of a substantial maternal antiviral immune response. Moreover, the newborn may not have gastric acid to inactivate HIV, which can be found in gastric aspirates (2784, 3258). In addition, some studies have suggested that cathepsin D in breast milk could modify HIV gp120 to increase its affinity for coreceptors and thus HIV transmission (1184).

Milk has also been a source of HIV-2 transmission in neonates. Oral, pharyngeal, and gastric aspirates from a large number of infants showed about 28% positive samples for HIV-2 RNA. Detection was related to high maternal plasma viral load (3595). Moreover, milk is a primary source of HTLV transmission to newborns (1838).

In a more recent study, blood and breast milk isolates were found to be similar, suggesting an equilibration of the blood and breast compartments (1805). However, as observed with genital fluids, several other reports suggest that there is a compartmentalization of HIV-1 between peripheral blood and breast milk. Thus, mother-child transmission by milk may not be predicted by high circulating plasma virus (289).

Milk has also been reported to have an antiviral substance that could be protective (3240); it is perhaps similar to that found in saliva (137) (see below). Some researchers suggest that the antiviral effects can come from α-lactalbumin, lactoferrin, and β-lactoglobulin A/B in milk (3109, 4346), and others report that natural anti-CCR5 antibodies in breast milk can prevent HIV infection (458). A role for secretory anti-HIV antibodies in preventing HIV transmission has not been well established (290). HAART will reduce free virus in breast milk

but not the number of virus-infected cells (4064). Thus, again, the HIV-infected cell could be a major means of transmission. Notably, some studies have found HIV-specific CD8$^+$ T cells in breast milk that might play a role in blocking transmission by this route (2656, 3857).

B. Saliva

Whereas blood, genital fluids, and milk can contain high levels of infectious virus or infected cells, other body fluids are not likely sources of HIV transmission (Table 2.1). Saliva, for example, yields infectious virus only on rare occasions (generally <10% of samples) and only in limited amounts (<1.0 IP/ml) (888, 1639, 1851, 2536). When studied, both free virus and infected cells were detected in saliva but at a low level (2536). By PCR techniques, virus-infected cells were rarely found, even in the presence of periodontal disease (4876), although in one study saliva-associated infected epithelial cells were detected in more than 80% of seropositive subjects (3639). In another study, low levels of free HIV-1 were detected by PCR in most saliva samples obtained from individuals with either high or low CD4$^+$ cell counts (2643). Nevertheless, as a source of transmission, it is the infectious virus titer that is important.

Because of the low level of infectious virus in this fluid, the risk of HIV infection following a human bite is extremely low. No infection was reported in more than 600 incidents of bites handled in U.S. hospitals (4402), although some cases of transmission by biting have been published (123, 276, 4603).

The low rate of recovery of infectious HIV from saliva could reflect not only relatively low virus content but also direct antiviral properties of saliva fluid, such as the secretory leukocyte protease inhibitor (2948), or non-HIV-specific inhibitory substances in the fluid (103, 137, 329, 888, 920, 2770, 3198, 4321). The latter can be fibronectins, glycoproteins, and mucins (e.g., MG1), which come primarily from gingival and not parotid salivary glands (103, 329, 888, 4321). Like dextran sulfate (190), MG1 blocks HIV infection at the cell surface (103) and could prevent cell-to-cell transfer of virus. Alternatively, saliva could aggregate HIV (2770) but not necessarily reduce infectivity unless these aggregates were removed. In addition, the oral epithelial cells can secrete β-defensins that have anti-HIV activity (3638). The presence of these inhibitory substances provides additional reasons to consider saliva an unlikely cause of transmission. Nevertheless, since infectious HIV has been recovered from the throats of infected children (2134), the extent of antiviral activity in the saliva of children compared to adults needs further study.

C. Other Body Fluids

Urine (2569, 4167), sweat (4819), bronchoalveolar lavage fluids (1019, 4972), amniotic fluid (3165), synovial fluid (4797), and tears (1384, 3889) have also been shown to contain no or only low levels of infectious HIV (2521, 2541) (Table 2.1), although viral RNA may be detected in some specimens. Thus, these fluids do not appear to be important sources of virus transmission. This conclusion is supported by the lack of HIV transmission in households or schools with infected children where there is exposure to body fluids (345, 1372, 3780).

In contrast to these body fluids, cerebrospinal fluid (CSF) contains large amounts of virus (e.g., 1,000 IP/ml), particularly in individuals with neurologic findings (1855, 1874, 2539, 4207; for a review, see reference 724) (see Chapters 4 and 8). It can be present in the CSF of asymptomatic individuals (1441). As noted with other localized fluids, simultaneous comparison of viral RNA sequences in CSF and plasma samples have indicated differences that support the conclusion that the brain is a distinct compartment (2173, 4385), particularly within the choroid plexus (559). CSF, however, would not be a natural source of transmission.

IV. HIV Transmission by Blood and Blood Products

A. Intravenous Drug Users

Among the first group of individuals showing evidence of HIV infection were intravenous drug users in the United States and Europe. The virus apparently entered this population in the mid-1970s and spread rapidly through 1985 (1053,

3137). The seroprevalence in this group has been estimated to be about 50 to 60% (1054). AIDS in intravenous drug users further confirmed the presence of HIV in blood and the high risk of infection through shared needles and syringes (1054). In this regard, infectious HIV can be recovered from syringes up to 4 weeks after blood contamination (6). The provision of sterile injection equipment (through needle and syringe exchanges and pharmacy sales) and stable attendance at methadone clinics have been major means of decreasing HIV infection among intravenous drug users. Such programs have led to definite decreases in the risk of HIV infection in people who inject illicit drugs (1054, 3137).

B. Transfusion Recipients and Hemophiliacs

Before the screening of blood and blood products (e.g., Factors VIII and IX), HIV could be transmitted to transfusion recipients and hemophiliacs. Screening of blood for anti-HIV antibodies reduced the chance of HIV transmission by transfusion in the United States 10 years ago to about 1 in 450,000 to 660,000 units (3997). Currently, with the sensitive viral RNA assays, the risk of transmission of HIV-1 and HCV is about 1 in 2 million units (4307). In rare cases, most likely in the first days of acute infection, very low virus levels in blood donations (<10 RNA molecules/ml) have been detected with recent highly sensitive RNA procedures (1286). The new techniques for inactivating HIV in blood and blood products (for a review, see reference 65) should provide even further safety to blood use.

For transfusion recipients, the potential risk of transmission depends on the virus load, defined as the number of free infectious viruses or HIV-infected cells in the blood (567). As noted above (Section I), the amount of virus in the blood is greatest during acute infection and as an infected individual (as donor) advances to disease (Tables 2.2 and 2.3). In one early study, the chance of infection was reported to rise substantially if the donor developed AIDS within 2 to 3 years (3474). Other studies have shown that individuals receiving blood from donors who subsequently develop AIDS within 29 months have a greater risk of progressing to disease than those who receive infected blood from donors who become symptomatic after 29 months (4683). Thus, these findings could reflect (i) the amount of virus present, (ii) the biologic properties of HIV in the donated blood (e.g., the fact that it replicates rapidly and is cytopathic), (iii) the need for virus-infected cells to be activated to release virus, and (iv) the potential existence of a strong antiviral immune response in the donor (see Chapters 9 to 11).

In the case of hemophiliacs without a history of blood transfusion, HIV transmission could only be caused by free virus and was associated with receipt of many vials of unheated clotting factors. The chance of an infectious HIV particle being present in a lyophilized product was thereby increased (1234, 1238, 1539). Retroviruses can survive lyophilization (2545). Nevertheless, evidence of virus particles in old clotting factor preparations has been substantiated only by PCR analysis (4045), in which viral RNA was detected. Attempts to isolate infectious HIV from these sources have been unsuccessful (J. A. Levy, unpublished observations).

When present in a Factor VIII or Factor IX preparation, the quantity of infectious HIV particles must have been relatively low (estimated at <10 IP/vial). The products prepared during the time of HIV transmission came from concentrates of 2,000 or more plasma collections (2521), obtained during 1980 to 1983, before HIV was recognized and when virus prevalence in the general population was low (1238). This assumption is supported by evidence showing that HIV infection in hemophiliacs is associated with receipt of multiple clotting factor preparations obtained from many donors (1238, 1539). Nevertheless, the amount of free virus needed to infect a human is not known; 4 IP (by tissue culture) administered intravenously to a chimpanzee caused infection (158). Moreover, studies of stored blood samples suggest that up to 50% of hemophiliacs were already infected by 1982 to 1983 (1539). Currently, heating Factor VIII and Factor IX to high temperatures (>60°C) either before (in the fluid phase) or after lyophilization (2545, 2546, 2919) has virtually prevented further infection of hemophiliacs.

C. Needlestick and Other Injuries

The estimated risk of HIV infection after percutaneous exposure to virus-infected blood is 1 in 300 to 400 (1494, 4443). The potential for infection is increased if it is a deep injury, if there is visible blood on the device causing injury, if the device has been in contact with the infected person's blood vessel, and if the infected person from whom the blood was taken died from AIDS within 2 months after the exposure (612, 656). The risk from mucosal membrane and skin exposure to infected blood is approximately 1 in 1,000 or less (1494) and is again influenced by the amount of blood and viral load. Precautions introduced into the hospital setting (sheathing devices for needles, correct disposal of sharps, prevention courses, and anti-HIV therapy) have helped to reduce this risk substantially (for a review, see reference 1495). An early trial of zidovudine (AZT) in needlestick injuries showed an eight-fold decrease in virus transmission (612). Finally, one report of HIV and HCV infection following a blow with a fist (8) indicates that transmission is possible following blood-related trauma.

V. Sexual Transmission of HIV

A. General Observations

AIDS was initially identified as a disease most likely transmitted by the sexual route. A high prevalence among homosexual men was reported. Subsequent studies indicated spread by heterosexual activity, which remains responsible for the majority of infections worldwide (3635) (for reviews, see references 2883 and 4527). A large community-based study in a rural district of Uganda indicated that viral load is the chief predictor of the risk of heterosexual transmission of HIV-1. HIV transmission was rare among people with plasma levels of <1,500 copies of HIV RNA/ml (3636). The findings add support to the conclusion that a reduction in plasma viral load could decrease the risk of HIV transmission. However, the relevance of these observations with untreated individuals to those people on antiviral drugs (in which HIV in genital fluids may not be as affected) remains to be determined.

As discussed above, the transmission of HIV by genital fluids is more likely through virus-infected cells than free virus (2517, 2521, 4958) (Section II.B) since cells can be present in higher numbers than free *infectious* virus in these body fluids. In this regard, whereas high levels of viral RNA may be detected in semen (878), infectious HIV is present in low levels (2521) (Table 2.1). Some investigators reported that rhesus macaques are infected intravaginally more readily by free virus than by SIV-infected cells (4195). However, the inocula were not delivered under conventional conditions (e.g., in semen). In this regard, prostaglandin E_2, a semen constituent, might increase HIV transmission directly (2350) or through immunosuppression (2349). In addition, cell culture studies suggest that the infected cells transfer HIV to epithelial cells most effectively when present in seminal fluid (Figures 2.4 and 2.5); cell-cell contact and virus production are most likely increased via factors (e.g., prostaglandins) in semen (1147, 3452). Most recently, SIV-infected PBMC, inoculated intravaginally at even very low levels (7 to 14 infected cells), gave rise to infection of cynomolgus macaques. Infection was more apparent with transient ulcerations of the female reproductive tract (2069a). In some cases, transcytosis of infected cells or virus through the mucosae could be involved (433) (see Chapter 4). Moreover, complement present in semen can enhance the infection of epithelial cells via HIV opsonization or direct interaction with complement receptors in the mucosa (457). The virus transmitted is usually of the R5 type (4957, 4958), reflecting, most likely, the predominance of this phenotype in genital fluids (see Section II and Chapter 13).

Several variables can be involved in the differences observed in virus transmission among sexual partners (for reviews, see references 877, 2883, and 3831) (Figure 2.5). For example, as noted above (Section II), different levels of infected cells in the genital fluids can be an important factor. Thus, it is not unexpected to find a higher risk of transmission in individuals who have sexually transmitted diseases (169, 1841, 1938, 2379, 3139), in whom large numbers of inflammatory cells containing virus-infected cells are present in genital fluids. Herpes simplex virus type 2 infection is associated with a high risk of HIV transmission (3705). Nonulcerative venereal diseases (chlamydia, gonorrhea, and trichomoniasis) are also associated with increased risk of HIV-1 transmission to women (2379). Moreover, activated neutrophils

during inflammation bind HIV-1 and can transfer virus to mucosal cells (1401). Vaginal fluids may also contain the protease cathepsin D, found in mik, which could increase HIV transmission (see Section III.A). It is noteworthy that vitamin A deficiency was not found to be associated with increased risk of HIV infection in men who had sexually transmitted diseases; those with this deficiency showed a decreased risk most likely because of reduced macrophages and lymphoid cell differentiation (2728).

A study of homosexual men showed that there was a greater potential for transmission close to or after the onset of disease (3351), when virus levels in the blood are high (Section I). Contact with symptomatic male partners positive for p24 antigenemia or with low CD4$^+$ cell counts also gave an increased risk of infection by heterosexual activity (2883, 3920). The relationship of these peripheral blood parameters to virus in genital fluids may be important. However, as noted above (Section II), a correlation between level of virus in blood and genital fluids has not been consistently found. Therapy directed at the cellular source could be helpful. In early studies, HIV-infected men treated with the antiviral drug AZT had a reduced incidence of heterosexual transmission compared to untreated males (3182), most likely reflecting an effect of this drug on virus load in the genital fluid (see Chapter 14).

Importantly, HIV transmission has been found to be associated with a lack of circumcision (1702, 1841, 1938, 3715). Several African and Asian countries with risk factors for heterosexual transmission similar to those of other countries have lower HIV infection rates associated with higher male circumcision prevalence (>80 versus <20%). This finding supports the suggestion that male circumcision protects from HIV infection (1702). Notably, uncircumcised men have more than a twofold-increased risk of acquiring HIV per heterosexual act compared to circumcised men (207). In a recent study in South Africa, where more than 3,000 non-HIV-infected males age 18 to 24 were randomized to be circumcised or not (both groups were counseled to use condoms), HIV acquisition was reduced by more than 60% among the men in the circumcision arm (180). The reasons for this increased risk of transmission

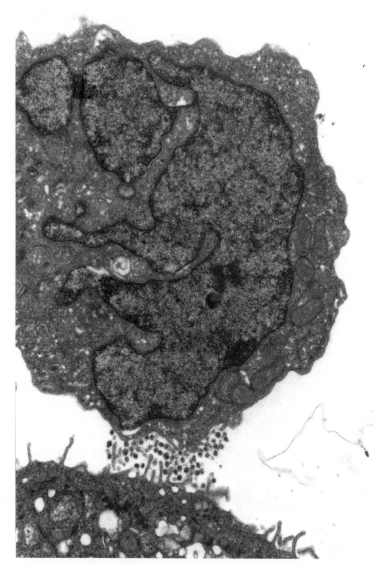

Figure 2.5 HIV-infected HUT 78 T cell (top) cocultivated for 1 h with an ME180 cervix-derived epithelial cell (bottom). Virus can be seen at the cell-cell interface (4375). It is noteworthy that virus is produced by the T-cell line only at the point of contact with the epithelial cells. A role for cytokines in this localized induction of virus production should be considered (see text). Magnification, ×10,000. Photomicrograph provided by D. Phillips.

associated with uncircumcised men is discussed in Section V.C.

Some individuals do not become infected by HIV, despite many unprotected exposures to the genital fluids of infected sexual partners (589, 3376) (see Chapter 13). In some cases, antibodies in the vaginal fluid appear to neutralize HIV and perhaps block virus infection via transcytosis (see Chapter 4). Antibody-dependent cell-mediated cytotoxicity directed against HIV-infected cells in vaginal/cervical fluids can be associated with a reduction in levels of infectious HIV (3197) (see Chapter 10). Moreover, treatment of venereal dis-

eases reduces the number of infected cells in seminal fluid (3139) (see Section II). In addition, other factors (e.g., immune response or virus subtypes) besides viral load (2521) may be involved in this lack of HIV transmission (see Chapter 13). Some studies suggested that neutralization-sensitive viruses were more readily transmitted during heterosexual activity (1050) (Section V.E). In contrast, in men having sex with men, very little correlation of transmission was noted in relation to virus neutralization sensitivity (1378). Moreover, mother-child transmission is reduced with the presence of maternal neutralizing antibodies (2239) (Section VI). The influence of antiviral antibodies on virus transmission needs further evaluation.

B. Infection of the Receptive Partner

1. OVERVIEW: RISK OF TRANSMISSION

As is well known, during heterosexual or homosexual activity, the receptive partner is more at risk for infection than the active partner. In some early studies of heterosexual activity, a two- to fivefold-greater risk of infection was observed in male-to-female transmission (1010, 3376) than in female-to-male transmission (2883, 3376). More recently, the transmission rates appear to be similar, although the receptive female partner is still at somewhat greater risk (Table 2.6). Female-to-male transmission appears to be increased during menses or when other bleeding is involved (3376). Not surprisingly, for a susceptible partner, transmission correlates directly with the number of exposures (3378), but transmission probably depends more on the number of different partners than the frequency of sexual contacts (1009, 1125). It is for this reason that long-term or serial monogamous relationships are encouraged (1926).

An early estimate of infection in females from one heterosexual contact with an infected male was 1 in 500 to 1,000 (1009). With homosexual activity, infection in a high-prevalence community was estimated to be 1 in 10 partners (i.e., infection status unknown) (4789) (for a review, see reference 3831). The apparent efficiency rates of contact transmission differ among the cohorts studied because of the variables involved (e.g., viral load in genital fluid and inflammatory diseases). In this regard, mathematical modeling has suggested that transmission from someone during primary infection, when viremia is high, can be 100- to 1,000-fold greater than that from a long-term asymptomatic person (1993). The evidence suggests that infectiousness is on the order of 1:10 to 1:20 per contact in the primary infection, and 1:1,000 and 1:10,000 in a chronic asymptomatic phase; it then increases to 1:100 to 1:1,000 during the pre-AIDS stage (1606, 1993, 4589, 4693). If the heterosexual transmission is not modeled according to a constant infectivity level, infection from a single contact with a randomly selected infected partner has been estimated to be about 1:60 (0.17) (1125) (Table 2.6).

For the receptive partner in sexual contact, early epidemiological data suggested that HIV needed a point of entry in the anal or vaginal canal. Lesions at these sites from venereal infections (e.g., herpesvirus or syphilis) presumably would increase transmission (1887). This assumption helped to explain the high rate of heterosexual

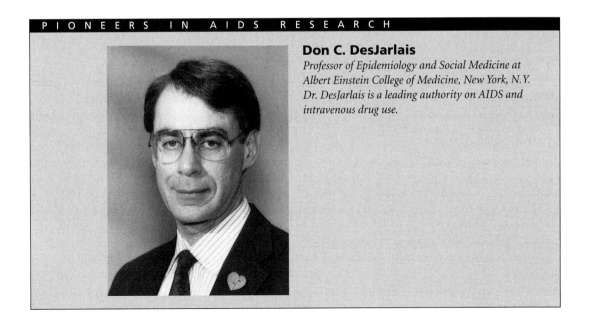

Don C. DesJarlais
Professor of Epidemiology and Social Medicine at Albert Einstein College of Medicine, New York, N.Y. Dr. DesJarlais is a leading authority on AIDS and intravenous drug use.

spread of HIV in Africa, where genital ulcers from venereal diseases (e.g., infection with *Herpesvirus* or *Haemophilus ducreyi*) are associated with increased HIV seroprevalence (589, 1841). Some studies suggest that genital ulcers not only are a possible point of entry for the virus but also could contain HIV and thus be the source of virus transmission (2326, 3950). Nevertheless, evaluation of biopsy tissues has shown that the bowel mucosa and perhaps the cervical epithelium can be infected directly by HIV (1792, 2544, 2870, 3234, 3567) without the need for ulcerations (see Chapters 4 and 8). Finally, the reported increased incidence of transmission associated with uncircumcised men could reflect the presence of inflammation with many infected cells associated with the prepuce (877, 1938) (see Section V.C).

These observations suggest a relationship of the clinical state to the viral load in genital fluid, but that finding is not conclusive (Section II); other factors can be involved. Importantly, while the risk of infection per contact can be estimated (Table 2.6), an accurate number is difficult to define because of the lack of information on variables that could influence HIV transmission. These variables include extent of viral load, presence of sexually transmitted infections, presence of erosions (cervical ectopy), circumcision, number of white cells in genital fluids, and, perhaps, age of the partner during sexual intercourse (Figure 2.6). Each parameter could be different, depending on the stage of infection and if the same or a different partner was involved (1125). Nevertheless, it is noteworthy that infection following only one sexual contact with an infected person has been reported (3378).

2. INFECTION OF WOMEN VIA THE GENITAL TRACT

Because the columnar and squamous cell epithelium of the vagina can be a barrier to virus infection, ulcerations caused by venereal diseases might be a prerequisite for efficient infection at this site. Nevertheless, transmission of HIV has been reported in a chimpanzee inoculated in the vaginal canal with high doses of the virus in culture fluid (1390). The factors involved in this infection, however, could be different from those in the natural state (i.e., in semen). In some cases, infection

of cells in the cervix might take place (797, 3294, 3567, 4375). Cervical ectopy (erosion) is associated significantly with HIV transmission to women (3138). Moreover, cell culture procedures have shown transmission of HIV from infected lymphocytes and macrophages to cervix-derived epithelial cells (4375) (Figure 2.5). Virus or infected cells coming into the uterus can infect CD4+ T cells and macrophages within the endometrium or could pass by transcytosis into the circulation (434, 1862) (see Chapter 4). Moreover, interleukin-8 (IL-8), a prominent cytokine in the female genital tract, can increase HIV replication in T cells and macrophages (3219).

Some studies have suggested that Langerhans cells (LC) in the vagina or cervix could serve as targets for HIV (4212). These CD4+ dendritic cells (DCs) are found within the superficial epithelial layers of the vagina and the foreskin (1940, 2244) and appear to express more CXCR4 than CCR5 (1848, 2893) (see Chapters 3 and 9). Thus, the initial dominance of R5 viruses after infection cannot be explained by this finding (see Chapter 13). However, both R5 and X4 viruses can be transmitted via the genital tract by DC:T-cell interactions (1848). In comparison to free virus, transmission from DCs to T cells has been shown to be more efficient and involve what has been called an infectious synapse (2044). Such an interaction of infected cells with the mucosae could also occur, as has been shown by electron microscopic pictures, suggesting that cellular structures (e.g., pseudopods) can play a role in HIV transmission (Figures 2.5 and 2.7).

Increased heterosexual transmission in women has been associated with contraceptive therapy in which increased shedding of HIV-infected cervical cells has been noted (4669). Apparently, the female hormones (particularly progesterone) can make the vaginal lining cells thinner and more susceptible to erosion, as shown in studies with SIV (2852). Thus, postmenopausal women and those who use progesterone-based contraceptives could have an increased risk of HIV infection. In this regard, a recent study has indicated an increased risk of HIV infection during pregnancy, perhaps reflecting hormonal changes in the cervicovaginal tract mucosae (1605). Other studies have indicated that estrogen-treated macaques can be protected from infection after intravaginal inoculation with SIV

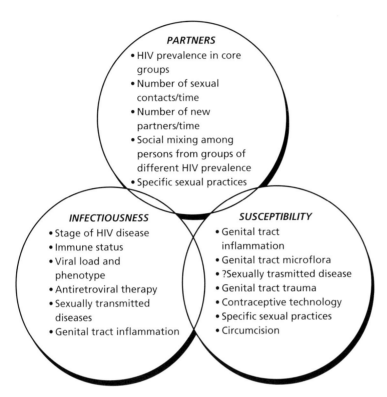

PARTNERS
- HIV prevalence in core groups
- Number of sexual contacts/time
- Number of new partners/time
- Social mixing among persons from groups of different HIV prevalence
- Specific sexual practices

INFECTIOUSNESS
- Stage of HIV disease
- Immune status
- Viral load and phenotype
- Antiretroviral therapy
- Sexually transmitted diseases
- Genital tract inflammation

SUSCEPTIBILITY
- Genital tract inflammation
- Genital tract microflora
- ?Sexually trasmitted disease
- Genital tract trauma
- Contraceptive technology
- Specific sexual practices
- Circumcision

Figure 2.6 Interconnected factors that influence the sexual spread of HIV. Adapted from reference 2883 with permission.

compared with untreated or progesterone-treated animals. A thickening of the vaginal walls takes place. Therefore, topical estrogen therapy to the vagina may be an effective antiviral approach in postmenopausal women (4189).

Some investigators have reported that women whose male sexual partners are uncircumcised have a threefold-increased risk of HIV infection (3831, 4517). This finding could reflect the increased infection rate in uncircumcised males (1702, 3715) (see Section V.A and below) and/or HIV transmission from infected cells associated with the foreskin (see above) (3012) (for a review, see reference 877). In terms of genetic predisposition to infection, certain *HLA-G* polymorphisms in women have been associated with an increased risk of infection, perhaps reflecting a reduction in cellular immune responses (2873). *HLA-DRB1* and *HLA-DQB1* alleles in men and women may be linked to heterosexual transmission (4380), reflecting differences in viral load (see Chapter 13). Moreover, the presence of HLA-Bw4 alleles in HIV-1-infected men has been associated with a decreased risk of transmission to women (4725a).

In the case of HIV transmission associated with artificial insemination (4295), virus-infected cells, along with spermatozoa, gained entry to the uterus when injected through the cervical os. Alternatively, infection of the cervix could have occurred from the presence of erosion (or ectopy) or during inflammatory conditions in the vagina (see above). In one early encouraging study, uninfected women, when inseminated with semen processed to remove free virus and infected cells, gave birth to infants who were all HIV seronegative (4046).

3. INFECTION VIA THE RECTUM
The finding of HIV infection in the rectal mucosa (see Chapters 4, 8, and 13) (Section II.D) provides another reason, besides abrasions, for the high risk of transmission associated with receptive anal/genital contact. This risk of direct infection of the bowel during sexual contact would appear to be the same for both male and female partners. Direct contact of the rectal mucosa with HIV-infected cells in semen could be responsible (467, 3452, 3497) (Figures 2.4 and 2.7). Infection could

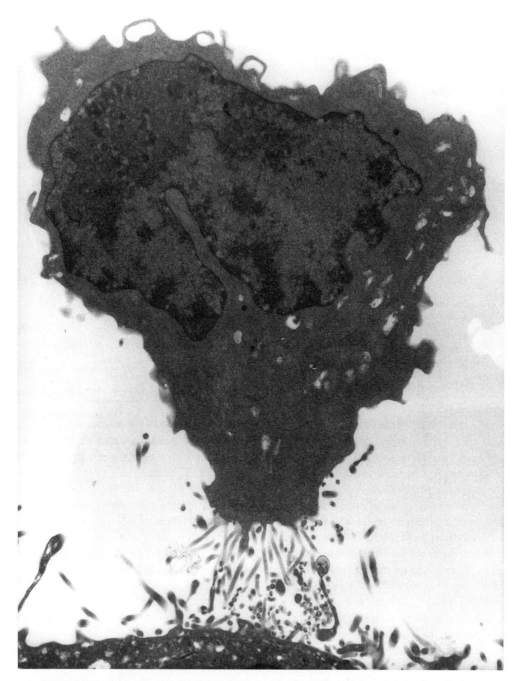

Figure 2.7 Transmission electron micrograph of HIV-infected U937 cells 3 h after addition to the I-407 intestinal epithelial cell line. Virus particles can be observed between the monocyte and the epithelial cell surface in the area of contact. Magnification, ×14,000. Reprinted with permission from reference 467. Photomicrograph provided by D. Phillips.

occur after interaction of the virus with cellular receptors (4841) or attachment of virus:antibody complexes to Fc receptors on the mucosal cells (1939) (see Chapters 3 and 10). Another possible means of HIV entry is via intestinal M cells present in the bowel epithelium (94). This transepithelial transport appears to require viral coreceptors (1337).

Epithelial cell transcytosis could be another major mechanism for free virus or virus-infected cells to infect mucosal lining cells and then spread through the body (434, 1862) (see Chapter 3). This transmigration of virus-infected cells through human epithelial cells is enhanced by intracellular adhesion molecule 2 (ICAM-2) and ICAM-3 on the membrane of epithelial cells. Proinflammatory cytokines increase the expression of these adhesion molecules (622).

HIV infection of the mucosa also supports the epidemiological data showing that douching of the anal canal before sexual contact increases the risk of infection (4789). Cleansing permits easier contact of infected cells with the mucosal epithelial cells. Thus, infection of the rectal mucosa could have been the portal of virus entry for many HIV-infected individuals. The number of sexual contacts with sufficient virus in the genital fluid can be the most important factor in determining sexual transmission.

C. Infection of the Insertive Partner

The insertive partner in sexual contact carries a relatively lower risk of infection, although it is not minimal (4789) (Table 2.6). In heterosexual contact, the infected woman could be most contagious during menses (3376, 3689), but this condition is not considered a major factor (see Section II.C). As noted above (Section V.A), lack of circumcision in males has correlated in several studies with increased risk of infection (up to twofold) (207, 589, 1702). Circumcision has not protected against other sexually transmitted diseases (3715), suggesting a biologic rather than behaviorial explanation for these observations. HIV transmission could take place through infection of LC in the prepuce or of macrophages or lymphocytes associated with the foreskin or along the urethral canal (for a review, see reference 877). In macaques, the macrophages associated with the foreskin or ure-

thral canal were found to be infected with SIV (3012). Thus, circumcision can reduce the chance of this transmission (180). HIV could also be transferred to the penis from infected cells (mostly macrophages or LC) in the cervix (3294) or in the intestinal mucosa (3234). The urethral epithelium also has Fc receptors that could mediate infection by HIV:antibody complexes (1940).

Heterosexual anal intercourse also causes an increased risk of infection for men (2400). Moreover, venereal diseases involving the foreskin could increase the chance of transmission of virus in vaginal fluids to inflammatory cells associated with the foreskin. Obviously, in all participants of sexual contact, an increased number of virus-infected cells in the genital fluids (e.g., resulting from venereal disease) would increase both transfer and receipt of the infectious virus.

D. Oral-Genital Contact

Oral-genital contact could also lead to HIV infection of either partner, albeit at a low frequency (1036, 3818, 4789). The oral cavity lacks $CD4^+$ LC and Fc receptors, suggesting that transmission is difficult by this route (1940). Moreover, saliva has several antiviral factors (see Section III.B). In one study, adult macaques exposed nontraumatically to high doses of SIV through the oral route developed AIDS (192). In other studies, however, chimpanzees receiving virus by the oral route were not infected (1390). Only a few cases of oral-genital transmission have been reported (for review, see reference 3818). Factors influencing transmission are oral trauma, sores, inflammation, allergy, sexually transmitted infections, ejaculation in the mouth, and immune system suppression (3757). The route may be via lymphoid tissues (e.g., tonsils or adenoids) in the oral cavity (B. Herndier and J. A. Levy, unpublished observations). HIV transmission by kissing occurs very rarely, if at all (see Section III.B).

E. Characteristics of the Virus Transmitted

Several studies have been directed at determining the factors that influence the particular virus transmitted. In primate studies, selected variants have been found to be transferred when an SIV preparation was inoculated via the vaginal canal (3230).

Most studies indicate that R5 viruses predominate shortly after acute infection (see Chapter 4), but both subtypes (X4 and R5) are capable of transmission. Therefore, other factors such as levels of virus subtypes in genital fluids and blood, the ability of viruses to infect certain cell types such as DCs and epithelial cells (2972), and, conceivably, selective immune responses against one subtype (1731) determine the ultimate dominance of a viral variant (see Chapter 13). In this regard, as noted above, some studies have suggested that a relatively unglycosylated neutralization-sensitive HIV strain is more likely to be transmitted by the heterosexual route (1050). That observation, however, has not been made with men having sex with men (1378) and requires further study.

In terms of biotype transmitted, DCs can express mRNA for the chemokine receptors CCR3 and CCR5 as well as CXCR4 (1095). This observation indicates that X4 viruses could also gain entry into a host through infection of DCs in the mucosal lining. These findings, together with the fact that most X4 viruses can probably infect DCs and macrophages to some extent (1294, 3268) (see Chapter 13), suggest that X4 viruses are not restricted in their ability to infect individuals through sexual contact. No apparent block to entry of the X4 virus variants occurs, but replication could be limited (see Chapter 5). R5 viruses may have the advantage during transmission because of their replicative ability in LC and macrophages in the vagina and DCs in the rectum (see Chapters 4 and 9). The relative ability to grow in resting versus activated lymphocytes could be a factor as well, since R5 viruses can induce cell activation and proliferation (1610, 2650) (for further discussion, see Chapters 4, 5, and 13). Nevertheless, transfer of infectious viruses from DCs to CD4$^+$ cells can take place without DC infection (see Chapters 3 and 9).

F. Summary: Preventive Measures for Sexual Transmission

All these observations on HIV transmission during sexual activity emphasize the importance of barrier techniques. The most common method is the use of condoms, which has been demonstrated by both in vitro and epidemiological studies to be effective in preventing the passage of virus (862, 3129, 3247). For women the use of spermicidal products (such as nonoxynol-9) against HIV is not recommended. Studies have demonstrated that vaginal and cervical irritations associated with the use of certain doses of these compounds could increase virus transmission (4542). Female condoms (1553), vaginal microbicides, or compounds that inhibit HIV adsorption and cell-to-cell contact (e.g., polycations) need further evaluation. Moreover, the use of a diaphragm in women might be helpful if indeed transmission occurs mostly by virus entry through the cervical os into the uterus. This approach is now under study in women, who could then protect themselves without the consent of their partners (4549). Since soap and water can readily destroy HIV (2571), washing of the penis before and after sexual contact might reduce transmission. However, women who perform vaginal washing with soap or other substances may have a greater risk for HIV infection than those who wash with water alone (2891). The findings most likely reflect the disturbance in natural antiviral factors present in vaginal mucosae.

Approaches for preventing sexual transmission have met with some success, including the 100% condom use policy of Thailand and the management of sexually transmitted diseases in Tanzania and Uganda (for a review, see reference 3831). In this regard, acyclovir used to suppress herpes simplex virus type infection is being evaluated (896). Moreover, if one can avoid sexual encounters during primary infection and have long-term serial monogamous rather than multiple concurrent contacts (1926), transmission can be reduced.

The search for an effective microbicide for women continues (232). More than 15 candidates are in clinical trials (for a review, see reference 1069). The product needs to be nonirritating to the vaginal canal. Certain gel formulations that cover mucosal linings and prevent contact with virus or virus-infected cells are under consideration (2155). In some countries, a substance that blocks HIV but is not a contraceptive is preferred. Administration of HAART in some studies decreased heterosexual transmission by 80% (636). HAART is also being evaluated as a postexposure prophylaxis (PEP) (3516) as well in high-risk individuals (837). Finally, environmental factors, such as mood-altering drugs and alcohol, can affect mental capacity and increase the risk of infection (see Chapter 13).

VI. Mother-Child Transmission of HIV

A. Prevalence of Transmission

The perinatal transmission of virus from untreated HIV-positive mothers is believed to occur in 11 to 60% of children (25, 3241; for a review, see reference 673). This prevalence is based primarily on PCR and virus culture studies; diagnosis by serologic testing is difficult because maternal antibodies are present in infants at birth. The reason for the wide variation in virus transmission rates is not known, and the answer could provide approaches for prevention. Nevertheless, some estimates on the risk of infection by mother-child transmission have been reported (Table 2.6).

Determining infection in the newborn can be difficult. Serologic evaluation at birth is not possible unless immunoglobulin A (IgA) antibodies are measured (2833, 4702). IgA does not pass the placenta and thus does not confer seropositivity to neonates, as other maternal antibodies do. Generally, maternal antibodies decline to background levels by 6 to 18 months (3427); IgG antibody synthesis in an infected infant has been estimated to occur 3 months after birth (3427). Anti-HIV IgA production should be specific for HIV infection in the newborn and could be explained in part by the swallowing of maternal blood or amniotic secretions by the infant in utero or during birth.

Another proposed serologic procedure for detecting an infected newborn is the induction of anti-HIV antibody production in the newborn's PBMC cultures by using a B-cell mitogen (3382). The two most helpful methods for detecting infection in newborns are PCR analysis for viral RNA and virus isolation procedures (1006, 3241, 3947). However, PCR can lack specificity, and virus culture can be time consuming and difficult to conduct routinely.

Currently the diagnosis of HIV infection in a child is best made by analyzing two blood samples in a single assay or in a combination of virus culture and PCR. By this protocol, two negative DNA PCR results for two consecutive blood samples at 6 months of age would establish noninfection (3445).

This conclusion may be misleading, as noted above, if no circulating infected white cells can be detected but virus is still present in lymphoid organs such as the liver or spleen. Therefore, RNA PCR could be a more reliable assay for detection of perinatal infection than is DNA PCR (4283).

B. Factors Influencing Mother-Child Transmission

The transfer of HIV from the mother to the newborn can be associated with several factors (Table 2.7), including a low $CD4^+$ cell count, high virus load (particularly measured by PCR), p24 antigenemia in the mother at the time of delivery (1007, 1009, 1082, 3814), a highly replicating cytopathic maternal virus (2240), and a large number of HIV-infected cervicovaginal cells (2036). A long duration of membrane rupture before delivery can

Table 2.7 Factors associated with mother-child transmission[a]

- Low $CD4^+$ cell count in the mother (1007, 3947)
- High viral load (p24 antigenemia) in the mother at time of delivery (1007, 3947)
- High-replicating, cytopathic virus in maternal blood (2240)
- High-level infection of cervicovaginal cells (2036)
- Long duration of membrane rupture before delivery (2337)
- Absence of secretory leukocyte protease inhibitor in vaginal fluids (3514)
- Low serum levels of a 90-kDa human glycoprotein (3463)
- Absence of anti-gp120 (V3 loop) antibodies in maternal sera (3814, 4521)
- Lack of neutralizing antibodies in maternal sera (2240, 4826)
- Enhancing antibodies in maternal sera (2240)
- HLA concordance (2726, 3565)
- Certain HLA-B alleles are increased (B*1302, B*3501) or reduced (B*4901, B*5301) (4788).
- Certain chemokine receptor polymorphisms in the newborn (2293)
- Ability of HIV-1 to infect placenta and be passed to the neonate (909, 2973, 3440)
- Number of virus-infected macrophages and T cells in colostrum and milk (291, 3928)
- Vitamin A deficiency (2035)
- Illicit drug use (2036, 3773)

[a]See Section VI for additional references.

increase the risk of mother-child transmission (2337). The presence of secretory leukocyte protease inhibitor in vaginal fluids (3514) or of high levels of a 90-KDa human serum glycoprotein in the serum of mothers and their newborns (3463) has been associated with a reduction in maternal HIV transmission. Presumably, these proteins act as antiviral substances.

Transmission of HIV to the newborn has also been reported to correlate with low levels or an absence of antibodies to the viral envelope, especially the third variable region (V3 loop) of gp120 (3814), and to the carboxyl region of gp41 (4521) in the mother. Neutralizing antibodies in maternal sera and, in some studies, inflammation of placenta membranes have correlated as well with protection from transmission (see below) (2240, 3944, 4244, 4826). Enhancing antibodies and the replicative ability of the maternal virus are associated with infection of the newborn (1222, 2240) (Section VI.D). These observations suggest that the level of free infectious virus in the maternal blood could predict the infectious status of the newborn.

Some genetic studies have suggested that class I and class II HLA specificities can influence mother-child transmission (see Chapter 13). While not confirmed by others (2874), a discordance in class I (e.g., *HLA-G*) has appeared to correlate with a reduced rate of perinatal transmission (41, 2726, 3565, 4380), most likely reflecting allogeneic immune responses (see Chapter 11). Moreover, certain maternal *HLA-B* alleles have been associated with increased (e.g., *HLA-B*1302* and *HLA-B*3501*) and others with reduced (e.g., *HLA-B*4901* and *-B*5301*) rates of mother-to-child transmission (4788).

Children with homologous *CCR5-59356* T mutation were also found to be at an increased risk of perinatal HIV-1 transmission (2293), as have children with a heterozygous SDF-1 genotype (*SDF-1 3' A/wt*) (particularly from postnatal breast milk) (2037). These genetic findings may reflect increased susceptibility because of reduced sensitivity of R5 and X4 viruses, respectively, to chemokines (see Chapter 3).

Some protection from infection may occur at the placenta level. In early studies, HIV was detected in the placentae of all infected women not treated with antiretroviral drugs (2973) (see Section VI.C). The infected cells were in both the syncytiotrophtoblasts and Hofbauer cell populations (2563) (see Chapter 4). Very few newborns were infected. The mechanism for blocking mother-to-fetus transmission could be production of the SDF-1 chemokine (909) or leukemia infectivity factor (LIF) (3440) by placental cells.

In resource-poor countries, maternal vitamin A deficiency has been associated with increased risk of infection for the newborn (2035, 4043), most likely resulting from reduced epithelial cell function in the gastrointestinal tract (3258). Some investigators have reported that mother-child transmission is higher with clades A and C rather than clade D infection (390a). Others report a greater transmission with clade D than with clade A viruses (4851). The differences perhaps reflect various in utero or postpartum factors (e.g., viral levels in plasma and vaginal fluids) (2039). In comparison to other clades, an increase in clade D transmission has also been noted in heterosexual risk groups (see Chapter 1). One mechanism could be enhanced transcytosis by certain viral species and subsequent infection (2380) (see also above and Chapter 4).

After delivery, HIV infection can result from infected breast milk (3387, 4544, 4962), particularly from mothers who acquired HIV postnatally (for review, see reference 1151). As noted above, during acute infection viremia levels are high (see Section III.A). This route of transmission has been associated with the presence of virus-infected cells and the absence of anti-HIV IgM and IgA antibodies in breast milk (291, 4543). In one study, breast milk transmission accounted for 16% of the infections, with the majority occurring soon after delivery (3226).

C. Time of Transmission and Source of Virus

The time of infection of the newborn and the source of HIV are controversial. In relation to the source of HIV in mother-child transmission, several observations, before the introduction of anti-HIV therapy, supported an in utero perinatal or postdelivery infection (2073, 2304) (for review, see references 673 and 1063) (see Table 2.8). Some researchers now propose that half of the infections take place in the days just before delivery when the

Table 2.8 Evidence for in utero, intrapartum, and breast feeding transmission of HIV-1[a]

In utero
- Positive DNA PCR in first 24–48 of life
- Maternofetal transfusion (proposed)
- Identification of HIV-1 in fetal tissue from 10 wks of gestation
- Placental membrane inflammation

Intrapartum
- Negative DNA PCR at birth, with subsequent positive results
- Increased risk in firstborn twin
- Isolation of HIV-1 in neonatal gastric aspirates
- Increased transmission risk with prolonged rupture of membranes
- Decreased transmission with elective Caesarean section

Breast-feeding
- Isolation of HIV-1 from cell-free breast milk
- HIV DNA detected in colostrum
- Increased risk of transmission compared with exclusively bottle-fed infants
- Breast-feeding was the only exposure of HIV-1-infected children

[a]Reproduced from reference 1063 with permission.

placenta begins to separate from the uterine wall. Another third occurs during labor and delivery when the newborn is exposed to maternal blood and genital fluids (2304). Recovery of HIV from cord blood or within 48 h of delivery certainly implies infection before delivery. Nevertheless, the exact time and source of the infection are not known. It could occur late in pregnancy, when maternal cells are most frequently found in the blood of the newborn and can carry HIV (981). HIV is often not isolated from cord blood, but is recovered from virus-infected infants after 1 month of age (557, 1006, 1180); a prepartum or postdelivery infection process would seem to be involved. In this regard, HIV has been detected in gastric aspirates from neonates (2784, 3258).

Infectious HIV has been found in amniotic fluid and uterine, placental, and fetal tissues, and virus can infect those cells in culture (48, 163, 971, 982, 2563, 3165, 4198). Neonatal monocytes and macrophages but not CD34+ cord stem cells (1729) may also have an increased susceptibility to HIV-1 infection (4228). However, the frequency of HIV infection of fetal tissues in utero has not been well documented. Some investigators have found no or very low-level virus infection in early-term fetal tissues (97, 527).

Placental cells, either expressing or lacking the CD4 protein, have been infected in vitro by virus or virus-infected cells. In one study examining the possible role of the Fc receptor on placental cells, infection was achieved with an antibody:virus complex (see Chapter 10), but only low-level replication took place (97, 4454). However, in some studies transfer of HIV from placental trophoblasts to CD4+ T cells has been shown via cell-to-cell contact involving LFA-1 (143). The relevance of these findings to the in vivo situation is not clear. In some studies, the presence of HIV-1 proviral DNA in the placenta has correlated with the detection of virus in the cord blood of newborns, but HIV-positive cord blood has also been found in the absence of detectable infection in the placenta (982). In addition, HIV-1 has been found in term placentae of all HIV-infected women in one study, but virus transmission to the newborn was not often found (2973). The reason for this block in virus transmission is not known (143) and could be the secretion of anti-HIV factors by placental cells (3440) such as LIF (3440), SDF-1 (909), or female hormones (466) (see above).

All these findings suggest that at least half the infant infections could occur during birth through contact with the genital secretions or blood of the mother. Such a route of infection could explain the increased risk of transmission when the fetal membrane ruptures more than 4 h before delivery (2397). Although not observed in one study (364), HIV transmission at the time of delivery could explain how only one monozygotic twin would be infected (2970), and why the firstborn of twins is at higher risk of infection (1538). The infected newborn twin could have been exposed to a higher concentration of virus. Caesarean delivery, moreover, has been associated with decreased HIV transmission (1228a, 3154).

Information on transmission of the other human pathogenic retrovirus, HTLV, might also have relevance to HIV. HTLV is not passed readily in utero (3929). This virus is transferred primarily from breast milk and genital fluids, most likely via infected cells (1838). Moreover, in one study on

HTLV transmission, approximately 22% of the placentae but only 7% of the infants were found to be infected. This observation suggests a defense mechanism at the maternal-fetal interface (1385), which may also be operating in HIV infection (see above). Perhaps this event is reflected in the inflammation of the placenta membrane that correlates with protection from HIV transmission (4244).

D. Characteristics of the Transmitted Virus

An important parameter in transmission could be the type of virus transferred from the mother (see also Chapter 4). Recent studies have suggested that HIV-1 clades can differ in the time of virus transmission (e.g., in utero versus during delivery) (3703). Furthermore, as noted above, the time during pregnancy at which HIV is transferred might determine the particular virus strain transmitted to the newborn (3703). In some cases, the heterogeneous sequences of the viruses recovered from the child suggest multiple virus transmission events (501). In this regard, different quasispecies from the mother could be detected in identical twins, reflecting transmission of multiple virus variants (365). Certain studies have indicated that maternal and newborn viruses can be distinguished by molecular and biologic properties (2238, 2240, 2389, 3946, 4808). As seen by PCR analysis, a dominant single maternal variant is usually found (2238, 4808). A specific virus transmission to the newborn may also occur when maternal cytotoxic-T-cell recognition is decreased (4782). The transferred virus, for example, could be a more virulent fast-replicating X4 strain found at a low frequency in the mother but readily transferred to the newborn. Maternal viruses with high replication kinetics and cytopathic properties associated with the X4 phenotype have been considered risk factors in transmission to the newborn (see below and Chapter 4) (2240, 3945). However, in one study a predominance of R5 viruses that replicate in the child's CD4$^+$ target cell was noted in transmitters (3334). In another study, all HIV-1 isolates from four infants were of the R5 phenotype (4227). Nevertheless, apparently, both X4 and R5 viruses can be transmitted (2240, 3945). In these cases, perhaps replicative ability and not syn-

cytium induction capacity is the major determinant (1222, 2240). These findings counter some suggestions that a noncytopathic macrophage-tropic R5 strain is primarily transmitted because it can infect placental macrophages (444). This route, if relevant, would only be involved in infections in utero.

In addition, serologic differences could be involved. A virus resistant to maternal antibodies or sensitive to enhancing antibodies in the mother's serum has been detected in newborns (2240, 4826). The presence of enhancing antibodies could explain the reports of increased transmission of HIV from mother to child in the presence of high levels of maternal antibodies to the V3 region of gp120 and the immunodominant domain of gp41 (2384, 2815).

In relation to breast-feeding, blood and breast milk isolates have been found to be similar, suggesting an equilibration of the blood and breast compartments (1805) (Section III.A). However, as observed with genital fluids, most studies suggest that there is a compartmentalization of HIV-1 between peripheral blood and breast milk, and thus mother-child transmission may not be predicted by increasing levels of plasma viruses (289). Finally, infection via breast milk could be predominantly with R5 virus because of the large number of infected macrophages in colostrum and early milk (3928).

E. Conclusions: Prevention of Mother-Child Transmission

In summary, mother-child transmission seems to occur in association with parameters observed during a poor clinical state: high virus load, fast-replicating HIV strains, and low CD4$^+$ cell numbers. If the factors influencing maternal transmission of HIV can be ascertained, approaches to avoid virus transfer could be better targeted. Fortunately, many trials have now established that antiviral therapy given to pregnant women, even as a short course around delivery, reduces dramatically the risk of perinatal transmission (3043, 4754) (see Chapter 14).

Early encouraging results were reported in blocking mother-child transmission with AZT treatment (076 study) (655). Reducing plasma virus RNA levels to <500 copies/ml decreased the risk of perinatal transmission substantially (3043).

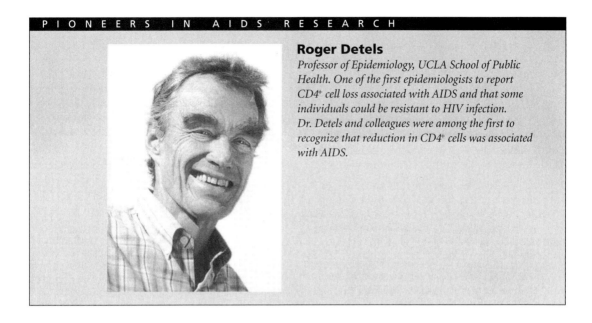

Roger Detels
Professor of Epidemiology, UCLA School of Public Health. One of the first epidemiologists to report CD4+ cell loss associated with AIDS and that some individuals could be resistant to HIV infection. Dr. Detels and colleagues were among the first to recognize that reduction in CD4+ cells was associated with AIDS.

However, in some cases, AZT-treated women with high HIV-1 levels have transmitted AZT-sensitive virus to newborns (1082). Most recently, combination antiretroviral therapy or even single-dose nevirapine (185, 1661) given alone to HIV-seropositive pregnant women or to the child as well within 3 days of birth (1661) dramatically reduced HIV transmission via the maternal route (1228). A single dose of nevirapine just to the infants has also offered protection to the child from infection (1603). Presently, with HAART administered to pregnant infected women, the incidence of HIV transmission by this route in several Western countries has been reduced dramatically, probably to <1% (1117) (see below) (see Chapter 14). In resource-poor countries, a shortened course of oral AZT during the peripartum period gave nearly a 40% reduction in HIV transmission even with breast-feeding (948, 4059). This approach helps but is less effective than a standard longer treatment period (2385).

Formula feeding over breast milk feeding in principle can be important for preventing postnatal transmission (3226). In a recent study, each 10-fold increase in cell-free virus and cell-associated virus in breast milk carried an almost 3-fold increase in transmission to the newborn child (2301).

Some studies, however, suggest that breast-feeding exclusively for 3 months or more, particularly soon after delivery (1953), does not increase the risk of infection over 6 months compared with the risk for newborns who are never breast-fed (910). The antimicrobial nutritional value of breast milk must be considered in developing countries, where breast-feeding can be important for survival of the newborn.

Besides antiviral therapy, other methods could include monitoring the mother during labor, cleansing the vaginal canal, and rapidly removing genital secretions and maternal blood from the newborn. In one report, however, cleansing of the birth canal before delivery did not significantly affect the risk of HIV transmission (366). Elective Caesarean section delivery does lower the risk of mother-child transmission (3154), even when mothers are receiving treatment with AZT (1228a). However, this procedure carries the risk of the surgery (4047). Thus, some of these procedures might at least reduce the transfer of HIV in the perinatal period. Importantly, where available, the administration of antiretroviral therapy shows the most promise in decreasing mother-child virus transmission substantially.

1. The risk of HIV transmission is increased with high levels of virus in the body fluids and the number of contacts an individual has with a body fluid.

2. Blood has the highest level of infectious virus that could serve as a source of transmission. The number of *infectious* viruses in body fluids is usually 1 in 60,000 to 1 in 100,000 of the virus particles detected. The amount of infectious virus in blood is lower than the number of virus-infected cells that could transfer virus to an individual.

3. Based on relative content of infectious viruses, HIV-infected cells in genital fluids appear to be the major source of transmission by the sexual route. Sexually transmitted diseases enhance the risk of virus transmission to either partner by increasing the presence of virus-infected cells. Lack of circumcision also increases the risk of sexual transmission.

4. The receptive partner in sexual transmission is most at risk. In women, cells in the cervix or within the endometrium can be infected. In men and women, the infection site can involve bowel mucosal cells or lymphocytes and macrophages present in the rectum. The insertive partner may be infected by cells along the urethral canal or associated with the prepuce.

5. Saliva, which contains HIV-inhibitory substances and only small amounts of infectious virus, is not a major source of transmission. Tears, urine, sweat, and other body fluids are not sources of virus infection.

6. Risk of HIV infection by blood depends on the level of infectious virus in this body fluid. Heating has eliminated the risk of infection from blood products. The estimated risk of HIV infection from needlestick injuries is 1 in 300 to 400, with deep injury carrying the greatest chance of infection. Risk from mucosal membrane and skin exposures is approximately 1 in 1,000 or less and is influenced by the amount of blood and viral load.

7. Condoms, male and female, should serve as efficient barrier techniques for sexual transmission of virus. Microbicides are being evaluated, but compounds that irritate the vaginal canal should be avoided. In women, trials in the use of diaphragms are being conducted as well as giving highly active antiretroviral therapy (HAART) shortly after HIV exposure.

8. Transmission of virus from mother to child can involve direct infection of the fetus in utero or, during birth, by exposure of the newborn to maternal blood and secretions. A variety of factors can influence this transmission, in particular, the level of infectious virus in the mother at the time of delivery.

9. Maternal milk can serve as a source of virus for the newborn, but this fluid also contains substances that can block virus infection. Virus-infected cells appear to be the major source of transmission.

10. Antiretroviral therapy and other preventive measures can greatly reduce the risk of mother-child transmission.

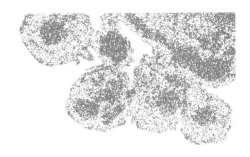

Steps Involved in HIV:Cell Interaction and Virus Entry

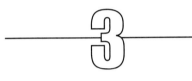

TRANSMISSION OF HIV requires the successful interaction of the virus with receptors on a cell surface. Subsequent processes facilitate the final penetration of the viral nucleocapsid through the cell membrane into the cell. The sites on the virus and on the cells that are involved in this interaction, and the events required for viral entry, are reviewed in this chapter.

I. CD4 Receptor

A. Virus Attachment Site

One of the first breakthroughs in the studies of HIV was the discovery that its major cellular receptor was the CD4 molecule. The reason for preferential growth of HIV in CD4+ lymphocytes was explained by its attachment to the CD4 protein on the cell surface (957, 2224, 2225). Subsequent studies have indicated that the D1 region of the CD4 molecule (particularly involving the Phe-43 amino acid in the complementarity-determining region 2 [CDR2] domain) (Figure 3.1) is involved in this virus binding (155, 1997, 3036, 3093; for a review, see reference 1107).

When the crystal structure of CD4 was revealed (3852, 4673), the binding site for the viral surface envelope protein gp120 was located on a protuberant ridge along one face of the D1 domain (Figure 3.1). Initially, the viral attachment site appeared to be separate from the major histocompatibility complex (MHC) binding site of CD4 (1311, 2386), but the location was delineated further by using viral mutants and high-resolution CD4 atomic structure (3042). These studies indicate that the class II MHC binding site appears to include the same CD4 region. Thus, this overlap might affect the use of inhibitors of the CD4:gp120 interaction.

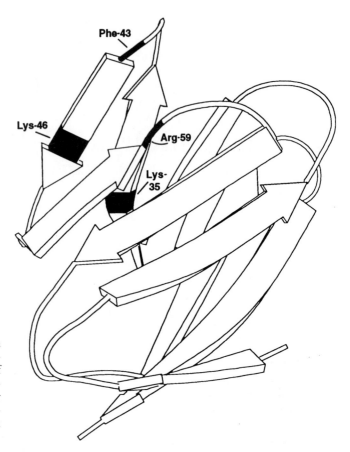

Figure 3.1 The gp120 binding sites on the CD4 molecule as determined by mutational analysis, displayed on this model of domain 1 (D1). The consensus is that Phe-43 and Arg-59 are likely contact sites for gp120, but there are various conclusions regarding Lys-35 and Lys-46. Reprinted from reference 3093 with permission.

On HIV, a major CD4 binding region is in the fourth conserved portion (C4) near the carboxyl-terminal end of the viral gp120 (2417, 3300; for a review, see reference 4347). The conformation of gp120 is important for CD4 binding (2918), and other noncontiguous regions of gp120 are now known to interact with sites on the CDR2 domain of the CD4 molecule (see Figure 3.1). The CD4 binding domain on gp120 appears to be a complex folded structure with sites from several regions coming in contact with the CD4 molecule (for a review, see reference 3093). Among these could be two hydrophobic domains in the conserved C2 and C4 regions of gp120 as well as hydrophilic domains in the C3 and C4 regions (2315, 3333; for reviews, see references 3093 and 4275) (Color Plate 1, following page 78) (see Chapter 10, Section II, for description of viral envelope structure).

In support of the involvement of an envelope conformational structure, several studies indicate that small changes in various regions of the HIV envelope can affect virus binding to the CD4 molecule and tropism (894, 895, 3333, 4128). In this regard, two highly conserved aspartic acid residues in the C4 and C5 domains of gp120 (in a predicted groove of this protein) contribute substantially to the binding (3333) (Color Plate 1, following page 78).

The CD4 molecule could also have a role in viral infection aside from its binding to the HIV envelope (588, 1756, 4489). For example, conformational changes in CD4 as a result of virus attachment could help in HIV entry through an enhanced interaction with coreceptors on the cell surface (4663) (for a review, see reference 3093) (see below). The participation of CD4 in virus:cell fusion, perhaps by means of flexibility in the D2-D3 hinge region (3852, 4673), has also been suggested (3593). Furthermore, certain domains of CD4 could be selectively involved in cell:cell fusion (3593, 4489) (see Chapter 6). The binding of HIV to the CD4 receptor also initiates signaling pathways and subsequent expression of cytokines and chemokines (3576) that can influence the infection process.

Another potential factor influencing the CD4:gp120 interaction is the glycosylation pattern of gp120 (2878, 3106), which can affect envelope conformation. Nonglycosylated envelope gp120 does not bind well to CD4 (4275). Moreover, the relationship of CD4 to chemokine receptors can influence the efficiency of HIV infection (2463) (see below). Recently, the need for only one Env trimer for HIV-1 entry was demonstrated (4860).

B. Studies with Soluble CD4

Biologic studies with soluble forms of CD4 (sCD4), produced in mammalian cells by molecular techniques, revealed some potentially important findings on the gp120:CD4 interaction, with differences noted among HIV isolates. After mixing with sCD4, the infection by many HIV-1 strains is inactivated to various extents (4714). Some, particularly macrophage-tropic R5 isolates, are relatively resistant (see below). Certain HIV-2 strains, and especially the SIV$_{agm}$ isolates, show an increase in infectivity, notably when low sCD4 concentrations are used (66, 787, 4729). In some studies, this interaction with sCD4 permits HIV-2 infection of CD4$^-$ human cells and nonhuman primate cells (787). Chemokine coreceptors may be involved (see Chapter 4). Moreover, sCD4 in low concentrations enhances infection of CD4$^+$ cells by some primary HIV-1 isolates (4333).

Although the reason for these diverse observations is not clear, a possible explanation for these various reactions to sCD4 is that sCD4 has differing affinities for the various gp120 proteins. With the inactivation of HIV infection, the sCD4 molecule apparently attaches to the viral envelope region and blocks receptor binding. Some experiments suggested that it causes removal of gp120 from the virus (1750, 3091) (Section II).

In contrast, with certain HIV-2 isolates, SIV$_{agm}$, and some HIV-1 isolates, sCD4 might bind at low affinities, and gp120 is not displaced on the virion. In this case, conformational changes could occur in the viral envelope, thereby permitting optimal virus:cell interactions (e.g., with chemokine coreceptors or gp41 fusion) (see Chapter 4). This possibility was suggested by early studies using sCD4

with antienvelope monoclonal antibodies (Section II) (2931, 3931).

This resistance of certain HIV-1 isolates to inactivation by sCD4 has been mapped to the V3 region of the virus envelope (1942, 3306). With different HIV-1 strains, sites outside the V3 loop but in the nearby regions (e.g., C2) appear to be responsible (4255). Since none of these portions of gp120 binds to CD4, the envelope conformation influencing this process seems to be involved. One explanation for the different effects of sCD4 on primary isolates might be a greater avidity of the macrophage-tropic R5 virus isolates for the cell surface CD4 receptors than for sCD4 (1975, 4255). Thus, in evaluating virus:cell interactions, the relative resistance of certain HIV-1 isolates to sCD4 can be a property reflecting a characteristic envelope conformation.

II. Postbinding Steps in Virus Entry into CD4$^+$ Cells

A. Envelope Displacement

During virus infection of a cell, the HIV envelope gp120 can be involved in steps other than binding. After attachment to the CD4 molecule, gp120 appears to be displaced, leading to the uncovering of domains on the envelope gp41 that are needed for virus:cell fusion (Figure 3.2) (3091, 3931). This displacement can result from a dissociation of a knob-and-socket-like structure involving the carboxyl-terminal region of gp120 and the central portion of gp41 (4008). It may involve gp120 cleavage (see below). Multimeric CD4 binding may be important for this release (1163), which can be demonstrated with sCD4 (Section I) and is related to specific CD4 binding to gp120 (322, 1750, 3090). Support for this phenomenon comes from the demonstration that certain V3 monoclonal antibodies can neutralize HIV-1 only in the presence of sCD4; the V3 epitope is exposed by this gp120:CD4 interaction (2931, 3931).

Whether a complete dissociation of gp120 from gp41 takes place during HIV infection is not clear. Total shedding does not appear to occur (1088) or to be necessary as long as the fusion domain on gp41 is exposed (3931).

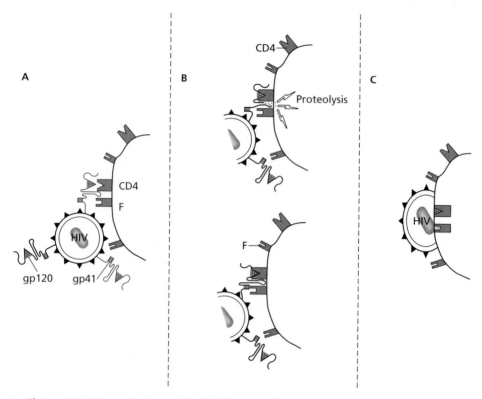

Figure 3.2 Proposed processes involved in HIV infection of cells. (A) HIV approaches a cell. A region on the viral surface envelope protein, gp120, interacts with a domain on a cell surface receptor (e.g., CD4). (B) Top, The interaction causes a conformational change in gp120 (and perhaps CD4), potentially resulting in a proteolytic cleavage of gp120, most likely in the V3 loop. Bottom, This process results in an interaction of the external portion of gp41 (fusion domain) with a proposed fusion receptor (F) on the cell surface. (C) HIV fuses with the cell. Alternatively, the interaction of gp120 with CD4 could lead to removal of gp120, with subsequent exposure of gp41 to the cell surface (see Section II.A).

B. Envelope Cleavage

Another possible event in virus infection is cleavage of the HIV envelope gp120 prior to HIV entry into cells. This process was very well explored several years ago but has received less attention recently. In the past studies, gp120 was found to have sites within the V3 loop that could be sensitive to selected cellular proteolytic enzymes (1760, 2181, 3174). These protease-sensitive sites included sequences (e.g., GPGR) that resembled trypsin inhibitors. Other aspartic protease cleavage sites have also been identified in the HIV-1, HIV-2, and SIV envelope regions (796). Moreover, HIV-1 gp120 was found to bind to a TL2-trypsin-like protease (2182). These observations suggested that these enzymes, when present on the cell, cleave gp120

after binding to CD4. This event could facilitate a conformational change in the envelope so that a viral region (e.g., on gp41) can subsequently fuse with the cell membrane (3931) (Figure 3.3). Thus, some CD4⁺ cells that cannot be infected by certain HIV strains might lack the necessary cellular proteases to cleave that particular virus envelope region when it is exposed.

The importance of envelope cleavage in infection gained some support from evidence demonstrating that gp120 can be digested by proteases and this activity can be blocked by neutralizing antibodies (796). Other studies showed that exposure of purified HIV to sCD4 leads to cleavage of gp120 by proteolytic activity (Figure 3.3) (4728). This phenomenon can be blocked by monoclonal

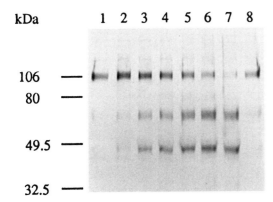

Figure 3.3 Purified HIV-1$_{SF2}$ was mixed with soluble CD4 and incubated for 1 to 8 h at 37°C. Subsequently, the viral envelope protein gp120 was extracted and examined by immunoblot procedures. Lanes 1 and 8, virus preparation without sCD4 incubated for 8 h; lane 2, virus preparation with 1 μg of sCD4 at time zero; lanes 3 to 7, virus and sCD4 mixed for 0.5, 1, 2, 4, and 8 h, respectively. After incubation with sCD4, the cleavage of the envelope gp120 into 50- and 70-kDa proteins is evident, and this process continues over time. The site of cleavage appears to be in the V3 loop (4728).

antibodies to the GPGR-containing regions of the V3 loop (4728). The cleavage therefore appears to involve the crown of the V3 loop. The explanation given for this observation is that an initial conformational change in gp120 (and perhaps CD4) takes place after attachment of gp120 to CD4, and this event exposes the V3 loop to the enzymatic activity. The source of the protease is not known but is most likely a cellular protein that copurifies with the virus.

The role of the proteolytic process in virus entry remains to be clarified. The fact that macrophage-tropic R5 isolates (see below) are relatively resistant to the cleavage of gp120 (1656, 4728) raises the question of the universality of this process for virus infection. Some researchers have considered that the lack of gp120 cleavage is a characteristic needed by a virus to infect monocytes/macrophages (1656).

C. Secondary Receptors for HIV Infection

1. GENERAL OBSERVATIONS

Several early studies examining the role of the CD4:virus interaction in HIV infection indicated that the CD4 receptor alone was neither sufficient

nor the sole means for viral entry (Table 3.1) (Section VI). Some human cells expressing high levels of the CD4 protein, including undifferentiated CD4+ monocytes, are not susceptible to HIV infection (741, 1230, 2184) (see Chapter 5, Section IV). Some animal cells, derived through molecular or somatic cell hybrid techniques to express human CD4 on the cell surface, could not be infected (786, 2753, 4406). Studies with somatic cell hybrids using human-human and human-CD4+ rodent cells suggested that another surface factor on certain human cells, besides CD4, was needed for HIV entry (517, 1129, 1740, 4406).

The search for the additional cell surface proteins that interact with HIV led to the discovery of the participation of chemokine receptors in virus entry. In this regard, several studies of viruses from different clades (Chapter 1) have confirmed the role of CCR5 as a coreceptor for macrophage-tropic isolates (727, 2009, 2736) and CXCR4 as a coreceptor for the T cell line-tropic strains (323) (Table 3.2). These two types of viruses can be distinguished and are now referred to as R5 and X4 viruses, respectively (321). Discussion of CCR5 and CXCR4 as well as other HIV receptors is included in the following section.

2. CHEMOKINE RECEPTORS AS CORECEPTORS

a. CXCR4

Based on the above observations, several investigators began searching for secondary cellular attachment sites for HIV on human cells. Berger and coworkers (1272) found a human cDNA clone that expressed a protein, which they termed fusin

Table 3.1 Evidence suggesting another cellular receptor for HIV

- CD4+ T-cell lines and CD4-expressing human cells can be resistant to infection by HIV (741, 2184).
- Animal cells expressing human CD4 are not infectible by HIV (786, 4406).
- CD4– cells can be infected by HIV (729, 4393).
- Some viruses incubated with soluble CD4 or antibodies to CD4 are not blocked from infecting certain CD4+ and CD4– cell lines (3711).
- A glycolipid, galactosyl ceramide has been detected as an alternative receptor on CD4– brain-derived and bowel-derived human cells (1730, 4841).

Table 3.2 Chemokine coreceptors of HIV infection

Receptor	Virus phenotype	Potential receptor[d]
CCR5[a]	R5	CCR8
CXCR4[a]	X4	CCR9
CCR3[a, b]	R5	US28
CCR2b[a]	X4	ChemR23
Bonzo/STRL33[b]	R5	CX3CR1 (V28)
BOB/GPR15[b]	R5	APJ[c]
CCR1[a]		D6[a, c]
CCR4[a]		RDC-1[c]
CXCR5/BLR1[a]		

[a]Major receptor for HIV-2 strains (1170, 3686). Generally HIV-2 isolates are dualtropic.
[b]Some HIV-1 isolates.
[c]Particularly brain cells.
[d]These other receptors have been reported for HIV infection, but their function is uncommon and not clearly defined (for reviews, see references 321, 1170, and 3684).

(formerly known as LESTR), that mediated fusion in the mouse-human CD4+ cell model. When the gene was introduced into HIV-resistant mouse cells expressing human CD4, the protein produced made the cells susceptible to HIV infection (1272). This molecule, now called CXCR4, was then shown to act as a coreceptor for HIV strains that are T-cell-line tropic (344, 1115; for an overview, see reference 2524). The receptor permits a close interaction between the virus and the cell surface (344, 1272, 2411, 2524) (Color Plate 2, following page 78).

The natural ligand for CXCR4 is the chemoattractant stromal-cell-derived factor 1 (SDF-1) (409, 3315), and this cytokine can block HIV infection of T cells (3315). SDF-1 is a member of a family of low-molecular-weight cytokines called chemokines that mediate inflammation by recruiting immune cells expressing the chemokine receptor to the site of injury or inflammation (3340, 4316) (Table 3.3). CXCR4 is a member of a seven-membrane-spanning protein family that includes many chemokine receptors. The amino-terminal domain of CXCR4 is involved in HIV binding, and intracellular signaling does not play an important role in virus entry (3590). However, the particular region of CXCR4 needed for HIV infection appears to be determined by the virus strain involved. Mutations introduced into the

amino-terminal extracellular domain of CXCR4 affected infection by some, but not all, HIV-1 strains (3504). In general, several CXCR4 domains appear to interact with X4 HIV, but especially the second extracellular loop structure (2684). The viral V3 loop is involved in this X4 virus infection (3883).

b. CCR5

The identification of CXCR4 as an HIV coreceptor occurred shortly before other investigators began examining chemokine receptors in HIV infection. The latter research was sparked by the observation that the β-chemokines RANTES, macrophage inflammatory protein 1α (MIP-1α), and MIP-1β, in combination, efficiently blocked HIV-1 infection of CD4+ lymphocytes (822). MIP-1α attracts a variety of white blood cells to the site of infection; MIP-1β attracts T cells, dendritic cells (DCs), macrophages, and NK cells (Table 3.3). Working with molecular clones of the β-chemokine receptors, particularly CXCR5 but also CCR3 and CCR2b, several investigators showed that these molecules help HIV enter cells (64, 758, 1049, 1115, 1130) (Table 3.2). The block of HIV infection by β-chemokines was shown to occur at an early cell surface binding step in the infection process, presumably by competitive interaction at the receptor site (3341). Expression of the β-chemokine receptors enhanced virus infection of cells, and the β-chemokines prevented the infection by primary HIV isolates, specifically, the macrophage-tropic R5 isolates (for overviews, see references 323 and 2524). CXCR5 is not used by the T-cell-line-tropic strains (Table 3.2).

In a cross-sectional study of HIV-infected and uninfected individual subjects, CXCR4 expression was found to be low in CD4+ and CD8+ T cells as well as CD14+ monocytes. CCR5 expression was up-regulated in CD4+ T cells in HIV-infected individuals compared to uninfected controls (3356). CXCR4 was expressed predominantly on quiescent (HLA-DR−) CD4+ T cells, and CCR5 was expressed on activated (HLA-DR+) T cells. With advanced disease and greater immune activation, higher expression of CCR5 was noted. With advanced disease, activation of CXCR4+ CD4+ cells was also noted (3356) (see also Chapter 4, Table 4.5).

Table 3.3 List of some of the chemokines associated with the hematopoietic system[a]

Chemokines	Receptors[b]					Chemoattracted cells											Source[c]											
C-X-C (α)	\(C-X-CR\)				Duffy Ag																							
	1	2	3	**4**		N	Eo	Ba	Ma	T	B	NK	M	Dc	Ec	F	N	Eo	Ba	Ma	T	B	NK	M	Dc	Ec	F	Pl
IL-8	★	★			★	★	★	★	★	★		★			★			★			★			★	★	★	★	
Groα		★			★	★		★		★														★		★	★	
Groβ		★				★		★								★								★		★	★	
Groγ		★				★		★																★		★	★	
ENA-78	★	★				★									★	★								★		★	★	
GCP-2		★				★																						
NAP-2		★				★																						
PF-4									★						★	★												★
MIG			★		★					★		★	★		★									★		★		
IP-10			★							★	★	★	★		★	★					★			★		★	★	
SDF-1α/β				★						★	★		★															[d]

Chemokines	Receptors[b]							Chemoattracted cells											Source[c]											
C-C (β)	\(CCR\)						Duffy Ag																							
	1	2a	**2b**	3	4	**5**		N	Eo	Ba	Ma	T	B	NK	M	Dc	Ec	F	N	Eo	Ba	Ma	T	B	NK	M	Dc	Ec	F	Pl
MIP-1α	★				★	★			★	★	★	★	★	★	★	★					★	★	★			★		★	★	★
MIP-1β	★					★			★	★	★	★	★	★	★	★					★	★	★			★		★	★	★
RANTES	★			★		★	★		★	★	★	★		★	★	★							★			★		★	★	
MCP-1		★	★				★		★	★	★	★		★	★	★							★			★		★	★	
MCP-2		★	★	★					★	★	★	★		★	★								★			★			★	
MCP-3	★	★	★	★					★	★	★	★		★	★	★							★			★				
MCP-4			★	★					★			★			★											★				
I-309															★															
Eotaxin				★					★											★								★		
C (γ)																							★							
Lymphotactin														★								★	★		★					

[a] Receptors for these chemokines, the cells affected by the chemokine (chemoattractant cells), and the source of the chemokine are also provided. Abbreviations: N, neutrophil; Eo, eosinophil; Ba, basophil; Ma, mast cell; T, T lymphocyte; B, B lymphocyte; NK, natural killer cell; M, monocyte; Dc, dendritic cell; Ec, endothelial cell; F, fibroblast; Pl, platelet. Information provided by G. Greco.

[b] HIV receptors are in boldface type.

[c] Only cells of the hematopoietic lineage are indicated.

[d] —, bone marrow stromal cells.

3. MECHANISMS INVOLVED IN INTERACTION OF HIV WITH CCR5

The region of CCR5 that participates in the interaction with the HIV-1 envelope involving, in part, the V3 loop is the amino-terminal domain or the first extracellular region (823, 3835, 4825). A highly conserved portion of gp120 that is located between the V1, V2, and V3 loops appears to take part in this coreceptor binding (3743). The importance of the V3 region for interaction with the chemokine coreceptors reflects early work showing that very few amino acid changes in this region of the envelope could determine whether the virus infected T-cell lines or macrophages (1942, 4113). A very small number of amino acid changes (as few as one) (4113) could affect the infection of certain cell lines (4107) (see Chapter 7).

The V1 and V2 envelope sequences, especially on R5 isolates, can also play an important part in HIV infection of macrophages, particularly when CD4 expression is low (4667). R5 viruses may have shorter V2 regions than X4 viruses, which could influence coreceptor use. The V2 region can be even smaller in R5 viruses associated with AIDS (2008).

The site on the coreceptor for HIV attachment has been found to be different from that involving the β-chemokines (168). Since chemokine receptors are G protein-coupled molecules, this distinction in binding site and other studies have indicated that signal transduction is also not required for CCR5 to act as an HIV coreceptor (1572).

Many unrelated viruses can use CCR5 for infection (e.g., HIV-1, HIV-2, and SIV), and several domains in gp120 (4477) and CCR5 (168) can participate in HIV entry. Differences among viral isolates in their interaction with CCR5 have been noted (3835), as was observed with CXCR4 (see above). Conformational changes in the coreceptors can influence the relative sensitivity of cells to virus infection (1106, 2576). Furthermore, the sensitivity of R5 viruses to β-chemokines can vary up to 100-fold (3083; C. E. Mackewicz and J. A. Levy, unpublished observations) (see Chapter 11). Thus, in general, the interaction of HIV with its coreceptors must be complex, as is observed with the CD4 receptor (Section I).

Table 3.4 Characteristics of R5 and X4 isolates of HIV[a]

Characteristic	Associated with:	
	R5	X4
Use of CD4 receptor	++	++
Chemokine coreceptor usage	CCR5	CXCR4
Growth in macrophages	++	±
Growth in T-cell lines	−	++
Cytopathicity[b]	−	++
Sensitivity to sCD4	−	++
Sensitivity to envelope cleavage	−	+
Net positive change in the V3 loop[c]	−	+
Associated with substantial loss of CD4+ cells	−	++
Associated with CNS[d] disease	++	−

[a]See Sections I and II for references. Further differences have been reported but need confirmation.
[b]Generally defined by induction of cytopathic effect in MT-2 cells (2279). Some R5 viruses can cause cytopathic effect in peripheral blood mononuclear cells.
[c]Observed in many, but not all, studies (1338).
[d]CNS, central nervous system.

4. VIRUS SUBTYPE CHARACTERISTICS

The different biologic characteristics of R5 and X4 viruses are listed in Table 3.4. Dualtropic HIV isolates (R5/X4), which are both macrophage tropic and T-cell-line tropic, have also been identified and can use either receptor (1115) depending on their relative density on a cell (727). In general, X4 viruses have an increase in their net positive charge in V3 (1338, 1638, 4113; see also references 2023, 2369, and 3707). Notably, coreceptors can compete for the association with CD4 and thus influence the type of HIV involved in the infection (2463). All the classification groups of HIV-1 can use the same coreceptors. Most clade C isolates are R5 viruses, even in AIDS patients, but some X4 and R5/X4 clade C viruses have been found in Zimbabwean patients on highly active antiretroviral therapy (2042).

The observation of CCR5 usage by R5 viruses has led to some contrasting findings on the effect of chemokines on infection, particularly of macrophages. Several studies indicated that HIV infection of macrophages and microglia (brain-derived macrophages) can be blocked by β-chemokines (1777, 4584). In other studies, the β-chemokines were found not to prevent infection of macrophages by macrophage-tropic R5 viruses (1130, 3977) despite the presence of CCR5 on the cell surface (3108). Moreover, in some studies, these cytokines appeared to enhance R5 virus replication in macrophages (3977). These differences could reflect the viruses and cell types examined (see Chapter 11). In addition, recent studies have suggested that infection of primary macrophages can vary up to 1,000-fold with R5 viruses from different tissues. The most macrophage-tropic viruses came from the brain, with less replicating capacity observed in the viruses from semen, blood, and lymph node specimens (3487). Thus, just a phenotype R5 virus may not indicate the cellular host range.

Macrophages also express CXCR4 but are not highly infectible by X4 viruses (4151) (see Chapter 4). Attachment may take place, but replication is limited compared to that of R5 viruses (1095, 4151, 4877) (see Chapter 5). Moreover, viruses that can use CCR5 may not always be macrophage tropic (1095). In addition, individuals whose macrophages do not express CCR5 on the cell surface (see below) are resistant to infection by both R5 and X4 viruses (871, 3661) but not dual-tropic viruses (3661). However, SIV_{mac} isolates that replicate in T-cell lines can infect human macrophages expressing or lacking the CCR5 receptor (3661). Thus, the use of a particular chemokine receptor does not always correlate with cell tropism.

These findings also suggest that virus entry into macrophages can involve CCR5 but probably also another, unidentified receptor (727, 1095, 3108) (see below). In this regard, a cell surface 75-kDa receptor (1817) and a transmembrane glycoprotein, CD63 (4631), have been considered potentially involved in this HIV-1 entry (see also Section VII.A).

5. CCR5 MUTANT STUDIES

A genetic variant involving a 12-bp deletion in CCR5 that introduces a frameshift mutation that results in a protein lacking the C-terminal domain (CCR5 Δ32) has been linked to resistance to HIV infection (1017, 2635, 3902). PBMC obtained from high-risk seropositive individuals, homozygous for the mutant chemokine receptor allele, were found to be resistant to infection with R5 viruses (871, 2635, 3661). In some studies, a delay in progression to disease in individuals who are heterozygous for the allele has been reported (1, 1017, 2635, 3902) (see Chapter 13). Moreover, the presence of a CCR5 promoter polymorphism (−2459 A/G) with CCR5 Δ32 heterozygosity is associated with decreased expression of CCR5 on CD4⁺ cells and reduced transmission (1849) (see Chapter 13). About 1 in 100 Caucasian people appear to be homozygous for this allele, but it is rarely detected in other racial groups (e.g., the black population from Western and Central Africa, and the Japanese population) (3902; for a review, see reference 2847) (Table 3.5).

These findings raise certain questions about resistance to HIV infection. It seems remarkable that the individuals homozygous for the deletion allele do not really come into contact with an X4 virus, since these viruses can also be transmitted (for a review, see reference 1578) (see Chapter 2). One study has suggested that the mutant CCR5 Δ32 protein also down-regulates expression of CXCR4 (32). Moreover, X4 virus are not commonly found in seminal fluid (see Chapter 2). Some findings suggest that individuals who lack CCR5 could be initially infected by an R5 virus that does not become well established in the host. It can, however, elicit cellular immune responses against HIV (4308). Subsequently, this immune response would have been able to ward off infections by other viruses (e.g., the X4 phenotype) (see Chapters 11 and 13). However, individuals homozygous for the CCR5 deletion have been found to be infected by X4 HIV-1 (384, 3305, 4416). And in subjects with only one CCR5 allele, X4 viruses were more commonly isolated than in

Table 3.5 Genotype frequencies of CCR5[a]

Ethnic group	No. of subjects	Genotype frequency (%)		
		+/+	+/Δ	Δ32/Δ32
Caucasian	235	75	23	2
African-American	238	97	3	<1
Hispanic	205	95	5	0

[a]Data from S. Y. Chang.

subjects with the wild-type CCR5/CCR5 homozygote phenotype (939). Evidently, since X4 viruses can be associated with primary infection (see Chapter 4), factors other than coreceptor expression (e.g., immune response) must also be involved in relative resistance of the host to HIV infection (see Chapters 10 and 11).

6. OTHER HIV CHEMOKINE RECEPTORS

Other HIV chemokine coreceptors have been identified, including CCR2b, CCR3, CCR8 (particularly in the thymus) (2464, 3834), CCR9, GPR15/BOB, STRL33/Bonzo, US28, CX3CR1 (V28), APJ, D6, and RDC-1 (particularly in cells of the brain) (758, 759, 1049, 1115, 3229, 4108, 4950) as well as ChemR23. Cytomegalovirus can induce the expression of chemokine receptor US28 (3834). These alternative receptors, however, are used less well than CCR5 and CXCR4 (for reviews, see references 323 and 1170) (Table 3.2).

HIV-2 strains have a wide coreceptor and usage, often are dualtropic, and can be CD4 independent, most likely via chemokine receptors (3684, 3686). The relationship of this finding to its reduced pathogenesis has not been elucidated. The range of coreceptors used by HIV-2 includes CCR1, CCR2b, CCR3, CCR4, CXCR5/BLR1, CCR5, D6, and CXCR4 (2086, 2938, 3229). The predominant one is CXCR4 (for reviews, see reference 1170 and 3685) (Table 3.2).

7. EFFECT OF CYTOKINES AND VIRAL PROTEINS

Certain cytokines (e.g., macrophage colony-stimulating factor [M-CSF], granulocyte CSF [G-CSF], and β-chemokines) can increase or decease chemokine receptor expression (1102, 2143, 2356, 2458), thus influencing virus infection and selection (Table 3.6). Interleukin-4 (IL-4) and transforming growth factor-β (TGF-β) can induce CXCR4 expression (4975), whereas IL-2 and IL-10 increase CCR5 expression on T cells (4217, 4980). IL-7 increases CXCR4 T-cell expression (4272). The type 1 interferons appear to inhibit CXCR4 expression on DCs, (4975), and IL-2 can down-modulate CD4 and CCR5 expression on macrophages, thereby reducing HIV infection (2357). Finally, in terms of viral proteins (see Chapter 7), HIV Tat can

Table 3.6 Effect of cytokines on CCR5 and CXCR4 chemokine receptor expression[a]

Cytokine(s)	Effect
IL-2	Increases CCR5 on T cells (410, 4980)
	Decreases CD4 and CXCR4 on macrophages (2357)
Type 1 interferons and IFN-γ	Increase CCR5 expression on monocytes (1728)
	Decreases CXCR4 on DC (4975)
	Decreases CCR5 on T cells (917)
TNF-α	Increases CCR5 expression on PBMC (1728, 3441)
IL-4	Increases CXCR4 on DC (4975)
IL-10	Increases CCR5 on monocytes (4217)
	Decreases CCR5 on CD4[+] lymphocytes (3441)
IL-7	Increases CXCR4 on T cells (4272)
IL-12	Increases CCR5 expression on PBMC (1728, 3441)
TGF-β	Increases CXCR4 and CCR5 on DC (3927, 4975)
M-CSF	Increases CCR5 and CXCR4 on macrophages (2458)
GM-CSF	Decreases CXCR4; increases CCR5 on macrophages (2458)
β-Chemokines	Decreases CCR5 (323, 2141, 4670)
PHA	Increases CXCR4 expression (410, 2458)
LPS	Down-regulates CCR5 expression on macrophages and (3898, 4127)

[a]See Section IIC for additional references. Table derived with assistance from K. Song and M. Roederer. IL-2, interleukin-2; IFN-γ, gamma interferon; TNF-α, tumor necrosis factor alpha; TGF-β, transcription growth factor β; M-CSF, macrophage colony-stimulating factor; GM-CSF, granulocyte-macrophage colony-stimulating factor; TGF-β, transforming growth factor beta; PHA, phytohemagglutinin; LPS, lipopolysaccharide; DC, dendritic cell; PBMC, peripheral blood mononuclear cell.

up-regulate the expression of CXCR4 on resting CD4+ lymphocytes, making them more susceptible to X4 infection (4029). gp41, most likely via CD4, can down-modulate the chemokine receptors on monocytes (4519).

8. OTHER OBSERVATIONS ON HIV CORECEPTORS

For both X4 and R5 viral phenotypes, the coreceptor seems necessary to ensure virus envelope binding to cells that have a small quantity of CD4 expressed (i.e., for R5 strains) or by viruses that bind weakly to CD4 (i.e., X4 viruses) (2319; for a review, see reference 1128). Important progress in defining the three-dimensional form of the HIV envelope has been made via crystallization (2369, 4830) and should help uncover the specific domains taking part in the virus entry process (see Chapter 10). The V3 loop is involved perhaps because it resembles a region of the chemokines (4072). Since additional chemokine receptors, as noted above, can also serve as coreceptors, still other sites for HIV interaction with the cell surface may soon be identified. In this regard, antibodies to CXCR4 have not blocked infection of T-cell lines by some HIV-1 and HIV-2 strains (2941), reflecting strain differences in the use of this receptor. Moreover, CXCR4 itself can act as a primary receptor (without the need for CD4) for infection of CD4- cells by certain isolates of HIV-2 (3686) (see Chapter 2). When this receptor was transferred to CD4- mink lung and feline kidney cells, infection by HIV-2 took place (1203). Other CD4-independent infections by HIV-1 or HIV-2 may be mediated by the chemokine coreceptors directly (see below).

T cells and macrophages express up to 10,000 copies of CCR5 or CXCR4 on the cell surface, with variations in levels (up to fivefold) depending on the individual cell type and growth conditions (2458). CD4 is found at approximately 65,000 molecules per CD4+ T cell (2458). Thus, coreceptor levels will probably be more important than CD4 in directing the cell susceptibility to virus infection and fusion (1106). In this regard, it is estimated that six CCR5 molecules that can interact with the viral envelope are necessary to elicit virus:cell fusion (2336). Similarly, three CD4 binding sites appear to be needed to activate optimally the HIV envelope trimers (1106). Thus, reductions in receptor expression on a cell can influence virus infection and the resultant low virus load (3713). Moreover, the avidity of the virus for its receptors can influence the replication efficiency of the virus itself and in competition with other viruses (2822).

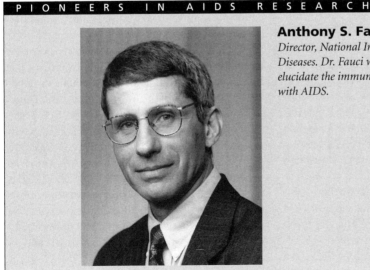

P I O N E E R S   I N   A I D S   R E S E A R C H

Anthony S. Fauci

Director, National Institutes of Allergy and Infectious Diseases. Dr. Fauci was one of the first scientists to elucidate the immunologic abnormalities associated with AIDS.

III. Virus:CD4⁺ Cell Fusion

A. Cell Surface Events

Enveloped viruses, such as HIV, following attachment, enter cells after fusion with the cell membrane. Thus, three major steps can be involved in infection: attachment, fusion, and entry (Figure 3.4). This fusion process can be measured by membrane fluorescence dequenching (4155). The full mechanism for this process in HIV infection is not yet known. In early studies, computer analysis of the amino-terminal external portion of the transmembrane gp41 HIV envelope demonstrated its similarity to fusion domains on paramyxoviruses, such as the Sendai and Newcastle disease viruses (1411, 1564; for a review, see reference 4745) (Color Plate 3, following page 78). This membrane-spanning region of gp41 is important in the fusion process (3034). These observations suggest that HIV entry involves viral gp120-CD4 receptor and coreceptor attachments and then fusion via gp41 with another cell surface molecule (1806, 3640, 4756; for a review, see reference 1106) (Color Plates 4 and 5, following page 78) (Sections II.C and VI). The loop domain of gp41 appears to bind and interact with phospholipid membranes during the viral fusion process (3431).

The role of gp41 in fusion has been supported by studies showing induction of syncytium formation by gp41 when expressed by both CD4⁺ and CD4⁻ cells (3473). For fusion to occur, the transition of gp41 from a coil-coil to a 6C helix bundle appears to be an important step (2964). This process could follow a conformational change in CD4 as well as dissociation of the envelope gp120 from the virion surface, perhaps following cleavage of the V3 loop (Figure 3.3) (Sections II.A and II.B) (324). The V3 loop, the V1/V2 domain, and gp41 could be important in this membrane fusion event (324, 328, 4105, 4274). Glycosphingolipids can help the formation of membrane fusion complexes (involving the envelope and CD4) and permit efficient HIV infection (1930).

The kinetics of the fusion reaction have suggested continued attachment of the virus to CD4 while fusion takes place (1088). Thus, complete gp120 shedding most likely does not occur, although some displacement, as described in Section II.A, might be involved. The virus interaction with

a chemokine receptor could bring the virus envelope closer to the cell membrane, permitting fusion (2524) (Color Plate 2, following page 78). Mutational studies with gp41 and with the V3 loop have suggested that cell:cell fusion and infectivity are linked, since in many cases these are affected by the same amino acid changes (see Chapter 6). HIV infectivity presumably reflects the virus:cell fusion event (328, 987, 1361, 1364, 1630) (Figure 3.4).

Recent evidence suggests that there are three processes involved in the entry of cell-attached infectious HIV (3536). The first is a rapid reversible association of the virus with the CD4 and chemokine coreceptor; the second involves the rate-limiting (up to 1 h) chemokine-dependent conformational change in gp41, and the third involves a rapid (within 5 to 10 min) step of viral entry. The third process includes virus:cell fusion and capsid entry (Figure 3.4 and Color Plate 5, following page 78). The V3 loop plays an important role in the rate-limiting coreceptor-dependent conformational change in gp41 (3536). Nevertheless, the fusogenic property of a virus may not be as important for infectivity as it is for cell syncytium formation (4274). These observations suggest that virus:cell and cell:cell fusion could involve distinct processes (see Chapter 6).

B. pH-Independent Entry

Experiments examining the mechanism for virus entry into cells have also evaluated the effect of changes in the relative acidity of the cytoplasmic endosomes. Enveloped viruses enter by either a pH-dependent or -independent process. If a low pH is needed, virus fusion most likely occurs in endocytotic vesicles. With those retroviruses that have been examined and many other enveloped viruses, an acidic environment in the cell is generally not needed for virus entry (1090, 1511, 4745). In the case of HIV, chloroquine and NH_4Cl, which raise the pH in cellular components, do not affect virus infection (4278). Thus, HIV entry is pH independent. This observation has suggested that the HIV envelope, after attachment and subsequent interactions with the cell surface, can fuse directly with the cell membrane and not necessarily within endocytotic vesicles (Figures 3.2 and 3.4 and Color Plate 2, following page 78). However, the possible entry of HIV through endosomes as

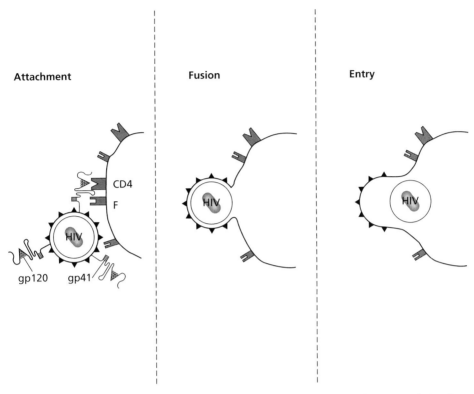

Figure 3.4   HIV entry into cells. Three major steps involved in virus infection are depicted based on observations in cell culture (3589, 4251). Adapted from reference 2520 with permission.

well has not been ruled out. Because HIV can enter by fusing directly with the plasma membrane, phagocytosis may also lead to infection in some cells (3448).

IV. Other Potential HIV:Cell Surface Interactions Involved in Virus Entry into CD4+ Cells

The possibility that other factors are involved in HIV infection of a cell, after the viral interaction with a receptor, has been suggested. Investigators have shown that after attachment to CD4 a delay in viral entry at the cell surface can influence the spread of HIV and the extent of virus production (2197). Different rates and efficiencies of entry are most likely linked to variations in the envelope protein (1281, 4112) (see Chapter 7). Other studies suggest that the cytoplasmic domain of gp41 might be partly involved in entry through a role

in virus uncoating or penetration (1402). Finally, nonprotein components (possibly glycolipids) could play a role in the envelope-CD4-mediated fusion needed for virus entry (1131).

The phenomenon of delayed entry has been associated in some studies with the absence of the D3 and D4 regions of the CD4 molecule (3593) and probably reflects inefficient conformational changes in the CD4 molecule associated with fusion (see Chapter 6). These observations support the notion that the CD4 protein could be involved not only in the binding but also in the fusion and perhaps penetration of the virion from the cell surface into the cytoplasm of the cell (1549). For a period of time, the virus might remain attached to CD4 without release of its viral core into the cytoplasm. Alternatively (although this hypothesis is highly conjectural), the core might be kept beneath the cell membrane bilayer without entry into the cytoplasm. In this regard, when certain

HIV-1 and SIV strains are used to infect a variety of CD4$^+$ or CD4$^-$ cells, attachment (measured by CD4 binding) and fusion (detected by fluorescence dequenching) may take place, but the presence of the viral core protein in the cell or the production of infectious virus cannot be detected (3589, 4254). Only after penetration and uncoating of the viral core would reverse transcription and the steps leading to viral production take place (Figure 3.4) (2524).

The exact mechanism for nucleocapsid entry is not known. One hypothesis is that the binding of the gp41 fusion domain with a fusion receptor (not yet identified) on the cell surface brings about an intermixing of the outer lipid membranes of the virus and the cell (i.e., hemifusion). However, unless the inner lipid membranes meet, nucleocapsid entry cannot take place (Color Plate 6, following page 78). The mixing of inner cell membranes may require other cellular or viral proteins that are yet to be defined. Another explanation could be the need for a particular process for core entry. A Gag protein is most likely involved in this step, since this viral protein (e.g., MA) plays an important role in the budding and release of HIV progeny at the end of the replicative cycle (4223, 4893) (see Chapter 7). This possibility has also been supported by SIV/HIV recombinant studies showing restricted replication of HIV-1 in rhesus macaque cells, in which a region encompassing the *gag* gene appears to be involved (1837).

V. Down-Modulation of the CD4 Protein

Another early observation made with HIV-1 replication in human T cells was the concomitant disappearance of the CD4 protein from the cell surface (1903, 2225, 4294). The extent and time of the down-modulation depend on the level of virus production (3593, 4294, 4898, 4907). Generally, a loss in CD4 expression in vitro is detected several days after HIV infection of cells, when sufficient progeny virions are produced. Restoration of CD4 expression can occur with a reduction in HIV-1 production by a Tat inhibitor or by CD8$^+$ cell anti-HIV immune responses (2543, 4061, 4658).

Table 3.7 Factors involved in modulation of CD4 protein expression

- Complexing of CD4 with envelope gp160 within the cell (918, 919, 1980)
- Vpu dissociates the CD4:gp160 complex and degrades CD4 (462, 4767).
- Down-modulation by Nef (1445, 2811)
- Block in transcription of CD4 mRNA (3899, 4290)
- Arrest in translation of the CD4 protein (1903, 4898)
- Masking of viral receptor by gp120 (88, 2918)
- Removal of CD4 from cell surface by replicating virions (1751, 2955)

The mechanism(s) involved in the altered expression of this cell surface receptor is still not clear (Table 3.7). The CD4 receptor does not necessarily internalize with HIV during infection, and CD4-related signal transduction events are not needed for virus entry (3346). Moreover, with some HIV strains (HIV-1$_{SF162}$ and HIV-2$_{UC1}$), infection with high levels of virus production does not affect CD4 expression (734, 1231). Differences in specific regions of the envelope gp120 could be involved. Using interviral recombinants of two HIV-1 strains differing in this biologic property, CD4 down-modulation was linked to the envelope region (4885). Some studies suggest a role of the complexing of envelope gp160 with CD4 in the endoplasmic reticulum of the cell (918, 919, 1980).

Vpu is also considered to be involved in this process, since this viral protein dissociates the gp160:CD4 complex by inducing degradation of CD4 (462, 4767) (see Chapter 7). This function could be needed to permit gp160 incorporation into virions and could certainly affect CD4 expression. In this regard, down-modulation of CD4 seems to be important for efficient HIV production, since CD4 can act at the cell surface to inhibit Vpu-enhanced virion release (462).

In other studies, the Nef protein has been implicated in down-modulation of the CD4 molecule (1445, 1676, 2811) (see Chapter 7). The mechanism has been linked to an endocytotoxic process in which CD4 is degraded in lysosomes (4485). Viruses that lack this activity appear to have a truncated Nef protein. With both Vpu and Nef, the cytoplasmic portion of the CD4 molecule is the major domain involved (116, 2490). It appears that

Env, Vpu, and Nef can all play a role in CD4 down-modulation. Nef down-modulates CD4 rapidly during the early steps in HIV infection; Env and Vpu function late in infection (712). In general, a combination of all three proteins is the most efficient in reducing CD4 expression (712).

Most studies have shown a decrease in CD4 protein expression, but some reports indicate reduced transcription of the CD4 mRNA (3899, 4294) or translation of the CD4 mRNA (1903, 4898). A few studies have suggested that masking of the CD4 binding site by the envelope gp120 (or gp120:antibody complexes) attached to the cell surface is involved (88, 2918, 3930). The latter phenomenon can be demonstrated by using an antibody to a different region of the CD4 molecule located outside the gp120 binding site. In addition, some investigators suggest that the CD4 molecule could be removed by budding virions (1751, 2955) (Table 3.7). The relative effect that each of these processes has on CD4 protein expression most likely depends on the virus and the cells infected.

The relevance of CD4 down-modulation to pathogenesis is unclear, since some viruses do not modulate expression of CD4 (734, 1231) (see Chapter 13). The removal of this HIV binding site on the CD4 molecule, however, does prevent superinfection of the cells by other HIV-1 strains (see Chapter 4) and permits higher levels of virus replication (462).

VI. Infection of Cells Lacking CD4 Expression

A. General Observations

Many CD4$^-$ cells can be infected by HIV (Table 3.8), including human skin fibroblasts, dental pulp fibroblasts, muscle and bone-derived fibroblastoid cell lines, human trophoblasts, follicular dendritic cells, brain-derived glial cells, brain capillary endothelial cells, bowel-derived cells, cervical epithelial cells, fetal adrenal cells, and human liver carcinoma cell lines (see Chapter 4). Evidence for the absence of a role of the CD4 receptor in virus entry of these cells comes from a variety of studies, including those involving monoclonal antibodies to CD4, incubation of virus with sCD4, and lack of detectable CD4 mRNA in the cells

Table 3.8 CD4$^-$ human cells susceptible to HIV infection^a

In vitro studies

Fetal astrocytes
Neuroblastoma cell lines (e.g., SK-N-Mc)
Brain-derived capillary endothelial cells
Brain microglia
NK cells
Osteosarcoma cell line (HOS)
Rhabdomyosarcoma cell line (e.g., RD)
Primary skin fibroblasts
Fetal adrenal cells
Follicular dendritic cells
Hepatic carcinoma cell line
Hepatic sinusoidal endothelial cells
Bowel adenocarcinoma cell lines
Trophoblast cell lines
Cervix-derived epithelial cell lines

In vivo studies

Bowel epithelium
Renal epithelium
Dental pulp fibroblasts
Brain astrocytes, oligodendrocytes

^{a}In vitro studies involve cell culture with HIV infection detected by reverse transcriptase, p24 antigen, and PCR assay procedures. In vivo studies include immunohistochemical and in situ hybridization methods. See text for references.

(249, 479, 605, 729, 788, 1533, 1734, 2569, 2965, 3443, 4026, 4249, 4375, 4393, 4901).

The extent of virus replication in CD4$^-$ cells is generally low, but where evaluated, HIV enters the cells in a pH-independent manner (4393), as it does in CD4$^+$ cells. The limited extent of virus production is due in part to inefficient viral entry and subsequent spread; usually less than 1% of cells initially become infected (479, 2965). Intracellular events can also limit steps leading to productive infection (see Chapter 5). Transfection experiments with DNA molecular clones of HIV suggest that once infection is established, substantial virus replication can occur in many of these cell types (2534). Thus, virus entry is the limiting step. To detect HIV production in several CD4$^-$ cell types, cocultivation of the cells with other sensitive target cells, such as PBMC, has been helpful (4393). Some studies suggest that cytokines produced by PBMC can enhance HIV production in CD4$^-$ cells, in particular those of brain origin (4350, 4451).

The cell surface molecule(s) responsible for viral entry into CD4⁻ cells is not known, but conceivably it could be a fusion receptor (4393) or a secondary binding site for HIV such as the CCR5 or CXCR4 receptor (1040, 1203, 1866, 3686) (Section II.C). Moreover, antibodies to HIV differ in their ability to neutralize HIV infection of lymphocytes and CD4⁻ fibroblasts (4393). A portion of the viral envelope that is different from that used for CD4⁺ cell entry seems to be involved. In this regard, the determinants for entry into CD4⁻ cells have been mapped outside the V1/V2 and V3 hypervariable loops (2260, 2371), which are usually involved in chemokine receptor interaction.

This alternative route of entry, however, is quite limited compared to the process mediated by CD4. One conclusion could be that with CD4⁺ cells, the attachment to CD4 enhances the interaction of the viral envelope with a cellular coreceptor (Section II.C) or a fusion receptor. CD4⁻ cells would use the same means of entry (a universal one involving fusion), but it would be much less efficient. Likewise, if the coreceptor or cell fusion receptor is absent, infection of CD4⁺ cells might not occur, as observed with some T-cell lines (2184). Some studies, however, indicate that HIV can enter certain CD4⁻ epithelial cells by a process not involving the viral envelope. These results suggest that the virus could infect certain tissues even in the presence of neutralizing antibodies (3403).

Finally, as discussed above, perhaps the third step of virus entry into the cell, the entry of the nucleocapsid (Figure 3.4 and Color Plate 2, following page 78), is blocked in CD4⁻ cells because of the lack of an appropriate cellular factor or interaction of a viral protein with a necessary intracellular factor.

B. Galactosyl Ceramide Receptor

A virus receptor on CD4⁻ brain-derived cells was identified by using rabbit polyclonal antibodies to the glycolipids galactosyl ceramide (GalC) and galactosyl sulfur (1730). Like a possible cellular fusion domain for paramyxoviruses (2819, 4745), a glycolipid could be involved in HIV infection of some CD4⁻ cells. The GalC receptor has also been linked to infection of bowel-derived cells and epithelial cells from the vagina (1399, 4841)

(Table 3.8). The chemokine receptor CXCR4 has also been identified as a possible coreceptor for HIV-1 entry into CD4⁻ GalC⁺ intestinal epithelial cells (1040). The interaction of HIV with all these cells appears to involve regions on gp120, such as the V3 loop and the V4 and V5 domains, that are different from those that interact with CD4 (1399, 1732, 4842).

The identification of GalC as a means of entry into brain and bowel cells might explain the reports of gastrointestinal disorders that accompany neurologic signs of HIV infection (1232); similar viral strains might use this cellular receptor. Whether the GalC mechanism for HIV entry of CD4⁻ cells is common is not known, but not all brain cells express this glycolipid.

VII. Other Possible HIV:Cell Surface Interactions

A. Additional Cellular Receptors for HIV

Several studies have indicated that HIV interacting with antibodies can enter cells via the Fc or complement receptor (Section VIII) (see Chapter 10). Antibodies to GalC do not block HIV infection of CD4⁻ fibroblasts and fetal adrenal cells (A. Barboza and J. A. Levy, unpublished observations), and thus other unidentified receptors must be involved. Moreover, human fetal astrocytes appear to utilize a mannose receptor (2639) (see Chapter 8), and a receptor of approximately 180 kDa distinct from GalC has been demonstrated on CD4⁻ glioma cells. Binding of recombinant gp120 to this protein receptor appears to induce tyrosine-specific protein kinase activity in the cells (3989) (Tables 3.9 and 3.10).

In addition, with the high mannose content in the HIV-1 envelope (1715), the macrophage mannose receptor (1240) could provide an alternative entry site for infection of macrophages by the virus. This possibility should be explored, particularly where the β-chemokine receptors do not appear to be involved (Section II.C). For example, cell surface heparin sulfate proteoglycans, particularly the syndecans, have been shown to serve as a major HIV attachment site on macrophages (3918), epithelial cells, and brain microvascular endothelial cells (414). In addition, galectin 1 (3363) and matrix

Table 3.9 HIV:cell surface binding interactions

Cellular receptor(s)	Major cell type(s)
CD4 (Section 1)	Lymphocytes, macrophages (2224)
Chemokine receptors (Table 3.2)	Lymphocytes, macrophages (320)
Galactosyl ceramide (Section VI)	Brain, intestinal, vaginal epithelial cells (1399, 1730, 4841)
Fc[a]	Macrophages, T cells (1882, 1883, 2933, 4363)
Complement[a]	Lymphocytes, macrophages (476, 1168, 3767)

[a]When virus is opsonized or complexed with antibody (see Section X and Chapters 9 and 10).

fibronectin (4398) can increase virus attachment to cells. Moreover, glycosphingolipids can enhance HIV infection by helping organize the membrane fusion complex (1930). CD4⁻ cells, such as neutrophils, erythrocytes, CD8⁺ cells and platelets (1827, 2530, 3330), and B cells (2772, 3048) can also bind HIV to the cell surface (see Chapter 2, Figure 2.3), and complement can increase this binding through immune complexes (1995, 3330). Finally, other C-type lectins (e.g., DC-SIGN [see below]) can bind HIV and help its transfer to CD4⁺ cells or virus entry into cells (see Chapter 9). In this regard, DC-SIGN expression on B cells appears to be involved in HIV transmission to T cells (3669).

B. Role of Cellular Proteins Associated with the HIV Envelope

The incorporation of MHC-related molecules as well as other cell surface proteins onto the viral envelope might help in attachment of HIV to the surface of cells (156, 1904, 3855; for review, see reference 4522) (Table 3.10). About 60 native HLA-II complexes per virion have been noted (4487). CD80 and CD86 may also be inserted into HIV virions and increase their infectivity by enhancing their attachment and entry following interactions with CD28 and CTLA-4 (1510). A possible role of the transmembrane receptor for hyaluronan, CD44, in productive infection by macrophage-tropic strains has been suggested (1146). HIV particles with CD44 associated with the viral envelope bind to T cells expressing hyaluronic acid (1666). This virion acquisition of cellular molecules appears to be determined by the viral isolate and the cells infected (600), and it has been associated with increased viral infectivity (599). Nevertheless, viruses grown in nonhuman cells are still highly infectious for human cells (2534).

Work demonstrating that the leukocyte function antigen 1 (LFA-1) cellular adhesion molecule can be a participant in HIV infection offers another alternative mechanism for virus attachment and viral entry, although its primary contribution appears to be in cell:cell fusion (1716, 1833, 2075, 3405) (see Chapter 6). Its ligands, the intercellular adhesion molecules 1 (ICAM-1), -2, and -3 incorporated onto virions via an interaction with Pr55 Gag protein (286), can increase virus infectivity of PBMC 2- to 10-fold as well as increase spread (460, 622, 1333; for a review, see reference 1839) and syncytium formation (1334). Perhaps adhesion molecules are important in the cell-to-cell transfer of virus. How these virus-associated cellular proteins make viruses sensitive to serum antibodies is discussed in Chapter 10.

Table 3.10 Other possible cellular binding proteins for HIV

- 75-kDa receptor (macrophages) (1817)
- 180-kDa receptor (glioma cells) (3989)
- CD44S (1146)
- Transmembrane glycoprotein CD63 (macrophages) (4631)
- C-type lections (e.g., mannose receptor) (1240, 2639), DC-SIGN (936)
- Heparin sulfate proteoglycans (e.g., syndecans) (3918)
- Galectin 1 (3363)
- Multimeric fibronectin (4398)
- Glycosphingolipids (1930)
- MHC (156, 1904, 3855)
- LFA-1[a] (1717, 1833, 4535)
- ICAM-1, -2, -3[a] (1839, 3742)
- CD80, CD86 (1510)

[a]On cells and/or virus (LFA:ICAM interaction). See Section VII.

It is noteworthy that the ICAM molecules bind to both LFA-1 and DC-SIGN (DC-specific ICAM-grabbing nonintegrin). DC-SIGN was originally noted to be a gp120 mannose-binding C-type lectin on CD4⁻ placental cells (936, 4199) (see below). The interaction of the DC-SIGN molecule with ICAMs helps cells bind to carbohydrate structures on the endothelium and elicit their transendothelial migration. Glyscosylation is therefore important for this binding to DC-SIGN (408). Virions carrying LFA-1 or ICAM can have better attachment to the cell surface, allowing concomitant interactions with specific cell surface receptors and virions and more efficient entry (4522). DC-SIGN may play a role in virus attachment to macrophages and certain DCs from which HIV can subsequently be transferred to sensitive target cells (e.g., CD4⁺ cells) or from mucosal surfaces to lymph nodes (408, 934, 1477, 1478) (see Chapter 9).

VIII. Other Possible Mechanisms Involved in Virus Entry

A. Fc and Complement Receptors

Besides entering cells via the direct interaction of the virus envelope with cell surface receptors, HIV can infect cells by other mechanisms. For example, during the course of studies on the humoral response to HIV-1 infection, the phenomenon of antibody-dependent enhancement (ADE) of HIV infection was discovered (see Chapter 10). ADE involves binding of the Fab portion of nonneutralizing antibodies to the surface of the virion and the transfer of virus into a cell through the complement or Fc receptor (Figure 10.1) (1882, 2430, 3700, 3766, 3767, 4366, 4464).

ADE of HIV highlights the potential role of herpesviruses as cofactors in HIV infection. These DNA viruses can induce both complement and Fc receptors on the surface of infected cells (280, 2933, 2947, 3654) that could serve as potential target cells for HIV infection (see Chapter 2). HIV was found to infect cytomegalovirus-infected human fibroblasts via virus:antibody complexes (2933). This observation confirmed the lack of participation by CD4 in HIV infection by the Fc receptor. Fc receptors have also been detected on rectal mucosal cells (1939). Conceivably, infection could take place in the anal canal via virus:antibody complexes in seminal fluid (see Chapter 2).

Other experiments have suggested that HIV alone can enter cells directly by the complement receptor (CR-2) after activation and binding to the C1 component (i.e., as opsonized particles) (475, 476, 1168). This mechanism, involving gp41, can lead to enhanced infection of cells by small amounts of virus (4418) and has also been suggested as the mechanism for the attachment of HIV-1 to follicular dendritic cells (see Chapter 9).

Martin S. Hirsch
Professor, Department of Medicine, and Director of Clinical AIDS Research, Harvard Medical School. Dr. Hirsch was among the first clinicians to note the presence of HIV in a variety of body fluids and its association with clinical syndromes associated with AIDS.

B. Phenotypic Mixing: Pseudotype Virion Formation

Another mechanism for HIV entry into cells is phenotypic mixing (1919). By this process, a viral genome can be placed in the envelope of a different virus and thus acquire the host range of that virus (Figure 3.5). Phenotypic mixing between HIV-1 and HIV-2 strains has been described (2474). Moreover, cells coinfected by HIV and murine retroviruses have demonstrated pseudotype virion formation in which the HIV genome can be found within the envelope of various mouse retroviruses (596, 2708). Subsequently, HIV could infect a wide variety of cells susceptible to these animal retroviruses (Figure 3.6).

HIV pseudotypes have also been produced in vitro with herpes- and rhabdoviruses (e.g., vesicular stomatitis virus [VSV]) (4960). VSV pseudotypes have been helpful in defining the cellular restrictions to HIV entry (4714). Cells exposed to a virus containing the VSV genome within the HIV envelope show VSV-induced lysis only if they are susceptible to HIV infection. Finally, in vitro phenotypic mixing among different human retrovirus groups (e.g., HTLV and HIV) has also been described (2393, 2474). In preliminary studies, however, phenotypic mixing during coinfection of cells with HIV and the human spumavirus has not been observed (J. A. Levy, unpublished observations). In summary, the following viruses have been shown to undergo phenotypic mixing with HIV-1: HIV-2; HTLV-1; murine xenotropic, amphotropic, and polytropic type C retroviruses; VSV; and herpesviruses.

Whether pseudotype virus formation occurs in nature is not known. HIV-infected individuals coinfected with herpesviruses or HTLV-1 could have virus populations representing phenotypic mixtures of the two viruses (2393, 4960), but this possibility has not been reported. Electron microscopic (EM) studies of nongenital herpes simplex virus type 1 (HSV-1) skin lesions have shown virions suggestive of phenotypically mixed particles (1810). The process may have facilitated HIV infection of the keratinocytes as well as HSV infection of the macrophages in the lesions. The findings, if confirmed, could have relevance to sexual transmission of HIV (see Chapter 2). Moreover, as noted above, infection in vitro by HIV-1 and HIV-2 can lead to phenotypic mixing (2474). The consequences of these events could include increased pathogenesis, but no evidence of this phenomenon occurring in vivo has been reported. Investigators using animal models to study HIV infection must also recognize that phenotypic mixing with an endogenous virus in the animal (e.g., rodents) (2077, 3130, 3131, 3210) might compromise the study objectives. This problem, however, has not been encountered in SCID/hu mice (D. Mosier, personal communication).

IX. Cell-to-Cell Transfer of HIV

Besides entering a cell as a free infectious particle, HIV can be passed during cell-to-cell contact (Color Plate 7, following page 78). In this process, multinucleated cells might result from syncytium formation (Figure 3.7), or cell-cell contact could take place by adherence without fusion of cell membranes (see Figures 2.5 and 2.7). The cell-to-cell mechanism of HIV transfer has been estimated to be up to 100 times more efficient than infection by free virus particles (3926). In some studies, evidence has been presented that HIV can

Phenotypic mixing

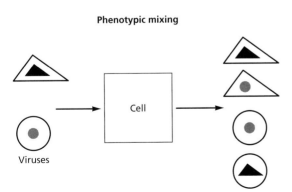

Figure 3.5 Phenotypic mixing. When two viruses of two different types enter the same cell, the progeny produced will consist of the initial viruses and also viruses that have exchanged their outside coat. These new viruses then have the host range of the virus from which they derived their envelope. Reprinted from reference 2512, copyright 1977, with permission from Elsevier.

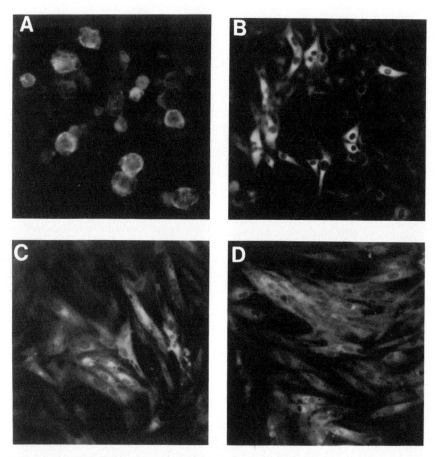

Figure 3.6 Coinfection of a human T-lymphocyte line with HIV-1 and the murine xenotropic retrovirus led to virus preparations that contained phenotypically mixed particles. Thus, the HIV genome enveloped in a xenotropic virus coat could infect a wide variety of animal cell lines previously resistant to HIV infection. (A) HUT 78 human T cells; (B) mink lung cells; (C) horse dermis cells; (D) goat esophagus cells (all magnifications, ×40). Reprinted from reference 596 with permission from Elsevier.

spread rapidly from one cell to another without formation of fully formed particles (3403, 3926). Conceivably, viral nucleocapsids are transferred to a new cell during cell-to-cell fusion with subsequent de novo reverse transcription (2573).

Macrophage-to-lymphocyte transfer of virus, presumably involving fusion, has been shown in the presence of neutralizing antibodies (1668). In cell culture studies involving cell-to-cell contact without cell fusion, HIV was also shown to be transmitted from monocytes or lymphocytes to epithelial cells in the presence of neutralizing antibodies (3452, 3497, 4375) (see Chapter 2). In these experiments, EM pictures revealed the transfer of complete virus particles that were present at the site of

the cell:cell interaction without cell fusion (Figures 2.5 and 2.7). In one report, time-lapse photography showed a migrating infected lymphocyte transferring virus particles to several different epithelial cells during short periods of contact (3452). In other EM studies of HIV-infected monocytes, virus was associated with pseudopods projecting from macrophages, suggesting another means of HIV transfer (Figure 3.8) (3477). Moreover, as noted above (Section VII.B), DCs or other cells can transfer virus to CD4+ T cells by cell:cell conjugates or via C-type lectins (934, 3574) (see Chapter 9). Thus, HIV spread in the host could result from cell-to-cell transfer (via cores or virions) as well as from circulating free virus.

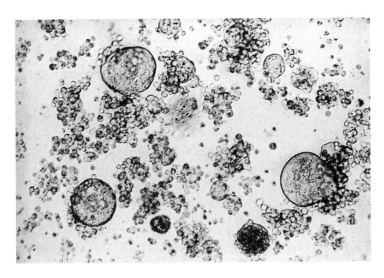

Figure 3.7 Multinucleated cell formation in peripheral blood mononuclear cells infected by HIV-1. Magnification, ×65.

X. Overview of Early Steps in HIV Infection

A key concept regarding the early events in HIV interaction with a cell (Table 3.11) is that attachment of HIV to the CD4 molecule most likely leads to some conformational changes in both gp120 and CD4. The initial attachment appears to be at two sites on the CDR2 domain of CD4 (Figure 3.1) and probably involves nonlinear epitopes of gp120 that come into contact with the CD4 receptor site through a specific conformational structure. Subsequent displacement of gp120 and/or cleavage of the envelope protein (e.g., in the V3 loop) by cellular enzymes (Figure 3.3) causes another alteration

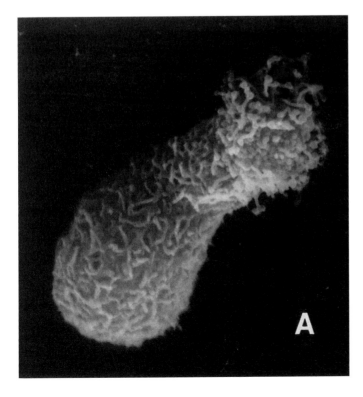

Figure 3.8 (A) Scanning electron micrograph of an HIV-infected, activated monocyte. The surface of most of the monocyte is characterized by irregular microvilli. However, the pseudopod of the monotype (top) is covered with small spherical structures which appear to be HIV virions. The bulges at the tips of these microvilli may be budding HIV virions. (From reference 3477 with permission.) (*Figure continues next page*)

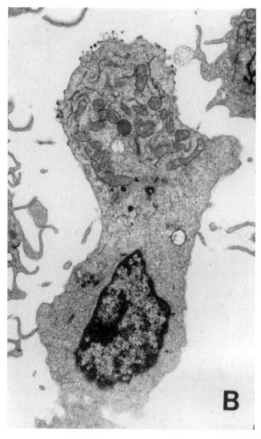

Figure 3.8 *(continued)* (B) Transmission electron micrograph of an activated monocyte showing a pseudopod with budding virus (top of figure). From reference 3477 with permission.

in the viral envelope. This alteration results in the conformational changes in gp120 and CD4 that give the viral envelope additional binding sites with the cell surface, such as through CXCR4, CXCR5, or other receptors (3191) (Tables 3.8, 3.9, and 3.10). This interaction will depend on the viral strain involved. Recent data show that the V3 loop is important in virus coreceptor usage and switching but is not the only portion of the envelope involved in receptor interaction (for a review, see reference 1752). In addition, there can be conformational changes in the coreceptors that influence cell sensitivity to virus infection (1106).

A subsequent process involves the gp41 fusion domain and the target cell membrane (possibly via another specific cell surface receptor). Virus:cell fusion, which is pH independent, then takes place (3931). The viral core subsequently enters the cell (Figures 3.2 and 3.4 and Color Plates 2, 5, and 6, following page 78) (Section III). Conformational changes in the CD4 molecule following gp120 binding may enhance virus entry (196). Other regions on CD4 and on gp120 (e.g., the V3 loop) could be involved in these processes.

In brief, this interaction of HIV with CD4 and subsequently its coreceptors can be influenced by several factors, including the following (for reviews, see references 1106 and 1549):

- the virus envelope proteins leading to fusion

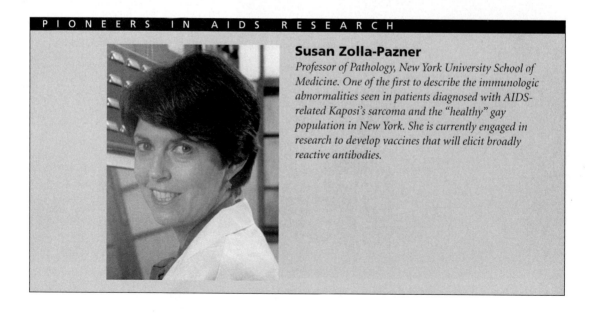

PIONEERS IN AIDS RESEARCH

Susan Zolla-Pazner
Professor of Pathology, New York University School of Medicine. One of the first to describe the immunologic abnormalities seen in patients diagnosed with AIDS-related Kaposi's sarcoma and the "healthy" gay population in New York. She is currently engaged in research to develop vaccines that will elicit broadly reactive antibodies.

Table 3.11 Steps involved in HIV infection of a cell[a]

1. Attachment of viral envelope gp120 to cell surface receptor (e.g., CD4) or alternative receptor
2. Conformational change in gp120 and perhaps CD4 (i.e., the cell receptor) following attachment
3. Binding of another gp120 region to a coreceptor
4. Displacement of gp120[b]
5. Proteolytic cleavage of the V3 loop or its envelope counterpart (i.e., for HIV-2)[b]
6. Interaction of the fusion domain of HIV (e.g., gp41) with a fusion receptor on the cell surface (conceivably a glycolipid)
7. Virus:cell fusion in a pH-independent fashion
8. Entry of viral RNA associated with core into the cytoplasm, uncoating of the core, and formation of reverse transcription complexes
9. Initiation of reverse transcriptase
10. Production of viral DNA copy (cDNA) from viral RNA and its duplication into a double-stranded DNA structure; generation of covalently bound circles and noncovalently bound circular forms
11. Transport of cDNA to the nucleus, in a preintegration complex (PR, RT, IN, Vpr) where integration of the noncovalently bound circular forms into chromosomal DNA takes place
12. Production of viral mRNA and viral genomic RNA from the integrated proviral DNA (extent of production depends on relative expression of HIV regulatory genes (3403) (see Chapter 5)
13. Production of viral proteins from full-length and spliced mRNA
14. Incorporation of viral genomic RNA into the capsid forming at the cell membrane (and in intracellular compartments)
15. Processing of Gag and Gag-Pol polyproteins at the cell surface or in budding virions (e.g., protease activity)
16. Budding of the viral capsid through the cell membrane, with incorporation of the processed viral envelope glycoproteins and other proteins present on the cell surface (can depend on viral *vpu* gene product)

[a]Summarized from discussions in the text (Section VIII). For a review, see reference 2476. Cell-to-cell transfer of HIV can also take place (3926).
[b]May or may not take place.

- posttranslational modification of the coreceptors
- the coreceptor density on the cell surface
- partitions of the receptors into lipid rafts that can associate and give enriched areas of expression
- the oxidative state of CD4, which may influence mostly the conformational changes required for coreceptor binding leading to fusion

Three major steps—attachment, fusion, and nucleocapsid entry—are thus part of HIV entry (Figure 3.4). Most likely, the virus:cell fusion mediated by gp41 and the nucleoid entry via the Gag protein represent other biologic steps in early HIV infection that need to be elucidated. Conceivably, specific viral and cellular factors are involved. Cellular proteins found on budding virions (e.g., MHC, LFA, and ICAM) could enhance the virus:cell interaction (Table 3.10). All these findings indicate the promiscuity of HIV in its interaction with the cell surface and the probability that several therapeutic approaches can be used to block infection at entry (see Chapter 14).

Following virus entry, subsequent events (e.g., nucleocapsid uncoating, reverse transcription, and nuclear transport) can determine the extent of virus replication in the acutely infected cell (see Chapter 5 for details) (2476). Expression of the CD4 molecule is generally reduced once substantial virus replication occurs (Table 3.7), but exceptions have been observed with some HIV strains. Finally, the spread of HIV in the host results from production of infectious progeny and also by cell-to-cell transfer of virus (see above) (Table 3.11) and possibly by non-envelope-mediated processes (3403).

1. The CD4 molecule is a major cellular receptor site for HIV infection. The viral regions binding to CD4 include the fourth conserved portion near the carboxyl-terminal end of the viral gp120, as well as other regions involved in the conformational structure of the envelope. The binding region on the CD4 molecule is located on a protuberant ridge along one face of the V1 domain. The binding site on CD4 appears to overlap with the class II major histocompatibility complex binding site.

2. Primary virus isolates, particularly R5 macrophage-tropic isolates, appear to be resistant to inactivation by soluble CD4 (sCD4). This resistance reflects the conformational structure of the envelope, particularly within the V3 region. Shedding of gp120, lack of envelope cleavage, and perhaps the avidity of the R5 strain for cell surface CD4 receptors rather than sCD4 could determine this process.

3. Binding of HIV to a cell may involve displacement of gp120, either completely or partially. Subsequently, cleavage of gp120 may take place (with X4 viruses), probably by a cellular protease. These two steps could permit the interaction of the fusion domain of HIV (in gp41) with a fusion receptor on the cell surface.

4. HIV generally uses chemokine receptors on cells for additional attachment before entry: CCR5 for macrophage-tropic viruses (R5 type) and CXCR4 for T-cell-line-tropic viruses (X4 type). The expression of these receptors can differ on CD4+ cells. Other chemokine receptors on different cells can be involved in HIV infection of some cells.

5. Individuals whose cells lack CCR5 expression are resistant to R5 virus infection but can be infected by X4 viruses.

6. R5 and X4 viruses show several biologic differences, including their effects on induction and the nature of the clinical disease.

7. Various cytokines and viral proteins can influence chemokine receptor expression.

8. Virus:cell fusion may take place as a separate step involving gp41 and a fusion domain on the cell.

9. Entry of the viral core into a cell is pH independent. This process may also represent a separate step involving different viral and cellular proteins.

10. Viruses can down-modulate CD4 expression (protein and mRNA) through the function of Vpu, Nef, and the envelope proteins.

11. CD4− cells can be infected via a variety of cell surface proteins.

12. Galactosyl ceramide can serve as a receptor for infection of cells in the brain, bowel, and vagina.

13. Cell surface molecules on the virion surface (e.g., HLA, LFA-1, and ICAM) can enhance HIV attachment to cells and virus infection.

14. Other cell surface proteins (e.g., C-type lectins and syndecans) can help HIV binding to cells and facilitate infection. They can mediate transfer of virus to susceptible cells (e.g., CD4+ cells).

15. After the virus interacts with antibodies, Fc and complement receptors can serve as alternative mechanisms for HIV entry into a cell. These receptors can be induced on cells by herpesviruses.

16. Phenotypic mixing with pseudotype virion formation could lead to further transfer of the HIV genome inside the envelope of a variety of other RNA and DNA viruses.

17. Cell-to-cell transfer of HIV appears to be a more rapid and efficient mechanism for infection of a cell than direct infection by free virus.

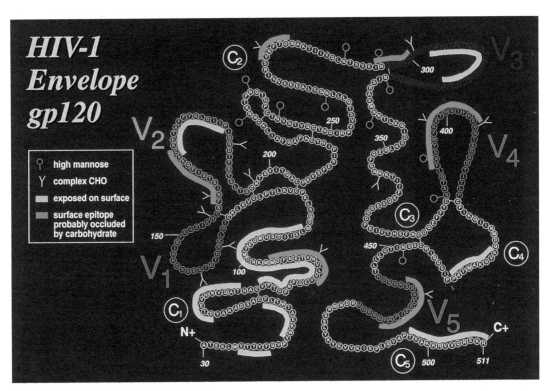

Color Plate 1 Schematic representation of gp120 HIV-1$_{LAI}$, showing disulfide and glycosylation sites. Glycosylation sites containing high-mannose-type and/or hybrid-type oligosaccharides are indicated, as well as the glycosylation sites with complex-type oligosaccharide structures. The variable regions are designated V1 to V5. The conserved regions are designated C1 to C5. Parts of the envelope exposed on the surface and those portions probably occluded by carbohydrates are demonstrated. The CD4 region contains a major attachment site for CD4 (2417). Also noted are other regions on gp120 that, according to studies with amino acid substitutions (3333), appear to be involved in binding to the CD4 molecule (3093). Reprinted from reference 2497 with permission. (See page 11.)

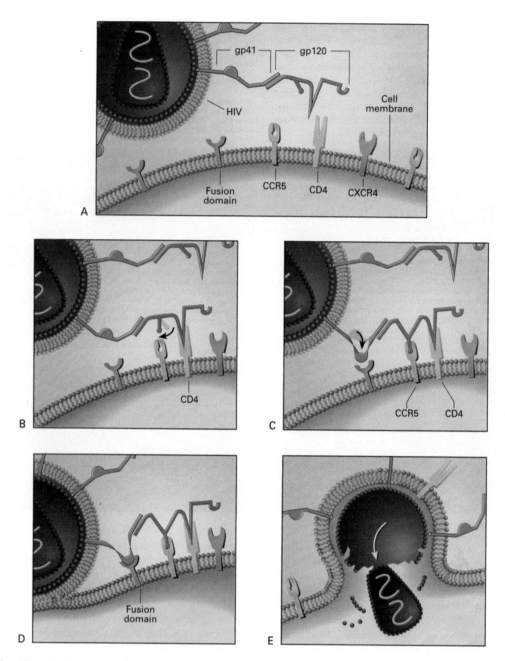

Color Plate 2 Interactions between HIV and the cell surface. (A) HIV interacts with a cell surface receptor, primarily CD4, and through conformational changes becomes more closely associated with the cell through interactions with other cell surface molecules, such as the chemokine receptors CXCR4 and CCR5. Alternatively, some viruses, such as certain strains of HIV-2, could attach to CXCR4 directly. (B to E) The likely steps in HIV infection are as follows. The CD4-binding site on HIV-1 gp120 interacts with the CD4 molecule on the cell surface. Conformational changes in both the viral envelope and the CD4 receptor permit the binding of gp120 to another cell surface receptor, such as CCR5. This attachment brings the viral envelope closer to the cell surface, allowing interaction between gp41 on the viral envelope and a fusion domain on the cell surface. HIV fuses with the cell. Subsequently, the viral nucleoid enters into the cell, most likely by means of other cellular events. Once this stage is achieved, the cycle of viral replication begins. Reprinted from reference 2524 with permission. Copyright © 1996 Massachusetts Medical Society. All rights reserved. (See page 60.)

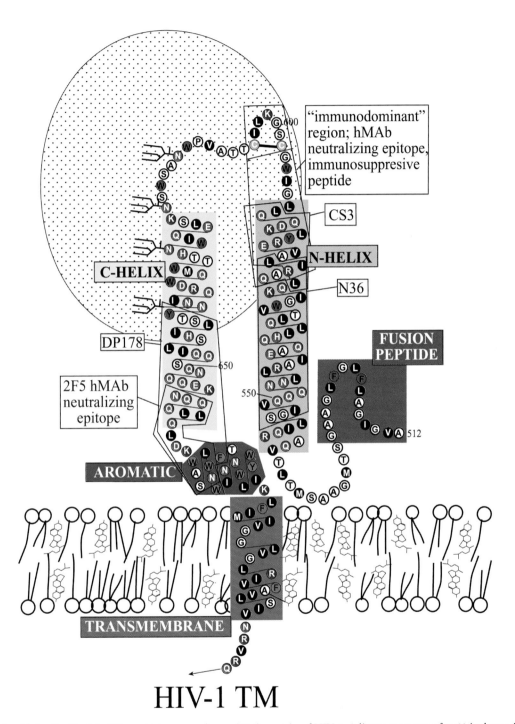

Color Plate 3   Model of the gp41 transmembrane (TM) protein of HIV-1. A linear sequence of gp41 is shown in a planar projection of the proposed structure derived from computer modeling and based on the influenza virus HA2 scaffold. α-Helices are depicted as modified helical nets alternating three and four amino acids per turn connected by single lines. Hydrophobic amino acids are indicated as solid circles, charged amino acids as open circles, and neutral amino acids as partly filled circles. Nonhelical regions are shown as loosely coiled extended chains; strong turns are indicated by a T, the proposed intramolecular disulfide bond by a double line. Specific functional regions are noted. Figure courtesy of R. Garry. Modified from reference 1412 with permission. (See page 66.)

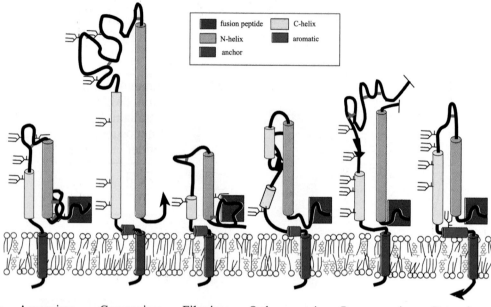

Family:	Arenavirus	Coronavirus	Filovirus	Orthomyxovirus	Paramyxovirus	Retrovirus
Example:	Lassa virus GP2	SARS coronavirus S2	Ebola virus GP2	Influenza virus HA2	Measles virus F1	HIV-1 TM

Color Plate 4   Common structural features of RNA virus fusion proteins. Similar motifs found in representatives of diverse virus families are depicted in "rainbow" order from amino terminus to carboxyl terminus. Each of these class I viral fusion proteins (α-penetrenes) has a fusion peptide (red) at the amino terminus and two extended α-helices (N-helix [orange-] and C-helix [yellow-]), and most have an aromatic rich domain (green) proximal to the transmembrane anchor (indigo). (Based on references 1412 and 1413.) Truncations: HIV gp41 transmembrane (TM) protein C-term; mumps virus F1 after N-helix; sudden acute respiratory syndrome-associated coronavirus (SARS CoV) S N-term. Provided by R. Garry. (See page 66.)

Color Plate 5   Hypothetical mechanism for HIV virion:cell fusion. (A) Binding of HIV-1 SU to the primary receptor (CD4) and coreceptor (chemokine receptor). (B) Rearrangement of the helical domains of TM. The rearrangement allows the putative fusion peptide (red) to interact with the cell plasma membrane. (C) The helical domains of TM "snap back," bringing the viral and cell membrane in closer proximity and resulting in membrane deformation or "nipple" formation (2009a). Alternatively, the rearrangement of the S2 protein into the six-helix bundle conformation does not result in nipple formation, but rather the virion itself is drawn closer to the cell surface. The fusion peptide, aromatic domain, and transmembrane anchor then constitute a contiguous track of sequences (black outline) that can facilitate the flow of lipid between the two membranes. (D) Six-helix bundle formation drives cellular and viral membrane closer together, resulting in spontaneous hemifusion. Peptide mimics (e.g., T20-like peptides) of the paired helices and/or the aromatic domain blocks six-helix formation in this step or as in panel C. (E) Fusion pore permits cytoplasmic entry of the HIV-1 core. SU, surface gp120 protein; TM, transmembrane gp41 protein. Provided by R. Garry. (See page 66.)

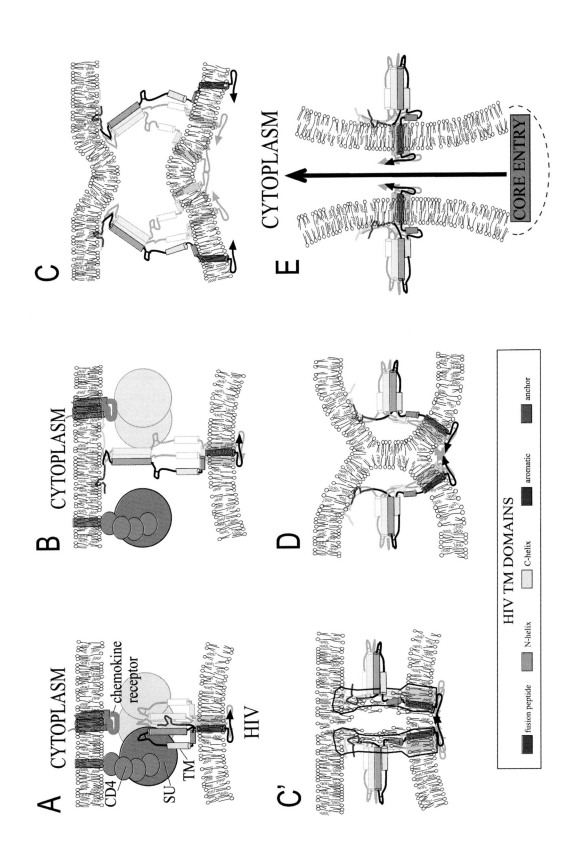

A CYTOPLASM

chemokine receptor

CD4

SU

TM

HIV

B CYTOPLASM

C

C'

D

E CYTOPLASM

CORE ENTRY

HIV TM DOMAINS

fusion peptide

N-helix

C-helix

aromatic

anchor

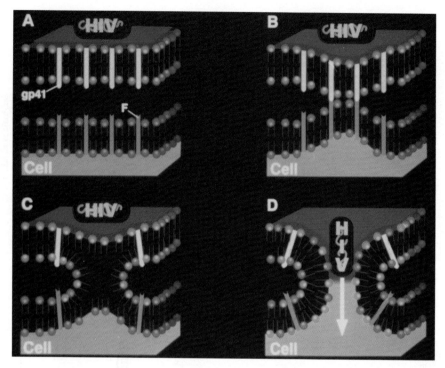

Color Plate 6 HIV:cell fusion. The fusion molecule on the HIV envelope (i.e., gp41) interacts with a fusion receptor (F) on the cell surface (A and B). This process leads to an intermixing of the inner lipid membranes (hemifusion) (C), but unless the outer lipid membranes also undergo intermixing (D), the HIV core cannot enter into the cell cytoplasm. This nucleocapsid entry may also depend on specific viral and cellular factors. Figure derived from a design provided by L. Stamatatos. (See page 68.)

Color Plate 7 An HIV-infected T lymphocyte (HUT 78 cell) shown by immunofluorescence staining fuses with an uninfected HUT 78 T cell. This interaction permits virus transfer to the uninfected cell. Magnification, ×65. Photo courtesy of E. Lennette. (See page 73.)

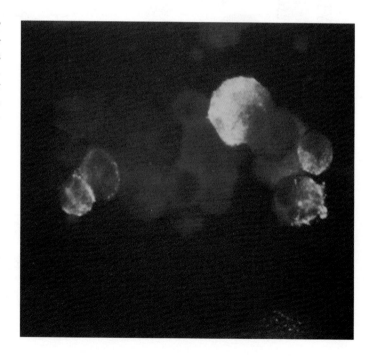

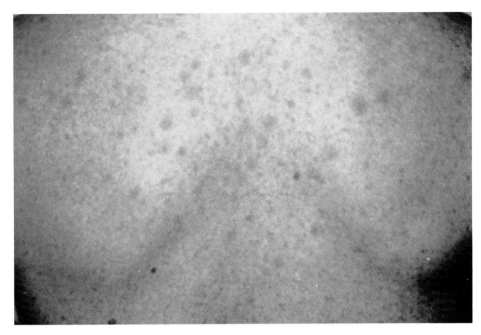

Color Plate 8 Typical macular-papular rash on the surface of the skin occurring within days after acute (primary) HIV infection. Photograph courtesy of R. Hutt and C. Farling. (See page 79.)

Color Plate 9 HIV infection of lymphoid tissue. Using both in situ DNA and RNA PCR procedures, the presence of HIV infection in cells of the lymph node was evaluated (1193). (A) A large number of cells are infected, as demonstrated by in situ DNA PCR procedures. Note the green grains (designating reaction with the HIV probe) over virus-infected cells. (B) In the same lymph node, evaluated by in situ RNA PCR, only two cells replicating virus particles (dark grains indicate viral RNA) can be detected. It has been estimated that 1 in 300 to 1 in 400 infected cells in the lymph node produce virus (4824). Photomicrographs courtesy of A. Haase. (See page 96.)

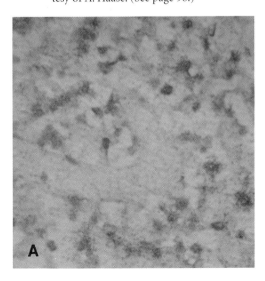

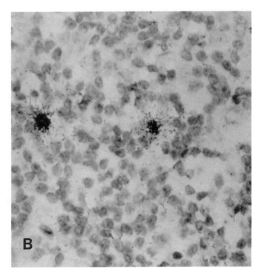

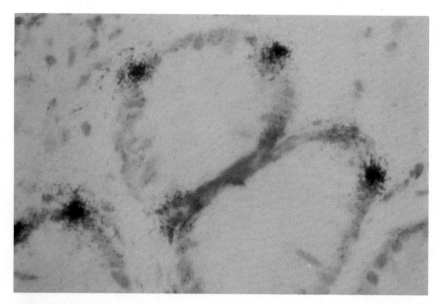

Color Plate 10 Histologic section of a colon biopsy sample from an HIV-infected individual with a gastrointestinal disorder. In situ hybridization shows the presence of HIV-1-infected cells in the bowel epithelium. The presence of grains of radioactivity designates reaction of cells with the viral protein. Photomicrograph courtesy of J. Nelson. (See page 98.)

Color Plate 11 Anti-HIV effect of APOBEC3G. APOBEC3G is encapsidated into the virions in the absence of HIV-encoded Vif protein. Following infection, the encapsidated APOBEC3G induces C⇒U deamination at the minus-strand viral DNA during reverse transcription. The C⇒U is converted into a plus-strand G⇒A mutation during plus-strand synthesis. The uracil-containing viral DNA is mostly degraded by cellular enzymes. Vif prevents the encapsidation of APOBEC3G into virions by directing APOBEC3G towards a ubiquitin-dependent degradation pathway. Figure provided by N. Landau. (See page 117.)

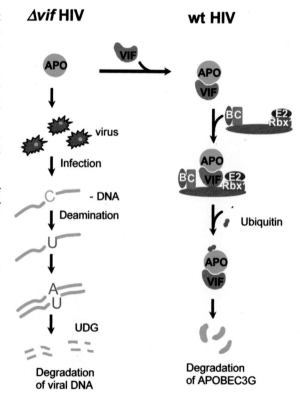

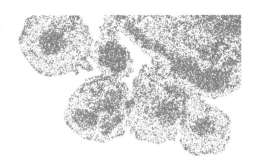

Acute HIV Infection and Cells Susceptible to HIV Infection

Acute HIV Infection

Cells and Tissues Infected by HIV

Differences in Cellular Host Range among HIV Isolates

Superinfection

Recombination

Τ HE IDENTIFICATION OF HIV, its mechanisms of transmission, and the early steps involved in the interaction of HIV with its target cells have been discussed. The selective transmission of HIV is considered in Chapters 2 and 13. This chapter covers the events surrounding acute HIV infection of the host following transmission. It reviews the clinical and laboratory findings in primary infection, the first cells infected, and the large variety of cells in the body that are susceptible to HIV infection.

I. Acute HIV Infection

A. Clinical Manifestations

Clinical manifestations of the initial HIV entry into the body might be expected, since symptoms commonly accompany acute infections by other viruses. Very early in the studies of AIDS, signs of acute HIV infection were described (881, 4434; for reviews, see references 2067, 2117, and 3511 (Table 4.1). Newly infected individuals may present, generally within 1 to 4 weeks, with a virus-like illness called the acute retroviral syndrome (ARS). Symptoms can include headache, retro-orbital pain, muscle aches, sore throat, low-grade or high-grade fever, swollen lymph nodes, and a nonpruritic macular erythematous rash involving the trunk and, later, the extremities (Table 4.1 and Color Plate 8, following page 78) (881, 2067, 2944). Fever, rash, swollen lymph nodes, muscle aches, and joint pains are most frequently seen (946, 1784). In some cases, oral candidiasis, ulcerations in the esophagus, anus, and vagina (3642, 3823), and central nervous system disorders (e.g., encephalitis) can be observed in patients (618, 1855). For some acutely infected individuals, pneumonitis as well as diarrhea and other

Table 4.1 Characteristics of acute HIV infection[a]

Clinical[b]
- Headache, retro-orbital pain
- Muscle aches and joint pains[c]
- Low-grade or high-grade fever[c]
- Swollen lymph nodes[c]
- Nonpruritic macular erythematous rash[c]
- Oral candidiasis
- Ulcerations of the esophagus or anal or vaginal canal
- Acute central nervous system disorders (e.g., encephalitis)
- Pneumonitis
- Diarrhea and other gastrointestinal complaints

Course
- Symptoms usually appear 1–4 weeks after acute infection
- Symptoms last 1–3 weeks
- Lymphadenopathy, lethargy, and malaise can persist for many months
- Generally followed by an asymptomatic period of months to years

Laboratory findings
- First week, lymphopenia and thrombocytopenia
- Second week, lymphocyte number rises secondary to an increase in CD8+ cells; CD4+/CD8+ cell ratio decreases
- Immune activation reflected by increased cytokine levels (e.g., IL-1β, TNF-α, and IFN-γ)
- Second week, atypical lymphocytes appear in the blood (generally <30%)
- HIV antigenemia and viremia detected within 3–10 days
- Virus can be present in CSF and in seminal fluid within 7–14 days
- Anti-HIV antibodies usually first detected within 1–3 weeks after acute infection
- Proinflammatory cytokines increased in blood (e.g., IL-15 and TNF-α)

[a]IL-1β, interleukin-1β; TNF-α, tumor necrosis factor alpha; IFN-γ, gamma interferon; CSF, cerebrospinal fluid.

[b]Some or all of these findings can be present in the acute retroviral syndrome. They usually appear after at least 1–4 weeks at the peak viremia levels before antibodies are detected.

[c]Most frequently seen (946, 1784).

gastrointestinal (GI) complaints have been reported (1118, 2435, 4434). These symptoms usually last from 1 to 3 weeks, although lymphadenopathy, lethargy, and malaise can persist for many months. These clinical features of ARS are similar for dif-ferent routes of transmission (3823) (i.e., sexual and through intravenous drug use) and usually appear before seroconversion (2067). The rash is a particularly valuable diagnostic sign since it can distinguish primary HIV infection from several other types of infections, but it can be difficult to diagnose. The cause of the rash is unknown, but it could reflect antigen:antibody complexes in the skin (2944).

At least 50% and in some series up to 90% of individuals infected by HIV will report a history of this acute mononucleosis-like illness (1346, 2067, 4434). An absence of ARS is generally associated with a delayed progression to disease (1118, 3952), whereas an occurrence and the severity of ARS with persistence of symptoms (particularly fever) are associated with the extent of disease progression (1118, 2147, 4159, 4570, 4594). Lower viral loads and fewer symptoms have been reported for primary infection in Senegalese women, suggesting an association with route of infection or viral subtype (3923). The symptoms may reflect a hyperresponding immune system with production of cytokines that give rise to the clinical signs (see below). This immune activation can enhance HIV spread and increase cell death by apoptosis (see Chapter 6).

In rare cases, a subject has a rapid disease course following acute infection, particularly when X4 viruses predominate (226). In one unusual case, AIDS-associated death occurred within 6 months of infection in which no HIV-specific cytotoxic T lymphocytes (CTLs) could be found (1046). The virus was of the R5 phenotype, and seroconversion took longer than commonly observed. In another, no seroconversion took place (2992). In a recent study, a subject progressed to AIDS within 4 to 20 months after acute infection. The virus proved to be dualtropic (R5/X4) and was resistant to all three major classes of antiretroviral therapies. This virus also did not show the usual reduced replicative capacity of drug-resistant viruses (2817) (see Chapter 14). The presence of a previous virus-like illness can, then, be determined only by taking a complete history. The use of therapy during primary infection is reviewed in Chapter 14. In general, primary HIV-1 infection is followed by an asymptomatic period of many months to years (see Chapter 13).

B. Laboratory Diagnosis of Acute and Primary HIV Infection

Acute HIV infection is defined as the first 1 to 4 weeks after virus transmission *before* antiviral antibodies are detected. At the time, circulating virus can be found in the blood. Primary or early HIV infection refers to the first 3 to 6 months following acute infection after the appearance of anti-HIV antibodies. Detection of plasma virus RNA, before seroconversion, helps diagnose acute infection. The nucleic acid amplification levels that measure viral RNA are more sensitive than p24 antigen tests previously used and are now utilized routinely in screening blood donations (1784, 4307) (see below) (see Chapter 2). In this regard, studies of serial samples collected before seroconversion from some acutely infected individuals have shown, within 2 to 4 days, the presence of low levels of viral RNA (sometimes in small blips) that become clearly evident by 7 to 10 days after the infection (1285, 1286). These individuals are in the very first stages of acute infection, with the early viremia most likely reflecting initial postexposure replication in mucosal or regional lymphoid tissue (see below).

The standard procedure for detection of anti-HIV antibodies is an enzyme-linked immunosorbent assay (ELISA) technique (see also Section I.G). The results are confirmed by supplemental testing, such as immunoblot (615), or by an indirect immunofluorescence assay (2081). The ELISAs have now gone through several generations and in most cases can detect antiviral antibodies within a few days after acute infection. Other serologic approaches to detect HIV infection in individuals without requiring blood samples include the examination of urine and saliva for antiviral antibodies (see below).

In general, the level of anti-HIV antibodies present in sera can help estimate the time of HIV transmission. A less sensitive (LS) ELISA that measures only high-affinity antibodies, which develop later, can approximate the date (see below) (2006, 2920). A negative LS ELISA and positive third- or fourth-generation ELISA can indicate that the infection occurred within 3 months. In addition, new assays for measuring anti-p24 IgG3 activity can give an estimate of infection within 1 to 4 months because of the transient nature of this antibody response (4786). A simple enzyme immunoassay that involves the gp41 immunodominant sequences for HIV-1 subtypes (clades) B, E, and D may provide a highly sensitive detection procedure for HIV-specific IgG antibodies to a variety of subtypes (3426). (For a review on assays for recent infection, see reference 2920.)

Other stages in HIV infection can be determined by the rapid growth phase of plasma viremia and the level of anti-HIV antibodies detected by Western immunoblot, ELISA, and other procedures (566, 715, 1285, 1286). Based on results from low- versus high-sensitivity ELISAs, measurements of p24 antigen, viral RNA levels, and Western blot analyses, a staging of primary HIV infection has been proposed (1286) (Table 4.2). Stage I usually occurs within 5 to 10 days of acute infection and refers to those subjects with detectable viral RNA in the blood only. The p24 antigen test becomes positive about 5 days later (stage II). Shortly after, a highly sensitive antibody ELISA can detect anti-HIV antibodies (stage III) (Table 4.2).

In resource-limited countries or rural communities, certain rapid antibody tests of saliva, urine, or blood (e.g., OraQuick, UniGold, Recombigen HIV, and Detune HIV-1/2) can be helpful for diagnosis and show excellent sensitivity (1317). Saliva testing gave up to 99% sensitivity in a large number of cases evaluated (1418), and urine testing has had similar accuracy (343). However, while encouraging, the sensitivity and specificity of detecting HIV antibodies in oral fluid or urine during early seroconversion has not been fully established, and their detection is likely delayed relative to the that of the initial antibodies found in plasma (3730a). A rapid assay is currently being used with pregnant women. It delivers timely results and provides HIV-positive women with immediate access to intrapartum and neonatal antiretroviral treatment. This approach has helped to reduce perinatal HIV transmission (553a).

Other methods for screening large numbers of individuals without requiring venipuncture have included a needlestick assay, in which blood is added to small cotton blots that are analyzed for antibodies by an enzyme reaction (293). This procedure is also sensitive and can be used for home

Table 4.2 Laboratory stages of primary HIV infection based on the emergence of viral markers[a]

| Stage | Virus | | Antibody EIA | | | Duration in days (95% CI)[b] | |
	RNA	p24 antigen	NS	S	Western blot	Individual	Cumulative
I	+	−	−	−	−	5.0 (3.1, 8.1)	5.0 (3.1, 8.1)
II	+	+	−	−	−	5.3 (3.7, 7.7)	10.3 (7/1, 13.5)
III	+	+	−	+	−	3.2 (2.1, 4.8)	13.5 (10.0, 17.0)
IV	+	+/−	−	+	ID	5.6 (3.8, 8.1)	19.1 (15.3, 22.9)
V	+	+/−	+/−	+	+[c]	69.5 (39.7, 121.7)	88.6 (47.4, 129.8)
VI	+	+/−	+/−	+	+	Open-ended	Open-ended

[a]CI, confidence interval; ID, indeterminate; NS, not sensitive (refers to second-generation not-IgM-sensitive enzyme immunoassay [EIA]); S, sensitive (refers to third-generation IgM-sensitive EIA). Reprinted from reference 1286 with permission.
[b]Calculations are based on a parametric Markov model.
[c]Without p31 band.

testing. Home testing, while controversial, is considered important for informing reluctant individuals of their infection status (2980, 4319) and may soon be approved in the United States. In brief, measurement of antibodies in plasma or serum by the very recent ELISAs is the most sensitive routine method for the detection of anti-HIV antibodies; viral RNA determination is the optimal approach for detecting acute HIV infection.

C. Immunologic Findings

Studies conducted on infected individuals during the first week following HIV infection usually show lymphopenia and thrombocytopenia (Table 4.1). In the second week, the number of lymphocytes increases, resulting primarily from a rise in the level of CD8[+] cells; the number of CD4[+] cells therefore appears to be reduced. Thus, during this period, the CD4[+]/CD8[+] cell ratio becomes inverted. Moreover, atypical lymphocytes (i.e., CD8[+] cells) can be present in the blood (882, 2538) but at a smaller number in primary HIV infection than with Epstein-Barr virus (EBV), cytomegalovirus, or other infections that elicit this response (2067). Within months following primary infection, the quantity of CD8[+] cells returns to a baseline or slightly higher level. This amount remains greater than that of CD4[+] cells, which increases somewhat; therefore, the inverted CD4[+]/CD8[+] cell ratio is maintained (4432). The targeting of specific CD4[+] cell subsets by HIV-1 is discussed in Section II.

During acute HIV infection, a large and preferential depletion of mucosal CD4[+] T cells compared with peripheral blood CD4[+] cells has been observed in studies of the GI tract (2957) (Section II.G). CD4 T-cell loss is predominantly in the short-lived effector T-cell compartment (i.e., lamina propria) of the GI mucosa and not in the inductive compartment (e.g., in Peyer's patches). This loss appears to be specific targeting of memory CD4[+] cells in the bowel by R5 viruses (2957, 2971, 2972) (see Chapter 8).

During the acute period of infection, levels of certain cytokines associated with immune activation, such as interleukin-1β (IL-1β), soluble CD8, tumor necrosis factor alpha (TNF-α), TNF receptors, and gamma interferon (IFN-γ), are increased in the plasma (368, 3279, 3739, 4159). Measurement of type 1 and type 2 cytokines during acute infection has also indicated that peripheral blood mononuclear cells (PBMC) express very low levels of both IL-2 and IL-4, although substantial levels of IL-2 can be noted in lymph node cells (1608). Production of IL-10 and TNF-α was consistently observed in all subjects studied, and the levels either were stable or increased over time (1608). Likewise, IFN-γ expression was found in all seroconverters, and the levels peaked early in primary infection along with the increase in CD8[+] cell numbers, probably induced by these cytokines (1608). The results indicate that high levels of proinflammatory cytokines are expressed with primary infection. This response, depending on the cytokine profile, could influence the CD8[+] cell expansion and the extent of ARS symptoms reflecting immune activation (see Chapters 6, 11, and 13).

Following acute infection, certain laboratory immune markers have been found to be associated

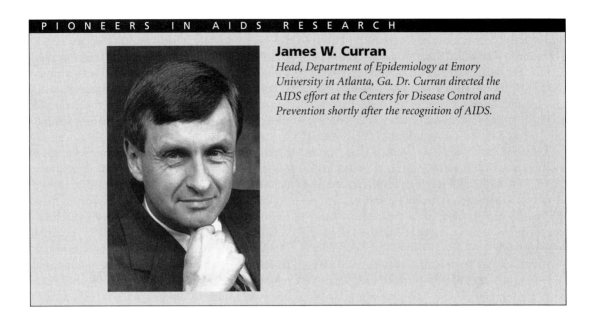

James W. Curran

Head, Department of Epidemiology at Emory University in Atlanta, Ga. Dr. Curran directed the AIDS effort at the Centers for Disease Control and Prevention shortly after the recognition of AIDS.

with rapid progression to AIDS (3958). These include persistent low CD4+ cell counts, high immunoglobulin levels, activation markers on lymphocyte subsets, and high CD8+ cell numbers (see Chapter 13).

D. Levels and Characteristics of the Transmitted Virus

During acute HIV infection, the individual becomes antigenemic and viremic, with very high levels of virus (10^6 to 10^7 RNA copies/ml) present in plasma (Table 2.3). Large quantities of infectious HIV can be detected in the peripheral blood after 7 to 14 days (568, 790, 947, 1408, 3266, 3502, 4634), with a peak of viremia observed by 21 days (2625a) (see Chapter 2, Table 2.2). Several billion viruses are produced daily by mostly activated CD4+ T cells (4931); over 10 million to 100 million infected CD4+ cells die daily (646). The viremia has a doubling time of approximately 0.3 day during the first 2 to 3 weeks of infection (1286, 2625a, 3511). Levels of baseline HIV RNA of more than 5 logs have predicted a greater risk for disease progression (2471). The time to reach a steady state of viral load (<0.5 $\log_{10}$ change), called the viral set point, ranges from 3 to 5 months (2123).

About 7% of seroconverters in one study achieved undetectable viremia following primary infection (866). Some of these infected individuals have been followed for up to 5 years and remained virus RNA negative (2754). This group of subjects most likely represents "elite controllers" (see Chapter 13). In studies of Kenyan adults, no gender difference in viral loads following acute infection was noted (3725). However, variations in viral loads in primary infection, depending on the viral clades, have been suggested (3923).

In pediatric studies, HIV RNA has been found in plasma in the first 10 days of life in about 25% of infected newborn infants. After 3 months, all of them showed evidence of infection (1037). The early plasma virus is relatively homogeneous in sequence (2104, 2341), probably indicating replication of a dominant virus strain. Some studies show that viral loads are higher in infants infected in utero or perinatally than in those acquiring the virus via breast milk (3724). The influence of a maturing immune system after birth is evident. Assays for proviral DNA in PBMC have also proved useful for early diagnosis of infection in newborns with passive maternal antibodies, although no commercial HIV DNA assays are currently available (see Chapter 2).

In acute infection, both R5 and syncytium-inducing (SI) X4 strains can be isolated initially, but R5 viruses dominate (see below and Chapter 13). In many cases, a variety of virus variants or quasispecies have been detected. When HIV-1 quasispecies diversity was studied with plasma donors who were very recently infected and thus antibody seronegative, R5 viruses were observed in 14 of the 17 infections (1042). Evidence for transmission of multiple variants was rarely obtained (1042). In some cases of seroconversion, however, infection by more than one isolate of HIV-1 has been documented (4959). Studies of blood samples within 1 to 5 months after infection showed that several women from Kenya were infected with multiple virus variants, in contrast to men (2659, 3870). How this finding reflected on HIV transmission or host immune response was not determined. Moreover, studies of some subjects 4 to 9 weeks after ARS have suggested initial infection with multiple virus quasispecies or perhaps superinfection (see Section IV) (2448).

During the early period, when there is an absence of immune response, the transmitted virus can replicate and spread, with isolates selected having increased growth potential (870, 1276). As noted above, in most studies, but not all, R5 viruses predominate in the acutely infected individuals. This observation led some researchers to conclude that in adults, R5 strains are the most transmissible (4957), perhaps via macrophages in the genital fluid (see below). Moreover, macrophages or dendritic cells (DCs) in the vagina, endocervix (4237), uterus, bowel mucosa, or penile urethra could be productively infected most readily by R5 strains (1596) (Sections I.E and II.B) (see also Chapters 2 and 13). Nevertheless, in other studies of transmission by sexual contact (homosexual and heterosexual), about one-third of the subjects had X4 viruses after acute infection (1294). Several other reports have shown that seroconverters can harbor X4 viruses (790, 1578, 3257, 3792, 3945). The possible reasons for a high prevalence of R5 viruses in primary infection are discussed in Chapter 13.

Quantitative heteroduplex tracking assays (Figure 1.8) on transmission pairs have supported the existence of various genomic complexities during acute infection. In chronically infected transmitters, HIV variants were detected in genital secretions that differed from those in the blood; the sequences of cell-associated virus also differed from those of free virus in the plasma (4958). These findings further indicate the heterogeneity of viruses found in asymptomatic subjects as well as support

the conclusions on the compartmentalization of the virus in different body sites (see Chapter 2). In contrast to the transmitters, the seroconverters showed relatively homogeneous virus populations, suggesting transmission of a limited number of variants. Furthermore, the virus present in the recent seroconverters represented only a minor species found in the semen of the transmitting partner. These results provide further evidence of selective transmission and virus growth after sexual contact (see Chapters 2 and 13).

Virus has been isolated as well from the cerebrospinal fluid (1855) and semen (4435) of individuals during the acute phase of HIV infection (Table 4.1). In many cases, the virus was very similar to that in the blood, indicating rapid dissemination (3735). These sources of the virus later, however, appear to reflect a separate evolution of HIV in cells of the brain (see Chapter 2). The finding of high levels of virus in semen during acute infection indicates the risk of transmission of the virus through sexual contact during this early period (836). Moreover, drug-resistant and CTL escape mutants can be transmitted (1588, 1785) (see below) and present challenges for therapy (see Chapter 14). Selective transmission of HIV isolates is considered in Chapter 2.

E. Initial Host Immune Responses in Acute Infection: Cellular Immunity

As noted in Chapter 2, within weeks after primary infection, the viremia usually is reduced, reflecting the strength of the host anti-HIV response. Cell immunity seems most important (Figure 4.1). Neutralizing antibodies do not appear to be involved (2067, 2749, 3729). Several studies of human and animal lentiviruses have shown that efficient control of virus replication soon after primary infection is the best predictor of a long-term asymptomatic course (2147, 2968, 3693) (see Chapter 13).

In terms of DC function, both myeloid dendritic cells (MDCs) and plasmacytoid dendritic cells (PDCs) are reduced in primary infection (26 to 57 days after transmission) (2187, 3375). This observation most likely reflects an active antiviral cellular innate immune response in the host (see Chapter 9). In early studies of T-cell proliferative responses, HIV peptide-specific T helper (TH) cells

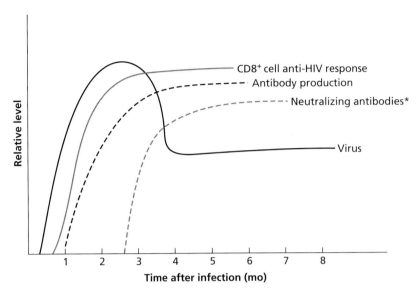

Figure 4.1 Estimated time course for host immune response to acute HIV infection. *, neutralizing antibodies are often directed at earlier virus and not the virus present in the blood at that time in the individual. CD8+ cell anti-HIV responses are both cytotoxic and noncytotoxic.

have been detected shortly after acute infection, before seroconversion takes place, and can be helpful in controlling infection (815, 3181, 3802) (see Chapter 11). Subjects who reach low viral set points without therapy have the strongest HIV-specific CD4+ T-cell responses (1534). These CD4+ cell responses are induced often against the Gag sequence and less frequently to Env-specific sequences (2778) (see Chapter 11).

In a study of T-cell responses in 39 untreated subjects with acute HIV infection, lymphoproliferative responses to mitogen, recall antigens, and HIV antigens were found to be impaired within the first 3 months (3181). After 69 months, responses to phytohemagglutinin (PHA) and recall antigens improved. Most HIV-specific CD4+ cell lymphoproliferation remained undetected throughout the infection. A number of additional studies subsequently confirmed the rapid loss of HIV-1-specific CD4+ T-cell lymphoproliferation following acute HIV-1 infection, and that early initiation of HAART can preserve this response (2587, 3801, 3802, 4888) (see Chapter 11). Those unusual individuals with persisting HIV-specific responses had lower plasma HIV RNA levels. The studies suggested that untreated individuals rarely recover

HIV-specific CD4+ T helper responses and perhaps should receive early therapeutic intervention. However, these results need further confirmation (see Chapter 14).

CD8+ CTLs have been detected by several groups during acute HIV infection (usually prior to seroconversion) (85, 446, 602, 2302, 4784) and SIV infection (4865). The response appears to help control virus replication. CD8+ cell anti-HIV noncytotoxic activity has been associated as well with a decrease in viremia in acutely infected individuals before seroconversion (2749) (see Chapter 11) (Figure 4.1). In comparison to other acute infections (e.g., EBV), the extent of the CTL response can be low (962). The function of these HIV-1-specific CD8+ T cells appears to be impaired early in HIV-1 infection (2587), and this lack of maintaining effective anti-HIV CTL activity may explain the inability to reduce viral loads dramatically and persistently (602). The initial CTL response usually is restricted to a limited number of viral epitopes in comparison to the broad CTL recognition in chronic infection (for a review, see reference 2589). Regions within Nef are preferentially recognized (79, 2588).

In general, untreated subjects with primary infection also have a broader HIV CTL response than those placed immediately on HAART (81). This anti-HIV reactivity in untreated subjects persists but can gradually decline. Moreover, several observations suggest that HIV-1 variants that escape CTL activity may be selected during acute infection (68, 2049, 3603) (see Chapter 11). Thus, cellular immunity must be a primary mechanism for control of HIV replication soon after infection.

The importance of the CTL response in affecting the viremia is suggested by specific HLA alleles that are associated with slow disease progression (1436, 2112, 2777) (see Chapter 13). In one study, antiviral CTL activity, after seroconversion, was noted only in those individuals who showed clinical symptoms of primary infection (2390). Importantly, the levels of viremia were reduced with both an oligoclonal and a polyclonal T-cell response, but the long-term follow-up suggested that the polyclonal response predicted a better clinical course (3408). The expansion in the number of CD8$^+$ T cells that occurs has shown T-cell receptor Vβ gene patterns that could predict the eventual clinical course (1698, 3409). A limited diversity of the T cells containing Vβ genes carries a poor prognosis (3408) (see Chapter 11). In some studies, the T-cell repertoire of CD8$^+$ cells has suggested a reduction in the initial responding cells (3417, 3965). The speed of the immune response and its pattern early in infection are valuable surrogate markers for a long-term asymptomatic infection (1600, 3408).

F. Production of Antiviral Antibodies

In most cases, ARS occurs before seroconversion (2067), suggesting that the symptoms come from cell-mediated immune responses and the secretion of proinflammatory cytokines (Section I.C). As noted above, antibodies to HIV generally appear in 1 to 2 weeks (1286, 1815), but seroconversion can sometimes be detected within a few days after infection (4434, 4436) (Figure 4.1 and Table 4.2). In a few cases, seroconversion has occurred after several weeks (see below). In some early studies, antiviral antibodies were first found in some subjects as soon as 6 days after infection by measuring the IgM response (881). Others have

also used IgM measurements to determine HIV infection (1409).

Current sensitive ELISAs can detect anti-HIV antibodies within 2 weeks for most infected people. In one study, serum anti-gp120 antibodies were first detected in HIV-infected subjects 4 to 23 days after ARS, when the viremia had declined to the viral set point (3094). Antibodies to the V3 loop were detected about the same time as or somewhat later than those directed at the CD4 binding site. Neutralizing antibodies appeared independently of levels of these antienvelope antibodies (3084). Generally, neutralizing antibodies appear some weeks after the anti-HIV antibodies are found (Figure 4.1) (2302, 2749, 3725, 3729), but in one well-documented case, they were present within 20 days after virus transmission (2420). As noted above, neutralizing antibodies may be responsible for the emergence of R5 viruses following the initial X4 replication (see 899, 2420). They can also select for escape mutants (3729) (see Chapter 10). In some well-documented studies, neutralizing antibodies against autologous contemporaneous strains were not noted following initial seroconversion. When identified, the neutralization response was usually evident against viruses present during an earlier phase of HIV infection (3076, 3729). This finding has been commonly observed (see Chapter 10).

Whether an infected individual can be antibody negative for longer than 3 months is still controversial. Before the development of the current sensitive ELISA kits, the "window" period before seroconversion had been estimated to be about 2 months, but some rare infections could take 6 to 12 months to show anti-HIV antibodies (568, 1892). In one case report of infection by needlestick injury, antibodies did not appear until after 8 months (2990). This long delay is rare and could reflect the delivery of a low virus inoculum by the percutaneous route and/or restricted virus replication. In other unusual cases, the patients developed AIDS without the presence of detectable antibody. The reason is not known (613, 2992, 3694). Moreover, in two individuals, virus was detected and cultured from the PBMC, but these individuals became seronegative along with loss of detectable virus in their blood (3874). Whether these cases reflect transient or an occult HIV infection is not known.

G. Summary

After HIV transmission, HIV RNA can be detected readily in 7 to 10 days and as low blips in 2 to 4 days (1285, 1286); however, there are false-positive rates as high as 1% with the latter highly sensitive tests (3511). In general, ARS is observed after about 1 to 4 weeks (usually before seroconversion) and can last days to weeks. Its occurrence can predict a more rapid clinical course. Seroconversion takes place 1 to 3 weeks after the initial HIV infection, and the virologic set point is reached usually after 3 to 5 months. In blood banks, donations are first screened simultaneously for the presence of anti-HIV antibody and viral RNA (usually in plasma pools). This monitoring of donors has dramatically reduced the risk of infection from transfusions and plasma derivatives (1 in 3 to 4 million units) (565, 905, 4307) (see Chapter 2).

In infants infected by mother-child transmission, the peak and set point viral loads are substantially higher than in adults (3724). Moreover, infants infected during the first 2 months of life have higher set points of HIV RNA levels than those infected after 2 months of age (e.g., breast milk transmission) (3724).

Many investigators believe that events occurring at the time of acute infection or shortly thereafter can determine the clinical course. For example, if the host can mount a strong cellular immune response against HIV, the infection can be maintained locally and perhaps even eliminated (see Chapters 8, 9, and 11). Antibodies are produced too late to play a major role in preventing the spread of virus. Preexisting inflammation may help in the transmission of virus. Therefore, studies are under way examining whether immediate use of HAART would protect cellular immune responses (e.g., CD4+ cell proliferative response) and permit the host to control the infection. In particular, CD4+ T memory cells in the GI tract would be preserved (see below and Chapters 8, 13, and 14).

Other important issues are how many different viruses are transmitted during acute infection and whether a large number of selected biologic subtypes can influence the clinical course. Furthermore, what correlates of immunity can help limit virus replication, essentially establishing the immunologic set point, are important questions in acute infection that are under study (http://www.aiedrp.org/).

II. Cells and Tissues Infected by HIV

A. Overview

The first cells to be infected by HIV may be present in the mucosa, in the blood, or in lymphoid tissue, depending on the route of transmission. After acute infection, the cellular host range of HIV can be extensive (Table 4.3). The cell types susceptible to HIV infection have been determined by techniques in cell culture, in situ hybridization, immunohistochemistry, electron microscopy, and PCR procedures using extracted tissues and individual cells (e.g., in situ PCR hybridization) (210, 211, 1193, 1194, 3294) (see below). These studies have shown that the extent of infection varies and can depend on the cell surface receptors expressed and the particular virus strain used. In general, CD4+ cells replicate HIV to the highest titers. Nevertheless, many CD4− cells can be infected (Tables 4.3 and 3.8). The in vitro studies indicate that successful virus infection is determined both by the efficiency of viral entry into the cell, reflecting cell surface interaction (e.g., receptor), and by postentry processes influenced by the intracellular milieu (see Chapters 3 and 5). Clinically, direct infection of the brain and bowel could be responsible for some of the signs and symptoms observed in individuals acutely infected with HIV.

B. Initial Cells Infected by HIV

Langerhans cells (LCs) and DCs in the blood, skin, and mucosae express CD4, CCR5, and CXCR4 and are susceptible to HIV infection (182, 405, 1096, 1596, 4908) (see Chapter 9). Because of their location in genital tracts, these cells have been considered the initial targets for HIV infection, particularly by R5 viruses. Their maturation can lead to a decrease in CCR5 expression, up-regulation of CXCR4, and infection by both virus biotypes (4908). Maturation of DCs also gives rise to a 10- to 100-fold-lower production of virus than observed in infected immature DCs (224, 598, 1596).

In the early stages of acute HIV infection following intravenous infection, the first cells infected

Table 4.3 Human cells susceptible to HIV infection[a]

Hematopoietic	Bowel
T lymphocytes	Columnar and goblet cells
B lymphocytes	Enterochromaffin cells
Macrophages	Colon carcinoma cells
NK cells	
Megakaryocytes	**Other**
Dendritic cells	Myocardium
Promyelocytes	Renal tubular cells
Stem cells	Synovial membrane
Thymic epithelium	Hepatic sinusoid endo-
Follicular dendritic cells	thelium
Bone marrow endothelial cells	Hepatic carcinoma cells
	Kupffer cells
Brain	Dental pulp fibroblasts
Capillary endothelial cells	Pulmonary fibroblasts
Astrocytes	Fetal adrenal cells
Macrophages (microglia)	Adrenal carcinoma cells
Oligodendrocytes	Retina
Choroid plexus	Cervix-derived epithelial cells
Ganglion cells	Prostate
Neuroblastoma cells	Testes
Glioma cell lines	Urethra
Neurons (?)	Osteosarcoma cells
	Rhabdomyosarcoma cells
Skin	Fetal chorionic villi
Langerhans cells	Trophoblasts
Fibroblasts	

[a]Susceptibility to HIV determined by in vitro or in vivo studies. See text for details and references.

would, most likely, be the CD4[+] T cells in both blood and lymph nodes (3948). Follicular dendritic cells (FDCs) in lymphoid tissue would subsequently be a source of abundant HIV particles (see below). HIV transmission by the mucosal route (vaginal and anal canals) seems to involve LCs and related DCs in the vaginal and rectal mucosae as well as CD4[+] T lymphocytes. Infection by the oral route, though rare, would most likely lead to infection first of the tonsil and adenoid glands (1357).

After intravaginal inoculation of high-dose SIV into rhesus macaques, viral DNA and RNA can be detected within 24 to 72 h in DCs, intraepithelial lymphocytes, and resting and activated CD4[+] T cells in the endocervical submucosa (1913, 3013, 3575, 4938) and then within 2 days in draining lymph nodes; in 5 to 7 days viremia occurs (3013, 4237, 4938) (Table 4.4). The results reflect the find-ing that a single layer of columnar epithelium in the endocervical surface is more easily infected and, with inflammation or ectopy, would be particularly susceptible to HIV infection (see Chapter 2).

Most recently, a high dose of SIV inoculated intravaginally gave rise to a small founder population of infected cells in the cervicovaginal canal. These susceptible cells appeared to be CD4[+] T cells, DCs, and macrophages. The small size of the infected cell population most likely reflects the low number of lymphocytes in the cervical canal, host innate immune defenses, or virus entrapment in cervical mucus (3013).

In experimental SIV infection of macaques via the rectum, the virus was found initially in lymph nodes draining the GI tract, and then later it spread through the host (908). Moreover, studies with SIV in monkeys have indicated that less than

Table 4.4 Timing of virus spread after intravaginal SIV inoculation

Tissue	Day 1	Day 3	Day 7	Day 13
Vagina	−	−	−	+++
Cervix	−	+	++	+++
Draining lymph node	−	−	−	+++
Distal lymph node	−	−	−	+++
Bone marrow	−	−	−	++

[a]Reprinted with permission from reference 4938. Copyright 1999 AAAS.

16 h after intradermal inoculation, newly infected cells can be found in the injection site of the skin and in the draining lymph node (4678). In general, the extent of virus replication and spread in the infected individual will depend on the local environment and the response of both the innate (e.g., interferons) and adaptive (cellular immunity) immune systems (see Chapters 9 to 11).

Similar observations on the short period of HIV transfer to other sites after initial infections via a mucosal site have been reported (3575). Virus can traverse the epithelial layer by transcytosis, epithelial cell capture, passage through lesions at the mucosal site, or direct infection (see below). The DCs in the region of HIV transmission can then transfer virus to other target cells (e.g., CD4+ lymphocytes) as well as transit to draining lymph nodes and other tissues (1848, 1913, 2067) (see Chapter 2).

HIV can infect or bind to C-type lectins on mucosal DCs and macrophages and pass through the mucosae and infect nearby CD4+ cells (934) (see Chapter 9). Low-level X4 virus replication within immature DCs has been documented, and this covert replication can increase the potential for transfer of this virus biotype (3268). Moreover, intestinal mucosal epithelial cells via DC-SIGN or CCR5 expression can selectively transfer R5 HIV-1 to CCR5-expressing CD4+ cells (1675, 2972). Within 2 days of infection, HIV-infected CD4+ cells can be found in nearby lymphoid tissue (3949). Finally, the infection of CD4+ cells can be facilitated through the formation of DC:T-cell conjugates (2914, 3574) (see Chapter 2).

As noted in Chapter 2 (Section V.B.3), when the mucosa is exposed to HIV, virus can be transmitted not only by DCs and M cells (94) but also by transcytosis. Transcytosis is a process by which proteins are transferred rapidly from the apical to the basolateral layer of an epithelial cell (432). By this mechanism virus can pass through a stratified squamous epithelium to get to underlying susceptible tissues. This intracellular transit can be blocked by immune complexes (296, 432) (see Chapter 10).

C. Hematopoietic Cells

For discussion of the infection of DCs, and other innate immune cells, see Chapter 9. Infection of lymphocytes, macrophages, and bone marrow is reviewed in this section.

1. CD4+ LYMPHOCYTES

Studies conducted soon after the initial recovery of HIV demonstrated that CD4+ T lymphocytes were the major target of HIV infection (2224). In lymphatic tissues, up to 100 million infected resting memory (HLA-DR− CD45RO+) CD4+ T cells can be found (4938) and about 5 billion to 50 billion virions are in immune complexes bound to FDCs (1193, 3410, 3414, 3575, 4941) (see below). Moreover, the large number of infected resting memory CD4+ T cells in lymphoid areas of the bowel must be considered (see Chapters 8 and 11).

In examining the relative sensitivity of activated CD4+ cells to HIV infection, great variability was observed unrelated to chemokine production (1609). When formed, CD4+ cells are predominantly resting naïve (HLA-DR− CD38− CD45RA+) cells that have not responded to antigen. They can become activated as effector and memory CD4+ cells (HLA-DR+ CD38hi CD45RO+) during acute infection. Certain activated memory CD4+ cells can return to a resting or central memory state (HLA-DR−; CD69−; CD45RO+) (see Chapter 11, Section II.C). Both activated and resting memory (CD45RO+) CD4+ cells are susceptible to HIV infection in vivo (see below). Although the thymus does not appear to be a major site of HIV infection (see Section II.E), the HIV provirus can be detected in naïve CD4+ CD45RA+ CD62+ T cells (3355). The reason could be the cytokine environment in the thymus. Cytokines such as IL-4, IL-6, IL-7, and IL-15 can render resting naïve CD4+ T cells susceptible to HIV infection (4527a). IL-2 treatment does not substantially change the susceptibility of the naïve (CD45RA+) cells to productive HIV infection, but IL-7 pretreatment has increased productive infection up to 58-fold (4272). IL-7 up-regulates surface expression of CXCR4 but not CCR5 and enhances the proliferation of naïve T cells.

In vivo, the activated CD4+ cells produce the largest amounts of infectious viruses, but the viral load also reflects the limited HIV replication in resting memory CD4+ cells (647, 1438, 4235, 4815). Infected activated CD4+ T cells can produce up to 5 times more virions than infected resting memory cells (4940). Importantly, >90% of the productively infected cells in acute infection are resting memory CD4+ T cells, and the turnover rate of these cells can be as long as 14 days (646, 4938); the half-life of an infected activated CD4+ cell is about a day (3471). Therefore, virus production over a longer period of time by resting

memory CD4+ cells would contribute most to the plasma viral load (for a review, see reference 3691a). The HIV-specific memory CD4+ T cells also contain more HIV DNA than other memory CD4+ T cells at all stages of HIV disease. These observations reflect their apparent enhanced sensitivity to infection and destruction (1120). The activated terminally differentiated CD4+ T cells that have poor proliferative properties have 10-fold-fewer copies of HIV DNA (491) (see Chapter 11). Some of the infected cells have latent integrated provirus; others have virus in a preintegration step (4141). Those cells with integrated HIV make up part of the long-lived reservoir and can live for up to 4 years (for review, see reference 4141) (see also Chapter 5).

In terms of chemokine receptor expression, the naïve (CD45RA+) CD4+ T lymphocytes as well as memory CD4+ cells have CXCR4, whereas CCR5 appears to be present predominantly on a subset of both activated and resting memory CD45RO+ T cells (410, 2458, 3898) (see Chapters 3 and 11) (Table 4.5). Therefore, CCR5 is normally expressed on far fewer T cells than CXCR4. These findings suggest that the R5 viruses can only infect the CCR5-expressing T cells, whereas the X4

Table 4.5 Chemokine receptor levels on CD4+ cells[a]

CD4+ cell subset	Chemokine receptor(s)[b]
Naïve (CD45RA+ CD62L+)	CXCR4, CCR7
Memory (CD45RO+ CD62L+)	CXCR3, CXCR5 CCR4, CCR5, CCR6, CCR7
Activated memory (CD45RO+ CD62L−)	CXCR3, CXCR6 CCR2, CCR3, CCRT, CCR5, CCR6 CX3CR1
TH1	CXCR3, CXCR6, CCR2, CCR5
TH2	CCR2, CCR3, CCR4, CCR5, CCR8
Skin-homing T cells	CCR4, CCR6, CCR8, CCR10
Gut-homing T cells	CCR9
Follicular helper T cells	CXCR5
Immature DC	High CCR5, CCR1, CCR2, and CCR6 and low CXCR4
Mature DC[c]	High CCR5 and CXCR4, CCR4, and CCR7

[a]Data from references 410, 438, 789, 2458, 3121, 3896, and 3898. Table prepared with assistance from K. Song and M. Roederer. See also Tables 11.3 and 11.4.
[b]Nearly all CD4+ cells express CXCR4.
[c]Maturation of peripheral blood dendritic cells (DCs) can give 3- and 40-fold increases in CCR5 and CXCR4 expression, respectively (2458).

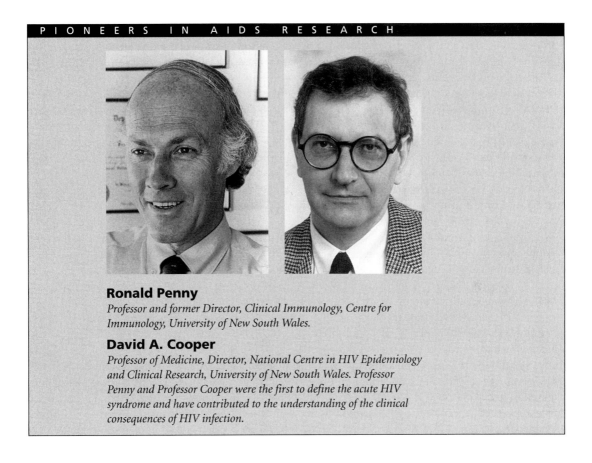

Ronald Penny
Professor and former Director, Clinical Immunology, Centre for Immunology, University of New South Wales.

David A. Cooper
Professor of Medicine, Director, National Centre in HIV Epidemiology and Clinical Research, University of New South Wales. Professor Penny and Professor Cooper were the first to define the acute HIV syndrome and have contributed to the understanding of the clinical consequences of HIV infection.

viruses can infect all CD4+ T cells, including naïve (CXCR4+) cells (2363). While not conclusive, this finding could be a cause of increased CD4+ cell loss after the emergence of X4 virus in the host.

Resting memory CD4+ cells (see Chapter 11) appear to be infected initially and predominantly by R5 viruses (491, 773, 3778, 3991, 4235, 4815). LFA-1 expression on these cells may help determine this preferential infection by HIV-1 (4388) (see Chapter 3). This finding could help explain the predominance of R5 virus in early infection (see Chapter 13). In addition, an increased ability of R5 viruses to replicate in permissive CD4+ CCR5+ CXCR4+ T cells could be responsible for the presence of the R5 biotype in acute or primary infection. Five to ten times more infectious R5 virus production per CCR5+ target cell has also been reported in comparison to levels of X4 HIV-1 isolates (3829, 4018). However, others have not observed an R5 versus X4 difference in replication using biologic virus clones (145). Possibly, the higher level of R5 virus replication reported reflects virus production that is less cytopathic (see Chapters 3 and 13).

CD4+ cells varying in cytokine expression (TH1 versus TH2) may also differ in coreceptor expression and sensitivity to HIV-1 infection (Table 4.5) (see Chapter 11 for discussion of TH cell subsets). CXCR3 and CCR5 are preferentially expressed on human TH1 cells. TH2 CD4+ cells express CXCR4, CCR3, and CCR5 (438, 3898). The two TH types have similar levels of expression of CXCR4; however, CCR5 expression has been found to be eightfold higher in TH1 cells than in TH2 cells (2652, 3898). HIV replication has also been reported to be fourfold higher in the TH1 than in the TH2 subset (3079). However, in other studies, TH2 cells replicated both R5 and X4 viruses at higher levels than TH1 cells (798, 3079, 4641). In some reports, R5 isolates appeared to infect all types of CD4+ lymphocytes, whereas X4 HIV isolates grew primarily in TH2-type cells (4377). This finding is surprising since, as noted above, all circulating naïve T cells express CXCR4 but only the activated memory T cells express CCR5 (332, 410) (see Chapter 3). In still other studies, both cell types were similarly susceptible to HIV infection but TH1 cells showed somewhat higher levels of virus replication (3007).

When unstimulated cord PBMC or CD4+ cell clones were used, some investigators have found that R5 isolates rather than X4 viruses replicate preferentially; with adult PBMC, opposite observations were made (3695, 4598). In contrast, X4 isolates have been shown to have a more consistent ability to infect primary CD4+ cell clones than have R5 isolates (1339). Some studies suggest that HIV-1 replicates threefold better in cord blood T lymphocytes than in adult blood lymphocytes and ninefold better in monocyte-derived macrophages (MDM) from cord blood than in adult MDM (4341a). The effect appears to be related to an increase in HIV-1 LTR-driven transcription.

Some CD4+ cell differences in susceptibility to infection, noted particularly in early studies, most likely reflect the virus used. The ability of certain cytokines to modulate the expression of these chemokine receptors (e.g., IL-2 and IL-7) (Table 4.5) can also influence CD4+ cell susceptibility to HIV infection (3898, 4272). Some of the findings could also reflect the ability of R5 virus infection to activate CD4+ T cells and increase their sensitivity to virus replication (1610, 2650, 3578, 4723). The process may involve signaling pathways via the CCR5 chemokine coreceptor (4598, 4723; for a review, see reference 3577). A relative effect on nuclear import of the preintegration complex could be responsible (3578). For example, the nuclear import of the R5 proviral DNA does not depend on CD3/CD28 activation of CD4+ T cells (3578) (see Chapter 13). These results could help explain the dominance of R5 isolates early in infection and the loss of TH1-type cells as a person advances to disease in the absence of a phenotypic virus switch (see Chapter 13).

Variations in virus production in PBMC (in which the major target cell is the CD4+ lymphocyte) from different individuals have also been reported. An HIV-1 or HIV-2 strain might grow to high titers in these cells from only certain individuals (Figure 4.2) (638, 821, 1230). In some cases, up to 1,000-fold differences in virus replication can be demonstrated (821). No HIV strain has been found

that grows well in PBMC from all individuals; likewise, PBMC from one individual have not shown equal susceptibilities to infection by all HIV isolates. In certain rare cases, as noted above, the PBMC (both CD4+ lymphocytes and macrophages) are resistant to infection by R5 viruses, since the cells lack the required CCR5 coreceptor (see Chapter 3) (871, 2635, 3661). Thus, it is conceivable that one virus infecting two individuals could induce different pathogenic pathways, depending on its ability to grow and spread in the peripheral lymphocytes of each person.

In summary, the susceptibility of CD4+ T cells to virus replication appears to be determined by the virus; by the genetic makeup of the host cell, which influences its cell surface molecules; and by intracellular factors (Table 4.6). A particular CD4+ cell subset does not appear to have a sensitivity to a particular HIV biotype (see Chapter 13).

2. MACROPHAGES

Macrophages, the target cells for other lentiviruses (1683), are also susceptible to HIV infection (1460, 2541, 2551). The macrophage-tropic R5 viruses replicate well in both peripheral blood macrophages and CD4+ lymphocytes (1486). In both cell types, the CD4 protein on the cell surface is the major receptor for entry (855, 924, 1486) and CCR5 is the coreceptor.

Macrophages, as observed with CD4+ lymphocytes (1230, 1609), show differences in ability to replicate HIV which are related to both the virus isolates and the particular cellular target involved (925, 4534). This finding may reflect CD4 and CCR5 expression levels, the relative affinity of the virus isolates for CCR5 (4078), and/or blocks in postentry steps (933, 4208, 4473) (see Chapters 2 and 5).

Often, in macrophage infection, only low-level production of virus takes place, and HIV can be found sequestered in intracellular vacuoles (1486). Intracellular mechanisms are involved in limiting HIV replication (see Chapter 5). In contrast to T cells, in which virus is released from the cell surface, HIV in infected macrophages usually buds into late endosomes or multivesicular bodies and is then released from the cell by fusion of these organelles with the plasma membrane (2324, 3462). Recent evidence suggests that HIV

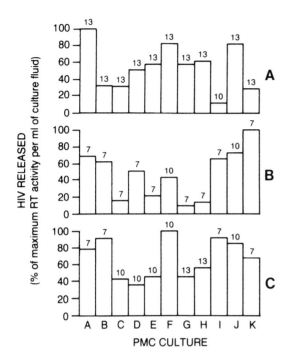

Figure 4.2 Variation in HIV replication in peripheral blood mononuclear cells (PBMC). The cells from 11 different donors of Asian (bars A to D), African-American (bars E, F, and G), and Caucasian (bars H to K) backgrounds were infected with three different strains of HIV-1 (SF2 [A], SF247 [B], and SF170 [C]). Reproducible differences in level of replication and time of maximum virus release (number above bar) were observed. Modified from reference 1230 with permission. Copyright 1987 The American Association of Immunologists, Inc.

resembles exosomes in using the late endosomal/multivesicular body pathway for budding from macrophages (740a, 1586). Exosomes are small (50- to 200-nm) membrane vesicles that are released into the extracellular milieu (see Chapter 5, Section I.A). R5 viruses are usually characterized as noncytopathic (see Chapter 3), but some of these HIV-1 isolates, especially those found in late-stage disease, grow to high titers in macrophages and can be cytopathic in these cells as well as CD4+ cells (319, 331, 2362) (see Chapter 13). In most cases, HIV-infected macrophages die by necrosis (319) (see Chapter 6).

X4 viruses can utilize macrophage CXCR4 for infection, but low-level replication usually takes place (3268, 4151, 4583, 4877). For instance, most X4 strains can be detected in macrophages after inocu-

lation or in macrophages within lymphoid tissue (2015) if PCR procedures or cocultivation of the cells with PBMC is conducted (3998). The lack of substantial X4 virus replication in macrophages can be related to a delay in reverse transcription and other postentry steps (3974). Virus production can also depend on appropriate function of the *vpr*, *vpu*, and *nef* genes (231) (Table 4.6) (see Chapter 5).

Usually, differentiation of monocytes to macrophages is needed for efficient infection (3722, 4005, 4473, 4537) (see also Chapter 5). However, macrophages are much less susceptible to HIV infection after several days in culture (4537; J. A. Levy, unpublished observations). Again, the variations observed can reflect the extent of CCR5 expression and/or envelope affinity (see Chapter 3).

HIV-1 isolates can differ in their ability to replicate in macrophages from different tissues (e.g., the lungs). Alveolar macrophages do not appear to be a major target of HIV-1 (3103). Macrophages from neonates can have an increased susceptibility to HIV-1 infection compared to macrophages from adults (4228). Cytokines can affect HIV replication in macrophages (223, 3110, 4672). For example, macrophage-derived colony-stimulating factor (M-CSF) or granulocyte-macrophage CSF (GM-CSF) produced by infected cells can increase the susceptibility of macrophages to R5 HIV infection (1487, 2356, 4672) via enhanced CCR5 expression (2458) (see Chapter 3). In contrast, some investigators have noted that GM-CSF induces macrophage differentiation that can cause a reduction in expression of chemokine coreceptors and decreased HIV entry (1072, 2143) (see Chapter 5). IL-2 can also inhibit the expression of CD4 and CCR5 on

Table 4.6 Factors influencing HIV infection and replication[a]

- Presence of cellular receptor(s) for the virus
- Virus envelope (structure, conformation, charge)
- Extent of viral envelope glycosylation
- Number of envelope spikes—extent of gp120 shedding
- Cellular proteases
- Interaction of intracellular factors with the viral LTR and viral proteins (e.g., Tat, Rev, and Nef)
- Extent of expression of viral regulatory and accessory genes (e.g., *tat*, *rev*, *nef*, *vif*, *vpu*, and *vpr*)

[a]These factors are discussed in Chapters 3, 4, and 8.

macrophages (2357) and reduce HIV infection (Table 3.6).

Activation of the macrophages with CD40 ligand can make the cells susceptible to replication of X4 viruses (223). Thus, the proinflammatory events occurring during ongoing HIV infection could enhance this process and contribute to the selection of X4 viruses in the late stages of the infection (see Chapter 13). However, IL-10 produced in advanced HIV infection can decrease X4 replication by macrophages (see Chapter 8). Obviously, as with CD4$^+$ cells, a variety of factors can influence the extent of infection of macrophages by different HIV isolates.

3. B CELLS AND CD8$^+$ CELLS

B cells and B-cell lines can be infected with HIV in cell culture but appear to be most susceptible if EBV is also present (955, 3058, 3060). They can transfer HIV to T cells (Figure 2.3) via expression of DC-SIGN (3668) (see Chapter 9).

CD8$^+$ cells can be infected in vitro, after previous infection with HTLV-1 (C. M. Walker and J. A. Levy, unpublished observations) and through the expression of CD4 on dually positive precursor T cells (4495). This susceptibility to HIV infection is commonly observed with neonatal CD4$^+$ CD8$^+$ lymphocytes (4853) and could explain the rapid progression to disease in newborn infants. Some researchers have suggested that infected CD8$^+$ T lymphocytes can be detected in seropositive individuals (2644, 2889, 3872, 3873, 4044). In most cases, the infection appears to reflect the presence of the CD4 molecule on the cell surface (i.e., CD4$^+$ CD8$^+$ precursor cells) (491, 4044) which can result from CD8$^+$ cell activation (825, 1305). Some investigators have noted HIV productive infection of CD4$^-$ CD8$^-$ T cells (2821), most likely reflecting an earlier expression of CD4 on the cell surface.

In other studies, a possible contamination of the cells with free virus should be considered, since only late-stage AIDS patients with high virus loads had evidence of HIV infection of CD8$^+$ cells (2644). By PCR assay, HIV infection has not been detected in CD8$^+$ cells recovered in vivo (L. Z. Pan and J. A. Levy, unpublished observations). Some reports on CD8-tropic viruses have appeared (3872) but need confirmation. The infection of CD8$^+$ cells by these viruses appears to occur only if some CD4

is expressed on the cell surface. The infection is blocked by anti-CD4 antibodies (B. Ashlock and J. Levy, unpublished observations).

4. BONE MARROW

Stromal fibroblasts (3943) and endothelial cells from the stroma of the bone marrow (3127) have been shown to be infected by HIV. The endothelial cell could be an important reservoir of the virus and pass HIV to CD4$^+$ lymphocytes. HIV infection can also influence the level of hematopoiesis in the bone marrow through disturbances in cytokine production (see Chapter 9). In this regard, after HIV infection, the BS-1 human stromal cell line did not support the proliferation and differentiation of cultured hematopoietic cells (4280). Some CD34$^+$ bone marrow cells have been found to be infected in certain seropositive individuals (4258) and at times have been susceptible to HIV-1 infection in vitro (i.e., when they express CD4) (710, 4670). Nevertheless, conclusive evidence for a major infection of CD34$^+$ stem cells is lacking (972, 992, 2798; for a review, see reference 3122) (see Chapter 8).

5. NUMBER OF CD4$^+$ LYMPHOCYTES INFECTED BY HIV

In the early period of research on the AIDS virus, in situ hybridization data suggested that only 1 in 10,000 or 1 in 100,000 peripheral leukocytes was infected by HIV (1736). The major target cell was the CD4$^+$ lymphocyte. These results raised questions about the viral pathogenic pathway, since the destruction of CD4$^+$ cells, which is characteristic of AIDS, could not be easily explained by the number of cells directly infected.

Subsequently, using quantitative competitive PCR, the number of virus-infected CD4$^+$ cells in the blood was reported to be as high as 1 in 10 in symptomatic patients and up to 1 in 1,000 in some asymptomatic individuals (211, 1907, 3611, 3990) (Table 2.1). This quantity greatly increases the target cell number considered infected by the virus and can explain in part the loss of CD4$^+$ cells in this infection (see Chapters 6, 8, and 13). Nevertheless, the number of cells actively replicating the virus (as revealed by in situ hybridization studies measuring viral RNA) can be quite small—only 10% of all PBMC containing the HIV genome

(4148). This observation most probably explains the long incubation period before disease onset often observed in this infection. It would not support the idea of productive infection by HIV as a major cause of CD4+ cell destruction (see Chapters 6 and 13).

Furthermore, as discussed in Section II.D, PCR studies have indicated potentially high levels of HIV predominantly in CD4+ lymphocytes in the lymph tissues of infected individuals (1194, 3412; for a review, see reference 1684), particularly in the GI tract (see Chapter 8 and below).

Since the PBMC represent only 1 to 3% of total lymphocytes (4737) in the body, the total number of infected CD4+ cells and the virus levels in blood could certainly be misleading. As noted above, many observations suggest that virus in the blood can be a poor reflection of total virus content in infected cells and lymph nodes and other tissues, particularly the bowel (see Chapter 8) (1256, 1686, 3413), and especially during the asymptomatic period (for a review, see reference 1684).

It is also important to remember that the CD4+ cell population includes macrophages, which are not readily killed by HIV (1486). However, many studies suggest that, aside from the spleen, relatively few infected macrophages are found in the host (216, 3442). This issue needs further clarification.

6. CONCLUSIONS

The hematopoietic cells now reported to be infectible, at least in cell culture, range from CD34+ stem cells to monocytes, macrophages, various types of DCs, B lymphocytes, megakaryocytes, natural killer (NK) cells, NK-T cells, γδ T lymphocytes (1956), eosinophils, thymic epithelial cells, mast cells or basophils (3628), and thymocytes (241, 639, 704, 709, 1365, 1771, 2353, 2581, 3288, 3443, 3876, 4026, 4637, 4943, 4982) (Table 4.3) (see Chapters 8 and 9). Nevertheless, infection of B cells, CD8+ cells, NK cells, CD34+ stem cells, and DCs in vivo, and in some cases in vitro, has not been consistently demonstrated (972, 992, 3052, 3680, 4086, 4630). In this regard, infection in vitro of an NK cell subset expressing CD4 has been reported (4026, 4536) (see Chapter 9) but may not be clinically relevant. Furthermore, the loss of CD34+ hematopoietic progenitor cells has been linked to apoptosis and not to direct infection (3680).

There is still controversy about whether DCs are directly infected by the virus or play a role in pathogenesis by carrying adherent virus in vivo to activated CD4+ lymphocytes (591, 592, 4720) (see Chapter 9). At this time, it appears that many types of DCs can be productively infected and, despite low-level virus replication, can pass HIV to other cells. Attachment of virus to the cell without infection does not seem to be a major means of transmission (Chapter 9). Some studies have demonstrated that mature DCs in the blood circulate in association with T cells (2244, 4720) and via conjugates can pass virus to CD4+ cells (2914, 3575). Importantly, HIV can also bind to a variety of CD4− cells without infecting them; these cell:virus complexes can pass virus to susceptible target CD4+ cells (Figure 2.3).

In summary, within the hematopoietic system, CD4+ lymphocytes are the most visibly infected cell type, since they can replicate high levels of virus. Increased envelope density on the surface of HIV leads to an improved virus production, most likely via signal transduction resulting from an envelope interaction at the cell surface (198, 4723). The genetic makeup of the CD4+ cells determines their susceptibility to a particular HIV isolate. Macrophages are infectible, but these HIV-infected cells are not found frequently in the blood or in the lymph nodes, where CD4+ lymphocytes are the predominant cell type infected (216, 1194). Nevertheless, infection of macrophages, as with DCs, may go undetected because of low virus production. Moreover, macrophages in some HIV transmissions may be the first cells infected because they exist in an activated state in lymphoid tissues (see below and Chapter 13). In the spleen, large numbers of infected macrophages can be detected (1686); this organ could be the primary source of tissue macrophages replicating HIV. Once the infection of a cell occurs, an independent evolution of virus progeny can take place depending on the cell type infected (1388) (see below).

D. Lymphoid Tissue

PCR and in situ PCR techniques have confirmed the widespread presence of HIV infection in lymphoid tissue even in healthy infected individuals. It has been estimated that in some asymptomatic individuals, HIV infection was up to 100 times more prevalent in lymph nodes than in peripheral blood (397, 3292, 3412, 3414). Similar observations have been made in healthy HIV-1-infected chimpanzees (3885). Several early studies showed HIV DNA in these tissues (1345, 3411, 3650, 4399). Most of the virus infection in lymph nodes is in CD4$^+$ lymphocytes (1194, 3948).

Histologic and electron microscopic examinations have indicated that in the early periods of HIV infection, viral particles can be visualized by electron microscopy in the villous processes of FDCs, in close contact with lymphocytes (for reviews, see references (3413 and 3414) (see Chapter 9). Several groups have not detected productive HIV infection of the FDCs (1193, 3413, 3696, 3981, 4502), while other investigators have reported that an average of 20% of these CD21$^+$ cells show HIV DNA (4230). Moreover, some investigators have reported in vitro infection of FDCs, probably by a CD4-independent mechanism (4249). Most evidence indicates, however, that these cells of mesenchymal origin (not from bone marrow) are not directly infected (2244) but can transfer virus to CD4$^+$ cells (1386).

HIV can persist on the FDCs as an infectious agent for at least 25 days in vitro. In studies using murine FDCs, virus was retained for up to 9 months with infectivity (4176). Most of the viruses found on FDCs are associated with antibody complexes. Certain studies, but not others (1386), suggest that this virus remains infectious even when neutralizing antibodies are present. These antibodies do not affect the transfer of virus to CD4$^+$ cells (1783, 4230). Lymphoid interdigitary DCs can be infected, but probably at a low level compared to other cells in these tissues (2927). In the oral cavity, gingival keratinocytes and adenoid epithelial cells have also been found to be susceptible to infection (particularly with R5 viruses) (2636, 3096).

The findings with lymphoid tissues led one group to conclude that HIV is trapped in the lymph node through the FDC network (perhaps complexed with HIV antibodies) and therefore the virus load, as reflected in the peripheral blood, appears to be reduced in the early stages of disease (for reviews, see references 1256 and 3413). By quantitative image analysis and in situ hybridization techniques, it was estimated that the amount of viral RNA in the FDCs was 100- to 10,000-fold greater than that in the blood (1686). FDC-associated virus in lymphoid tissue is also in much larger quantities than virus associated with other infected cells (1686). At first, the virus associated with FDCs did not appear to be affected by antiviral monotherapy (1686). However, later studies with HAART have shown in 6 months a several-log decrease in levels of FDC-associated virus (646, 4941) (see Chapter 14).

As infection progresses, CD4$^+$ cells are depleted, follicles are destroyed, and the lymph node architecture is increasingly disrupted by collagen deposition, further contributing to CD4$^+$ cell depletion and somewhat limiting reconstitution with antiviral therapy (3953). The mechanisms responsible for this depletion of cells in the lymphoid tissues and for the destruction of FDCs have yet to be fully defined (see Chapter 13), but both the CD4$^+$ cell depletion and destruction of lymphoid follicles are partially reversible with antiviral therapy over an extended period (3954, 4939, 4941). The high viral infection in lymph nodes (estimated to be 25% of white cells or 200 billion CD4$^+$ cells in some cases) primarily represents cells with low virus replication, latent, or defective infection (Color Plate 9, following page 78) (1194, 1686, 3295, 3413, 3807) (see Section II.C.1).

With about 500 billion to 1 trillion leukocytes in the body, primarily in lymphoid tissue, some estimate that in asymptomatic infected individuals, 20 to 30% of these cells (mostly CD4$^+$ lymphocytes) could be infected by HIV (1194). Moreover, many of these infected CD4$^+$ cells are not producing virus when transcription of viral RNA is measured. Only 1 in 300 to 400 infected cells in the lymph nodes of asymptomatic individuals appeared to be releasing virus (Color Plate 9, following page 78) (1193, 1194, 3807), and perhaps even fewer (772). Nevertheless, in one study, the number of CD4$^+$ T cells carrying replication-competent HIV-1 was approximately 40 times higher in tonsillar tissue than in peripheral blood (3807).

The findings on viral latency in the lymphoid tissue resemble those noted above for peripheral blood lymphocytes (775, 3442, 4140, 4148) and could reflect the antiviral activity of CD8$^+$ cells, both in the blood and in the lymphoid tissues (397) (see below and Chapters 5 and 11). Nevertheless, conclusions about relative levels of infected CD4$^+$ cells in lymph nodes and blood and the number of cells capable of releasing infectious virus still cannot be drawn.

In these studies of lymph nodes, about 0.5% of the resting CD4$^+$ cells contained HIV DNA, but only 1/10 of these cells carried integrated provirus. Thus, many of these cells seemed to have an abortive infection characterized by a full-length linear unintegrated DNA (552, 4383, 4903). Moreover, only 10% of the latter cells were capable of releasing HIV virions. Thus, of a total of 10^9 CD4$^+$ "resting" lymphocytes containing HIV, 10^7 had latent provirus and 10^6 had the potential to produce infectious virus. When activated cells were included, a two- to threefold-greater number of infected cells could be detected (772, 4140). These studies suggested that a large number of infected cells (up to 10-fold) in the lymph node contain a defective provirus that is unable to produce infectious virions. This presence of HIV latency in vivo has also been noted in peripheral blood cells (214, 771, 1193, 3442, 4141). The mechanisms involved are considered in Chapter 5.

When the number of infected macrophages in lymphoid tissue was determined, integrated DNA was found at a very low number (1 per 20,000 cells) (772). Thus, a great deal of the viral DNA detected in lymph nodes by standard PCR represents unintegrated virus, perhaps in an arrested state that cannot be replicated. As noted above, these observations counter the quantitative studies on viral load in lymphoid tissue reported earlier (1194), but the number of infected cells in lymph nodes may be much greater than these most recent findings suggest (3948). This issue remains to be resolved. In any case, the number of cells in the lymphoid compartment that can carry infectious virus, particularly in the lymphoid tissue of the bowel (see below), still presents a major challenge to antiviral therapies (see Chapter 14).

E. Thymus

HIV infection of the thymus is another important area of study. All thymic cell subsets, immature and mature, are targets for HIV infection by a CD4-dependent mechanism (for a review, see reference 1466). Most infected cells detected in the thymus are of the early CD4$^+$ CD8$^+$ precursor cell type (4538) (see Chapter 8). In some studies, the mature T cells seemed most susceptible, perhaps influenced by the presence of TNF-α and IL-2 in the thymic tissue (720). Epithelial cells as well as lymphocytes in this organ have been found to be susceptible to HIV (581, 1771, 3288, 4538), but the extent of infection of epithelial cells and DCs in vivo requires further evaluation. In one study, recovery of a cytopathic thymotropic virus variant was reported (581). Cell death in the thymus can occur by direct cell killing by HIV and by the induction of apoptosis (1466). The importance of the thymus in the immune response is discussed in Chapter 11.

F. Brain

In the brain, resident macrophages and microglia have been the major cells showing the presence of virus (514, 1500, 2252, 2986, 3233, 3622, 4077, 4759; for a review, see reference 1563). However, the hypothesis that microglia (which can express CD4) (1080) are targets for HIV has been challenged (see Chapter 8). Some investigators (3493) were unable to infect microglia from the fetal brain, and microglia can be confused with peripheral blood macrophages infiltrating the brain. These two cell types can be distinguished by specific antigens (514, 3493), and both do appear to be susceptible particularly to R5 virus isolates (1500).

Reports of other infected brain-derived cell types, including astrocytes, oligodendrocytes, capillary endothelial cells, and perhaps neurons, have appeared in the literature (Table 4.3) (1679, 2535, 2986, 3158, 3295, 3622, 4759). By in situ PCR hybridization and laser capture microdissection procedures, many infected astrocytes and some neurons have been detected in patients with dementia (3295, 4422). Whether neurons can be infected is controversial. Infection of astrocytes, oligodendrocytes, and brain-derived endothelial cells has been demonstrated in cell culture (56, 729, 1171, 2535, 3123). Perivascular macrophages expressing CD163 are major targets for HIV (2198) (see Chapter 8). IFN-α can facilitate infection of astrocytes (628). In some cases this infection occurs by a CD4 and chemokine coreceptor-independent mechanism (3862), perhaps via the mannose receptor (2639). The consistency of these findings on infected cells in the brain and the prevalence of cells infected needs further evaluation.

Several studies have indicated the ability to infect brain microvascular endothelial cells with HIV (3123). These cells express CXCR5 and CCR5 as well as DC-SIGN (3158). The virus can enter by a mechanism involving lipid rafts (2632). This infection could explain the passage of the virus into the brain (see Chapter 8). It is noteworthy that in contrast to brain-derived endothelial cells, endothelial cells from umbilical or saphenous veins do not appear to be susceptible to HIV (3123). Finally, the sequence differences observed with brain-derived versus blood-derived isolates (681, 2173, 4065, 4422) do suggest distinct cell targets and a separate evolution for HIV in the central nervous system (see Chapter 13).

G. Gastrointestinal System

CD4$^+$ lymphocytes in the lamina propria of intestinal tissues are the cells primarily infected by HIV (187, 1308, 1344, 2296, 2971, 3234) (see Chapter 8). This region of the bowel contains effector T cells. HIV infection can lead to substantial losses in these T cells (1657, 2957, 4186) that are not evident in measuring circulating CD4$^+$ cell numbers (see above). These bowel CD4$^+$ cells predominantly express CCR5 but also have CXCR4 on their surface (2971, 4185, 4186). Such T cells represent about half of the total body T cells (3150), whereas only 15% of blood and lymph node T cells express CCR5 (1640, 2348). The CD4$^+$ cells in the mucosae that are primarily lost in acute infection are the CCR5$^+$ effector memory cells that have come from secondary lymphoid tissue (3150). R5 virus infection is therefore the most dominant in the bowel (187), destroying up to 80% of CD4$^+$ cells rapidly (2957) (see Chapter 13). In blood and lymphoid tissues, a similar percentage of CCR5-expressing CD4$^+$ memory cells are lost, but these cells represent a much smaller number of the circulating T lymphocytes (2957).

Intestinal epithelial cells expressing CCR5 can also selectively transfer R5 HIV-1 to CCR5-expressing cells (2972), thus increasing this CD4$^+$ cell infection. DCs are rarely found in GI lymphoid tissue (2971), and infected macrophages are not seen as frequently until the CD4$^+$ T cells have

been diminished (4185). Once they are eliminated, the replacement of CD4$^+$ cells should come from lymphoid tissues, but replacement does not occur very readily, even after antiretroviral therapy (1657, 1658) (see Chapters 13 and 14).

In the bowel, the presence of HIV in mucosal cells has been detected by cell culture, in situ hybridization, and PCR studies of all regions of the GI tract (1515, 1792, 2296, 2870, 3234) (Color Plate 10, following page 78). The bowel cell types considered infectible include goblet and columnar epithelial cells and enterochromaffin cells (1792, 2544, 3234) (Table 4.3). The enterochromaffin cells are cytokine- and hormone-producing cells that regulate cell motility and function (3553). In rhesus macaques, enterocytes have also been found to be infected by SIV (1792).

HIV also infects cultured bowel explants and transformed bowel carcinoma cell lines (19, 166, 262, 279, 1249, 1250, 1308, 3153). In vitro infection can cause impaired function in human colon epithelial cells (1249). These in vitro findings on infection of bowel cells require further confirmation, particularly in vivo with in situ PCR hybridization studies (for a review, see reference 2267).

In the liver, infection of cultured CD4$^+$ endothelial cells from human liver sinusoids has been reported (4019, 4270). Other observations suggest that Kupffer cells and hepatocytes can be infected by HIV-1 in vivo (604, 1897, 1928, 3979) and in vitro (3979). Infection of hepatic cells can cause selective impairment in function (2377). The above results showing infection of liver parenchymal cells lacking CD4 expression are supported by the finding that CD4$^-$ cell lines derived from hepatocellular carcinomas are susceptible to HIV (605). The virus receptor on these cells has not been reported.

H. Other Cells and Tissues

HIV has also been detected in the synovial membrane in the joints of AIDS patients (1224, 1933). In the skin, fibroblasts and most likely LC can be infected by the virus, as shown by in situ hybridization, immunohistochemistry, PCR analysis, and cell culture studies (783, 788, 1950, 2965, 3667, 3887, 4393, 4494) (see above). Evidence of widespread infection of LC by HIV in vivo, however, is lacking (see Chapter 9). Some early studies have not detected infection of these cells in the tissues examined

(2090). Certainly, epidemiological studies do not support the idea of infected skin as a means of HIV transmission (345, 1498, 3780). Fibroblasts in dental pulp removed from HIV-positive patients have also been found to contain virus (Tables 3.8 and 4.3) (1533). Many of the above-cited cell types lack CD4 expression and emphasize the use of other receptors by HIV for infection (see Chapter 3).

Finally, in vivo or in vitro infection of other cells and tissues from organs such as the kidney, heart, lung, muscle, eye, placenta, cervix, vagina, uterus, fallopian tube, prostate, testes, mammary epithelial cells, oral epithelial cells, and adrenal glands has been reported (Table 4.3) (163, 249, 597, 601, 680, 701, 788, 831, 944, 1103, 1399, 1613, 1634, 1902, 2093, 2449, 2621, 2823, 2879, 2965, 3096, 3294, 3535, 3567, 3568, 3639, 3811, 3889, 4447, 4773, 4793) and could be clinically relevant (see Chapters 2 and 8). In patients with myopathy, HIV could be involved. HIV antigen and viral nucleic acid have been detected in muscle macrophages and myocytes (666, 4035). Placenta trophoblasts can be infected by HIV following interaction of T cells with placental cells. The transfer from placental cells to T cells involves an up-regulation of adhesion molecules, such as ICAM-1, that can be blocked by LFA antibodies (143). Moreover, full-term trophoblasts expressing CXCR4 but not CCR5 or CD4 can be infected by CD4-independent CXCR4-utilizing X4 viruses (48). Infection of placenta and fetal tissues is further discussed in Chapter 2.

In all these tissues studied, the cells infected could either lack or express the CD4 molecule (see Chapter 3). In several instances, confirmation of the infection is needed (245, 1068, 3166, 3196). Nevertheless, the studies of HIV infection of human cells consistently indicate that this agent is polytropic and not solely T lymphotropic.

III. Differences in Cellular Host Range among HIV Isolates

A. General Observations

The variety of cells and cell lines susceptible to HIV-1 infection in vitro and in vivo has been reviewed. Ongoing studies continually demonstrate the wide and varied cellular host range of both HIV-1 and HIV-2 strains (Table 4.3). When HIV-1 was initially recovered, the virus was grown in mitogen-stimulated normal PBMC (272). Because with time the cells died, fresh PBMC had to be added on a regular basis. After a few months of study, however, the virus was shown to infect and grow persistently in established lines of T and B cells that were not killed by the virus. These lines were useful in growing large quantities of HIV-1 through cell culture procedures (2537, 2551, 3060, 3580). Established cell lines soon became the source of screening tests used for detecting antibodies to HIV (1418, 2081).

The early observations on HIV diversity, however, indicated that many HIV-1 strains could not be propagated in established human T-cell lines (165, 1230, 2535). Subsequent studies with several independent HIV-1 isolates then demonstrated that some viruses can grow well in certain established human T-cell, B-cell, and monocyte lines and others cannot (165, 639, 821, 1230, 1274, 2551, 3880, 4015, 4403). Some were SI and highly cytopathic; others were not (NSI). Nearly all the isolates could replicate in peripheral blood CD4$^+$ lymphocytes, except for cells lacking CCR5 expression (e.g., R5 isolates) (see Chapter 3). Certain viruses, the NSI type, replicated well in primary macrophages, whereas others grew efficiently only in peripheral blood CD4$^+$ T cells (see below) (639, 1486, 4015, 4625). Variations in infection of these primary cell types were also noted (924, 1230, 1609) (see Section II) (Figure 4.2).

The basis for the major differences in cell tropisms has now been explained by the specific coreceptor used by R5 NSI macrophage-tropic (CCR5) and X4 SI T-cell-line-tropic (CXCR4) isolates (Tables 3.2, 3.5, and 4.7). Moreover, some SI isolates are both macrophage and T-cell-line tropic (731) and considered dualtropic (R5/X4) (see Chapter 3). Obviously, besides coreceptor interactions, intracellular processes can also affect the viral replicative cycle (see Chapter 5).

Some HIV-1 (usually X4) isolates can infect CD4$^+$ B-cell lines and even primary B lymphocytes in culture, particularly if EBV is present (954, 1804, 3060). Viruses can also be distinguished by their relative ability to grow in bowel- and brain-derived cell lines as well as in primary cells from fetal and adult organs (262, 734, 1274, 4015; for a review, see reference 639) (see Chapter 8).

Table 4.7 Classification of HIV isolates by biologic properties

Subtypes

- Virulent versus nonvirulent (731)
- Syncytium-inducing versus non-syncytium-inducing (2279, 4394)
- Rapid/high versus slow/low (1274)
- Groups a–d (for lymphocytes) or α–γ (for macrophages)[a] (4625)
- Macrophage tropic versus T-cell-line tropic; now recognized as CCR5-utilizing (R5) and CXCR4-utilizing (X4) HIV isolates

Phenotype considered

- Host range is defined by replication in macrophages vs established human T-cell lines. Some differences in growth in CD4+ lymphocytes and established T-cell, B-cell, and monocyte lines have been used.
- Replication is defined by how soon virus is released from the cell (kinetics, i.e., rapid versus slow) and to what levels it is produced at peak virus replication (titer, i.e., high versus low). In the infected individual, the replicative ability is often referred to as "fitness," reflecting the ability of the virus to grow in the presence of many variables within the in vivo environment.
- Cytopathology is defined by cell killing as well as induction of syncytia in cells.

[a]Kinetics is not a parameter.

In summary, both HIV-1 and HIV-2 can also be distinguished by their ability to form syncytia and to grow rapidly to high titer or slowly to low titer in CD4+ cells (53) (Table 4.7). Most HIV-2 isolates appear to be dualtropic (R5/X4), and some can enter cells by a CD4-independent mechanism (3685) (see Chapters 1 and 3). The relationship of these host range differences to HIV pathogenesis is discussed in Chapter 13.

B. Kinetics and Level of Virus Replication

The difference in ability of HIV strains to infect cells is reflected not only in virus entry, as discussed above, but also in the rate of virus replication (kinetics) and the extent of viral progeny production (titer) in various cell types. In part, the virus titer over short periods can indicate the level of HIV-1 spread among the cells inoculated. The relative ability of HIV-1 to replicate in vivo, which reflects the influence of many host variables, has been termed "fitness."

These measures of kinetics and titer were used in early studies by some investigators to categorize HIV into slow/low (now mostly R5) and rapid/high strains (X4 virus) (165, 1274) (Table 4.7) (see Chapter 13). The rapid/high strains were associated with disease in infected individuals, as are X4 viruses (731) (Figure 13.4). In general, these distinctions in kinetics and titer fit most isolates; however, some low-titer viruses have been found to replicate rapidly, and certain slowly replicating viruses can eventually grow to high titers after a prolonged period in culture (4625; J. A. Levy, unpublished observations). Moreover, in some studies, slow infection kinetics was found to reflect low production and spread of infectious virus rather than a long replication time (1089).

From the virus perspective, X4 viruses appear to replicate more rapidly than R5 isolates but may produce less progeny than R5 viruses (4018). However, R5 viruses isolated from AIDS patients show high replication kinetics (2362, 4020) and thus differ from R5 viruses from healthy infected individuals (see Chapter 13). In this regard, a particular *tat* gene could influence the extent of virus replication (see below and Chapter 7). Measuring a virus' protease and reverse transcriptase (*pol*) functions, particularly in the context of antiretroviral treatment, has more recently been used to reflect relative replication ability (247).

All these findings, as well as those on virus entry and intracellular differences (see Chapter 5), emphasize again how both external and internal cellular factors, interacting with various viral gene products, can influence the extent of infection and replication by individual HIV isolates (Table 4.6).

C. Influence of Glycosylation on Cellular Host Range

Two early studies (730, 3453) demonstrated that HIV-1 isolates passed through a variety of cell types were modified in their cellular host range properties. Although selection of a variant could be involved, posttranslational modification of the infecting virus strain should be considered. For example, some HIV-1 isolates grown in the HUT 78 T-cell line, in contrast to PBMC, take on biologic features permitting infection of a variety of other established T-cell and macrophage lines. When the virus is passed back in PBMC, this expanded host

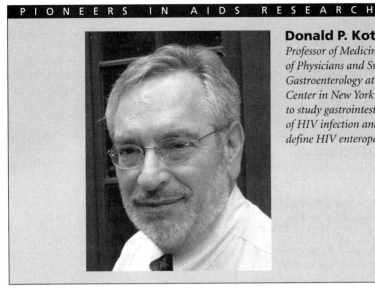

Donald P. Kotler

Professor of Medicine, Columbia University College of Physicians and Surgeons, and Chief of Gastroenterology at St. Luke's-Roosevelt Hospital Center in New York City. Dr. Kotler was among the first to study gastrointestinal and nutritional complications of HIV infection and AIDS. His findings helped to define HIV enteropathy.

range disappears. The only viral proteins that appear to be changed during this transfer of HIV-1 are the envelope glycoproteins. On exposure to tunicamycin, the nonglycosylated envelope proteins for all the viruses studied have the same size (730); it is the extent of glycosylation that differs. The results strongly suggest that the glycosylation pattern of the envelope protein determined by events within the cell (1268) can affect the host range of the progeny virions. One hypothesis considers that carbohydrate binding proteins on the cell surface or a macrophage endocytosis receptor (1240) can interact with oligosaccharides on HIV-1 and affect its infectivity and cellular host range (1268) (see also Chapter 3). However, it is equally possible that the extent or arrangement of potential N-linked glycosylation sites on viral envelope glycoproteins modulates its conformation (2497, 4829) and, hence, its interaction with CD4 and coreceptors. Other studies suggest that only some N-linked glycosylation sites might be important for infectivity (2468, 2710, 2775). This posttranslational alteration of viral proteins is another example of the influence that intracellular factors could have on HIV infection and spread (Table 4.6) (see Chapter 5).

Recently, glycoprotein differences in the V3 loop have correlated with the virus' cellular host range (1752). The extent of glycosylation can also influence HIV binding to C-type lectins (408, 934)

(see Chapter 9). Glycosylation can affect the sensitivity of certain HIV strains to antiviral antibodies as well (721, 4699) (see Chapter 10). Therefore, envelope glycosylation differences should be added to the general features of HIV that might determine pathogenesis in individuals infected by the same HIV isolate.

D. Modulation of CD4 Protein Expression

In early studies of HIV-1, infection of CD4+ cells was associated with elimination of CD4 protein expression on the cell surface (see Chapter 3). In subsequent evaluations of HIV-1 and HIV-2 strains, some viruses were found that did not down-modulate the CD4 receptor. One HIV-2 strain (UC1) (1231), which is also generally noncytopathic, replicates to high titer in CD4+ lymphocytes without disturbing the expression or intensity of the CD4 molecule on the cell surface. Another HIV-2 strain (ST) (2345) has also been shown to have minimal effects on CD4 protein expression. This variation in extent of CD4 expression can be seen with diverse HIV-1 isolates (2535), and lack of CD4 down-modulation is one notable property of R5 viruses recovered from the brain (734) (Section II.F) (Table 3.4) (see Chapters 8 and 13). It appears that X4 viruses and R5/X4 viruses consistently reduce CD4 expression (735), whereas R5 viruses do so only after chronic infection (735). Whether this feature, which varies among viral strains, plays any role in the pathogenic pathway is still unknown. The mechanism for this process is discussed in Chapter 3, and the potential viral protein determinants of this process are reviewed in Chapters 3 and 7.

E. Cell Culture Changes

Molecular approaches have suggested the presence of HIV-1 diversity in infected hosts that is not appreciated after isolation of viruses in vitro (2354, 2987). In certain studies, the system used for virus cultivation appeared to select for various genetic variants within the PBMC from individuals. The genotype most frequently found in uncultured PBMC resembled that in the plasma. However, when peripheral lymphocytes, macrophages, or mixed cultures were analyzed in culture, certain variants appeared that were underrepresented in the uncultured PBMC (4626). Thus, the virus cultivation system may not reflect all the genotypes present in PBMC.

In addition, CCR5 is up-regulated in PBMC after exposure to lectins such as PHA (410). Thus, selection of R5 viruses in cell culture may be misleading as to the type(s) of viruses present in the infected individual. Moreover, fresh (primary) HIV-1 isolates, particularly from plasma, might not readily infect cultured PBMC, perhaps reflecting a reduced affinity for the CD4$^+$ lymphocyte in culture or the use of a specific coreceptor (see Chapter 3). For these reasons, some investigators warn about artifacts introduced by in vitro techniques that can affect the biologic characterization of HIV-1 (2354, 2996). Furthermore, prolonged growth in vitro of a virus from an individual could select for a more rapidly growing X4 variant (2694) when both R5 and X4 viruses are present (3907). Nevertheless, studies using the same approaches for isolation, short-term culture, and comparison among strains should help control for these variables.

Finally, evaluation of viral strains directly in tissues and PBMC (e.g., by PCR) carries the risk of studying defective virions (3906). Most measurements indicate the presence of up to 1,000-fold more noninfectious than infectious viruses in HIV preparations (2201) and up to 100,000-fold more noninfectious than infectious particles in

Table 4.8 Factors involved in resistance to virus superinfection

The cell
- Loss of cell surface receptors (e.g., CD4) (741, 2474)
- Arrest in reverse transcription (4358, 4623)
- Block by noninfectious HIV particles (339)

The host
- Different sensitivity to virus strains
- Differences in viral input levels
- Down-modulation of virus receptors in sensitive cells (2474)
- Neutralizing antibody or ADCC^a activity (4465)
- Cell-mediated immune response (e.g., CD8$^+$ cell anti-HIV noncytotoxic response) (257, 2095)

^{a}ADCC, antibody-dependent cellular cytotoxicity.

the plasma of seropositive individuals (2438, 3502). Nevertheless, some studies have indicated that limited cell culture procedures for isolation of HIV-1 (7 to 10 days) can provide a good indication of the major infectious virus variant present in the specimen studied (3860).

IV. Superinfection

A. Cellular Level

After the initial infection with most retroviruses, the cell becomes resistant to superinfection by a similar virus (Table 4.8). The mechanism for this interference appears to be the elimination or covering of the cell surface receptor needed for viral entry (4267, 4621). This process is observed in the HIV system, in which superinfection cannot occur if the CD4 molecule is down-modulated or blocked by antibody (742, 1745, 2194, 2474) (see Chapter 3). Yet the previously infected cells can replicate a different HIV-1 strain if its DNA molecular clone is transfected in vitro into the already infected cells (2474). The block to superinfection is primarily at the cell surface and not intracellular.

In some studies, however, superinfection has been shown to occur in certain chronically infected cells (e.g., HUT 78). In these examples, replication of the superinfecting virus was blocked at a point in reverse transcription (4358). A similar mechanism for resistance to superinfection has been observed in some infected human cells before CD4 is down-modulated (4623). Further experiments using PCR techniques should determine the universality of these findings. In this regard, a potential role for the complementarity-determining region 3 (CDR3) domain of the CD4 molecule in superinfection has been suggested. Infection of cells has been reported if CDR3 is still expressed after the initial infection when the major CD4 receptor epitope for HIV-1 (i.e., OKT4A) is absent (3322).

The lack of viral interference has been proposed as one cause for cytopathology by HIV isolates. Before cells down-modulate CD4, continual infection of these cells by the progeny HIV can take place. This superinfection can lead to an accumulation of unintegrated viral DNA that is associated with cell death (see Chapter 6) (349, 3447, 3762, 4907). However, cells infected by the relatively noncytopathic HIV-2$_{UCl}$ strain continually express CD4, produce high titers of virus, and remain viable (266, 1231, 2474). Whether these cells lack an accumulation of extrachromosomal viral DNA copies is not known. They can be superinfected by an HIV-1 isolate, leading to production of both virus types as well as mixed-pseudotype viruses (2474) (see Chapter 2). These observations suggest that the relatively slow decrease or lack of elimination of the major viral receptor could lead to superinfection of cells by the same or other HIV isolates.

Finally, some in vitro studies (339) suggest that noninfectious HIV-1 virions can block HIV replication, as observed with other viruses (1919). A defective interfering viral effect on HIV spread takes place and could play a role in preventing de novo infection in the host. Despite these reasons for a block in superinfection of a previously infected cell, the process must be taking place. Recombinant virions that can only form by dual infection of a cell are becoming much more common (see Section V).

B. Within the Host

1. MULTIPLE HIV INFECTIONS

Superinfection is a term also used for infection of an individual by more than one HIV isolate. Infections of individuals with both HIV-1 and HIV-2 have been documented (1232, 2498, 3677), but the time at which the infections occurred (i.e., simultaneously or sequentially) is an important question. Whether superinfection or dual infection takes place requires documentation of the partner providing the second virus. Otherwise, both viruses could have been present during the time of initial transmission but one did not become evident until later. In terms of dual infection, two distinct HIV-1 isolates as well as recombinant viruses were identified in a concurrently transfused infant (1079). The latter most likely reflected coinfection of a cell (see below). In contrast, in an adult exposed to two viruses, only one HIV-1 type was detected (1079). The reason for this finding could be the relative viral load or differences in sensitivity of the host for infection by particular virus isolates (see Chapters 2 and 3).

The prevalence of infection by more than one strain of HIV-1 in vivo has not been commonly noted (153) or clinically evident. However, molecular studies suggest that multiple infections are possible (2083, 3887, 4369, 4959), perhaps even with up to three different HIV-1 clades (4369). In studies of spleen cells in HIV-infected subjects, an average of three or four proviruses per cell was noted, and evidence of a large number of recombinant viruses with extensive genetic variations was found (2055). This evidence indicates that multiple virus infections have occurred and that cells were infected by more than one virus (potentially generating recombinants), most likely *prior* to the down-modulation of CD4. However, the time at which the event takes place and the clinical importance of a second or third strain are the key questions. One HIV-1 type usually dominates and must influence the pathogenic course; generally, in both early and late stages of infection of the same individual, the viruses studied by PCR procedures seem related to a dominant strain (2341, 2945).

Even if the initial infection potentially involved several viral isolates (e.g., recipients of many Factor VIII units or multiple blood transfusions), a predominant HIV-1 strain seems to emerge and play an important role in pathogenesis. Other isolates, if present, are presumably suppressed or are eliminated by the dominant virus and/or the host immune response (2521) (see Chapters 3 and 11). At most, a different isolate(s) might remain as a minor component(s) of the viral load, particularly in lymph nodes. Over time, fluctuations in the circulating viruses can be observed, most likely reflecting immune selection as noted in other HIV infections (2908). The mechanism for emergence of a predominant strain has not been elucidated but could reflect less efficient recognition of the virus by the antiviral immune response or death of cells infected by other viral isolates, permitting sufficient spread of the alternative virus type to additional cells.

In some reports, initial infection of individuals by HIV-2 has been linked to resistance to subsequent HIV-1 infection (4462), but this finding is controversial (148) and is not usually observed. Encouraging evidence has come from studies with macaques showing that after seroconversion the animals were protected from secondary challenge (3359). The immune response seemed to be important. However, in one noteworthy study, superinfection of macaques with SIV took place and reactivated the HIV-2 initially used to infect the animals (3492). Both HIV-2 and SIV were present, but the animals were protected from the pathogenic course. A similar observation was made with baboons infected initially and then at later times with distinct isolates of HIV-2 (2649).

2. PREVALENCE OF SUPERINFECTION

Currently, it seems, as with other viral infections, that superinfection can occur in vivo (2531) but is influenced by the host immune system (i.e., immature or compromised) (see below). CD4-expressing cells infected with HIV but not those producing the virus have been recovered from separated PBMC of infected individuals (3611, 4658). Conceivably, these represent nonactivated cells that carry virus for a short time (see Chapter 5), cells suppressed in virus replication by CD8+ cells (2543), or cells having HIV in a latent state (see Chapter 5). These cells could be superinfected before the initial virus infection is aborted or suppressed, or prior to HIV production. The resulting progeny virions might consist of phenotypically mixed particles and even recombinant viruses (Section V).

Case reports have suggested that superinfection could take place after the initial infection and that certain conditions could influence this process. Chimpanzees can be superinfected (640, 1394), most likely reflecting a limited spread of the initial

virus in the animals and the subsequent challenge with high doses of a second HIV isolate and infected cells. Nevertheless, resistance to challenge by heterologous virus strains in chimpanzees has been observed (4102).

Most recently, superinfection in humans has become recognized as a real possibility (495, 1247, 1912, 2790). In an extensive study of more than 1,000 intravenous drug users (IVDU), 126 recent seroconverters were followed, among whom 20% were infected by subtype B virus and 80% were infected with the recombinant virus, subtype E. No dual-subtype infection was detected. After a year, superinfection was noted at 1.5 to 3.9 per 100 person years, suggesting that this process is not uncommon in an HIV high-incidence population (1912). In addition, infected IVDUs have shown evidence of superinfection which in one patient appeared to be transient (4874). Moreover, superinfection was reported at a prevalence of 5% per year for individuals during primary infection (4179, 4180).

In some cases, superinfection seemed to occur during primary infection shortly after seroconversion (3659). Conceivably, the initial immunologic response was not sufficient to prevent subsequent infection. This importance of the immune response in preventing superinfection could be inferred from another case in which an individual placed early on treatment after acute HIV infection subsequently had evidence of superinfection (84). Despite a substantial CD8+ T-cell antiviral response, the superinfecting virus appeared to be resistant to this immunologic response. Conceivably, the antiviral therapy, which is known to reduce anti-HIV immune responses (4309) (see Chapter 14), could have made the individual more susceptible to the superinfection. Nevertheless, a study using antiretroviral therapy in macaques showed that treatment during a primary infection induced protection from a later heterologous virus challenge (3805).

An additional study in Cameroon found several mixed infections involving a variety of HIV-1 clades (A, C, D, and F) as well as HIV-2. These mixed infections could represent coinfections instead of superinfections but highlight the particular possibility for recombination and development of new HIV strains (4367) (see below). Recombinant viruses found in an individual who was originally infected by one clade (4368) suggested that superinfection of the infected individual at the cellular level took place, since recombination can only occur within the cell (Section V).

In contrast to the findings with primary infection are results from a study of 14 HIV seroconcordant couples with a high risk of reexposure to virus in which no evidence of superinfection was noted (672). Similar findings were reported in studies of 37 HIV-infected IVDUs with samples collected after 1 to 12 years on therapy. A level of protection against superinfection seemed to be involved (4496). Moreover, in a study of 1,718 infected individuals, no evidence of superinfection was noted in 1,072 individuals during the first year of observation (1560). All these observations suggest that superinfection is uncommon in chronic infection but can occur in primary infection (4179).

C. Potential Factors Influencing Superinfection and Its Clinical Relevance

Most evidence supports the concept of a predominant virus strain in the infected host despite superinfection. The number of incoming virus particles would be quite small compared to the amount of virus already present in the blood and lymph nodes of the individual (2521) (see Chapter 2). Thus, establishing an infection with another strain would seem unlikely. Moreover, to some extent, down-modulation of CD4 on the surface of infected cells would block the extent of superinfection (2474). Nevertheless, as noted above, it could occur in cells with latent HIV infection that express CD4 (4661) (see Chapter 5, Figure 5.5).

An active immune system should be capable of eliminating or suppressing virus superinfection of the host through neutralizing antibodies, by antibody-dependent cellular cytotoxicity, and particularly by antiviral CD8$^+$ cells (see Chapter 11). As shown in cell culture studies with PBMC, antiviral antibodies produced in the host might prevent superinfection (1686). Moreover, CD8$^+$ cells can establish a state of resistance in the PBMC so that superinfection of the host is limited (257). A second virus can infect, but its replication is suppressed (257, 2095). Moreover, other immunologic responses may be involved in protection from superinfection besides CD8$^+$ cell cytotoxic and noncytotoxic activities. In a study of superinfection with wild-type pathogenic SIV following vaccination with live attenuated SIV, removal of CD8$^+$ lymphocytes with anti-CD8 antibodies did not dramatically change the resistance of the rhesus macaques to superinfection (4266). The role of the innate immune system should be considered (see Chapter 9).

The issue of superinfection becomes important if the superinfecting virus comes from a person receiving HAART. A resistant virus could be passed and remain relatively silent until the recipient of the virus began the drugs involved in this viral resistance. Preferential outgrowth of the transferred drug-resistant virus would take place (4181). That possibility is a major reason to encourage risk-free behavior between two HIV-infected people.

Importantly, superinfection with formation of a recombinant virus could produce HIV progeny with more cytopathic properties, with resistance to drugs or immune responses, and with a wider host range. The clinical consequences of this process occurring more frequently as the epidemic spreads need to be appreciated (for reviews, see references 390 and 495). It is still uncertain what impact superinfection has on the course of HIV infection. In some cases an accelerated disease progression was shown after presumed superinfection (1574). However, whether the virus or an already compromised immune system was responsible cannot be determined (for a review, see reference 4179).

Some researchers believe that the occurrence of superinfection suggests that development of an HIV vaccine will be very difficult or impossible (1391). However, superinfections occur with most viral infections (2531) despite previous infections or vaccinations. Past experiences with vaccines indicate that an efficient immune system can be induced that can block the transmission and spread in the host of related viruses (2531).

V. Recombination

During initial virus:cell interactions, the possibility of recombination between the genomes of two different viruses infecting the same cell should be considered. This process can take place if heterotypic viruses form (i.e., if the two RNA species within a virion core come from different viruses) (1918). The event could produce new viruses with different biologic and pathogenic properties. Recombination is detected in an HIV isolate by the appearance of genetic differences in specific regions of the viral genome (e.g., Gag and Env).

The first HIV-1 isolate to be identified as a recombinant was MAL (H2231), a clade A/D strain obtained from a 1976 blood sample from the Democratic Republic of Congo (63; for reviews, see references 2906 and 4601). Currently, circulating recombinant forms (CRFs) indicating the spread of recombinant viruses comprise 10 to 40% of clinical isolates in Africa (L. Demeter, personal communication) (see Chapter 1).

Recombination appears to occur within all regions of the viral genome but particularly the *gag* and envelope domains (897, 2083, 2906, 3756, 4961). It takes place primarily among viral subtypes. It has been reported with Chinese isolates between clade B and C viruses in the *tat* region (4322) and between B and F in several genomic regions (619). We now know that the former clades E and I represent recombinant viruses (see Chapter 1, Figure 1.10). Recombinant viruses from South America have shown evidence of recombination with A, G, J, and K clades and other unknown subtypes (3201, 4601). Obviously, the viral recombination event will be recognized only when regions having breakpoints do not interrupt gene expression.

Recent findings indicated that in vitro intraclade recombination among clade C viruses and clade B viruses occurred at similar rates but that an interclade recombination between clades B and C was much lower (747). A three-nucleotide sequence difference in the dimerization initiation signal region between clades B and C appeared to be responsible for this reduction in interclade recombination. Recombination obviously depends on matched sequences in the dimerization initiation signal region. Nevertheless, even recombinant viruses involving different groups of HIV-1 (M, N, and O) have been found (4368).

Several recombinants, often of three different clades (2762), have been identified. Some of these isolates represent secondary recombinations (e.g., CRF07-BC recombined with other strains) (4857). However, recombination of HIV-1 and HIV-2 does not seem feasible because their RNA dimer initiation hairpin sites are sufficiently different that they cannot form RNA heterodimers within the capsid (818, 1094).

As noted above (Section IV), recombination can occur if the cell is infected simultaneously by more than one virus, or if a cell is superinfected before the CD4 molecule is down-modulated and resistance is established (Section IV). This phenomenon could take place early in the infection process (the first 1 to 3 days), with a latently infected cell or a cell in which virus is suppressed (3611, 4661), or with cells infected by viruses that do not reduce CD4 protein expression on the cell surface (1231, 2474).

Some studies have indicated that HIV-1 can recombine approximately two or three times per genome per replication cycle, giving it a much higher rate of recombination than observed with other retroviruses (2024, 4961). Using a method employing different reporter viruses in vitro, a single round of HIV replication in T lymphocytes was found to give an average of nine recombination events per virus and even more in infected macrophages (2510). The genetic recombination rates, however, generally appear to be similar in T cells and macrophages (747). Essentially, under conditions in which the template is degraded efficiently by the RNase H enzyme (which can occur during transcription pausing), recombination is promoted (1160). Homopolymeric nucleotide tracks cause pausing of the reverse transcriptase enzyme and can thereby promote template switching and recombination (1160) (Figure 4.3).

Some studies have indicated that recombination in the Gag region occurs during reverse transcription at the early part of the coding region, which is unusually G rich and promotes extensive pausing by reverse transcriptase in vitro (1160) (Figure 4.3). Other studies suggest local hot spots for recombination throughout the HIV genome (4961). The C2 envelope domain appears to be a

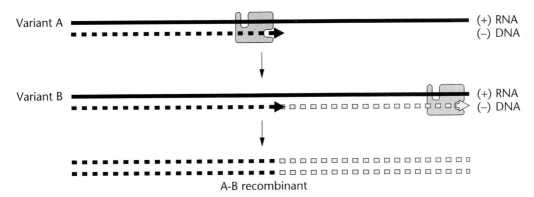

Figure 4.3 Steps involved in recombination. This diagram illustrates how recombinants can be generated during reverse transcription through strand transfer. The plus-strand genomic RNAs of two genetically distinct HIV variants coinfecting a cell are shown. In the example shown here, reverse transcriptase (represented as a gray rectangle) initiates synthesis using the plus-strand genomic RNA of variant A as a template. As synthesis proceeds, conditions may arise that cause the reverse transcription and the nascent minus-strand DNA copied from variant A (shown as a dotted black line) to transfer to the variant B genomic RNA. Synthesis then proceeds, using the variant B genomic RNA as a template (shown as a dotted line). The resultant proviral DNA contains sequence information from both variants A and B. The process outlined here is referred to as strand transfer and can be carried out by reverse transcriptase in vitro. Provided by L. Demeter.

"hot region." Moreover, the secondary structure of RNA may enhance recombination (e.g., hairpin structures) (2024). In addition, G-to-A mutations occur at a high frequency within runs of G residues. Highly G-rich regions can both promote recombination and be sensitive to G-to-A substitutions (perhaps reflecting APOBEC3G activity; see Chapter 5) (1160).

The process of homologous recombination could allow two defective viruses to become cytopathic (2216) and could introduce new strains into the population, thereby challenging therapy (via drug resistance) and vaccine approaches (1635,

2083, 3756, 3860). In one experiment involving the inoculation of two poorly replicating mutant SIV strains into a monkey, competent recombinant virus was recovered within 2 weeks (4817). In another SIV study, selected mutant viruses with deletions in *vpx, vpr,* and *nef* were administered simultaneously or sequentially by intravaginal inoculation. Recombination occurred in vivo (2193). However, if a more highly replicating mutant was given first, recombinants did not form (2193). The latter finding most likely reflected the dominance of the first virus that prevented conditions that would permit superinfection (Section IV).

SALIENT FEATURES • CHAPTER 4

1. Acute virus infection is characterized by a clinical state (the acute retroviral syndrome) that involves a flu-like illness and often a macular-papular rash. This clinical syndrome occurs in 50 to 90% of infected people and generally predicts a more rapid clinical course.

2. Acute infection is defined as the first 1 to 4 weeks after virus transmission before antiviral antibodies are detected. Virus RNA can be found in the blood within 2 to 14 days. Peak viremia occurs after about 3 weeks.

3. Primary or early HIV infection refers to the first 3 to 6 months following acute infection when HIV antibodies appear.

4. Detection of anti-HIV antibodies is performed by an enzyme-linked immunosorbent assay technique and confirmed by supplemental testing (e.g., immunoblotting or indirect immunofluorescence assay).

5. HIV infection can also be detected by examining urine and saliva for antiviral antibodies, but the sensitivity is less than that of measuring serum antibodies. The level of anti-HIV antibodies in sera can estimate the time of HIV transmission.

6. Based on the presence of RNA levels with or without anti-HIV antibodies, a staging of primary HIV infection has been proposed.

7. During acute infection, levels of certain cytokines associated with immune activation are increased in the plasma and can be involved in the acute retroviral syndrome.

8. During acute HIV infection, the individual can have very high levels of plasma virus (e.g., 10^7 RNA copies/ml). Several billion viruses are produced daily, primarily by activated CD4$^+$ T cells. Generally, the R5-type virus predominates in early infection. Virus can also be found in the cerebrospinal fluid and genital fluids of infected individuals.

9. HIV can be transmitted from the mucosae by trancytosis involving the basolateral layer of epithelial cells.

10. Dendritic cells (DCs) as well as CD4$^+$ T lymphocytes and macrophages in the mucosae are the first cells infected. Virus replication in DCs is generally at a low level. In some cases, a transfer of HIV from infected and uninfected DCs takes place. Within 2 days, regional lymph nodes show evidence of HIV infection.

11. In lymphoid tissues, CD4$^+$ T cells, DCs, and differentiated macrophages are the first sites of virus replication. Virus is also found associated with follicular dendritic cells (most probably not infected) and can be passed by these cells to activated CD4$^+$ cells present in the lymphoid tissue.

12. During acute infection, CD4$^+$ cell numbers are reduced and CD8$^+$ cell numbers are increased. The decrease in CD4$^+$ cell number is very prominent in the gastrointestinal tract. Subsequently, in the blood, the CD4$^+$ cell number may return to a near-normal level but remain reduced in relation to the CD8$^+$ cell number. CD4$^+$ cells do not generally return to normal levels in the blood.

13. High viral replication during the acute syndrome is subsequently reduced, most probably reflecting cell-mediated immune activities. A polyclonal CD8$^+$ cell response reflected by the T-cell repertoire is associated with a better prognostic course. Neutralizing antibodies are not frequently detected in primary infection.

14. HIV is a polytropic virus and can infect many cells in the body. CD4$^+$ lymphocytes produce the highest levels of the virus, and the extent of virus replication can depend on the specific CD4$^+$ cell subset infected. Variations in virus production can be observed in cells from different individuals. These variations reflect levels of receptor expression, intracellular factors, and the virus isolate involved.

15. Infected macrophages can remain as reservoirs of HIV, continually producing virus, although some cytopathic virus strains destroy these cells.

16. The number of circulating CD4$^+$ lymphocytes infected by HIV can vary from 1 in several million in asymptomatic and long-term survivors and from 1 in 10 in symptomatic individuals. In the bowel, this number during acute infection can reach 80% of CD4$^+$ cells. After primary infection, most infected cells in the blood and lymph nodes are in a latent state that eventually can be activated to release virus.

17. In the brain, the major cells infected are the macrophages and microglia, but astrocytes, oligodendrocytes, and capillary endothelial cells can also be infected at various frequencies. Perivascular macrophages expressing CD163 are major targets of HIV infection.

18. In the bowel, a variety of mucosal cells can be infected, but they may be detected at a low level in comparison to the large number of infected CD4$^+$ lymphocytes and macrophages infected in the gastrointestinal tract.

19. HIV isolates can differ in their kinetics and level of replication in different cell types. How a virus replicates in vivo has been termed as its relative fitness.

20. In the host, superinfection can occur but resistance may be established once the immune system has responded effectively (i.e., in chronic infection). Coinfection of individuals with two HIV-1 isolates, or with HIV-1 and HIV-2, can take place and appears to be most common in acute or primary infection. The immune response, particularly by CD8$^+$ cells, most probably controls the relative ability to have more than one dominant strain within an infected host.

21. Recombination occurs when two viruses infect the same cell. It can take place within all regions of the viral genome.

22. Recombination takes place with virus from the same clade, other clades, or other virus groups.

23. Recombination does not involve an HIV-1 and HIV-2 isolate because the RNA dimer initiation hairpin sites are different.

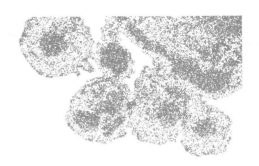

Intracellular Control of HIV Replication

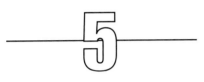

Early Intracellular Events in HIV Infection

Natural Intracellular Resistance to HIV Replication

Interaction of Cytokines and Viral Proteins with Cellular Factors

Virus Infection of Quiescent Cells

Latency

T HE DISCUSSION THUS FAR HAS FOCUSED on early events involved in HIV interaction with the cell. This interaction can be influenced by the specific virus involved, the cellular receptors expressed (see Chapter 3), and the nature of the cells infected (see Chapter 4). Once virus entry takes place, various functions of the virus determine its ability to replicate. The infectious cycle is also influenced by intracellular proteins, which may vary for different cell types. Thus, virus entry alone does not necessarily signify productive infection. In this chapter, the virus:cell interactions that take place within the intracellular compartment are considered. Details on the molecular events involved can be obtained from recent reviews (571, 1618, 1620).

I. Early Intracellular Events in HIV Infection

A. Overview of HIV Replicative Cycle

After HIV has entered the cell as a ribonucleocapsid, several intracellular events take place that lead to the integration of a proviral form into the cell chromosome (Figure 5.1). In an early step, the HIV RNA exits from the viral capsid with the help of the capsid protein, p24, in association with cyclophilins (2686; for review, see reference 931). Cyclophilin A (CypA) is a peptidylprolyl isomerase that binds to the capsid protein (CA) and can help with HIV replication. It is present in HIV virions because of its direct interaction with the Gag protein during virion assembly (see below). Its facilitating role in virus production is dependent on its presence in the target cells (1762). This process is sensitive to the inhibitory effects of cyclosporine (4340, 4410) (Section II.B).

Still associated with core proteins (primarily MA), the viral RNA undergoes reverse transcription by using its RNA- and

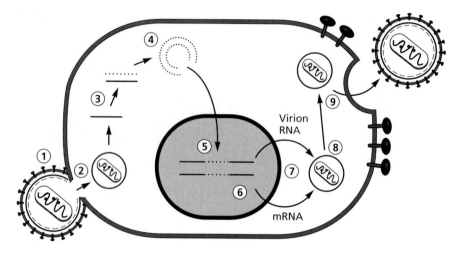

Figure 5.1 The HIV infection cycle. The steps are as follows: 1, attachment; 2, uncoating; 3, reverse transcription; 4, circularization; 5, integration; 6, transcription; 7, translation; 8, core particle assembly; and 9, final assembly and budding. In steps 3 to 5, some viral core proteins are associated with the viral genome (——, RNA, - - - -, DNA). Double-stranded circular forms can be found both covalently and noncovalently bound. The latter are the forms that integrate into the cell chromosome. Antiviral therapies can be directed against each step and can potentially interrupt virus replication and spread. Figure provided by H. Kessler.

DNA-dependent DNA polymerase and RNase H activities and eventually forms a double-stranded DNA copy of its genome (cDNA) (for reviews, see references 571, 3362, and 3483). For efficient reverse transcription, the nucleocapsid (NC) protein p7 appears to act like a chaperone protein (1273, 2685). It increases the proportion of long cDNA transcripts produced by reverse transcription (1273) and later, before budding, plays a role in the efficient packaging of genomic RNA (334, 2685). This NC protein contains two retroviral zinc fingers that are essential for its function (1136).

The resulting cDNA is part of the preintegration complex (PIC) that has been reported to contain the viral MA, Vpr, and integrase (IN) proteins (551, 1791). The MA protein may not be required in the PIC (1254, 3691). Moreover, Vpr in the PIC may help in virus nuclear import (see Chapter 8) but also is not required (469, 3691). The IN protein has a short nuclear localization signal sequence which is needed for PIC entry but is not involved in the protein's enzymatic activity (469). The PIC is transported to the nucleus as a nuclear pore complex. The linear viral DNA then becomes integrated into the cell chromosome via a process involving integrase and host cell factors (for reviews,

see references 931 and 2476). In this regard, recent studies show that emerin, an integral inner nuclear envelope protein, may be necessary for HIV replication (1992). Without emerin, the interaction of the viral cDNA with chromatin and subsequent integration may not take place (see Chapter 7).

This integration of the HIV provirus appears to occur primarily in transcriptionally active regions of the host genome, particularly those activated by HIV infection (442, 3030, 4000). The integration could involve a specific nuclear complex of viral integrase with the human lens epithelium-derived growth factor/transcription coactivator p75 (LEDGE/p75) protein. LEDGE/p75 is a chromatin-associated cellular protein that appears to protect cells from stress-induced apoptosis (737) and is a major chromatin-tethering factor for integrase (737, 784). LEDGE/p75 appears to target HIV integration at transcription sites, particularly those having less GC-rich sequences (784). However, whether tethering of integrase to chromatin via LEDGE/p75 determines the selection site for integration is still under study (784, 2757).

The karyophilic transport of the PIC can depend on an interaction of MA and Vpr with a cellular karyopherin complex containing cyclophilins

(1415). As noted above, the cellular protein CypA, found to be associated with Gag within the virion, is involved early in the replicative cycle of HIV-1. This function, however, does not seem to be required, since the Gag proteins of other replicating retroviruses, including HIV-2, SIV, and HIV-1 group O isolates, do not bind to CypA (478, 1354, 4410). In addition, using green fluorescent protein-labeled viral particles, some investigators (2913) were able to show that HIV, after entry, associates with cytoplasmic cytoskeletal components and moves possibly to the microtubular network, where it undergoes reverse transcription before the capsid protein is lost. Then after its formation, the PIC travels to the nuclear membrane, where it enters through nuclear pore structures (see also Chapter 7 for the role of Vpr). Generally, cell activation enhances HIV infection (2807) by permitting an easier entry of the PIC into the nucleus.

Following virus integration, the earliest mRNA species made in the infected cell are doubly spliced transcripts encoded by the major regulatory genes, particularly *tat*, *rev*, and *nef* (1620, 3362). The *nef* mRNA represents the majority (80%) of these species (3750), although it is not known which viral protein is made first.

Whether infectious HIV can be produced without integration of the provirus into the cell chromosome is still not certain. In several studies, HIV integration was found to be necessary for efficient virus progeny production (1204, 3879). In one study with an SIV *int/nef* mutant, SIV replication was greatly reduced (4617), although some expression of viral antigen took place. Currently, integration is considered necessary for virus progeny production, but HIV protein expression (e.g., Nef or Gag) may take place (4827).

The regulating cell proteins are needed in the initial steps of infection of resting cells, and thus their early transcription is important and could explain the Nef and Tat epitopes predominantly recognized by cytotoxic T lymphocytes in acutely infected subjects (see Chapter 11) (3362). Presumably, the extent of production of viral proteins can determine whether HIV infection leads to a productive or latent state. High-level expression of Tat will activate substantial virus production (980, 1300). Nef has a pleiotropic role and usually increases virus replication depending on the cells infected and the particular Nef allele involved (for review, see reference 1620) (see Chapter 7).

The Rev protein appears to provide a balance in the expression of regulatory and structural proteins of HIV. Rev encourages the transport into the cytoplasm of large, unspliced mRNA species responsible for the viral structural gene products and enzymes that give rise to infectious viruses (1266, 4197). Its function depends on certain cellular factors (e.g., CRM-1 and hRIP) (4896; for a review, see reference 1620) (see Chapter 7). Early studies with Mason-Pfizer monkey virus identified a viral gene that can substitute for Rev by interact-

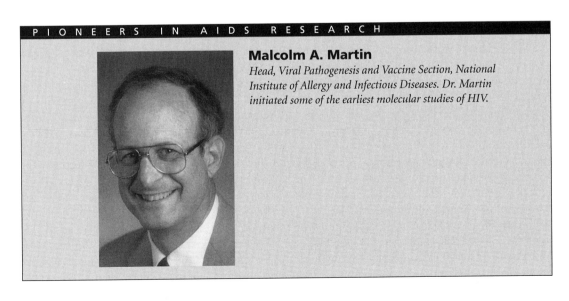

P I O N E E R S   I N   A I D S   R E S E A R C H

Malcolm A. Martin

Head, Viral Pathogenesis and Vaccine Section, National Institute of Allergy and Infectious Diseases. Dr. Martin initiated some of the earliest molecular studies of HIV.

ing with a cellular factor involved in mRNA transport (487). In the late stages of the virus replicative cycle (Figure 5.1), Rev could down-regulate its own production and cause decreased progeny virus formation and perhaps latency. In cells not fully permissive to HIV replication, the relative expression of the regulatory proteins can differ, leading to abortive infection, low persistence, or a latent state (3569) (Section V).

Viral assembly takes place at the cell membrane, where viral RNA is incorporated into capsids that bud from the cell surface, taking up the viral envelope protein. The incorporation of gp120 and gp41 into the virion envelope involves the association of the cytoplasmic tail of gp41 with the Gag (Pr55) protein (3173, 4831). There are two major models for HIV-1 budding (1555). One involves lipid "rafts" on the plasma membrane that are enriched in sphingolipids and cholesterol. Gag and Gag/Pol precursors localize to these rafts, and HIV preferentially buds from these regions (3249). This attachment of the virion to rafts is influenced by sufficient amounts of cholesterol and appears to be important for HIV assembly and release (2785, 3337; for a review, see reference 595). Nef may play a role in increasing the synthesis of cholesterol and its incorporation into virions (4947).

The other model is called the Trojan exosome hypothesis (1586). It appears to be a process more common in macrophages and involves the assembly of HIV in multivesicular bodies to which the virus buds. These bodies come to the cell surface and fuse with the plasma membrane, releasing the virus as an exosome.

For virus budding to take place, the cell membrane is broken and then resealed to form discrete viral and cellular membranes. The virus recruits cellular proteins to assist in this process, and the docking site for the Gag protein, which drives HIV-1 assembly, is p6. Since this Gag protein is most important at the very late stages, it is considered part of the L domain (see above). One of the proteins that participates in the disruption of the cell membrane for the release of the virus is the product of the human tumor susceptibility gene 101 (Tsg101). It is related to the ubiquitin-conjugating (E2) enzymes and binds p6. It facilitates HIV budding by trafficking Gag to the cell membrane and helping particle maturation and virus

release from the cell. Tsg101 may also prevent Gag polyubiquitination and degradation (1454a, 4592a).

The mature capsid at the time of budding resembles a fullerene cone (2575). Final maturation of the virion proteins, mediated by the viral protease, occurs within the budding particle. The capsid p2 protein as well as Vpu (see Chapter 7) is involved in the final steps of virus particle assembly (14; for reviews, see references 1360 and 4633). As noted above, for many HIV-1 isolates, cyclophilins can also play an important role in the assembly process through their association with the capsid protein (2685; for a review, see reference 931).

B. Differences in Virus Production: Role of Intracellular Factors

T-cell activation and monocyte differentiation can influence the extent of viral expression (see Chapter 4). These observations emphasize the role of intracellular factors in the HIV replicative cycle. Although the HIV long terminal repeat (LTR) alone can be its own promoter, early mRNA transcription appears to rely primarily on binding to the LTR by cellular transcription factors such as nuclear factor kappa B (NF-κB), NFAT, AP-1, SP-1, and the Tat binding proteins (for reviews, see references 1620 and 3362) (Figure 7.2). Thus, the intracellular milieu can determine the relative dominance of viral regulatory proteins in an infected cell. In this regard, cDNA microarrays conducted on acutely infected CD4+ T cells indicated that genes involved in T-cell signaling, subcellular trafficking, and transcriptional regulation are differentially regulated (1479).

Further evidence of this intracellular control is provided by biologic studies showing variations in replication of HIV isolates in different cell lines and peripheral blood mononuclear cells (PBMC) from various donors (Figure 4.2) (638, 639, 821, 1230, 2551, 4625). Variations in the infectibility of macrophages from different sites in the body have also been reported (925, 3327) (see Chapter 4). Viral binding and entry can be similar, but the post-entry events differ, so titers of the progeny viruses produced vary widely (see below). The data with HIV infection of PBMC are most dramatic, and the various viral and intracellular factors responsible could influence virus spread and pathogenesis in the host (see Chapter 13).

Intracellular blocks can affect early and late steps in reverse transcription, formation of the PIC, and transport of the PIC to the cell nucleus. With peripheral blood T lymphocytes arrested in cell division, for example, virus infection is abortive at steps prior to integration, primarily reflecting a block in PIC entry into the nucleus (Section II.C). In nondividing macrophages or epithelial cells, progeny virus production can take place (Section II.D) because the PIC passes the nuclear membrane. CD4$^+$ cells become sensitive to infection after they have moved into the G_{1b} stage of the cell cycle. CD3 activation alone results in a G_{1a} transition only with incomplete HIV-1 reverse transcription. Costimulation involving the CD3 and CD28 molecules permits a completed virus transcription process (2285). In astrocytes, the decrease in translation of viral proteins appears to be mediated by high levels of a double-stranded RNA binding protein kinase that results from low expression of a PKR antagonist, the transactivating response region (TAR) RNA binding protein (TRBP) (3336).

In permissive activated T cells, HIV undergoes integration and replication within 24 h (2197). In macrophages, the process is similar, but progeny production may take 36 to 48 h (3167). The latter result could reflect the slower incorporation of nucleotide precursors in these nondividing cells (3310). However, under conditions of stimulation with macrophage colony-stimulating factor (M-CSF), replication in macrophages is more rapid and very efficient (1790, 2356).

These differences in intracellular replication of HIV can be studied after virus entry by transfecting molecular cDNA clones of HIV-1 into cells. The results again show variations depending on cell type. In general, human cells replicate HIV to the highest levels, compared with cells of other animal species, particularly the mouse (2534). Similar observations are made with phenotypically mixed particles that introduce the HIV genome into heterologous cells via a different viral envelope (596) (see Chapter 3, Section VIII). After undergoing reverse transcription from their own RNA genome, the respective viruses replicate to various degrees in cells. Intracellular control of virus replication has also been observed with other retroviruses (2513). These observations indicate either the presence of a cellular inhibitory factor or the relative lack of a cellular product needed for viral replication (see below).

Some studies with human:animal cell hybrids have suggested the dominance of the permissive state for virus replication. Thus, the absence of a particular cellular protein appears to limit viral production. Human:hamster and human:mouse cell hybrids have implicated human chromosome 12 in coding for a permissivity factor that enhances Tat activity (1747, 3244). Several candidate cellular proteins participating in Tat activity have been considered (1055, 1825, 3231, 4104) (see Chapter 7, Section II). An 83-kDa TAR RNA loop binding protein has been identified (1748).

Other experiments have demonstrated that resistance of a cell to HIV infection can be dominant, and a factor in murine cells that acts against the *rev* gene has been described (4486). These inhibitors of Tat and Rev activities in murine cells act by independent mechanisms (4792) and could be considered in potential approaches to antiviral therapy. The discovery of the antiviral effects of TRIM5α also has relevance to these findings (Section II.B).

C. Replication in T Cells

In T cells, activation is important for HIV replication and involves the conventional interaction of intracellular factors with regions in the viral LTR (2048, 3193; for reviews, see references 1620 and 3362). The viral Tat protein is involved (see below). This cell activation is part of a signal transduction process by which the binding of mitogens or antigens within the major histocompatibility complex molecules to the surface T-cell receptor (TCR [CD3]), coupled with costimulation via the interaction of CD28 with B7 molecules, affects gene expression in the cell (for reviews, see references 2618 and 3698). LFA-3 interaction with CD2 can also activate lymphocytes in a costimulatory manner (3429). The process is mirrored by an increase in the concentration of intracellular free calcium and depends on the activation of calcium-dependent protein kinase C and other phosphorylation events (Figure 5.2) (2210, 3362, 4445).

During steps in this T-cell stimulation, transcriptional factors are activated. For example, NF-κB is normally associated with its inhibitor, IκB (for a review, see reference 261). However, phosphorylation

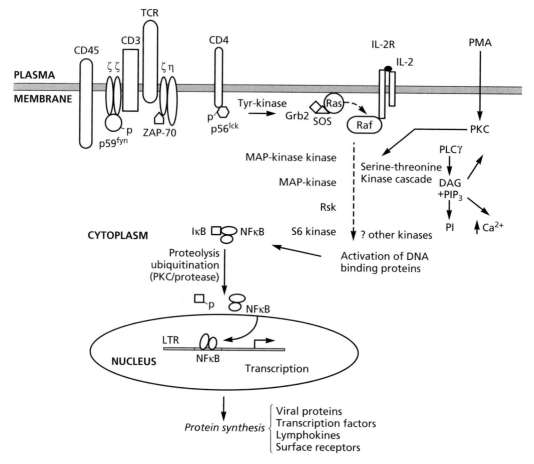

Figure 5.2 Schematic diagram of intracellular signaling events that occur during T-cell activation. The activation process begins with the generation of a signal at the plasma membrane (top of figure) mediated by receptor-ligand interactions, e.g., interleukin-2 receptor (IL-2R) + IL-2, a receptor-linking T-cell receptor (TCR) + CD4 interaction, or passage of membrane-permeating molecules (e.g., phorbol myristate acetate [PMA]) across the membrane. In the case of the TCR, stimulation results in the activation of tyrosine kinases (top left of figure), such as Fyn (p59^{fyn}), ZAP-70, and Lck (p56^{lck}). This action is probably regulated by tyrosine phosphatases such as CD45. The activated tyrosine kinases phosphorylate a number of different cytoplasmic substrates that initiate a chain of signaling events. These steps usually involve the association of intermediate signaling molecules. As an example, Ras (top middle of figure) can be activated upon binding to Grb2 and SOS. This action results in the activation of cytoplasmic serine kinases such as Raf, which initates a cascade of serine-threonine kinases (e.g., MAP kinase kinase, MAP kinase, Rsk, and S6 kinase), thereby propagating the activation signal. The serine-threonine kinase cascade results in the activation of DNA-binding proteins and transcription factors which regulate gene expression. Phosphorylation and/or proteolysis of IκB in the cytoplasm (bottom left of figure) dissociates it from NF-κB and permits the translocation of NF-κB across the nuclear membrane so that it can bind to DNA and activate transcription and protein synthesis. This signal transduction process can also be initiated by the stimulation of protein kinase C (PKC) by phorbol esters (e.g., PMA) (top right of figure). Activated PKC stimulates phospholipase Cγ (PLCγ) to generate the secondary messengers diacylglycerol (DAG) and phosphoinositol trisphosphate (PIP3), a process which results in the mobilization of intracellular calcium (Ca^{2+}) and liberation of phosphoinositol (PI). Figure and legend provided by E. Sawai.

of IκB by protein kinase C dissociates IκB from NF-κB and allows the translocation of NF-κB into the nucleus, where it binds to a region of the LTR sequence of the HIV provirus (3272) (Figure 7.2). The interaction of these cellular transcriptional factors with viral LTR domains can up-regulate viral replication (3362) or repress it (e.g., YYI) (2809). With some X4 virus mutants, a loss in expression of NF-κB DNA binding proteins was shown to be associated with a reduction in HIV replication (3629). Nevertheless, some HIV-1 isolates and an SIV mutant lacking the LTR NF-κB site can replicate well in PBMC (1954, 2499, 4936). Moreover, an NF-κB SIV mutant can induce AIDS in monkeys (1954). Identification of all the cellular factors involved in the replicative cycle is an ongoing endeavor (for reviews, see references 1556 and 3362). Certain cytokines and hormones, as well as transactivating proteins from other viruses, can also increase HIV production via these intracellular events (1501, 2210, 3232) (Section III).

After HIV infection of a CD4$^+$ cell, displacement of the Src family tyrosine kinase p56^{lck} from the CD4 molecule could take place, leading to activation of protein kinase C and increased virus production (Figure 5.2) (3362, 4445). Since p56^{lck} appears to have a variety of intracellular targets such as the interleukin-2 (IL-2) receptor (1757), it could either directly or indirectly affect the activity of cellular factors binding to the HIV LTR.

In some early studies, attachment of native gp120 to CD4 alone activated CD4$^+$ lymphocytes, as measured by an increase in intracellular levels of inositol triphosphate and calcium, as well as induction of expression of the IL-2 receptor (1287, 2287). This observation, however, was not confirmed by others, who have reported no effect of HIV binding on cellular or CD4 phosphorylation patterns, CD4-associated p56^{lck} kinase activity, or calcium influx (3345, 4645). Furthermore, the calcium channel inhibitor verapamil has shown no effect on HIV entry (3345). Thus, a role for calcium influx in the initial events in HIV infection of T cells is not established. Nevertheless, as discussed in Chapter 8, gp120 can induce calcium influx in certain neural cell lines by a mechanism blocked by verapamil, but not involving the CD4 protein (1133). In brief, signaling via CD4 does not seem to be important in HIV production.

It is noteworthy that memory CD4$^+$ cells in some studies have shown a postentry block to R5 HIV-1 replication which is not observed with X4 viruses (3578, 4640). The mechanism is not known but could explain a lower pathogenicity of the R5 viruses for CD4$^+$ memory T cells. In addition, resting CD4$^+$ cells seem to be resistant to HIV infection via a function of the intracellular protein APOBEC3G (Section II.A).

D. HIV Replication in Monocytes/Macrophages

Studies of peripheral blood monocytes indicate that intracellular events also influence the extent of productive infection. A selective intracellular block in replication of certain HIV-1 isolates in macrophages can be demonstrated (Table 5.1). For example, by PCR techniques, non-macrophage-tropic (X4) virus isolates have been shown to enter macrophages but to undergo only limited reverse transcription (1924, 3105, 3589, 3975, 4473). A delay in reverse transcription and nuclear import of the PIC takes place (1182, 3974) (see Chapter 4).

With monocytes, differentiation into macrophages (e.g., via CD40 ligand [CD40L]) rather than activation is most important for susceptibility to HIV infection (4208). An increase in CD4 and chemokine coreceptor expression could be involved (223, 318). Recent studies suggest a role for APOBEC3G in this process (755) (Section II.A). Uncultured, freshly isolated blood monocytes show no evidence of reverse transcription after inoculation with HIV-1. In contrast, cells cultured for at least 24 h show reverse transcripts as well as evidence of virus integration (4208).

Some studies suggest that monocyte differentiation affects susceptibility by inducing NF-κB components with transcriptionally active heterodimers (2556). These observations provide molecular evidence that blood monocytes, despite the expression of HLA-DR, do not appear to be permissive to viral entry (3722, 4005, 4208, 4382, 4537) and thus are not susceptible to infection in vivo unless differentiation into macrophages has taken place (see also Chapter 4). Most studies indicate that HIV can infect a nondividing differentiated macrophage (4382, 4706) in which integration takes place (318, 4208). Terminally differentiated macrophages cultured for a long time are not very susceptible to HIV infection

Table 5.1 Level of arrest of virus replication in different cell types[a]

Cell	Virus	Level of block	Possible mechanism	Reference(s)
Macrophages	X4	Envelope processing	Intracellular factors	4284
		Reverse transcription (RT)	Intracellular factors	1182, 1924, 3105, 3974, 3975, 4003, 4473
		Nuclear import		1182, 3974, 4473
Monocytes[b]	R5	Entry	Cell surface receptor	223, 318, 4208
Monocytes	R5 and X4	Pre-RT[c]	APOBEC3G	755
GM-CSF-derived MDM	R5	Posttranscription[d]	Relative Hck:C/EBP-β levels	2269
Resting CD4+ cells	R5 and X4	Pre-RT or limited RT	ABOBEC3G, intracellular factors	755, 4293, 4383, 4903
T-cell line	R5	RT	Intracellular factors	1924

[a]GM-CSF, granulocyte-macrophage colony-stimulating factor; MDM, monocyte-derived macrophages; RT, reverse transcription.
[b]Undifferentiated macrophages.
[c]May involve binding to viral capsid or RNA.
[d]In contrast, M-CSF-induced MDM replicate R5 viruses.

(4537); the reason has not been elucidated but could involve low expression of cell surface receptors.

In some early studies, monocytes in the blood were found by PCR techniques to be infected (2057), but this observation has also only been reported in a few cases and in a low number of cells (216, 2921). By in situ PCR procedures, most infected monocytes/macrophages in the blood were shown not to produce virus (214). These findings place further emphasis on differentiated tissue macrophages as a primary site of virus infection. These cells could certainly be a source of virus replication in the spleen (see Chapter 4).

In terms of cytotoxic effects, granulocyte-macrophage CSF (GM-CSF)-induced monocyte-derived macrophages (MDM) are susceptible to R5 HIV infection, but replication is inhibited posttranscription (2269). In contrast, M-CSF-induced MDM are susceptible to high HIV production (2269). The difference observed can be explained by the relative expression of the Src-like tyrosine kinase human hematopoietic cellular kinase (Hck), which can bind to HIV Nef to make it active (3884). The relative resistance of macrophages to HIV-1 appears to be related to levels of Hck and the CCAAT-enhancer binding protein beta (C/EBP β). C/EBP β is expressed in the cell as large and small isoforms. High levels of Hck and the large C/EBP β isoform are found in M-CSF-induced macrophages. The small form is

found with low levels of Hck in GM-CSF-induced MDM in association with reduced virus replication. Thus, in the macrophage, the large C/EBP β form and Hck enhance virus production (2269). It is noteworthy that the small form can be induced by *Mycobacterium tuberculosis* infection and beta interferon (IFN-β), resulting in inhibition of HIV replication in macrophages (1552, 1885, 4703). These observations support previous findings that M-CSF produced during HIV infection of macrophages increases HIV replication (1487, 2356), whereas GM-CSF inhibits HIV production by macrophages (2143).

The particular macrophage cell factor(s) responsible for the block of X4 virus replication in macrophages is not yet known. Some viruses, particularly dualtropic ones, appear to be able to infect macrophages and replicate substantially (3200). These findings strongly suggest that the intracellular control of X4 viruses represents a particular pathway that can be avoided by R5 and R5/X4 viruses. Perhaps the X4 virus PIC is placed postentry into a compartment which does not have an efficient nuclear import. Macrophages exposed to lipopolysaccharides from gram-negative bacteria or other bacterial wall components will become susceptible to X4 viruses. This finding partly reflects an up-regulation of CXCR4 expression and the production of β-chemokines that can reduce R5 virus infection (340, 3110).

Work with SIV infection of macrophages has uncovered other potential roles of the envelope region in virus replication besides the interaction with cell surface receptors. Envelope recombinant mutants that replicate poorly in macrophages were found to enter with an efficiency similar to that of macrophage-tropic viruses, but steps involved in the late stages of reverse transcription were inhibited (3105). The mechanisms responsible could be induction of cytokines, signal transduction (i.e., following viral envelope interaction with the cell membrane), or events involving the processing of Env. In some studies of macrophage-tropic (R5) and non-macrophage-tropic (X4) isolates, the processing of the Env and Gag precursor proteins of an envelope chimeric virus was blocked (2033). Alternatively, some viral envelopes may not be processed appropriately (4284). A similar finding of an arrest in the reverse transcription process was reported with infection of a T-cell line by a macrophage-tropic R5 HIV-1 isolate (1924).

Following acute HIV infection, tissue macrophages in turn could pass the virus to T cells, but only after the lymphocytes are activated. Resting CD4$^+$ cells in the G_0/G_1 phase and lacking HLA-DR expression cannot be infected when cocultured with virus-releasing macrophages (S. B. Tang and J. A. Levy, unpublished observations). Moreover, direct cell-to-cell interactions appear to be necessary for efficient cell transfer to take place (1083, 3999). Similarly, the induction of monocyte-to-macrophage differentiation that increases HIV replication can depend on CD4$^+$ cell-monocyte contact (1083), most likely involving CD40L. These findings indicate that macrophages in tissues, particularly lymphoid organs, can be a major target and reservoir for HIV and help the spread of HIV in the host. This concept, however, does not explain why in situ PCR studies thus far have not shown many infected macrophages in lymphoid tissue (1194, 3292).

II. Natural Intracellular Resistance to HIV Replication

A. APOBEC3G

1. DISCOVERY AND FUNCTION

Several years ago, Malim and coworkers described a potential function of Vif that counteracted an intracellular anti-HIV activity in human cells. The cell resistance appeared to involve steps in the virus replicative cycle sensitive to an innate intracellular factor (4154). The findings were based on studies comparing HIV-1 variants lacking *vif* and wild-type HIV-1 having the *vif* gene. In selected cells it was shown that some T cells (e.g., the CEM-SS cell line) were fully permissive to both viruses but, more frequently, T-cell lines such as HUT 78 as well as PBMC were nonpermissive to the Vif– viruses. In the latter cells, the virus with the Vif deletion replicated up to 50-fold less. Vif seemed to interact with a cellular protein early in the infection process to enhance virus infectivity (2176).

Subsequent studies uncovered a human cellular gene initially called CEM-15 which inhibited HIV replication; its effect was abrogated by the Vif protein (4083). CEM-15 was then found to represent a known human cellular gene coding for the protein apolipoprotein B mRNA editing enzyme, catalytic polypeptide-like 3G (APOBEC3G), which causes DNA deamination (for a review of the APOBEC family of genes, see reference 932). APOBEC3G induces G-to-A mutations in newly synthesized viral DNA (1742, 2788, 4927). The activity leads to replacement of cytosine by uracil in the retroviral minus-strand DNA. Thus, this change creates an increased frequency of G-to-A mutations in the plus-strand DNA (Color Plate 11, following page 78). Inactivated progeny viruses result either because of the mutations or because of DNA degradation triggered by viral *N*-glycosidases and a basic nuclease. Vif, through its interaction with APOBEC3G, prevents the accumulation of these genetic mutations (2451) and ensures production of infectious HIV (for reviews, see references 1618, 2327, and 4890).

The catalytic domain of APOBEC3G is important for its function, and the zinc binding region is essential for its cytidine deaminase activity and antiviral effects. Another domain (CD1) is responsible for RNA binding and is required for incapsulation of APOBEC3G into viral particles (3222). Whether the viral genome RNA is needed for the incorporation of APOBEC3G into virions is not certain (2177, 3222), but the nucleocapsid domain of HIV Gag is essential (for a review, see reference 2327).

Vif induces the ubiquitization and degradation of APOBEC3G via the cellular proteins Cullen5

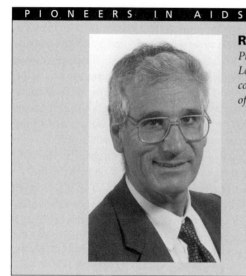

Robin A. Weiss

Professor of Viral Oncology, University College, London, England. Professor Weiss was one of the first to conduct studies on the cellular host range and biology of HIV.

(CUL5), elongens b and c, and RBX1 (2812, 4894) (Color Plate 11, following page 78). Two different domains of Vif appear to be involved in these functions: one that binds APOBEC3G and another that mediates its degradation via a proteosome-dependent pathway (2626, 2812). Vif also prevents the incorporation of APOBEC3G into virions, and thus new infections by the virus progeny can proceed without deamination (4084). The HIV viral RNA helps stabilize the association of APOBEC3G with the HIV-1 nuclear protein complex within the virion (2177). Once APOBEC3G is within virions, Vif may be less effective in blocking its antiviral activity (2626). APOBEC3F has been noted to have the same antiviral function as APOBEC3G and can be countered by Vif (4946). Most recently, another member of the human APOBEC family, APOBEC3DE, has been found to inhibit both HIV-1 and SIV via cytidine deaminase activity with some novel target site specificity (964b).

2. PRESENCE AND INTERACTION OF OTHER APOBEC3G PROTEINS

A similar activity for SIV is observed in monkey cells via the SIV_{mac} Vif protein, which is only 30% similar to HIV-1 Vif. Vif proteins from distantly related primate lentiviruses (SIV_{agm}) do not work against the human APOBEC3G because of the lack of their interaction with the human protein (2069). The functions of the human and monkey

APOBEC3G proteins are therefore species specific. A single amino acid change in APOBEC3G can switch the resistance patterns for HIV and SIV in monkey and human cells, respectively. Replacement of aspartic acid in the human APOBEC3G with a lysine in African green monkey (AGM) APOBEC3G (423) makes the resulting protein sensitive to SIV_{agm} Vif and resistant to HIV-1 Vif (4001) (Table 5.2). A reverse change in the AGM APOBEC3G makes it sensitive to HIV-1 Vif. Moreover, a single amino acid substitution in the conserved region of Vif can reduce its function (423, 2626, 4001).

On another note, human APOBEC3G shows antiviral activity with both HIV and murine retrovirus vectors produced from human and murine cells (2250) (Table 5.3). In contrast, murine APOBEC3G does not suppress infectivity of murine retroviral vectors but shows antiviral activity with both wild-type and *vif*-deleted virions of HIV-1 in human cells. The absence of an effect on murine retroviruses could be a lack of binding of murine leukemia virus (MLV) Gag to murine APOBEC3G (1100). These results suggest that the murine homologue has a different mechanism for blocking HIV-1. An interaction of the cellular protein with the virus seems to be involved. Moreover, an HIV-2 isolate lacking *vif* can grow in cell lines nonpermissive for HIV-1 *vif*-negative viruses (3719). These results most likely reflect other intracellular mechanisms for restricting HIV-2.

Table 5.2 Host-specific interactions of the cellular protein APOBEC3G with viral Vif proteins[a]

		Vif	
APOBEC3G	**Genetic change**	**HIV-1**	**SIV$_{agm}$**
Human	D128	+	−
	D128-K	−	+
Monkey (AGM)	K128	−	+
	K128-D	+	−

[a]Human APOBEC3G encodes aspartate (D) at position 128 and functionally interacts with HIV-1 Vif but not with SIV$_{agm}$ Vif. African green monkey (AGM) APOBEC3G encodes a lysine (K) at position 128 and functionally interacts with SIV$_{agm}$ Vif but not with HIV-1 Vif. The functional interactions can be reversed by mutating human APOBEC3G to K at position 128 and by mutating AGM APOBEC3G to D at position 128. A plus sign indicates that APOBEC3G will be sensitive to Vif, and a minus sign indicates resistance. Adapted from reference 2069 with permission. Copyright 2004 National Acadamy of Sciences, U.S.A.

In this regard, further evidence suggests that APOBEC3G can also affect RNA editing and non-editing pathways (381). Notably, this cellular protein deaminates single-stranded DNA but not double-stranded DNA or RNA/DNA hybrids (4890). APOBEC3G can inhibit hepatitis B virus and HTLV replication as well (3924, 4505), and the mechanism appears to be different from a cytidine deaminase activity (3806). In this regard, recent studies suggest that APOBEC3G and APOBEC3F may also have other roles in preventing HIV repli-cation besides hypermutation. Their ability to prevent the accumulation of reverse transcripts could be involved (380a). Other studies show that IFN-α can upregulate APOBEC3G in liver cells and macrophages but not in T lymphoid cells. The process does not involve the induction of STAT-1. These findings suggest that the interaction of IFN-α with APOBEC3G can elicit additional antiviral effects in liver cells and macrophages (3921a).

Finally, besides APOBEC3F, APOBEC3G, and APOBEC3DE, APOBEC3B when expressed in cells has been found to suppress the infectivity of both HIV with a Vif deletion and wild-type HIV prior to integration (424). It binds to the nucleocapsid domain of HIV Gag and can be packaged into progeny virions. APOBEC3B does not bind to HIV-1 Vif and therefore is not affected by Vif expression. It is not made in lymphocytes, but its activation in these cells might inhibit HIV infection (381, 1099).

3. OTHER POTENTIAL ROLES IN NATURE

The inability of the SIV Vif to block APOBEC3G in human cells could be a factor in SIV zoonotic infection. APOBEC3G may be a mechanism for prevention of transmission of monkey viruses to humans. The chimpanzee virus, SIV$_{cpz}$, a recombinant of the red-capped mangabey (*Cercocbus torquatus*) (SIV$_{rcm}$) and the greater spot-nosed monkey (*Cercopithecus nictitans*) (SIV$_{gsn}$) (220),

Table 5.3 Intracellular retrovirus restriction factors[a]

Restriction	Gene	Cell specificity[b]	Restriction site	Viral proteins involved[c]
HIV Vif⁻ virus	APOBEC3G	Primate cells (HIV)	RT at cytidine deaminase[d]	Vif
Ref-1	Trim 5α	Human cells (N-MLV, EIAV)	Prior to RT, binds to viral capsid[d]	Gag
Lv-1	Trim 5α	Rhesus macaque (HIV-1, N-MLV)	Prior to RT, binds to viral capsid[d]	Gag
Lv-1	Trim 5α	African green monkey (HIV-1, HIV-2, SIV$_{mac}$, N-MLV, EIAV)	Prior to RT, binds to viral capsid[d]	Gag
Lv-2	Trim 5α	Rhesus macaque (HIV-2)	After RT, binds to viral integration complex	Gag and Env
Fv-1	Endogenous MLV	Mouse cells (N-tropic and B-tropic MLV)	After RT and prior to provirus formation, binds to viral capsid	Gag

[a]RT, reverse transcription; N-MLV, NIH mouse cell-tropic murine leukemia virus; EIAV, equine infectious anemia virus.
[b]The virus(es) inhibited is in parentheses.
[c]Known or proposed.
[d]Other processes may be involved.

appears to have the *vif* gene of SIV$_{rcm}$ (see Chapter 1). Both SIV$_{cpz}$ and SIV$_{rcm}$ can grow in human cells.

The observations on APOBEC3G also seem to indicate that it could be a general defense mechanism against retroviruses, retrotransposons, and other mobile genetic elements (for a review, see reference 1941). In this regard, mice transgenic for deletion of the APOBEC enzyme have shown evidence of a greatly enhanced presence of endogenous transposons (1223). (For a review on the large family of cytidine deaminases and their potential role in various tissues, see reference 4506.)

Moreover, a role for APOBEC3G in preventing HIV infection of immature DCs (3523a) and of resting CD4$^+$ T cells and monocytes (755) has been suggested (755) (Table 5.1). Resting CD4$^+$ cells have a large quantity of APOBEC3G in a lower-molecular-weight mass (LMM) that can block virus replication by a different process. Upon activation, this LMM is transferred to a high-molecular-weight mass (HMM) in which the APOBEC3G now functions as a cytidine deaminase. While the HMM APOBEC3G is sensitive to Vif, the low-molecular-weight APOBEC3G has a different function unaffected by Vif that may involve binding to the incoming viral capsid or viral RNA (755, 3242).

The LMM of APOBEC3G predominates in unstimulated CD4$^+$ cells and monocytes and appears to block HIV replication. This LMM prevents replication of both the wild type and *vif* mutants. After cell activation, the LMM becomes part of the HMM and becomes inactive (755). Moreover, when monocytes are induced to differentiate to macrophages, the LMM is replaced by a high-molecular-weight complex (755) and replication of wild-type virus (containing Vif) can take place. This finding could explain the early postentry block to virus replication in monocytes and resting CD4$^+$ T cells. In resting primary CD4$^+$ cells, IFN-α can enhance the expression of APOBEC3G in association with the LMM. Thus, this process is another means by which interferon can block HIV replication (715a).

B. TRIM5α

Several early studies indicated a natural antiviral resistance in primate cells that limited, up to 50-fold, NIH mouse cell-tropic murine leukemia virus

(N-MLV) replication in human cells and HIV replication in rhesus macaque cells (1837, 4100). In human cells the gene responsible for blocking the replication of N-MLV as well as equine infectious anemia virus (EIAV) was named *Ref-1* for resistance factor 1 (4457). *Ref-1* appeared to act before reverse transcription. In monkey cells, the gene named *Lv-1* (911), for lentivirus susceptibility factor 1, was considered responsible for a block in HIV DNA synthesis prior to reverse transcription (1837, 3168, 3366). Both the *Ref-1*-restricted MLV replication in human cells and *Lv-1*-restricted HIV replication in monkey cells appeared to involve the virus capsid, and both restrictions could be countered by a high input of virus (350, 3366).

Differences in these intracellular restrictions could be appreciated depending on the cell lines tested and the viruses used (1761). These inhibitions of primate virus replication resembled that of the *Fv-1* locus in mice, which determines the tropism of different MLVs. *Fv-1* codes for a cellular protein that interacts with the MLV capsid to prevent virus replication (1541, 2318). This *Fv-1* gene appears to be derived from an endogenous retrovirus (352) and blocks MLV replication in mouse cells prior to reverse transcription (1541).

The solution to these primate intracellular blocks in retrovirus replication was solved with the finding that TRIM5α (tripartite motif protein 5α), a cytoplasm component, was the intracellular factor (4304, 4314) (Table 5.3; Figure 5.3). The TRIM family proteins are composed of an N-terminal RING domain, one or two B box type 1 or type 2 domains, and a coiled-coil region (for a review, see reference 3265).

The TRIM5α genes were found to be responsible for the *Ref-1* restriction of N-MLV and EIAV replication in human cells and the *Lv-1* block of HIV replication in monkey cells (1763, 2139, 4861). Notably, TRIM5α from rhesus monkey cells restricts HIV-1 replication but not SIV$_{mac}$ (4880). TRIM5α in human cells does not inhibit replication by HIV or other primate retroviruses (for a review, see reference 3265). In addition, AGM cells were found to block replication of HIV-1, HIV-2, SIV$_{mac}$, N-MLV, and EIAV but not SIV$_{agm}$. Again, a TRIM5α gene product was found to be responsible (1761, 2139, 4457). This innate cellular resistance is species specific (as is APOBEC3G), involving,

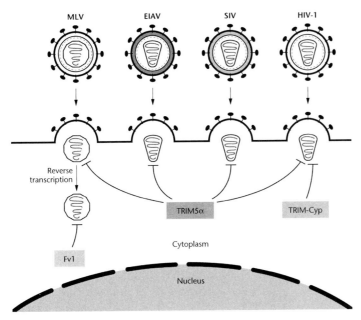

Figure 5.3 Capsid-specific restriction factors. After entry into the cytoplasm, retroviral capsids can be recognized and infection can be blocked by one of many factors. Fv-1, unique to the mouse, blocks infection by murine leukemia virus (MLV) only, in an Fv-1 allele- and MLV strain-specific way. TRIM5α, which is present in most primates, can block infection by a range of retroviruses, including N-tropic N-MLV, equine infectious anemia virus (EIAV), simian immunodeficiency virus (SIV), and HIV-1. The precise spectrum of TRIM5α antiretroviral activity depends on its species of origin. A unique form of TRIM5 exists in owl monkeys, due to transposition of a CypA pseudogene, and the resulting fusion protein inhibits HIV-1 because of the latter's CypA-core binding activity. Reprinted with permission from Macmillan Publishers: *Nature Immunology* (361), © 2004. CypA, cyclophilin A.

most likely, a block in the uncoating of the retroviral core (3366, 4315). In this regard, it resembles the activity of Fv-1 (1541). Another possible mechanism of TRIM5α action could be targeting viral particles for degradation (for a review, see reference 3265). TRIM5α acts at an earlier stage of reverse transcription than APOBEC3G and is not packaged in the virions.

This restriction of HIV replication in primate cells involves a differential interaction of the viral capsid with CypA. This host cellular protein binds to the HIV-1 CA protein (4458) and helps in the replication of many HIV-1 isolates (e.g., group M) (see above and Chapters 1 and 4). When cyclosporine, an antagonist of CypA, is used to treat monkey and human cells, different effects are seen. With monkey cells, the cyclosporine prevents the CA:CypA interaction and can increase HIV replication in these primate cells more than 100-fold. Therefore, this compound prevents the effect of Lv-1 (4458). In contrast, with human cells, cyclosporine blocks replication of HIV, most likely by also disrupting the CA:CypA complex. In this case, however, the complex appears to be important in preventing the effect of the TRIM5α restriction factor (*Ref-1*) in human cells (4458). The observation with cyclosporine suggests that HIV uses a cellular

protein to counteract the restriction factor expressed by human cells (4458).

These findings illustrate the dynamic interactions between the viral capsid protein, CypA, and TRIM5α. How the cyclophilin in rhesus macaque monkey cells is involved in the restriction of HIV-1 is not known, but it could be by bringing the viral core into contact with the rhesus TRIM5α. In this regard, the TRIM5α expressed in owl monkeys has been reported to have a CypA fusion protein that plays a role in the resistance of its cells to HIV-1 infection (3264) (Figure 5.3).

Similar to findings of a single amino acid change affecting APOBEC3G function (423), one amino acid difference in the SPRY domain of human TRIM5α can make it resemble the primate cell counterpart and confer a restriction to HIV-1 replication in human cells (3208, 4001, 4862). There is also a block to HIV-2 infection occurring after reverse transcription and before nuclear entry. This *Lv-2* restriction is mediated by the viral capsid and envelope (3980). Recent studies suggest that this postentry restriction is dependent on a lipid raft-dependent pH-independent endocytic pathway in which the viral envelope is the major determinant (2800).

Besides TRIM5α, other TRIM protein family members are involved in a variety of cellular pro-

Table 5.4 Natural intracellular resistance to HIV replication

Cellular protein	Mechanism of action[a]
APOBEC3G	Cytosine deaminase
TRIM5α (Lv-1/Ref-1)	Blocks HIV-1 capsid uncoating; affects reverse transcription
Lv-2	Blocks nuclear entry of HIV-2
Murr-1	Inhibits degradation of IκB
Unknown	Inhibits virus assembly[b]

[a]Other activities may be involved.
[b]Countered by Vpu.

cesses, including cell proliferation, differentiation, development, and oncogenesis (for a review, see reference 3265). Nearly 70 genes in the human genome appear to code for TRIM proteins (3265). Only a few have been fully characterized. One TRIM protein, TRIM32, has been shown to bind to the activation domain of the Tat protein (1371), although its function is not known. Another member of the TRIM family, TRIM22, was found to be an interferon-induced factor that can repress HIV LTR expression (4438). Its effect on HIV replication is not yet established (for a review, see reference 3265).

C. Other Processes

In studies on cellular host range sensitivities, a block of HIV replication in murine cells appeared to be at virion assembly (2810), not at the reverse transcription step. Another type of intracellular anti-HIV activity could be responsible. Moreover, Murr-1 has been recognized as a protein that can induce latent infection by inhibiting the degradation of IκB (1423). In addition, an intracellular factor has been detected that inhibits HIV assembly. It appears to be countered by Vpu (4571). This identification of natural intracellular resistances to HIV replication (Table 5.4) provides novel approaches for antiviral therapy.

III. Interaction of Cytokines and Viral Proteins with Cellular Factors

A. Cytokines and Intracellular Pathways of HIV Replication

Cytokines, particularly TNF-α, have been shown to affect intracellular transactivating factors within the viral LTR, particularly NF-κB (see Chapter 11) (1144, 1721, 2317, 3350, 3559) (for a review, see reference 3557) and can substantially increase HIV production (2871; for a review, see reference 3397) (see Chapter 8). Moreover, some viruses, such as cytomegalovirus and herpes simplex virus, can enhance HIV production through activation of the viral LTR, a process that can be mediated by a cytokine (3117, 3488) (see Chapter 13, Section III). Moreover, certain cytokines (e.g., IL-2 and IL-10) can modify the expression of CD4 and chemokine receptors and thus affect virus replication and viral isolates at the entry level (2357) (see Chapter 3, Table 3.6).

B. Effect of HIV Proteins

Tat binds to the TAR element of the viral LTR in conjunction with cellular RNA binding proteins (1825, 2080, 4822) that may be phosphorylated (1712) (see Chapter 7). Viral expression is subsequently up-regulated, following interactions of cellular proteins with other regions of the LTR (1825). Cellular proteins involved with Tat activity could increase Tat binding to the TAR region (75) or to promoters, such as AP-1, upstream from TAR (1825). Thus, two interactions of Tat with the viral LTR could be required to up-regulate HIV replication. The induction of TNF-α production in T cells by HIV Tat could also increase virus production (555, 3675). Other early experiments also suggested that two related cellular Tat binding proteins might compete to up-regulate (e.g., MSSI) or down-regulate (e.g., TBP-1) Tat activity and thereby affect HIV production (3231, 4104).

In this regard, cellular factors such as cyclin T1, hexim, and 7SK RNA can influence the extent of Tat activity by activating or inactivating the positive transcription elongation factor b (P-TEFb)-mediated mRNA elongation process (Figure 5.4). This complex, in association with Tat, helps in RNA transcription from the viral LTR (4859; for reviews, see references 246, 1620, 2619, and 3483). The Nef protein could also affect virus replication by interacting with cellular factors that may be involved in cellular activation (283, 3937). The role of viral proteins in HIV replication is further discussed in Chapter 7. The effect of other infectious agents on intracellular

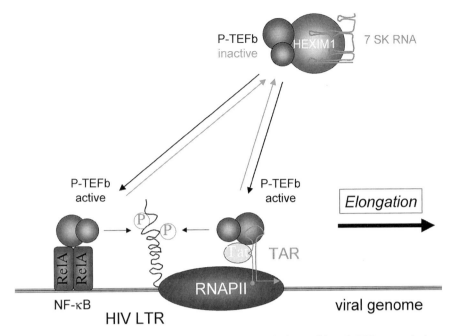

Figure 5.4 Positive transcription elongation factor b (P-TEFb) and HIV transcription. The viral promoter contains many common promoter elements, as well as enhancer sequences and the transactivation response (TAR) element. They recruit and position RNA polymerase II (RNAPII) on the HIV long terminal repeat (LTR). RNAPII then clears the promoter but stalls at or near TAR. P-TEFb, which consists of cyclin T1 (CycT1) and cyclin-dependent kinase 9 (CDK9), is necessary for transcription complexes to elongate. It phosphorylates the C-terminal domain of RNAPII. This change removes initiation and negative transcription factors from RNAPII and replaces them with capping, splicing, and polyadenylation machineries. P-TEFb exists in two forms in cells. The larger, inactive complex contains CycT1, inactive CDK9 kinase, HEXIM1, and 7SK RNA. The smaller, active complex contains only CycT1 and CDK9 and is required for effects of NF-κB and Tat. Most cells contain sufficient amounts of active P-TEFb to support HIV replication. The binding between NF-κB and P-TEFb allows for initial rounds of viral transcription. However, when sufficient amounts of Tat are made, then Tat and P-TEFb bind TAR with high affinity and lead to greatly increased rates of viral replication. Importantly, both NF-κB and Tat ensure that viral genes are copied and processed correctly. Figure provided by M. Peterlin.

processes governing HIV replication is discussed in Chapter 13.

IV. Virus Infection of Quiescent Cells

A. CD4⁺ Lymphocytes

The steps leading to productive viral infection and the consequences of that infection have been discussed. What happens when HIV encounters a "resting" lymphocyte is another important question. The initial experiments with HIV infection of lymphocytes indicated that virus replication occurred best with antigen- or mitogen-induced activation (272, 2807). When established T-cell lines were arrested in growth by drug treatment, HIV replication was blocked in some cells (4384) but unaffected in others (2568). These systems, however, did not reflect what may occur under normal conditions with peripheral blood CD4⁺ lymphocytes (135). In some studies, a previously activated CD4⁺ cell infected by HIV was shown to return to a resting infected cell state as defined by cell surface markers (e.g., CD69⁻ CD25⁻ Ki67⁻)

Anthony J. Pinching
Associate Dean (Cornwall) & Professor, Peninsula Medical School, University of Plymouth, United Kingdom. Dr. Pinching was one of the first physicians to establish clinical programs for HIV-infected individuals in Europe.

(690). This observation in cell culture merits further evaluation as a model for studying HIV latency in primary CD4+ lymphocytes.

1. PERIPHERAL BLOOD CD4+ CELLS: IN VITRO STUDIES

Early studies using nondividing peripheral blood CD4+ T cells have provided valuable information on the events involved in efficient virus infection and progeny production (Tables 5.1 and 5.4). The results indicate that the level of cell activation (expression of HLA-DR and CD25) can influence the extent of viral reverse transcription and release of infectious virus from the cell (3657, 4383). The processes required are discussed in Section I.A and below (Section IV.A.3).

CD4+ cells completely blocked in DNA synthesis and kept nonactivated (at G_0/G_1) (e.g., no HLA-DR and low CD25 expression) cannot be productively infected by HIV (1591, 4383). Despite the expression of CD4, these cells show no evidence of viral infection when subjected to subsequent cell activation procedures that can induce infectious virus production in culture. Molecular studies have shown that the virus enters the cell but usually only short transcripts of viral DNA are made; reverse transcription is either slow or not completed and cannot be induced after virus entry (4383). Preintegration forms are labile. Thus, the infection is abortive and decay processes in the cell

reduce the replicative competency of an infectious virus within 1 to 2 days (3509, 4952).

In contrast to the above observations on nondividing cells, some investigators have reported that resting CD4+ lymphocytes can be infected in vitro, and that virus replication is arrested but can be induced. The definition of "resting" is important since these cells may have previously been activated and still have intracellular factors expressed that help in HIV infection (Section I). Unintegrated viral cDNA forms can be detected by PCR in these resting T cells from a few days to 2 weeks after the initial infection (4293, 4383, 4903). Upon activation, these cells can then be induced to release infectious progeny viruses. These studies have suggested that HIV enters the "quiescent" cells, but only limited transcription of the viral gene takes place (4902, 4903). The virus is not integrated, and no viral proteins are produced. In certain cases, if these cells are not fully activated within 3 to 5 days, the infection is aborted (4903). In other situations, long cDNA viral forms may be made in the cell, and this unproductive viral infection can persist for 2 to 4 weeks (4293, 4383). In this type of infection, the PIC remains in the cytoplasmic compartment until activation leads to its rapid transport to the nucleus by a process requiring ATP and not cell division (552) (see Section I). Upon activation, full-length viral DNA is formed (4340) and integrated, followed by production of virus.

Again, the resting versus activation level in the cell needs to be considered. Quiescent cells lacking CD25 expression have been found to be completely resistant to HIV infection, most likely at the stage of entry, since no viral transcripts are detected (765). If cultured with CD25$^+$ CD4$^+$ cells, however, a nonproductive infection of the resting CD25$^-$ cells takes place, similar to those described above (4293, 4903). Some factors produced by CD25$^+$ cells (e.g., IL-2) must influence this process to place the target cells in a more responsive state.

Other experiments have shown that HIV can enter purified CD45RA$^+$ (resting) or CD45RO$^+$ (memory) CD4$^+$ cells, but only the CD45RO$^+$ CD4$^+$ (memory) cell cultures produced virus over time (4815). The studies suggested that the virus enters the CD45RA$^+$ naïve cell, but unless the cell is stimulated and activated, the infection is aborted, most likely because the PIC is not transported to the nucleus. These results conflict somewhat with those cited in Chapter 4 suggesting that chemokine receptor expression on naïve (CXCR4$^+$) versus memory (CCR5$^+$) cells can influence virus infection. In the cited studies, both cell types appear to express CXCR4 and are susceptible to X4 virus. However, activation determines the extent of HIV replication, as observed in the other studies described above. The data confirm and help explain previous work suggesting preferential infection of memory CD4$^+$ cells by HIV-1 (3778, 3991, 4235) (see Chapter 4).

In other studies with quiescent CD4$^-$ cells, HIV infection of macrophages appears to release factors that when interacting with B cells cause secretion of IL-6 that can make a resting CD4$^+$ cell sensitive to virus replication (4349). While these observations need confirmation, they do provide possible pathways by which resting cells could be infected even if not in a fully activated state; they can remain as long-term cellular reservoirs for HIV in the body.

2. QUIESCENT CD4$^+$ CELLS: IN VIVO STUDIES

The observations in vitro with purified quiescent CD4$^+$ cells have also been applied to clinical specimens. Purified CD4$^+$ cells from asymptomatic individuals consisted of a large percentage of resting cells that contained primarily unintegrated viral

DNA forms (553). These cells were reported to lack HLA-DR expression, but a low level of HLA-DR$^+$ cells was present in the cell population (0.3%) (553). Phenotypic analyses of the latently infected cells showed very little if any distinguishing evidence of virus infection (526). Thus, recognition by the immune system would be difficult. In subjects on highly active antiretroviral therapy, the number of latent CD4$^+$ cells can be reduced to levels of 1 million to 10 million cells (772, 774, 776, 1292); a small percentage of these cells will replicate virus when treatment is stopped (see Chapter 14). These latent cells are established early in acute HIV infection even in the treated subjects (774).

The findings on resting cells support the conclusion that in many CD4$^+$ cells of asymptomatic individuals, HIV can be present in an unintegrated noninfectious form after entry for perhaps many more days than suggested by studies in cell culture. Other cells in the blood, as discussed in Chapter 4, can also be present with integrated but nonexpressed viral mRNA or protein (3442, 3886, 4148). Possibly the CD8$^+$ cell producing the anti-HIV factor that suppresses virus replication contributes to this arrest in viral replication in quiescent cells in vivo (see Chapter 11). Conceivably, the free virus in the plasma (see Chapter 2) could be the source of repeated infection of quiescent cells that, unless activated, eventually lose the viral cDNA forms. If virus replication does not take place, CD4 expression on cells could remain intact and reinfection or superinfection would be possible (see Chapter 4). Thus, cycles of fluctuation in virus infection and loss could characterize a dynamic situation within an infected individual (Figure 5.5). Under these conditions, there is a chance of recombination from multiple infections of a cell (see Chapter 4).

3. INTRACELLULAR MECHANISM

The intracellular factors that might influence the extent of virus production in resting CD4$^+$ cells are being defined. They could involve cellular proteins that bind to DNA (e.g., NF-κB) and/or RNA and inhibit HIV replication (Section I.B). Moreover, as noted above, results with R5 and X4 HIV-1 isolates showing a block in reverse transcription in activated T-cell lines (1924) and in macrophages (1924, 3975) (Sections I.C and I.D), respectively, suggest

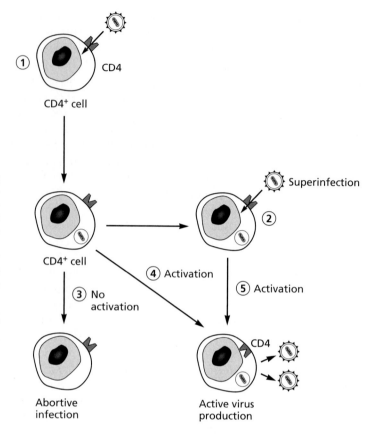

Figure 5.5 HIV can infect a resting CD4+ cell that expresses the CD4 molecule (step 1). If that cell is not activated, virus replication cannot take place. Because the CD4 molecule is still expressed on a resting cell, superinfection by another virus can occur (step 2). With no activation of the resting cell after infection, an abortive infection takes place (step 3). With activation, active virus replication takes place (step 4). Similarly, activation of the superinfected cell can lead to virus production, and both type viruses and recombinants might be found. Following activation and virus production (step 5), the CD4 molecule is downmodulated so superinfection cannot occur.

that similar intracellular mechanisms could be involved (Table 5.1).

Some of the in vitro and in vivo observations on limited reverse transcription of HIV in quiescent cells could have other explanations. For example, heterogeneous viral DNA species have been found in HIV virions, resulting from partial reverse transcription within the virus particles (2669, 4484, 4928). This DNA might be responsible for the low-level DNA detected by PCR in the experiments with resting cells (4903). The partial reverse transcripts in the cells could be those associated with viruses bound to the cell and not internalized, or those failing to continue their replicative cycle. This possibility, however, does not seem feasible because of the control cultures used in the experiments in which the infection of resting cells was evaluated. Most recently the block in virus replication in resting CD4+ cells has been linked to high expression of a subspecies of APOBEC3G (755) (Section II.A). Resting cells

have a large quantity of APOBEC3G in an LMM that blocks virus replication via a process not yet defined. Upon activation, this LMM complex is transferred to an HMM in which the APOBEC3G now functions under normal conditions (Section II.A).

4. CONCLUSIONS

The difficulty in resolving the various findings on resting cells revolves around the definition of quiescence. Most immunologists would insist that such cells should lack CD25 expression (3657). Others emphasize an absence of CD69, Ki67, and HLA-DR expression as well. If a small number of HLA-DR+ cells were present in the inoculated cell population in vitro, they would be permissive to HIV infection and could misleadingly suggest, by the PCR analysis used, successful infection of all cells. This possibility can be ruled out by the elimination of all HLA-DR+ cells (4383). The findings support the conclusion that virus entry and expression can be influenced by the state of cell activation (Sections I.A and I.B). The length of time a cell could carry the unintegrated viral DNA must also reflect the level of its activation (553, 4293, 4903).

How quiescent CD4$^+$ cells lacking HLA-DR expression are infected in vivo is also unknown (553). Whether an HLA-DR$^+$ CD4$^+$ lymphocyte can, after infection, return to a quiescent nonproductive HLA-DR$^-$ state needs to be determined. Some studies have suggested that it can take place (690) but is probably a rare event (776). Conceivably, the infection could take place when resting CD4$^+$ cells are exposed to certain cytokines (4272, 4349, 4527a) (see Chapter 4, Section II.C.1). Alternatively, as noted above, the few quiescent CD4$^+$ cells found infected in vivo (553) could be those few HLA-DR$^+$ cells that are present in the resting cell population (0.3%). Finally, the clinical relevance of these studies on resting T cells needs to be considered. Most CD4$^+$ cells in vivo are in a relatively quiescent state but are still susceptible to productive virus infection. It seems more important, therefore, to focus on activation events that establish the infection in these cells.

B. Other Quiescent Cells

Nondividing human epithelial cells expressing the human CD4 molecule can be infected by HIV, and virus integration can take place (Table 5.5) (2561). The murine type C retroviruses that can infect human cells do not show this biologic activity, and infection does not occur. Thus, productive infection of resting cells seems to be cell type specific. The reason for the productive infection of the nondividing epithelial cells by HIV is not known but does not appear to involve any of the regulatory or accessory genes. It could depend on the MA (p17) and Vpr proteins (1791) that direct the PIC to the nucleus (551, 1415). The large PIC of other retroviruses may not be able to enter the intact nucleus of resting cells via nuclear pores (551) (see Chapter 3). This event appears to depend on tyrosine phosphorylation of MA (1416), the function of Vpr (998) mitosis (2562), and an interaction of the PIC with cellular karyopherins (1415) (see Chapter 3). The findings have suggested directions for utilizing lentivirus vectors in gene therapy of resting human stem cells (3699).

V. Latency

A. Cellular Latency

The preceding discussion on HIV infection indicated that some nonactivated cells can harbor the HIV genome in an unintegrated state for several days without evidence of virus replication. This type of silent infection in cells differs from the classic state of viral latency in which the full viral genome is in the cell but expression is completely suppressed. In the case of retroviruses, very little, if any, viral RNA or protein would be made from the integrated provirus in the cell chromosome (1320). Subsequently, conditions occurring within the cell would alter its state so that HIV replication, spread, and cell death would follow. The induction of retroviruses from a latent state has been studied in many different systems, and a variety of approaches can be used (2513) (Table 5.6).

The presence of cellular latency for HIV has been supported by biologic and molecular studies (1291; for reviews, see references 2899 and 3566). HIV latency can be generated during normal T-cell differentiation within the thymus and results from a decrease in cellular RNA transcription (525). These latently infected CD4$^+$ T cells have predominantly R5 viruses, but X4 viruses have also been identified (3508). Coculture studies suggest that direct infection of naïve T cells occurs rarely and the latency is predominantly in resting memory cells, which are the major source of HIV progeny virus (3508) (see above and Chapter 4, Section II). Most analyses suggest that the latent integrated provirus in resting CD4$^+$ lymphocytes in vivo is suppressed at RNA transcription and only a small

Table 5.5 Studies of quiescent cells^a

- Virus replication is blocked at virus entry; only short transcripts are made (765, 1591, 4383).
- Virus enters but is blocked in reverse transcription (4293, 4383, 4903).
- Virus enters and is reverse transcribed, but is blocked at viral integration (552, 4293, 4903).
- Virus enters and integrates into nondividing cell (e.g., epithelial cell), with subsequent virus replication (2561) or induction of latency (4140).

^{a}In examples 2 to 4, HIV can be produced after activation of the cell (Table 5.6). See the text for discussion.

Table 5.6 Induction of retroviruses from a latent state[a]

- Halogenated pyrimidines (e.g., iododeoxyuridine and bromodeoxyuridine)
- Nucleic acid analogs (e.g., 5-azacytidine)
- Protein inhibitors (e.g., cycloheximide)
- B-cell mitogens (e.g., lipopolysaccharides)
- T-cell mitogens (e.g., phytohemagglutinin and concanavalin A)
- Amino acid analogs (e.g., L-canavanine)
- Cytokines (e.g., TNF-α and granulocyte colony-stimulating factor)
- Inhibitors of histone deacetylase (HDAC)
- Graft-versus-host reaction
- UV irradiation
- Heat shock
- Infection by other viruses (e.g., herpesvirus and retrovirus)

[a]These approaches have been used with a variety of retroviruses, including HIV. TNF-α, tumor necrosis factor alpha.

subset (1%) can be induced by cell activation to release infectious virus (1822) (Section IV.A).

Some groups have observed that virus-producing established cell lines can have gradually decreased virus production over time (2081, 2580, 4205). In both CD4[+] lymphocytes and established CD4[+] T-cell lines, temporal changes in the steady-state levels of viral mRNA were associated with a shutdown of HIV transcription, and enhanced production of spliced mRNAs was observed (2580).

In other studies of cells in vivo, the presence of HIV DNA but not RNA has been noted in PBMC, as well as in lymphoid tissue (776, 1193, 1194, 3292, 3442, 4140) (see Chapter 4). Moreover, CD4[+] lymphocytes carrying HIV-1 DNA can be recovered from the PBMC of infected individuals, and these cells express the CD4 molecule, conceivably because they are not producing progeny virus (3993, 4658). This state is reflected as well by an excess of multiply spliced or singly spliced viral RNA compared to unspliced RNA in infected cells recovered in vivo (3442, 3886, 4055) (Section I). As noted above, high levels of viral mRNA species in peripheral blood cells have predicted progression to disease (3886), presumably reflecting the onset of virus replication.

In one of the first experimental studies of HIV latency in cells from an infected individual, the long-term culture of naturally infected human CD4[+] lymphocytes did not express much virus until several weeks after culture. Then, high levels of HIV were spontaneously produced, followed by cell death (1905). These observations were subsequently confirmed by using purified resting CD4[+] T cells from infected individuals (776). Moreover, as noted above, clones of CD4[+] lymphocytes derived from seronegative donors have been shown to harbor virus in a latent state after infection with HIV-1 in vitro (690). Thus, a state of postintegration latency appears to occur.

Some researchers have used established cell lines such as the infected U-1 and ACH-2 cell lines to study cellular latency; these cells produce very low levels of HIV (1319, 1321, 3559). The lines were derived from established monocyte (U-1) or T (ACH-2)-cell lines chronically infected with HIV-1$_{LAI}$ and generally show only 2-kb mRNA (2995, 3569). After activation by a variety of approaches, HIV transcription increases, mirrored by a shift in mRNA patterns with a reduction in spliced mRNA and an increase in unspliced mRNA (2995). These cells appear to have deletions in the Tat or TAR region (1196) (Section V.B). A block in Rev function has also been linked to restricted HIV-1 production by human astrocytoma cells (3238).

Silent infection of monocytes has been reported with mutant HIV-1 strains lacking *vpu* or *vpr* functions (4738). Virus can be recovered from these cells by cocultivation with uninfected PBMC. A similar observation on the amplification of HIV release by adding PBMC to the cultures has been made with established T-cell and monocyte lines, as well as HIV-infected macrophages (1230, 1320, 3998) and fibroblasts (4393). Thus, the "latent" state in monocytes and other cells could reflect an arrest in virus release rather than earlier events. Nevertheless, the role of cytokines or cell-to-cell activation should be considered; the mechanism has not yet been elucidated.

In studies to activate virus from a latent state, halogenated pyrimidines, UV rays, and heat shock have been used (645, 4257, 4277) and are effective, perhaps secondary to DNA damage (4540) (Table 5.6i Figure 5.6). Other viral infections can reactivate a latent HIV infection in vitro, most probably via effects on the viral LTR (3117) (see Chapter 13). Moreover, proinflammatory cytokines such

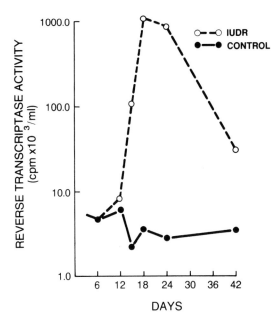

Figure 5.6 Latent HIV infection of an established T-cell line. The HIV-1$_{SF247}$ strain, obtained from a patient of Dr. E. Koenig from the Dominican Republic, was used to infect the Jurkat T-cell line. After 6 days in culture, very little virus replication was detected by the reverse transcriptase assay. After the addition on day 6 of iododeoxyuridine (IUDR) (50 μg/ml), HIV-1 was released to high levels, as measured by particle-associated reverse transcriptase activity. Within 2 weeks, virus replication decreased to almost a latent state. Reproduced from reference (2535) with permission.

as IL-6 and TNF-α as well as IL-2 can induce HIV from latency. Some investigators believe that this strategy might help eradicate the virus from immune reservoirs (775) (see Chapter 14). Recently, the histone deacetylase (HDAC) inhibitor valproic acid (Section V.B) was shown to reduce the level of resting infected CD4+ cells in three patients (2481). This approach will receive more attention, but it must be recognized that virus in other long-lived latent reservoirs (e.g., the brain and bowel) may remain (Table 4.3) (775).

It is also important to recognize that nearly all these in vitro studies of cellular latency have used established cell lines with integrated HIV genomes and not infected normal lymphocytes, which would be more relevant to the in vivo situation (690). Moreover, observations on cells that have viruses with known mutations (e.g., the U-1 and

ACH-2 cell lines) do not mirror latent cells infected by wild-type viruses.

B. Mechanism of Cellular Latency

1. POSSIBLE PROCESSES

Several hypotheses have been presented to explain the mechanism of cellular latency with HIV (Table 5.7) (for reviews, see references 1320, 2899, and 4290). Each may relate to certain processes within a specific cell type and to particular viral strains (1139). The latency could reflect the site of virus integation (2050, 4791) in which methylation of certain portions of the integrated viral LTR needed for induction of the replicative process may be involved (292) or methylation of extra-chromosomal viral DNA sequences (4158). It could result from regulating sequences in noncoding DNA (2558) or chromatin interaction with

Table 5.7 Possible mechanisms of HIV latency[a]

- Site of virus integration (2050, 4791)
- Methylation of viral DNA (292, 4158)
- Regulatory sequences in noncoding DNA (2557)
- Chromatin interaction with the HIV promoter (4553)
- Lack of sufficient viral Tat expression (1196, 1274, 1747)
- TAR mutation (1196)
- Lack of expression of Rev (3238, 3569, 4484)
- Histone suppression of gene expression (HDAC-1 activity) (2423, 4092, 4879)
- Inhibition of intracellular factors that interact with the NF-κB protein or other regions on the viral LTR (3193, 3362)
- Inhibition by human cell transcription factors (YY1, LSF) (3789)
- Expression of viral Nef protein (479, 723, 2689, 3256, 4449)
- Lack of viral Vpu and Vpr expression (4738)
- Cellular block to Vpu function (4571)
- Effect of heat shock protein 70 (hsp70) (1962)
- Effect of Murr-1 (1423)
- A block in the IFN stimulating element (ISRE) in the HIV LTR (4425)
- Inhibition of virus expression by CD8+ cell anti-HIV factor (CAF) (2532, 4659)

[a]See the text for other references and discussion. TAR, trans-activating response region; LTR, long terminal repeat.

the HIV-1 promoter (4553). Inactivation of the *tat* or *rev* gene (164, 1137, 1320, 1747, 4486) or a TAR mutation (1197) could be responsible. In one early study, the viral genes responsible for the arrest in a T-cell line were mapped primarily to the 3' LTR, but *tat, rev,* and *vpu* also seemed to be involved in the process (4205).

Histone suppression of gene expression could be responsible (2423). In this regard, HIV-infected resting CD4$^+$ T cells can be induced to release virus following inhibition of HDAC. The latency of HIV in these cells appears to reflect effects on chromatin structure (4879) in which this silencing of the HIV genome is linked to HDAC-1 activity. Thus, inhibition of HDAC (4553) and histone deacetyl transferases, promoting acetylation of histones and other transcription factors, can play a role in enhancing HIV replication (4092). Another mechanism may be through human cell transcription factors, which can inhibit HIV-1 LTRs and virus production (e.g., YY1 and LSF) (3789).

Early studies in cell culture suggested that the virus itself produces a protein, such as Nef, that interacts with cellular factors and establishes the silent infection (37, 723, 2689, 3256). This effect, however, seems linked to certain *nef* alleles and cell lines (see Chapter 7). As noted above, suppression of *vpu* or *vpr* function could be responsible for cellular latency (2511, 4738) but needs further evaluation.

In this regard, Vpu enhances particle assembly and release in human cells, and recent studies indicate that Vpu overcomes a cellular block to this assembly of virions (4571) (See Chapter 7). The nature of the mechanism remains to be elucidated. Moreover, heat shock protein 70 (hsp70) has been shown to inhibit the nuclear translocation of HIV Vpr in macrophages and can be found in association with this viral protein (1962). Potentially functioning as an innate antiviral factor, hsp70 could reduce replication in macrophages or even induce latent infection via this inhibitory mechanism. With Vpr-negative viruses, hsp70 stimulated nuclear import and virus replication. Thus, these two proteins may have similar roles but compete intracellularly when both are present. As a further example cited above (Section III.C), the cellular gene product Murr-1 can inhibit HIV replication

in resting CD4$^+$ cells (1423). This protein blocks NF-κB activity and could be responsible for HIV latency.

Moreover, in some cases a block in HIV replication by IFN-α production can be reversed by a sequence in the viral LTR which resembles the interferon stimulatory element (ISRE). Interferon regulatory factors can bind to this region and enhance HIV transcription (4425). A block in ISRE could be involved. Finally, cellular latency could reflect the activity of CD8$^+$ cell HIV-suppressing activity (2543) (see Chapter 11).

2. CONCLUSION

The mechanisms involved in the induction of a state of latency with HIV have not yet been fully defined (Table 5.7), and the reason that certain viral strains can enter latency more readily than others is unexplained. Moreover, whether the in vitro studies of viral latency have relevance in vivo has yet to be determined (Section V.A). Nevertheless, the HIV regulatory proteins, Tat, Rev, and Nef, and certain intracellular factors certainly could be involved either positively or negatively in inducing this biologic process.

C. Clinical Latency

The interval between infection and clinical disease in an individual has often been called latency. This state is quite different from the latent state within the cell. The factors influencing this clinical condition not only are cellular but also, most importantly, involve the immunologic response of the host against the virus (discussed in Chapters 9 to 11). By following individuals whose time of infection has been documented, it has been estimated that it takes 8 to 10 years to show signs of HIV infection

Table 5.8 Retrovirus latency and persistence

- Cellular—lack of viral RNA and protein expression after integration
- Clinical—interval between infection and onset of symptoms
- Abortive infection—lack of virus integration (e.g., in a resting CD4$^+$ cell)
- Low persistent infection—only low levels of virus production are detected. Often cocultivation with other target cells is needed to demonstrate virus replication.

(see Chapter 13). This absence of symptoms has been considered a clinical latency, but virus replication can remain active in the host (see Chapter 3). Individuals identified as long-term survivors (infected for more than 10 years with no symptoms) reflect this "silent" infection in which the presence of

HIV might not be suspected if serology tests were not conducted. Clinical latency essentially reflects the length of time it takes for HIV to infect and compromise the immune system and/or other tissues, leading to disease. Thus, biologic latency and clinical latency are quite distinct (Table 5.8).

SALIENT FEATURES • CHAPTER 5

1. The replicative cycle of HIV involves the intracellular interaction of a variety of viral, structural, and regulatory gene products with cellular genes. Some regulatory genes (e.g., *tat*) up-regulate virus replication, and others may suppress virus expression.

2. Differences in virus production can be noted in PBMC and appear to be related to intracellular differences. In the productive infection of cells, coreceptors on the cell surface as well as intracellular factors and the particular virus involved need to be considered.

3. Activation is important for HIV replication and involves several intracellular factors that interact with regions of the viral long terminal repeat. Intracellular blocks may be responsible for the lack of replication of some X4 viruses in macrophages and R5 viruses in T-cell lines.

4. Differentiated macrophages are most susceptible to virus replication. The reason may be the up-regulation of NF-κB transcriptionally active proteins. Certain cytokines (e.g., macrophage colony-stimulating factor) can influence the extent of virus production in these cells.

5. Nondividing macrophages, as well as certain other human cells, can be infected by HIV, with integration of virus into the cell chromosome. This process, different from that of many other retroviruses, appears to involve the MA and Vpr viral proteins that help direct the preintegration complex to the nucleus.

6. APOBEC3G is a species-specific intracellular protein that can block HIV replication if the viral Vif protein is not expressed. This cellular protein acts primarily as a

cytokine deaminase, causing production of defective particles, but can have other antiviral functions.

7. TRIM5α is a member of a family of species-specific intracellular proteins that can block murine leukemia virus infection of human cells and HIV infection of nonhuman primate cells. It acts principally by binding to the viral core before reverse transcription.

8. Quiescent CD4+ cells are resistant to productive infection by HIV. Either limited transcripts of the viral RNA are made or virus entry is completely blocked. Unless the cells are activated, the virus infection can be aborted. The intracellular mechanisms may involve APOBEC3G.

9. A state of cellular latency has been found in HIV infection in which CD4+ cells or other cells can contain unexpressed HIV that can be activated under certain conditions.

10. Many different approaches, including irradiation, halogenated pyrimidines, and coinfection of a cell with other viruses, can activate latent HIV infection.

11. Cellular latency may be explained by an inactivation of certain viral genes (e.g., *tat*, *rev*, and *vpu*) and effects of the virus integration site and its transcriptional ability.

12. Clinical latency defines an individual who has not developed disease. These individuals may have complete control of virus replication, although most evidence suggests that low-level virus replication takes place continually. Low virus expression in infected individuals correlates with a long-term asymptomatic clinical course.

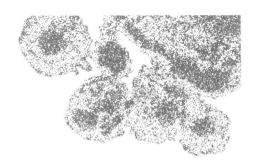

Cytopathic Properties of HIV

HIV Induction of Cell:Cell Fusion

Accumulation of Extrachromosomal Viral DNA and Cell Death

Direct Cellular Toxicity of HIV and Viral Proteins

Apoptosis

Activation

Role of Superantigens

A N IMPORTANT PART OF OUR UNDERSTANDING of the pathogenesis of HIV in the host should come from studying the cytopathic effects of the virus or its proteins on individual cells. As reviewed in Chapter 4, certain HIV-1 isolates (i.e., X4 viruses), particularly those recovered when the infected individual is advancing to disease, have a greater capacity for killing infected CD4$^+$ cells in culture than do strains isolated in the clinically asymptomatic period. Cell death appears to result from formation of multinucleated cells, necrosis, and apoptosis and can occur from direct or indirect mechanisms. Some investigators have provided evidence that apoptosis or related cell death processes may be the major killing mechanisms of CD4$^+$ cells and other cells in HIV-infected persons (1451, 1875, 2578, 3002). Other studies suggest that necrosis can be the mechanism for cell death reflecting single-cell lysis (603, 2489, 3539). Macrophages appear to die by necrosis (319). In addition, rapid cell lysis could result from the contact of normal CD4$^+$ cells with HIV-1-infected cells in the absence of syncytium formation (1788). The extent of this cytopathology produced by HIV-1 and HIV-2 in vitro can differ substantially (107, 731, 2279, 4291, 4394).

The SI and NSI strains, now termed X4 and R5 viruses, respectively, were first distinguished by the induction of syncytia in T-cell lines by X4 viruses (SI characteristics) (2279, 4394, 4403) (Figure 3.7). Moreover, some HIV-2 isolates have been recovered that replicate to high titer in PBMC but do not induce any cytopathology, as defined by syncytium formation and reduction in cell viability (1232, 2271). Many R5 HIV-1 isolates show limited cytopathic properties in PBMC, but these observations in cell culture may not reflect the observed cytotoxic effects of R5 virus in vivo (see Chapter 13). For example, a marked depletion in CD4+ cells occurs in the gastrointestinal tract during early infection in which R5 viruses are responsible (493) (see Chapter 8). Both direct and indirect processes appear to be involved.

This chapter reviews various processes associated with the cytopathic effects of HIV (Table 6.1).

I. HIV Induction of Cell:Cell Fusion

A. Features of Syncytium Formation

An important biologic feature of HIV infection is the formation of multinucleated cells (syncytia) in culture (and perhaps in the host) as a result of the fusion of infected cells with uninfected CD4+ cells (Figures 3.7 and 6.1) (2599, 2604). Syncytium formation is often the first sign of HIV infection of PBMC in culture and can appear in these cells within 2 to 3 days; accompanying this cytopathic effect is balloon degeneration of the cells, most probably resulting from changes in membrane permeability (Section III) (Figure 6.2). In culture, cell:cell fusion can be observed within 2 h (4382) and can be monitored by redistribution of fluorescent

Table 6.1 Possible mechanisms of cytopathology by HIV or its proteins[a]

- Syncytium formation
- Accumulation of unintegrated viral DNA
- Virus release causing changes in membrane integrity
- Alteration of plasma membrane permeability
- Decrease in synthesis of membrane lipids
- Decrease in "second messenger" (diacylglycerol) activity
- Interference with cellular heteronuclear RNA processing
- Degradation of cellular mRNA and reduction in cellular protein synthesis
- Induction of apoptosis[b]
- Release of toxic cytokines by infected cells and/or uninfected cells (Table 6.3)
- Destruction by immunologic responses (ADCC, CTL)
- Inhibition by HIV of normal growth factors (e.g., in the brain)

[a]The viral proteins gp120, gp41, Tat, Nef, and Vif have been considered potentially responsible for cell death (Table 6.3). ADCC, antibody-dependent cellular cytotoxicity; CTL, cytotoxic T lymphocytes.
[b]Cytokines might be involved, as well as superantigens.

Figure 6.1 Multinucleated giant cells formed by cell:cell fusion during acute infection of peripheral blood mononuclear cells by HIV-1. Balloon degeneration of the cells is also evident. Phase microscopy; magnification, ×80.

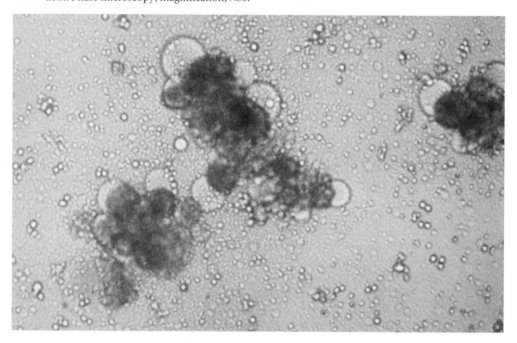

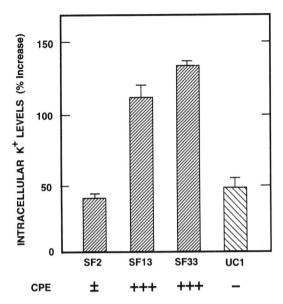

Figure 6.2 Membrane permeability changes resulting from HIV infection. Peripheral blood mononuclear cells were infected with HIV strains with different cytopathic effects (CPE), and the influx of radioactive potassium (K^+) was measured by standard procedures. A correlation of cytopathology with a greater ingress of K^+ was noted. UC1 is from a relatively noncytopathic HIV-2 isolate (1231). Experiments conducted with R. Garry.

dyes (Color Plate 12, following page 366) (1087, 4709). As noted above, HIV isolates can be distinguished by their ability to induce cell fusion (or syncytia) in established T-cell lines (e.g., MT-2 cells) (2279, 4394).

This cell:cell fusion is temperature dependent (1369) and does not require cellular DNA, RNA, or protein synthesis (1717, 4382); it appears to involve cell surface carbohydrates (1717, 2878, 4382) and glycolipids (1131) (Table 6.2). Some studies suggest that a certain number of gp120:CD4 complexes are required for the process, which most probably involves multiple envelope:CD4 molecule interactions (1369).

Whether the process of syncytium formation is similar to that of virus:cell fusion is not clear. For example, certain receptors for HIV entry, which were discovered by using cell fusion assays (see Chapter 3), are not directly involved in the virus:cell membrane fusion process (Color Plates 2 and 4, following page 78). In contrast, the cell:cell

fusion event, as shown by specific antibodies, involves the CD4 molecule as well as both the HIV gp120 and gp41 envelope proteins (1361, 1717, 2599, 3473) (Figures 3.7 and 6.1; Table 6.2) (see below). Results with interviral recombinants have indicated that syncytium formation can be linked to specific regions of gp120 (see Chapter 7) (728, 4251, 4885).

Conformational changes in gp120 or gp41 of the virus occur after envelope binding to CD4 and appear to be important in rapid fusion (1547) (Color Plates 1, 2, and 4, following page 78). Shedding of HIV-1 gp120 has been observed but is probably not necessary for cell:cell fusion (1380) (see Chapter 3). Moreover, cell fusion can be influenced by the pattern of viral envelope glycosylation (1268), as well as by the extent of proteolytic cleavage of gp160 within the cell (450) (Table 6.2).

B. Mechanisms of Cell:Cell Fusion

Regions of CD4 and the virus envelope (e.g., gp120) different from those used for viral attachment can play a role in the cell:cell fusion (121, 588, 2603, 3593). As discussed in Chapter 3, certain anti-CD4 monoclonal antibodies will not block virus binding to cells but will prevent cell:cell fusion and HIV infection (649, 1780, 4489). In studies with HIV-1 and HIV-2, gp41 has been noted to contain the fusion peptide, the major determinant for cell fusion (Section III) (1361, 1363, 4274) (Color Plate

Table 6.2 Factors influencing cell:cell fusion in HIV infection

Cell
- Temperature dependent (1369)
- Does not require DNA, RNA, or protein synthesis (1717, 4382)
- Involves surface carbohydrates and glycolipids (1131, 1717, 4382)
- Involves CD4 expression (1369, 4382)
- Involves surface adhesion molecules (e.g., LFA-1 and CD7 glycoprotein) (1833, 3925)

Virus
- Envelope gp120 and gp41 proteins (1363, 1717, 2599)
- Pattern of gp120 glycosylation (1268, 2878)
- Extent of proteolytic cleavage of gp160 within the cell (450)

3, following page 78). The membrane-spanning domain of gp41 seems to be very important in this process (3034), and additional regions of gp41 also appear to be critical for fusion, including portions of the molecule in the extended "cytoplasmic tail" (743, 3102, 4833). Formation of a six-helix bundle (trimeric coiled coil) is involved (2964) (Color Plate 4, following page 78). The prefusogenic conformation of gp41 is unknown, but it appears to be distinct from that of a six-helix bundle (3026). Thus, the central gp41 coiled coil is formed during the transition of the HIV-1 envelope glycoproteins from the precursor state to the receptor-bound intermediate. Whether gp41 alone via a fusion domain can mediate this activity is not yet clear (2803). Moreover, it is still not certain which viral gp41 epitopes are directly involved in cell:cell fusion and which only influence this biologic event.

The possible role of cellular membrane proteins such as the integrin, lymphocyte functional antigen 1 (LFA-1) (1833), or the CD7 glycoprotein (3925) in cell:cell fusion has been considered (see Chapter 3). Monoclonal antibodies to these cell surface proteins block cell aggregation and/or syncytium formation. Those directed against LFA-1 do not prevent virus infection (3405), but anti-CD7 antibodies do (3925). Finally, the absence of fusogenic activity when murine cells that express the human CD4 molecule were mixed with HIV-infected cells appears to reflect the lack of a human cell factor

(516, 1129, 4406). In one study, this factor appeared to be a glycolipid (1131). These findings underline possible differences between cell:cell fusion and virus:cell fusion.

C. Cell Death

The process of cell membrane fusion has been linked to viral cytopathicity and cell death (603, 2370, 2599). Some investigators believe that cell fusion is important in the depletion of CD4$^+$ cells resulting from single-cell lysis and perhaps multinucleated-cell formation (603, 1455, 1788). The mechanisms can involve disturbance in cell membrane integrity (Section III.C). Evidence for multinucleated cells in vivo is lacking except in the brain (3401, 4067). Moreover, in other retroviral systems, multinucleated cells can remain viable for long periods (2513).

II. Accumulation of Extrachromosomal Viral DNA and Cell Death

Besides cell:cell fusion, the cytopathology and cell death that occur during acute HIV infection in vitro can be associated with an accumulation of unintegrated viral DNA in the cytoplasm of the cells (2541, 4076). Whether this process occurs during virus infection in vivo is not known. Neurologic damage has been found to be associated with large amounts of unintegrated HIV DNA

Bruce L. Evatt
Chief, Hematologic Disease Branch, Centers for Disease Control and Prevention, Atlanta, Ga., and Clinical Professor of Medicine, Emory University School of Medicine. Dr. Evatt was one of the first researchers to study HIV infection in hemophiliacs. He alerted the scientific community about the possible transmission of HIV through blood products and has continued to work in the area of safety in blood and blood products.

in cells in the brain (3401). Similar observations have been made with infected T cells arrested in division (4384). In this case, continued production of the unintegrated cDNA could be the cause of cell death, since viral progeny are not produced. The same phenomenon linked to cytopathology has been previously reported with in vitro infection of cells by the avian spleen necrosis virus (2166).

These observations support the conclusion that high levels of intracellular DNA can be toxic to the cell and could contribute to the initial cell killing observed in the early stages of infection (2541, 4076). Nevertheless, single-cell killing is not always associated with the accumulation of viral DNA in the cytoplasm (327, 4203) (see Chapter 8). Moreover, accumulation of extrachromosomal viral DNA sequences during a noncytopathic latent HIV infection of a monocyte line has been reported, although in that case, the DNA was methylated (4158).

III. Direct Cellular Toxicity of HIV and Viral Proteins

A. General Observations

Several observations link cell death with direct toxicity of the virus or viral envelope proteins (for reviews, see references 1455 and 1687) (Table 6.3). The mechanism of cell death is not always specified in the studies reported but can involve a disturbance of cell membrane integrity (Section I; see also below) (Figure 6.2) and/or apoptosis (Section IV). The relative quantities of the viral envelope protein produced by the cell (2315, 2600, 3670,

Table 6.3 Viral proteins that can be cytotoxic[a]

gp120 (235, 780, 1133, 2433, 2599)
gp41 (3017, 3323, 3473)
Nef (1383, 4731)
Vpr (1990, 4296)
Vpu (44)
Tat (2565, 3856, 4736)
Vif and Vpr coexpression can cause cell necrosis (3881)

[a]Direct killing or induction of apoptosis is involved. Other references can be found in Section III. Some viral proteins (e.g., Vpu, Vpr, and Tat) can inhibit apoptosis under certain conditions (Section III.G).

4196, 4292), as well as the extent of glycosylation of the viral envelope (3073, 4291), can determine cytopathicity. Presumably, the cytopathic effect of irradiated HIV (3670) also results from the viral envelope proteins.

B. Cell Interaction with Virus Envelope Proteins

1. gp120

In interviral recombinants, cytopathicity, including cell:cell fusion (as noted above), has been mapped to regions in gp120 (121, 728, 987, 4885) (see Chapter 7). Moreover, the cell:cell fusion that often leads to cell death can be induced directly by gp120 (732, 2600, 2601, 4196). In one study, just a doubling in the production of gp120 following HIV infection gave rise to cytopathology and cell death (4292). In another, two changes in the N-linked glycosylation sequences of gp120 produced a cytopathic strain (4291). In one study, the accumulation of gp160 without secretion of the processed envelope proteins (gp120 and gp41) led to single-cell death (2253), linked to apoptosis (Section IV) (2683). Moreover, adding gp120 to PBMC or cultured brain cells caused cell killing in a dose-dependent manner (494, 1133, 2068) (see Chapter 8). Finally, some studies suggest that gp120 on the surface of CD4$^+$ cells (uninfected or infected) can activate complement components, leading to cell death (4342) (Section IV.E).

2. gp41

gp41 can also be toxic to cells, most probably through induction of alterations in membrane permeability (3017). Mutations in the viral gp41 (1301) have modified the extent of cytopathicity or produced cytopathic variants. As noted above, gp41 alone can induce the cell:cell fusion that accompanies cell death (3473, 4172) (see also Section IV.E).

C. Cell Membrane Disturbances and Cell Death

The mechanisms for the induction of cell death by the viral envelope proteins are not yet defined. Disturbances in membrane integrity could be involved, as reflected by the balloon degeneration of cells in vitro (Figure 6.1). HIV binding to and

entry into cells have shown membrane discontinuities and pores in association with ballooning
(1279). For example, cells producing cytopathic
HIV are unable to control the influx of monovalent and divalent cations that accumulate in the
cell along with water (820, 1455, 2713, 4636) (Figure 6.2). The resulting loss in intracellular ionic
strength not only leads to cell death, visualized by
balloon cells, when carried to its extreme (Figure
6.1), but also, at relatively noncytopathic levels,
could change the electrical potential of the cell,
thereby compromising normal cell function.

The phenomenon of direct damage to the cell
membrane has been demonstrated with cultured
brain cells exposed to HIV gp120 (see Chapter
8). There was a high influx of calcium concomitant with a disturbance in membrane integrity
and cell function (1133). The toxic effect of the
viral envelope was reversed by the calcium channel antagonist nimoptene (1133). Conceivably, the
glycosylated HIV protein expressed on the surface of the infected cell disturbs membrane permeability in some manner, leading to cell death.
Alternatively, the viral envelope could induce N-
methyl-D-aspartate (NMDA) receptor-mediated
neurotoxicity (2623).

Changes in cell membrane potential have also
been demonstrated after exposure to the Nef
protein, which contains a small region with some
sequence homology to scorpion toxin (4731).
Soluble Nef can be cytotoxic for human CD4+ T
cells (1383). This viral protein, if expressed on
the cell surface, could cause the death of normal
uninfected CD4+ cells by cell contact (1382). Domains on other viral proteins (e.g., Tat and gp41)
have shown similarities to a neurotoxin as well
(1457). Moreover, the Tat protein causes the death
of neuronal cells in culture (3856) and can induce apoptosis of CD4+ cells (2565) (see Chapter
8). In addition, Vpu and Vpr could influence
processes affecting cell viability through their ion
channel activities (for a review, see reference
2387) (see Chapter 7). These viral proteins as
well as the envelope proteins can be involved in
apoptosis (Section IV.E).

The cytopathic effects of HIV have also been
linked to a cellular activation process involving
gp41 and CD4 in which tyrosine phosphorylation of a 30-kDa protein was detected (832).

Inhibition of this phosphorylation led to reduced
syncytium formation, apparently related to a
block in cell mitosis. This mechanism resembles
the effect of HIV envelope and Vpr on CD4+
cells, in which a block in cell replication at the G_2
phase can result in apoptosis (1778, 2261, 3679)
(Section IV). The question of whether modifying
specific intracellular signals would decrease CD4+
cell loss via this process merits further study. Moreover, some evidence suggested that cellular protein synthesis is reduced during HIV infection of
cells; a degradation of cellular mRNA may be involved (34).

IV. Apoptosis

A. General Observations

Apoptosis is an alternative general mechanism for
cell death besides necrosis (Figure 6.3). The phenomenon is a normal physiological response during
embryogenesis, thymocyte maturation, and other
differentiation processes and can be elicited in cells
by a variety of stimuli, including virus infection
(835, 2163, 2164; for reviews, see references 302 and
1585). Apoptosis requires cell activation, protein
synthesis, and the function of a Ca^{2+}-dependent
endogenous endonuclease that fragments the cellular DNA into small, measurable nucleotide units
(Figure 6.4). It may involve cells sensitized by
interleukin-2 (IL-2) to antigen recognition (3678)
(Section IV.D). The process can be blocked, however, by the administration of IL-2, which appears to
prevent the reduction in expression of the antiapoptotic protein Bcl-2 (20). The extent of apoptosis
correlates with the stage of HIV infection (3438,
3905), the extent of immune activation, and disease progression (1583, 1585). A number of observations correlate the intensity of T-cell apoptosis
and the pathogenicity of the infection, including the
following: (i) long-term survivors (nonprogressors)
have low levels of T-cell apoptosis (1348, 2596)
(see Chapter 13), and (ii) infection with HIV-2,
which is less pathogenic than HIV-1, is associated
with a lower level of immune activation and T-cell
apoptosis (3000) (see Chapters 1 and 3). Comparative studies of pathogenic models of lentivirus
infection indicate that increased apoptosis of lymphocytes is only observed in pathogenic lentivirus
infections (1225, 1582) (see Chapter 13).

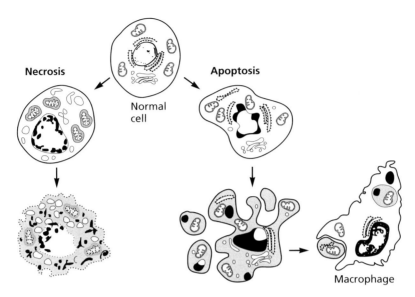

Figure 6.3 Processes of cell death. The sequential ultrastructural changes occurring in apoptosis and necrosis are shown. In apoptosis (right), a normal cell undergoes compaction and segregation of chromatin into sharply delineated masses that lie against the nuclear envelope. Condensation of the cytoplasm and convolution of the nuclear and cellular outlines occur. Rapid progression of the process is associated within minutes with nuclear fragmentation, marked convolution of the cellular surface, and the development of pedunculative protuberances. The protuberances then separate to produce membrane-bound apoptotic bodies which are phagocytized and digested by macrophages. In necrosis (left), chromatin is clumped into ill-defined masses and gross volume organelles, and folliculin densities appear in the matrix. Membranes break down and the cell disintegrates at the late stages. Figure modified from reference 2163 with permission.

B. Mechanisms

Two major mechanisms appear to be responsible for the HIV-associated CD4+ T-cell apoptosis: direct infection by HIV and indirect effects, which include interference with T-cell renewal by HIV; bystander killing induced by HIV gene products; activation-induced cell death, which depends on death receptors (extrinsic pathway); and activated T-cell autonomous death, which is mediated by Bcl-2-related proteins (intrinsic pathway) (for review, see references 203 and 1585) (Table 6.4). The latter can be induced by an interaction of uninfected CD4+ cells with antigen-presenting cells such as macrophages (1818) (see below). Some studies suggest that death by apoptosis of the uninfected CD4+ cells is mostly involved (811, 1290).

Several cellular death receptors are involved in apoptosis, including the Fas (CD95) receptor, the p55 tumor necrosis factor alpha (TNF-α) receptor, and TRAIL/APO-2-L (TNF-related apoptosis-

inducing ligand) receptors 1 and 2 (e.g., DR5) (for reviews, see references 203 and 2436). Ligation of the receptors (via the Fas ligand, TNF-α or TRAIL) causes the activation of a family of cysteine proteases called *caspases* that cleave aspartate residues (i.e., cysteine-dependent aspartate-specific proteases). These enzymes (which number up to 15) are activated by proteolytic removal of their terminal pro-domain. Some of them function in cytokine processing and inflammation, and at least seven (caspases 2, 3, 6, 7, 8, 9, and 10) contribute to cell death.

Caspases that participate in apoptosis can be divided into the initiator caspase group, which includes caspases 2, 8, 9, and 10, and the effector caspase group, to which caspases 3, 6, and 7 belong (2425). In general, caspase 8 (FLICE) and caspase 3 are involved in many of the apoptosis pathways. The activated caspases cleave other caspases, which sets in motion the endonucleosis

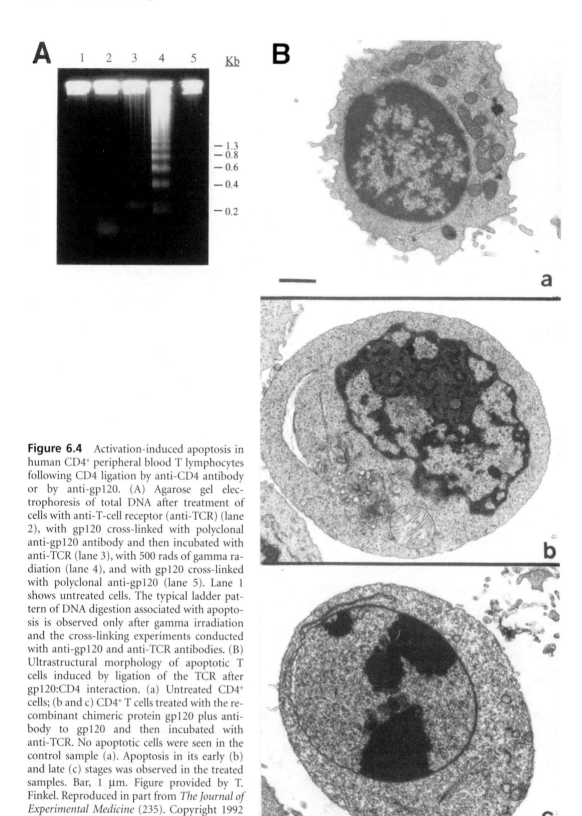

Figure 6.4 Activation-induced apoptosis in human CD4[+] peripheral blood T lymphocytes following CD4 ligation by anti-CD4 antibody or by anti-gp120. (A) Agarose gel electrophoresis of total DNA after treatment of cells with anti-T-cell receptor (anti-TCR) (lane 2), with gp120 cross-linked with polyclonal anti-gp120 antibody and then incubated with anti-TCR (lane 3), with 500 rads of gamma radiation (lane 4), and with gp120 cross-linked with polyclonal anti-gp120 (lane 5). Lane 1 shows untreated cells. The typical ladder pattern of DNA digestion associated with apoptosis is observed only after gamma irradiation and the cross-linking experiments conducted with anti-gp120 and anti-TCR antibodies. (B) Ultrastructural morphology of apoptotic T cells induced by ligation of the TCR after gp120:CD4 interaction. (a) Untreated CD4[+] cells; (b and c) CD4[+] T cells treated with the recombinant chimeric protein gp120 plus antibody to gp120 and then incubated with anti-TCR. No apoptotic cells were seen in the control sample (a). Apoptosis in its early (b) and late (c) stages was observed in the treated samples. Bar, 1 μm. Figure provided by T. Finkel. Reproduced in part from *The Journal of Experimental Medicine* (235). Copyright 1992 The Rockefeller University Press.

Table 6.4 Causes of apoptosis in HIV infection[a]

- Direct HIV infection—cytopathic effect (1585, 2432, 4401)
- Immune activation (1585, 3176); TCR-triggered activation-induced cell death (1643, 3373)
- Interaction of HIV envelope protein with the CD4 molecule (cross-linking) (235, 780) or chemokine coreceptor (338, 4616)
- Exposure to viral proteins (e.g., Nef, Tat, Vpu, and Vpr) (874, 1383, 1556, 1778, 1990, 2433, 2565, 2579, 2765, 3473) (Table 6.3)
- Increased cell expression of death receptors: Fas (CD95), p55 TNF-αR, TRAIL/APO-2-LR1, APO-2-LR2 (203, 999, 1226, 2436, 4146)
- Interaction of cytokines or ligands (e.g., TNF-α, FasL, and TRAIL) with specific receptors (e.g., Fas, TNF receptors, and DR5) (15, 811, 1819)
- Expression of TNF-α and FasL by HIV-infected macrophages (203, 760, 1818, 2098)
- Release of cytochrome *c* by mitochondria (1289) or alterations in Bcl-2 regulatory protein expression (455, 1236)
- Granulolysin release by NK cells or CTL (2115)
- Interaction of CXCR4 with CD4 (338) or SDF-1 (1816)
- Superantigen activity (Section V)

[a]For other references, see Section IV and reference 1585. Table provided by M.-L. Gougeon. TCR, T-cell receptor; TNF, tumor necrosis factor.

that results in nuclear DNA fragments giving the morphological, karyotypic, and molecular changes characteristic of apoptosis (203) (Figure 6.4). Mitochondria play an important role in apoptosis, particularly via the release of cytochrome *c* (for a review, see reference 1289). Moreover, the Bcl-2 family of regulatory proteins that are either proapoptotic (such as Bax or Bid) or antiapoptotic (such as Bcl-2 or Bcl-x$_L$) are released from mitochondria (1236).

Accelerated T-cell apoptosis in HIV infection can be related to a variety of processes (for reviews, see references 203 and 1585). They include induction by specific viral proteins (e.g., Tat), interaction of the HIV envelope protein with the CD4 molecule (cross-linking), and interactions of cytokines with specific receptors (particularly the Fas ligand [FasL], TNF, and TRAIL) (Table 6.4). In addition, disorders in antigen-presenting cells (e.g., macrophages and dendritic cells) leading to defects in T-cell activity as

well as superantigen activity (Section V) can be involved. In general, whether in the peripheral blood or lymph nodes, apoptosis is increased in immune cells (B and T lymphocytes) during HIV infection, concomitant with a state of immune activation (1098, 1583, 3176) (Section V). These studies support the observation that enhanced apoptosis is related to a high sensitivity to death receptors, including Fas, in both T and B lymphocytes (1226, 3050, 4146).

In this connection, most studies show that cell proliferation alone does not lead to apoptosis of CD4$^+$ cells from HIV-infected individuals; cell-activation is needed. In support of this conclusion, cross-linking CD4 or stimulation with major histocompatibility complex (MHC)-restricted class II recall antigens (e.g., tetanus toxin) or pokeweed mitogen causes cell activation and up to 40% cell death by apoptosis in CD4$^+$ cells from asymptomatic HIV-infected subjects (235, 1643, 3373).

In general, the Fas/Fas ligand pathway (CD95/CD95L) appears to be most important in HIV-associated CD4$^+$ cell death via apoptosis but perhaps not in direct killing of cells by the virus (1422, 3275; for reviews, see references 203 and 2098). Thus, enhanced expression of the Fas ligand and TNF-α production by HIV-infected macrophages and DCs (2590a) can increase apoptosis of infected and uninfected CD4$^+$ T lymphocytes expressing CD95 (202, 760, 1818) (Table 6.3). Granulolysin released by NK cells or CTLs can also activate the caspase 3 pathway and induce apoptosis in cells (2115). The apoptosis can be inhibited by anti-CD95 neutralizing antibodies or antibodies to the CD95 ligand.

C. Cell Subsets and Apoptosis

Both CD4$^+$ and CD8$^+$ lymphocytes of HIV-infected individuals can undergo apoptosis, but the process appears to be most evident in CD4$^+$ cells (1581, 1643, 2432, 2984, 3275); it can occur as well in B cells (3050, 3176). Apoptosis has been linked to active HIV-1 replication (2432, 2834, 4401) and disease progression (1583, 3398), which will reflect an enhanced immune-activated state (see Chapter 13). In this regard, antiviral therapy, particularly with protease inhibitors, reduces apoptosis (426, 700, 2040), activation, and disease (see Chapter 14). Most likely, uninfected cells more than infected cells are the major targets of this process (811, 1290),

Table 6.5 Effect of cytokines on CD4$^+$ cell and CD8$^+$ cell apoptosis^a

- Type 1 cytokines, IL-2, IL-12, and IFN-γ, can prevent in vitro TCR-programmed death of HIV-infected CD4$^+$ T cells (i.e., TH1) (812).
- Type 2 cytokines, IL-4 and IL-10, accelerate apoptosis (812, 2456).
- IL-15 prevents spontaneous apoptosis of T cells from HIV-infected patients (3211) and Fas-induced apoptosis of HIV-specific memory CD8$^+$ T cells (3491).
- TNF-α and FasL induce macrophage-dependent apoptosis of CD4$^+$ T cells (201) and of CD8$^+$ T cells expressing TNFRII (999, 1816).
- TGF-β rescues cortical neurons from gp120-induced apoptosis (4022).
- Binding of gp120 or SDF-1 to CXCR4 induces apoptosis of CD8$^+$ T cells (1816) and death of neuronal cells (1828).
- Granulolysin activates a novel pathway of CTL- and NK cell-mediated death distinct from granzyme- and death receptor-induced apoptosis. It may also contribute to apoptosis of infected CD4$^+$ T cells (2115).

^{a}Table provided by M.-L. Gougeon. TCR, T-cell receptor: IL-4, interleukin-4; TNFRII, tumor necrosis factor receptor II.

which is affected by viral proteins and cytokines (Tables 6.3 and 6.5). As noted above, apoptosis has been reported in T cells during other viral infections (e.g., EBV and lymphocytic choriomeningitis virus) (3678, 4520). Furthermore, enhanced CD8$^+$ cell apoptosis has been noted in HIV-infected children in whom EBV is reactivated (2422).

In studies of CD4$^+$ cell subsets, memory T cells (see Chapter 4) were found to be more susceptible to the cytopathic effects of an X4 virus (773), whereas both naïve and memory cells could be infected similarly by these viruses. Cell death appeared to result in part from apoptosis, but the mechanism was not determined. It could be mediated by a particular viral envelope. In this regard, the interaction of CXCR4 with CD4 has been noted to mediate CD95-independent apoptosis of CD4$^+$ cells (338).

D. Role of Cytokines

The apoptotic process involving CD4$^+$ cells is related in part to alterations in cytokine synthesis during HIV infection (Table 6.5). Some results have suggested that the type 1 cytokines (e.g., IL-2, IL-12, and IFN-γ) prevent CD4$^+$ cell apoptosis,

whereas type 2 cytokines (e.g., IL-4 and IL-10) can accelerate this process (20, 798, 812, 1226, 2456) (see Chapter 8, Section I.H, and Chapter 11, Section II). In addition, IL-15 decreases T-cell apoptosis, most likely via its induction of Bcl-2 expression (705, 3211, 3491).

Transforming growth factor β (TGF-β) can prevent gp120-induced apoptosis of cortical neurons (4022). In some studies, IL-1α and IL-2 used together (but not alone) prevented apoptosis of CD4$^+$ cells from HIV-infected individuals (1581). In other studies, selective rescue from glucocorticoid-induced apoptosis was observed with cytokines and different CD4$^+$ cell helper subsets: IL-4 protects TH2 cells, whereas IL-2 protects TH1 cells (4981). In this regard, IL-2-producing CD4$^+$ cells were found to be less susceptible to apoptosis than those producing IFN-γ or TNF-α (2456). As noted above, the protection is linked to Bcl-2 expressions.

T cells from HIV-infected subjects are susceptible to TNF-α-mediated apoptosis (999). Moreover, TNF-α and FasL can cause macrophage-dependent apopotosis of CD4$^+$ cells (201) and of CD8$^+$ T cells expressing TNFRII (1818). Some cytokines (e.g., IL-4) can increase apoptosis in macrophages by countering the protective effects of other cytokines (e.g., TNF-α and IFN-γ) (2787). Granulolysin can also cause CD4$^+$ cell death by apoptosis (2115) (Table 6.5). Finally, both HIV-1 gp120 and the SDF-1 chemokine can induce apoptosis of neuronal cells via CXCR4 (1828), and SDF-1 binding to CXCR4 can cause CD8$^+$ T-cell apoptosis (1818).

E. Effect of Viral Proteins

1. ENVELOPE PROTEINS

Besides the direct cytopathic effect of viral envelope proteins on cell membrane integrity (Sections III.B and III.C), these viral products can induce apoptosis (Table 6.3). The envelope glycoprotein complex (gp120:gp41) can cause apoptosis of both infected and uninfected cells. Env that is expressed on the plasma membrane of infected cells can interact with a CD4 molecule and a suitable coreceptor to trigger cell-to-cell fusion mediated by gp41; the resulting syncytia subsequently undergo apoptosis. Apoptosis of syncytia is not mediated by the Fas or TNFRI pathways (3323), but HIV-infected T cells become more susceptible to CD95-induced apoptosis. Syncytia that arise from the fusion of Env-expressing cells with cells that express the CD4:CXCR4 complex undergo apoptosis through a mitochondrion-dependent pathway. This pathway is initiated by the up-regulation of the cyclin B-CDK1 (cyclin-dependent kinase 1) pathway and nuclear translocation of the mammalian target of rapamycin (mTOR). This process leads to p53-dependent up-regulation of expression of Bax, subsequent release of cytochrome c, and apoptosis (634).

The envelope viral protein gp120 alone can elicit apoptosis through virus:antibody complexes (4401), or via a gp120:CD4 interaction (2433). In this process CXCR4 can also be involved (203, 1828). Circulating gp120 can induce apoptosis in uninfected cells by this interaction with CD4, causing the activation of caspase 3 and caspase 6 (780). Cross-linking of the gp120 bound to human CD4+ lymphocytes followed by T-cell activation with anti-CD3 antibodies has also caused apoptosis of these cells (Figure 6.4) (235).

Other studies suggest that this process involving a signal transduction pathway requires the cytoplasmic tail of CD4 and is most efficient when p56 on the CD4 molecule is intact (889). The rapid induction of apoptosis by the interaction of the viral envelope with CD4 can be demonstrated as well in the cell-cell transmission of HIV (2774). Finally, the HIV envelope and Vpr (see below) can also cause apoptosis of CD4+ cells by blocking their replication at the G_2 phase of the cell cycle (1778, 2261). Importantly, some studies suggest that the HIV envelope can facilitate virus replication within CD4 cells without inducing an activation state (2211). These cells could then avoid activation-induced apoptosis.

Apoptosis could be involved with cell death following the emergence of X4 viruses. Both CD4 and CXCR4 can be involved in CD95-independent apoptosis (not via the caspase pathway) of CD4+ cells (338). The X4 virus envelope interaction with CD4 induces caspase-dependent cell death (780), whereas its interaction with CXCR4 gives caspase-independent cell death (4616). The R5 HIV envelope via CCR5 also causes caspase 8-dependent death (4616). Moreover, studies with SCID/hu mice reconstituted with human PBMC

indicated that R5 viruses and not cytopathic X4 viruses induced the greatest CD4+ cell loss (3132). The reason is not known but could involve relative levels of cytokines produced (e.g., TNF-α) and their influence on CD4+ cell apoptosis (Table 6.5; Figure 6.5).

The interaction of the X4 envelope with CXCR4 on CD8+ cells can cause cell death as well. TNF-α appears to be involved in this caspase-independent process (1816). Importantly, CD8+ cells are greatly activated in HIV infection and are more sensitive to apoptosis-inducing events. Moreover, with activation these cells express the CD4 receptor and can become susceptible to direct HIV infection (1305, 2217) (see Chapter 4). Apoptosis of CD8+ T cells appears to take place when the HIV gp120 X4 virus activates CXCR4 expression on macrophages and CD8+ T cells. Concomitant expression of TNF-α and its receptor leads to cell death. The findings can help explain why X4 virus infection shows lower levels of CD8+ cells (1816) and a more rapid clinical course (see Chapter 13). The CD8+ T-cell rebound, however, occurs earlier than that of CD4+ T cells, so apoptosis of CD8+ cells may not be as evident in the peripheral blood.

2. Nef, Vpu, Vpr, AND Tat PROTEINS

Certain other HIV proteins can trigger mitochondrion-associated cell death processes (Table 6.3). These include Nef, Vpu, Vpr, and Tat, which can induce apoptosis at an early time period; however, higher-level expression of these proteins can prevent this cell death process (874; for a review, see reference 1236). Nef can enhance cell susceptibility to apoptosis via activation and also induce this process in infected and uninfected cells through a Fas-independent pathway (2765, 3325). Activation also increases the expression of HIV coreceptors, particularly CCR5, making them more susceptible to HIV infection (802). Vpu can induce apoptosis by blocking expression of anti-apoptotic factors (44). Vpr can induce apoptosis through cell cycle arrest and rapid disintegration of the mitochondrial transmembrane potential in intact cells, as well as the release of cytochome c by effects on mitochondria (1990, 4296). However, under some conditions, this viral protein can inhibit this cell death process (186, 1387) (see Chap-

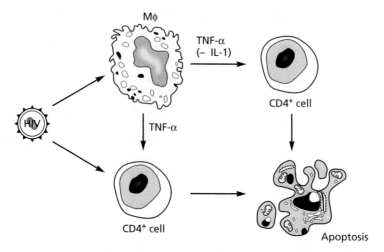

Figure 6.5   Cell killing by noncytopathic HIV-1 isolates. A proposed mechanism for indirect loss of CD4+ cells is shown. HIV-1 infection of macrophages can lead to the production of cytokines (e.g., tumor necrosis factor alpha [TNF-α]) that can induce programmed cell death (apoptosis) of CD4+ cells (infected or uninfected) (835). Moreover, the loss of interleukin-1 (IL-1) production by infected macrophages (1209, 3830) can cause apoptosis of CD4+ cells, particularly in the presence of antigen. In some cases, infection of CD4+ cells may increase this process of programmed cell death. Reprinted from reference 2520 with permission.

ter 8). Recent evidence suggests that the necrotic form of cell death that can occur in HIV infection is related to the direct coexpression of Vpr and Vif (3881).

Tat can induce apoptosis in uninfected and infected CD4+ lymphocytes in association with an increased Fas ligand expression and an activation of cyclin-dependent kinases and the caspase pathway (277, 2565, 4736). Tat suppresses cell function and can cause cytotoxicity and apoptosis (2565). The second exon of Tat is associated with increased expression of caspase 8 (277). Tat in infected cells, as well as pure protein, can also enhance the apoptosis of T cells exposed to antibodies to CD3, Fas, and TNF-α (2892, 4915). In addition, Tat alters the cellular redox state of noninfected cells, leading to cell death (4736), and this alteration is not observed in T cells from chimpanzees, a nonhuman primate model of resistance to HIV disease (1179). Nevertheless, in some studies, Tat-expressing cells appeared to be resistant to the cytopathic effect of Tat as well as to other inducers of apoptosis (2892). Moreover, the Tat protein has been found to protect human T cells and epithelial cells, as well as rat neuronal cells, from

apoptosis, most likely via Bcl-2 induction (2892, 4916).

F. T-Cell Apoptosis and Susceptibility to Disease Progression in Primates

Apparently, CD4+ cells from HIV-1-infected chimpanzees or SIV-infected African green monkeys do not undergo apoptosis (1581, 1582, 4006), even after exposure to Tat (1179). These animals do not generally develop disease. In contrast, apoptosis was observed in CD4+ cells from SIV-infected macaques that can advance to AIDS (1581). This distinction was most evident when CD4+ cells and not CD8+ cells were compared (1225), even under conditions of activation (1582). Thus, the lack of a pathogenic course in some animals could be explained by the absence of the apoptotic pathway, most likely related to the extent of immune system activation (Section V) (see Chapter 13). Levels of expression of activation markers on CD4+ and CD8+ cells are not usually increased in HIV-1-infected chimpanzees (1582). In this regard, the only reported cases of HIV pathogenicity in chimpanzees involved two females that received an inoculation of HIV-1 isolated from a chimpanzee

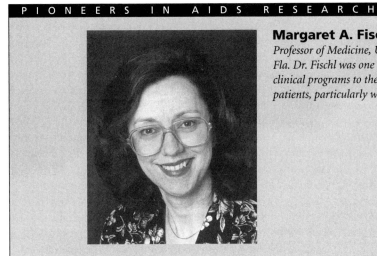

Margaret A. Fischl
Professor of Medicine, University of Miami, Miami, Fla. Dr. Fischl was one of the first physicians to devote clinical programs to the diagnosis and care of AIDS patients, particularly women and Haitians.

that was infected 8 years earlier (975). They showed a progressive loss of CD4+ T cells that was associated with high virus loads, hyper-immune activation, and increased levels of CD4+ T-cell apoptosis.

G. Conclusions

Considering all these features of apoptosis, it is evident that this process as well as its inhibitors plays an important role in HIV pathogenesis. However, because studies thus far conducted have used different techniques and different cell populations, consistent results are not always available. For example, unstimulated CD4+ cells removed from infected individuals do not undergo apoptosis (2984), but PBMC do (3373). Thus, the potential factors influencing apoptosis (Table 6.5), and the extent of this process in vivo (from activation) (3176), are not yet fully defined. Importantly, approaches to prevent apoptosis in CD4+ cells (e.g., up-regulation of Bcl-2 expression, and IL-2 administration) (129, 3912) could sustain the viability of uninfected CD4+ cells and might allow immune control (e.g., by CD8+ cells) of virus production by the infected cells (see Chapter 11). Perhaps normal function could return to the infected cells in which virus has been sufficiently suppressed.

Other data suggest that cell death does not always occur by apoptosis, but by a necrotic or lytic form dependent on caspase l activation in directly infected cells (431, 2489). HIV-1 isolates cyto-pathic for macrophages appear to induce the death of these cells by necrosis (319). They can, however, cause apoptosis of CD4+ cells via cytokine production (Figure 6.5). The Nef and Env proteins do not seem necessary for this effect (2489). The coexpression of Vpr and Vif may be responsible (3881). The relevance of these findings to levels of CD4 cells is not known.

Apparently HIV and its proteins can affect processes that either enhance or inhibit apoptosis depending on the stage in the replication cycle. For example, prolonged cell viability would give increased virus production, whereas cell death would be helpful if that involved anti-HIV CD8+ cells (2098). An example of this dual biologic role is TNF-α, which induces HIV replication but also apoptosis (2098). Whereas several HIV gene products have been shown to be associated with apoptosis (Table 6.3) (Section IV.E), some of these can have antiapoptotic activity. For example, Nef, gp120, and Vpu contribute to the down-regulation of expression of the CD4 receptor by infected cells, thereby preventing subsequent gp120:CD4-mediated apoptosis. Nef down-modulates the expression of MHC class I molecules and up-regulates the expression of CD95L by infected cells, a strategy that might function to protect infected cells from cytolysis by CTLs or NK cells (854, 4014). Low-level constitutive expression of Vpr inhibits apoptosis by causing the up-regulation of Bcl-2 and the down-modulation of Bax. Tat can promote cell cycle progression, inhibiting apoptosis and allowing the cells to increase the production of virus (2892). Thus, cell death depends on the cellular state and its environment.

Finally, besides the occurrence of T-cell death by well-known processes of apoptosis or necrosis, another pathway may be involved. In the stimulation of CD4+ and CD8+ cells with phytohemagglutinin or anti-CD3 antibodies, cell death by apoptosis can occur first and later through a process by which ribonucelotides cannot be synthesized (419). This inability to synthesize new proteins or to complete the cell cycle leads to cell necrosis. The features of necrosis observed include membrane leakage and degraded nuclei. The extent of this activation-associated necrosis can range from 10% to more than 90% and can correlate with advancement to AIDS (419).

V. Activation

Because activation makes a cell more sensitive to apoptosis, the events involved in causing cell activation should be considered. The reduction in CD4+ T cells (infected and uninfected) (2492, 4216) and progression to disease correlates with immune activation (for reviews, see references 160, 1122, and 1641) (see also Chapter 13, sections V and VI). CD4+ cell loss can involve activation-induced cell death via death receptors (the extrinsic pathway) or the activated T-cell autonomous death via an intrinsic pathway involving Bcl-2. Down-regulation of Bcl-2 can induce a cell to undergo apoptosis (for review, see reference 236a). Uninfected CD4+ T cells can die by bystander activation. This process involves induction of cell activation without interaction with the T cell receptor (TCR). Soluble factors (e.g., IFN-α or IFN-γ) (2076a) as well as membrane-bound molecules and receptors other than the TCR can bring about this cell death (for review, see reference 236a). In primary infection, a high level of immune activation (measured by CD38 expression) is associated with a more severe CD4+ cell loss over time (1029). The role of cofactors such as other infections in increasing CD4+ cell loss may reflect the immune activation resulting from these infections (310), particularly in the bowel (493).

Activation of lymphocytes requires two signals, which help to distinguish a response to a foreign antigen vs a self-antigen (4). The first signal involves antigen recognition and the second a costimulatory stimulus, which is mediated through the B7 family of surface molecules (4, 497). Activation-induced cell death takes place in previously activated cells, as can occur with repeated antigen stimulation (4733). Thus, with the high level of T-cell activation in HIV infection, a subsequent stimulus can induce CD8+ cell apoptosis and their loss. This process can reflect an enhanced sensitivity to apoptosis via the interaction of Fas ligand with an increased expression of Fas on the cell surface or the effect of TNF-α via the TNF (or TRAIL/APO-2) receptor (Section IV). In this regard, a reduction in immune cell activation appears to be related to the lower rate of disease progression in HIV-2-infected individuals (1718, 4216), particularly those with antigen-specific CD8+ T-cell responses (1718). As noted above, activation-induced apoptosis could result from a reduction in the expression of the antiapoptotic Bcl-2 protein and an increase in the proapoptotic Bim protein (1832).

CD38 is a type 2 surface glycoprotein (45 kDa) that was initially identified over 25 years ago (3697). This protein plays a role in cell:cell adhesion via CD31 detected on human endothelial cells (1077). Its expression on T cells is linked with activation (for a review, see reference 3936). The value in measuring CD38 expression as an indication of immune activation and faster progression to AIDS was first highlighted by Giorgi and coworkers (1521, 1522). Higher numbers of activated CD8+ CD38+ cells predicted a loss of CD4+ T cells (421, 1029, 3038). Moreover, the enhanced susceptibility of HIV-specific CD8+ cells to apoptosis may reflect their increased expression of CD38 (776a).

CD38 can be found on both infected and uninfected cells. In the latter case, the enhanced expression most likely reflects the production of inflammatory cytokines (3936). Soluble CD8 levels in blood and CD38 expression, particularly on CD8+ memory CD45RO+ cells, are excellent markers of T-cell activation (421, 2493, 3936) (see Chapters 11 and 13). Naïve resting T cells (CD8+ CD45RA+ T cells) can express CD38 normally. Other markers of cell activation include CD69 and HLA-DR.

Finally, by another process leading to loss of T cells, acute HIV infection can induce activation of

PIONEERS IN AIDS RESEARCH

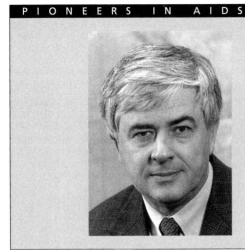

Myron (Max) Essex
Professor of Infectious Diseases, Department of Immunology and Infectious Diseases, Harvard School of Public Health and Chairman, Department of Immunology and Infectious Diseases, Harvard School of Public Health. Dr. Essex was one of the early researchers involved in determining whether a retrovirus was the cause of AIDS.

CD4+ cells as well as CD8+ T cells, which become advanced in cell differentiation. This activation-induced change can cause replicative senescence (i.e., loss of telomerase activity) and play a role in the decline in T-cell function in infected individuals (1173, 3419).

VI. Role of Superantigens

HIV may have a peptide that acts like a superantigen that can attach to CD4+ lymphocytes by one portion of the MHC class II molecule (e.g., the α but not the β chain) and the β-chain region on the T-cell receptor (Color Plate 13, following page 366; see also Chapter 11 and Color Plate 18 following page 366 for a description of viral antigen interaction with the TCR). This phenomenon could induce cell death by the process of apoptosis just described (828, 1581; for a review, see reference 900). Importantly, it could lead to an imbalance in the T-cell repertoire by expansions and deletions with "gaps" that may compromise the robustness of the immune response (see Chapter 11). Some support for this concept comes from the observation that individuals with AIDS show a disproportionate loss of T cells that have certain T-cell receptor beta chains (960, 1955, 2429, 3965). Furthermore, in many HIV-1-infected individuals, a Vβ-specific (Vβ8) anergy has been found in both CD4+ and CD8+ lympho-

cytes (949). One report suggested that HIV replicates more efficiently in CD4+ cells that express certain Vβ genes (e.g., Vβ12), presumably because they are influenced by a superantigen-like activity (1097).

Some studies do not support a role for superantigens in Vβ deletion and loss of CD4+ cells in HIV infection (902, 3263, 3587). Moreover, whether the alterations in the PBMC reflect changes in the lymphoid tissue needs to be examined (900). If there is a superantigen-induced loss of T cells in HIV infection, the particular antigen involved has not been determined. Conceivably, it might come from other organisms or foreign proteins present during HIV infection.

A reduction in B cells expressing the immunoglobulin VH3 gene product was also described in some early studies. This subpopulation of normal B cells was found to bind to HIV gp120 by a membrane IgM. This interaction induced immunoglobulin secretion, suggesting functional activation (316). A portion of gp120 identified as a discontinuous epitope spanning the V4 domain and the amino-terminal region flanking the C4 domain could serve as a superantigen for the VH3 B cells (2109). This interaction, which requires further evaluation, could induce some of the B-cell responses observed in HIV infection (see Chapter 8).

1. Several processes are involved in the induction of cell death by HIV, including syncytium formation, cell membrane changes, necrosis, and apoptosis.

2. HIV induces cell:cell fusion by an interaction of its envelope gp120 with CD4. Coreceptors on the cell surface may help in enabling this virus envelope:cell membrane fusion, which involves gp41 and can result in cell death.

3. Accumulation of viral extrachromosomal DNA can be responsible for cell death.

4. HIV envelope proteins can induce cell death through changes in cell membrane integrity, permitting an influx of monovalent and divalent cations with water, leading to balloon degeneration.

5. HIV infection can be associated with apoptosis, resulting from the direct action of viral proteins (e.g., Nef, Vpu, Vpr, and Tat), gp120 binding to the CD4 molecule, disorders in antigen-presenting cells, and superantigens.

6. Apoptosis may be more common in uninfected ("bystander effect") than infected CD4+ cells. The process can be observed in other cells, including CD8+ T lymphocytes, B lymphocytes, and neuronal cells.

7. Apoptosis is influenced by cytokine alterations. Type 1 cytokines can prevent apoptosis, whereas type 2 cytokines can increase the process. Other cytokines can also mediate antigen-stimulated CD4+ cell apoptosis.

8. The Tat protein is associated with the induction of apoptosis but can protect human T cells, epithelial cells, and neuronal cells from this process. The role of this protein appears to be pleiotropic, as demonstrated by its ability to suppress cell function and to prevent cell death, as well as to induce cytotoxicity and apoptosis.

9. HIV gp120 and Vpr can cause apoptosis of CD4+ cells by blocking replication at the G_2 stage of the cell cycle.

10. Some R5 HIV isolates can induce the death of macrophages by necrosis. Coexpression of Vpr and Vif can cause cell necrosis. R5 virus infection can cause CD4+ cell loss by apoptosis via induction of cytokine production (e.g., tumor necrosis factor alpha).

11. Immune system activation is associated with the induction of apoptosis.

12. Superantigens can play a role in up-regulating cell replication and inducing cell activation associated with apoptosis. A portion of gp120 can serve as a superantigen for VH3 B cells and thus could induce some of the B-cell responses observed in HIV infection.

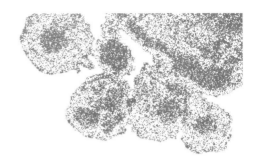

Viral Proteins Determining Biologic Features of HIV

7

INITIAL MOLECULAR STUDIES OF THE HIV genome defined in general the relative importance of various viral genes for infection and replication. The influence of the viral envelope on cell tropism and cytotoxicity was appreciated. These approaches led to the recognition of several regulatory genes affecting virus production (for reviews, see references 1620, 3362, and 3483) (see Chapter 1). Subsequent studies have emphasized how these genetic regions in the virus, interacting with intracellular factors, can be responsible for various biologic and serologic properties (for reviews, see references 361, 1542, 1620, and 3362). The findings on the viral proteins associated with many of these features of both HIV-1 and HIV-2 infection are summarized in this chapter.

I. Envelope Region and Cell Tropism

A. Genetic Studies

1. GENERAL OBSERVATIONS

Several reports initially demonstrated that the envelope region contains the primary genetic sequences responsible for cell tropism (i.e., T-cell-line and macrophage tropism), cytopathology, CD4 protein modulation, and virus neutralization (see Chapter 10) (728, 732, 894, 1942, 2642, 3308, 4111, 4885). In all these studies and others cited in this book, it is important to recognize that differences in the ability of HIV isolates to infect established (transformed) T-cell lines do not necessarily indicate variations in tropism for primary CD4$^+$ lymphocytes. All viral mutants, except those losing infectivity in general, maintain the ability to infect peripheral blood CD4$^+$ cells, assuming that the appropriate coreceptor is present (see Chapter 3).

Moreover, most, if not all, HIV isolates can infect macrophages, but the extent of replication varies. Thus, macrophage tropism primarily refers to R5 viruses that grow to substantial titer in macrophages. Moreover, dualtropic viruses can be identified (R5/X4 isolates) that replicate well in macrophages and T-cell lines (see Chapter 3). Several viruses have been found to grow well only in CD4+ lymphocytes and not in macrophages or T-cell lines (see below and Chapters 3 and 4). Finally, tropism for primary macrophages does not correlate with infection of transformed monocytic cell lines. Thus, results from cell culture studies may not have direct relevance in vivo, but the observations do reveal the importance of certain genetic regions and envelope conformation in cell tropism.

With the current recognition that specific cellular coreceptors can define cell tropism, the early findings reviewed in the following section are particularly relevant to understanding the interaction of macrophage-tropic (R5) or T-cell-line-tropic (X4) viruses with cell surface receptors (Table 3.2). For example, for CCR5 and CXCR4, the V3 loop appears to be an important determinant (823, 4224; for a review, see reference 1752) (see Chapters 3 and 13). However, the diversity of strains that use this receptor (different clades of HIV-1, HIV-2, and SIV) implies that regions other than this variable envelope domain are also involved. Nevertheless, some studies have suggested that a similarity between domains of the V3 loop and chemokines can explain a common means of entry (4072).

2. MACROPHAGE TROPISM

Certain experiments conducted several years ago considerably narrowed down the region(s) of the virus responsible for macrophage tropism. Studies with recombinant viruses derived from two unrelated HIV-1 isolates (the T-cell-line-tropic X4 SF2 virus and the macrophage-tropic R5 SF162 virus) initially showed that infection of primary macrophages was associated with a 159-amino-acid region in the 3' portion of gp120 (4111). A similar finding was made with two other viral isolates (3308). Subsequently, the involvement of the V3 loop alone (amino acids ~304 to 324 of the viral gp120 protein examined) in macrophage

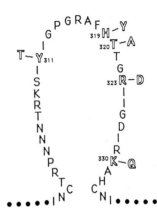

Figure 7.1   Comparison of the amino acid sequence of the V3 regions of the HIV-1$_{SF2}$ and HIV-2$_{SF162}$ strains. The complete V3 sequence of a molecular clone of HIV-1$_{SF2}$ is shown, and the five amino acid residues that differ in HIV-1$_{SF162}$ are designated. The positions of amino acid residues are relative to the HIV-1$_{SF2}$ genome referenced in the Los Alamos AIDS and Human Retroviruses database. Reprinted from reference 4112 with permission.

tropism was demonstrated (1942, 4112). As few as three amino acid changes in the V3 domain (positions 319, 320, and 323) were found to confer macrophage tropism on an X4 virus (4112) (Figure 7.1; Table 7.1). Nevertheless, conversion of an X4 virus such as HIV-1$_{SF2}$ to an R5 virus with replicative properties equal to those of HIV-1$_{SF162}$ required the transfer of the V1 and V2 regions as well as the V3 loop (2257). Similar observations on the importance of the V1 and V2 regions for efficient replication in cultured macrophages were made with other virus recombinants (4448).

In other mutant virus studies, elimination of two N-linked glycosylation sites in the V2 region of SF2 conferred macrophage tropism and eliminated the T-cell-line tropism of HIV-1$_{SF2}$ (2258). This dramatic finding appeared to reflect the importance of envelope conformation (i.e., epitope accessibility) and/or charge on viral entry (Section I.B). Finally, certain studies suggested that productive infection of macrophages involves two distinct genetic regions and mechanisms: the envelope gene for virus entry, and *vif* and *vpr* for efficient virus replication (1843) (see below).

3. T-CELL-LINE TROPISM

For T-cell-line tropism, the V3 loop was also found to be important (1942, 4112). The SF2

Table 7.1 Cellular host range of HIV-2$_{SF2mc}$ and HIV-1SF$_{162mc}$ mutant viruses[a]

HIV-1 strain	V3 region sequence	PBMC	Macrophages	HUT 78 cells	MT-4 cells
		Virus replication in[b]:			
SF2					
WT[c]	iYigpgrafHTtgRiigdirKA	+++	−	+++	+++
Mu1	–T-------YA--D------Q–	+++	+	−	−
Mu2	–T-------YA--D--------	+++	+	−	−
Mu3	---------YA--D--------	+++	+	−	−
Mu8	------------D--------	+++	−	+++	−
R19	–T-------YA--D------Q–	+++	+	−	−
SF162					
WT	iTigpgraf YAtgDiigdirQa	+++	++	−	−
Mu10	–Y-------HT--R------K–	+++	+	−	−
Mu11	–Y-------HT--R--------	+++	+	−	−

[a]Mutant proviral DNAs were generated from molecular clones (mc) by site-directed mutagenesis using mutant oligodeoxynucleotides as primers. Mutant viruses were recovered by transfection of mutagenized proviral DNA into human RD4 cells followed by cocultivation with peripheral blood mononuclear cells (PBMC) from seronegative individuals. These viruses were inoculated at 10^6 cpm of reverse transcriptase activity onto PBMC, primary macrophages, and the HUT 78 and MT-4 T-cell lines. Adapted from reference 4112.

[b]The relative extent of virus replication is represented by plus signs. A minus sign indicates no detectable virus production.

[c]WT, wild type.

recombinant virus with the SF162-like V3 domain described above lost its T-cell-line tropism when it gained macrophage tropism (4112). Moreover, replacing the five different amino acids in the V3 loop of HIV-1$_{SF162}$ with the amino acids of HIV-1$_{SF2}$ did not convert the HIV-1$_{SF162}$ recombinant to an X4 virus. However, in one SF2 mutant (Mu8), a single amino acid change in the V3 loop (position 323 [Figure 7.1]) eliminated the ability of the SF2 mutant virus to infect one particular T-cell line (MT-4) but not others (4112) (Table 7.1).

4. THE V3 LOOP

Focusing on the V3 loop (for a review, see reference 1752), mutations made in the crown (GPGRA) of this HIV envelope region have generally induced a loss of infectivity and changes in the fusogenic potential of the viruses examined (1630, 3381, 4251) without affecting CD4 binding. Furthermore, in certain experiments, the envelope charge in the V3 loop (e.g., the presence of a positively charged amino acid at position 11 or 28) was found to be associated with efficient T-cell-line infection, syncytium formation, and virus replication (1338, 4112). In some cases, however, this correlation of X4 viruses with specific amino acids in the V3 sequence was not confirmed (3861, 3946). Further-

more, differences among HIV-1 clades in terms of concordance with these molecular findings have been noted (3861). With HIV-2, the association of cell tropism with the V3 loop has also been reported (53). As noted above, the common use of the V3 loop for virus entry could be explained by domains in this envelope region that resemble chemokines (4072).

Finally, as discussed in Chapter 3, other viral regions besides gp120, particularly gp41 (677, 4172), have envelope domains needed for postbinding steps (e.g., virus:cell fusion) involved in virus entry (Figures 3.2 and 3.4 and Color Plates 2 and 5, following page 78).

5. TROPISM FOR BRAIN-DERIVED CELLS

Studies of infection of CD4$^+$ brain-derived fibroblasts with other isolates of HIV-1 (e.g., the GUN viruses) showed that a single amino acid in the V3 loop (amino acid 311) can affect HIV infection (4370). The results demonstrated that changes in this region of the virus can affect cell tropism and sensitivity to neutralizing antibodies (2940). Moreover, perhaps as expected, using the JR-FL virus (R5) and NL4-3 virus (X4), the infection of brain-derived microglia was linked to the same envelope region controlling macrophage tropism

(4075). In this regard, certain amino acids in the V1/V2 domain have been associated with syncytium formation in microglia (4105). In other early studies, the pattern of envelope N-linked glycosylation appeared to be important for this infection (2468).

In addition, as noted with T-cell and macrophage tropisms, changes within the crown of the V3 loop were found to be needed for infection of brain-derived cells (e.g., meningiomas) (4109). Moreover, sequences regulating the tropism of HIV-1 for brain capillary endothelial cells were localized to a region encompassing the C1 portion of Env and overlapping reading frames for Vpr, Vpu, Tat, and Rev. This domain does not cosegregate with either macrophage or T-cell-line tropism (3126). Nevertheless, the sensitivity of brain capillary endothelial cells to HIV-1 infection correlated best with X4 tropism and not with R5 tropism (see Chapter 8). In addition, sequences in either V3 or V4/V5 appear to determine the tropism of some viruses for neural cell lines, in which entry can be mediated by galactosyl ceramide (GalC) (1730, 1732) (see Chapter 3). The relevance of these findings to other brain isolates requires further study.

6. INFECTION OF CELLS NOT EXPRESSING CD4

The CD4-independent tropisms of HIV-1 and HIV-2 also involve certain regions in the envelope protein. With HIV-1, as noted above, domains within the V3 loop that interact with GalC on CD4⁻ brain- and bowel-derived cells have been identified (1730, 1732, 4842). With HIV-2, sequences in portions of the transmembrane protein and the V3 loop as well as areas flanking the base of the V4 loop appear to be responsible (1203, 3688). In some cells the chemokine coreceptors interacting with primarily the V3 loop provide the means for HIV infection (787, 1172; for a review, see reference 251) (see Chapter 3, Table 3.2).

B. Role of Envelope Conformation in Cell Tropism

All the results have indicated that generally more than three amino acid changes are required to affect cell tropism, particularly if substantial replication is measured. Nevertheless, in some cases, one modification has affected the infection of a single cell line (894, 4112) (Table 7.1). The findings emphasize the importance for HIV entry of a variety of viral epitopes, determined most probably by the conformation of gp120, particularly in the V3 loop. In support of this conclusion, additional regions of the envelope gp120 outside the V3 loop were found to enhance the extent of virus replication in T-cell lines and macrophages, probably by increasing the efficiency of virus entry via the V3 loop (624, 625, 4111, 4251). In this connection, certain studies have suggested that the V1 and V2 domains, together with the V3 loop, can increase viral infectivity and replication in macrophages (2257). Moreover, conserved regions in gp120 (such as the C4 region) can influence HIV infection of certain cell types; with the help of V1/V2, these additional domains can determine syncytium formation in culture and affect viral tropism (2156). It seems likely that the envelope of each viral isolate, depending on the amino acid makeup of the envelope, will have a different conformational structure. Therefore, various envelope regions for specific viruses could affect their ability to infect cells.

Several viral properties reflect the importance of envelope conformation (Table 7.2). Among these, cell tropism and antibody binding (including serum neutralization) appear to be most important (1167, 3095, 4255) (see Chapter 10). The influence of gp120 glycosylation on cell tropism also supports the role of envelope conformation

Table 7.2 HIV properties reflecting envelope conformation[a]

- Host range: macrophage versus T-cell-line tropism
- Antibody neutralization; conformation-dependent epitopes
- Antibody binding efficiency[b]
- Envelope cleavage
- Envelope glycosylation
- Virus:cell fusion
- Soluble CD4 inactivation
- Virus-CD4⁺ binding and virus-coreceptor binding
- Spontaneous gp120 shedding

[a]Most of the parameters do not appear together consistently.
[b]Measured by monoclonal antibodies.

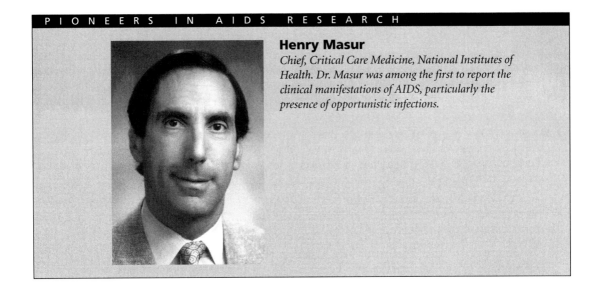

Henry Masur
Chief, Critical Care Medicine, National Institutes of Health. Dr. Masur was among the first to report the clinical manifestations of AIDS, particularly the presence of opportunistic infections.

in this process (2258, 2468) (see Chapter 3). These properties do not necessarily occur together and do not reflect specific variations responsible for a particular conformation.

The susceptibility of HIV-1 isolates to monoclonal antibodies appears to distinguish R5 from X4 isolates very well (1167, 4255; for a review, see reference 563) (see Chapter 10). Such antibodies can detect conformational changes in gp120 that occur after virus-receptor binding and that distinguish viruses with different cell tropisms (4252). Other studies reflecting the role of envelope conformation have shown that certain genetic changes that reduce the infectivity of one HIV strain may not have any effect on the infectivity of another virus if the sequences surrounding the mutated site are different (3381). Moreover, certain amino acid changes in the C2 and V3 loop regions of the SF2/SF13 mutant viruses discussed earlier can increase the extent of gp120 shedding by the viral envelope without affecting binding to the CD4 cell surface protein. In this case, virus infectivity of T-cell lines can be increased, perhaps secondary to enhanced exposure of the gp41 fusion molecule (see Chapter 3, Figure 3.2, and Color Plate 2, following page 78). The effect of amino acid substitutions in the V3 loop on the virion gp120:gp41 envelope complex has been noted in other studies on cell tropism (4772; for a review, see reference 1752).

II. Influence of Accessory Proteins on HIV Replication

A. Introduction

The HIV genes that encode accessory or regulatory proteins that help in HIV replication are considered in this section. Vif is discussed in Chapter 5. Several reports have suggested that small changes in *vif*, as well as *vpr* and *vpu*, can affect the extent of virus infectivity and replication (3882) (see Chapter 5). Thus far, however, alterations in other accessory viral genes, besides *nef* and *tat*, have not correlated with the rate of disease progression or a long-term asymptomatic course (see Chapter 13).

B. Long Terminal Repeat (LTR)

The LTR region of HIV contains many genetic elements involved in viral transcription (3362) (Figure 7.2). It is the major viral region determining the extent of HIV replication. The downstream core promoter/enhancing region of the LTR is generally conserved among clades. Nevertheless, a series of experiments comparing in vitro and in vivo chimeric HIV-1 viruses on the same background (SIV_{mac}) (i.e., SHIV strains) revealed differences in the virus replicative capacity associated with the LTR. The findings indicated the heterogeneity of this region in terms of its influence on virus replication (661). For example, the

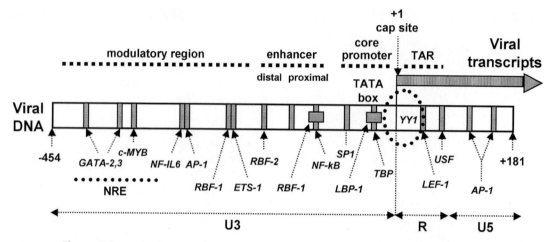

Figure 7.2   Major features of the HIV-1 LTR in viral DNA. The LTR contains *cis*-acting sequences that function in either integration or transcription of the provirus, and is divided into three regions (U3, R, and U5), which are generated from the single-stranded viral RNA genome by the reverse transcription process. The convention uses +1 to identify the 5' ends of viral transcripts, which are capped at initiation of viral RNA synthesis. The 5' LTR of HIV-1 contains the single promoter for transcription of all viral genes and is divided into four functional regions: the modulatory region (-454 to -104), the enhancer region (-105 to -79), the core or basal promoter (-78 to -1), and the transactivation response element (TAR) (+1 to +60). Deletions in a portion of the U3 region augment initiation of viral transcription; accordingly, this region has been designated the negative regulatory element (NRE) (-340 to -184). This figure identifies the sites for binding of selected cellular transcription factors, labeled in italics, that provide for positive regulation of viral transcription: GATA-2,3 (-441 to -373, -343 to -338), c-MYB (-304 to -299), NF-IL6 (-258 to -238), RBF-1 (-151 to -141), ETS-1 (-160 to -140), RBF-2 (-131 to -121), ETS-2 (-104 to -95), RBF-1 (-104 to -80), NF-κB (-104 to -95, -91 to -81), SP1 (three sites, -78 to -46), TBP (TATA box at -27 to -23), LBP-1 (-39 to -16), LEF-1 (+17 to +32), USF (+35 to +60), and AP-1 (+92 to +102, +160 to +167). The dotted circle shows the location of a nucleosome (nuc-1), which is remodeled in chromatin during transcriptional activation of the 5' LTR. Host factors, such as YY1, recruit histone deacetylases to maintain nuc-1 in a hypoacetylated state and thereby inhibit transcription. A hexamer site for addition of poly-(A) tails to viral transcripts is located at +73 to +78; this site, although contained in both LTRs, is functional in the 3' LTR. The transcription factor binding sites mediate combinatorial DNA:protein and protein:protein interactions and thereby produce a complex regulatory network to regulate HIV transcription in various cell types in response to different extracellular stimuli. This figure is based on a more comprehensive list of transcription factors that interact with the HIV-1 LTR. For references and further discussion, see reference 3469a. Figure provided by P. Luciw.

promoter for clade C viruses, in comparison to that for the B and E clade viruses, appears to be better adapted for early replicating properties. Moreover, the HIV-1 clade C promoter is associated with increased viral loads, perhaps reflecting an enhanced sensitivity to TNF-α (2016, 3064). High cytokine levels, particularly in mucosal sites, could increase viral loads and therefore transmission (see Chapter 2). When the core promoter element of HIV-1 subtype E was placed within an infectious molecular clone of LAI (clade B), the virus showed higher levels of replication (2016). These data, along with those observed with Tat (see below), indicate the importance of the LTR promoter in eliciting early or persistent virus replication.

Other studies have shown differences in replication and cytokine production depending on the number of NF-κB sites that appear in the viral LTR (2016). Subtype E has one site, subtype C has three sites, and other clades have two. The LTR of HIV-2 has one site (4446). The response to TNF-α, reflected by virus replication, correlates with the

NF-κB sites. Moreover, HIV-1 clade C viruses were found to be more transcriptionally active than HIV E isolates (3065). The differences could explain the increasing spread of this HIV clade through Asia (3064). Nevertheless, in the in vitro studies, subtype E replicated in cell cultures better than the subtype C viruses (2016) (see Chapter 1).

C. Rev

Rev, a 19-kDa protein, is very important in the transfer of viral mRNA to the cytoplasm for translation into viral proteins. The 9-kb genomic transcript of HIV-1 serves as the mRNA for Env and Gag proteins and can be spliced in multiple alternative ways to give rise to nearly 50 subgenomic mRNAs (951, 1620) (see Chapter 1). The unspliced RNA and many singly spliced viral mRNAs are unable to exit the nucleus in the absence of the viral protein Rev (1266, 4197). Rev promotes the export and stability of these incompletely spliced viral mRNAs by binding directly to them in the nucleus. The binding occurs at a highly structured *cis*-acting element within an intron-containing viral RNA, known as the Rev responsive element (RRE), found in the viral envelope transcript. It is present in all Rev responsive RNAs but is excised as an intron from all others. After the initial high-affinity binding of Rev to the RRE, multimers of Rev attach to the RRE and elicit its function (for a review, see reference 1620). Besides its arginine-rich RNA binding region, the Rev protein has a nuclear localization signal (NLS) and a nuclear export signal (NES) that take the viral mRNAs to the cytoplasm (for a review, see reference 4211). Through the NLS and NES domains, Rev can shuttle between the nucleus and the cytoplasm, but it accumulates primarily in the nucleus. Rev utilizes the CRM-1/export 1 pathway (3239); other unrelated viruses have proteins with similar functions but use different pathways (3214). Several cellular proteins interacting with Rev have been reported (1620, 4896).

D. Tat

Tat is a 23-kDa protein named because of its primary role in transactivation of HIV transcription. By interacting with cellular proteins, Tat helps in the transcription of viral RNA from the LTR via the transactivation response element (TAR) (see Chapter 3) (1355; for a review, see reference 1620). This viral protein functions primarily by promoter elongation of the mRNA messages (1620, 4445). The interaction of a positive transcription elongation factor b complex (P-TEFb) with the Tat:TAR complex enhances transcription substantially (1620, 4445). P-TEFb is composed of cyclin T1, CDK9, and 7 SK snRNA (for a review, see reference 246) (see also Chapter 5).

Using interviral SF2/SF13 recombinants, the biologic propterties of Tat were substantiated. Increased virus replication in PBMC and in the HUT 78 T-cell line was linked to the first exon coding region of *tat* and reflected only two amino acid differences (732, 733). A change in one of these two amino acid differences in Tat$_{SF13}$ reduced the extent of replication of the dualtropic SF13 strain to that of the related X4 SF2 strain (2475). While initially Tat was thought to regulate the kinetics of virus replication, close examination showed that the effect was on the level of virus production (1089). HIV-1$_{SF13}$ produces nearly twice as many infectious viruses as does HIV-1$_{SF2}$. Thus, faster kinetics reflected increased number and spread of progeny viruses in culture. The results indicate that for some isolates, limited modifications in the Tat regulatory protein can greatly affect virus production.

Additional studies with chimeric viruses using the chloramphenicol acetyltransferase (CAT) assay supports the effect of Tat proteins on their respective LTRs (2475). The results showed that the cell type can influence the effect of Tat and that the LTRs from high-virus producer isolates (SF13 and SF33) were more sensitive to Tat$_{SF2}$ than was the LTR from a low-replicating SF2 isolate (2475). Moreover, no substantial difference was observed in the extent of transactivation by Tat$_{SF13}$ when using the LTR from the three different viruses. Despite these findings in the laboratory, however, studies of viruses from HIV-infected individuals with different rates of progression to disease have not revealed a major influence of the TAR and *tat* regions (2215).

Differences in function of Tat proteins from various clades have also been observed (1057). HIV-1 clades C and E had Tat proteins with strong transactivation, and Tat E had a longer half-life within the cell and interacted more efficiently with the TAR. The extent of cyclin T1 association with

Tat appeared to be important in this transactivation efficiency (1057).

Tat has been implicated in many biologic processes (Table 7.3) and appears to function early in the infection process (4445). The Tat protein is released by infected cells and can be readily taken up by other cells and influence their function. It has sequences similar to the β-chemokines and thus can be a potent chemoattractant for monocytes (54), basophils, and mast cells (2032). The Tat protein shares cell surface receptors with MCP-1, MCP-3, and eotaxin (2378), and it can also enhance virus spread by up-regulating the expression of CCR5 and CXCR4 (1920, 4029). Soluble Tat inhibits the interaction of X4 viruses with CXCR4 and could be involved in the selection of R5 viruses during HIV infection (4836). Some investigators have reported the presence of Tat in the cell membrane that could help HIV-1 cell binding and/or entry (2802).

In terms of the immune system, Tat up-regulates the major histocompatibility complex (MHC) and can enhance production of IL-12, TNF-α, and the β-chemokines (1245). It promotes the maturation and antigen-presenting functions of monocyte-derived dendritic cells, leading to a type 1 immune response. Through infection or by contact with soluble Tat protein, B- and T-cell functions can be enhanced in antigen processing and in expression of CTL epitopes (1467). With regard to B-cell functions, whereas Tat has been shown to inhibit proliferation of naïve and memory B cells, it enhances the germinal-center B-cell proliferation induced by CD40 antibody and IL-4 (2470). Thus, it could play a role in the hypergammaglobulinemia observed in HIV infection and perhaps the development of B-cell lymphomas (see Chapter 12).

Table 7.3 Potential functions of Tat in HIV infection

- Enhances transcription of viral RNA from the LTR via TAR by promoter elongation of the mRNA messages (2097, 4445)
- Chemoattractant for monocytes, basophils, and mast cells (54, 2032)
- Up-regulates expression of CCR5 and CXCR4 (1920, 4029)
- Can inhibit the interaction of X4 viruses with CXCR4 (4836)
- Presence in the cell membrane could help HIV cell binding and/or entry (2802)
- Up-regulates MHC and enhances production of IL-12, TNF-α, and β-chemokines (1245)
- Promotes maturation and antigen-presenting functions of monocyte-derived dendritic cells
- Can enhance B- and T-cell functions in antigen processing and in expression of CTL epitopes (1467)
- Inhibits proliferation of naïve and memory B cells
- Enhances germinal-cell and B-cell proliferation (2470)
- Reduces the mannose receptor expression on monocytes (584)
- Induces IL-10 production by peripheral blood monocytes (204) that reduces immune responses (816)
- Can suppress IL-12 production (1970)
- Can block PKR function and affect IFN-α production (579)
- Induces apoptosis (2565, 4736)
- Blocks NK cell activity (4974)
- Induces MCP-1, IL-8, and IL-10 expression by astrocytes (861, 2355)
- Activates vascular endothelial growth factor receptors, leading to increased cell permeability (142)
- Interacts with low-density lipoprotein receptor on neurons (2638)
- Inhibits neuronal endopeptidase, which could lead to dementia (3702)
- Suppresses a natural intercellular RNA silencing function (307)

Tat has known immunosuppressing activities (842). It reduces the mannose receptor expression on monocytes through an effect on the promoter. Thus, this HIV protein could contribute to an impaired response to *Pneumocystis jiroveci* (*carinii*) phagocytosis by macrophages as well as other cellular functions (584). Tat can induce IL-10 production by peripheral blood monocytes (204) and reduce immune responses (816). When added to PBMC, soluble Tat suppresses IL-12 production (1970). Again, in view of the studies on IL-12 cited above (1245), the relative amounts of Tat expressed appear to determine its effect on IL-12 production. Tat can also block protein kinase R (PKR) function and reduce interferon production in HIV replication (579). In some studies, Tat has induced apoptosis (2565, 4736) and blocked NK cell activity (4974).

Tat can also induce MCP-1, IL-8, and IL-10 expression by astrocytes (861, 2355) and has been evaluated for its role in HIV-related neurologic disease either through its chemoattractant property (2355) or through its interaction with a low-density lipoprotein receptor on neurons (2638). In this regard, Tat can activate vascular endothelial growth factor receptors, leading to increased cell permeability (142). Moreover, Tat can inhibit neuronal endopeptidase (neoprosin) (3702), which degrades amyloid-β and prevents its accumulation and dementia (see Chapter 8).

In general, the specific function of Tat in cells seems to depend on its level of expression and the cell types infected. Different domains of the Tat protein are responsible for its role in transactivation versus suppression of immune responses (532). The clinical importance of these reported activities of Tat is unknown. Expression of human Tat in transgenic mice has not led to any detectable pathology in the animals (2610). Most recently, some evidence has shown that the Tat protein suppresses a natural intracellular RNA silencing function by affecting the ability of Dicer to process precursor double-stranded RNA (short hairpin RNA) (307) (see Chapter 14, Section II.D.3). The mechanism does not appear to be binding of Tat to the shRNA but may be by directly interacting with Dicer. Since small interfering RNAs are not affected by Tat, this type of strategy may be necessary if RNA silencing is to be used for antiviral therapy (307) (see Chapter 14).

E. Nef

The pleiotropic function of Nef, a 27-kDa protein, is reflected in many research laboratory investigations showing its influence on virus infection and replication as well as on the immune response (Table 7.4). The sequences in the Nef region are highly heterogeneous (1038), and differences in activity can be found among various alleles and in different cell types (e.g., T-cell lines versus CD4$^+$ lymphocytes) (see below) (1240a, 3851). A role for Nef in virus entry has been proposed (2702, 3955). Some studies with viral pseudotypes suggested that Nef can enhance fusion of the cell surface by a neutral pH mechanism (702), but most results define only intracellular functions of Nef in HIV replication (see below). Similar to cyclophilin, Nef is found inside the virion (478, 846, 1354, 2298, 3400, 4725) and appears to participate in an early postentry step by helping in the disassembly of the viral core (40, 1329, 2175, 4440); it also enhances reverse transcription (40). Recent studies suggest that incorporation of Nef into virions is not necessary for its role in enhancing infectivity and HIV replication (1240a).

Within the cell, Nef has been found to down-regulate the expression of the MHC class I molecule (854) and CD4 (1445, 1676) as well as the beta chain of the CD8 $\alpha\beta$ receptor (4303). Nef increases their endocytosis by binding to these cellular cytoplasmic domains (4014, 4776). The down-modulation of MHC class I and CD4 appears to involve Nef when bound to lipid rafts (60). The decrease in MHC class I expression occurs by its accumulation into intracellular organelles (4345). Nef also can impair MHC class II expression (4320) and increases CD28 endocytosis, causing a reduction in CD28 expression (4348). These effects of Nef on MHC, CD4, CD3, and CD28 all appear to involve separate domains on the viral protein (4348, 4776; for a review, see reference 151).

The CD4 down-modulation occurs rapidly early in infection as a result of Nef, but the later expression of Vpu (116) and the viral envelope gives the optimal reduction in CD4 expression (712). This influence of Nef on CD4 can enhance HIV infection since the association of gp120 with gp41 remains stable (2700) (see below). Nef has

Table 7.4 Potential functions of Nef in HIV infection

- Could have a role in virus entry (2702, 3955)
- Enhances fusion of the cell surface by a neutral pH mechanism (702)
- Has a role in an early postentry step by helping in the disassembly of the viral core (2175, 4440)
- Enhances reverse transcription (40)
- Enhances virus replication (767, 1004, 3019, 4013, 4921)
- Down-regulates MHC class I expression (854, 4014)
- Impairs MHC class II expression (4320)
- Down-modulates CD4 expression in some T cells (1445, 1676, 2811)
- Decreases expression of the beta chain of the CD8$^+$ cell $\alpha\beta$ receptor (4303)
- Increases CD28 endocytosis with reduction in CD28 expression (4348, 4776)
- Reduces TCR-initiated signaling by interfering with the CD3:TCR complex (1945, 2703)
- Transports newly synthesized cholesterol to sites of viral budding (4947)
- Plays a role in T-cell activation (283, 2797, 4169)
- Modulates proteins involved in calcium signaling pathways in T cells (283, 2679)
- Can suppress HIV replication in T-cell lines (723, 726) and possibly in astrocytes (479, 4449)
- May down-regulate virus replication in T cells and monocytes via competition for factors interacting with the LTR, thereby decreasing cell activation and transcription (37, 2692, 3255, 4501)
- Binds viral p6 in Gag/Pol that retains Nef in the virion and helps in the budding process (904)
- Enhances incorporation of envelope glycoproteins on the virion (3911)
- Induces proteins that up-regulate B-cell receptor expression and can make resting CD4$^+$ lymphocytes susceptible to HIV infection (4349)
- Nef released by infected cells can suppress B-cell IgM switching to IgG and IgA (3630)
- Induces CD4$^+$ T-cell death by apoptosis (1383, 1996)
- Can inhibit apoptosis via ASK-1 (1485) or binding to p53 protein (1626)
- Blocks production of IL-2 and IFN-γ (851, 1723, 2703)
- Induces MIP-1α and MIP-1β production (4349)
- Induces IL-10 production (507)

been shown to transport newly synthesized cholesterol to sites of viral budding (4947), which would help in the formation of infectious virions. In this regard, Nef has been observed to bind to p6 in Gag/Pol, which is important for retention of Nef in the virion and also helps in the budding process (904). Nef has also been found to enhance virion incorporation of retroviral envelope glycoproteins by increasing their localization in late endosomes (3911). Recently the potential role of a secreted Nef in preventing immunoglobulin class switching by B cells (e.g., immunoglobulin M [IgM] or IgG) has been reported (3630).

Likewise, the finding of Nef within virions (3399, 3400, 4725), its association with protein kinase activity (3937), and its potential function in activating CD4$^+$ lymphocytes (see below) suggested that it plays a role in inducing a permissive state for virus replication early in infection. Nef appears to associate with a 65-kDa protein that is serologically and functionally related to the p21-activated kinases that are involved in signal transduction (3289).

A possible role for the *nef* gene in cell latency was initially proposed because deletion of this viral gene from the molecular clone of the HIV-1$_{SF2}$ strain produced a variant that replicated to a high titer and was more cytopathic than the original SF2 isolate (2689). In further studies, the HIV-1$_{SF2}$ *nef* gene (linked to the viral LTR or the simian virus 40 promoter) transfected in T-cell lines suppressed virus replication (723). However, Nef from a highly cytopathic X4 virus did not have this effect (726). Moreover, HIV-infected human astrocyte lines have demonstrated a correlation between an arrest in virus replication and high-level Nef expression (479, 4450). Similarly, biopsy specimens from brains of children and adults have shown high expression of Nef in non-virus-producing cells (3875, 4449). Down-modulation of HIV LTR activity by a portion of the *nef* gene has been detected (2692) (see also below). Thus, Nef might play an inhibitory role in astrocytes, but the mechanism(s) is not known (see Chapter 8). Work in T-cell lines with other HIV isolates, and with SIV, supported the finding that the *nef* gene can down-regulate virus replication in T cells and monocytes, most notably via the LTR (NF-κB and AP-1 sites) (37, 3254, 3256, 4407, 4501).

Despite these early observations, the suggestion that Nef reduces virus production has not been confirmed by others. Several studies have shown that viruses with *nef* deletions replicate to a limited extent and appear to be attenuated (1999, 2170) (see below). Importantly, different results on Nef activity are obtained when normal CD4+ lymphocytes are used instead of transformed human T-cell lines. In this regard, some viruses with *nef* mutations were shown to replicate better in macrophages than in T-cell lines (4408), whereas the *nef* allele of other viruses was associated with acceleration in virus replication in CD4+ lymphocytes and also T-cell lines (1004, 4922). This heterogeneity of the viral *nef* allele could explain why investigators initially did not find a silencing effect of Nef on HIV expression (1709, 2196).

Notably, animal experiments do not support a virus-suppressing role for Nef. In rhesus macaques, the mutant virus with the *nef* deletion is less pathogenic than its wild-type counterpart (2170). The requirement for Nef in pathogenicity was also inferred from studies in the SCID mouse system, in which *nef* deletion mutants of HIV-1 strains had attenuated growth properties and did not induce depletion of human CD4+ cells in the animals (1999). This role of Nef becomes most evident in nonstimulated CD4+ lymphocytes (3019, 4230, 4234). In these cells, most viruses with *nef* deletions do not replicate substantially, although they grow efficiently in activated CD4+ lymphocytes. In addition, a deletion in the *nef* gene has been found in some HIV-1 isolates from long-term survivors (see Chapter 13) (2447) and in viruses recovered from transfusion recipients who did not progress to disease (2993). These studies suggest that Nef could play a role in delaying disease progression in some cases (see Chapter 13). However, over time some of these subjects later developed AIDS (371).

The observed importance of Nef for high-level virus production can be secondary to its influence on early steps in virus entry of cells and/or reverse transcription (40, 767, 3019, 4013, 4230). Nef modulates the proteins involved in calcium signaling pathways in T cells such as BAK and PAK kinase (283, 2679) and can cause cell activation via NFAT-1 (2797). Nef also reduces the TCR-initiated signaling within the cell by interfering with the CD3:TCR complex (298, 1901, 1945, 2703). This potential effect of Nef on T-cell activation (283, 4169) and its association with serine kinase activity (3937, 3938) suggest that its importance for HIV replication is linked to signal transduction (Figure 5.3). Thus, how Nef affects the intracellular milieu could determine its ultimate effect on the replication in a cell by a particular HIV isolate. Conceivably, the reduction in CD4 expression by Nef described above helps virus replication by preventing cell death by fusion or other CD4-mediated events (see Chapter 6). Nevertheless, studies have demonstrated that the down-modulation of CD4 by Nef can be separated from its enhancing effects on virus replication (1550).

In terms of immune cell responses, Nef can block the efficient production of IL-2 and IFN-γ (851, 1723) and induce IL-10 production (507) that can suppress type 1 immune activities. Thus, the relative effect of Nef on cytokines could affect immune function and the extent of HIV replication. During infection, Nef has been found to induce MIP-1α and MIP-1β production associated with chemotaxis. This function appeared to be linked to macrophage infection by R5 viruses

(4351). Nef can also have an influence on resting CD4$^+$ cells after infection of macrophages. Proteins (soluble CD23 and soluble ICAM) which up-regulate B-cell receptor expression are induced by Nef and can make CD4$^+$ lymphocytes (even in a resting stage) susceptible to HIV-1 infection (4349). This mechanism could be involved in HIV infection of resting CD4$^+$ cells (see Chapter 5).

Nef in cell culture studies has been shown to induce CD4$^+$ cell death by apoptosis (1383, 1996) (see Chapter 6). In some studies, this process, associated with the beta chain of the TCR, is enhanced (4839), probably by an up-regulation of the Fas ligand. However, Nef, in other studies, has been shown to inhibit apoptosis through its association with the apoptosis signal-regulating kinase 1 (ASK-1), a threonine kinase involved in the Fas-Fas ligand signaling pathway (1485). Moreover, Nef can bind to the tumor suppressor 53 protein and inhibit apoptosis (1626). This effect of the viral protein could allow a longer period of HIV replication in infected cells.

In summary, the various effects of Nef proteins (Table 7.4) most likely reflect its interaction with cellular proteins (numbering over 30), probably via phosphorylation events yet to be fully defined (1676, 1677, 3289, 3594, 3937, 3938, 4801; for a review, see reference 151). Its overall influence on HIV replication depends on the particular *nef* allele, the cell type infected, and perhaps the location of Nef in the cell. Also, conceivably, specific domains in the *nef* gene differ in their biologic function (1240a). Most investigators currently consider that the major function of this viral protein carried within the virion (4725) is to induce activation and promote virus replication rather than suppress virus replication (for reviews, see references 151 and 1620). Nevertheless, the exceptions reviewed above continue to suggest a possible role for certain Nef alleles in viral latency in some cells.

F. Vpr and Vpx

HIV-1 Vpr, a 96-amino-acid (12- to 14-kDa) protein produced late in virus replication, is also found within the virion. It can play a role in HIV-1 entry, cell cycling, and apoptosis as well as other processes (Table 7.5) (see below). Vpr was recognized early as a protein needed for efficient infection of monocytes and macrophages (869),

Table 7.5 Potential functions of Vpr in HIV infection[a]

- May be part of the preintegration complex, which helps entry into the nucleus of cells (2076, 2562, 4093)
- Arrests cell proliferation in the late G_2/M stage of the cell cycle (874, 2561)
- Can increase LTR transcription (1544, 1906, 3571)
- Enhances or reduces apoptosis of infected cells (874)

[a]Similar functions have been described in part for Vpx of HIV-2.

most likely reflecting its role in the nuclear transport of the preintegration complex (PIC). Certain cellular proteins were found to be associated with Vpr, one of which could influence early steps in HIV reverse transcription (4264). Several studies have also indicated that Vpr can increase LTR transcription early after infection, even prior to virus integration, and in nondividing cells (3571). Its presence can enhance transcription from integrase-defective viruses (3571). Importantly, Vpr can also transactivate the viral LTR in the integrated viral DNA, a function that requires G_2 cell arrest (1544).

HIV-2 expresses two genes with homology to HIV-1 Vpr: the HIV-2 Vpr and Vpx genes. These HIV-2 genes are thought to have arisen as a duplication of a common ancestral gene because both genes share sequence and functional conservation and are located in tandem in the retroviral genome (4475). The HIV-1 Vpr gene and its counterpart, the Vpx gene in HIV-2, are present in high copy numbers in virus particles (840, 4891). In the virion core, Vpr is found in association with the p6 Gag protein (3450). It has been estimated that the stoichiometry of the HIV-1 Vpr and Gag proteins in viral particles is 1 to 7 (3160). Vpx is associated with the capsid protein and is expressed on the outside of the core particle (4891). Functions that are performed by HIV-1 Vpr have been segregated in HIV-2 as follows: HIV-2 Vpr maintains the ability to induce G_2 arrest, whereas Vpx retains the ability to enhance infection of nondividing cells (1309, 3532).

Vpr is another HIV protein, along with MA, that has been considered part of the PIC and helps its entry into the nuclei of dividing and nondividing

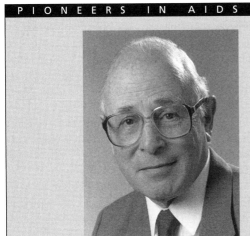

Herbert A. Perkins
Past Director, Irwin Memorial Blood Centers,
San Francisco, Calif. Dr. Perkins was one of the
pioneers in screening blood for HIV and recognizing
the transmission of the disease by blood.

cells (2562) (see above). This viral protein shuttles between the nucleus and the cytoplasm (4093) and interacts with importin α to promote passage of the PIC into the nucleus (2076, 3579). Vpr appears to help in the docking of the PIC at the nuclear membrane and interacts with components in the nuclear pore complex (i.e., the nuclear pore and hCG1, a nucleoporin) (2445, 3579). In this regard, the PIC, which measures about 56 nm (3018), is too large to pass through the nuclear pores, which measure 25 nm (for reviews, see references 4573 and 4852). Thus, it is noteworthy that Vpr was found to disrupt the nuclear envelope, which could allow entry of the PIC by a means that is distinct from the nuclear pore (998). The importance of this process is still not conclusive, since other viral proteins help the PIC gain entry into the nucleus and they do not involve nuclear envelope disruption. Moreover, Vpr-negative vectors can replicate in nondividing cells (4984) such as macrophages (1309). In addition, some HIV-2 and SIV isolates that lack the Vpr and Vpx genes, respectively, still induce AIDS in primates (265, 1507). Vpx in HIV-2 may be necessary for replication in macrophages (1309).

When HIV infects a cell, HIV-1 and HIV-2 Vpr arrest cell proliferation in the G_2/M stage of the cell cycle (1309, 3532). This effect can increase virus expression via LTR transcription and increase virus production (1544). It can enhance or reduce apoptosis of infected cells (874). Its in-

duction of apoptosis may be related to its association and inactivation of the antiapoptotic mitochondrial protein HAX-1 (4869). In this regard, recent studies have shown that the expression of HIV-1 Vpr activates the ataxia telangiectasia-and-Rad3-related kinase (ATR), a cellular protein whose normal function is to detect certain forms of DNA damage and, in turn, induce blockade of the cell cycle (4969). Subsequently, ATR was shown to be required for the induction of G_2 cell cycle arrest by Vpr (110). Therefore, it appears that G_2 arrest, induction of apoptosis, and transactivation of the LTR are functionally related effects of Vpr.

G. Vpu

Vpu, a 16-kDa membrane protein, is encoded by an envelope precursor bicistronic mRNA (4016; for a review, see reference 1898). It is expressed late in virus production and enhances HIV replication, most likely through formation of membrane pores (461, 463, 1628). High-level production of viral particles depends on Vpu for HIV-1 and two regions of the HIV-2 envelope (both the cytoplasmic tail and the ectodomain) (3). The counterpart for Vpu in HIV-2 is in the KDA envelope region (3, 463). Some studies suggest that a region in the HIV-1 envelope can also have Vpu function (4002).

Vpu has been associated with several other activities (Table 7.6). Along with the HIV-1 envelope and Nef, Vpu can down-regulate expression and

Table 7.6 Potential functions of Vpu in
HIV infection

- Enhances HIV replication through formation of
  membrane pores (461, 463, 1628)
- Down-regulates expression of CD4 (462, 2490)
- Interacts with K^+ channels in release of viral particles
  from the cell (1909)
- Promotes apoptosis in HIV-infected cells (44)
- Increases VCAM expression of endothelial cells
  (1809)
- May counter inhibitory effects of certain cellular
  proteins on HIV-1 budding process (4571)

enhance degradation of CD4 (462, 2490). By this
role in CD4 elimination, it causes a release of
gp160 from the CD4 envelope complex in the
endoplasmic reticulum (4767). The observations
have suggested that the cytoplasmic domain of
CD4 contains one determinant susceptible to this
Vpu-inducing degradation (2490). The removal
of CD4 increases HIV replication (462), since continual expression of CD4 on the cell surface inhibits the action of Vpu (462) and can reduce viral
particle production up to fivefold. Vpu can help in
the release of viral particles by interacting with K^+
channels (1909). Vpu also promotes apoptosis in
HIV-infected cells and increases VCAM-1 expression on endothelial cells (44, 1809). Some findings
suggest that Vpu counters an inhibitory effect of
a certain cellular protein(s) on the HIV-1 budding
process (4571). The cellular protein involved has
not yet been identified.

III. Envelope Region and Cytopathicity, CD4 Protein Modulation, and Soluble CD4 Neutralization

Besides defining the role of Env in cell tropism
(Section I), observations with interviral recombinants have identified, to some extent, the specific
regions in the viral envelope that can determine
induction of cell death (see Chapter 6), down-
modulation of CD4 expression on cells, and sensitivity of HIV to sCD4 inactivation. The genetic
regions influencing these biologic properties are
described below.

A. Cytopathicity

Cytopathicity as measured by syncytium formation
(728, 4251, 4885) usually leads to cell death (see
Chapter 6). Using the SF2/SF13 HIV-1 recombinants described above (Section I), a region that includes X4 virus tropism but not the V3 loop (4251)
was found to be involved. The role of the V1, V2, or
V3 loop in HIV-1 and HIV-2 cytopathicity has also
been identified in other mutational studies (121,
987, 1362–1364, 3381, 4334).

The V1 and V2 regions can influence the extent of syncytium formation (1636, 4334), perhaps through a functional interaction with the
C4 region of gp120 (1362). This potential interaction between the V1/V2 domain and C4 has
also been suggested by studies with monoclonal
antibodies (2934). The important role of gp41 in
this process reflecting cell:cell fusion has been
considered as well (see Chapter 6) (1301, 1363,
2314, 3473, 4172). Most cytopathic X4 viruses
have a positive charge near the crown of the V3
loop (1338). Therefore, in evaluating viral cytopathicity, some studies demonstrated that the introduction of one positively charged amino acid
(e.g., arginine) into a specific region of the V3
loop can, in some cases, produce an X4 virus
(986). Nevertheless, some X4 isolates, particularly of the HIV-2 type, do not show this characteristic (3861) (Section I.A).

In terms of gp120, only two glycosylation sites
in this viral envelope protein can determine the
extent of cell death resulting from lysis, independent of cell fusion (4291). This observation supports the role for glycosylation in cytopathicity
(3073) (see Chapter 6). Moreover, in other studies
of cytopathicity, a more cytopathic HIV-1 isolate
was Vpu deficient and during infection led to the
accumulation of envelope glycoproteins at the cell
surface. This phenomenon suggested that the cellular retention of virions, which are usually released with the help of Vpu (see above), could be
partly responsible for the cytopathic effects of
HIV-1 (1977).

B. CD4 Protein Down-Modulation

CD4 down-modulation was mapped to the envelope region of HIV (728, 4885). In this case, most

probably the CD4 binding region of gp120 was involved. Isolates from the brain showed this property (725), and some HIV-2 isolates do not affect CD4 expression (1231). Nevertheless, the potential role of Nef (1444, 1677) and Vpu in this process must also be appreciated (see above and Chapter 3, Table 3.7).

C. Soluble CD4 Neutralization

The structural basis for HIV heterogeneity with regard to sensitivity to sCD4 has been examined. In general, R5 viruses are resistant to sCD4 and appear to bind this molecule less avidly (see Chapter 2). Early studies showed that sCD4 resistance and macrophage tropism are associated with the V3 and flanking regions of gp120 (1943). With molecular clones of R5 and X4 viruses, sCD4 sensitivity corresponded to a rapid shedding of gp120 after interaction with sCD4. The sCD4 sensitivity is temperature related, since there is increased shedding of gp120 and inactivation of the R5 viruses at 4°C, whereas at that temperature the sensitivity to sCD4 for the X4 viruses is reduced (3309). The number of gp120 molecules on R5 viruses appears to be about four times greater than that on the X4 viruses (3309) (see Chapter 2). Thus, potential posttranslational changes to the virion occurring within a cell can affect not only cell tropism and sensitivity to antibody neutralization but also sensitivity to sCD4 neutralization. The results support previous studies showing that adaptation of R5 viruses to T-cell lines increases their binding to sCD4 (3095). Nevertheless, some studies have suggested that gp120 density and stability are not involved in resistance to sCD4 (2105).

IV. Conclusions

The initial studies on the viral genetic determinants of cell tropism provide insights into the domains on the envelope of HIV that determine their interaction with CCR5 and CXCR4. While the V3 loop in many of the genetic studies appears to be required for the virus:cell interaction, the diversity of viral isolates interacting with CD4 and coreceptors suggests that other regions are necessary and can be very important. Moreover, the studies of brain-derived cells and CD4$^-$ cells indicate that other genetic regions can control HIV infection. In general, the envelope conformation appears to be the major determinant of several biologic properties of HIV, particularly cell tropism (Section I.B) (Table 7.2) (3381, 4251).

A great deal of new information has also been obtained on the function of the accessory genes of HIV-1. Most of them have a large number and variety of activities influencing HIV infection, cell function, apoptosis, and immune response. They interact with many different cellular proteins that can affect their function. The relative importance of these pleiotropic effects of the viral regulatory proteins, particularly Tat and Nef, depends on the cell type infected, the specific allele, and the level of protein expression. Moreover, it is important to note that many functions attributed to these viral proteins were determined by cell culture studies and may not reflect their true activities in the infected cell and host. The findings have been valuable not only for understanding the steps involved in HIV infection but also for providing insights into normal cell function (e.g., Tat and Rev). The new processes defined also present novel strategies for antiviral therapy (see Chapter 14).

1. The cellular host range of HIV is determined to a great extent by linear and conformational epitopes of the viral envelope region. The conformation of the viral envelope appears to be the major determinant for cell tropism.

2. Small differences (as few as two or three amino acids) can determine whether a virus is macrophage tropic or T-cell-line tropic. Both types of viruses have the capacity to infect CD4+ lymphocytes.

3. The V3 loop of the viral envelope is a major determinant for infection of cells, most probably through its role in the interaction with coreceptors on the cell surface (see Chapter 3).

4. Tropism for brain-derived cells is also determined by the envelope region but can involve other viral regions, including the HIV regulatory proteins.

5. Infection of CD4− cells involves in part the V3 loop as well as other regions of the viral envelope.

6. The long terminal repeat (LTR) region and the viral regulatory proteins (i.e., Rev, Tat, Nef, Vpr/Vpx, and Vpu) are involved in the kinetics of virus replication and level of HIV production. They can influence cell proliferation, activation, expression of CD4 and the major histocompatibility complex molecules, and cell death.

7. Tat and Nef proteins have shown many different effects on HIV infection in cell culture. Their roles in infection in vivo appear to be less diverse.

8. Nef, Vpu, and gp120 can reduce the expression of CD4 on the cell surface.

9. The envelope region is also an important determinant of viral cytopathicity and sensitivity of HIV isolates to sCD4 neutralization.

10. The heterogeneity of HIV, resulting from its error-prone reverse transcription, can lead to the emergence of viral strains with differing biologic features involving virus:cell interactions, induction of cell death, and modulation in CD4 expression on the cell surface.

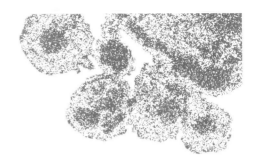

Effect of HIV on Various Tissues and Organ Systems in the Host

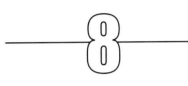

HIV INFECTION, EITHER DIRECTLY OR INDIRECTLY, can affect a wide variety of tissues in the host. This chapter reviews the major organ systems that appear to be affected by the virus. Its influence on the immune system is also discussed in Chapters 4, 9, 10, and 11.

I. Hematopoietic System

A. Bone Marrow

Many AIDS patients have anemia, leukopenia, and thrombocytopenia. The anemia is caused by decreased erythrocyte production, increased erythrocyte destruction, and blood loss (3498). The thrombocytopenia in HIV infection results from a shorter life span of platelets (4639), increased sequestration of platelets in the spleen, and reduced platelet formation by bone marrow megakaryocytes (843). Autoantibodies (Chapter 10) or a virus isolate that has special effects on certain hematopoietic cells (4638, 4639) might also be involved. Some data suggest that the reduction in bone marrow function results from an increase in CD8[+] (e.g., γδ) T cells that inhibit the growth of progenitor cells (1480).

HIV replication has been considered a major cause of the bone marrow dysfunction (2259, 2798; for a review, see reference 3498). Although early bone marrow progenitor cells have been infected in vitro, most data indicate that CD34[+] stem cells are not directly infectible (for reviews, see references 992, 3122, and 3228). Infected CD34[+] cells have been found in some HIV-infected subjects in vivo (1322, 4258), but not in others (972, 2798), and are not usually infected prior to expression of CD4. Variations in the extent of virus expression and replication could explain the differences.

The HIV-1 envelope gp120 or gp160 protein may cause the lack of proliferation of stem cells and their death (4917, 4918). Infection of cells that support CD34⁺ cell differentiation and function could also be responsible (e.g., T cells, macrophages, and stromal cells) (3122). In addition, bone marrow microvascular endothelial cells can be infected in HIV-infected subjects (3127), and this infection could affect production of hematopoietic growth factors such as erythropoietin (4680), leading to clinical disorders (e.g., anemia). Impaired telomerase activity reflecting an aging process has also been detected in hematopoietic cells of HIV-1-infected patients (4608). Thus, bone marrow dysfunction can come from a lack of progenitor cells, dysfunction of the cells that control differentiation and the release of hematopoietic growth factors, or activation of genes that inhibit these functions (3122).

Suppression of myeloid activity in the bone marrow, as measured in cell culture, has been attributed to gp120 (4608) and to the viral Gag p24 protein (3656). The effect appears to result from the induction of soluble toxic factors released by bone marrow cells or stroma such as TNF-α (2732). The findings have clinical relevance, since levels of p24 that can suppress bone marrow activity in vitro can be found circulating in the blood of AIDS patients (3656).

B. Immune System: Overview

A simplified presentation of the major cells involved in immunologic activities is provided in Figure 8.1. The different T-cell subsets and their functions are discussed in Chapter 11 (see Tables 11.3 and 11.4). The immune responses to HIV infection are discussed in Chapters 9 to 11, and disorders in innate immune cell function (e.g., DCs and NK and NK-T cells) are considered in Chapter 9. The role of HIV in the destruction of lymphoid tissues (including the thymus) and its effect on immune-cell subsets and cytokines are discussed in this chapter. Precisely how HIV causes disorders in the immune system (Table 8.1) is still not fully understood.

Immune abnormalities can be observed in T cells, B cells, and NK cells early in infection, before the loss of CD4⁺ cells begins (578, 815, 2399, 3004, 3792, 4079) (see Chapters 3 and 9) (Table 8.1). Decreases in macrophage function occur, as well as the eventual destruction of lymphoid tissues. These disorders could result from direct cytopathic or

noncytopathic effects of HIV or its proteins (Table 8.2) on the cells or from the enhanced activated state in the infection (see Chapter 6). In addition, a reduction in the function of polymorphonuclear leukocytes (neutrophils) can develop soon after HIV infection (3528), perhaps related to interleukin-4 (IL-4) and IL-10 production (4392) (see Chapter 11). HIV-1 can also induce damage to neutrophils through binding of the viral envelope components to the cell membrane. In some cases, there are decreased chemotactic responses, phagocytic activity, and superoxide production (3170). The result could explain the serious bacterial infections encountered.

Besides the known reduction in total CD4⁺ cell numbers and the rise in CD8⁺ cell levels with HIV infection, certain subsets of these cells can reflect abnormalities in immune status (see Chapter 11). In terms of both CD4⁺ and CD8⁺ cells, a loss in the number of naïve cells (CD45RA⁺), which are important for the primary immune response, has been consistently noted with disease progression (303, 3778) (see below). In this regard, CD4⁺ T helper lymphocytes are important for inducing and maintaining an effective CD8⁺ T-cell antiviral response and play a role in inducing CD8⁺ memory cell development (4338) (see Chapter 11).

C. CD4⁺ T-Lymphocyte Abnormalities

The primary abnormality in HIV infection is the marked reduction in CD4⁺ cell number and function. Potential reasons for this immunologic disorder, reflecting cell death, reduced cell proliferation, and limited cell regeneration, are listed in Table 8.3 (see Table 11.3 for description of CD4⁺ T cell subsets).

1. DIRECT AND INDIRECT EFFECTS OF HIV INFECTION ON CD4⁺ CELL NUMBER

The first immunologic disorder recognized in AIDS was a loss of CD4⁺ lymphocytes of the helper (inducer) cell type (1576, 3008, 4246). The definitive cause(s) of this finding is still not clear. The processes involved are reflected in the observed inversion of the CD4⁺ cell/CD8⁺ T-cell ratio in HIV infection. As noted previously, the loss of CD4⁺ cells could reflect direct cell destruction by the virus or its proteins, immune activation with apoptosis (1290), a secondary effect of an immune system disorder (e.g., anticellular effects of

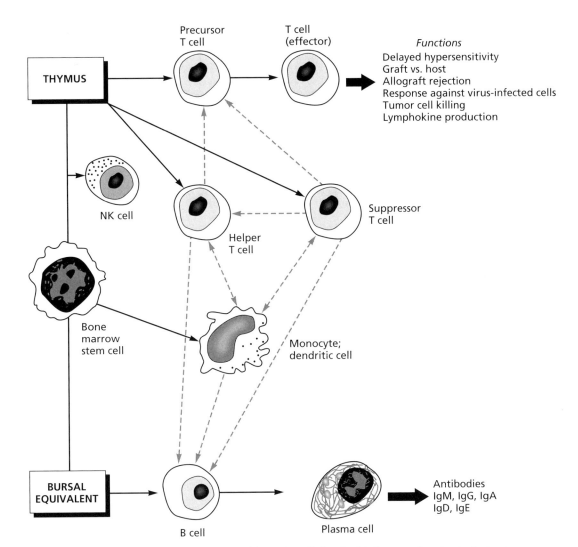

Figure 8.1 A simplified version of the major cells involved in immune function in the host. Bone marrow stem cells circulating through the thymus give rise to T cells that can have helper or suppressor/cytotoxic cell functions. Monocytes or dendritic cells (antigen-presenting cells) are derived from the bone marrow and interact with T-cell subsets to present antigens to induce an immune response. B cells from bone marrow pass through the bursal equivalent in humans to evolve into B cells that produce antibodies (plasma cells). All these functions entail interactions with several different members of the immune system, particularly antigen-presenting cells. The CD4 helper cells can assist in both cell-mediated and humoral immune responses. Their separation into type 1 or type 2 cells provides some distinction in these cell types (Table 11.2). Moreover, CD4$^+$ CD25$^+$ cells have been identified with suppressor or regulatory function (see Chapter 11). The final result is a balance in both arms of the immune system with functions used in defending against incoming organisms. The complex interaction of the cytokines produced by the various immune and other cells in the body is illustrated in Figure 8.3. Cells derived from a particular precursor cell are designated with a solid-line arrow; the influence of a cell on another cell is designated with a broken-line arrow.

Table 8.1 Abnormalities of the immune system in HIV infection

CD4+ lymphocytes[a]

Loss of CD4+ cell number

Decreased proliferation to recall and alloantigens, and subsequently mitogens

Decreased antigen-specific response

Decreased production of IL-2 and other cytokines

Disturbance in memory cell number and function

Decreased cell diversity (e.g., T-cell receptor repertoire)

CD8+ cells

Decreased antigen-specific proliferation

Decreased antigen-specific cytotoxic activity

Decreased redirected cytotoxic activity

Decreased anti-HIV responses (cytotoxic and suppressing)

Decreased diversity (e.g., T-cell receptor repertoire)

B lymphocytes

Polyclonal activation

Hypergammaglobulinemia

Lack of response to T-cell-independent antigens

Production of autoantibodies

Macrophages

Decreased chemotaxis

Decreased IL-1 production (or production of IL-1 inhibitor)

Decreased microbicidal activity

Reduced antigen-presenting activity

Dendritic cells

Decreased cell number (PDC and MDC)

Decreased cytokine production (e.g., IFN-α, IL-12, and IL-15)

Decreased ability to function as antigen-presenting cells (↓ MHC class I expression)

Decreased ability to stimulate primary T-cell proliferative response

NK cells

Decreased cytotoxic activity

Decreased number

Thymus

Decreased production of new lymphocytes

Neutrophil dysfunction

Decreased chemokine response

Decreased phagocytic activity

Decreased intracellular superoxide production

General disorders

Activation with increased proinflammatory cytokine production

Increased lymphocyte apoptosis

Lymphoid tissue disorders: destruction of germinal centers

[a]Details on these and other immune system abnormalities are discussed in the text and Chapters 9 to 11. PDC, plasmacytoid dendritic cells; MDC, myeloid dendritic cells.

CTLs), or the loss of de novo cell production (see Chapters 6 and 11). Another reason for this reduction in circulating CD4+ T cells could be that after activation within the lymph node, these cells remain in this tissue, whereas CD8+ T cells are induced to enter the circulation (3803). In addition, HIV can elicit CD62L expression on CD4+ T cells (4810) and have them traffic to the lymph node. The reduction in CD4+ cell number is reflected by disruptions in the CD4+ as well as CD8+ T-cell receptor repertoire (1471, 1571) (Table 8.1). Subjects who respond to antiviral therapy show improvement in the repertoires (see Chapter 14).

The total number of mature CD4+ T cells in healthy young adults (<30 years) is 2×10^{11} cells (1684). In HIV infection, when the CD4+ cell count falls to 200 cells/μl, this number can be reduced by half (1684). Moreover, as a person advances to disease, a decrease in the naïve (CD45RA+ CD62L+) T

cells is observed and an increase in the activated effector/memory and central memory (CD45RO+) T cells occurs. In addition, as noted below, several of these activated cells may not function efficiently (see Table 11.3 for distribution of CD4+ cell subsets). For example, some studies suggest a preferential infection of CCR5+ CD127+ long-term memory cells during primary infection (4919a), and most of the HIV-specific CD4+ cells express CTLA-4 and respond poorly to antigen stimulation (4919a).

Importantly, the level of CD4+ cells in the blood may not reflect the true number in the infected individuals, since the most extensive loss in CD4+ T cells is in the gastrointestinal (GI) tract. Studies in rhesus macaques and humans have shown that the greatest number of CD4+ CCR5+ resting memory cells can be found in the lymphoid tissues of the GI tract and many are infected. Up to an 80% reduction in these cells occurs during early infection

Table 8.2 Potential detrimental effect of viral proteins on immune response

Protein	Effect
T cell	
gp120	Cytotoxic; increases apoptosis (235); suppresses T-cell responses (689, 1075)
	Inhibits IL-2 production (3372); induces IL-10 production by monocytes (3994); blocks T-cell activation (751)
Gag	Decreases function by binding to cyclophilin (2686)
Tat	Decreases CD4$^+$ cell proliferative responses to antigen (4613); induces apoptosis (2565)
Nef	Decreases MHC expression (4014, 4320)
B cell	
gp41	Increases B-cell activation and immunoglobulin production (749, 3383)
gp120	Induces IgE production via IL-4 (1142)
Tat	Causes B-cell depletion (2470)
Nef	Causes B-cell depletion (3630)
APC[a]	
Tat	Reduces mannose receptor expression (584)
Nef	Decreases MHC expression (4014, 4320)

[a]APC, antigen-presenting cells (e.g., macrophages and dendritic cells).

Table 8.3 Potential factors involved in HIV-induced loss of CD4$^+$ lymphocyte number and immune function[a]

- Direct cytopathic effects of HIV and its proteins on CD4$^+$ cells and progenitor cells
- Effect of HIV on cell membrane permeability; enhanced fragility of CD4$^+$ cells
- Induction of apoptosis via immune activation
- Decreased cell proliferation
- Decreased lymphocyte function
- Effect of HIV on production of cytokines needed for CD4$^+$ cell function
- Preferential destruction of CD4$^+$ memory cells
- Destruction of bone marrow (e.g., stem cells and stromal cells)
- Effect of HIV on signal transduction
- Suppressive effects of immune complexes
- Immune suppression by viral proteins (e.g., gp120, Gag, Tat, and gp41) (Table 8.2)
- Cytokine cytotoxicity
- Trafficking and maintenance in the lymphoid tissues
- Destruction of lymphoid tissue (e.g., thymus) and reduced production of new cells
- Cell destruction via circulating envelope gp120 attachment to normal CD4$^+$ cells: ADCC and CTL
- Anti-CD4$^+$ cell cytotoxic activity (by CD8$^+$ cells, CD4$^+$ cells, NK cells)
- CD8$^+$ cell anti-CD4$^+$ cell suppressor factors
- Anti-CD4$^+$ cell autoantibodies
- Opportunistic infection of bone marrow (e.g., CMV and *Mycobacterium avium-M. intracellulare*)
- Infiltrating malignancies
- Nutritional deficiencies

[a]See Section I.C for discussion and references (for a review, see reference 2901). ADCC, antibody-dependent cellular cytotoxicity; CTL, cytotoxic T lymphocytes.

with an R5 virus (HIV or SHIV) (493, 2957) (Section IV.B). This loss could be responsible for the reduced viremia observed in early infection (i.e., decreased target cells) as well as the onset of opportunistic infections and other GI conditions. In contrast, naïve and memory CD4$^+$ cells that express CXCR4 (see Chapter 3) are found predominantly in lymph nodes and are targeted primarily by X4 viruses (1731, 1860) (see Section I.F).

An explanation for the low CD4$^+$ T-cell levels in HIV infection is that the enhanced destruction of CD4$^+$ T cells cannot be compensated for by an increased production of these cells, either from replication of effector memory cells present in the tissues or from production of naïve cells derived from the thymus (1312) (Section I.G). Advanced HIV infection is characterized by both a shortened average life span of T cells and a failure to produce enough cells in compensation. In this regard, because CD8$^+$ T-cell division and death rates are almost as high as those for CD4$^+$ T cells (1797, 3047), the reduction in CD4$^+$ cell number appears to reflect a selective suppressive effect on CD4$^+$ cell re-

plenishment. In this regard, HIV infection is associated with decreased expression of IL-7 receptor α (IL-7Rα), and decreased sensitivity to IL-7-induced cell proliferation can result (3710) (see Chapter 13).

Cell labeling studies (2901) have indicated that CD4$^+$ and CD8$^+$ T cells in healthy HIV uninfected subjects have half-lives of about 84 and 95 days, respectively, with absolute production rates of 10 CD4$^+$ T cells/μl per day and 6 CD8$^+$ T cells /μl per day. In HIV-infected subjects with CD4$^+$ T-cell levels of ≥350, the half-life of each cell population is about 30% less (1797, 2901, 2902), without any increase in the production rate of CD4$^+$ T cells (Table 8.4). Detailed kinetic analyses of T-cell subsets as

Table 8.4 Half-life of circulating CD4+ and CD8+ T cells[a]

| Cell type | Uninfected | HIV infected | |
		>350[b]	<350
CD4+	84	65 (men), 78 (women)	23
CD8+	95	58 (men), 77 (women)	25

[a]Provided by M. Hellerstein (1797, 2901, 2902). Values are estimated number of days.

[b]Number of CD4+ cells/microliter in the HIV-infected individual.

HIV infection progresses have revealed an impaired capacity to produce new CD4+ T cells with long-lived behavioral phenotypes, i.e., naïve and central memory T cells. A higher proportion of newly formed effector memory CD4+ T cells exhibit "effector-type" kinetics against HIV-1. These cells are characteristically short lived and die within 3 weeks of dividing (1798). Since these cells are usually targeted by HIV (1120), their early destruction does not markedly affect the overall half-life of CD4+ cells.

In advanced infection (<350 CD4+ cells/μl), however, the average life span of CD4+ and CD8+ T cells becomes shorter, with half-lives of around 20 days, reflecting the loss of long-lived CD4+ cells (e.g., naïve and memory) (Table 8.4). The inability to produce new, long-lived CD4+ cells may be due to activation-induced cell death, direct viral killing, or altered developmental pathways for the new cells. The consequence is a failure to replenish the CD4+ T-cell pool. Notably, even in asymptomatic infection, repopulation of CD4+ T cells in the bowel is markedly delayed in comparison to that in the blood (Section IV).

Studies evaluating the life span of specific lymphocyte subsets in humans have projected various survival curves, with some memory cells lasting for several years (1366, 1798, 2733, 3001, 4239). Older studies monitoring the persistence of T cells with chromosomal damage following radiation therapy have also provided estimates of cell turnover rates. Naïve lymphocytes by this approach divide once every 3.5 years, and central memory lymphocytes divide every 22 weeks (2733). It also appears that in the absence of persistent exposure to antigen, some memory lymphocytes can revert to a naïve phenotype (1796, 3001) but only, on average, after

3.5 years in the central memory cell class (see Chapter 11).

After HAART for only 12 weeks (1312, 1797), the production and presence of CD4+ and CD8+ T cells may increase in some locations (Section I.D) but not necessarily in the GI tract (Section III). The newly dividing cells exhibit a longer life span (1798). After several months of therapy, the proliferation of CD4+ T cells decreases, suggesting that a homeostatic mechanism is in place (1312). Thus, the higher levels of CD4+ cells observed with treatment result from increased production of cells that are capable of a long half-life (1797).

These findings are supported by studies of subjects 1 to 3 years after HAART (2902). The half-life of naïve CD4+ and CD8+ T cells was 116 to 365 days, whereas the half-life of short-lived effector memory cells was 22 to 79 days. Therefore, the naïve T cells had become more abundant than in untreated infected subjects (Table 8.4). The total T-cell half-life was increased with HAART in association with enhanced cell production as reflected by abundant thymic tissue (2266, 2901). Variations among subjects were seen and may be related to the type of therapy or extent of thymic output (2902).

In brief, studies determining the loss of HIV-infected cells over time during combination antiviral therapy suggest that there are two phases (see also Chapter 14). The data also support some estimates on the potential turnover rate of infected T cells in the host (Table 8.5). Plasma virus levels drop in a biphasic fashion when HAART is initiated. If HAART stops all new infection of susceptible cells, the decay of plasma virus levels would reflect the turnover of virus-producing cells. The first phase reflects the rapid loss of productively infected cells within 2 days (646, 3470, 3471). These cells are likely to be activated CD4+ T cells that have been infected by the virus. After this initial phase, there is a second phase that has been estimated to have a half-life of up to 2 weeks (3470, 3471). This time period reflects the slower decay of another population of infected cells, perhaps (3470) infected macrophages/DCs or resting memory CD4+ T cells, which may decay with a half-life of 2 weeks (3470, 3471, 3691a) (Table 8.5). Some HIV production by infected CD4+ cells can persist, reflecting the release of virus from stable reservoirs. The best-understood reservoir for HIV

Table 8.5 Estimated turnover rate of infected CD4$^+$ cells in HIV-infected individuals[a]

Cell type	Half-life (days)
Productively infected CD4$^+$ lymphocytes	1.1
Latently infected CD4$^+$ lymphocytes	1,320
CD4$^+$ lymphocytes with defective virus	145
Virus-infected macrophages/ dendritic cells[b]	14.4

[a]Summarized from references 1292, 3470, and 3471. The mean plasma virus half-life has been estimated at 2.3 days (1177).

[b]Or other long-lived cells, such as some infected resting memory CD4$^+$ T cells (3691a).

is a small pool of latently infected resting memory CD4$^+$ T cells that can persist for years (half-life, 44 months) and that represent a major barrier to HIV eradication (1292, 1293). Removal of HIV from this and other reservoirs in other tissues (e.g., the brain) could take considerably longer or be unattainable (see below). The accuracy of these estimates requires further study.

For asymptomatic HIV infection, the extent of HIV replication and cell turnover can vary substantially. Whereas cell-free virus is found to undergo rapid turnover (see Chapter 4), noncytopathic infection of latently infected CD4$^+$ T cells has a much lower rate of turnover and can therefore maintain viral persistence during therapy (1293, 4811) (see Chapter 14). Thus, recent studies suggest that the decay of the infected immune cell compartments can take decades versus years (up to 60 years) for the long-lived infected cell population and years versus weeks for short-lived infected cell populations (1293, 4140). Infected cell reservoirs may show little decay over several years, most likely reflecting the intrinsic stability of the memory T cells that harbor latent HIV. In the face of low-level viremia (<50 copies/ml) during HAART, the virus detected appears to be archival, coming from stable reservoirs rather than from ongoing new infections (1821, 3236). Nevertheless, whether virus continues to infect cells in subjects under HAART is controversial (see Chapter 14). In any case, as discussed in Chapter 14, elimination of HIV infection from the immune system by current antiviral therapies is not achievable.

The relevance of all these findings to the potential role of the thymus (i.e., when therapy is not used) needs to be considered (Section I.G). Some studies suggest that a lack of production of new naïve cells in the thymus, from which viable memory cells are generated, plays a role in the reduction of CD4$^+$ T-cell number and function (1773). Other studies have suggested a reduced proliferation of peripheral blood CD4$^+$ T cells during HIV infection with therapy (4439). An increase could be observed only in subjects with less than 100 CD4$^+$ T cells/µl, but the major site of T-cell proliferation was the lymph nodes. Moreover, through thymectomy studies in rhesus macaques, the major reduction in CD4$^+$ cell counts appeared to come from cell destruction or a lack of cell proliferation rather than a loss in thymus output (152).

2. EFFECT OF HIV ON CD4$^+$ CELL PROLIFERATION

Studies have shown that subjects with viremia have increased rates of division of CD4$^+$ and CD8$^+$ T cells (2488) resulting from immune activation. This rapid proliferation can lead to cell death, most likely by activation-induced apoptosis (1583, 2309) (see Chapter 6). The level of virus replication directly affects this cell proliferation, as it does polyclonal activation. In some studies, however, HIV-infected subjects have not shown a difference in numbers of proliferating CD4$^+$ T lymphocytes (cell cycling measured by Ki67) compared to HIV-negative subjects, but the CD8$^+$ T lymphocytes showed increased proliferation (Ki67$^+$) in the HIV-infected subjects (2488). With HAART, the CD4$^+$ T-cell proliferation in lymph nodes and PBMC has been found to be increased in some studies in association with the egress of more naïve and memory CD4$^+$ T cells. This response shows a maximum of a twofold increase after 9 months (1312). In other studies, HAART has been associated with reduced cell proliferation, reflecting a decrease in immune activation (2488) (see above).

In HIV-infected individuals who progress to disease, the ability of CD4$^+$ cells to proliferate in response to HIV proteins is markedly reduced (4785). IFN-γ production by the cells is observed, but not cell proliferation (2950). In addition, CD4$^+$ cell proliferative responses to T-cell receptor antibodies is greatly decreased in HIV-infected individuals, particularly those with high viral loads (4132). Thus, a lack of CD4+ cell proliferation can also be a reason for the low cell number in HIV infection. In some studies, the reduction in CD4+ T cells was found to be accompanied by an increased presence of IL-7 (3212), believed to be produced in response to the loss of T-cell homeostasis (3970). Other data suggest that IL-7 levels are increased because of the low number of CD4+ T cells that do not absorb this cytokine (C. Mackall, personal communication).

Nevertheless, in studies using genetically marked lymphocytes of an uninfected syngeneic twin, the marked cells were found after 6 months in lymphoid tissue at a level similar to that in the peripheral blood. The data indicated that the fresh CD4+ T cells persisted in the individual for several weeks and that the CD4+ T-cell population in the infected twin was maintained by the proliferation of these T cells rather than new emigrants from the thymus (4664).

Moreover, since the circulation of lymphocytes in the blood represents only 1 to 3% of the total population in the body (4737), the loss of stem cells or early precursor cells would influence the replenishment of circulating normal CD4+ cells required to maintain a steady state. As noted above, hematopoiesis can be suppressed with HIV infection. In addition, the formation of antibody:viral antigen complexes (3115) could "tie up" the reticuloendothelial system, affect cytokine production (e.g., IL-1), and influence CD4+ cell proliferation and function (Table 8.3).

3. HIV EFFECT ON CD4+ CELL FUNCTION

The function of CD4+ cells, measured by proliferative responses to specific stimuli, was found to be reduced before a loss in cell number was noted (815, 1655, 2398, 3004, 4079, 4555), perhaps related to DC function (see Chapter 11). The earliest abnormality reported in CD4+ cells was a reduced response to recall antigens followed by a decreased proliferation in response to alloantigens and, finally, a loss of response to lectins (e.g., phytohemagglutinin) (Figure 8.2; Table 8.1). Those subjects who showed a reduction in all three responses progressed much more rapidly to disease than did those who had all or some of these immunologic functions (815, 4079). In most studies,

**LOSS OF CD4+ CELL FUNCTION
IN HIV INFECTION**

Recall antigen (e.g., flu)

⇩

Alloantigen (MHC)

⇩

Mitogens (e.g., PHA, Con A)

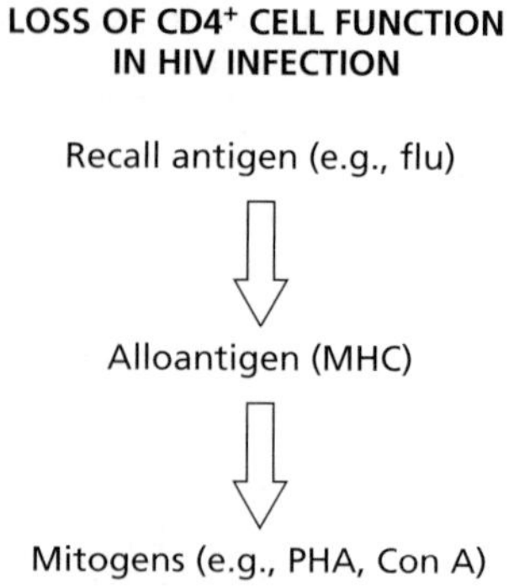

Figure 8.2 The earliest abnormality noted in CD4+ cell function has been the inability to respond to recall antigens (e.g., tetanus and influenza), followed by a reduced proliferation to alloantigens and finally to mitogens (e.g., Phytohemagglutinin [PHA] and concanavalin A [Con A]). This progression in loss of response by CD4+ cells has correlated with a more rapid progression to disease (809, 4079).

the HIV-specific CD4+ T-cell proliferative responses are low in HIV infection (3506, 4079), but early antiviral treatment in acute infections may maintain this activity, which could be important for a beneficial clinical course (3802) (see Chapter 11).

Some investigators believe, based on cell culture studies, that a preferential infection of CD45RO+ memory CD4+ T cells (3991, 4235) causes immune dysfunction. This infection is dominated usually by R5 viruses (see Chapters 4 and 13). In this regard, virus entry appears to be the same in both naïve CD45RA+ and memory CD45RO+ CD4+ cells, but virus replication occurs primarily in the CD45RO+ cells (4235, 4815), and these memory cells are more susceptible to the cytotoxic effects of HIV (773). Importantly, over time the naïve T cell is found at a reduced frequency (3777), perhaps because IL-7 can make naïve CD4+ T cells sensitive to HIV infection (4272). Whether selective infection occurs in vivo in the host and has relevance to the immune dysfunction or the naïve T cells become memory CD4+ cells needs further study. HIV can be detected in CD4+ CD45RO cells in vivo (3991) (see Chapter 4).

4. OTHER EFFECTS OF HIV ON CD4+ T CELLS

Other direct effects of HIV-1 replication, besides cell destruction, might contribute to the reduction in CD4+ cell number and function (Table 8.3). For example, infection of T-cell clones by HIV has led to disorders in cytokine production (2723). Moreover, despite the inability to detect HIV-1 replication in a large number of CD4+ cells, particularly in asymptomatic individuals (see Chapter 2), HIV could be present in a latent or "silent" state; the virus could then affect the function, long-term viability, and growth of these cells. The presence of this covert cellular state is supported by studies using in situ DNA and RNA PCR methods (1193, 1194, 3292, 3442) (see Chapter 5). Thus, HIV, even if not replicating to high levels, might alter cytokine production and the membrane integrity of CD4+ cells sufficiently not only to affect normal function (see Chapter 6), including cell proliferation, but also to increase their sensitivity to the toxic effects of certain cellular factors (cytokines) (Section II).

5. EFFECT OF VIRAL PROTEINS

HIV proteins can have a detrimental effect on T cells, B cells, and antigen-presenting cells (APC) (e.g., DCs, and macrophages) (Table 8.2). Several investigators demonstrated in early studies that the viral envelope proteins (e.g., glycosylated gp120 and gp41) have immunosuppressive effects on the mitogenic responses of T lymphocytes (689, 1075, 2792, 3372, 3383, 4646, 4708). Considering the

role of CD4+ T cells in B-cell function, gp120 could interfere with normal T-cell helper function via a block in contact-dependent interactions (752). Some cell culture studies suggest that gp120, through its interaction with CD4, inhibits IL-2 production by CD4+ lymphocytes (3372) and can increase apoptosis (235) (see Chapter 6). The effects could result from the induction of IL-10 production by monocytes (3994). In addition, gp120 could block T-cell activation and function by interfering with costimulation (751). However, sufficient amounts of soluble gp120 may not be present in vivo to give these effects (2223).

Initial studies with the envelope gp41 placed particular emphasis on portions of this protein that could suppress immune responses (689, 3838, 3839), most probably by inhibition of activation pathways (3839). A related protein in other animal retrovirus systems (i.e., p15 in murine and feline retroviruses) causes depressed immune reactions (779). In addition, gp41 and gp120 can be directly toxic to CD4+ cells through other processes (see Chapter 6).

The HIV Gag protein might also affect normal intracellular activities and function through binding to cellular cyclophilins (2686) (see Chapter 5). Moreover, the HIV *tat* gene, expressed in infected cells, can reduce in vitro the proliferative responses of CD4+ cells to recall antigens (e.g., tetanus)

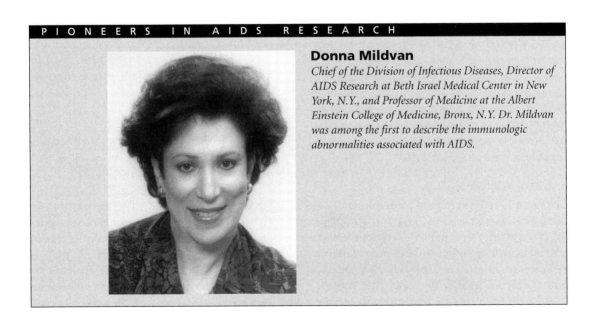

PIONEERS IN AIDS RESEARCH

Donna Mildvan

Chief of the Division of Infectious Diseases, Director of AIDS Research at Beth Israel Medical Center in New York, N.Y., and Professor of Medicine at the Albert Einstein College of Medicine, Bronx, N.Y. Dr. Mildvan was among the first to describe the immunologic abnormalities associated with AIDS.

(4613). This potential effect on immune function would be most evident via transfer of extracellular Tat to uninfected CD4+ cells (4613). The above mechanism, if present, could involve CD26 and an interference with a signal necessary for IL-2 production (4326). In this regard, restoration of the recall antigen response can be achieved in vitro by the addition of soluble CD26 (3984). Moreover, Tat as well as gp120 has been implicated in the induction of apoptosis of CD4+ T cells (2565) (see Chapters 6 and 7) (Table 7.3).

6. DISTURBANCE IN SIGNAL TRANSDUCTION

Besides certain indirect effects of HIV and its proteins on CD4+ lymphocytes and their precursor cells, infection of these cells by HIV could interfere with the normal events in signal transduction. This process, as discussed previously (see Chapter 5), involves an extracellular signal that affects the activity of sequence-specific intracellular transcription factors (Figure 5.3). These events lead to an information transfer within the cell involving a protein kinase cascade and protein phosphorylation. It occurs when natural ligands bind to the CD4 antigen or interact with other membrane surface proteins to bring about T-cell activation and an effective immune response (for a review, see reference 3362).

HIV-1 gp120 has been found to form an intracellular complex with CD4 and p56^{lck} in the endoplasmic reticulum (919). The retention of this tyrosine kinase in the cytoplasm could be toxic to the cell or affect its function. In addition, both HIV and envelope gp120 have been reported to inhibit the early steps of lymphocyte activation (1868, 2613). Thus, the function of these cells could be compromised by HIV even if they are not directly infected. Moreover, induction of the phosphorylation of a 30-kDa protein has been linked to CD4+ cell death by apoptosis (832, 4427), mostly ascribed to a block in mitosis (4427).

7. BYSTANDER EFFECT

The death of uninfected CD4+ cells can occur as a result of indirect effects of HIV. For example, as discussed in Chapter 6, immune activation and the resultant cytokine production can induce apoptosis of more uninfected CD4+ cells than infected ones (1290, 1583, 1875; for review, see reference 236a). In addition, uninfected CD4+ cells could be covered by gp120 released by infected cells. In this case, the gp120 peptides would be associated with MHC class II and not class I molecules (648). These uninfected cells are recognized as virus-infected cells by NK effector cells or CTLs (2409, 4142, 4707, 4708) and are subsequently destroyed (see below). This killing process, because it involves presentation by MHC class II molecules, would be most evident with CD4+ cytotoxic cells (1710, 2796). Proof of this hypothesis would require the detection of circulating gp120 in the blood of individuals or on uninfected cells. While some gp120 released from cells has been found in in vitro studies (1512, 3985), circulating levels of gp120 are not high (2223). This type of cell death process has not been well documented in vivo.

8. CYTOTOXIC CD8+ CELLS AND IMMUNE SUPPRESSOR FACTORS

Cytotoxic CD8+ cells recovered from the blood of infected individuals have shown the ability to kill normal CD4+ cells as well as those infected with HIV (363, 3280, 3343, 4707, 4914). A role for these cells in alveolar disease of the lung has been suggested (178) (see Chapter 11). This process may also result from contact of normal CD4+ T cells with HIV-infected cells, in which rapid cell lysis can occur (1788). In addition, NK cytotoxicity has been cited as a possible cause of CD4+ T-cell loss (4604).

In some early studies, the induction of immune suppressor factors, several of which block IL-2 activity and reduce cell proliferation, has been described (101, 1807, 2428, 4138), although none has been well characterized. A factor produced by CD8+ cells has been found to reduce the response of CD4+ cells to certain recall antigens (810) but has not been further characterized. This effect could explain the early abnormalities observed in CD4+ cell function (815, 3004, 4079) (see above) (Table 8.3).

D. CD8+ T-Lymphocyte Abnormalities

CD8+ T-cell numbers are increased during acute HIV infection, as is observed in many viral diseases (412). Their number eventually returns to a near-normal range but then increases with the loss of CD4+ cells. In some cases, a homeostatic mechanism may be involved. Activation markers on CD8+ T lymphocytes are consistently observed from the early stages of infection, and changes in certain

T-cell subpopulations can then be noted over time (1522, 2394, 4690). The initial proliferation of CD8$^+$ T cells most likely reflects the results of immune activation rather than a compensatory homeostatic response (4144). Moreover, progression to AIDS is associated with an increase not only in the total number of circulating CD8$^+$ cells but also in the subpopulations of activated cells (CD38$^+$ HLA-DR$^+$), memory cells (CD45RO$^+$), and CD8$^+$ cells showing the cytotoxic phenotype (CD11b$^+$ CD28) (303, 1522, 2394, 2396, 4569) (Table 11.4). In contrast, in AIDS, the number of activated CD8$^+$ cells with the CD28$^+$ phenotype associated with anti-HIV noncytotoxic suppressing activity is reduced (2396) (see Chapter 11). These findings appear to correlate with observations on clonogenicity (3415) and functional studies with cultured CD8$^+$ cells (2396).

In this regard, during immune activation, naïve CD8$^+$ T cells can differentiate into two major functioning cell types: effector and memory cells (see Chapter 11). Sometimes the term "memory" is used to distinguish two cell types: effector memory and central memory. The central memory cells are characteristically long-lived and persist as reservoirs until antigen-specific activation converts them into T effector memory cells (Tem) with a high proliferative potential (1798) (see Chapter 11). The effector cells with strong antigen-specific responses are then derived from these Tem cells. As noted above, labeling studies conducted with deuterated water (for long term) or glucose (for short term) have shown that the effector CD8$^+$ T cells are generally short-lived and function to eliminate the cause of their activation (e.g., a pathogen) (1798). Naïve CD8$^+$ T and memory T cells have a long life span. In advanced HIV infection, the long-lived CD8$^+$ T-cell (central) memory cell production is reduced in comparison to the presence of the short-lived effector cells (1798). As noted above with CD4$^+$ cells, HAART restores the balance of these two cell types (see Chapter 14). In HIV infection, the virus-specific function of these CD8$^+$ T cells can be greatly compromised (see Chapter 11).

E. Antilymphocyte Antibodies

Autoantibodies to lymphocytes could also contribute to the immune deficiency of HIV infection (see Chapter 10). In some early HIV studies, anti-bodies to both T helper and T suppressor lymphocytes were detected, and their presence was later confirmed (139, 1119, 2243, 3161, 4705). In general, the anti-CD4$^+$ cell antibodies appear first, but autoantibodies to both CD4$^+$ and CD8$^+$ lymphocyte subsets can be noted as symptoms of disease appear. Even antibodies to B lymphocytes have been detected (D. Kiprov, personal communication). Some of these antibodies could result from anti-MHC responses induced by the HIV proteins (see Chapter 10). Moreover, autoantibodies to the CD4 protein itself (although not to the HIV binding site) have been detected in HIV-infected individuals (675, 4419); these antibodies could be responsible for the death of some CD4$^+$ lymphocytes.

Some studies suggest a link of these antilymphocyte autoantibodies to CD4$^+$ helper cell defects (4705) and disease (2221, 3161). However, all the early observations suggesting that this humoral immune response could affect the immune system have not been further evaluated. For instance, plasmapheresis, which eliminates autoantibodies and can result in clinical improvement (e.g., in conditions involving losses of platelets and neutrophils, and in peripheral neuropathy) (2213), did not change the CD4$^+$ cell number.

F. HIV Effects on Lymphoid Tissue

The effects of HIV on the immune system, defined mostly through studies of the peripheral blood, have also been described for the lymph node. Lymphoid tissues may, in fact, be the first sites for virus replication following acute infection (see Chapter 4) (2375). Initially, with primary infection, lymph nodes show reactive hyperplasia and high levels of virus replication (for a review, see reference 839). The tissue enlarges, with particular increases in secondary germinal centers (or follicles) filled with the ingress of small activated mature B cells (560) (Color Plates 14 and 15, following page 366) that cause disruption to the normal follicular architecture and compromise the function of lymphoid tissue cells (4814). This event reflects the polyclonal B-cell activation and hypergammaglobulinemia found early in HIV infection (Section I.B). The paracortical areas also become increased in size (Color Plate 12A) and show damage with collagen deposition (3953) that can limit the extent of CD4+ cell recovery with antiviral therapy. The fibrosis in lymphoid tissue may result from transforming growth factor β (TGF-β) production by CD8+ T cells (1226a). An entry of CD8+ cells reflected by the expanding number of CD8+ cells in the peripheral blood (1199, 3650) may be responding to enhanced production of β-chemokines by resident macrophages (420, 4396). Many appear to be short-lived CD8+ cells (420). In this acute period, the follicular mantle and paracortical regions can show many infected CD4+ cells (1194, 4941).

During the subsequent asymptomatic clinical period, the lymph node may contain a large number of virus-infected CD4+ cells, particularly in the mantle regions (see Chapter 4), but most of these cells are latently infected (1194) (see Chapter 5) (Color Plate 9, following page 78, and Color Plate 15, following page 366). Germinal-center CD4+ T cells are also an important site of HIV infection (1929). Despite this infection, the CD4+ T-cell number in lymphoid tissue in asymptomatic HIV-infected individuals may be maintained at normal levels, even when CD4+ T-cell counts are reduced in the peripheral blood. By molecular techniques (PCR procedures) and by electron microscopy, virus particles can be best visualized in close contact with follicular dendritic cells (FDCs) (149, 1199, 4399) (Color Plate 15, following page 366), but very few, if any, of the FDCs are infected (3696). The binding of HIV to FDCs appears mediated by ICAM and LFA-1 adhesion molecules (1386). Evidence suggests that FDCs, localized to germinal centers, facilitate the transfer of HIV to CD4+ cells (4230) (see Chapter 2).

In situ hybridization and quantitative image analysis have indicated that early in infection and maintained during HIV infection is the presence of >7 log units of HIV RNA/gram of lymphoid tissue (3949). This virus load occurs within 2 to 4 days of the onset of the acute retroviral syndrome. The virus particles appear bound in germinal centers to the FDCs in a complement (C3)-dependent manner (2043). Antibodies to the virus can increase this effect of complement. A role for gp41 in the binding of complement to virions has been considered (1168) (see Chapter 3, Section VIII). These complexes are infectious (239). Some evidence also suggests that neutralizing antibodies are associated with virions on FDCs but do not block the infection of CD4+ cells by the complexes (1783).

In studies of lymphoid tissue from HIV-infected individuals at different clinical states, only symptomatic patients showed extensive ongoing virus replication as detected by in situ RNA hybridization techniques (397). Importantly, the number of virus-infected cells was substantially higher (up to 100-fold) in lymph node mononuclear cells than in PBMC. Moreover, the percentage of cells that contained infectious virus (detected by infectious-center assays after cell activation) ranged from 1 to 10%. Since up to 25% of CD4+ lymphoid cells could contain HIV as detected by DNA PCR (1193, 1194), probably about half of these infected cells have defective nonreplicating viruses, but the others could have infectious viruses under tight cellular control (see Chapters 4 and 5) (Color Plate 9, following page 78, and Color Plate 15, following page 366). CD8+ cells appear to play a role in suppressing HIV replication in the lymphoid tissue (397) (see Chapter 13). With advanced disease, the CD8+ CTLs have reduced antiviral function (1323) (see below).

A noteworthy finding is the relatively small number of infected macrophages detected in lymphoid tissue (1193, 1686, 4941), although a large number of these infected cells can be found in the spleen (A. Haase, personal communication) (see Chapter 13).

Over the course of the infection, the lymph node gradually loses its normal architecture owing to the slow but persistent destruction of CD4+ cells, deterioration of the stromal elements (e.g., FDCs), and release of virus from intercellular trappings in the FDCs or from infected lymphoid cells producing virus (Color Plates 14B, and 15, following page 366) (1256, 3416, 3696). According to some studies, a loss of CD4+ cells may not be evident in some lymphoid tissues at the time the number of these cells in the blood is reduced (3807, 3809). The causes of these findings are unknown but most probably resemble those suggested for loss of immune cells in the blood (see Chapter 13): an inability to control virus replication, a reduction in CD4+ and CD8+ cell function (117), and a lack of substantial T-lymphocyte renewal. As the FDCs undergo destruction, immune function falters, and the HIV-infected subject advances to disease concomitant with a return to high levels of virus replication (3406) (Color Plate 14, following page 366).

The end-stage lymph node shows typical atrophy (Color Plate 14C, following page 366), with marked depletion of CD4+ cells and destruction of FDCs, resulting from the virus itself (1256, 3292, 3416, 4230), from cytokine production by cells in response to increased virus replication (1199), or, conceivably, from activated CD8+ cells (2543, 4971). In studies of lymph nodes from SIV-infected macaques and HIV-infected patients, a possible detrimental role for CD8+ cells in destruction of lymphoid tissue and induction of fibrosis via TGF-β secretion has been considered, (1226a, 2277, 3804) (see Chapter 13).

At the late stages of infection, a large percentage of the remaining CD4+ cells show active HIV replication (Color Plate 15, following page 366). Moreover, a loss of the FDCs reduces efficient antigen presentation and the ability of the host to generate strong antiviral immune responses (2722, 4360; for a review, see reference 2244). In some studies, a further increase in the percentage of CD8+ cells has been described for the late-stage lymphoid tissue (2789), reflecting in part the loss of CD4+ cells. Similar T-cell alterations are seen in Peyer's patches, the lymphoid structures in the bowel (2972). Major losses in CD4+ cell numbers are noted (Section III). The antiviral function of the CD8+ cells in the lymphoid tissue appears to be markedly decreased (see Chapter 13) (117, 397, 1323). Finally, infected CD4+ lymphocytes producing virus emerge from the lymph node and become a large part of the virus-expressing cells found in the blood.

G. Thymus

HIV can infect and induce damage to precursor cells or stromal cells in the thymus (58, 441, 1771, 4259, 4523, 4538; for a review, see reference 1466), with a resultant decrease in intrathymic cell proliferation (1092). Thymocytes are usually both CD4+ and CD8+ initially and have both HIV chemokine receptors, although expressed at a low level; the presence of CCR5 is low compared to the presence of peripheral blood CD4+ T cells (331). The CD4+ intrathymic T progenitor cells that give rise to the double positive thymocytes are most susceptible to HIV infection by X4 viruses, since these cells express CXCR4 but not CCR5 (332). Thymic DCs also can produce high levels of HIV, particularly R5 viruses (3972). Precursor T cells and thymocyte infection can affect the production and release of fresh T lymphocytes, particularly naïve cells, that then reside in lymphoid tissue throughout the body. These cells are vital for response to new antigens (Sections I. C and I. D). Studies using the SCID/hu Thy/Liv mouse model support the conclusion that HIV infection depletes hematopoietic progenitor cells as well as thymocytes (58, 441, 4259). Toxic effects in the thymus appear to be caused primarily by cellular factors and not the virus itself (2021).

The adult thymus can contribute naïve functioning T cells to the peripheral lymphocyte pool.

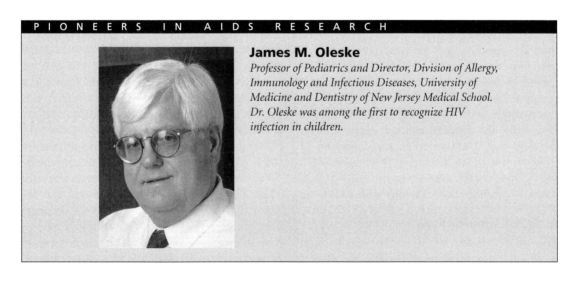

James M. Oleske

Professor of Pediatrics and Director, Division of Allergy, Immunology and Infectious Diseases, University of Medicine and Dentistry of New Jersey Medical School. Dr. Oleske was among the first to recognize HIV infection in children.

Thus, as noted above, T-cell loss can reflect damage to the thymus. Previously, the thymus gland in adults had been considered inactive and thus unable to contribute to restoration of T cells following anti-HIV treatment. Several studies have now changed that view. One of the first showed that thymus tissue could be detected, particularly in young adults with CD4$^+$ cell counts in the range of 300 to 500 cells/μl. The gland also appeared induced to grow in older infected subjects without clinical disease (2903).

Thymus production of lymphocytes is reflected by recent thymic emigrants, which have episomal DNA circles generated through excisional rearrangements of TCR genes. These TCR rearranged excision circles (TRECs) are not duplicated and are diluted out with each cell division. Thus, TRECs are indicative of recent thymic emigrants. In chickens, TRECs have a half-life of about 2 weeks (2270); however, the half-life of TRECs in humans remains unclear (for a review, see reference 1775). An active thymus gland with thymopoiesis shows the presence of TRECs with a diverse T-cell receptor β repertoire (2000). In HIV infection, the decrease in CD4$^+$ and CD8$^+$ naïve T cells is reflected in the reduced TRECs detected in circulating T lymphocytes (1092, 4930).

The restoration of thymic function can be detected by an increase in size and return of lymphatic proliferation as well as the presence of TRECs in the circulating lymphocytes. TREC$^+$ cells are observed during the use of antiretroviral therapy (1121, 4182, 4273). The levels of circulating TREC-containing cells, however, can be influenced by other processes such as lymphocyte distribution, proliferation, and cell death. These factors need to be considered along with assays for apoptosis and cell cycle (1775, 4273). With some restoration of thymic function, a reconstitution of the immune system is possible. Several studies have shown that thymic function is associated with the degree of T-cell recovery after initiation of effective antiretroviral therapy (989, 4182, 4397, 4607). Other studies suggest that the use of growth hormone can help restore thymus tissue (3213).

H. B-Cell Abnormalities

Abnormal activation of B lymphocytes is found in HIV infection, leading to B-cell dysregulation (100, 749, 1982, 2399, 3992) (Table 8.1). Viremia is associated with the inability of B cells to induce CD4$^+$ T-cell activity (2771). Moreover, these B cells are defective in their proliferative response to a variety of stimuli (3049). A CD21 low subpopulation seems to be primarily involved that has increased immunoglobulin production (3049). Evidence for HIV-mediated polyclonal hyperactivation of B cells is also suggested from several longitudinal and cross-sectional studies where effective antiretroviral therapy was found to reverse B-cell dysfunction (1988, 3050, 3112, 4325).

Evidence from several laboratories indicates that the viral envelope proteins, particularly gp41, can induce this polyclonal B-cell activation (749, 3383, 3992) and hypergammaglobulinemia, which are particularly evident in HIV-infected children (98). Whether the antibody response is general or virus specific is still not clear, but most probably both activities are involved (89, 4116). This proliferation of B cells may be mediated by IL-7 (3867) or by the production of IL-6 or IL-10 by monocytes (90, 490); the activation can be shown in cell culture by spontaneous production of antibodies to HIV as well as to other proteins (90). Moreover, HIV envelope gp120 (and gp160) can induce IL-4 release, which leads to IgE production (1142) (Table 8.2). The hypergammaglobulinemia observed early in infection also correlates with increased amounts of immune complexes in the blood (2399) (see above). HIV Nef and Tat have also been implicated in the dysfunction of B cells both in vivo and in vitro (2470, 3630).

The polyclonal B-cell response can be reflected by a persistent generalized lymphadenopathy (1982). Histologically, the adenopathy shows reactive follicular hyperplasia of B cells with an increase in the number of secondary germinal centers (561) (Section I.F). In early studies, binding of gp120 to B cells expressing the V$_H$3 immunoglobulin was reported to be associated with the induction of immunoglobulin synthesis by the B cells (316). The role of this interaction in B-cell abnormalities needs further evaluation. The activation of B cells has been linked to a defect in the ability of infected individuals to mount a novel immune response to immunization with new antigens, as well as to an impaired response of individuals to T-cell-independent antigens, such as lipopolysaccharides (100). This presumed anergy to new antigens may be related to a reduced number of naïve CD4$^+$ cells or the poor function of the CD4$^+$ helper T cell (815, 3004, 4079) (Section I.D). Importantly, memory B cells appear to be lost at all stages of HIV infection (764, 997, 2773, 4527a).

I. Macrophage Abnormalities

Monocyte/macrophage functions that appear to be impaired in HIV infection include chemotaxis (4390, 4646), phagocytosis (367, 699, 2141, 2143, 2144), intracellular killing (367), and cytokine production (2142; for a review, see reference 2141) (see below). HIV-1 is known to impair FcR-mediated phagocytosis (2144). The latter appears to be related to the down-modulation of the gamma signaling chain of the Fc-gamma R receptor in the HIV-infected macrophages (2142) (Table 8.1).

Several studies, however, have not shown a substantial effect of HIV on phagocytic function (236, 3285). For example, certain reports have indicated a deficiency in macrophage binding to yeasts, but normal ingestion of the organism takes place. Nevertheless, the yeast cells show increased intracellular growth (699). A similar finding was noted with *Cryptococcus neoformans* infection, and the impaired intracellular degradation activity appeared to be related to defects in both oxidative and nonoxidative effector pathways (1743). Other studies have also suggested that infected macrophages from the peritoneum and the blood but not the lungs (590) have reduced antifungal activity. In some cases, a reduction in phagocytotic activity has been reported in association with the presence of circulating immune complexes (4468). The lack of a consistent finding of a major defect in macrophage activity could reflect the relatively small number of these cells infected by HIV in vivo (211, 3442).

Most of the evidence on macrophage function in HIV infection suggests reduced antigen-presenting function (e.g., decreased ability to induce lymphocyte proliferation) (1140, 1209, 3053, 4062, 4884), reduced response to chemoattractants (3556, 4187), and a disruption in normal cytokine production (3053, 3830; for reviews, see references 1486 and 4884) (see Chapter 11). CD154 is the

CD40 ligand (CD40L), a type II membrane glycoprotein of 39 kDa with an extracellular domain similar to TNF-α and -β (1863). CD40L is predominantly expressed by CD4$^+$ T cells. An interaction of CD40 with CD154 on macrophages is required for macrophages to be activated and produce IL-12, an important cytokine involved in the development of immune responses to viral infections (Section II.A). This interaction may be reduced in HIV infection (1863).

Part of this decreased function of macrophages (and other APC) could be the HIV-induced loss of expression of MHC class II (3564) and of B7 molecules needed for costimulation (1140) (Section I.D) (Tables 8.1 and 8.2). In certain studies, the decreased proliferative response of CD4$^+$ cells on contact with HIV-infected macrophages in culture appeared to be mediated by a cytokine released by macrophages (2963). The abnormalities may result directly from HIV infection (590, 4646, 4820) or from an abnormal cross-communication among cytokines produced by other cells (Section II).

II. Induction of Cytokines and Their Effect on Immune Function and HIV Replication

A. Cytokine Production

A great deal of information has indicated the influence of various cytokines on the activity of the immune system (see Chapters 9 to 11) (for a review, see references 422 and 2141; nomenclature and the biologic roles of several cytokines can be found in reference 2605). The cytotoxic effects of cytokines are also described in Chapter 6. Their production is induced by HIV infection (and its immune activation) as well as by virus production (Table 8.6).

Depending on their cytokine production, CD4$^+$ cells have been classified into TH1 (or type 1) and TH2 (or type 2) cells, and certain cytokines can induce the differential production of cytokines by these cells (see Chapters 4 and 11 and Table 11.1). For example, IL-12 enhances the development of TH1 cells, which produce IL-2 and IFN-γ, important for cell-mediated immunity. IL-4 promotes the emergence of TH2 cells, which produce IL-4 and IL-10 (3134, 3135, 3786), linked to antibody

Table 8.6 Effect of HIV infection and HIV proteins on cytokine production

Cell type or viral protein	Cytokine(s) produced	Reference(s)[a]
Cell types		
CD4⁺ lymphocyte	IL-2, IFN-γ, TNF-α, IL-4, IL-6, IL-10[b]	555, 814, 3135, 3787
Macrophage	IL-10, IL-12, IL-1, TNF-α	2977
B lymphocyte	IL-6, IL-10	456
Dendritic cell	IFN-α, IL-10, IL-12	See Chapter 9
Viral protein		
gp120	IL-1, TNF-α	2977
gp41	IL-10	250
Tat	TNF-α, IL-1γ	555
Nef	IL-10	507

[a]See text for additional references. Some of the observations listed need to be confirmed.
[b]These cytokines have been used to classify CD4⁺ cells as TH1 or TH2 cells (3135).

production (for reviews, see references 814, 3135, and 3786).

Macrophages (and DCs) produce IL-1, IL-12, and other cytokines that permit CD4⁺ cells to reach the level of maturation to produce IL-2 (2605). IL-2 is needed for self-replication of the CD4⁺ cell population and for growth and function of CD8⁺ cells (4341). IFN-α (produced by plasmacytoid DCs) and IL-12 enhance NK cell function (for review, see references 377 and 4470) (see Chapter 9).

HIV infection and viral proteins can disturb this production of cytokines and their usual interactions, which maintain normal immune function (Tables 8.2, 8.3, and 8.6; Figure 8.3) (see Chapter 7). Production of IL-1 and TNF-α by macrophages infected by HIV or exposed to the viral gp120 has been observed (2977). Other studies (Section I) suggest that HIV-infected macrophages, on stimulation, release diminished amounts of cytokines or have no change in production of these cellular factors (3053, 3830). The gp41 envelope protein induces IL-10 secretion by monocytes/macrophages and can decrease IL-2 and IFN-γ production by PBMC (250). Moreover, increased production of TNF-α, but not IL-1 or IL-6, has been reported with Tat expression by HIV-infected T cells (555). TNF-α increases the production of IL-1 and IL-6, and these cytokines can in turn enhance HIV expression (Table 8.7) (see below). In this connection, the reported increased levels of TNF-α in serum of patients with AIDS and not asymptomatic individuals (175, 2381) are noteworthy.

Moreover, the ability of these cellular products to act as cofactors influencing the destruction of CD4⁺ cells or compromising their function needs to be considered (Section II.C).

HIV induction of IL-6 production by human B lymphocytes has also been described (456). This event can contribute to the polyclonal activation of these cells (Section I.B) and to toxic effects in the bowel (Section IV). Recombinant Nef has also been shown to induce IL-10 production in PBMC (507) (Table 8.6). Whether sufficient extracellular Nef is made to affect the immune response (particularly B-cell proliferation) via this cytokine production remains to be studied (see Chapter 7).

B. Effect on Immune Function

Studies with CD4⁺ cell populations have suggested that over time, the TH1 response is replaced by a TH2 response, leading to a marked reduction in cellular anti-HIV immunity (810, 2233). A decrease in IL-2- and IFN-γ-producing CD4⁺ cells and an increase in the percentage of IL-4- and IL-10-producing CD4⁺ cells are observed. This change can decrease the CD8⁺ cell immune response (e.g., via reduction in IL-2) and encourage antibody production (805, 817). The reduction in IL-12 and IFN-γ in HIV infection appears to be related to this loss of IL-2 and IFN-γ production by CD4⁺ T cells (707). These cytokine changes affect the viability as well as the function of CD4⁺ T cells (see Chapter 11).

The type 1 cytokines (e.g., IL-2, IL-12, and IFN-γ), for example, can protect against apoptosis

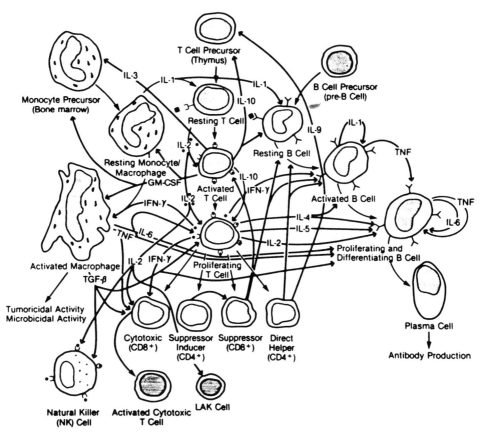

Figure 8.3   Early rendition of the complex interactions among cells in the immune system and their secreted cellular factors (cytokines). Each represents a process of checks and balances to ensure a normal functioning immune system. More recent findings add further complexity to this network system. Figure courtesy of A. Fauci.

of CD4+ cells, whereas type 2 cytokines (e.g., IL-4 and IL-10) encourage this process (812). IL-4 can increase apoptosis by inhibiting the function of other cytokines that prevent this process (e.g., IL-2, and IFN-γ in macrophages) (2787) (see Chapter 6) (Table 6.5).

IFN-γ, a type 1 cytokine, particularly with CD40 ligand can restore IL-12 production by PBMC from HIV-infected individuals (766, 1744). This cytokine also helps to maintain the cellular immune response. Other cytokines, such as IL-6 and IL-10, which enhance B-cell growth and function, and IL-4, which induces T-cell maturation, can affect the relative dominance of the CD4+ cell helper immune response (for reviews, see references 814 and 3786). Moreover, IL-7 can restore the numbers of CD4+ and CD8+ T lymphocytes through increased proliferation of peripheral lymphocytes. This cytokine, as noted above, is known to have a thymopoietic effect (1379, 3326). Moreover, IL-13 appears to increase CD4+ T-cell responses via an affect on the APC function of monocytes (3420).

Importantly, PBMC production of IL-15 is decreased in HIV-infected subjects and restored with antiviral therapy (941). Produced by monocytes/macrophages and DC, IL-15 can activate and expand CD8+ T effector cells (30; for a review, see reference 4656). This cytokine enhances NK cell activity (2961) and the CD8+ cell noncytotoxic antiviral response (CNAR) without necessarily increasing cell proliferation (635) (see Chapters 9 and 11). IL-15 also activates antigen-specific lymphocyte proliferation without inducing HIV-1

Table 8.7 Effect of cytokines on HIV-1 replication[a]

Cytokine	Major source(s)	T-cell line	PBMC	Primary macrophages	CD4+ cells
		Effect on HIV replication in:			
TNF-α	Macrophage, T cell, B cell, keratinocyte	↑↑	↑↑	↑↑	↓+ or ↑
TNF-β	T cell, B cell	↑↑	↑↑	NT	↑
GM-CSF	Macrophage, T cell	–	↑↑	NT	↑
IL-1	Macrophage, fibroblast, endothelial cell	↑ or –	NT	NT	–
IL-2	T cell	–	↑	NT	–
IL-3	T cell	–	NT	↑↑	–
IL-4	T cell	–	NT	↑↑	–
IL-5		NT	NT	NT	↑ or ↓
IL-6	Macrophage, T cell, glia, fibroblast	–	NT	↑↑	↑
IL-7	Bone marrow stromal cell	NT	NT	↓	↑
IL-8	T cell, monocyte, keratinocyte, fibroblast, endothelial cell	NT	NT	NT	↓
IL-9	CD4+ T cell	NT	NT	NT	↑
IL-10	T cell, B cell, mast cell	NT	NT	NT	↓
IL-12	Macrophage, B cell	NT	NT	NT	–
IFN-α	B cell	↓↓	↓↓	↓↓	↓↓
IFN-β	Fibroblast, B cell	↓	↓↓	NT	↓↓
IFN-γ	T cell, NK cell	↓ or –	↑ or –	↑	↑
TGF-β	Platelet, macrophage, T cell	–	↓	↓↓	↓+ or ↑

[a]Data on the effect of cytokines on acute infection of the cells listed are presented (2744, 2871, 4204). Results show by number of arrows an increase (↑) or decrease (↓) in virus production. A line through the arrow indicates a slight effect. In limited studies, macrophage colony-stimulating factor increased HIV replication in primary macrophages, and granulocyte colony-stimulating factor enhanced HIV production in CD4+ cells. IL-13 has been shown to inhibit HIV replication in peripheral blood macrophages but not in CD4+ lymphocytes (3063). Symbols and abbreviations: +, high concentration only; –, no effect; NT, not tested; GM-CSF, granulocyte-macrophage colony-stimulating factor.

expression (3439). It can stimulate HIV-infected macrophages to produce chemokines (e.g., IL-8 and MCP-1) that bring neutrophils and monocytes to the site of inflammation, which can help in the immune response to different pathogens (941). IL-15 can also enhance the function of neutrophils, as reflected by an increase in neutrophil chemotaxis and fungicidal activity and less apoptosis (2866).

TNF-α can also be a major regulator of chemokine production and thus play a role in attracting white cells to areas of infection. It induces the production of chemokines from stromal cells (4032). TNF-α helps maintain a balance in production of several lymphokines but can be toxic to T cells and induce apoptosis (see Chapter 6). To some investigators, TNF-α is a major cause of HIV pathology (2871, 4820), and its level has correlated with immune activation and low CD4+

cell counts (2452). Nevertheless, early studies of lymphoid tissue did not find any correlation between TNF-α gene expression and the level of HIV-1 production (2573). These results differ from those obtained with brain cells from patients with dementia (4734); high levels of TNF-α RNA were detected (Section II.C).

C. Effect on HIV Replication

In addition to their potential effects on immune function, several cytokines, produced by immune cells activated during infection, can affect HIV replication, as observed by in vitro studies (Table 8.7) (2744, 3063; for a review, see reference 868) (see also Chapter 3). Among these, TNF-α and IL-2 are important in inducing and maintaining HIV replication (1321, 2209, 2317) (see Chapter 11). IL-7 can make naïve CD4+ T cells susceptible to HIV infection (4272). In certain cases, virus production is affected in some cells by certain cytokines (e.g., decrease in replication in macrophages by IL-10 and IL-12) and not in others (e.g., CD4+ lymphocytes). (Table 8.7) (47, 1291, 2280, 3063). Moreover, IL-2 can increase HIV replication by CD4+ cells (2206) but inhibit virus replication in macrophages via a reduction in CD4 and CCR5 expression (2357). In one study, the enhancement of HIV replication noted in vitro with granulocyte-macrophage colony-stimulating factor (1487) was also observed in vivo (2374), and this effect can be blocked by antiviral therapy (3942).

Cytokines could cause cell death via enhanced HIV growth or by direct toxicity. For example, TNF-α increases HIV production and can be toxic for cells, leading to apoptosis (see above and Chapter 6). In other situations, the relative amounts of cytokines produced can influence the results. For instance, high levels of IL-10 reduce HIV replication in macrophages, probably secondary to a decrease in TNF-α production (4721). Low levels can increase virus production in the presence of other cytokines (4722). Moreover, HIV replication has been inhibited in the SCID/hu mouse by the administration of IL-10 (2264).

β-Chemokines and IL-16 have been reported to suppress HIV replication (219, 822). These cellular factors produced during HIV infection, particularly immune activation, have therefore been considered potential immune antiviral factors affecting pathogenesis. IL-16 via the CD4 receptor also induces high-affinity IL-2R (CD25) expression on CD4+ T cells. It could then be used together with IL-2 therapy for immune reconstitution (3421). These cellular factors are made by a wide variety of cells, including CD8+, CD4+, NK, and B cells. Importantly, whether the observations in vitro reflect a role for these cytokines in vivo remains to be shown (see Chapters 9 to 11).

D. Summary

As mentioned above and discussed in detail in other chapters, cytokines can influence the extent of cell-mediated versus humoral immune responses (see Chapters 10 and 11), affect HIV replication (Table 8.7), influence cell viability (see Chapter 6), and induce symptoms in the infected host. A balance in secretion of certain of these cellular factors is needed for the normal functioning of the immune system (2688, 4080, 4091). Their interactions are very complex, as illustrated in Figure 8.3. The known importance of cytokines for intercellular activities emphasizes their potential role in modulating or enhancing HIV pathogenesis.

III. Central Nervous System

A. General Observations

Lentiviruses are associated with encephalopathies and other brain disorders (1683, 2514), and similar conditions are observed with HIV infection (2998, 3490, 3605). Encephalopathy can also be the presenting symptom of acute HIV infection (618, 1855). HIV has been readily isolated, even early in infection, from the central nervous system (CNS) (see Chapter 4) (724, 725). In some cases, CNS disorders may be the only manifestation of HIV infection (2535, 3223), but HIV-induced CNS disease generally is a late feature of the infection (Table 8.8). About 25% of subjects with AIDS have neurologic symptoms (4872), particularly HIV encephalitis, which can occur despite the use of HAART (2861, 2888, 4423). Generally, but not always (452), a correlation is found between high levels of HIV RNA in the cerebrospinal fluid (CSF) and the presence of neurologic disorders (1074), including dementia (1812) (see below).

Chronic HIV infection can contribute to an increase in amyloid deposition in the brain of subjects of older age (1612); an increase in amyloid-β has been shown to correlate with years of HIV infection (3702). Older age also has been associated with increased HIV-related dementia (4531). Moreover, with reduced immune response, opportunistic infections such as cytomegalovirus (CMV) and JC virus can give serious neurologic complications

Table 8.8 Features of neuropathogenesis

- Multinucleated giant cell encephalitis
- Astocytosis (gliosis)
- Macrophage/microglial activation and proliferation
- Neuron loss
- Sensory neuropathy
- Vacuolar myelopathy
- Dementia

(e.g., progressive multifocal leukoencephalopathy) in HIV-infected subjects (for a review, see reference 326). These observations suggest that an increase in neurologic problems can occur in people living longer as a result of HAART (see Chapters 13 and 14).

The findings of brain pathology in conjunction with immunologic disease are not surprising when one appreciates the many shared features of these two systems, particularly cell surface markers and cytokines (4281) (Table 8.9). General pathologic conditions include gliosis, reflecting increased numbers of astrocytes (primarily in the white matter) (Figure 8.4), and perivascular infiltration of lymphocytes and macrophages (549, 1214, 3606, 4066). The clinical disorders range from acute encephalopathies to the AIDS dementia complex (3606) (also called HIV dementia or the HIV-associated cognitive/motor complex) (549) (Table 8.8).

Dementia has correlated with high levels of β_2-microglobulin and neopterin in the CSF (500) and the presence of CD69$^+$ macrophages in the peripheral blood (3618). These cells appear to release products toxic to brain cells (Section III.D). (For a review on HIV infection and dementia, see reference 1459.) The CSF of patients with HIV-associated dementia complex also have factors such as HIV proteins or cytokines that interfere with astrocyte function (2263) (see below). HIV infection is also associated with neuropathies. These include distal sensory neuropathies, mononeuritis multiplex, inflammatory demyelinating polyradiculoneuropathies, and progressive polyradiculopathy

(2171; for reviews, see references 2171 and 2888). Their etiology is not well defined but most likely results from the effects of both cellular and viral products as well as harmful immune responses.

In animal model systems (e.g., visna/maedi virus and caprine arthritis-encephalitis virus (Table 1.1), CNS disease usually results from direct infection of the brain parenchyma, particularly glial cells, astrocytes, and possibly microglia (1682). Microglia, as noted above, form the macrophage counterpart in the brain compartment. Most observations indicate that these cells become part of the CNS only during embryonic development; after birth, peripheral blood macrophages circulate but generally do not take up residence in the CNS (2418, 2615, 3478). The cause of neurologic disease with HIV infection is not yet defined but obviously depends first on HIV entry into the CNS.

Six major concepts can be considered to explain how HIV enters and causes pathology in the CNS (Table 8.10): (i) transfer of free virus or infected cells into the brain directly or through infection of endothelial cells with effects on the blood-brain barrier, (ii) specific HIV neurotropism, (iii) the toxic effects of viral proteins, (iv) the induction of toxic cellular factors (e.g., cytokines), (v) autoimmune and other immunologic phenomena, and (vi) potential copathogens (e.g., herpesviruses and papovaviruses). These concepts are considered below.

B. HIV Entry into the Brain

1. TRANSFER BY VIRUSES OR INFECTED CELLS

The mechanism(s) by which HIV gains entry into the CNS is not known, but entry occurs obviously by free virus or by infected cells (Table 8.11). Multinucleated giant cells (presumably of microglial origin) are an important component in this infection of the CNS, particularly in children (Figure 8.5) (2986; for reviews, see references 1214 and 4066). These cells are the only HIV-specific pathologic finding associated with this infection of the brain. Moreover, studies with HIV-associated CNS disorders have indicated that the one cell type that readily shows evidence of HIV infection is the macrophage, particularly macrophages that have come into perivascular areas (2252, 3606, 4759). There are conflicting data on whether these cells

Table 8.9 Surface molecules present in the nervous and immune systems^a

- Neural cell adhesion molecule (N-CAM)
- L1
- Axonal glycoprotein 1 (TAG-1)
- Contactin
- Neuroglycan
- Fasciclins II and III
- Thy-1
- CD4
- Myelin/oligodendrocyte glycoprotein (MOG)

^{a}These cell surface molecules are members of the immunoglobulin superfamily.

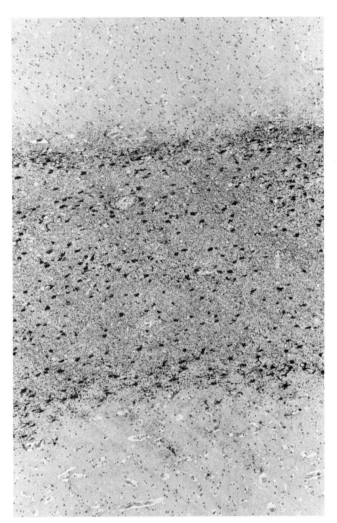

Figure 8.4   Reactive astrocytes in intragyral white matter of the cerebral hemisphere of a 25-month-old boy with AIDS and severe progressive encephalopathy. Astrocytes stain dark in this photograph. Glial fibrillary acidic protein (GFAP) avidin-biotin immunoperoxidase reaction, with light hematoxylin counterstain; magnification, ×64. Photomicrograph provided by L. Sharer. Reprinted from reference 1214 with permission.

resembling macrophages are brain microglia. Many investigators believe that the infected cells in the brain are resident peripheral blood macrophages (3493, 4688) (see Chapter 4), but infection of both cell types seems to be possible. Most recently, CD163, a monocyte/macrophage marker not present on microglia, has identified perivascular macrophages that can be major targets of HIV infection (3752). CD163 high/CD16⁺ monocytes in the blood appear to migrate to the brain vessels and can carry HIV into the CNS (1297, 2198). These cells are increased in the blood in association with viral loads and could predict CNS disease (2198).

Based on these early CNS findings on macrophage infection by HIV, many researchers concluded that peripheral blood macrophages

brought the virus into the brain and thereby caused neurologic disease (2252, 3606). Nevertheless, studies with animals have indicated that activated T cells as well as some macrophages

Table 8.10 Concepts in HIV neuropathogenesis

- Virus entry: effects on blood/brain barrier (endothelial cells, astrocytes)
- HIV neurotropism: glial cells, microglia, astrocytes
- Toxic effects of viral proteins (gp120, gp41, Tat, Nef)
- Effects of toxic cellular factors produced by macrophages and astrocytes (e.g., TNF-α and quinolinic acid)
- Immune response: autoimmunity, cytotoxic cells
- Viral cofactors: herpesviruses, papovavirus

Table 8.11 HIV entry into the central nervous system

Sources
- Infected CD4+ lymphocytes
- Infected macrophages
- Infected endothelial cells
- Virus passage through fenestrations in brain endothelium
- Transcytosis of free virus through endothelial cells

Mechanisms
- Adhesion molecules on infected cells (and endothelial cells) help in cell attachment and transendothelial migration into the CNS (1070, 1831).
- Cytokines (e.g., TNF-α, IL-6, and IL-10) up-regulate adhesion molecules on brain endothelial cells (985, 3284, 3480).
- Tat production up-regulates adhesion molecules on endothelial cells and alters the permeability of the blood-brain barrier (1867, 2378).
- Tat and gp41 can increase the permeability of the blood-brain barrier (125, 2378).
- Cytokines (e.g., TNF-α) produced by infected macrophages or endothelial cells cause endothelial cell leakage (1270); passage of virus and virus-infected cells can occur.

continuously circulate in the CNS (1831, 2418, 3478, 4724). The role of these lymphocytes merits attention. Cell activation appears to be a prerequisite for this trafficking in the brain (1831), since cytokines produced by the activated cells (e.g., TNF-α, IL-6, and IL-10) up-regulate cell adhesion molecules on brain endothelial cells (3284, 3480). These adhesion proteins help in cell attachment and migration but are not necessary on the endothelium for cell trafficking. Individuals

Figure 8.5 Multinucleated giant cell (arrow) and inflammatory cells surrounding a blood vessel in the brain of a 6-year-old boy with AIDS and severe progressive encephalopathy. Hematoxylin and eosin; magnification, ×555. Photomicrograph courtesy of L. Sharer.

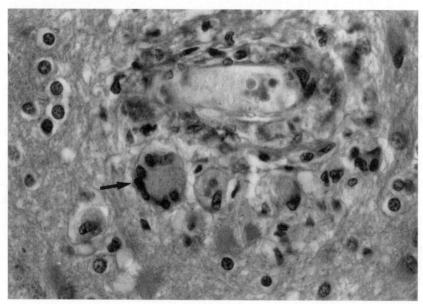

on HAART but with high viral loads have a decrease in circulating monocytes that produce inflammatory cytokines but continue to express activation markers, including the chemokine MCP-1 (3620). Moreover, HIV infection can elevate levels of adhesion molecules on monocytes (1070).

Activated infected cells enter the CNS by attachment and diapedesis between endothelial cells (1831) (Figure 8.6). Both types of peripheral blood cells (macrophages and CD4$^+$ T cells) could, therefore, be the initial source of HIV infection, although in vitro studies suggest that infected CD4$^+$ lymphocytes preferentially migrate to the brain through the endothelium (372).

Some investigators believe that Tat released from infected cells activates endothelial cells and alters the permeability of the blood-brain barrier (1867). Other studies suggest that TNF-α released by infected macrophages can cause endothelial cell leakage (1270), as well as an enhanced expression of adhesion molecules (985, 3284). This process can cause destruction to the endothelial cell structures (2378) and affect the integrity of the blood-brain barrier (Sections II.C and II.D). All these changes can promote the entry of the infected cells into the CNS.

How HIV establishes infection in the brain is also not known. In acute HIV infection (and in asymptomatic individuals), free virus and mild pleocytosis can be found in the CSF without any signs of neurologic disorder (1855, 1874) (see Chapter 4). In one case study, HIV-1 was isolated from the brain of a man 15 days after accidental transfusion with contaminated infected PBMC (976). Therefore, conceivably, free virus can readily enter the CSF and brain from the blood via the vascular endothelium. Then, infection of brain cells might be established if a "neurotropic strain" is present (Section III.C).

2. THE BLOOD-BRAIN BARRIER: INFECTION OF ENDOTHELIAL CELLS AND ASTROCYTES

Both detection of HIV in brain capillary endothelial cells (4759) and the ability of the virus to infect these cells in vitro (3123, 3554) suggest that the endothelium could serve as an initial portal of entry for HIV. Subsequently, as observed with cultured glioma (astrocyte) cell lines (Section III.C), HIV could infect the astrocytes associated with the blood-brain barrier. Thus, circulating HIV from the

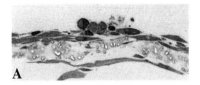
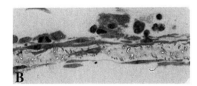
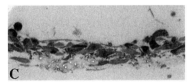
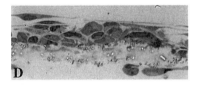

Figure 8.6 Light microscopic analyses of migration of HIV-1-infected and uninfected monocytes through a blood-brain barrier model system involving bone marrow microvascular endothelium (3480). (A) Uninfected control monocytes. (B) HIV-infected cells added to the blood-brain barrier; they attack but do not alter the bone marrow microvascular epithelial cells, and the astrocyte portion remains intact. Lipopolysaccharide-stimulated uninfected (C) and HIV-infected (D) monocytes modify the morphology of endothelial cells, and the monocytes penetrate the barrier system. Astrocytes are found partially detached from the membrane in sites of active monocyte transmigration; magnification, ×126,000. Reprinted from reference 3480 with permission. Copyright 1997 The American Association of Immunologists, Inc.

blood might first infect the vascular endothelial lining cells in the brain and then bud from the basolateral surface layer (Figure 8.7) (3367) to infect astrocytes. Alternatively, astrocytes could be infected via diapedesis of infected cells or by HIV passage through the endothelial cells by transcytosis without infecting these cells (432) (see Chapter 4). Recent studies suggest that the viral envelope plays a role in this process (240). Subsequent mutational changes in the virus could determine its ability to spread from astrocytes and cause disease in the CNS (i.e., as a neurovirulent strain) (Section III.C).

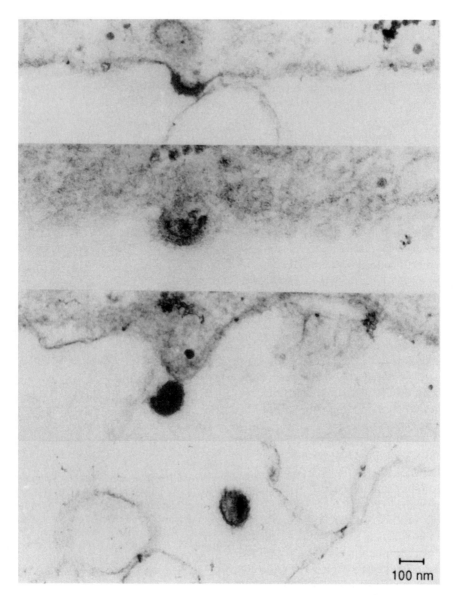

100 nm

Figure 8.7   HIV-1 maturation at basolateral surfaces of polarized epithelial cells. Vero monkey monolayer cells were grown to confluency on Millicel-HA filters and prepared for electron microscopy. All stages of virus assembly were observed from the first signs of budding (top) to the final release of progeny virions (bottom). Reprinted from reference 3367 with permission.

Early observations in the SIV system support the conclusion that the virus must penetrate through the blood-brain barrier to infect the brain. Lymphocyte-tropic SIV strains cannot replicate in the brain (4069), and certain macrophage-tropic viral isolates cannot induce CNS disease in primates unless they are injected directly into the brain. It is also noteworthy that replication of these macrophage-tropic SIV strains in the blood and other tissues of the animals studied did not induce disease (e.g., via circulating cytokines) and that infected T cells and macrophages were not found in the CNS (4070). Thus, entry of free virus seems to be the initial step in neuropathogenesis in this animal model. Subsequently, emergence of a neurotropic strain would occur.

Intraviral recombinant studies with SIV have confirmed that macrophage tropism alone is not sufficient for the development of neurologic disease. Portions of the transmembrane envelope protein and/or *nef* conferred neurovirulence (2791). This evolution of the virus seems to be necessary, since some studies suggest that certain SIV strains can be neuroinvasive but not pathogenic (2034). Moreover, neuropathogenic viruses do not necessarily have the capacity to pass through the blood-brain barrier (2827, 4070). Therefore, the inability of viruses to infect the brain endothelial cells (or to pass through their fenestrations) and their ability to infect certain brain cells (e.g., microglia and astrocytes) could be the important determining factors in neurotropism.

Some studies indicate that passage of macrophage-tropic SIV strains in vivo can select a virus that readily goes from the blood into the brain compartment of monkeys, causing CNS disease to develop. A certain group of macrophage-tropic (R5) neurovirulent SIVs appears to cause disease in the brain after entry through the blood-brain barrier (194). Some SIVs that prove to be neurotropic have been noted to infect endothelial cells (2791). In this regard, neuropathogenesis of a murine leukemia virus is determined by its ability to infect brain capillary endothelial cells (2867).

Since astrocytes help to maintain the integrity of the blood-brain barrier (1325), this proposed infection of brain endothelium and subsequently of astrocytes (see below) could cause a disturbance within the blood-brain barrier. The infection of endothelial cells could also result in the release of TNF-α, which can induce endothelial cell leakage (1270), increase adhesion molecule expression, and permit entry of virus-infected cells. Moreover, other proinflammatory cytokines, such as IL-6 and IL-10, secreted by activated immune cells can contribute to a transendothelial migration of infected or uninfected monocytes (3480). Tat and gp41 can also increase the permeability of the blood-brain barrier and affect its integrity (125, 1867, 2378). Toxic products as well as infected cells could enter the brain and might induce the dementia and other neurologic disorders observed. Arguments against this concept include

the fact that other viruses, such as CMV, can infect endothelial cells and astrocytes but do not appear to give rise to certain neurologic conditions found in HIV infection, such as vacuolar myelopathy (3490). CMV can, however, cause a virulent encephalitis in AIDS patients.

C. Neurotropism

The term neurotropic designates a virus that infects brain-derived cells. It does not necessarily indicate the extent of virus replication in these cells. In some cases, HIV could remain latent in the cell. Also, the virus infecting CNS cells may not be neurovirulent but most likely, over time, would cause neuropathology. Another important factor in CNS disease is neuroinvasiveness: whether HIV passes readily through the blood-brain barrier or enters via infected cells.

Once transmitted to the brain compartment by one of the processes described above, a neurotropic HIV strain seems to emerge, as indicated by the consistent recovery from the CNS of viruses with certain biologic properties such as macrophage tropism (i.e., R5 viruses) (725, 3599) (see below) (Tables 8.12 and 8.13). Recent studies suggest that the R5 viruses isolated from the brain replicate to higher levels in macrophages than viruses from the blood (3487) (see Chapter 4). Moreover, HIV can be detected in glial cells (e.g., microglia and oligodendrocytes) and astrocytes and perhaps even neurons (213, 2535, 2986, 3295, 3622, 4759; for reviews, see references 725, 2782, and 3606) (see Chapter 4) (Figure 8.8). Infection could occur via the CD4 molecule, which can be expressed on glial cells and neurons in the brain (1396), but this observation still needs confirmation. A cellular receptor for HIV-1 other than CD4, galactosyl ceramide (GalC), has been found on some brain-derived cells (1730) and could be involved in HIV infection (see Chapter 3).

In addition, cell culture, immunohistochemical techniques, and ultrastructural examination have indicated that brain-derived cells, including astrocytes, oligodendrocytes, and fetal neuronal cells (many lacking CD4 expression), can be directly infected by HIV (56, 514, 729, 1679, 1734, 1735, 1777, 2051, 2351, 2986, 3493, 3622, 3875, 4075, 4206, 4449, 4688, 4694, 4753; for reviews, see references 2325 and 2782) (Table 8.14). Recent studies

Table 8.12 Recovery of HIV from CSF and brain tissues

Clinical condition	No. positive/total (%)
Neurologic disorder[a]	74/96 (77)
Asymptomatic	36/68 (53)

[a]Meningitis, myelopathy, peripheral neuropathy, encephalopathy, and dementia. See reference 725. All the virus isolates are R5 biotype.

Table 8.13 Evidence for a neurotropic virus

- Separate evolution of virus in the brain (193, 2173)
- R5 viruses associated with neurologic disease (194, 725)
- HIV detected in glial cells and astrocytes (213, 2782, 3295)
- Ability to infect certain cells (macrophages and astrocytes) (2791) and brain-derived endothelial cells (3123)
- LTR from CNS-derived virus and not T-cell-derived virus gives gene expression in transgenic murine brain cells (573, 893, 2325, 2782)
- Macrophage infection by CNS isolates induces production of factors that are toxic to brain cells (3599)

suggest that there are at least two pathways for HIV infection and transmission from astrocytes (791). In one, there is mostly a restricted replication of virus with very low-level production. By the other, HIV enters the astrocyte by phagocytosis or macropinocytosis and is released without replication, although in some cases replication may take place.

The identification of certain HIV-1 isolates in the CSF that show biologic and serologic properties distinct from those of blood-derived isolates (see Chapter 13, Table 13.16) supports the idea that a neurotropic strain exists (725, 734). For example, CNS isolates in contrast to blood isolates from the same person can be resistant to antiviral therapy (4305). Some SIVs that prove to be neurotropic have been selected to infect endothelial cells (2791). In recent studies with pig-tailed macaques, the recovered inoculated SIV was similar in the brain and PBMC in the early stages of infection, but a separate evolution occurred later in which neurovirulent genotypes appeared (193).

In another study, certain HIV-1 isolates were found that preferentially grew in microglia compared to macrophages (4317). The viruses induced cytopathic effects in microglial cultures and had a V3 loop sequence similar to those isolated from patients with HIV dementia. The findings place further emphasis on the selection for a virus in the CNS and one that is cytopathic. In this regard, PCR studies of viral envelope sequences have supported the possibility (see Chapters 2, 4, and 14) that a viral strain in the same host can evolve independently in the brain and in the blood and can be distinguished by molecular as well as biologic features (Figure 8.9) (1213, 1932, 2173, 2251, 2283, 3402, 3598, 4288). Some genomic differences correlate with neurologic disorders (3598). For example, the envelope of certain viruses appears to induce in infected macrophages the production of factors that

are toxic to cultured fetal human neuronal cells (3599) (Section III.D).

In terms of a brain-specific HIV, observations with transgenic mice containing the long terminal repeat (LTR) of either a CNS-derived strain or a T-cell-line-tropic strain of HIV are noteworthy (893). Only animals generated with the CNS-derived LTR showed gene expression in the brain, particularly in neurons. In newborns, this HIV-1 expression was noted in endothelial cells and macrophages as well as in neurons (573). These findings support the concept of differential ability of brain-derived strains to replicate in the CNS and the presence of temporarily regulated cellular transcription factors in the CNS (Table 8.13). The results also suggest that neurons could be involved in a neuropathic process in infected individuals (1235, 2172, 3295).

In further support of HIV neurotropism is the observation that persistent noncytopathic low-level virus infection of glial cells can occur. This infection cannot be detected by in situ hybridization studies but can be demonstrated after exposure of the cells to infected lymphocytes, cytokines, or culture fluids of PBMC (4451) or by in situ PCR procedures (3295). Without killing the cell, such a phenomenon in HIV-infected oligodendrocytes, for example, could reduce myelin production by these cells and thus affect normal nerve transmission.

Once infection takes place, as has been observed in other tissues, the cytopathicity of HIV itself in the brain could be related to viral proteins or individual cellular products which affect the permeability or function of the cell membrane (see Chapter 6).

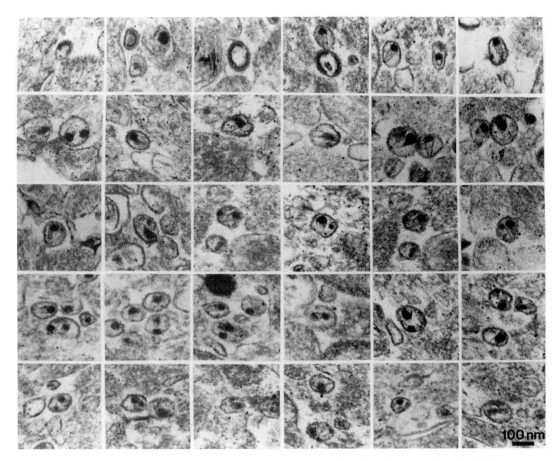

Figure 8.8   Montage of HIV-1 particles within multinucleated and mononucleated cells in the brain of a 6-year-old boy with AIDS and severe progressive encephalopathy (same patient as in Figure 8.5). Several types of particles are present, including immature particles and mature particles. Other particles have an atypical morphology, which suggests that they may be defective. Scale bar, 100 nm. Reprinted from reference 2986 with permission.

Table 8.14   Cultured brain-derived cells susceptible to HIV infection[a]

Cells	CD4 expression[b]
Astrocytes (fetal)	±
Microglia	±
Dorsal root ganglia (glia)	−
Choroid plexus	−
Glioma cell lines	±
Medulloblastoma[c]	−
Neuroblastoma	−

[a]Generally, low virus replication takes place and is amplified with addition of PBMC. See Section III.C for references.
[b]Symbols: +, CD4 detected in some cells or cell lines; −, no CD4 expression.
[c]Expresses glial and neuronal cell markers.

Accumulation of unintegrated HIV-1 DNA in brain tissue could also be responsible (3401) (see below).

D. Toxic Viral Proteins

1. gp120

A consequence of macrophage or microglial infection could be the production of high levels of HIV-1 proteins in the CNS. HIV infection of primary brain cell cultures induces apoptosis in neurons and astrocytes once virus production is at its peak (3320, 4097). As noted previously, the envelope protein gp120 in particular appears to be involved by a number of potential processes (Table 8.15). gp120 has been found to be toxic to cultured

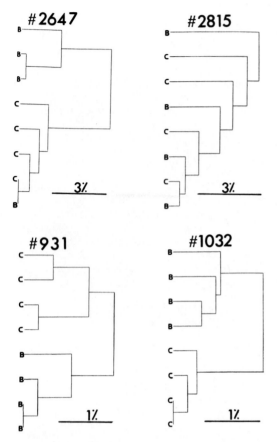

Figure 8.9 Relationship of nucleotide sequences of viruses isolated from the blood (B) or cerebrospinal fluid (C) of the same infected individual. Results with viruses from asymptomatic carriers (#2647, #2815), one patient with persistent generalized lymphadenopathy (#931), and one patient with AIDS (#1032) are shown. The lines at the bottom of each phylogenetic tree indicate the percentage of sequence differences for comparison. A separation of blood and brain isolates by genome sequence analyses is apparent for the symptomatic patients. Reprinted from reference 2173 with permission from Elsevier.

brain-derived cells, including neurons (308, 494, 2623, 3320, 3621, 4839, 4875). Distinct changes in the ultrastructure of the cells, particularly tubular fibrils, can be seen (3621). Envelope gp120 could be responsible for the endothelial cell apoptosis observed in the brains of AIDS patients (4097). The toxic effect may reflect gp120 induction of IL-6 and TGF-α, which are known to cause damage in the CNS (4875) (Section III.E). gp120 can induce the neuronal cell damage via an interaction with CXCR4 on macrophages/microglia. This process causes release of factors such as SDF-1, which can induce apoptosis (2124).

Moreover, the HIV envelope could be involved in inducing membrane damage directly (1279, 1455) or in activating, via a receptor, toxic tyrosine kinase activity in brain cells (3989) (see Chapter 6). This viral protein can affect the permeability of the cell membrane and its electrical potential via an effect on ion transport and calcium channels (308, 1133, 2068, 2622) (see Chapter 6). The effect can be exacerbated in cultured cells by glucocorticoids or abrogated by estradiols (524).

The toxicity from gp120 can involve production of nitric oxide (978) and can act via the N-methyl-D-aspartate (NMDA) receptor (2623). Quinolinic acid has also been implicated in this process (Section III.E). Thus, NMDA antagonists can reduce the toxic effect of gp120 (2623).

Perturbations in astrocyte function induced by gp120 could also affect neurons (3621). A detrimental effect of gp120 on the β-adrenergic regulation of astrocytes and microglia has been suggested from studies of rat cells (2506). Moreover, gp120 can stimulate secretion of TNF-α, endothelin 1, and other potentially neurotoxic factors (1178, 1530). The increased expression of adhesion molecules and changes in signal transduction induced by gp120 (as well as Tat) in astrocytes and microglia have been cited as possible pathogenic factors because of enhanced binding of monocytes to these cells (2378, 4123).

Finally, potential toxicity of gp120 on the CNS (Table 8.15) was demonstrated in studies of transgenic mice expressing the HIV-1 envelope under the control of the glial fibrillary acid protein (GFAP) promoter or neurofilament light gene promoter (341, 4442). Extensive vacuolization of dendrites and a reduction in the number of neurons were found in animals expressing gp120. Furthermore, the brain showed a widespread reactive astrocytosis, particularly in areas of high gp120 mRNA expression. As noted above, this pathological finding is common to individuals infected with HIV-1 (549).

2. Tat

The Tat protein has been found to be toxic to brain-derived cells in culture (2763, 3016, 3017, 3856)

Table 8.15 Potential role of gp120 in HIV neuropathogenesis[a]

- Kills cultured human brain cells (308, 2623, 3619)
- Kills cultured rodent neuronal cells (494, 1834, 3014)
- Intracerebral injection induced cell death in rat brain neurons (217, 1834).
- Induces IL-6 and TNF-α in brain cultures (astrocytes and macrophages) (4875) that can be cytotoxic and induce endothelial cell apoptosis (4097)
- Interacts with CXCR4 on monocytes/macrophages, leading to neuronal cell damage via SDF-1 production (2129)
- Activates, via a receptor, tyrosine kinase activity that is toxic to brain cells (3989)
- Increases permeability of the cell membrane (308, 1133, 1279, 1455)
- Induces production of nitrate oxide (978) that is toxic via the NMDA receptor (2623)
- Causes alterations in membrane integrity and astrocyte function (e.g., GFAP expression and ion transport) (308, 1133, 2068, 2622, 3621)
- Inhibits β-adrenergic regulation of astrocytes and microglial function (2506)
- Stimulates secretion of endothelin 1 (also TNF-α) by macrophages (1178)
- Stimulates monocytes to release neurotoxic factors (1530)
- Increases ICAM-1 levels in glial cells, leading to enhanced binding of monocytes (2378, 4123)
- Transgenic mouse expression of gp120 through the GFAP promoter caused astrocytosis and neuron loss (341, 4442).

[a]See Section III.D for discussion and additional references. NMDA, N-methyl-D-aspartate. ICAM-1, intracellular adhesion molecule 1.

(Table 8.16) (see Chapter 6). Tat was neurotoxic when inoculated intracerebrally into mice (3856). In addition, a Tat region, different from its transactivation domain, was found to cause aggregation and fascicle formation in cultures of primary rat cortical brain cells (2265). Moreover, the Tat protein has been implicated in neuronal cell death by binding to the lipoprotein receptor-related protein (LRP). Subsequently, Tat entering the neuron can be toxic to the cells (2638). This viral protein, like gp120, can cause an increase in expression of adhesion molecules on endothelial cells (see above), depolarization of cells, and degeneration of cell membranes. The mechanisms remain to be elucidated, but Tat is neuroexcitatory (via the NMDA receptor) and induces a decrease in cell membrane resistance (2763). It has been reported to show some homology to a neurotoxin (see below) (1457) and can affect cell permeability (1867).

Tat can also induce MCP-1, IL-8, and IP-10 expression in astrocytes. These proteins cause chemotaxis of lymphocytes and monocytes to the brain (861, 2355). Finally, this viral protein has also been found to inhibit the amyloid-β-degrading enzyme neprilysin. Thus, enhanced amyloid-β accumulates, which is associated with dementia (3702).

3. gp41 AND Nef

Sequence similarity between the HIV Nef protein and perhaps a portion of gp41 to scorpion toxin has been noted as well (1458, 4731). gp41 has been linked to increased expression of nitric oxide synthase with the possible toxic effects of nitric oxide (23). Immunohistochemical studies have confirmed that the AIDS dementia complex is associated with increased cellular production of superoxide ions and nitric acid, which give rise to perioxynitrite, a neurotoxic substance (470).

The Nef protein can affect normal cellular transmembrane conduction (4731) and appears to be selectively expressed in astrocytes in vitro (197, 479, 4450) and in vivo (3664, 3875, 4449). Nef could compromise the electrical potential and function of these cells.

Moreover, the cause of vacuolar myelopathy is not known, but in a transgenic mouse model showing low levels of Nef in oligodendrocytes, this pathological condition occurred (3651). Nef appears to affect the differentiation of the oliogodendrocytes. These observations are worthy since studies in the primate system have shown that Nef is important for SIV infection of astrocytes (3365).

Table 8.16 Neurotoxic effects of Tat

- Kills cultured rodent glioma and neuroblastoma cells (2763, 3856)
- Neurotoxic after intracerebroventricular injection of mice (3856)
- Causes aggregation and fascicle formation in cultured rodent cortical brain cells (2265)
- Binds to the lipoprotein receptor-related protein and can cause toxicity to neurons (2638)
- Increases expression of adhesion molecules on endothelial cells (like gp120) (2378)
- Neuroexcitatory via the NMDA receptor and neurotoxic (2763)
- Shows homology to a neurotoxin (1457)
- Affects cell permeability (1867)
- Induces MCP-1, IL-8, and IP-10 expression in astrocytes, causing chemotaxis of lymphocytes and monocytes to the brain (861, 2355)
- Inhibits the amyloid-β-degrading enzyme, neprilysin, which can lead to dementia (3702)

In summary, gp120, Tat, gp41, and Nef might play a role in the neurologic conditions observed with HIV infection. It is important to note, however, that some studies have not shown any cell toxicity with recombinant HIV-1 proteins, including gp120, p24, Nef, protease, and reverse transcriptase (1529, 1530, 4739).

E. Toxic Cellular Factors

1. OVERVIEW

HIV infection of the brain could induce a high production of toxic cellular products that have neuropathic effects (for a review, see reference 2782). Apoptosis of neurons and astrocytes has been detected in brain tissue of AIDS patients; most of the apoptotic cells were found near HIV-infected cells but did not involve them (4097). These observations, mirroring those noted in lymph nodes (1290), provide further support for the role of soluble cellular factors in CNS disorders. Several cytokines are produced by cells in the CNS (2591) (Table 8.17). Moreover, high levels of quinolinic acid have been found in the CSF of HIV-1-infected patients (530, 1830). A direct relationship of this protein to CNS disease has not been shown in adults (4757) but was reported to occur in children (530). Which cells make this excitatoxin, an NMDA agonist, is not known, but work with poliovirus suggests that macrophages and microglia are involved (1830).

Many investigators believe that after HIV infection or exposure to viral envelope proteins, the microglia and macrophages within the brain are induced to produce certain cytokines (e.g., TNF-α, IL-1β, and IL-6), including chemokines (e.g., SDF-1) (2124, 2658, 3976) or oncostatin M (1212), which can be directly toxic to the CNS (594, 1419, 2978, 4518, 4734, 4875) (Figure 8.10). Essentially, activated cells (whether infected or not) could produce these toxic products. In this regard, cysteine, a neurotoxin acting on the NMDA subtype of glutamate receptor, can contribute to the neurologic disorders. Cysteine appears to be released by activated macrophages and not virus-infected cells (4872). Astrocytes eliminate extracellular cysteine and glutamate, which are toxic to the brain. Infection of astocytes could therefore compromise this function (4889) (see below).

Table 8.17 Cytokine production in the brain

Cells	Cytokines[a]
Astrocytes	TNF-α, lymphotoxin, IL-1, IL-6, IFN-α, IFN-β, TGF-β
Microglia (macrophages)	IL-1, TNF-α, TGF-β, IL-6, low-molecular-weight cytotoxins (?), SDF-1, quinolinic acid, endothelin 1
T cells	Lymphotoxin (TNF-β), neuroleukin

[a]The potential neurotoxicity of these cytokines is discussed in Section III.E.

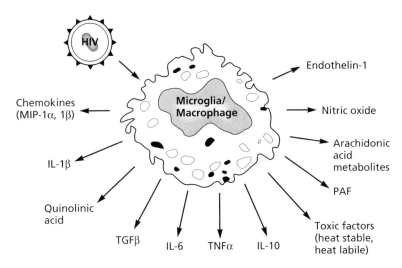

Figure 8.10 Role of infected microglia/macrophages in neuropathogenesis.

2. TNF-α

Most notably, TNF-α mRNA has been found in high levels in brain cells from infected patients with dementia (4734) and by in situ PCR techniques in infected astrocytes and microglial cells in the brain (3295). In addition, some studies suggest that stimulated astrocytes (perhaps via HIV infection or exposure to viral envelope proteins) produce TNF-α, which can be toxic to brain cells such as oligodendrocytes (2978, 3745), astrocytes (3339, 4039), and neurons (1481) (Table 8.18). TNF-α and lymphotoxin (TNF-β) have been found to be cytotoxic for bovine oligodendrocytes but not astrocytes (4038). The mechanism of this cell destruction appears to be by apoptosis, perhaps by activation of AMPA (α-amino-3-hydroxy-5-methylisoxazole-4-proprionic acid) receptors (1481).

At high concentrations, TNF-α has been shown to destroy rodent neurons and human fetal neurons (1481). TNF-α is toxic for myelin and human brain-derived cell lines (3850, 4040, 4739). TNF-α can also induce the production of β-chemokines that could have anti-HIV activity in the brain (2658) but most probably cause harmful inflammatory effects. Whether these cytokines could be damaging to the CNS in vivo is not known. In some studies, relatively low levels of TNF-α have been found in CSF (1631, 4518). However, elevated amounts of TNF-α and quinolinic acid have been detected in some brain tissue (16).

3. OTHER CYTOKINES

IL-1 production has also been linked to CNS disease, although IL-1 mRNA was not detected by in situ PCR techniques in infected cells in the brain (3295). This cytokine, which is secreted by monocytes, microglia, and endothelial cells, can be cytotoxic and can induce proliferation of astrocytes in vitro (3339), as do TNF-α and IL-6 (4039). Thus, the role of these cellular factors in the gliosis observed in HIV-associated infection should be considered.

Table 8.18 Toxic effects of TNF-α in the brain

- Is cytotoxic and causes astrocyte proliferation (gliosis) (4039)
- Induces IL-1 secretion that can be cytotoxic and induce astrocyte proliferation (3339)
- Can destroy oligodendrocytes and neurons (1481, 2978, 3745, 4038)
- Can cause degeneration of myelin (direct and indirect) (3850, 4739)
- Is toxic for human brain-derived cell lines (3850, 4040)
- Induces β-chemokines with potentially harmful inflammatory effects (2658)
- Can act synergistically with IL-1 and IFN-γ to augment monocyte/macrophage cytotoxicity

Induction of transforming growth factor β (TGF-β) production by macrophages and astrocytes has been linked as well to CNS disorders (4647). Expression of TGF-β was found in the brain, and purified human monocytes infected with HIV were shown to secrete increased levels of this cytokine. Moreover, infected macrophages release substances that induce uninfected cultured astrocytes to secrete TGF-β. Since TGF-β is a very potent chemotactic factor and can augment the production of other cytokines, including TNF-α, its role in CNS disease deserves further attention. Another monocyte-derived cellular factor with potential neuropathic effects is endothelin 1, which has potent vasoconstricting activity in the brain (1251). One study showed increased production of this cytokine by monocytes after exposure to gp120 in vitro (1178) (see below).

4. ROLE OF MACROPHAGES

In further support of the role of toxic cellular factors in neuropathogenesis is the early observation that HIV-infected macrophages, in contrast to uninfected macrophages, release factors (in addition to TGF-α and TGF-β) that are destructive to rodent neuronal cells and to cultured human brain cells (1529, 3619) (Figure 8.10) (Table 8.17). Macrophages recovered from the PBMC of HIV-infected individuals also can induce damage in cultured human brain cells (3619). Low-molecular-weight substances produced by infected macrophages appear to mediate the effects. One is heat labile (L. Pulliam, personal communication); the other is heat stable and protease resistant (1529, 1530). The heat-stable factor can be blocked by antagonists to NMDA receptors and by soluble CD4 (1530). In this regard, HIV-infected patients with dementia had significantly elevated CD69+ monocytes that, when cultured, produced factors toxic to brain cells (1140). In the era of HAART, the number of these CD69+ monocyte-derived macrophages is decreased and they no longer produce neurotoxic factors (3620).

Certainly, the induction of brain pathology by macrophage-tropic (R5) and not T-cell-tropic (X4) isolates of SIV does suggest a major role in human CNS disorders for infected macrophages (or the microglial counterparts) and their production of toxic cellular factors (4069) (Table 8.19). The hypothesis is also supported by studies showing pathology in human neural xenografts only when HIV-infected macrophages are present (937). Moreover, coculturing HIV-infected macrophages with astrocytes leads to production of high levels of the neurotoxins IL-1 and TNF-α. Arachidonic acid metabolites (eicosinoids) and platelet-activating factor (PAF), produced by activated macrophages, have also been implicated in the observed toxicity to astrocytes and neurons (1482, 1489, 4739). All these results could explain the cell death described in human neural cells after direct contact with infected macrophages (4387).

Table 8.19 Evidence that macrophage tropism is associated with neuropathogenesis

- Virus isolated from the CSF and brain in neurologic disease is macrophage tropic (R5) (725)
- Intracerebral inoculation of macrophage-tropic SIV gives rise to severe encephalitis (4070)
- HIV-infected macrophages produce high levels of neurotoxins (Table 8.17; Figure 8.10) (3619)
- Dementia is associated with a high number of CD69+ monocytes (1140)
- Induction of pathology in human neural xenografts when HIV-infected macrophages are present (937)
- Neuroadaptation of SIV$_{mac239}$ in macaques leads to encephalitis, and that virus is a macrophage tropic virus (194)
- Lymphotropic, non-macrophage-tropic SIV can cause persistent infection of the brain without disease
- Virus isolated from the brain in animals dying of AIDS without neurologic disease is not macrophage tropic

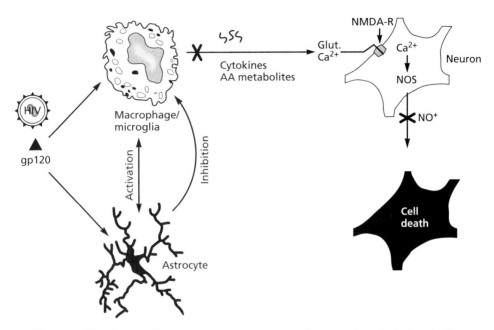

Figure 8.11   Some evidence suggests that astrocytes play an active role in inactivating toxic substances entering the CNS (3286). The cells, by interacting with macrophages and microglia, can inhibit their production of cellular products that are toxic to neurons. This toxicity can be mediated by the *N*-methyl-D-aspartate receptor (NMDA-R). Thus, a balance is established by which astrocytes can either synthesize neurotoxins or remove them from the CNS (Section III.E).

5. ROLE OF ASTROCYTES

Astrocytes, as well as microglia, play an important role in antigen presentation and can have phagocytic activity (4124). They can induce type 2 immune responses (74). These cells are a key factor in CNS disorders. They produce cytokines that help maintain the blood-brain barrier or could be harmful to the brain (e.g., IL-1β and TNF-α), and they inactivate neurotoxins (Figure 8.11; Table 8.17). In the latter case, the overexpression of eicosinoids, PAF, and TGF-α by activated monocytes during HIV infection of the brain (Figure 8.10) can be countered by the function of astrocytes that inactivates these substances in the CNS (3286; for a review, see reference 3444). Thus, a balance seems to be established, with astrocytes either synthesizing neurotoxins or removing them from the CNS. The end result of this activity could determine the pathogenic pathway. Nevertheless, as mentioned above, whether any of these cytokines detected by in vitro studies are produced in the brain in sufficient quantities to cause pathology is not yet known.

F. Autoimmunity

Autoimmune responses induced as a result of molecular mimicry (3328) could play a role in CNS disease (see Chapter 10), because HIV proteins resemble normal cellular proteins. Autoantibodies to peripheral nerves have been found in this infection (988, 2212) and appear to be responsible for peripheral neuropathy (2212; for a review, see reference 2171) (Table 10.4). Levels of antibody to myelin basic protein in the CSF have also correlated with the severity of dementia (2693). The reported cross-reactivity of anti-gp41 antibodies with certain proteins in astrocytes (but not GFAP) could compromise the function of these brain cells (4225, 4844). Moreover, the reaction of a V3 loop monoclonal antibody with human brain proteins (4488) suggests that molecular mimicry could be part of a pathogenic pathway. Furthermore, brain-reactive antibodies have been detected in the sera of infected patients (2344), particularly those with neurologic disease. The presence of these antibodies in immune complexes within the CSF has been noted as well (325). In addition, antiviral or anticellular CTLs that are harmful to the brain could be generated in the CNS (2011).

G. Copathogens

Several investigators have reported the presence in the CNS of other infectious agents, such as herpesviruses (e.g., CMV) and papovaviruses (e.g., JC virus), that could exacerbate the neuropathologic condition (3232, 3233, 4760). Cells coinfected with HIV and CMV have been found (3233). Nevertheless, whereas herpesviruses and papovaviruses have been shown to activate the HIV LTR in a conventional chloramphenicol acetyltransferase (CAT) assay (977, 1488, 1519, 1861, 2426, 3117, 3354, 3662) (see Chapter 13), whether their infection in the brain has biologic importance in terms of HIV replication and pathology is not known. In some cell culture studies, for example, CMV increased HIV replication (4168); in others, the opposite effect was noted (2313). Many findings suggest that opportunistic infection, when present, can be the primary cause of the neurologic disease. Other early observations, however, such as the improvement in a patient's dementia after zidovudine (AZT) therapy (227, 1022, 3584, 3585), suggest that HIV directly or indirectly can play a major role as well.

H. Conclusions

Because certain neurologic findings are primarily found to be associated with HIV infection (e.g., multinucleated cells and vacuolar myelopathy) (3490), the concept that neuropathogenesis depends on infection of the brain by a neurotropic HIV strain should be considered. This virus would evolve from a circulating virus that replicates sufficiently in endothelial cells and particularly in astrocytes to cause damage to the blood-brain barrier (Figure 8.12). Nevertheless, how an R5 macrophage-tropic virus emerges as a pathogenic isolate in the brain when X4 viruses preferentially infect brain-derived endothelial cells and astrocytes is not known (729, 3123). Conceivably, the R5 virus does not enter the brain via infection of the blood-brain barrier but passes through by diapedesis of infected cells or via viral transcytosis (432). Evolution of an X4 virus within the brain compartment seems a much less feasible possibility than such a selective transfer. Activated in-

fected CD4+ lymphocytes and macrophages (e.g., CD163+) can traffic through the CNS and introduce virus (most likely R5 type) to the brain by this means (1297, 2198). The recovery of R5 virus from the CNS supports this conclusion (725, 734).

The compromise in the function of the blood-brain barrier brought about by HIV infection also leads to disease within the CNS through the ingress of toxic products as well as virus and infected cells (Figure 8.12). Subsequently, through mutations, the neurotropic strain that replicates well in macrophages, and perhaps microglia and other brain cells (see Chapter 4), emerges and produces viral proteins (e.g., gp120, gp41, Tat, and Nef) that can be toxic to cells (Tables 8.15, 8.16, and 8.17). Moreover, these viral products could compete with neurotropic factors to inhibit cell-to-cell communication. The loss of neurons observed in the frontal cortex in HIV disease (1235, 2172) could result from the viral infection itself (3295) or its sequelae.

The macrophage-tropic R5 viruses might also pass most easily to other brain cells such as oligodendrocytes, producers of myelin needed for nerve transmission, and even to neurons. A macrophage-tropic R5 virus has several features that associate it with neurovirulence (Table 8.19). Specific infection of macrophages or other cells in the brain (e.g., astrocytes) could also favor enhanced production of toxic cellular factors (Figures 8.10 and 8.11; Tables 8.17 and 8.19) that damage other brain cells and myelin. HIV infection of astrocytes could induce many of the sequelae leading to neuropathogenesis because of their importance in detoxification of the CNS (Table 8.20; Figures 8.11 and 8.12). Therefore, the role of these innate immune cells in diseases of the brain merits increased attention (for a review, see reference 2782) (see Chapter 9). In addition, the potential role of complement in preventing HIV infection in the brain or exacerbating the neuropathogenesis has been appreciated (1461, 4229) (see Chapter 9, Figure 9.8).

Eventually, any approach to limiting HIV replication and spread should decrease neurologic symptoms. Such a response was reported in early studies of patients receiving antiviral therapy treatment; symptoms of AIDS-related dementia were markedly reduced, at least for some time (227, 3585). This

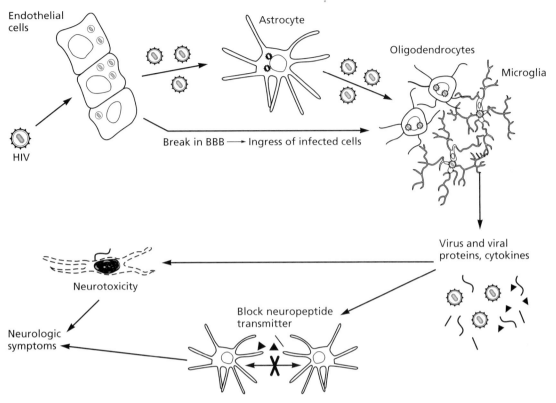

Figure 8.12 HIV neuropathogenesis. It is proposed that the virus infects capillary endothelial cells of the brain and passes via the basolateral surface of these cells to astrocytes
lining the blood-brain barrier (BBB). Infection of both these cell types leads to a breakdown
in the BBB and ingress of infected T cells and macrophages. The ultimate result is an infection of other brain cells (e.g., oligodendrocytes and microglia) by HIV. Production of HIV
and its viral proteins ensues, as does the release of various cytokines (e.g., TNF-α and low-
molecular-weight substances). These products could lead to an interruption of cell-to-cell
transmission through a blockage of neurotropic factors. Direct infection of cells, as well as
high levels of viral proteins (e.g., envelope glycoproteins, Tat, and Nef) and cytokines, could
lead to direct neurotoxicity through detrimental effects on the cell membrane.

encouraging observation has been attributed to an
anti-HIV and/or anticytokine effect of HAART. The
fact that the dementia is reversible with AZT argues
for at least an initial noncytotoxic effect of HIV (and
its proteins) or the presumed induced cytokines.
With the introduction of HAART, more control of
HIV in the brain should be achieved (2888) as long
as good drug penetration of the blood-brain barrier
can occur. Nevertheless, CNS disease is still evident,
despite a reduced incidence, and the prevalence of
brain-related disorders is increasing in infected patients on HAART (2888, 4423).

   Autoantibodies also appear to be involved in
some neurologic disorders, primarily peripheral

neuropathy, as shown by immunohistochemical
staining and successful treatment by plasmapheresis (2213). The role of other viruses, if not primary,
could also be contributory in many cases. Finally,

Table 8.20 Role of astrocytes in the CNS

- Antigen presentation
- Phagocyte activity
- Induction of type 2 immune responses
- Cytokine production (e.g., PGE[a] and IL-1β)
- Maintenance of the blood-brain barrier
- Decrease the effect of neurotoxins

[a]PGE, prostaglandin E.

abnormal vitamin B_{12} metabolism in HIV infection has led some investigators to suggest that this deficiency can be responsible for some abnormal neurologic findings (2227).

IV. Gastrointestinal System

A. Clinical and Pathologic Findings

HIV enteropathy, reflecting direct HIV infection of the bowel, is a clinical condition that affects >75% of people with HIV infection (2294). Just as CNS disorders can be observed during some acute HIV infections, bowel symptoms have been reported soon after infection, when HIV destroys many intestinal CD4$^+$ cells (2971), (see below), but then they subside (4434). The subsequent chronic malabsorption, malnutrition, and diarrhea occurring several years later have largely been attributed to opportunistic infections in the bowel as a result of immune deficiency (1138, 2295). The extent of diarrhea and malabsorption then depends on which organism is responsible. Whether these infections cause the pathology or are superimposed on the background of HIV infection needs more study.

HIV pathogenesis in the bowel has not yet been fully explained. As with HIV infection of the CNS, certain mechanisms have been considered (Table 8.21), including direct HIV infection as well as toxic effects of HIV proteins and induced cytokines (2294). The enteropathy is characterized by disturbances in the intestinal cell permeability, loss of immune protection, and disruption in epithlial microtubular function (2294, 2297).

Histochemical studies of the GI tract in HIV infection usually show chronic mild inflammation

Table 8.21 Factors potentially involved in HIV pathogenesis in the bowel[a]

- HIV infection of bowel cells (128, 1792, 3234)
- Toxicity of viral proteins (e.g., gp120 and Tat) (794)
- Induction of toxic cytokines (e.g., IL-1β and IL-6) (4271)
- CTL activity (4192)
- Malnutrition (4681)
- Opportunistic infections

[a]See Section IV.A for additional references.

(2294, 2295, 3234) that is not unlike that in bowel disorders caused by a variety of infections and toxic agents (Figure 8.13). Nevertheless, the extensive diarrhea and malabsorption observed in AIDS do suggest a direct effect of the virus on intestinal cell membrane integrity, perhaps in the handling of sodium ions and water (see Chapter 6). The watery diarrhea often observed could be the effect of a toxin, perhaps a product of infected cells or a viral protein. As in the CNS disease, the potential role of the envelope glycoproteins, or of Tat or Nef, in cell viability and physiologic function should be considered (Section III.D). Finally, increased numbers of CTLs have been found in the small intestines of HIV-infected patients (4192). Although no relationship between the cell number and the presence of diarrhea has been found, some tissue injury may result from the presence of these cells (see Chapter 11).

A GI problem, first described in Africa, has been termed "Slim's disease" (4053) because of the substantial loss of weight resulting from HIV infection. Generally, the GI tract shows only subtle histologic changes during this infection (Figure 8.13), unless an opportunistic infection such as CMV infection, cryptosporidiosis, *Mycobacterium avium* complex, or microsporidial infection is present (2294, 2295). Thus, the permeability changes reflected by diarrhea and malabsorption may not be readily apparent in a bowel biopsy. Moreover, these processes can occur in the duodenum, for which documentation of HIV infection is limited (2294, 2991).

Malnutrition is considered to be present in a patient with a weight loss of more than 10% and greater protein wasting than is observed in other cases of starvation (756, 2295). This malnourishment in HIV infection can result from anorexia or nutrient malabsorption secondary to intestinal damage and inflammation (1138, 2294, 2295). Deficiencies in micronutrients, particularly vitamins A and B_{12}, have been associated with disease progression (282, 4378; for reviews, see references 1546 and 4378). The administration of these nutrients to improve clinical outcome is discussed in Chapter 14.

Metabolic abnormalities, such as hypertriglyceridemia, have also been observed in HIV-infected individuals (1651) and are particularly

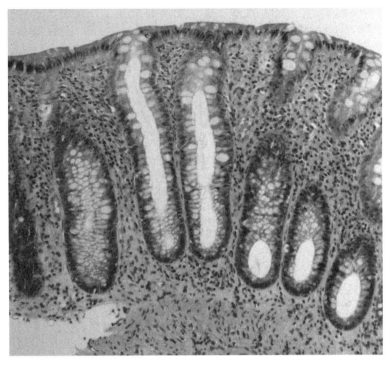

Figure 8.13   Histology of bowel. Colonic biopsy sample from an HIV-infected subject with chronic diarrhea and no detectable pathogens. The biopsy sample shows only mild chronic inflammation, without epithelial cell damage or acute inflammation. (Hematoxylin and eosin; original magnification, ×125. Figure provided by D. Kotler.

evident in subjects taking HAART (see Chapter 14). Without therapy, this condition is likely related to the high cytokine production in HIV infection (1652, 3869).

B. HIV Infection

Studies investigating the cause of GI disturbances have demonstrated the presence of HIV itself in the bowel mucosa from patients with intestinal disorders, as well as from infected asymptomatic individuals (128, 1792, 2294, 2296, 2870, 3234) (Color Plate 10, following page 78). Some studies have demonstrated that certain HIV-1 isolates can infect intestinal cells by a CD4-independent mechanism (736). In this regard, it is important to note that epithelial cells contain chemokine receptors and other potential sites for attachment and possible cellular uptake. In many cases, especially in people with CD4+ lymphocyte counts above 200 cells/µl, HIV is the only pathogen found in the bowel. Thus, the virus can "home out" in this organ as well as in the brain. Complement can enhance this infection of epithelial cells and can play a role in its transmission via the bowel and the cervix (457). The presence of HIV in enterochromaffin cells in the bowel mucosa (2544, 3234) is noteworthy. These cytokine- and hormone-producing cells are distributed throughout the intestinal tract and are responsible for normal motility and bowel function (3553).

HIV infection of the bowel is particularly evident in the lymphoid tissues lining the GI tract. They make up the largest lymphoid organ system in the body, consisting of areas of gut-associated lymphoid tissue (GALT) with follicular (e.g., Peyer's patches) (inductive) and lamina propria (effector) T-cell functions (3150). CD4+ cells, activated by antigens, express CCR5 and migrate to the lamina propria as intestinal effector cells. With reduction in antigen, they become resting memory CCR5+ cells. One process for CD4 T-cell transit to the bowel is expression of mucosal addressin cell

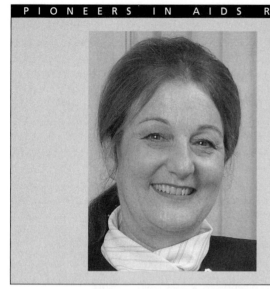

Alexandra Levine

Professor of Medicine and Chief of Hematology and Medical Director of USC/Norris Cancer Hospital. Dr. Levine was among the first to recognize lymphomas in AIDS patients. She is an internationally known expert on lymphoma, Hodgkin's disease, and AIDS-related malignancies.

adhesion molecule 1 that is induced during intestinal opportunistic infection (2991). Recent studies suggest that within days after acute infection, the entering R5 virus targets the activated and resting memory CCR5-expressing CD4$^+$ T cells in the lamina propria (491, 1657, 1658, 2957). The resting cells appear to be a recently activated cell population that has returned to a resting state (CD25$^-$Ki67$^-$). They have sufficient levels of CCR5 coreceptors, nucleotide pools, and transcriptional activators to enable them, unlike truly quiescent CD4$^+$ T cells, to support productive HIV infection (4940) (see also Section I.C and Chapter 4).

As observed with SIV infection (1493, 2872, 4574), these CD4$^+$ cells in the bowel are infected and destroyed very early by the R5 subtype of HIV (262, 1731, 2410, 2572, 4185) and throughout the course of the infection (2972). This loss of CD4$^+$ cells in the bowel, first noted several years ago (2606), could also involve R5 virus-induced apoptosis (Figure 6.5). In some studies, a selective transfer of R5 virus to CD4$^+$ cells via intestinal epithelial cells expressing DC-SIGN and CCR5 has been suggested (1675, 2972, 4185). Intestinal infection is ongoing because of continual recruitment of CD4$^+$ T cells from the circulation.

Estimates suggest that nearly 80% of resting memory CD4$^+$ T cells in the intestinal tract (particularly the lamina propria) and elsewhere in the body (i.e., blood and lymphoid tissues) are destroyed within 4 to 10 days after virus transmission. These cells die by direct infection, CTL anticellular activity, or Fas/Fas ligand-mediated apoptosis activated most likely through the viral envelope (2574, 2872, 4574). More CD4$^+$ cells than CD8$^+$ cells are observed undergoing apoptosis (2872) (see Chapter 6). The loss of CD4$^+$ cells is most dramatic in the GI tract since the majority of CD4$^+$ cells in the lamina propria are resting memory cells. In this tissue, both infected and uninfected cells appear to be lost, as is observed in peripheral lymph nodes (Section I.F). The CCR5$^+$ CD4$^+$ T cells, expressing the intestinal homing receptor integrin $\alpha 4\beta 7$, have shown the major decrease in number; these CD4$^+$ cells are among the only ones restored by antiretroviral therapy (2334) (see Chapter 14). The loss of CD4$^+$ cells in the bowel could be partially responsible for the reduction in viremia observed after acute infection (i.e., loss of target cells).

As a result of virus infection, monkeys chronically infected with SIV have only 1 to 3% of the usual number of mucosal CD4$^+$ T cells present; in disease, the figure is 0.5% (3505, 3507). These observations in the primate system also suggest that in the very early days after infection, the cellular immune component of the immune system, which should respond to various pathogens in the body, is either quickly eliminated or not induced. A similar finding was recently made in studies with SIV inoculated intravaginally (3013); the CD8$^+$ cell antiviral response was markedly delayed (3714). In some cases, where studied, opportunistic infections in the bowel of animals have been noted. In those monkeys in which the amount of virus in the GI tract was limited, a better prognostic course was observed. The extent of CD4$^+$ cell return, which appears to be delayed, can determine the clinical outcome (3505).

In many cases of HIV infection, some T cells are found in the GI tract during the chronic phase of infection, but in general very few CD4$^+$ T cells are there. The observations underline the appreciation that the peripheral blood may not give a correct reflection of what is occurring within the body. Already known was the fact, noted above, that the number of CD4$^+$ cells circulating in the blood, where only 15% may be memory cells, may not reflect what is present in the lymph nodes. Now this fact becomes even more apparent when recognizing the extent of infection in the GI lymphoid tissue, where a large number of memory CD4$^+$ cells are located. Moreover, the low number of CD4$^+$ T cells does not readily reflect the ongoing recruitment, infection, and loss of CD4$^+$ cells.

Importantly, CD4$^+$ cell repopulation of the bowel does not usually occur rapidly even after HAART (1658) despite the increase in the number of circulating CD4$^+$ cells. Part of this lack of CD4$^+$ cell restoration is the ongoing viral replication in the GALT (128, 1658) resulting, most likely, from limited access of HAART to the mucosal tissue. With successful antiretroviral therapy given in the SIV model during early infection, complete restoration of the GALT was achieved (1492). HAART has also reduced HIV RNA levels and apoptosis as well as clinical symptoms of virus infection in the bowel (2297).

The findings of CD4$^+$ cell loss have argued for an early treatment of HIV infection (within days after the acute phase) before seroconversion. Otherwise, most of the damage to GALT that occurs early cannot be prevented (1492, 1657). Moreover, since individuals on HAART do not see a great restoration of CD4$^+$ T cells in the GI tract (1657), approaches are being strongly advocated to help bring these cells back to this important lymphoid organ. Some have suggested that therapies protecting CCR5$^+$ cells in particular would be helpful in this case. This issue needs further evaluation (see Chapter 14).

While the lamina propria CD4$^+$ cell is considered the primary target for HIV in the GI tract (2971), some studies in humans have shown evidence of HIV infection in infected macrophages (1344, 2296, 3234, 4185), particularly at the time of bowel symptoms (548, 2606, 2607, 4271). Blood monocytes migrate to the mucosa, where they differentiate into lamina propria macrophages in the presence of stromal-cell-derived factors (4185). The infected macrophages, though at low numbers (0.06% of lamina propria mononuclear cells), can be an important virus reservoir and source for some of the toxic cytokines (4185) (see below). They most likely represent the cells remaining in the GI tract after the large reduction in CD4$^+$ cells takes place.

In support of these findings on HIV infection in the GI tract, bowel-derived HIV strains with some properties that can distinguish them from viruses recovered from the blood of the same individual have been described (Table 13.16). As noted above, these viruses are usually R5 macrophage tropic (262). Moreover, SIV isolates from the bowel and the brain of the same monkey have shown genetic features that suggest independent evolution of the virus variants in these tissues of the animal (2251). The same phenomenon can be expected with HIV (see Chapter 4).

C. Role of Viral Products and Cytokines

As with CNS disease, several investigators believe that an indirect effect of HIV infection is involved in the clinical conditions. For example, the pathology in the intestine could be related to HIV gp120, which causes calcium release (794), perhaps via an interaction with GalC on the mucosal cell surface (979, 2799). The effect appears to be related to particular HIV isolates (795). In this regard, recent data suggest, in the SIV system, that the enteropathy is related in part to the V3 loop region of the virus envelope (4344). Studies of this animal model might uncover the direct cause of GI disorders associated with HIV infection in humans. Moreover, as shown with the HT29 bowel cell line, an interaction of gp120 with the chemokine receptor Bob/GPR15 shows microtubular changes similar to those observed with HIV enteropathy. The disorder also resembles findings with other inhibitors of tubulin polymerization, such as colchicines (795), pharmacological agents known to promote diarrhea. In addition, HIV infection of macrophages and T cells in the intestines of HIV-infected patients could induce production of cytokines that affect intestinal permeability at moderate concentrations and give toxic effects at high concentrations. Such activities of cytokines have been considered the cause of CNS disorders (Section III.E) (Table 8.17).

In the primate model, SIV infection of intestinal lymphoid tissue (macrophages and T lymphocytes) was associated with abnormalities in absorption, even before the onset of clinical disease (1793). The results may reflect the known effect of cytokines such as IL-6 (378) (presumably produced by the infected cells) on the morphology and function of GI cells (2729). The R5 HIV strains readily isolated from bowel tissue (262) could influence the cytokines produced.

Differences in cytokine secretion by intestinal mononuclear cells from AIDS patients and uninfected subjects have been noted (4271). However, in these cases, IL-1β and IL-6 production was increased but levels of TNF-α (generally a toxic cytokine) were decreased. In these studies, the number of CD4+ cells in the lamina propria of the AIDS patients was reduced, but the possible role of cytokines released by other cells in the intestinal mucosa was not considered. Furthermore, the reduced level of APC (e.g., activated DCs) and CD4+ cells in the bowel of HIV-infected individuals could contribute to a loss of immune function and the occurrence of opportunistic infections in these tissues (2607).

V. HIV-Associated Nephropathy

A. Pathology

HIV disease of the kidney, known as HIV-associated nephropathy (HIVAN), is now the third leading cause of end-stage renal disease (ESRD) in African-Americans between the ages of 20 and 64 (3812). Over 90% of affected patients are of African descent (3811), suggesting a role for genetic factors. HIVAN is classically characterized by heavy proteinuria and a rapid progression to ESRD in infected individuals (536, 3811). The kidney shows glomerulosclerosis and tubular interstitial lesions with damage to epithelial cells and microcystic tubular dilation (536). Hyperplasia of the tubular or glomerular epithelium is observed, as well as a process of extracellular matrix formation in the mesangium and interstitium of the tubules. While nephropathy usually develops late in the course of HIV infection, some patients may have this clinical condition after acute infection (4793). A variety of potential virologic and immunologic mechanisms for HIV-associated nephrology have been considered (3666). It can be seen in HIV-2 as well as HIV-1 infection (1979).

B. Etiology

The cause of HIVAN has been questioned and, as in CNS and bowel disorders, is considered secondary to either HIV infection itself or toxic cellular factors. The virus has been found in cells of kidneys of HIV-infected subjects (537, 831, 1613, 2199, 2200, 3665). Using laser-captured microdissection, HIV was detected in individual renal epithelial cells, where it resembled the virus circulating in the blood (2823) but still seemed to indicate its own reservoir (Figure 8.14). Even in subjects on antiviral therapy, HIV has been found in renal epithelial cells (4793). Moreover, the susceptibility of renal epithelial cells to infection has been found to be mediated by a CD4-independent pathway (3676). A specific HIV subtype might be involved (3676). The cells infected were limited in their growth and survival (3676).

Others have demonstrated that HIV infection of proximal tubular epithelial cells leads to apoptosis via caspase activation and Fas up-regulation (859). Human mesangial and tubular cells were permissive to the virus infection and appeared to express CD4 and the chemokine coreceptors. For those studies, infection by an X4 virus caused the death of the tubular cells. The process was not induced by gp120, gp41, or Tat (859). The means of cell entry was not determined. Expression of the chemokine coreceptors is not generally detected in renal epithelium (1183) despite their presence in cell culture.

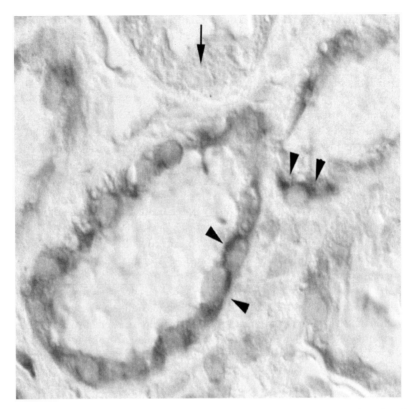

Figure 8.14 In situ hybridization of renal biopsy sample from an HIV-infected patient showing tubular epithelial cell expression of viral mRNA (arrowheads). Magnification, ×200. Reprinted from reference 3811 with permission.

X4 virus infection of primary and immortalized cultures of glomerular endothelial and mesangial cells and of glomerular epithelial cells has also been shown (860). Cytokines were produced that are known to be involved in the development of glomerulosclerosis (e.g., platelet-derived growth factor, TGF-β, IL-6, TNF-α, and IL-8). In further support of a viral etiology, nephropathy has been induced in mice expressing the HIV transgene in renal epithelial cells (536, 1081). Moreover, in the primate model, rhesus macaques have developed glomerulosclerosis and other kidney disorders and an R5 virus has been detected in the glomeruli (4285). While HIVAN is the predominant kidney disease associated with HIV infection, immune complex glomerulonephritis has also been described. Unlike with HIVAN, however, the severity of immune complex kidney disease does not appear to correlate with the viral load or CD4+ T-cell number, and the disease does not appear more common in patients of African descent (2200).

VI. Heart

Most cardiac conditions in HIV infection are not clinically evident, but some can have fatal outcomes. Pericardial effusion and myocarditis are among the most commonly found (4899). The disease could be due to direct infection of cardiac myocytes (2621, 3774) or to the presence of infected macrophages and/or T cells releasing toxic products (2634). In the latter studies, viral proteins have been found in the macrophages and T cells but not in cardiomyocytes (2634). Cardiomyocyte apoptosis has been noted with the presence of macrophages and TNF-α in the heart (4515). Moreover, HIV-infected macrophages and CD4+ T cells infiltrating the myocardium in association with myocarditis have been found with progression to cardiomyopathy (2634). Moreover, the known effects of gp120 on membrane permeability (Section II.D and Chapter 6) could explain some of the electrophysiologic abnormalities that accompany heart disease. In addition, some cardiovascular abnormalities have been reported in infected newborns (2620).

Coronary artery calcifications, as well as carotid vessel intimal thickening, have been found more commonly in patients with HIV infection (1910a). These observations can be predictive of cardiac symptoms (4166). An increased risk of disease results from endothelial dysfunction and increased inflammation in the heart as well as metabolic abnormalities that alter fat distribution (for a review on cardiovascular disease, see reference 2079). Lipodystrophies are often observed in patients on HAART (see Chapter 14). Some of the cardiovascular problems, however, could reflect behavioral practices such as smoking and a diet leading to high cholesterol. The latter finding is an important side effect of antiviral therapy.

VII. Other Organ Systems

HIV has been detected in the lungs of HIV-infected people with pneumonia (1019) and in the joint fluid of arthritis patients (4797). In the lung, changes in permeability or other toxic effects of viral proteins should be considered, especially in the childhood pneumonias. A role of anti-HIV CTL in this tissue could be involved (178, 3534). Visna/maedi virus causes pneumonitis in sheep (Table 1.1) (3331). Moreover, lung fibroblasts can be infected by HIV (3535), and HIV isolates from the lung and blood of the same individual can be distinguished (1969). This finding suggests a possible pathogenic role for certain HIV strains in this tissue. Clinical symptoms related to pulmonary disorders have been recently reviewed (1644).

The presence of HIV antigens in joint fluid and synovial membranes (1224, 4797) also merits further consideration of the potential role of HIV in associated arthropathies. The caprine lentivirus counterpart, caprine arthritis-encephalitis virus, causes rheumatoid arthritis-like disease in goats (916, 2926).

HIV has been recovered as well from the adrenal glands of infected individuals (C. Walker and J. A. Levy, unpublished observation), and fetal adrenal cells in culture are susceptible to HIV infection (249). In the adrenal glands, cytokines expressed by infected hematopoietic cells could be involved in the decreased adrenal gland function (1632). Most evidence suggests, however, that in vivo, CMV and not HIV causes the cell destruction noted in this tissue (1617, 3615). Nevertheless, a role of HIV in other endocrine disorders by a variety of mechanisms merits further study (1632).

SALIENT FEATURES • CHAPTER 8

1. HIV infection is associated with suppression of hematopoiesis, as reflected by reduced growth of bone marrow cells in culture. The infection of bone marrow endothelial cells and stroma could be involved.

2. HIV infection is reflected by changes in the subset number and phenotype of lymphocytes. Activated cells are increased, CD4$^+$ cells are reduced, and a loss of naïve lymphocytes occurs over time.

3. B-cell abnormalities include polyclonal activation and a lack of antibody responses to new antigens.

4. Abnormalities in the function of macrophages, natural killer (NK) cells, and dendritic cells (DCs) are reflected in cytokine production, reduced phagocytosis, cytotoxicity, and decreased antigen presentation ability. Loss of expression of the B7 costimulatory molecule on DCs and macrophages can be involved.

5. A decrease in CD4$^+$ lymphocyte function is demonstrated by the reduced proliferative responses to recall antigens, alloantigens, and mitogens. Potential reasons for the loss in CD4$^+$ cell number and function include both direct and indirect mechanisms, such as the effect of viral proteins, disturbance in signal transduction, loss of noninfected cells (e.g., bystander effects), cytotoxic cells, immune suppressor factors, and antilymphocyte antibodies.

6. Cytokines released as a result of HIV infection can determine the maturation of CD4$^+$ cells and their function. They can influence the extent of HIV replication and the strength of the antiretroviral immune response.

7. HIV, after transmission, most probably infects lymphoid tissues very early in infection and gradually causes a disruption in the architecture and function of this organ system. Virus particles are visualized on follicular dendritic cells, and eventually germinal centers are destroyed, leading to the decrease in immune activity. Destruction in the normal function of lymphoid tissue presages progression to disease.

8. HIV infection in the central nervous system (CNS) is determined by a variety of factors, including how the virus enters cells through the blood-brain barrier, which cells it infects, development of neuropathic strains, toxic viral and cellular products, autoimmune phenomena, and other cofactors, such as concurrent viral infections. Infection of astrocytes may cause CNS disorders by disturbing their function in antigen presentation and inactivation of neurotoxins.

9. HIV infection causes a massive loss of memory CD4+ T cells in the gastrointestinal (GI) tract 4 to 10 days after acute infection. This loss of potential target cells for HIV could explain, in part, the reduced viremia observed after acute infection and also the clinical conditions affecting the bowel.

10. Infection of the GI system may also result from direct HIV infection of bowel cells or from a disturbance in cytokine production, leading to poor absorption with malnutrition and a lack of control in handling of electrolytes and water.

11. HIV may have effects on several organ systems, such as the kidneys, heart, lungs, joints, and adrenal glands. HIV has been isolated from several of these tissues. Cytokine production and immune responses to the virus could play a role in the disorders observed.

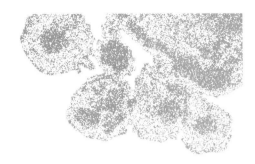

Innate Immune Responses in HIV Infection

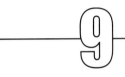

I. Introduction

A great deal of attention has been given to the role of adaptive immunity in HIV infection. Studies of CD4[+] and CD8[+] T-cell anti-HIV-specific responses (see Chapter 11) and anti-HIV antibody production (see Chapter 10) have approached one major component of the immune system. The potential role of the other, innate immunity, has only recently been appreciated (2528, 2549). The innate immune system represents the first line of defense against infectious organisms. Its earliest origin and presence in primordial organisms indicate that it was the precursor to the adaptive immune system (2001, 2953). Being the first reaction to the entry of pathogens and injury, this immune response is most important for preventing HIV infection (e.g., via vaccine or natural exposure) and for maintaining control of the infection (2528, 2549). The large number of participants in the innate immune system in relation to the adaptive immune system (Table 9.1) seems to reflect the longer existence of innate immunity. The role of various innate immune cells and soluble factors in HIV infection is covered in this chapter. Most cytokines, as well as substances in body fluids such as saliva, tears, and milk and the placenta (3440), are part of the innate immune system (2528) (see Chapters 2 and 5). A discussion on macrophages, which, like DCs, bridge innate and adaptive immunity, can be found in Chapters 4 and 8, and the CD8[+] cell noncytotoxic anti-HIV response is reviewed in Chapter 11. The latter has many characteristics of an innate immune response (Table 11.9).

Table 9.1 Components of the innate and adaptive immune systems

Innate immune system
Dendritic cells
Macrophages
Neutrophils
NK cells
γδ T cells
NK-T cells
CD8+ lymphocytes[a]
B-1 cells
Cytokines (e.g., IFN)
Chemokines
Defensins
Complement
Lectin-binding proteins (collectins)
Fever (acute-phase reactants: cathelicidins, pentraxins)

Adaptive immune system
Dendritic cells
Macrophages
B lymphocytes
CD8+ lymphocytes[b]
CD4+ lymphocytes

[a]Noncytotoxic antiviral activity.
[b]Cytotoxic activity.

II. Characteristics of Innate Immunity

A. Overview

Innate immunity differs in several ways from adaptive immunity. Innate cells respond very rapidly (minutes to days) to a pathogen and can act without MHC restriction. Participants in innate immunity recognize a conformational pattern of an organism rather than a specific epitope (2001) (Table 9.2). The innate immune system also produces cytokines (e.g., interferon-α [IFN-α]) that can have direct antipathogen effects (Figure 9.1) as well as activate innate (e.g., natural killer [NK] cells) and adaptive (e.g., T cells) cellular immune responses (2528). Whereas most studies indicate that innate immunity does not have memory, recent observations do suggest that antigen-specific memory responses can be observed with NK cells (3328a) as well with immune systems found in lower organisms (2353a).

Table 9.2 Comparison of immune systems[a]

Parameter	Innate	Adaptive
Quick response (minutes–days)	+	−
Delayed response (days–weeks)	−	+
Antigen specific	−	+
Memory responses	−	+
Gene rearrangement	−	+
Conserved through evolution	++	+

[a]Reprinted from reference 2528 with permission from Elsevier.

The innate immune system recognizes incoming microbial organisms via evolutionarily conserved pathogen-associated molecular patterns (PAMPs) and responds through intracellular signaling and subsequent cytokine production. Pattern recognition receptors (PRRs), through nonphagocytic and phagocytic processes, serve as pathogen sensors. These PRRs include the Toll-like receptors (TLRs) and the nucleotide-binding oligomization domain (NOD) protein-like receptors (NLRs) (1348a). Several RNA helicases such as retinoic acid-inducible gene 1 (RIG-1) and MDA-5 (melanoma differentiation associated 5) can also be intracellular PRRs. The pathogens recognized by these RIG-1-like receptors (RLRs) are associated with RNA viruses that enter by endocytosis or fusion (2131; for reviews, see references 46a and 916a). These viruses release products such as double-stranded RNA which can be recognized by the helicase PRRs and elicit cytokine (e.g., IFN) production. Another pathogen sensor may exist in the cytoplasm that recognizes double-stranded DNA viruses (1964a).

The NLRs detect bacteria, whereas the response from RLRs is essentially directed at eliminating replicating viruses (for reviews, see references 916a and 2131). NLRs and RLRs are located solely intracellularly. The TLRs can be on the cell surface or within endosomes (e.g., TLR-3 and TLR-7 to -9) (for reviews, see references 46a and 916a). PRR signaling activates transcription factors, such as NF-κB and IFN regulatory factors 3 and 7 (IRF-3 and IRF-7), which induce inflammatory responses and stimulate the immune system. NF-κB elicits proinflammatory cytokines such as interleukin-1β (IL-1β) and TNF-α; IRF-3 leads to the production of IFNs as well as a variety of chemokines (46).

NLRs participate primarily in the intracellular recognition of bacterial pathogens and their prod-

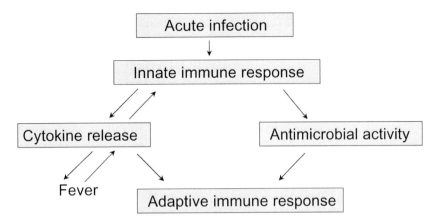

Figure 9.1 Interaction of the innate and adaptive immune systems. Following acute infection by a microorganism, the components of the innate immune system respond rapidly, releasing cytokines that induce fever and initiating antimicrobial activity by innate immune cells (e.g., neutrophils and natural killer cells). The cytokines and the antimicrobial activity also elicit the subsequent responses of T and B cells of the adaptive immune system. Thus, a close interaction between the innate and adaptive immune systems exists, and the early activity of innate immune cells can have influence on both innate and adaptive immune responses. Adapted from reference 2528 with permission from Elsevier.

ucts (e.g., muramyl dipeptide peptidoglycans). Similar to TLRs, the NLRs, after interacting with their ligands, activate NF-κB, a process involving intracellular kinases leading to the expression of cytokines and chemokines (Color Plate 16, following page 366). Some evidence suggests that an interplay can take place between TLRs and NLRs in the induction of cytokine production (916a). Another family of PRRs is the TREM (triggering receptors expressed on myeloid cells) proteins found on myeloid as well as other cells. They function as modulators of the cellular immune response and can affect activities of other innate immune sensors. They can have a positive and negative function in regulating the activation and differentiation of myeloid cells (2237a).

In addition, other PRRs involved in phagocytosis include the C-type lectin-like receptors (CLRs) (see below; Table 9.3) that help clear destructive self molecules as well as pathogens (46a, 1566, 3762a). Examples of CLRs, of which there are more than 50, are the beta-glucan receptor (1566) and the mannose receptors (MRs) that interact with mannose-containing organisms (e.g., HIV) and encourage engulfment by macrophages. Another ligand is the mannose-binding lectin, produced by the liver (1240) (See Section V.A).

Finally, circulating lipoproteins may also be part of the innate immune system. They represent a nonspecific antiviral response to infection (4156a). A serum apolipoprotein has been reported to inhibit HIV infection (3365a).

B. Toll-Like Receptors

TLRs, named after their counterpart initially discovered in *Drosophila*, are type 1 integral membrane glycoproteins with cytoplasmic, transmembrane, and extracellular domains. There are 11 human TLRs currently identified (Table 9.3). The nonphagocytic receptors recognize the PAMPs extracellularly (e.g., via TLR-1, -2, and -4 to -6) or intracellularly (e.g., TLR-3 and -7 to -9), leading to signal transduction (for reviews, see references 46 and 3433). The TLR-associated cytoplasmic domain has homology to the IL-1 receptor and is known as the Toll IL-1 receptor (TIR) domain. Following interaction with ligands, it recruits signal adaptor molecules to respond to chemicals, peptides, and nucleic acid ligands (2953, 3433).

The TLRs can be found on macrophages, DCs, neutrophils, B cells, epithelial cells, endothelial cells, and T cells (1890; for a review, see reference 4343a). The cytokines or chemokines produced in response to TLR signaling can elicit migration

Table 9.3 Pattern recognition receptors[a]

Pattern recognition receptor(s)[b]	Ligands
TLR-1[c]	Bacterial lipoproteins from *Mycobacteria* and *Neisseria*
TLR-2[c]	Zymosan yeast particles, peptidoglycan, lipoproteins, glycolipids, lipopolysaccharide
TLR-3	Viral double-stranded RNA, poly(I·C)C
TLR-4	Bacterial lipopolysaccharides, plant product taxol
TLR-5	Bacterial flagellins
TLR-6[c]	Yeast zymosan particles, lipotechoic acid, ipopeptides from mycoplasma
TLR-7	Single-stranded RNA, R-837 and R848,[d] other synthetic compounds such as loxoribine and bropirimine
TLR-8	Single-stranded RNA; R848
TLR-9[e]	CpG oligonucleotides (ODN)
TLR-10	Unknown
TLR-11	Bacterial components from uropathogenic bacteria
NLRs	Peptidoglycans
RLRs	Double-stranded RNA
Scavenger receptors[f]	Acetylated/malelylated proteins; modified low-density lipoproteins and other polyanionic ligands
Macrophage MR and other CLRs	Sulfated sugars, mannose-, fucose- and galactose-modified polysaccharides and proteins
Type 3 complement receptors and lectin type receptors	Zymosan particles, beta-glucan

[a]Reproduced with permission from Macmillan Publishers Ltd.: *Nature Medicine* (3433), © 2005. Information on RLRs has been added. See references 46, 46a, and 1566.

[b]TLR, Toll-like receptor; NLR, NOD-like receptor; RLR, RIG-1-like receptor; MR, mannose receptor; CLR, C-type lectin-like receptor.

[c]TLRs can form heterodimers, which further changes their specificity. For example, TLR-2 and TLR-6 form heterodimers that recognize a mycoplasmal lipoprotein. TLR-1 and TLR-2 have similarly been shown to cooperatively recognize a mycobacterial lipoprotein.

[d]R-837 (imiquimod) and R-848 (resiquimod) are the first small-molecule synthetic TLR ligands to be identified. R-837 is licensed for use as a topical cream (Aldara) against anogenital warts caused by human papillomavirus.

[e]TLR-9 from human and mouse shows CpG oligodeoxynucleotides (ODN) sequence specificity.

[f]Scavenger receptors are further subdivided into SR-A, SR-B, SR-D, and SR-F, depending on structure and ligand recognition.

of new immune cells to an area of infection or inflammation and can help in the maturation of DCs to present antigens to the adaptive immune system. Part of this presentation results from the up-regulation of MHC molecules on the cell surface through production of innate cytokines such as type 1 IFNs (375, 2335) (Sections III.C and III.G). This type of process is important since immature DCs are located at various mucosal sites in the body. Upon stimulation through their PRRs, they mature, migrate, and can help induce adaptive as well as innate immune responses (Figure 9.1 and Color Plate 16, following page 366).

All TLRs except TLR-3 have a common signaling pathway that uses the adaptor protein MyD 88 (myeloid differentiation factor 88) (Color Plate 16, following page 366). In some cases there is direct binding through a TIR domain; in others (e.g., TLR-2 and TLR-4) another adaptor molecule such as TIRAP (TIR domain-containing adaptive protein) can be involved (46, 2131, 2953, 3433). The ultimate result of these interactions is the activation of transcription factors such as NF-κB and the production of cytokines, including the IFNs and the chemokines (46). The activation of the innate immune system, particularly at sites of infection or inflammation, can prepare the immune system for the induction of appropriate adaptive immune responses (1976).

TLR-7 recognizes synthetic single-stranded RNA as well as RNA from influenza virus and perhaps HIV (295, 1787, 1800, 2699). TLR-3, -7, -8, and -9 are located only in endosomal compartments

PIONEERS IN AIDS RESEARCH

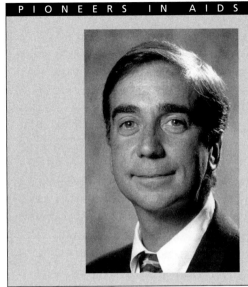

Donald I. Abrams
Professor of Clinical Medicine, Department of Medicine, University of California, San Francisco (UCSF), Chief of Hematology/Oncology, San Francisco General Hospital. Dr. Abrams pioneered the early studies of persistent lymphadenopathy syndrome in HIV-infected homosexual men. He also initiated community-based trials of antiviral drugs.

(1976, 2421). Chloroquine, which blocks endosomal acidification, can therefore prevent the responses of these TLRs (1891) (see below). Activation of a particular innate molecule receptor by a specific ligand can also lead to preferential type 1 or type 2 immune responses. For example, lipopolysaccharide-induced TLR-4 activation can lead to type 1 cellular immune responses (3617).

III. Dendritic Cells

A. Types of Dendritic Cells

DCs were first identified in the 1970s (4282) and have been shown to play a major role in the induction of immune responses (Figure 9.2). They share a stem cell precursor origin with macrophages. The DCs are widely distributed in the body (except in the brain) and are called Langerhans cells (LC) in the skin and genital tract; interdigitary cells and follicular dendritic cells (FDCs) in the lymph nodes; DCs in the thymus; interstitial DCs in the heart, lungs, and intestine; and blood DCs in the peripheral circulation (see below) (Table 9.4). The presence of DCs in the genital mucosa (1940) identifies them as potentially the first cell infected by HIV (see below and Chapter 4). DCs generally take up antigens and present them to the immune system via MHC peptide complexes on their cell surface (for a review, see reference 234), a process not generally used by other immune cells.

DCs appear to be the major cells for stimulating resting T cells efficiently. The whole balance of the immune system may be regulated by signals provided initially by DCs to both T cells and B cells, perhaps in lymphoid tissue through collaboration via signaling with FDCs (234). DCs have the unique property of aggregating naïve resting T cells as well as memory cells nonspecifically and stimulating primary T-cell responses (233). In contrast, macrophages and other tissue cells bearing MHC molecules are less efficient at priming naïve T cells. DCs and macrophages are important antigen-presenting cells (APC). Costimulation of T lymphocytes through the interaction of CD28 on T cells with B7 on DCs enhances the T-cell response (see Chapter 11). Other T-lymphocyte cell surface markers can play a role in enabling the efficient communication between a T cell and an APC (Figure 9.3). Some of these cell surface molecules are found on virus particles (e.g., LFA and ICAM) and may serve as an alternative method for virus attachment to cells (see Chapter 3).

If B7 expression is decreased on the APC (1140) or if DCs are removed more quickly from the blood and tissues than they can be renewed (2247), a compromise in immune function could result. Thus, approaches for restoring APC function may

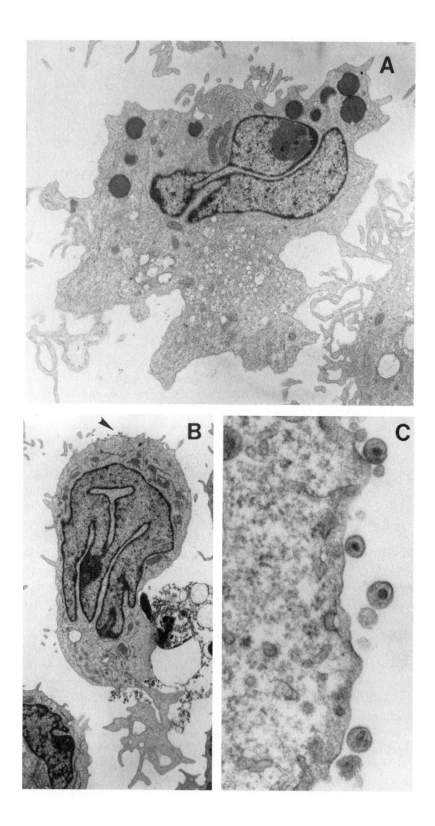

Table 9.4 Distribution of dendritic cells[a]

DC type	Location
Langerhans cells	Skin and genital tract
Interdigitary cells	Lymph nodes
Follicular dendritic cells	Lymph nodes
Dendritic cells	Thymus
Interstitial dendritic cells	Heart, lung, and intestine
MDC, PDC	Blood

[a]All these dendritic cells (DC) are susceptible to HIV infection to various extents (see Section III). MDC, myeloid dendritic cells; PDC, plasmacytoid dendritic cells.

be very important in regaining anti-HIV immune function (see Chapter 14). In HIV infection, the DC number is decreased (see below), most likely reflecting a variety of biologic processes, including the following:

- HIV infection
- Cytokine dysregulation
- Decreased expression of costimulatory molecules (e.g., B7)
- Cytotoxic T lymphocytes (CTLs)

B. Blood Dendritic Cells

Two major types of blood DCs have been recognized and make up about 1% of PBMC: the lymphoid-derived cells, known as plasmacytoid dendritic cells (PDCs), and myeloid dendritic cells (MDCs) (Table 9.4; Figure 9.4). Both cell types function as APC, express CD4, and have the chemokine coreceptors. They lack the markers of other types of whole-blood cells and are considered "lineage negative." The MDCs, not PDCs, express the integrin CD11c (Table 9.5). PDCs on stimulation are the major producers of type 1 IFN (4133) (for reviews see references 1972 and 2641). They also produce TNF-α, β-chemokines, and, in some cases, IL-10. MDCs are the primary produc-ers of IL-12 (1972). Prior to the discovery of PDCs (which represent a small percentage of blood DCs), the MDC was the cell type studied as a blood DC (3312, 4362). Therefore, previous blood DC observations in HIV infection have generally involved MDCs.

The MDCs mature into APC after exposure to IFN-γ (e.g., secreted by CD8[+] cells or NK cells) or to IFN-α produced by PDCs (see below). By interacting with TLRs on the DC surface, the maturation of these cells takes place (402, 1976). Thus, many different immune cells can affect the function of MDCs. Mature DCs (MDCs and PDCs) also stimulate NK-T and γδ T cells via cytokine production (3172). This interaction of DCs and the innate immune system lymphocytes occurs primarily in secondary lymphoid organs. Therefore, by enhancing the maturation of DCs, the innate lymphocytes can be helped in their function via an interaction with cells and cytokines.

DCs, after maturation, can migrate to various tissues and play a role in both innate and adaptive immunity. Their secretion of cytokines such as IFN-α up-regulates MHC class I and II expression, which enables efficient presentation of antigen to lymphocytes (234, 376, 2335). Various lymphocyte populations (NK, NK-T, and γδ T cells) can induce DC maturation as reflected by increased expression of CD86, IL-12 production, and priming of T-cell responses (3172). TNF-α is a major inducer of this maturation as well as the interaction of CD40/CD40 ligand via both cytokine and cell contact mechanisms (3172).

The monocyte-derived dendritic cells (MDDCs), obtained with cytokine treatment (e.g., with GM-CSF and IL-4) from peripheral blood monocytes (926, 3312, 4362), can also be active APC but vary in their phenotype and function (Figure 9.2). The exact relationship of the MDDC to MDC is not clear (for a review, see reference 233). For example,

Figure 9.2 Dendritic cells, uninfected and infected with HIV-1. (A) Purified dendritic cells were obtained from PBMC cultured for 6 days in GM-CSF and TNF-α. Magnification, ×9,000. (B) CD4[+] cord blood cells were cultured with GM-CSF, TNF-α, and stem cell factor. After 7 days, the derived cells were infected with HIV-1$_{BAL}$, washed, and cultured for a further 8 days. A mature dendritic cell with a very indented nucleus and HIV on the surface (arrowhead) is shown. Magnification, ×4,500. (C) Further magnification of the dendritic cell in panel B, showing HIV-1$_{BAL}$ particles on the cell surface. Magnification, ×60,000. All panels provided by S. Knight and R. English.

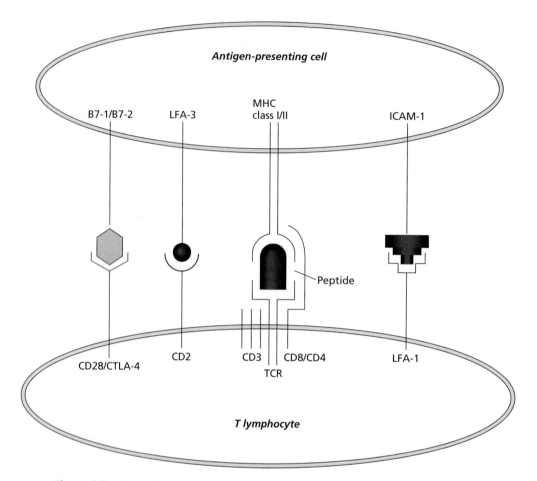

Figure 9.3 T-lymphocyte surface markers and their corresponding ligands on the antigen-presenting cell. Cell-to-cell contact between a CD8+ (MHC class I-restricted) or a CD4+ (MHC class II-restricted) T lymphocyte and an APC involves the binding of several surface molecules with their specific ligands on the APC surface. Figure provided by S. Stranford.

studies comparing MDDCs to blood DC (i.e., MDCs) have shown that the immature MDDCs are larger and have a dominance of CLRs that bind to HIV gp120 (e.g., DC-SIGN, MR, and another trypsin-resistant CLR); the MDCs bind gp120 by CD4 (4510). MDDCs, like monocytes, express TLR-1 to 6 and -8 but not TLR-7 (for a review, see reference 1976) (Section III.D) (Table 9.6).

C. Plasmacytoid Dendritic Cells

The identification of PDCs comes from initial studies examining indirect methods for assessing the HIV-infected clinical state. Siegal and coworkers noted that the production of type 1 IFNs after exposure of peripheral blood mononuclear cells

(PBMC) to irradiated herpes simplex virus (HSV) could predict clinical outcome (2666, 4134). HIV-infected individuals whose PBMC produced more than 300 U of IFN-α per ml in culture fluids, after exposure to HSV, had a good prognosis for survival with a reduced risk of opportunistic infections and cancer (4138).

Several researchers sought to identify in the PBMC the particular cell responsible for high-level type 1 IFN production that was originally referred to as the natural IFN-α-producing cell (1303, 1304). Initially recognized as a CD4+ CD11c− lineage-negative PBMC, it was shown to grow in culture in the presence of IL-3. Moreover, the addition of CD40 ligand (CD40L) resulted in its differentiation morphologically into a DC (1642, 3734). Finally, in 1999 two groups (651, 4133) demonstrated that a plasmacytoid type cell, present in the blood at low levels (2 to 10 cells/µl), could produce 200 to 1,000 times more IFN-α than any other human cell type (Figure 9.4). The cell identified, initially recognized as a pre-DC-2 cell (see below) (1642), had actually been described in lymph nodes 25 years previously and considered a plasmacytoid T cell (2494). The PDCs are found in the mantle of the CD4+ cell region of lymphoid tissue. The counterpart to human PDCs was subsequently identified in mice (167, 385, 3204).

Initially, the PDC was identified as a precursor of a cell that gives rise to mature DCs that stimulate a type 2 immune response (pre-DC-2 cells) (1642, 3734). Others subsequently observed that pre-DC-2, activated by influenza virus and CD40L, can also give a potent type 1 immune response mediated by the effects of IL-12 and type 1 IFNs (650). Essentially, human pre-DC-2 can induce ei-

ther type 1 or type 2 immune responses depending on their exposure to viruses or IL-3, respectively (1971). A preferential priming of TH2-type cells occurs through Sendai virus stimulation in which OX4OL is expressed during maturation and type 1 IFN production is down-regulated (1971).

In human peripheral blood, PDCs can be distinguished from MDCs by the absence of CD11c expression (Tables 9.5 and 9.6). Moreover, the PDCs have a low-level expression of CCR7 and the PDCs react with two monoclonal antibodies against blood dendritic cell antigen 2 (BDCA-2) and BDCA-4 (1161), now classified as CD303 and CD304, respectively. CD304 can be found on a small number of MDCs. The use of BDCA-2 and BDCA-4 antibodies (1161) has expedited the purification of these cells by sorting and their identification by cell surface markers using flow cytometry (3971). When the PDC matures, after release of IFN, expression of BDCA-2 is lost (J. A. Levy, unpublished observations). PDCs have TLR-7

Figure 9.4 Morphology of PDCs and MDCs. By electron microscopy (a), PDCs appear as lymphoblasts with a medium to large diameter; a lightly eccentric, indented, round or oval nucleus; lightly stained perinuclear areas; and well developed rough endoplasmic reticulum. By scanning electron microscopy, resting PDCs have a spherical shape (b), whereas CD40L-activated PDCs have a dendritic cell-like morphology (c). Original magnifications, ×7,000 (a) and ×3,000 (b, c). By Giemsa staining, the PDC have a plasmacytoid morphology (d). The CD11c+ blood MDCs display dendrites by Giemsa staining (e) and electron microscopy (f). Reproduced from references 1642 and 4133 with permission.

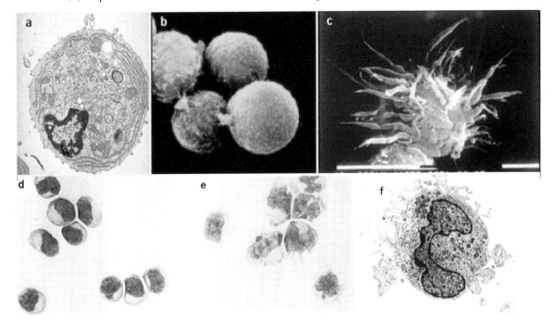

Table 9.5 Comparison of blood dendritic cells[a]

Marker	PDC	MDC
Lineage	−	−
CD11c	−	+
CD4	++	+
HLA-DR	++	++
CCR5/CXCR4	+	+
CCR7	±	−
IL-3 receptor (CD123)	++	−
BDCA-2, -4	++	−[b]
DC-SIGN	−	−[c]
Growth factor	IL-3	GM-CSF
Phagocytosis	+/−	+
TLR-7, -9	+	−[d]
TLR-2 to -6, -8	−	+
Major cytokine production	IFN-α TNF-α β-Chemokines	IL-12

[a]PDC, plasmacytoid dendritic cells; MDC, myeloid dendritic cells; GM-CSF, granulocyte-macrophage colony-stimulating factor.
[b]Some expression of BDCA-4 can be detected.
[c]Expressed on monocyte-derived DC (MDDC), which are similar to MDC but are larger and have a dominance of C-type lectin-like receptors (see also Table 9.6).
[d]Some evidence of TLR-7 expression.

and -9 (2062) and perhaps TLR-10 (1890), whereas MDCs express TLR-2 to -6; some report expression of TLR-7 as well (1972, 2062). PDCs can be grown in culture in the presence of IL-3 since they express CD123 (IL-3 receptor) (2640, 2935) (Tables 9.5 and 9.7).

PDCs are therefore lineage-negative, CD11c⁻ CD4⁺ cells and make up 0.1 to 0.6% of circulating white blood cells (compared with up to 40% CD4⁺ cells) (for reviews, see references 2641 and 2935). This percentage comes to about 2 to 10 PDC/μl of blood (4133, 4215). PDCs are generated from CD34⁺ hematopoietic stem cells (411, 4238) (Table 9.7).

PDCs produce type 1 IFNs in response to enveloped viruses such as HSV and HIV; Sendai virus infection stimulates IFN production primarily by monocytes (1884). The induction of IFN by HSV in PDCs is inhibited by several monosaccharides as well as antiserum to the mannose receptor. Thus, certain sugars on viruses can influence the extent of IFN production by PDC (3022).

The above results would reflect CLR expression on PDCs, but only a few of these cells appear to have these receptors (4511) (Table 9.6) (Section III. D). IFN-α production by PDCs has been found to be associated with infection or entry of single-stranded RNA viruses (1787, 1891, 2699). Recently, a PDC line on exposure to influenza virus acquired TNF-related apoptosis-inducing ligand (TRAIL) and killer activity against TRAIL-sensitive target cells. Since IFN-α induces TRAIL on CD4⁺ cells (1819), activation of PDCs could induce them to have cytotoxic activity against infected cells (691). However, a CTL function of primary PDCs has not been noted (M. Colonna, personal communication).

As noted above, PDCs, via cytokine production, can influence both innate and adaptive immunity (for reviews, see references 856, 2641, and 2935). Essentially, by secreting IFN-α, the PDCs can have a direct anti-HIV activity and encourage NK cell responses (377) (Figure 9.1). They enhance CTL activity by their induction via IFN of increased MHC class I molecule synthesis and expression on APC (422, 2335).

G-CSF and flt-3 ligand can increase the number of PDCs in the blood (3616). Thrombopoietin with flt-3 ligand can also enhance the generation of PDC precursors (716), and IL-18 can act as a chemoattractant for PDC (2110). This cytokine is produced by DC-1 cells and can influence the type 1 immune response (2110). PDCs activated by CpG can induce the generation of CD4⁺ CD25⁺ T regulatory cells. This activity requires direct contact of PDCs with the CD4⁺ CD25⁺ cells. The mechanism is not known but does not appear to be via type 1 IFN production (3119). Other DC can also produce IFN-α in response to double-stranded RNAs, but this response is lower than that produced by PDCs (1884). Recently, IFN production by human PDCs, following stimulation with HSV but not other inducers, resulted in the development of CD4⁺ T cells with enhanced cytotoxic activity and T regulatory function. Thus, PDCs may play a role in controlling inflammatory responses in chronic viral infection (2132).

D. Dendritic Cells, C-Type Lectin-Like Receptors, and HIV Infection

Whereas virus:cell fusion predominates in the infection of CD4⁺ lymphocytes, the endocytic

Table 9.6 Characteristics of dendritic cells[a]

Marker or receptor	Myeloid DCs				Blood plasmacytoid DCs
	Blood myeloid DCs	Langerhans cells	Interstitial DCs	Monocyte-derived DCs	
DC-specific markers					
BDCA-1/CD1c	+	+	+	+	−
BDCA-4	−	−	−	+	+
CD1a	−	+	+/−	+	−
E-cadherin	−	+	−	−	−
Birbeck granules	−	+	−	−	−
C-type lectin-like receptors					
DC-SIGN	+	−	+	+	−
Langerin	−	++	−	−	−
Mannose receptor	−	−	+	+	−
BDCA-2	−	−	−	−	+
Myeloid markers					
CD13	+	+	+	+	−
CD14	−	−	−	−	−
CD33	+	+	+	+	−
Lymphoid markers					
CD4	+	+	+/−	+/−	++
CD36	+	−	+	+	+
CD68	+	−	+	?	+
Adhesion molecules					
CD11b	+	+/−	+	+	−
CD11c	+	+	+	+	−
Cytokine/chemokine receptors					
CCR5	+	+	+	+	+
CXCR4	+/−	+/−	+	+	+/−
CCR6	−	+	−	−	
CD123	−	−	−	−	+
Miscellaneous markers					
MHC class II	++	++	++	++	++
CD45RA	−	−	−	−	+
CD45RO	+	+	+	+	−
Toll like receptors					
TLR-1	++			−	+
TLR-2	++	+		+	−
TLR-3	−			−	−
TLR-4	++	+		+	−
TLR-5	++			+	−
TLR-6	+			−	+
TLR-7	−	−			++
TLR-8	++			+/−	−
TLR-9	−	+		+	++
TLR-10	−			−	+/−

[a]Adapted from *The Journal of Leukocyte Biology* (1109) with permission. CD40, CD80, and CD86 are at low expression on all unactivated dendritic cells (DCs).

Table 9.7 Characteristics of plasmacytoid dendritic cells[a]

- CD4[+]/lin[-]/CD11c[-]; dendritic cell precursor (1642, 3734)
- Plasmacytoid morphology
- Generated from CD34[+] hematopoietic stem cells (411, 4238)
- Found in CD4[+] cell mantle region of lymphoid tissue (2494)
- Present in very low numbers in blood (4133)[b]
- Express CCR5, CXCR4, and CD123 (2641)
- Express TLR-7 and TLR-9 (2062)
- Identified by BDCA-2 and BDCA-4 antibodies (1161)
- Secrete high levels of type 1 interferon with exposure to herpes simplex virus and other pathogens (2641, 4133)[c]
- Generally reduced with HIV infection (4215)
- Loss usually mirrors CD4[+] cell reduction (4215)
- Increase in number with flt-3 ligand, G-CSF, and thrombopoietin (716, 3616)
- Can induce generation of CD4[+] CD25[+] T regulatory cells after CpG activation (3119)

[a]For reviews, see references 2641 and 2935. See text for other references. G-CSF, granulocyte colony-stimulating factor.
[b]Present in the blood at 2 to 10 PDC/μl. See Section III.C.
[c]Two hundred to 1,000 U/ml of cell culture fluid (4133).

uptake of HIV occurs primarily in DCs (934) and is facilitated by C-type lectin receptors (CLR) and not CD4. Essentially, two processes can be involved in CLR:HIV interaction: (i) endocytosis without infection, in which the virus can remain infectious for a short period (6 to 12 h) (4512) before its degradation, and (ii) direct infection, in which virus can be continually passed by the infected DCs after 24 h. Thus, the suggested persistent infectivity of HIV within DC endosomes initially reported (2366) has not been confirmed (4193, 4512). The transfer of HIV by DCs to CD4[+] cells would then seem more likely to occur by infected cells than by free virus. Nevertheless, the short-term internalization of HIV via DC-SIGN may be involved in virus transfer from B cells to CD4[+] cells (3668). Moreover, with low viral titers, the CLR can be important in concentrating virus on the DCs to be transferred to T cells. Differences in virus envelope glycosylation can determine the relative ability of HIV to bind to different C- type lectins (934).

Two types of CLR (type 1 and 2) can be distinguished by the placement of the N terminus of the lectin receptor and the number of carbohydrate recognition domains (CRDs). The type 1 CLR has an N terminus distal to multiple CRDs and is represented by the MR (CD206). Type 2 CLR have the lectin receptor N terminus within the cytoplasm and a single CRD. Its members include dendritic cell ICAM-3 grabbing non-integrin (DC-SIGN; CD209) as well as langerlin (CD207) (1288) (Table 9.6).

The MR was the first CLR identified, but DC-SIGN, initially described for placental cells (936) and found on MDDCs, has been studied more frequently in terms of its binding to HIV gp120 (1476) (see below). MR is on macrophages, DC subsets, and epithelial and endothelial cells but not LC (Table 9.6). It provides an entry receptor for HIV on macrophages as well as for transfer of virus from these cells to T cells (1240, 3248). Circulating DCs do not express CLRs except for a small amount of MR on PDCs (4511).

DC-SIGN is present on MDDCs in vitro and usually not on DCs in vivo except for dermal and lamina propria DCs. Also, LC and the superficial epithelium do not express DC-SIGN. LC have langerlin. Thus, DC-SIGN is not found on MDCs or PDCs circulating in the blood (1324, 4215) (Table 9.5) or on DCs in noninflamed lymph nodes; only macrophages in vivo show the presence of DC-SIGN (934, 1597). Much of the experimental evidence for HIV binding to DC-SIGN comes from studies from MDDCs, and this in vitro DC phenotype may be a counterpart for monocytes in inflamed tissue in vivo (2724). Some studies have, however, reported DC-SIGN on immature DCs in humans (4200). A related lectin, DC-SIGNR, has been found expressed on endothelial cells and has a presumed similar role (3546). Differences in the ability of these two CLR to bind and transfer various HIV isolates have been noted (3545, 3546).

Therefore, prevention of sexual transmission of HIV inhibition via DC-SIGN and other CLR, including langerlin and the MR, needs to be considered in addition to CD4 and the chemokine coreceptors (see Chapter 3). Targeting the CLR is important since HIV binds to these structures with higher affinity than its natural receptors (CD4 and CCR5). DCs carrying the virus can also stimulate high-level replication of CD4$^+$ T cells (934).

E. HIV Infection of Dendritic Cells

As noted above, DCs are involved in a number of HIV infection processes, including uptake of the virus by endocytosis and serving as target cells for direct infection in the mucosae. DCs then transfer the virus to lymphoid tissue, where infection of T cells occurs and priming of the HIV-specific CD4$^+$ and CD8$^+$ T-cell immune responses takes place. In stratified epithelium, the major DCs are epidermal LC and dermal DCs. In the rectum, the DCs in the lamina propria are similar to dermal DCs (934).

LC are probably the first DCs to interact with HIV. They are found in large amounts in the foreskin and at great frequency in the ectocervical epithelium and the vaginal epithelium. LC infection probably takes place at a low level (around 5% [2133], but HIV infection of DCs by less than 1% could still give effective virus transfer to CD4$^+$ lymphocytes) (934).

While perhaps only small numbers of DCs in various tissues of the body show HIV infection, reports of infected DCs in lymph nodes, blood, and the myocardium (3774) are noteworthy (for a review, see reference 2244). The DCs from several tissues appear to be susceptible to HIV infection (2405, 2720, 2721, 3443), but probably not all DCs in the blood are sensitive to the virus (591, 4719) (for a review, see reference 2244). Moreover, within lymphoid tissue are found FDCs that play a role

in activating B and T cells (see Chapters 9 and 11). FDCs, as well as B cells, can have infectious HIV on their surface alone or via trapped complement (239) (see below and Chapter 2, Figure 2.3).

Apparently, selective subpopulations of blood DCs are susceptible to HIV infection in vitro (4719). Cultured DCs derived from CD34$^+$ progenitor cells in the bone marrow and blood have been shown to produce high levels of the virus after infection (2405). Other cell culture studies have demonstrated HIV infection of both MDDCs and MDCs obtained directly from blood (926, 1207, 3443, 4500) (Figure 9.2). In a recent study, a subset of MDCs expressing BDCA-1 were shown to be susceptible to HIV infection. These cells have CD4 and low levels of CCR5 and CXCR4 coreceptors on their cell surface but not DC-SIGN (1598). The infected cells were unable to stimulate T-cell-mediated immune responses.

Early evidence suggested that MDCs are productively infected only as they mature (2244, 4720). Other reports indicate that immature MDCs can be most susceptible to HIV infection, perhaps because they express higher levels of CCR5 than mature DCs (934). Moreover, immature DCs can also engulf virus without the need for CD4$^+$ cell interaction. Nevertheless, studies have shown sensitivity to infection of both immature and mature DCs (598, 3268). Low-level HIV replication in MDCs (immature and mature) can provide a reservoir for transfer of virus to activated CD4$^+$ lymphocytes and subsequent high-titer virus replication (3268, 3574). Thus, the controversy over the infectibility of these cells may be related to the particular cell subtype examined, the level of virus production, and the state of maturation/differentiation.

Differences in sensitivity to HIV infection between MDCs and PDCs have been noted (1304, 2641, 2935, 4174) (see below and Chapters 4 and 13). Both subsets are susceptible to X4 and R5 viruses, although MDCs replicate R5 isolates best; moreover, HIV replicates to higher levels in MDCs than in PDCs (4174). Infection of MDCs appears to depend on CD4 expression, but CD4-independent infection has also been described (706, 926). CCR5, CXCR4, and SDF-1-sensitive non-CXCR4 receptors have been identified on these cells (3832). PDCs, as noted below (Section II.F), are susceptible to both R5 and X4 HIV infection via CD4 and coreceptors but at the low level characteristic of resting CD4$^+$ cells (3973). Nevertheless, as with MDCs, these cells, replicating virus at low levels, can readily transfer HIV to target CD4$^+$ cells.

Several studies demonstrated that macrophage-tropic (R5) viruses preferentially infect DCs (2244, 2246, 2247, 2405, 3832, 4212). However, other observations with DCs and monocytes derived from the same population of CD34$^+$ progenitor cells suggested that X4 viruses can also replicate in DCs (3268, 4685). X4 viruses have been found to grow at a low level in immature DC, and the cells can transfer the virus directly to CD4$^+$ cells after attachment for a short time (2 h) to the cell surface (3268). The latter transfer differs from that described for R5 viruses (1207) that can productively infect DCs (see below). Some reports have shown that in DCs and macrophages, IL-10 up-regulates CXCR4 expression, which favors X4 HIV replication. These observations require further investigation but could explain how X4 viruses can also be transmitted via the mucosae (see Chapter 3).

F. Plasmacytoid Dendritic Cells and HIV Infection

PDCs were found to express CD4 as well as CXCR4 and CCR5 and can be infected by both X4 and R5 viruses without any evidence of cytotoxicity (1324, 3973). The extent of infection resembles that of unactivated CD4$^+$ cells (3973). However, once PDCs mature into DCs, after exposure to CD40 ligand, the virus replicates to a higher level and cytopathology is noted (1324, 3973). Treatment of PDCs with anti-IFN-α antibody also makes them more sensitive to HIV infection (1324, 3973). This effect of HIV-1, in addition to CCR7 expression (see below), could explain the reduction in PDC levels in the blood of HIV-infected individuals.

PDC levels present in HIV-infected individuals are found to vary depending on the clinical state (4215) (Figure 9.5). This loss in number and qualitative dysfunction of PDCs correlate with decreased CD4$^+$ cell numbers (274, 1269, 3972). As a person advances to disease, the number of PDCs is reduced, reflecting as well the decrease in CD4$^+$ cells and high viral loads (4215). Importantly, those infected individuals who are long-term survivors (LTS) have higher levels of PDCs circulat-

ing in the blood than healthy controls (2549, 4215) (Figure 9.5). LTS are individuals who have been infected for at least 10 years, remain healthy without therapy, and have a normal CD4$^+$ cell count (see Chapter 13). When subjects with acute infection are studied, those with low viral loads in the early period following virus transmission are found to have higher PDC levels than those with high viral loads (2187, 3374). These findings may indicate that those individuals who present with high PDC levels will become LTS.

An early recovery of PDC number before CD4$^+$ cell counts has been observed in subjects receiving HAART (3972, 4136). Moreover, after treatment interruption, the PDC count and not the CD4$^+$ T-cell count has correlated inversely with plasma viral load (2187). In addition, some untreated HIV-infected subjects who remain asymptomatic have very low numbers of CD4$^+$ cells (<100 cells/µl), with normal or elevated numbers of PDCs (2549, 4215).

Certain studies indicated that HIV itself, and in some cases HIV gp120 but not gp41, could induce IFN production by PDCs (1032, 1269, 1324, 1327, 3971, 4883). However, in these studies, high concentrations of HIV were used that are not clinically relevant (3971). The interaction of PDCs with HIV-infected cells is the most potent mechanism for inducing type 1 IFN production. Up to threefold-greater levels are induced by virus-infected cells than by free virus (3971). After exposure to HIV-infected cells, PDCs mature (CD83$^+$ and CD86$^+$) (1327, 3971, 4883) and express CCR7, suggesting that they then migrate to lymphoid tissues (523, 1021). This activity, besides direct HIV infection, could help explain their low number in HIV infection.

The IFN induction appears to be mediated by CD4 on the PDC surface and an interaction requiring a strong affinity of viral gp120 (3971). The chemokine coreceptors and direct infection seem to be involved (3971). Chloroquine blocks the induction of IFN by CpG (the TLR-9 ligand) and by HIV-infected cells to a greater extent than by a synthetic TLR-7 ligand (3971). The same approach of blocking endosomal acidification with chloroquine has indicated that TLR-9 mediates HSV induction of IFN production by murine PDCs (1787, 2698). Thus, the major TLR involved

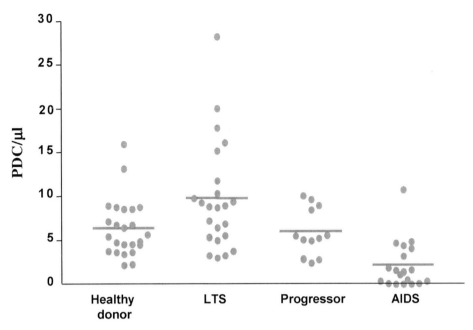

Figure 9.5 Relationship of plasmacytoid dendritic cell (PDC) number to clinical state. Each circle represents a value for a different study subject. Horizontal bars indicate the median. The number of blood PDCs is increased in long-term survivors (LTS) ($P < 0.05$ for all group comparisons versus LTS) and decreased in AIDS patients ($P < 0.01$ for all group comparisons versus AIDS). Most of the progressors had received antiretroviral therapy for several months; no substantial difference in PDC number was observed between these subjects and those who were untreated. Reprinted from reference 4215 with permission.

in human PDC activation by HIV could be TLR-9. Others have suggested that TLR-7 is primarily responsible for IFN-α induction by HIV (295).

When HIV-infected CD4+ cells are cocultured with PDCs, the production of IFN-α suppresses virus replication in the CD4+ cells (3971). In addition, when CD8+ cells from HIV-infected subjects are cocultured with PDCs, an increase in the CD8+ cell noncytotoxic antiviral response (CNAR) is observed. This activity, demonstrated by suppression of HIV replication in CD4+ cells in the absence of cell killing (2543), can also be enhanced by IFN-α alone (see Chapter 11). When this cytokine is added to CD8+ cells, restoration of CNAR can be observed in CD8+ cells that have lost the anti-HIV response (J. Castelli and J. Levy, unpublished observations) (see Chapter 11). The findings again emphasize how this innate cell can be important via cytokine production in protection from HIV infection and disease progression.

Some studies have indicated that PDCs from HIV-infected individuals can differ in their production of type 1 IFN after exposure to various stimuli (1269; G. Wortzman-Show and J. A. Levy, unpublished observations). PDCs from healthy infected individuals produce lower amounts of IFN-α in comparison to healthy uninfected controls, but a higher amount than that produced by PDCs from HIV-infected patients with low CD4+ cell counts. Thus, the number of PDCs can be reduced in HIV infection and their level in the blood may not reflect their actual function, which can be further compromised as an individual shows signs of HIV infection (1269).

G. Role of IFN-α in HIV Infection

The beneficial role of type 1 IFNs in HIV infection was suggested in early studies of antiviral drugs. IFN-α and -β were shown to directly inhibit HIV infection in vitro (2997, 3560, 4849) (see above). Essentially, the type I IFNs are critical in antiviral

Table 9.8 Roles of type 1 interferons

- Interfere with virus replication (3482, 3903)
- Increase antiviral activity of NK cells (377)
- Induce adaptive antiviral T- and B-cell responses (375, 2442)
- Enhance cytotoxic T-cell activity through increased MHC class I expression on APC[a] (422, 2335)
- Increase function of dendritic cells as APC (377)
- Increase IFN-γ production by CD4+ T cells (515)
- Promote a type 1 immune response (3782)

[a]APC, antigen-presenting cells.

immunity (Table 9.8) because (i) they can directly interfere with virus replication, an activity mediated by IFN-stimulated genes (3482, 3903), (ii) they increase the antiviral activity of NK cells (375, 377), and (iii) they are critical for the induction of adaptive antiviral T- and B-cell responses (375, 1153, 1842, 2442).

IFN-α activates MDCs, causing the up-regulation of MHC and costimulatory molecules, and this process increases their functional capacity as APC. In some circumstances, the activation of MDCs can lead to a type 2 immune response. In addition, type 1 IFNs increase IFN-γ production by CD4+ T cells (515) and promote a type 1 immune response (3782). As noted above, following maturation into DCs with the CD40 ligand, which would occur after interaction with CD4+ cells (1324, 3971), PDCs can become DC-2 cells that produce cytokines such as IL-4, IL-5, and IL-10 and enhance antibody production (for a review, see reference 2641).

IFN-α can favor the growth of T lymphocytes, but also their death, depending upon the time of exposure to the cytokine (1109a). This cytokine delays the entry of T lymphocytes into the G_1 phase of the cell cycling and increases Bcl-2 expression early after activation. Later these cells express enhanced levels of surface Fas, making them sensitive to apoptosis. In this regard, type 1 IFNs can have an antiapoptotic effect on uninfected CD4+ and CD8+ lymphocytes, but not on CD4+ T cells from HIV-infected individuals (3772a), most likely reflecting the extent of T-cell activation. Moreover, IFN-α has induced the expression of TRAIL on CD4+ T cells from HIV-infected subjects. This process was associated with CD4+ T-cell death (1819). Whether this observation

on the detrimental effect of IFN-α has clinical relevance merits further attention.

H. Effect of HIV on Dendritic Cell Function

In HIV infection, there is a progressive depletion of both the PDC and MDC populations that correlates with an increased HIV-1 viremia (1108, 1269, 3972, 4215) (Table 9.9). Moreover, PDCs and MDCs are important mediators of defense against HIV infection (2528) and were noted in early reports to have reduced function in HIV infection (2246, 2720, 2721). The DC number in skin, bone marrow, and PBMC is decreased in individuals with HIV infection (2720) (Table 9.4). The number of cells infected, however, seems too small to suggest that infection itself causes much dysfunction. These cells could be affected indirectly by certain viral or cellular proteins (Section II.E).

The processes responsible for the loss of DCs during acute and chronic HIV infection have not yet been clearly elucidated, but they most likely resemble those involved in CD4+ cell loss: direct HIV infection, activation-induced apoptosis, and killing by CTLs (2244, 2247) (see Chapters 4, 8, and 11). The earliest report on potential compromise in DC function by HIV infection showed a reduction in ATPase and MHC class II antigens on LC of the skin (300). These cells are also decreased in the oral cavity in association in some cases with hairy leukoplakia (1625). Importantly, besides cell number, DCs from HIV-infected individuals, as well as cells infected in vitro, have a decreased ability to stimulate primary T-cell proliferation responses, to act as APC, and to increase B-cell antibody production (2244, 2719, 2721) (Table 9.9). This reduced MDC activity could help explain the decrease in CD4+ cell numbers (1796). Moreover, MDCs in HIV viremic patients are impaired in

Table 9.9 Effect of HIV infection on dendritic cells[a]

- Decreased cell number
- Decreased function as antigen-presenting cells
- Decreased ability to stimulate primary T-cell proliferative responses
- Decreased ability to increase B-cell antibody production
- Defect in cell renewal

[a]See references 2244 and 2247.

their ability to secrete IL-10 and IL-12, and these cytokines are needed for the function of NK cells (2881a) (see Section IV.A).

The effect of HIV on DCs may relate to CTL antiviral responses. Viral antigen presentation by these APC might elicit cytotoxic effects of CTLs that kill the DCs (2543, 4971) (see Chapters 11 and 13). Thus, the number of DCs will be decreased if fresh cells cannot be replenished at an equal rate by CD34+ progenitor cells. A defect in DC renewal appears to be present in HIV infection (2245) but needs further substantiation. This possible process of DC destruction is supported by observations with infection by lymphocytic choriomeningitis virus in mice. Destruction by CTLs of lymphocytic choriomeningitis virus-associated DCs leads to immune deficiency (445).

IV. Other Cellular Components of the Innate Immune System

A. Natural Killer (NK) Cells

1. OVERVIEW

NK cells are an important part of the innate immune system and represent about 15% of the PBMC (883). These cells recognize and in many cases kill virus-infected cells in a non-MHC-dependent manner. The function of NK cells is determined by interactions with cell surface inhibitory or activating molecules (2408) (Table 9.10). The extent of decreased MHC class I expression on virus-infected cells can determine the susceptibility of these cells to NK cell killing (540). In this regard, their function is blocked when (i) HLA-A, -B, and -C are recognized by the killer cell immunoglobulin-like receptors (KIRs); (ii) HLA-E interacts with the C-type lectin superfamily, including CD94 and NKG2A; and (iii) CD85j recognizes HLA-A, -B, and -G (2408). There are also several non-MHC class I molecules which can inhibit NK cells, such as CEA (CD66e) (2813).

The NK cell defense against microbes includes their production of immune regulatory cytokines as well as cytotoxic activity (for reviews, see references 883 and 2408) (Table 9.11). They help adaptive immunity through production of cytokines (e.g., IFN-γ) and have been reported to induce CD8+ CTLs, perhaps via CD56 (2288).

Table 9.10 Natural killer (NK) cell receptors and their ligands[a]

Receptor	Ligand
Transmembrane activating	
CD16 (FcγRIII)	IgG
KIR2DS1	HLA-C
KIR3DS1	HLA-Bw4 (?)
CD94/NKG2C/E[b]	HLA-E
NKG2D	MICA/B, ULBP-1, -2, and -3
NKp30	?
NKp44	?
NKp46	?
Transmembrane coactivating	
2B4	CD48
NTB-A	NTB-A
LFA-1	ICAM-1, -2, and -3
NKp80	?
DNAM	PVR/nectin-2
Transmembrane inhibitory	
KIR2DL1	HLA-Cw1, -Cw3, -Cw7, -Cw8
KIR2DL2	HLA-Cw2, -Cw4, -Cw5, -Cw6
KIR3DL1	HLA-Bw4
KIR3DL2	HLA-A3, -A11
ILT-2	HLA-A, -B, -G
CD94/NKG2A	HLA-E

[a]Provided by E. Barker.
[b]Coreceptors play a role in NK cell function (543).

Normal NK cells can produce TNF-α, GM-CSF, IFN-γ, IL-5, IL-12, and the β-chemokines (for reviews, see references 377, 1265, and 2408). These cytokines, especially IFN-γ, not only are involved in the cytotoxic function of NK cells but also, more importantly, promote the activation of other immune effector cells, particularly CD8+ cells. In this regard, IFN-γ contributes to MDC activation and has been shown to prime for type 1 immune responses (3896).

2. FUNCTION IN HIV INFECTION

Some evidence has suggested that down-regulation of MHC class I by HIV proteins (e.g., Tat, Vpu, and Nef) (for a review, see reference 2082) (see Chapter 8) protects HIV-infected cells from CD8+ cell cytotoxic activity (3779). These effects noted in

Table 9.11 NK cell function[a]

- Kill virus-infected cells and tumor cells
- Produce cytokines (e.g., IFN-γ and IL-2) (377, 883, 3896)
- Produce a variety of cytokines that help cytotoxic function of CD8[+] cells and NK cells (377, 2408)
- Produce cytokines that promote activation of other immune effector cells

[a]For reviews, see references 377 and 2408.

T-cell lines may not be observed in primary CD4[+] cells (435). This MHC down-regulation, however, would classically permit the cell to be recognized and killed by NK cells. However, whereas the expression of conventional HLA class A and B molecules can be reduced in HIV-infected cells (2082) (see Chapter 8), HLA classes C and E, which prevent NK cell killing, can still be expressed (436, 833). The presence of HLA-C and HLA-E molecules on HIV-infected cells can also protect them from antibody-dependent NK cell killing of autologous CD4[+] cells (435, 4682). Certain NK cells that lack the HLA-C and -E inhibitory receptors, however, can kill the infected CD4[+] cells having this MHC class I expression (4682). Moreover, NK cells have been shown to produce β-chemokines and other soluble factors that can inhibit HIV-1 infection (1265).

NK cell number and function are decreased in HIV infection (1326, 2121, 2779, 2961, 4524; for reviews, see references 377 and 1258) (Table 9.12). The reduced cell number correlates with low CD4[+] T-cell counts (1123). Notably, NK cell function appears to be normal in healthy HIV-2-infected individuals in association with high CD4[+] T-cell counts but decreased with reduction in CD4[+] cell levels (3296). In one study, LTS had normal NK cell numbers and cytotoxic function (1963). An increase in inhibitory receptors and a loss of activating receptors are associated with decreased NK cell function (2962). In some studies, the expression of natural cytotoxicity receptors and NK cell function (e.g., IFN-γ production) were found to be decreased in viremic patients (994, 2881, 2881a). Furthermore, the capacity of NK cells to lyse immature dendritic cells has been reported to be impaired (2881a, 4391).

HIV viremia is also associated with an enhanced expression of the NK cell inhibitory receptors (Table 9.12) and may be responsible for the loss of NK cell function (2300, 2962) if any MHC class I molecules are expressed on cells. In HIV viremic individuals, the major activating NK receptors (except NKG2D), including NKG2A and CD94, are down-modulated on NK cells (2881). NKG2A and CD94 together recognize HLA-E (543). In addition, an induction of the nonclassical MHC class I molecule, HLA-G, by HIV can occur on infected cells and prevent NK cell killing (436, 3451; E. Barker, personal communication) (Table 9.12). This molecule, for example, expressed on placental cells is known to reduce maternal NK cell responses (3045). HLA-G appears to be resistant to Nef-induced cell surface down-regulation, primarily because of the length of its intracytoplasmic domain (3529).

Cytokines increase NK cytotoxic responses through their ability to activate the cells and to trigger the expression of the NK activation receptor NKp44. Recently, it was shown that NK cells kill CD4[+] cells from HIV-infected individuals through recognition of NKp44 ligands on the cell surface. NKp44 expression on CD4[+] T cells is induced by gp41 peptides (4604). Nevertheless, the relevance of these findings to the in vivo situation is not known. HIV-infected cells do not express NKp44 (E. Barker, personal communication).

In contrast to the above findings, some investigators report that NK cells, although reduced in number in subjects with HIV viremia, secrete more

Table 9.12 Effects of HIV on NK cell function

- Decreased NK cell number and function (377, 1258, 1326, 2299, 2961)
- Reduced natural cytotoxicity receptors (994, 2881)
- Impaired ability to lyse immature dendritic cells (4391)
- Enhanced expression of NK cell inhibitory receptors and loss of activating receptors (2300, 2962)
- Induction of MHC class I HLA-G (436)
- Reduced expression of NKG2A and CD94, which recognize HLA-E (2881)
- Reduced ADCC (2026, 4516) (see Chapter 10)
- Secretion of high levels of IFN-γ and TNF-α (78)[a]
- Reduced perforin production (437)
- Reduced ability to respond to IFN-α (4524)
- Alterations in NK cell subpopulations (78, 883)

[a]Some report a decreased production (188).

IFN-γ and TNF-α than NK cells from nonviremic subjects or HIV-negative controls (78). Notably, the NK cells in viremic patients have a higher level of expression of CD107a, a marker of lysosomal granule exocytosis. This marker can reflect active cytotoxic function of NK cells. Other investigators have shown that NK cells, despite an increase in number following antiretroviral therapy (4696), continue to show impaired IFN-γ production (188) and an inability to respond to IFN-α (4524). Other studies show an improvement in NK cell function with HAART (for a review, see reference 1258). These differing observations require further study.

NK cells eliminate HIV-infected cells through ADCC as well. By this process, HIV-infected cells are killed by NK cells through the recognition of antibodies bound to the viral envelope proteins on the infected cell surface. Most ADCC studies measuring levels of antibodies to the HIV envelope proteins have not shown a correlation with the clinical state; anti-gp120 antibody levels do not differ substantially in most symptomatic or healthy HIV-infected individuals (see Chapter 10). If, however, the number of active effector cells (e.g., neutrophils and NK cells) in the infected individual is considered, a reduction in ADCC can be demonstrated with disease progression (496, 4356, 4516) (see Chapter 10). Finally, as noted previously, NK cells carrying complement receptors may kill infected as well as uninfected cells through an interaction with complement on the cell surface (4871) (see below). Importantly, some studies suggest that NK cells can be lost during ADCC, either directly or via apoptosis (2026).

3. MECHANISM OF DECREASED NK CELL FUNCTION IN HIV INFECTION

The reduction in NK cell function could result from direct infection of NK cells by HIV (704, 4536) or indirect effects of the virus (1981). In this regard,

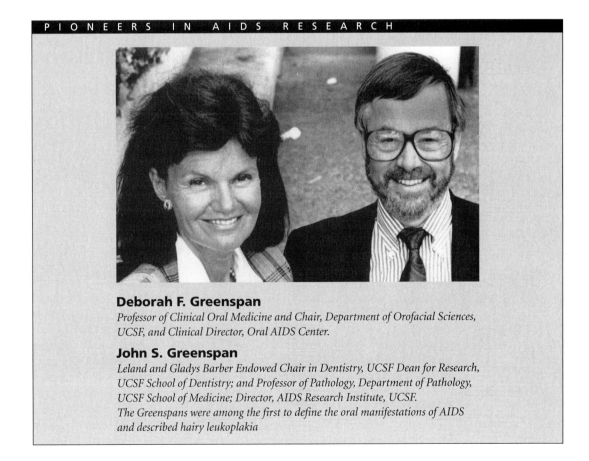

PIONEERS IN AIDS RESEARCH

Deborah F. Greenspan
Professor of Clinical Oral Medicine and Chair, Department of Orofacial Sciences, UCSF, and Clinical Director, Oral AIDS Center.

John S. Greenspan
Leland and Gladys Barber Endowed Chair in Dentistry, UCSF Dean for Research, UCSF School of Dentistry; and Professor of Pathology, Department of Pathology, UCSF School of Medicine; Director, AIDS Research Institute, UCSF.
The Greenspans were among the first to define the oral manifestations of AIDS and described hairy leukoplakia

immune activation increases the expression of CCR5 on NK cells, making them more susceptible to HIV infection. However, the number of infected NK cells in the infected person is too low to account for the overall disruption in function of these cells. Moreover, in viremic patients, NK cells do not contain HIV proviral DNA. The loss of function is associated with a trend towards an increased expression of inhibitory NK receptors and a reduction in activating NK receptors. Suppressive effects of the viral envelope could also be responsible for loss of cell function (644, 3481). In addition, some evidence suggests that HIV-1 Tat inhibits NK cell cytotoxic activity by blocking calcium channels (4974). Nevertheless, it would appear to be unlikely that viral products secreted by HIV-infected cells prevent NK cell killing of the infected cell since these cells are able to kill HIV-infected CD4+ T-cell lines to the same extent as an uninfected T-cell line (435).

The loss of NK cell activity, which is not necessarily related to cell number, probably mirrors a reduction in perforin production (79a, 437), perhaps affected by a decrease in the presence of certain cytokines such as IL-12, IL-2 (708), IL-15 (2961), and IL-10 (3424) or a reduced responsiveness to IFN-α (4524) (Figure 9.6). In HIV-infected individuals, the reduced perforin expression in NK cells can be reversed with IFN-α treatment (377, 3583); IL-15 (705, 2961) and IL-2 can enhance NK cell activity, including IL-12 secretion (3790). Since PDCs are the major cells producing type 1 IFNs (Section I.C), these innate cells appear to be involved in NK cell activity. Impaired DC secretion of IL-15 and IL-12 can reduce the function of NK cells (1278, 2881a, 2961).

The reduced NK cell function in HIV infection has also been countered in vitro by the addition of IL-12 to the assay mixture (708). Production of this

Figure 9.6   Regulation of NK cell activation and function during viral infections. Soon after many acute viral infections, IFN-α/β is induced by infected cells to activate NK cell-mediated cytotoxicity and blastogenesis (open arrows pointing to the right in the top pathway). Some, but not all, viral infections also spontaneously elicit detectable IL-12 production (broken arrows pointing to the right in the bottom pathway). If IL-12 is present, NK cell production of IFN-γ is induced. The IFN-γ response has been conclusively shown to contribute to antiviral defense primarily by activating cell-mediated immune responses. IFN-α/β acts to block or inhibit IL-12 expression and can cause a lack of detectable IL-12 during certain viral infections. This process, by reducing IFN-γ, could affect the extent of cell-mediated response induced by IFN-γ. Once T-cell responses are activated, they can then act to turn off the NK cell response. Reprinted from reference 374 with permission.

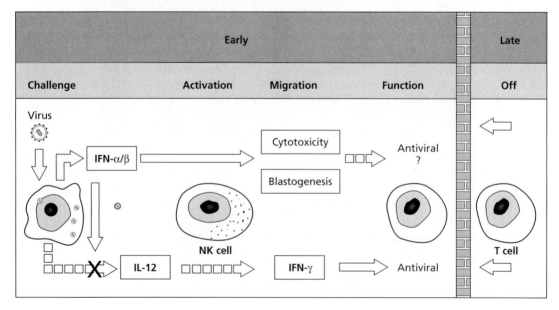

cytokine may be reduced because of HIV infection of DCs and macrophages (see Chapters 4 and 8). Alternatively, the decreased production of IL-12 may result from a direct effect of the increased levels of IFN-α and IFN-β found in HIV infection (4635). These cytokines, while enhancing the NK response, can down-regulate IL-12 expression (4727; for a review, see reference 377) (Figure 9.6).

IFN-γ is needed for NK cell function (4895), and cocultivation of NK cells with DCs enhances NK cell cytotoxicity with production of IFN-γ. Cell-to-cell contact and IL-18 and IL-12 appear to be required for this DC activity. The results suggest that by cell-to-cell contact and cytokine production, DCs enhance NK cell cytotoxicity by up-regulating both perforin/granzyme B- and FasL/Fas-based pathways (4895).

In some studies, the decrease in NK cell function has correlated with alterations in subpopulations of these cells. Two major NK cell subsets have been distinguished according to their expression of cell surface molecules. About 10% of the NK cells are CD56[bright] CD16[−] cells that are primarily immunoregulatory and the major producers of cytokines; they have low cytotoxic activity (78, 883). The other subset, CD56[dim] CD16[+], has cytotoxic activity (78; for a review, see reference 883). In chronic HIV infection, the mature CD3[−] CD16[+] CD56[bright] cells are decreased, whereas the CD16[+] CD56[dim] or CD56[−] cells are increased (78, 80, 1123, 2881, 4386). In lymphoid tissue, the NK cells are predominantly the CD56[bright] type cell that produces IFN-γ (883).

In acute HIV-1 infection, an early loss of immune regulatory cytokine-secreting CD56[bright] cells has been reported (80). This loss is associated with a reduction in the cytotoxic CD56[dim] cells, paralleled by an accumulation of functionally anergic CD56[−] cells (80). This presence of poorly cytotoxic perforin-low, NK cells in chronic infection is mimicked by similar low-functioning CD8[+] T cells, perhaps reflecting immune activation (132, 4925) (see Chapter 11). After HAART, the cytotoxic NK cell population returns to a normal level (4696) (see above).

B. Natural Killer T Cells

Natural killer T (NK-T) cells have both NK and T-cell markers (1536, 2191). Most findings now suggest that NK-T cells are involved in responses to bacterial and parasitic pathogens, whereas NK cells play a role in controlling viral infection (3172). NK-T cells are a subpopulation of αβ T cells, and the major subset (the invariant [iNK-T]) interacts with DCs expressing the antigen-presenting molecule, CD1d (2469). These iNK-T cells, which will be referred to in this book as NK-T cells, have a conserved TCR (Vα24Jα18-Vβ11) that is believed to recognize self-antigens or microbial antigens resembling synthetic glycolipids such as galactoceramide (α-Gal/Cer) (4787) through the nonclassical MHC class I molecule of CD1d (for a review, see reference 508). Four subpopulations of NK-T cells can be distinguished by their differential expression of CD4 or CD8 or the absence of both (4787). About half the NK-T cells express CD4 and some have CXCR4 and CCR5 on their cell surface (2191). NK-T cells are present in high numbers in human liver, spleen, and the gastrointestinal tract and are found in about 1 cell per 100 to 1,000 PBMC (1536). Their immunologic effect comes from secretion of type 1 and type 2 cytokines. About 10% of NK-T cells express CCR7 and traffic to secondary lymph nodes (2191).

The CD4[+] NK-T cells produce IL-4 and IL-13, whereas the CD4[−] cells have a type 1 immune profile (IFN-γ and TNF-α). G-CSF can direct NK-T cells towards a type 2 (IL-4) immune response following α-Gal/Cer stimulation and expansion of the CD4[+] cell subset (923). NK-T cells have cytotoxic properties related to perforin and granzyme B (4190) as well as Fas/FasL-induced apoptosis (136).

The CD4[+] Vα24 NK-T cells can be infected by HIV primarily of the R5 type using the CCR5 coreceptor; the infection is cytopathic (1310, 3144, 3909). In HIV infection, this cell type is reduced, and the lowest numbers of CD4[+] NK-T cells in HIV-infected people have been associated with the highest viral loads (3909). This depletion is particularly evident soon after infection (4550). Some studies have shown that Nef can reduce CD1d expression on infected cells and affect NK-T cell function (757). Nevertheless, an effect of NK-T cell infection by HIV on the clinical state has not been elucidated.

C. γδ T Cells

γδ T cells differ from the conventional αβ T cells in that their TCR is encoded by different gene

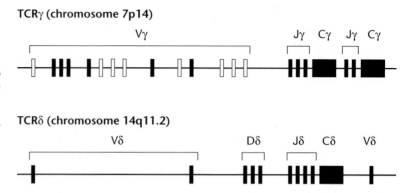

Figure 9.7 Gene arrangement at the TCR-γ and TCR-δ loci of γδ T cells. Approximate location of V, (D), J, and C segments are illustrated. Pseudogenes are indicated by empty boxes. Adapted from the International Immunogenetics Information System (http://imgt.cines.fr). Provided by D. Pauza.

segments (Figure 9.7). The γδ cells develop in the thymus and are classified primarily by their δ subset (Table 9.13). The Vδ1+ cells migrate into body tissues, particularly the mucosal lining cells of the intestine, vagina, and skin. The Vδ2 cell subset is found in blood and lymph nodes. Other subsets are rare. The majority of circulating cells are Vγ2Vδ2 cells, and they represent 1 to 10% of the T cells in the blood and are even rarer in lymph nodes (2061). Like NK and NK-T cells, this cell population has effector functions, including cytotoxic activity and cytokine production.

Via their TCR, γδ cells bind to antigens that can be intact proteins as well as other types of organic molecules (prenylphosphates). Antigen recognition is MHC independent and does not require APC. In humans, the Vδ1+ subpopulation of γδ T cells is restricted by the nonclassical MHC class I molecule CD1c found on epithelial cells, which can present microbial glycolipids or lipopeptides (for a review, see reference 1766). The Vδ2Vδ2 subset (also called Vδ9Vδ2 in an alternate nomenclature) (Table 9.13) can also recognize heat shock protein 60 (hsp60) molecules and appears to be a first line of defense against certain invading pathogens, particularly *Mycobacterium tuberculosis* and the malaria pathogen. Both of these infections also reduce the number of γδ cells (2564, 2843, 4818) and

Table 9.13 Official and alternative nomenclatures for common TCR-γ and TCR-δ genes of γδ T cells

TCR	WHO-IUS[b] (138, 4749)	Huck and Lefranc (1925)	Strauss et al. (4311)	Takihara et al. (4372)
TCR-γ	TCRGV1S2	Vγ2	Vγ1.2	
	TCRGV1S3	Vγ3	Vγ1.3	
	TCRGV1S4	Vγ4	Vγ1.4	
	TCRGV1S5	Vγ5	Vγ1.5	
	TCRGV1S8	Vγ8	Vγ1.8	
	TCRG(V2S1	**Vγ9**	**Vγ2**	
	TCRGJ1S2	**JγP**	**Jγ1.2**	
	TCRGJ1S3	J1	Jγ1.3	
	RCRGJ2S2	Jγ2	Jγ2.3	
	TCRGC1	**Cγ1**	**Cγ1**	
	TCRGC2	Cγ2	Cγ2	
TCR-δ	TCRDV101S1			Vδ1
	TCRDV102S1			**Vδ2**
	TCRDV103S1			Vδ3
	TCRDC1			**Cδ1**

Nomenclature according to indicated source[a]

[a]The segments marked with bold letters highlight the most common TCR rearrangements in blood γδ T cells. Table provided by D. Pauza and A. Hebbeler.
[b]WHO-IUS, World Health Organization/International Union of Immunological Societies.

thus, as cofactors, could enhance HIV pathogenesis. Intestinal epithelial lymphocytes contain a large number of γδ T cells (up to 50%). Recently, their role as APC eliciting adaptive immune responses has been described (485).

γδ T cells, after activation, can express CCR7 and thus can migrate to HIV-infected lymph nodes and show anti-HIV activity (485; for a review, see reference 3120). Moreover, the Vδ2 positive γδ T cells can act as APC for CD8$^+$ T cells, reflecting an up-regulation of APC molecules after their activation (for a review, see reference 3120).

Some reports indicate a decrease in the Vδ2 subset of γδ T cells and an increase in the Vδ1 subpopulation in HIV infection (179, 1000, 2845, 3544, 3555, 4156). The loss is due to specific depletion of cells expressing the Vγ2-Jγ1.2 Vδ2 TCR (1202). Some recovery has been noted in the ratio of Vγ2 to Vγ1 cells with HAART (2844, 2845), particularly when viremia is controlled (443). Decreased function of γδ T cells in HIV-infected subjects has been seen in their response to tumor cells and mycobacterial proteins (3541, 4665). Cytokine production (e.g., IFN-γ) has also been reduced but restored with HAART (2844, 2845). Moreover, some investigators suggest that an expansion of cytotoxic γδ Vδ1 cells that is associated with increased viral loads may contribute to HIV pathogenesis by depletion of bystander CD4$^+$ T cells (4156). This possibility needs further evaluation in terms of the role of γδ T cells in infectious disease (for a review, see reference 3469).

Recent evidence suggests that a subpopulation of γδ T cells express CD4 as well CCR5 and CXCR4 and can be infected by HIV-1 (1956). Most γδ cells do not express CD4 or CD8. These cells can play a role in HIV infection directly by cytotoxic responses, including perforin and granzymes or Fas/FasL-induced apoptosis (459). Notably, γδ T cells have also been reported to produce β-chemokines and perhaps other anti-HIV factors that suppress replication of both XY and R5 viruses (459, 3540, 3542) (see Chapter 13). They also produce IFN-γ and TNF-α, which can affect HIV pathogenesis (459).

V. Soluble Innate Factors

A. Mannose-Binding Lectin

Mannose-binding lectin (MBL), made in the liver, is a C-type lectin that binds to carbohydrates on gp120 (for reviews, see references 1240 and 2027). MBL reacts with both R5 and X4 viruses, since end-linked complex and high-mannose carbohydrates make up about half of the molecular weight of HIV (1749). The MBL interaction with HIV-1 leads to virus inactivation by opsonization, not neutralization (4878). MBL is an acute-phase protein, and its levels and the ability to activate complement are increased in HIV-infected individuals with advanced disease. In the presence of HAART, large amounts of MBL are associated with the most variable virologic response (1786). Moreover, polymorphisms in the MBL 2 promoter, particularly a 6-bp deletion, are associated with high levels of MBL and correlate with resistance to HIV infection in children (439). However, after infection, the high MBL levels are associated with progression to AIDS, perhaps reflecting activation of the classical complement pathway that enhances viral infection (439).

B. Anti-Tat Immunoglobulin M Antibodies

Natural antibodies often made by CD45$^+$ B cells can be part of an innate response to pathogens (for a review, see reference 3316). In the serum of infected or uninfected individuals, natural immunoglobulin M (IgM) antibodies can be detected that bind to the Tat protein. They are found at lower titers as HIV infection progresses to disease (3770). These innate IgM antibodies that react with two defined sequences of Tat (3772), are capable of inhibiting Tat-induced apoptosis, and are found in both human and chimpanzee IgM pools (3769; for a review, see reference 3771).

C. Complement

Complement can participate in several processes associated with HIV infection (Table 9.14), and serum levels of complement components appear to be stable throughout the course of HIV infection (for a review, see reference 1400). Activation of complement is reflected by the presence of complement by-products (e.g., C4d, Ba, and C3d) that are elevated in HIV-infected individuals as well as the by-products from both the alternative and classical pathways regardless of the stages of infection. These complement components, made in the liver, are activated during HIV infection and can lead to destruction of the virus by two antibody-independent mechanisms. By the first process, the complement components can bind to the virion or infected cells

Table 9.14 Potential role of complement in HIV infection

Direct
- Lysis of virions in association with antibodies (4221, 4222)
- Binding to virions and activation of the alternative complement pathway (4201)
- Binding to gp120 and activation of the classical complement pathway (4342)
- Increased HIV binding to cells via immune complexes (1995, 3330)

Indirect
- Lysis of CD4+ cells carrying envelope proteins (1400, 2825, 4342)
- Participation in antibody-dependent neutralization of HIV (4219, 4220)
- Participation in antibody-dependent enhancement of HIV replication (3767)
- Induction of direct lysis of cells expressing complement receptors through interaction with NK cells (4871)
- Lysis of cells via attachment with antibodies (i.e., ADC[a]) (3216)

[a]ADC, antibody-dependent cytotoxicity.

and become activated by the alternative pathway (4201). During HIV infection, this process is increased because molecules that inhibit complement activation (e.g., decay-accelerating factor [DAF] and CD59) are made in lower concentrations in infected individuals than in seronegative ones (2453, 4712). Neverless, DAF and the human complement factor H can inactivate the anti-HIV effect of complement (4298). By the second mechanism, activation of complement by the classical pathway can occur directly from an interaction with gp120 (4342). The viral lysis appears to occur in vivo from antibody binding to complement proteins on virions. This process could be a reason for the rapid virus clearance from plasma (4332).

Complement can also increase HIV binding to CD4+ and CD4− cells through immune complexes (1995, 3330) (see Chapter 2). This process can be a means of virus transfer as well as infection. Complement can also affect the HIV virion by several other mechanisms besides direct interaction (Table 9.14), primarily via processes involving cells. First, if the viral envelope proteins (particularly gp41) are bound to the surface of uninfected CD4+ cells, complement can fix to the cells and lyse them (1400, 2825, 4342). Any mechanism by which gp120 ex-

pression on infected cells is increased will enhance complement-mediated lysis (for reviews, see references 4218 and 4871). Second, complement can play a role in antibody-dependent enhancement of HIV infection through the interaction of immune complexes with the complement receptor (see Chapter 10). Third, by opsonizing virus particles, complement can facilitate HIV infection via the complement receptors on cells. Such a process has been suggested for virus transmission via semen (457) (see Chapter 2). Finally, complement activated by the alternative pathway can induce direct lysis of cells (infected and uninfected) expressing complement receptors through their interaction with NK cells (4871). This process appears to result from the decreased levels of complement inhibitors in the blood of infected people (2453, 4712).

VI. Conclusions

Whereas the importance of the adaptive immune system has received a great deal of attention for its response to HIV infection, only recently has the innate immune system been appreciated for its potential role in controlling HIV pathogenesis (2528, 2549). Included in this recognition have been studies of innate immunity in the brain (for a review, see reference 4229). Astrocytes, DCs, macrophages, and microglial cells, as well as several soluble factors (e.g., complement and chemokines), play a role in this immune response. Astrocytes express TLR-3, which can mediate an intracellular block to HIV replication (4328) (Table 9.15). Both PDCs and MDCs can be found in cerebrospinal fluids of individuals with CNS disorders such as multiple sclerosis. Very small amounts of cells are found unless there is inflammation. For example, PDCs range from 0 to 60

Table 9.15 Features of innate immunity in the central nervous system

- Role of microglia as a viral reservoir and in the immune response (e.g., cytokines)
- Role of chemokines and cytokines in response to HIV and in interacting with adaptive immunity
- Response of astrocytes to viral infection
- Role of dendritic cells (PDCs, MDCs)
- Effect of activation of local complement system

[a]For a review, see reference 4229. PDCs, plasmacytoid dendritic cells; MDCs, myeloid dendritic cells.

Table 9.16 Potential role of complement in HIV neuropathogenesis

- Complement factors synthesized in the brain
- Complement receptors present in the brain
    CR-1 and CR-2 on astrocytes
    CR-3 on microglia
- Complement cascade pathways can be activated by HIV (with or without antibody)
- Complement synthesis and activation can cause immune and virologic effects
    Opsonized particles enter microglia and astrocytes
    Lysis of virion and cells expressing gp120 (with or without antibody)
- Complement products induce astrocytosis, microgliosis, and neurodegeneration
- Chronically activated complement factors contribute to neurodegeneration

[a]For a review, see reference 4229.

Table 9.17 Interactions of HIV with the innate immune system

- Reduces innate cell numbers and function; causes changes in cell subpopulations
- Infects innate immune cells (e.g., macrophages, dendritic cells and NK, NK-T, and γδ T cells)
- Uses chemokine receptors for cell attachment
- Can be affected by soluble innate immune components such as mannose-binding ligands, complement, and anti-HIV factors in body fluids
- Affects production of innate cytokines
- Can activate plasmacytoid dendritic cells and induce type 1 interferon production
- Elicits NK cell responses and can reduce NK cell function
- Elicits the CD8+ cell noncytotoxic antiviral responses (see Chapter 11)

cells per ml and MDCs from 0 to 60 cells per ml in individuals with noninflammatory neurologic disease (3432). Most recently, the production of IFN-β in the brain during acute SIV infection was documented. This cytokine not only suppressed the virus but also showed the ability to induce a latent cellular state for SIV (and presumably HIV) in the brain (244). The potential roles of complement and complement factors in preventing HIV infection of the brain or exacerbating neuropathogenesis have also been considered (4229). A variety of effects, including complement factor synthesis in the brain (1461), can influence the result (Table 9.16).

Thus, the interactions of HIV with the innate immune system are multiple (Table 9.17). Besides

Figure 9.8 Functional network of innate immunity elements in the brain. Reprinted from reference 4229 with permission from Elsevier. MNGC, multinucleated giant cells.

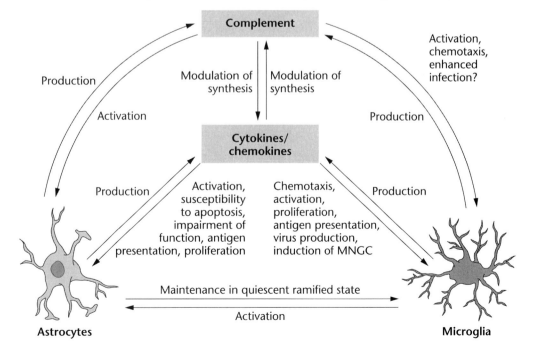

affecting general HIV pathogenesis, three major components of the innate immune system—astrocytes, microglia/macrophages, and complement—can interact and influence HIV CNS disease (Figure 9.8). Importantly, the immediate response to HIV by this arm of the immune system can help prevent infection and dramatically reduce the progression to disease (see also Chapter 11). Nevertheless, some components, both

soluble (e.g., complement) and cellular (NK cells), can contribute to disease progression. Approaches for eliciting this response in a vaccine are under consideration (see Chapter 15), as is the use of certain cytokines and compounds to increase innate immune activity (see Chapter 14). In all cases, beneficial immune activities must be elicited with minimal detrimental inflammatory or pathologic responses.

SALIENT FEATURES • CHAPTER 9

1. The innate immune system responds very rapidly (minutes to days) to a pathogen. It recognizes the conformational pattern of an organism rather than a specific epitope. It produces cytokines (e.g., IFN-α) that can have a direct antimicrobial effect as well as activate innate and adaptive immune responses.

2. The innate immune system recognizes incoming pathogens through pattern recognition receptors (PRRs). Among these are Toll-like receptors (TLRs), nucleotide-binding oligomerization domain (NOD)-like receptors (NLRs), and RIG-1-like receptors (RLRs). C-type lectin-like receptors (CLRs) also interact with carbohydrate-containing organisms.

3. Following interaction with ligands, the PRRs recruit signal adaptor molecules to respond, leading to cytokine production via activation of transcription factors such as NF-κB.

4. At least 11 (perhaps 12) human TLRs have been recognized that respond to different stimuli (e.g., ligands).

5. Dendritic cells (DCs) play an important role in innate immunity by their induction of immune responses. A variety of subtypes of these cells are distributed throughout the body. DCs take up antigens and present them to the immune system via MHC peptide complexes on their cell surface. CLRs can participate in this process.

6. DCs express a variety of C-type lectins that can play a role in HIV attachment and infection.

7. DCs in the blood are the myeloid dendritic cells (MDCs) and plasmacytoid dendritic cells (PDCs). The majority of DCs are MDCs. PDCs represent <1% of the blood DCs.

8. MDCs can be distinguished from PDCs by cytokine production (e.g., IL-12) and by their major role as APC in inducing immune responses.

9. PDCs respond to pathogens by production of large amounts of type 1 IFNs. After activation, they up-regulate CCR7 and can migrate to lymph nodes.

10. HIV infects DCs and usually shows low-level virus replication. MDCs are more susceptible than PDCs to virus infection and replication. The DCs can pass infectious virus to CD4+ cells.

11. NK cells function through the interaction of cell surface inhibitory or activating molecules. They respond against virus-infected cells having decreased MHC class I expression.

12. NK cell response against microbes includes production of immune regulatory cytokines (e.g., TNF-α and IFN-γ) as well as cytotoxic activity.

13. HIV infection reduces NK cell function. A subset of NK cells can be infected by HIV.

14. NK-T cells have both NK and T-cell markers and are involved in responses to bacterial and parasitic pathogens. The major subset (the invariant [iNK-T]) interacts with DCs expressing the antigen-presenting molecule CD1d.

15. NK-T cells are present in high numbers in the human liver, spleen, and gastrointestinal tract and are at low levels (<1%) in PBMC. Some can be infected by HIV.

16. $\gamma\delta$ T cells differ from the conventional $\alpha\beta$ T cells in that their T-cell receptor is encoded by different gene segments. These cells, which can be infected by HIV, are present in several body tissues, but particularly in mucosae. Like NK and NK-T cells, $\gamma\delta$ T cells have effector functions, including cytotoxic activity and cytokine production.

17. $\gamma\delta$ T cells bind antigens that can be intact proteins through an MHC-independent mechanism that does not require antigen-presenting cells. In some cases, the γδ T cells recognize compounds in the context of a nonclassical MHC class I molecule, CD1c, on epithelial cells.

18. Other components of the innate immune system include soluble factors such as mannose-binding lectin (MBL) and anti-Tat IgM. MBL can react with both R5 and X4 viruses and lead to their inactivation.

19. Innate complement factors are associated with several processes affecting HIV infection, including direct lysis of cells and killing of virus-infected cells. They also can facilitate virus infection of cells via the complement receptor.

20. Innate immunity plays a role in controlling HIV infection in the central nervous system.

21. HIV has many interactions with the innate immune system and affects immune cell number and function as well as the production of innate cytokines and soluble components.

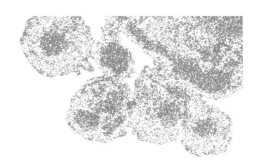

Humoral Immune Responses to HIV Infection

10

THUS FAR, THE BASIC BIOLOGIC FEATURES of HIV and its heterogeneity have been discussed. How certain characteristics could play a part in the pathogenic pathway has been considered. The role of the innate immune system was reviewed in the previous chapter. The next two chapters will cover the adaptive immune responses of the host that could influence HIV-induced disease. The effect of HIV on the immune system was considered in Chapter 8. This chapter describes four processes involving circulating antibodies that react against HIV and HIV-infected cells: neutralizing antibodies, antibody-dependent cellular cytotoxicity (ADCC), antibody-dependent cytotoxicity (ADC), and complement binding antibodies.

I. Detection of Anti-HIV Antibodies

Shortly after the discovery of HIV, different tests were developed to detect antibodies to the virus. As noted in Chapter 4, these antibodies are made soon after the acute infection (within 1 to 2 weeks). The isotype distribution of these HIV-specific antibodies can reflect their function. ADCC, complement-dependent cytotoxicity, and neutralizing and blocking abilities reflect specific antibody classes (e.g., IgG1). These molecules circulate in the blood or are secreted at mucosal surfaces. They can be detected in genital as well as other body fluids.

The evolution of antibody responses in HIV infection begins with the early presence of antibodies to the Gag protein followed by Nef, Rev, and finally Env. Subsequently, there is a stable peripheral B-cell repertoire during the first year of infection (1188). Following the development of IgG antibodies, HIV-1 IgA antibodies can be detected with higher prevalence rates in individuals who are recent seroconverters or who have progressed to

AIDS (2805) than in asymptomatic HIV-infected persons. Generally these antibodies are at a much lower level than IgG (2323, 4082). Thus, an association of high viral load with IgA antibodies may indicate advancement of HIV infection (2321) (see Section III) (for further discussion of anti-HIV IgA and IgG neutralizing antibodies that can prevent virus entry by transcytosis at the mucosal surface, see Chapter 3).

Antibodies to a variety of viral proteins can differ in their isotype. For some antiviral responses (e.g., Gag), several subclasses may be present in infected individuals. In others, such as anti-envelope-specific antibodies, one major type (e.g., IgG1) is usually found (254). Cytokines present at the time of exposure of B cells to a specific viral protein can influence the type of antibodies produced (254). In general, IgG antibody levels in serum are lower in AIDS patients than in asymptomatic infected individuals (171, 2916). IgG1 is the dominant subclass in all clinical stages and can be found at similar titers (2646). Levels of other antibody classes (e.g., IgM, IgA, IgG2, IgG4, and IgD) can vary depending on the clinical stage (for a review, see reference 254). IgM and IgA levels can be higher in AIDS patients.

II. Neutralizing Antibodies

A. General Observations

A conventional response of the host against viral infection is the production of antibodies that attach to the virus and inactivate (neutralize) it. Generally neutralization by IgG is higher than that by IgA (2322). The HIV envelope is the major target for such humoral antibody responses. The viral proteins primarily involved in antibody neutralization have been localized to the envelope gp120 and the external portion of the transmembrane envelope protein, gp41 (370, 521, 688, 1696, 2877, 3765, 4243) (Table 10.1) (for a list of neutralizing antibodies, see http://hiv-web.lanl.gov/content/immunology/tables/ab_summary.html). In a large study analyzing a panel of anti-HIV-1 monoclonal antibodies (MAb), the anti-gp120 antibody showed selective reactivity against clade B viruses, whereas anti-gp41 antibodies had broader interclade activity (370). In these studies, five neutralizing immunotypes, not necessarily correlating

Table 10.1 Regions of HIV sensitive to antibody neutralization[a]

Viral envelope gp120

V3 loop

CD4-binding domain

V1 region

V2 region

Region uncovered after CD4 binding

Viral envelope gp41 (MPER)

Envelope carbohydrate moieties

Cell surface proteins (e.g., LFA-1, ICAM, and HLA) on the envelope

[a]All regions can have linear or conformational epitopes, but the CD4 binding domain is generally conformational and the epitopes in gp41 are usually linear. MPER, membrane-proximal external region.

with genotype, were found involving a variety of clades. Moreover, certain broadly reactive MAb (e.g., b12) have been identified directed against the CD4 binding site epitope. This information on virus diversity provides an important insight into approaches for vaccine development (370) (see Chapter 15).

The presence of anti-HIV neutralizing antibodies in infected individuals has been reported by several investigators. Whereas some sera show high levels of antiviral activity against common laboratory strains, sera from infected individuals have not consistently demonstrated strong neutralizing activity against their autologous isolate (722, 1881, 4715). In early studies using HIV-1 infection of PBMC, these antibodies were found at titers of 1:10 to 1:1,000 (722, 1881) (Table 10.2). In these analyses at least four serologic subtypes of HIV-1 could be proposed (see below). The differences in sensitivity to neutralization observed could reflect an "escape" from the humoral immune response (51, 141, 2932, 3701), a greater affinity of the virus for its cellular receptor than for antiviral antibodies, or the method used to assay for virus neutralization (4977) (see Section II.G).

B. Methods for Measuring Neutralizing Antibodies

For many of the early studies on virus neutralization, laboratory isolates and T-cell lines were used with sera from infected subjects. In many cases,

Table 10.2 Neutralization of HIV-1 infectivity by anti-HIV-1 sera[a]

Proposed subtype	HIV-1$_{SF}$ strain	Source	Serum Activity		
			1	2	3
A	2	PBMC	>1,000	100	10
	4	PBMC	>1,000	100	100
	13	PBMC	>1,000	100	10
	33	PBMC	>1,000	100	10
	66	PBMC	>1,000	100	10
	113	PBMC	>1,000	100	100
	117	PBMC	>1,000	100	10
	301A	CNS	>1,000	100	100
	315	PBMC	100	10	10
B	97	PBMC	80	20	–
	171	PBMC	20	10	–
C	98	CNS	20	–	–
	128A	CNS	20	–	–
	161B	CNS	100	–	–
	162	CNS	100	–	–
	178	CNS	20	–	–
	185	CNS	20	–	–
	153	PBMC	20	–	–
	247	PBMC	100	–	–
D	170[b]	PBMC	–	–	–

[a]Tenfold and twofold dilutions of anti-HIV-1 sera (1, 2, and 3) were tested for their ability to neutralize infectivity of PBMC by 20 different HIV-1 isolates from individuals in the United States, the Dominican Republic (SF247), and Africa (SF170 and SF171). Numbers represent the reciprocal of the highest serum dilution causing a reduction of at least 67% in reverse transcriptase activity in the culture fluid. A minus sign indicates no virus neutralization at a 1:10 serum dilution. Reprinted from reference 722 with permission.
[b]Rarely neutralized by sera from individuals outside Africa.

virus neutralization was more readily observed using T-cell-line-adapted virus with T-cell lines rather than primary isolates in PBMC (3087). Importantly, to replicate the in vivo situation, it would seem necessary to measure neutralizing antibodies by procedures utilizing autologous primary virus isolates and normal PBMC. These components of the assay come closest to being the clinically relevant for measuring the potential for HIV neutralization in vivo. A definition of a primary isolate has not been formally made, but it conventionally represents a virus that has been replicated only in cultured PBMC for no more than three passages and preferably for less than 2

months after initial recovery. Some investigators have recommended using unstimulated PBMC for neutralization assays, since cells in vivo would not be activated (4977). The value of this procedure needs further study (4949), particularly since unactivated cells may express different viral coreceptors (see Chapter 4) (410).

More recent assays using recombinant virus technology and single-cycle virus assays can detect much higher levels of neutralizing antibodies (3729). Their relevance to the clinical state needs to be assessed. For example, recent studies have shown that HIV envelope pseudotype viral vectors and infectious molecular clones of HIV having the same envelope glycoproteins show similar neutralization sensitivities. Culture of the infectious molecular cloned virus in PBMC, however, showed a substantial decrease in this sensitivity (2671). The result may reflect an increase in the envelope glycoprotein on the surface of the PBMC-grown virus. This observation has obvious relevance to the clinical significance of neutralizing antibodies when measured by these more rapid assays. Nevertheless, the difference was quantitative and not qualitative and the envelope pseudoviruses appear to have a sensitivity similar to that of primary isolates of HIV-1. Importantly, with progression to disease, neutralizing antibodies can be replaced by enhancing antibodies (1881) (see Section III). Most recently, certain methods and viruses have been recommended for assessing neutralizing antibody responses, particularly when induced by a vaccine (2856).

C. Mechanism of Virus Neutralization

The mechanism for antibody-mediated neutralization of HIV has not yet been well defined. Some studies suggested that it did not involve agglutination of virus or dissociation of the envelope protein (4256) as has been described for this reaction with other virions (1091). Several studies have indicated that HIV neutralization can involve virus attachment, fusion, or a step following virus:cell fusion (2928). Possibly a disturbance in the flexibility of the envelope occurs that is required for virus entry into the cell (2917). The ability to neutralize HIV appears to depend on the number of surface envelope glycoprotein molecules (or spikes), which is generally about 7 to 14 envelope knobs per virion (740, 2438, 3910), but that number can vary (see Chapter 1). Shedding of gp120 can also reduce the virus infection (3091, 3548). Thus, the ability of the antibody to cover or detach the envelope protein from the virion (2438) could determine its neutralizing potential. Moreover, the kinetic rate of antibody binding to the virion may be more important than the affinity of the antiviral antibodies (4268).

Somewhat unexpected are the recent observations that all the envelope proteins on a virion must be targeted by at least one antibody (e.g., b12) to get sufficient neutralization (4860). Moreover, structural studies on an antibody directed against the HIV-1 gp120 CD4 binding site (see below) indicated that the antiviral activity depended on the antibody's ability to penetrate a recessed CD4 binding site on the gp120 (3919).

D. Factors Influencing HIV Sensitivity to Antibody-Mediated Neutralization

Why certain laboratory strains, passaged for months or years in vitro, are very sensitive to neutralization by a variety of heterologous sera is not clear. With some HIV-1 isolates (e.g., SF2 and MN) a common envelope epitope (i.e., in the V3 loop) can be involved, but with others (e.g., IIIB/LAI) an antigenic similarity among many isolates is not evident. Moreover, some long-passaged laboratory strains are resistant to neutralization and others are more sensitive to antibody-mediated enhancement (Section III) (1881, 1883, 2239). Different antibody binding affinities seem to be involved (2239, 4567). Thus, other factors besides prolonged growth in culture can determine the sensitivities of various HIV strains to antibody neutralization (Table 10.3).

Usually, sera from HIV-1-infected individuals can neutralize HIV-1 but not HIV-2 strains. In contrast, sera from HIV-2-infected individuals have been reported to cross-react and neutralize some HIV-1 strains (4716); they also cross-neutralize SIV strains (3748). This finding emphasizes further the reported similarities in envelope structure of these two human lentiviruses (see Chapter 1). In some cases, the addition of soluble CD4 (sCD4) will help in neutralization of HIV-2 isolates by HIV-1 sera (787, 1023) (see Chapter 4) (see also Section II.F.2).

Table 10.3 Factors influencing virus sensitivity to neutralization[a]

Genetic
- Linear epitope on viral envelope protein
- Conformational epitope on viral envelope protein

Nongenetic
- Glycosylation differences
- Virus envelope stability (e.g., gp120 shedding)
- Cellular proteins on the virion surface (e.g., LFA-1, ICAM, HLA, blood group antigens)
- Age of virus preparation
- Immune dominance

[a]See Sections II.D, II.E, and II.G.

Immunization of animal species (e.g., rodents, guinea pigs, rabbits, goats, monkeys, and baboons) with HIV envelope proteins has induced antibodies that neutralize the immunizing virus and are type specific. With several booster inoculations, the antibodies produced can cross-react with other diverse HIV-1 strains, reflecting a broadening of the humoral immune response (1694, 2012). Such serum cross-neutralization has been observed with HIV-1 isolates from different clades (173, 3297). What governs neutralization cross-reactivity is not clear, but this cross-reactivity could reflect antibodies to conformational epitopes on the viral envelope, especially those related to the CD4 binding site (see Sections II.E and II.F) (4243, 4276). Finally, some data indicate that sera from subjects soon after seroconversion can neutralize virus infection of macrophages but not CD4+ lymphocytes (3843). The reason for this observation has not been addressed but did not involve β-chemokines.

E. Neutralization Epitopes on HIV

1. OVERVIEW

By comparing the genetic sequences of the envelope gp120 from HIV-1 virus isolates, conserved (C) and divergent or variable (V) regions have been identified (2497, 4263, 4766, 4769). Five C and V domains have been recognized (Color Plate 1, following page 78). Furthermore, by using MAb, the structure of gp120 can be defined in terms of naturally exposed or covered epitopes (3092; for reviews, see references 563 and 3194). The latter appear to be primarily conserved determinants (3092) (Color Plate 17, following page 366). (For an up-to-date summary of envelope regions involved in neutralization and ADCC, see http://hiv-web.lanl.gov/content/immunology/ tables/ab_summary.html). Recognition of these regions has helped to identify domains in the envelope gp120 that are sensitive to neutralizing antibodies. In general, these epitopes are associated with gp120 oligomers and not monomeric forms of the viral envelope (562, 563, 3932; for a review, see reference 4243) (Color Plate 17, following page 366).

The regions of gp120 targeted by antibodies have been defined by X-ray crystallography (4829). The structure of a deglycosylated HIV-1 gp120 complexed with CD4 and a neutralizing antibody has also been defined (2368). The data provide insight into the conformation steps involved in HIV attachment and entry that can be blocked by antiviral antibodies (Color Plate 17, following page 366). Other observations suggest that additional linear or conformational envelope epitopes sensitive to neutralization will be detected. Moreover, the pattern of glycosylation could influence the results of HIV neutralization (304, 1268, 1462) (Table 10.3). Some antibodies interact with a carbohydrate-dependent epitope on the surface of gp120 (e.g., MAb 2G12) (582, 3910), particularly V1/V2 domains (3517). Moreover, carbohydrate properties on gp120 can block access to reactivity with neutralizing antibodies (200, 2775).

2. VIRAL REGIONS MEDIATING SENSITIVITY TO NEUTRALIZATION

Most studies of neutralization sites on HIV indicate that at least five regions of the viral envelope could be involved in HIV neutralization: four portions of gp120 and an immunodominant region of gp41 (Table 10.1) (688, 3183, 4483) (Color Plate 1, following page 78) (see http:// hiv-web.lanl.gov/content/immunology/tables/ab_ summary.html). Also called the membrane-proximal external region (MPER), this envelope domain of gp41 participates in viral entry and is highly conserved (for a review, see reference 4988). Antibodies to this region are difficult to detect in sera (1768) (see above), but certain broadly reacting MAb have been derived (e.g., 2F5 and 4E10) (521, 1768, 4481). Studies have suggested

that these MAb also react against regions of the virus that resemble normal human proteins (1768). Thus, in a conventional infection the epitopes may be recognized as self and not induce an antibody response (see Chapter 15).

The gp120 regions include the V3 loop and the CD4 binding domain (1630, 1752, 2012, 2013, 2415, 3518, 4276, 4339). In this regard, a region in the conserved C4 domain of gp120 (3203) may be involved since it contains a major CD4 binding site (2417, 3203) (see also http://hiv-web.lanl.gov/ content/immunology/tables/ab_summary.html and Chapter 3). Other variable regions of gp120 such as V1 and V2 may also be targeted by antienvelope antibodies. Further potential neutralizing epitopes on gp120 may be revealed best after HIV binds to CD4 (2088, 2756, 3931, 4256, 4413; for a review, see reference 4243) (see Section II.F.2).

3. V3 LOOP

An important immunodominant neutralizing domain of gp120, also called the principal neutralizing domain (PND), is found in the central portion or crown of the third variable region (V3 loop), located approximately in the mid-portion of gp120 (521, 522, 2012, 2013, 2415, 2877). The V3 loop is involved in a post-CD4 binding step (i.e., with a coreceptor) needed for HIV entry into cells (see Chapter 3). Although V3 is a variable region, the PNDs of many strains differ only slightly in amino acid structure (Figure 7.1). The cysteine-bound V3 region has a central portion with certain amino acid sequences (e.g., GPGRAF) that are shared by many HIV-1 isolates (e.g., HIV-1$_{SF2}$), particularly those found in the United States and Europe (2012, 2415). Thus, immunization with this region of gp120 can, with time, induce antibodies that neutralize a large number of HIV-1 strains that share this envelope domain (336, 1570, 2012). As a corollary, related isolates with different sequences in the PND are resistant to neutralization by the same MAb (943). The recent crystal structure of HIV-1 gp120 complexed to the CD4 receptor shows the V3 coreceptor binding tip protruding from the envelope core. This observation suggests an antibody accessibility that could explain the immunodominance of the V3 loop (1922).

The V3 loop can have both neutralizing and nonneutralizing epitopes, since sera with high-titer antibodies to V3 peptides do not always neutralize the homologous HIV-1 strain (4686). Moreover, work with neutralizing "escape" mutants has indicated that regions within the V3 loop (4807) or outside it (2932, 3701, 4689, 4766) (Figure 3.1) can reduce antibody neutralization (4275). Some of these mutants have the same V3 loop sequence but bear changes distal to this envelope region (2222, 4766). The other sites can apparently alter the conformation of the V3 loop, permitting escape of the virion from neutralization. Thus, the V3 region can present both linear and conformational determinants for antibody recognition (for a review, see reference 1752).

The neutralization could result from inhibition by the antibodies of the V3 envelope cleavage (4728) that may be required for virus attachment to cells (see Chapter 3). The V3 loop-directed neutralization does not appear to involve the CD4 binding domain (4165), but importantly, changes in this domain and other envelope regions might alter the antibody interaction with the V3 loop and vice versa (3519). In some cases, neutralization is enhanced; in others, it is reduced (3519). In this regard, a synergy in neutralization has been demonstrated by using antibodies against the CD4 binding region and the V3 domain (4429).

4. CD4 BINDING SITE

A second major neutralizing region on gp120 is the CD4 binding domain, a large complex conformational region of the envelope (2930) (see Chapter 3). Polyclonal antibodies that cross-neutralize a large number of strains (both primary and laboratory adapted), including those with different V3 regions, are directed against this domain (2089, 2417, 3518, 4276, 4339). The determinant is generally conformation dependent, and antibodies are frequently found in sera of infected individuals (3086, 4276).

Neutralizing MAb that recognize discontinuous epitopes on gp120 that are involved with CD4 receptor interaction have been derived from HIV-infected individuals (4412). The antibodies are thought to block the ability of the HIV strains to attach to CD4. Because several regions of the HIV envelope are involved, neutralization by one MAb may not show a broad antiviral activity (1568) and several may be needed (943). Moreover, early

studies indicated that point mutations in gp41 as well as in the V3 loop can affect this neutralization (via the CD4 binding domain), most likely as a result of conformational changes in gp120 (199, 2222, 2930).

5. V1 AND V2 REGIONS

The third and fourth major neutralizing sites on gp120 can be found in the V1 and V2 regions (1395, 1696, 2934, 4121). As with the V3 loop, both linear and conformational determinants appear to be involved (2934, 4121). These regions are recognized by antibodies directed at both glycosylated (3517) and nonglycosylated (1852) epitopes. It is noteworthy that in studies with mutants of an R5 virus (HIV-1$_{SF162}$), a V2 loop deletion enhanced the virus' susceptibility to neutralization and increased its sensitivity to antiviral activity of sera from subjects infected by other HIV-1 clades (4253). Removal of the V2 loop appeared to uncover epitopes on the envelope conserved among a variety of HIV-1 clades that were sensitive to neutralizing antibodies (see Chapter 15). In contrast, deletion of the V1 loop has made some viruses resistant to neutralization (3935), particularly by antibodies blocking the CD4 binding site. Whether the V4 and V5 regions also contain domains that induce neutralizing antibodies, as was suggested by early work with other deletion mutants (1696), remains to be determined.

6. gp41

Neutralizing antibodies directed against gp41 are receiving more attention because of common sites on the external portion of this protein involved in virus:cell fusion (Figure 3.4) (Color Plates 3 and 5, following pages 78). In early studies, immunization of laboratory animals with the amino-terminal portion of this protein envelope (a common fusion domain, the membrane proximal region [MPER]) elicited antibodies to the homologous and to heterologous isolates (688, 958). MAb to gp41 have also shown anti-HIV activity; they interact with the ectodomain (amino-terminal region) of this viral protein (3183) and can have broad reactivity (3625). The immunodominant portion of gp41 has been recognized particularly after HIV interaction with CD4; the removal or displacement of gp120 is assumed to have occurred (3931, 3933) (see Chapter 3). As described above, the MPER of gp41 is recognized by broadly neutralizing mAb (e.g., 2F5 and 4E10) and has been recommended as a target for anti-HIV vaccines (for a review, see reference 4988) (see Chapter 15). However, as noted above, their recognition as autoantibodies reacting with normal cellular proteins (e.g., cardiolipin) poses the problem of autoantigen mimicry in vaccine development (1768). Anti-idiotype neutralizing antibodies have been made as well by using portions of gp41 (4948).

7. CD4-INDUCED NEUTRALIZING ANTIBODIES

Antibodies that bind to HIV-1 gp120 after its interaction with CD4 are referred to as CD4-induced or CD4i antibodies. They can compete with coreceptor binding and may broadly neutralize different HIV-1 isolates (3743, 3900, 4834). Recent studies assaying for these HIV-1 antibodies with CD4 have shown efficient neutralization of HIV-2 in which the envelope glycoprotein differs by at least 40% from that of HIV-1 (1023, 2340). The findings support the earlier studies with human sera and sCD4 (787) (see above). The cross-reacting neutralization observed is encouraging since it indicates the high degree of antigenic conservation linked to coreceptor binding by these two viral subtypes (1023). The results can have relevance to vaccine development.

8. HIV-2

A region suggestive of a V3 loop in HIV-2 strains has been identified (387, 418, 1014). Studies with the HIV-2 envelope protein have also defined epitopes in the C1, V1/V2, and V3 envelope regions that react with neutralizing antibodies. As with HIV-1, some of them are conformation dependent; others react to linear regions of the envelope (2939). As noted above, in some studies, antibody-mediated neutralization of HIV-2 can be increased by the use of sCD4 (787, 1023).

F. Relative Sensitivity of HIV to Antibodies Mediating Neutralization

Initially, evidence for neutralizing antibodies against HIV was limited, most likely because of the viral assays employed. Subsequently, a number of laboratories using different approaches demonstrated that sera from HIV-infected individuals from many parts of the world could neutralize HIV-1 and HIV-2 isolates to various extents (see below) (722, 1856, 2877, 4715, 4716). Some viruses, such as HIV-1$_{SF2}$, are easily neutralized by many sera, particularly from the United States. Often high titers of serum neutralizing antibodies can be detected with this isolate (722, 1883, 4715). One explanation for these observations is that SF2 is a member of the North American sequence subtype, clade B (see Section VI and also Chapter 1) and shares envelope properties with many HIV-1 isolates. The HIV-1$_{MN}$ isolate is a similar antigenic type (2013, 2415). Another possibility is that the high sensitivity of these isolates to neutralization could reflect the increased release of their envelope gp120 from the virion and/or the reduced number of gp120-bearing knobs on the virion surface (2929). These properties could have resulted from culturing the virus for a long time in the laboratory.

As noted above, early studies of HIV-1 neutralization suggested at least four subgroups, depending on their sensitivity to three different sera (Table 10.2) (722). Viruses recovered from the brain, in contrast to those from the blood, were not very sensitive to neutralization, a characteristic of central nervous system (CNS)-derived isolates (see Chapters 8 and 13). Also noteworthy is the fact that an isolate from Africa (SF170) was resistant to neutralization by these sera as well as many other North American sera, but could be neutralized by African sera.

Several later studies employing sera from individuals infected with different HIV-1 isolates have indicated that cross-neutralization of a variety of HIV genomic subtypes (including clades A to F and O) can be achieved (2858, 3085, 4695), and even with some human MAb (3298, 4482). Nevertheless, clade-specific reactivity has been noted (746, 1149, 1947, 2857, 3085). In extensive neutralization studies using diverse HIV-1 isolates and sera from people infected with either group M (A to H) or group O type HIV-1 isolates, cross-neutralization was found among the M group of clades and some clade O isolates (3298, 3299). In contrast, antibodies from individuals infected with HIV-1 group O showed a reduced ability to neutralize primary isolates from the group M genotype (3298).

Importantly, these results and others obtained, using many different HIV-1 clades with human MAb to the V3, C5, and gp41 regions, have suggested a lower number of immunotypes than genotypes (3297). What controls the breadth of this immune response (e.g., host or antigenicity of the virus) remains to be determined, but it can reflect conformation-dependent neutralizing antibodies (1568, 4276). This potential sharing of conserved neutralizing epitopes among group M and group O viruses offers some encouragement for vaccine development.

Variations in sensitivity to neutralizing antibodies have been found as well with viruses recovered over time from the same individual. Generally, the sera from infected individuals do not neutralize the homologous virus (the isolate replicating in the person at the time of serum collection) as effectively as they neutralize previous autologous isolates or other heterologous HIV-1 isolates, especially those grown in the laboratory (1719, 1881, 4627). Importantly, differences can be seen when T-cell lines instead of PBMC are used (1719, 3087) (Section I.G). This finding on neutralization sensitivity, particularly noted in individuals after acute or primary infection or after development of disease, suggests that the virus mutates and escapes the immune antiviral responses in the host (51, 141, 2932, 3701, 3729, 4493, 4699) (see below). It further emphasizes the serologic diversity of isolates even within the same individual.

With HIV-2 isolates, specific neutralizing domains of the viral envelope have been suggested by some reports (387, 418, 1014). Essentially, neutralization studies have also demonstrated heterogeneity in antibody responses against HIV-2 isolates (638, 4716). Cross-neutralization of HIV-1 and HIV-2 isolates has been described with HIV-1 sera but not HIV-2 sera (4716). In general, however, the neutralizing capacity against HIV-2 isolates is low (3299), reflecting important serologic or antigenic differences between these two virus types.

G. Factors Influencing HIV Neutralization

A variety of genetic and nongenetic factors can affect the sensitivity of HIV to antibody-mediated neutralization (Section II.E) (Table 10.3). Genetic changes that affect linear and conformational changes in the envelope can be involved, as well as other factors described in this section.

1. CARBOHYDRATE MOIETIES

As noted above, some reports indicate broad neutralizing activity against carbohydrate regions of the viral envelope, including results with MAb 2G12 (304, 1268, 1714, 3910). Whether the response to these antibodies reflects conformational epitopes or true anticarbohydrate reactions is not clear. However, the broad antiviral activity of the human MAb 2G12 has been linked to its recognition of carbohydrates on gp120 (582) (Table 10.3). Glycosylated forms of the HIV-1 envelope can be better recognized by immune sera and antibodies than by nonglycosylated proteins (973, 1694, 3517, 3910, 4275, 4276). Nevertheless, carbohydrate side chains (e.g., N-glycans) may also interfere with the interaction of virus with neutralizing antibodies (61, 200, 2775, 4699). Since intracellular modification of HIV envelope glycosylation has been observed (730) (see Chapter 7), escape variants might emerge by this mechanism.

2. CELL SURFACE NONVIRAL PROTEINS

Some researchers have noted a variation in sensitivity to neutralizing antibodies with viruses grown in PBMC versus those grown in macrophages or T-cell lines (3940, 4770; for a review, see reference 3087). The possible mechanisms for these differences could be selection in the target cells of different subpopulations within a virus preparation, cellular posttranslational modifications of the virus such as glycosylation (973, 1268, 1462, 1714, 4770), envelope stability, genetic mutation during passaging in culture, or incorporation of different host cell proteins on the virion surface (Table 10.3).

In this regard, antibodies to a variety of molecules, such as the adhesion molecule LFA-1, detected on the surface of virions (see Chapter 3) can enhance the neutralization of HIV-1 by antiviral antibodies (1557). The activity depends on the anti-gp120 antibody used. Some antibodies to the intracellular adhesion molecules (ICAM) can increase or decrease a virus' sensitivity to anti-gp120 neutralizing antibodies (1335, 1557, 1840, 3742). Sensitivity is enhanced, particularly with antibodies directed at the V3 loop and the CD4 binding domain (1840, 3742).

Other nongenetic factors can reveal differences in serologic responses to HIV-1 isolates as noted above. Viruses cultivated in one cell line in a laboratory, for example, can yield progeny that become more or less sensitive to neutralization by specific sera (see below) (4770). In some instances, the serologic effect could be due to reactivity with cell surface proteins (e.g., human leukocyte antigen [HLA]) on the virions (156, 1904) (see Chapter 5), carbohydrate moieties (1714), or differences in viral envelope stability.

HLA molecules on the surface of the virus may serve as binding sites for anti-HLA antibodies that lyse or neutralize the virus, particularly in the presence of complement (4220). This mechanism appeared to protect macaques from SIV grown in human cells (4302). In this regard, polytransfused patients who had anti-HLA antibodies were found to have sera that neutralized HIV in vitro, particularly in the presence of complement (4241) (see Sections V and VI). These findings support suggestions that alloimmunization might be beneficial in preventing HIV infection (see Chapter 15, Section X). In addition, antibodies to the histo-blood group A antigen have been reported to neutralize HIV-1 produced by lymphocytes from blood group A donors (140). Similar results were obtained when complement was used with antibodies to blood group antigens (3229).

3. AGE OF VIRUS PREPARATION

The age of the virus preparation can also affect antibody sensitivity. With time in culture, the envelope region of the virion becomes less stable and detaches early; neutralization becomes more effective (2439, 2929). Thus, it has been recommended that viruses for serologic study preferably come from the individual being evaluated, and that they be taken from culture fluids 2 days old or less. Moreover, as noted above, for the most clinically relevant results, the immunologic assays should be performed in PBMC and not in established T-cell lines.

4. IMMUNE DOMINANCE

Some concern has been raised about whether antibodies made against one viral strain will suppress the ability of B cells to make antibodies to a different viral strain. This concept of "original sin"

was first described by Francis (1351) and has been recognized with a variety of viruses, including the toga-, paramyxo-, and enteroviruses, as well as influenza virus (3215). The humoral immune response to a variety of antigens may be limited in HIV-1 infection, as revealed by some evidence in animal models (2254, 3215). The mechanism appears to be a paralysis by B-cell clonal dominance resulting from the reaction of B cells to the initial infecting virion (2255). The hypothesis deserves further study, particularly in relation to HIV vaccine development (see Chapter 15).

H. Neutralization-Resistant Virus Isolates

The emergence of viruses that have escaped neutralization by serum antibodies was demonstrated in early studies using cell culture. HIV-1 isolates grown in the presence of neutralizing MAb were found to become resistant to neutralization (2932, 3701, 3751). Most likely selection for resistant viruses took place. In these studies, an alteration within (2222, 2239, 2932) or outside the epitope identified by the MAb was associated with this resistance (4411, 4771, 4781). Such a modification, for example, was found in gp41 (2222, 3701, 4411, 4769, 4771). A change from alanine to threonine at position 582 in gp41 conferred resistance to neutralization by antibodies on the CD4 binding site of gp120 (4411).

A single amino acid substitution in the conserved region of gp120 was noted to confer virus resistance against a broadly reactive antiserum (4689). This change apparently affected several regions of the envelope that were involved in antibody neutralization. A single amino acid change within the V2 domain was found to be responsible for escape from neutralization by an anti-V2 region MAb (1569, 4886). Changes in the V3 region can also affect the neutralization sensitivity (2239; for a review, see reference 3085). On another note, mutations in gp41 conferred a neutralization-sensitive phenotype to HIV-1, by affecting the interactions of antibodies with gp120 (199).

These observations on resistance to antibody-mediated neutralization emphasize the influence of other envelope domains on the overall conformation of the viral envelope that can determine effective antibody binding. This conclusion has been reached as well by studies of fractionated antibody preparations (4276) and MAb (1166, 2239, 3081, 3082). Thus, viral escape from anti-HIV responses most likely occurs by multiple mechanisms, including changes in the linear and conformational epitopes in the envelope and gp120 shedding (Table 10.3). For example, studies of virus sensitivity to sCD4 inactivation have suggested that the resistance of primary isolates could reflect the density and stability of the envelope gp120 (see Chapters 4 and 8). Moreover, recently it has been appreciated that nonfunctional forms of the envelope appearing on virions can bind to antiviral antibodies and help HIV evade neutralization (3097). Development of successful envelope-based vaccines, therefore, will most likely require the identification of conserved regions in the viral envelope that are critical for function so that any alteration within them would render the virus inactive (4689).

I. Clinical Relevance

The clinical relevance of neutralizing antibodies remains unclear. They appear to be important in preventing mother-to-child transmission (2240, 4826). In many infected subjects, neutralizing antibodies against earlier virus isolates and not against the isolate present at the time of plasma collection have been found (1881, 3076, 3729, 4466, 4627, 4699). The results suggest selective pressure or delayed recognition of HIV-1 by the immune system (1378, 3729, 4699, 4821). These findings were demonstrated recently using a recombinant-virus single-cycle assay to measure neutralizing antibodies to HIV-1 during acute infection. In these studies, neutralizing antibodies against the autologous virus could be detected within 4 to 8 weeks of primary infection (4699). Low-level activity against heterologous isolates was observed. In some cases, the initial virus was resistant to serum neutralization, whereas later viruses were sensitive (3729, 4699). Selective immunologic pressure appeared to be involved. Essentially, the neutralizing antibodies seemed to influence the emergence of the dominant viruses in the host. Such selection of virus immunotype has been made as well with neutralizing antibodies to equine infectious anemia virus (EIAV) (3074, 3892).

Neutralizing antibodies against autologous and heterologous viruses have been found in chronically infected individuals with low viremia. In acutely infected individuals, antibodies against autologous viruses were absent in the face of high viremia; antibodies against heterologous viruses could be detected. The observations suggested that HIV replication induces the early production of antibodies that can cross-neutralize a variety of HIV isolates but not the autologous virus. Nevertheless, these antibodies may protect against superinfection (1030). In chronic infection, both types of antibodies are maintained. The results suggest that HIV has a limited capacity to generate new epitope-specific regions in the face of the host immune response.

In early studies, levels of neutralizing activity against laboratory HIV-1 strains appeared to correlate with the clinical state (3749, 4034, 4627), but some patients, including those with AIDS, were found to have substantial titers of these neutralizing antibodies (3749). In most cases, however, their antiviral response to the autologous virus, which would be clinically relevant, was not evaluated. In a few studies with autologous isolates, a loss of neutralizing antibodies was found with progression to disease (1881, 4466). In a recent study, viruses present in plasma samples from two infected patients were analyzed for susceptibility to antibody-mediated neutralization. A variety of viruses coexisted in one sample that was heterogeneous in terms of sensitivity to neutralization. The strength of the antiviral activity for both autologous and heterologous viruses increased with duration of the infection (4170).

Some observations (1881) suggest that AIDS patients often elicit antibodies that enhance rather than neutralize infection by the virus found in the patient (Section III). Moreover, as discussed above (Section II.H), the virus undergoes changes during immunologic responses that provide resistance to neutralization (141, 1881, 2932, 3066, 3217, 3749). This escape from neutralization generally has been linked to amino acid changes in the V3 loop (2239) but can also be related to changes within other envelope regions (e.g., C2) (940). The resistance may be related to conformational masking of the envelope receptor binding site on the virion (2367).

In certain studies, anti-SIV antibodies delayed progression of disease (1695). In other SIV studies, however, passive immunization had no effect and may have enhanced the infection (see below) (1447). Neutralizing MAb have also protected

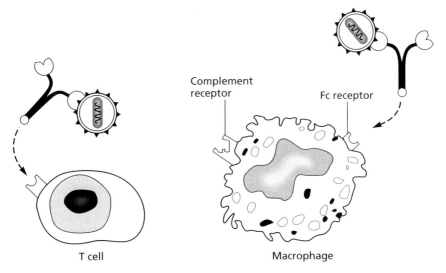

Figure 10.1 Mechanism of antibody-dependent enhancement of HIV infection. The antiviral antibody binds to the viral envelope glycoprotein. This virus-antibody complex can then enter cells (T cells and macrophages shown here) through an interaction of the Fc portion of the antibody with either the cellular Fc receptor or the complement receptor (after complexing with complement). Reprinted from reference 2519 with permission.

neonatal macaques from oral infection by SHIV (1282) (see Chapter 14).

An effective antiviral antibody response would have the best value when elicited by a vaccine, but the potential effect of neutralizing antibodies in controlling viral spread after early infection is not known. Moreover, the sensitivity of the various clades (see Chapter 1) to cross-neutralization has relevance to future vaccine development. Fortunately, the HIV-1 genotype does not necessarily correspond to the neutralization phenotype (3085, 3297) (see above). This cross-reactivity can reflect a linear epitope as well as a nonlinear conformational structure common to many viral strains (Table 10.3). The latter can be recognized by a wide variety of conformation-dependent neutralizing antibodies.

III. Enhancing Antibodies

A. Complement- and Fc-Mediated Responses

Enhancing antibodies were recognized during evaluation of sera for neutralizing activity against HIV (see Chapter 3). Two types of antibody-dependent enhancement (ADE) were detected: complement mediated and Fc mediated. Both involve binding of antiviral antibodies to the virion and infection of cells by this immune complex via the complement or Fc receptor (Figure 10.1). In one, complement in the presence of HIV-1 seropositive sera enhanced the infection of the MT-2 T-cell line by certain HIV-1 isolates (3766, 3767) (Figure 10.1). The other was recognized when sera from guinea pigs immunized with various HIV-1 isolates enhanced HIV infection in PBMC in the absence of complement (1882, 1883). Virus replication in CD4$^+$ lymphocytes as well as macrophages doubled or tripled after exposure of the HIV inoculum to the sera or to purified immunoglobulins from the immunized animals, as well as from chimpanzees infected with HIV. Notably, sera from HIV-infected individuals also showed similar results (1883, 4366). Depending on the viral isolate used and the serum selected, virus infection was neutralized or enhanced (1883).

Most important was the observation that a viral isolate within the same individual can change over time from showing sensitivity to serum neutralization to showing sensitivity to enhancement

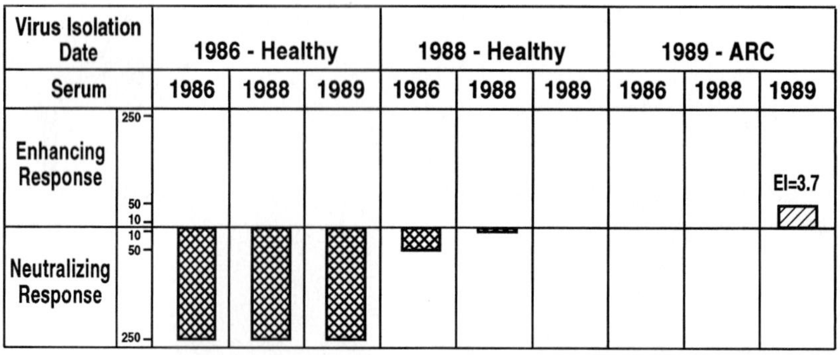

Virus Isolation Date	1986 - Healthy			1988 - Healthy			1989 - ARC		
Serum	1986	1988	1989	1986	1988	1989	1986	1988	1989
Enhancing Response									EI=3.7
Neutralizing Response									

Figure 10.2 Neutralization or enhancement of infection by sequential homotypic HIV-1 isolates. HIV-1 strains recovered from the same individual were tested for enhancement or neutralization by the corresponding sera obtained early or late in the infection. The sera were evaluated at fivefold dilutions (1:10 to 1:1,250). Normal control serum was used at similar dilutions. The clinical status of the individual at the different time points is indicated (ARC, AIDS-related complex). The extent of neutralization is shown below the bar; the enhancement index (EI) is shown above the bar. The response is defined as the ratio of the viral reverse transcriptase activity in supernatants of cultures receiving virus preincubated with homotypic serum to that in supernatants of cultures receiving virus preincubated with control serum. Modified from reference 1881.

(1881) (Figure 10.2). Generally, this modification in HIV is associated with progression to disease (see Chapter 13). Other studies suggest that very few amino acid substitutions in the V3 loop can bring about this alteration in the serologic sensitivity of the virus (2239) (see below). The variations in response to antibodies could result from distribution of the viral gp120 on the virion surface and its stability. The relative binding affinity of the gp120 to the antibodies can also be involved (2239) (see below). Enhancement of infection by some HIV-2 isolates has also been noted with certain sera (B. Castro and J. Levy, unpublished) or sCD4 (787). Thus, this immunologic phenomenon, which also reflects viral heterogeneity, could have relevance for pathogenesis by either HIV type.

Enhancing antibodies are often evident after dilution of serum past the level showing virus neutralization. This observation may reflect a greater population of antibody species with less binding affinity for the viral target (2239). That possibility, if proved, would suggest that as antibody levels decrease in an infected individual over time, the enhancing antibody might be preferentially conserved. The results with various sera also suggest that at any given dilution, the overall effect on the virus in cell culture would reflect the net effect of neutralizing and enhancing antibodies. With some sera, however, only a neutralizing antibody or an enhancing antibody for a specific virus strain has been noted (173, 1882, 1883, 2239).

IgA-mediated enhancement of virus infection has also been demonstrated with sera from HIV-infected patients (2002, 2321). Some studies suggest that these patients produce more IgA than IgG antibodies with enhancing activity (2321). This response may be important at the mucosal level of infection.

B. Mechanisms of Antibody-Mediated Enhancement of HIV Infection

In complement-mediated ADE, complement receptor 1 (CR-1), CR-2, and CR-3 appear to be involved (3767, 4417). In Fc-mediated ADE, two receptors for the antibody have been identified: FcRI in the U937 monocyte cell line (4365) and the FcRIII receptor in primary macrophages (1882). The latter receptor, identified by antibodies to CD16, is found on natural killer (NK) cells and a variety of other human cells (including T cells) that conceivably could also be infected by antibody: HIV complexes.

The role of CD4 in ADE is controversial. Some studies (3476, 3767, 4924) have suggested that

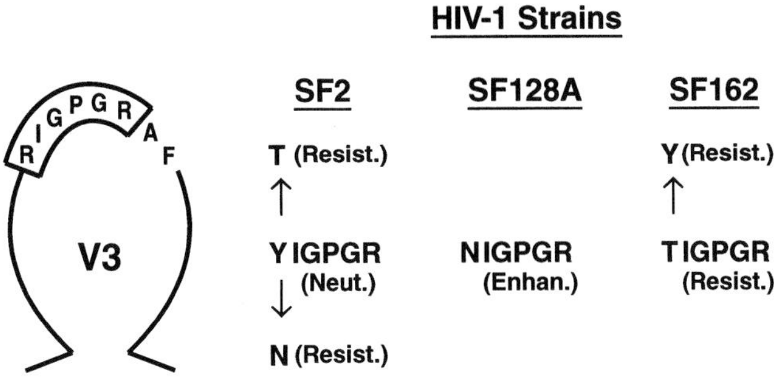

HIV-1 Strains

Figure 10.3   The V3 loop in virus-antibody neutralization versus enhancement. Using a monoclonal antibody to a small epitope in the HIV-1 V3 loop, differences in response of various virus strains can be appreciated. Some are neutralized (Neut.), others are enhanced (Enhan.), and still others are resistant (Resist.). As demonstrated, only one amino acid change appears to affect the serologic response, but the results are strain specific. If the amino acid is modified by site-directed mutagenesis (arrows), the mutant virus appears to become resistant. Data from reference 2239.

enhancement via the complement receptor depends on CD4, since MAb to CD4 can block viral enhancement. Others (4365) drew the same conclusion with Fc-mediated enhancement. In contrast, in studies with peripheral blood macrophages, ADE via the Fc receptor took place in the presence of blocking antibodies to CD4 (Leu 3a) as well as after pretreatment of the virus with large quantities of sCD4 (1882). Likewise, studies of ADE in cultured human syncytiotrophoblasts showed that complement-mediated enhancement of infection required CD4 but the Fc-dependent process did not (4454). Thus, different mechanisms on the same cells can be involved in these two ADE processes observed with HIV infection in vitro. In further support of a non-CD4 mechanism is the experiment with HIV:antibody complexes demonstrating that HIV can replicate in CMV-infected fibroblasts lacking CD4 but expressing the Fc receptor (2933).

Most investigators conclude that if CD4 is involved in ADE, the enhancement occurs because the virus:antibody complexes are brought closer to the CD4 molecule after attachment to Fc or complement receptors. Alternatively, if CD4 is not involved, HIV could be brought to the cell surface via Fc receptor binding. Then the virus interacts with a coreceptor or fuses directly with the cell membrane (see Chapter 3). These observations on ADE differ from those showing an enhancement of virus entry with sCD4 (see Chapter 3).

C. Virus Epitope Determinants of Antibody-Dependent Enhancement

In contrast to the identification of several viral domains involved in neutralization (Section II), only limited regions on the virion thus far have been linked to ADE. Antisera made in animals to peptides have suggested that the process can be mediated by certain regions on envelope gp120 and gp41 (2029, 4474). However, the relevance of these induced antibodies to naturally produced antibodies requires further evaluation. In the complement-mediated ADE process, two domains (amino acids ~579 to 613 and ~644 to 663 for the isolate studied) at the amino-terminal end of gp41 appeared to be the reactive sites (3763, 3764).

For studies of Fc-mediated ADE, polyclonal antibodies against regions in gp120 and MAb directed against the V3 region of some HIV-1 strains have been helpful (4976). Polyclonal anti-gp120 and anti-V3 loop antibodies have shown both neutralizing and enhancing effects, depending on the HIV-1 strain and on the concentration of the antibodies used (943, 2030, 2239). Moreover, a human MAb that also reacts with the amino-terminal region of gp41 has been found to enhance HIV-1 infection in the absence of complement (1165).

A noteworthy observation was the presence in some human and animal sera of antibodies that neutralize one HIV-1 strain and enhance another

(1883, 2239). MAb that can distinguish between those serotype properties have been described (2239, 4364). Two human MAb and one murine MAb that react with the V3 domain of HIV-1$_{MN}$ were found to neutralize the SF2 and MN strains of HIV-1 but to enhance the SF128A strain (2239) (Figure 10.3). They had no effect on the SF162 strain, which was resistant. These MAb were shown to bind to gp120 cloned from all of these viral strains, but the affinity of the binding was reduced with the viral strains that were resistant or enhanced in infectivity (2239). Among the three affected strains (SF2, SF162, and SF128A), only one amino acid differed in the epitope on the V3 loop recognized by the MAb (Figure 10.3). Subsequently, one amino acid change made in the V3 loop of the viral envelope was found to reduce the virus sensitivity to enhancement or neutralization (2239); three changes in the carboxyl-terminal portion of the V3 loop of SF162 to those of SF2 elicited antibody sensitivity (Figure 10.4). The results indicated how very few modifications in the viral envelope can affect the reaction of HIV to antiviral antibodies (2239).

An important consideration coming from the studies undertaken is that high-affinity binding of the antibody leads to virus neutralization (2239), perhaps through removal or displacement of gp120 (3091) (see above). In contrast, low-affinity binding might bring HIV to the cell surface (e.g., via the Fc receptor) and subsequent detachment of the virus from the antibody would permit infection of the cell and thus enhancement (Figure 10.5).

Figure 10.4   The V$_3$ loop of HIV-1$_{SF162}$ with the amino acid substitutions (present on HIV-1$_{SF2}$) that make this strain neutralizable by an anti-HIV-1$_{SF2}$ monoclonal antibody (see Figure 10.3).

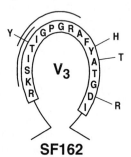

SF162

In some ways, this hypothesis involving gp120 binding mirrors the one proposed for inactivation versus enhancement of HIV infection with sCD4 (787, 3091, 3097) (see Chapter 3). However, in the latter process, the affinity of the gp120:CD4 attachment seems most important.

D. Clinical Relevance

The clinical importance of ADE is not known, but its association with HIV disease (see Chapter 13 and Figure 10.2) (1397, 1881) suggests a role in pathogenesis. Complement-mediated ADE has correlated with high plasma viral loads (4353) and has been found in patients with low CD4$^+$ cell counts (4324). Circulating infectious virus:antibody complexes have been described in HIV infection (2249, 3115). It is surprising that these virus:antibody complexes are infectious rather than being destroyed in the macrophage lysosomes. The reason could be the relative affinity of antibodies for the HIV envelope protein and how the complexes are dissociated within the cell.

The potential clinical relevance of ADE in vivo has been evaluated in animal model systems. In EIAV infection, ADE was recognized in vaccine studies. Horses immunized with a baculovirus-expressed recombinant envelope glycoprotein of one strain were protected from infection by that strain, but disease developed more rapidly when a heterologous strain was used as the challenge strain (4675) (see Chapter 15). Enhancement of virus infection was also found in cats immunized with certain envelope glycoprotein subunits of the feline immunodeficiency virus (3726, 4131). The presence or absence of enhancing antibodies also correlated with clinical disease in primates infected with SIV (3072) and in one study reduced the beneficial effects of an SIV gp160 vaccine (3031). High-titer enhancing antibodies also correlated with failure of passive immunization to protect from SIV infection (1447). Complement-mediated ADE was noted in acute primary infection of macaques and was detected before the appearance of neutralizing antibodies (3071). As the extent of ADE activity decreased, neutralizing antibodies appeared, reflecting the comment, noted above, that a balance between these two responses determines the overall immunologic effect.

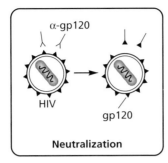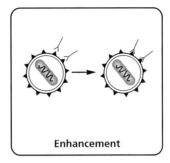

Figure 10.5 Mechanisms for neutralization versus enhancement. The concept is proposed that neutralization involves a strong binding of antibody to the viral envelope with the subsequent removal of gp120, resulting in virus inactivation. Enhancement would involve binding to the virus without removal of the envelope glycoprotein. Conformational changes would subsequently occur that enhance infection by the virus, presumably via virus:cell fusion.

Results have been presented showing no clinical significance of ADE (4058) or no correlation with disease progression (3069). Nevertheless, an increase in symptoms of disease linked to ADE has been observed with dengue virus, coronaviruses, and other viruses (273, 1703, 3252, 3454, 3461, 3600). The process has been reported with retroviruses (2473), including, most convincingly, the caprine (2926), feline (3726, 4131), and equine (EIAV) lentiviruses (4675). Thus, the risk of this type of immune response should be considered in treatment approaches and vaccine development (3067). In this regard, ADE did not appear to be induced in the latest VaxGen phase III trials (1514) (see Chapter 15).

E. Significance of Anti-HIV-Neutralizing versus -Enhancing Antibodies

Certain important conclusions can be drawn from these early findings on antibody responses to HIV infection:

- Neutralizable HIV strains can mutate to be resistant to or enhanced by the same antibody species.
- Immunization of individuals with a particular viral strain might induce neutralizing antibodies to the immunizing virus but enhancing antibodies to a different viral strain.
- Defining envelope regions that will induce only neutralizing antibody responses and

not enhancing antibody responses could be very difficult. A highly conserved envelope domain, without which HIV infection could not take place, must be identified.
- Changes in linear as well as conformational domains (e.g., glyscosylation) of the virus can determine its sensitivity to anti-HIV antibodies.

Thus far, regions in gp120, as well as gp41, have been associated with both neutralizing and enhancing humoral immune anti-HIV reactions. It is particularly noteworthy that some studies suggest that only a small change at a critical region, perhaps in one amino acid, might determine the sensitivity of a virus to neutralization or enhancement by an antibody. Nevertheless, the overall conformation of the viral envelope appears to be the most important determinant, and in the immune sera a variety of antibody species are present, one or several of which can conceivably recognize a mutated virus.

IV. Antibody-Dependent Cellular Cytotoxicity (ADCC) and Antibody-Dependent Cytotoxicity (ADC)

Antibodies (primarily IgG1 isotypes) to both the gp120 and gp41 envelope proteins induce ADCC (1233, 2645, 2646, 3277, 3791). In this process, the antibody-antigen-coated cells are recognized by effector NK cells or by monocytes/macrophages

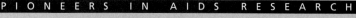
P I O N E E R S   I N   A I D S   R E S E A R C H

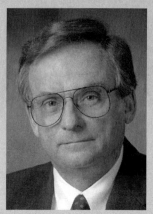

Arthur J. Ammann
*President of Global Strategies for HIV Prevention, and
formerly Professor, Department of Pediatrics,
University of California, San Francisco. Dr. Ammann
was one of the first to recognize AIDS in children.*

(2025) bearing Fc receptors (see Chapter 9). They are killed by a cytolytic mechanism, either perforin mediated or via apoptosis (for a review, see reference 4840). The relative binding of the antibodies to the viral antigenic determinant on the surface of cells infected by a variety of isolates can differ depending on the specific gp120 and gp41 proteins expressed (2645).

Certain epitopes on HIV envelope proteins must induce this response, since not all anti-Env antibodies produce this activity. The ADCC immunoglobulins can be distinguished from neutralizing antibodies (454, 4629), but not in all cases (4629). This observation most probably reflects the presence or absence of a neutralization epitope on the viral envelope expressed on the cell surface. Cross-reactivity of antibodies mediating ADCC with HIV-1 and HIV-2 strains has been demonstrated (3277). Nef-specific ADCC activity has also been observed in the presence of plasma and PBMC derived from long-term nonprogressors (4845), suggesting that ADCC is also directed against nonenvelope HIV proteins expressed on the surface of HIV-infected cells.

The ADCC process is active in destroying herpesvirus-infected cells early after virus transmission (4120). This process induced by a vaccine has also correlated with protection of rhesus macaques from SIV challenge (1558). Whether ADCC is clinically relevant in HIV infection is not known; conflicting data on its association with an asymptomatic state have been presented (1233,

2646, 3939; for a review, see reference 35). The activity can be detected in acute infection prior to development of neutralizing antibodies (3939). It is low in subjects with reduced CD4+ cell counts (1331, 4324). Some reports have shown a close association of ADCC with a healthy state and loss of this response with progression of disease (38, 281). This activity is found in long-term survivors (36). Since antienvelope antibodies are present at substantial titers throughout the course of the infection (1233) and before development of neutralizing antibodies, the extent of effector cell function (e.g., NK cell) would appear to be the most important parameter influencing the ability of the ADCC process to control HIV infection (1332, 4356, 4516). One detrimental effect of this process during HIV infection could be the release, by cell destruction, of large quantities of infectious particles, with subsequent spread in the host. At that time, neutralizing antibodies should play an important antiviral role.

In principle, ADCC would seem most valuable soon after infection to kill incoming or postentry virus-infected cells. Induction of the ADCC response by vaccines, which has shown promising results in primates (1558), would then be an important objective. This response might be helpful in preventing mother-to-child transmission. Thus, ADCC could be another reason to consider passive immunization with anti-HIV envelope antibodies for recently exposed individuals or infected mothers before delivery. This process might explain in part the protection from SIV (SHIV) infection observed with administration of antibodies to macaques post-exposure (see Chapter 14).

By another process, anti-HIV antibodies in chimpanzees directly killed infected cells via a complement-mediated mechanism (3216). Antibody and complement attach to virus-infected cells and can bring about cell death without effector cells. This ADC has not been generally observed in humans, although studies with certain cell lines lacking CD55 and CD59 expression have demonstrated this activity (3982). The general absence of this process in humans has been cited as one possible reason that infected chimpanzees have not developed HIV-induced disease (see Chapter 13).

V. Complement-Fixing Antiviral Antibodies

As reviewed above, complement can play a role in both innate and adaptive immune responses (see Chapter 9, Table 9.16). Some studies have indicated that certain neutralizing and nonneutraliz-ing antibodies can lyse HIV via complement fixation (4221). With neutralizing antibodies, the antiviral titer can sometimes be increased up to 10-fold by the addition of high levels of complement to the assay (4219, 4220, 4324). More recent studies have detected this IgG-mediated activity against autologous and heterologous HIV-1 isolates early in acute infection (2). This response could counter the ADE observed, since only low levels of complement initiate this immune response.

VI. Autoimmunity

A. Overview

Since HIV disturbs the balance of the immune system, it is not surprising that autoimmune disorders (e.g., Reiter's syndrome, psoriatic arthritis, systemic lupus erythematosus, Sjögren's syndrome, vasculitis, and polymyositis) can accompany this viral infection (580, 4539; for reviews, see references 3114, 3475, and 4966) (Table 10.4).

Table 10.4 Autoantibodies detected in HIV infection and associated clinical condition[a]

Antibodies to	Clinical condition
Lymphocytes	Loss of CD4+ and CD8+ cells and B lymphocytes
Platelets	Thrombocytopenia
Neutrophils	Neutropenia
Erythrocytes	Anemia
Nerves (myelin)	Peripheral neuropathy
Nuclear protein (antinuclear antibody)	Autoimmune symptoms
Sperm, seminal plasma	Aspermia
Lupus anticoagulant (phospholipids, cardiolipin)	Neurologic disease (?), thrombosis (?)
Myelin basic protein	Dementia, demyelination
Collagen	Arthritis (?)
CD4	CD4+ cell loss
HLA	Lymphocyte depletion
Hydrocortisone	Addison's-like disease
Thymic hormone	Immune disorder
Cellular components (Golgi complex, centriole, vimentin)	Immune disorder
Thyroglobulin	Thyroid disease

[a]See Section VI for references.

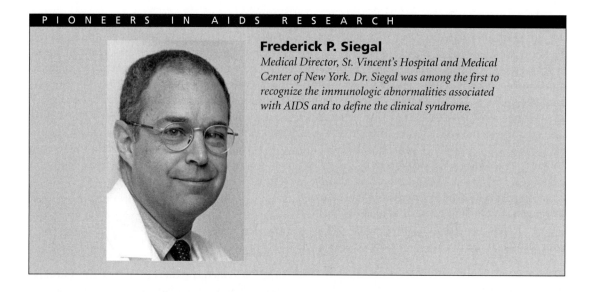

Frederick P. Siegal
Medical Director, St. Vincent's Hospital and Medical Center of New York. Dr. Siegal was among the first to recognize the immunologic abnormalities associated with AIDS and to define the clinical syndrome.

Vasculitis has been linked in HIV infection to immune complexes (580), but immune complex glomerulonephritis is not commonly found (see Chapter 8, Section V). Moreover, the ingress of CD8$^+$ T cells in the salivary glands giving rise to the diffuse infiltrative lymphocytosis syndrome could reflect an autoimmune reaction (see Chapter 11).

In early studies of AIDS patients, antibodies, often associated with clinical disorders, against platelets, T cells, and peripheral nerves were detected (see also Chapter 9) (for a review, see reference 3114). Later, autoantibodies to a large number of normal cellular proteins were found in HIV-infected individuals (Table 10.4) (22, 139, 413, 675, 1490, 1601, 2212, 2220, 2693, 2751, 3891), including erythropoietin (4161). Their role in disease has been considered (e.g., anemia) but has been documented in only a few cases. The reason for these autoimmune sequelae is not clear, but they could reflect T-cell dysregulation, B-cell activation, and the presence of cellular membrane proteins on HIV particles (156, 1751, 1904, 2956, 3995), molecular mimicry or anti-idiotype antibodies (Table 10.5). The potential influence of these cellular products on virus neutralization is discussed in Section II and on vaccine development is considered in Chapter 15. Some of these processes potentially involved in autoimmunity are discussed below.

B. B-Cell Proliferation

A lack of T-cell regulation during HIV infection can lead to a proliferation of B cells, with resultant polyclonal activation and antibody production (see Chapter 8). These kinds of reactions have been reported in other viral infections (e.g., Epstein-Barr Virus) in which hypergammaglobulinemia and autoimmune disorders are described (1814). Polyclonal B-cell activity has been observed in HIV-infected individuals (1982, 3383) and is associated with high levels of antibody production, particularly in children (98). These hyper-B-cell responses can result from the presence of viral proteins or from increased production of cytokines (interleukin-6 [IL-6] and IL-7) by HIV-infected or reactive macrophages or B cells (490, 3867). Tat can induce TNF-α and IL-6 production by T lymphocytes (555, 3674). B-cell growth can result from TNF-α production (175), particularly if this cytokine, like TNF-β, is expressed on the cell sur-

Table 10.5 Potential mechanisms for induction of autoimmunity by retroviruses

- T-cell dysregulation
- B-cell activation
- Cellular proteins on viruses
- Molecular mimicry
- Carrier hapten
- Anti-idiotype antibodies

Table 10.6 Regions of HIV that resemble normal cellular proteins[a]

Normal cellular protein	HIV region	Relation
Astrocytes	p17, gp41	Serology
Brain	Env (V3 loop)	Serology
Epithelial cells	p17	Serology
Fas	gp120	Sequence
HLA (MHC)	gp120	Sequence
	gp41	Serology
	nef, p17	Sequence
IL-2	gp41	Sequence
	LTR	Sequence
IL-2R	*nef*	Sequence
Immunoglobulin	gp120	Sequence
Interferon	LTR	Sequence
Neuroleukin (phosphohexose)	gp120	Sequence; serology
Neurotoxin	*nef, tat*, gp41	Sequence
Cardiolipin	gp41	Serology
Platelet glycoprotein	gp120	Serology
Platelets	p24	Serology
Protein kinase	*nef*	Sequence
Thymosin	p17	Serology
Vasoactive intestinal polypeptide	gp120 (peptide T)	Sequence; serology

[a]See Section VI.C for references and discussion.

face (2149). Finally, some of the altered B-cell functions could be secondary to enhanced production of type 2 cytokines (4091) (see Chapter 11). Among the immunoglobulins released by the activated B cells are autoantibodies.

C. Molecular Mimicry

When an organism shares nucleotide sequence, amino acid homology, or conformational form with a normal cellular component, molecular mimicry can result (3328). In this regard, similarities between HIV proteins and normal cellular proteins could elicit antiviral antibodies or cellular immune responses that cross-react with normal cellular proteins (386, 3328) (Table 10.6). Evidence in favor of this possibility includes the presence of IL-1, IL-2 receptor, major histocompatibility complex (MHC) classes I and II, and interferon-like sequences in the HIV genome as well as epitopes on certain portions of the viral envelope (960, 1457, 1548, 2518, 2663, 3225, 3690) (Figure 10.6). Molecular mimicry could explain the loss of platelets in HIV infection.

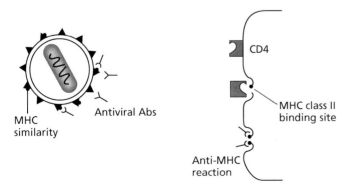

Figure 10.6 HIV molecular mimicry and autoimmunity. If the viral envelope protein has a similarity to an MHC domain (class I or II), antibodies to this portion of the viral envelope could induce an anti-MHC reaction at the cell surface even with uninfected cells.

Cross-reactive antibodies recognizing the HIV gp120 envelope protein and a platelet glycoprotein have been observed in individuals with thrombocytopenia purpura (353). A murine anti-Gag (p24) MAb has reacted with human platelets (1873). Sequence homology between gp120 of HIV-1 and Fas, a protein involved in apoptosis (4355), may also have clinical relevance if anti-Fas antibodies are found in infected individuals. Similarities of some regions of the viral Gag, Tat, and Nef proteins to normal proteins have been described as well (1456, 1458, 3430, 3904, 3988) (Table 10.6).

Most notable are the studies showing that some antibodies to the carboxyl-terminal domain in HIV gp41 cross-react with regions found on the HLA class II molecule, particularly the beta chain (398, 1548). Antibodies to HLA class II proteins are found in HIV-infected individuals. They bind to native class II HLA antigens and interfere with normal activation of CD4$^+$ T cells; they also have the potential to induce lysis of MHC class II-expressing cells by ADCC (Figure 10.6) (398). The presence of these anti-HLA antibodies in asymptomatic individuals correlates with a subsequent loss of CD4$^+$ cells (398). Some studies have suggested that in advanced stages of HIV infection, immunoglobulins reacting with CD8$^+$ T cells can cause their destruction (4830). In addition to molecular mimicry with gp120 cited above, thrombocytopenia in HIV infection could be caused by antibodies to a portion of gp41 that resembles a platelet glycoprotein (1105).

Figure 10.7 Possible mechanisms for autoimmune responses in HIV infection. HIV infection of T cells could lead to T-cell disorders (step 1), with subsequent loss of T-cell control of B-cell proliferation. Similarly, infection of macrophages by HIV could lead to enhanced production of IL-6, with resultant B-cell proliferation (step 2). B-cell proliferation could eventually lead to lymphomas through chromosome changes and establishment of a transformed state (see Chapter 12). The presence of cellular antigens on the surface of HIV virions or expressed together with viral antigens on the cell surface (step 3) might induce immune responses (e.g., antibodies) against normal cellular antigens (step 3) in a carrier-hapten fashion (2612) (step 4), leading to autoimmune cellular reactions. Antiviral responses by B cells could also lead to autoantibodies through molecular mimicry (step 5) (Table 10.6). By this phenomenon, viral proteins may resemble normal cellular proteins sufficiently to cause an autoimmune response against these cellular components.

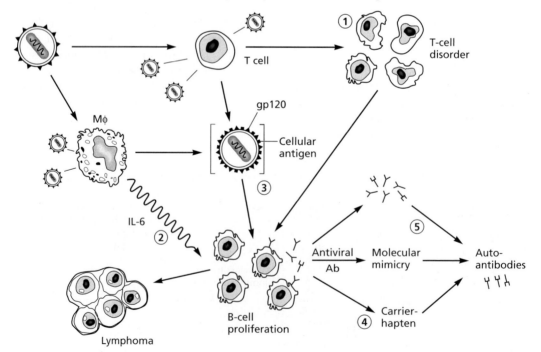

In terms of neurologic disease, antibodies to the amino-terminal region of gp41 have been found to react with normal rodent brain astrocytes (4844). Moreover, antibodies to the immunodominant region of HIV-1 gp41 have been demonstrated to bind to a 100-kDa protein on the surface of human astrocytes (4225), and the reaction of the broadly neutralizing anti-gp41 MAb with cardiolipin could be associated with neurologic discord (1768). In addition, a MAb to an epitope in the V3 region cross-reacts with a human brain protein (4488). All these observations do suggest that molecular mimicry could represent a possible source of some pathogenic autoimmune responses.

Finally, HIV replicating in normal cells could induce antibody responses against normal cellular epitopes via a carrier hapten mechanism (2612). By this process, normal cellular proteins are recognized in the context of the expression of viral proteins on the surface of infected cells. Autoantibodies are induced directly against the cellular proteins, either alone or because of their association with virion proteins.

D. Anti-Idiotype Antibodies

One concept that had received some support as a mechanism for autoimmunity involves the network of antibodies produced after introduction of an antigen into the host. Besides making antibodies to the incoming antigen, antibodies to the antiantigen antibodies may be induced. These anti-idiotype antibodies should be mirror images of the epitope against which the initial antibody was produced (1132). Thus, antibodies to the HIV envelope gp120 might induce autoantibodies against the CD4 epitope to which the gp120 attaches. While the possibility for these antibodies to form and be detrimental to the host has been proposed, evidence for such a phenomenon has not been shown. The anti-CD4 antibodies produced (675) are not against the epitopes involved in the site of binding to HIV-1 gp120. Nevertheless, anti-idiotype antibodies mirroring a region on the envelope gp120 have been implicated in autoimmune thrombocytopenia (2108).

E. Conclusions: Potential Importance of Autoimmune Responses

Autoimmunity should be considered a potential cofactor in HIV pathogenesis. The possible mechanisms involving both humoral and cellular activities are reviewed in Figure 10.7. Autoimmune responses have been linked to the loss of neutrophils and platelets and to peripheral neuropathy (2212, 2213). One explanation for the reduction in CD4$^+$ cells in HIV infection has also been the induction of anti-T-cell antibodies or antibodies to CD4 (675, 1119). The use of plasmapheresis in HIV-infected patients has supported the role of autoantibodies in the loss of neutrophils and platelets and in peripheral neuropathy but not in the loss of T cells (2213). In treated individuals, neutrophils and platelets return and the neuropathy is ameliorated; no change in CD4$^+$ cell count is observed (D. Kiprov, personal communication). The potential contribution of autoreactive cells in HIV infection also merits further study.

On another note, a potential danger in vaccination with HIV proteins could be eliciting via molecular mimicry immune responses that deplete CD4$^+$ cells, compromise the immune system further, or induce autoimmune pathology in other tissues. Monitoring a possible autoimmune response should be part of the evaluation of any approach at preventing HIV infection (see Chapter 15).

SALIENT FEATURES • CHAPTER 10

1. Antibodies appear usually within 1 to 2 weeks after acute infection. Gag is the earliest viral protein recognized, followed by Nef, Rev, and then Env. The IgG1 subclass is dominant in all clinical stages. Other antibody classes can vary depending on the clinical stage.

2. Neutralizing antibodies to the autologous virus strain provides the most clinically relevant response. Generally, these antibodies are at low levels and appear often at a time when the initial autologous virus has changed.

3. Neutralizing antibodies could have relevance for vaccines to prevent entry of infectious virions. After infection, antibodies might be helpful in killing cells by antibody-dependent cellular cytotoxicity (ADCC). Generally, levels of antibodies in the host have not correlated with a particular clinical state.

4. Antibodies that bind to the virus and enhance virus replication have been demonstrated, particularly in individuals who progress to disease. The mechanism can involve the complement and Fc receptors.

5. The difference between neutralization, enhancement, and resistance to both processes appears to be related to the affinity of binding of the antibody to the virion.

6. HIV can mutate and become resistant to neutralization and enhancement and can undergo changes and become sensitive to antibody-mediated enhancement. Both linear and conformational changes in the viral envelope can be involved.

7. ADCC can have clinical relevance by destroying virus-infected cells, but the process appears to depend mostly on the function of host effector cells (e.g., macrophages and NK cells).

8. Complement can play a role in the antiviral response by enhancing antibody-mediated lysis of virions or by destroying virus and virus-infected cells through binding and activation by the classical or alternative pathways. Complement can also interact with complement receptors on NK cells to cause direct lysis of both infected and uninfected cells. This protein can also enhance the antiviral effect of neutralizing antibodies.

9. HIV is associated with a variety of autoimmune disorders, particularly those involving blood vessels, muscles, and joints.

10. Autoimmunity can occur as a result of B-cell proliferation, molecular mimicry, or carrier hapten mechanisms. Autoantibodies can be made to several normal cellular proteins and can produce clinical symptoms such as reduction in platelets and neutrophils and a peripheral neuropathy.

11. Anti-idiotype antibody production might also play a role in autoimmune disease syndromes.

12. Plasmapheresis of HIV-infected patients has produced reduction of symptoms in people who have decreased levels of neutrophils and platelets or have neuropathy associated with autoantibody production.

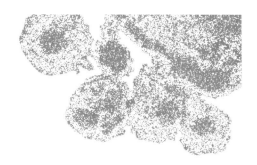

T-Lymphocyte Immune Responses in HIV Infection

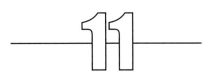

I. Introduction

In most viral infections, the cell-mediated immune response plays a vital role in arresting or eliminating the infectious agent. For HIV, this antiviral activity involves both the innate and adaptive immune systems. Reviewed in this chapter are the adaptive T-cell immune responses that appear to be directed against HIV through recognition of viral proteins associated with HIV or virus-infected cells. Since HIV infection disturbs the immune system, some of the findings cited in Chapter 8 also have direct relevance to this discussion. In addition, the noncytotoxic anti-HIV activity of CD8+ cells that appears to be an innate immune activity is reviewed. Other innate cellular anti-HIV immune responses of NK cells, NK-T cells, and $\gamma\delta$ T cells are discussed in Chapter 9. Importantly, effective innate and adaptive cellular immune activities depend on efficient functioning of antigen-presenting cells (APC), particularly macrophages and dendritic cells (DC) (see Chapter 9).

II. T Lymphocyte Anti-HIV Activities

A. General Observations on T Lymphocytes

Two major categories of CD4+ and CD8+ T lymphocytes exist: antigen-naïve (naïve) and antigen-experienced (memory) cells. The memory T cells are a phenotypically heterogeneous population that can be broadly divided into two types. (i) Central memory (Tcm) cells that circulate among secondary lymphoid tissue through the blood and lymph channels. They express CCR7 and CD62L, which permit trafficking to lymphoid tissue and recirculation (523, 1021). (ii) Effector memory T cells (Tem) that migrate from secondary lymphoid tissue into extra-lymphoid effector

259

sites such as the intestine, lamina propria, and epithelium (3897). The latter cells lack CCR7 and CD62L expression, can actively respond to an antigen (e.g., HIV), and become effector cells; these cells, after reduction in antigen, survive about 1 week or become Tcm cells (for a review, see reference 3015a) (see also Sections II.C and II.D). Some investigators use the term "resting" with central memory cells to indicate a difference in size (small) from activated memory cells and the lack of some cell surface markers (e.g., HLA-DR, CD69). Resting memory cells therefore appear to be T lymphocytes that have encountered antigen as Tem cells but, with reduction in antigen, can enter into a resting state. They are induced to return to being effector memory cells after reexposure to the antigen. Thus, the resting memory cell has the characteristics of the Tcm cell (see Chapter 8, Section I.C).

The Tcm cells rapidly produce cytokines after restimulation by antigen exposure. They reduce

their expression of CCR7, proliferate, and traffic to peripheral organs and become Tem cells. The Tem cells remain at the site of the microbial infection to combat the organism. In responding to antigens, the Tem cells are activated and become effector cells and then evolve into the short-lived terminal effector cells (Figure 11.1) (1340). Some may revert to a Tcm (resting memory) state. The Tcm and Tem cells (especially CD8+ cells) apparently can most likely go back and forth in their functional phenotype. The Tem cells have a limited replicative capacity, whereas naïve and Tcm cells live longer, having many more replicative cycles. For example, some studies have suggested the persistence of vaccinia virus-specific CD4+ Tcm cells for over 70 years after vaccination (1706).

CD8+ and CD4+ T lymphocytes showing cytotoxic T-lymphocyte (CTL) activity usually respond to the presentation of epitopes by APC (see Chapter 9, Figure 9.3) in association with MHC class I

Figure 11.1 Differentiation of CD4+ lymphocytes. This overall development of various T-cell subsets is mirrored as well in the formation of CD8+ T-cell subsets. Naïve cells after exposure to antigen develop into effector cells, which in terms of CD4+ cells are of the TH1 or TH2 type (Table 11.2). Effector cells can revert to effector/memory cells or resting (central) memory cells in the presence of low antigen. With reexposure to antigens, the T effector memory cells quickly respond and evolve into terminal effector cells. These cells are short-lived with high antigen specificity and, particularly in the case of CD8+ cells, show cytotoxic activity. Figure from reference 1340.

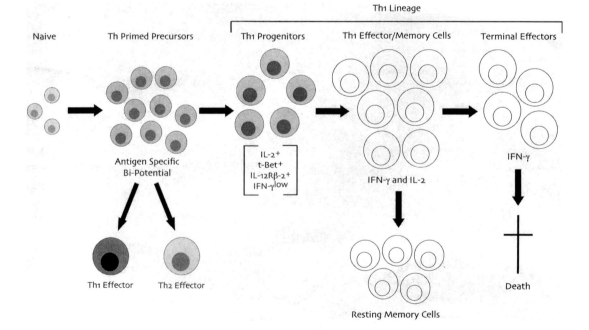

or class II molecules, respectively. An antigen is recognized by means of the T-cell receptor (TCR), which is a heterodimeric cell surface molecule that interacts with the foreign antigen presented as short peptides with MHC class I or class II molecules on the cell surface (Color Plate 18, following page 366). The TCR is composed of either α, β, γ, or δ chains, although the vast majority of circulating T lymphocytes express αβ (see Chapter 9 for a description of γδ T cells). Recognition of viral pathogens with class I molecules appears to be more precise, not only because of limitations to the length of the peptides (8 to 10 residues) but also because the ends of the peptide (amino-terminal and carboxyl-terminal) must fit into defined pockets at opposite sides of the grooves in the MHC class I locus (for reviews, see references 648 and 3658) (Color Plate 18, following page 366). The peptides in the MHC class II grooves can be longer (12 to 24 residues) and thus more heterogeneous. Therefore, the diversity of antigenic determinants presented to CD4$^+$ cells by MHC class II molecules can be greater than that presented to CD8$^+$ cells by class I molecules (648).

The human leukocyte antigen (HLA) genetic background (i.e., MHC) and environmental factors can influence the mature T-cell repertoire, which, if diverse, can be beneficial to the host (for a review, see reference 4735). Alterations in the T-cell repertoire (as reflected by different TCR subunits) can also come about in HIV infection by (i) expression of other viral antigens that induce selective cell expansion or cell death, (ii) molecular mimicry by regions of gp120 that resemble HLA (4577) (see Chapters 4 and 10), (iii) HLA molecules incorporated into the viral envelope, and (iv) superantigen effects of HIV (see Chapter 6, Section V, and Color Plate 13, following page 78) (156). The overall result is an imbalance in the diversity of the CD8$^+$ cell or CD4$^+$ cell responses, which could have detrimental consequences (4735).

When the CD4$^+$ cell and CD8$^+$ cell repertoires are limited, immunologic responses can be compromised, particularly when new antigens are encountered (1195, 3408, 3783). Thus, the extent of diversity of the T-cell repertoire response during primary infection may predict the clinical outcome (see Chapter 4) (3408). In particular, in studies of HIV-infected people, CD4$^+$ and CD8$^+$ cell expan-

sions can be clonal or oligoclonal. Because these expansions are not necessarily concomitant, spaces or "gaps" in the T-cell repertoire can exist and become exaggerated with disease progression (3783). Nevertheless, some flexibility in this response is possible (Figure 11.2).

The repertoire alterations result in either protective or deleterious responses if the cells have CTL or other anti-HIV activity (3783, 3965). An absence of, or reduction in, certain T-cell specifications may decrease the resistance to infection and malignancy (3783, 4735). Also noteworthy, the T-cell repertoire in the peripheral blood may change but the distribution in lymphoid tissue (e.g., tonsil) may not (3157). This finding can reflect the observation that peripheral blood CD4$^+$ T-cell reduction may not be seen in lymphoid tissues (509, 3809) except perhaps for the dramatic loss of T lymphocytes in the gastrointestinal tract (493, 2957, 2971) (Chapters 4 and 8).

Early studies had suggested that there may be a physiological regulation of T lymphocytes in the host (26). A loss of CD4$^+$ lymphocytes appears to be compensated for by an increase in the number of CD8$^+$ lymphocytes. This CD8$^+$ cell lymphocytosis could interfere with regeneration of CD4$^+$ cells (2806). If such homeostatic mechanisms exist, approaches in HIV-infected individuals to increase the number of CD4$^+$ cells by modulating CD8$^+$ cell numbers might be possible.

B. Measurements of HIV-Specific T-Cell Responses

A variety of procedures can be used to detect CD4$^+$ and CD8$^+$ T-cell responses to HIV (Table 11.1). Using the tetramer technique, HIV-specific CD4$^+$ and CD8$^+$ T cells can be measured by flow cytometry with reagents for specific HLA subtypes (87). Enzyme-linked immunospot assays and intracellular cytokine assays using flow cytometry are utilized after short-term in vitro stimulation with HIV peptides in which cytokine (e.g., Il-2 and IFN-γ) production is measured with specific antibodies (2592). Another assay, using carboxyl fluorescein diacetate succinimidyl, (CFSE), assesses cell proliferation by flow cytometry. It gives information similar to that provided by the lymphocyte proliferation assay that detects cell division by incorporation of radioactive precursor DNA ([^{3}H]thymi-

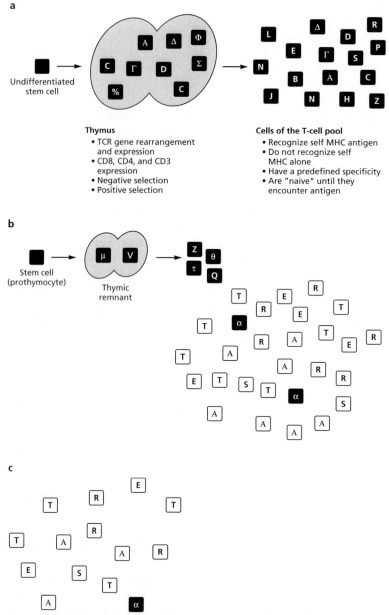

Figure 11.2 Generation of the T-cell repertoire. (a) Undifferentiated lymphoid stem cells (prothymocytes), as they pass through the thymus, express CD4 and CD8 molecules. Their T-cell receptor (TCR) genes are rearranged and expressed, and the resulting thymocytes undergo negative and positive selection. T-cell clones released into circulation have a diverse TCR pattern, indicating their potential for polyclonal responses. (b) With destruction of T cells by HIV, a limited T-cell repertoire may exist which, when allowed to regenerate through a variety of therapeutic interventions, may not recover the entire repertoire initially present in the host. (c) The end-stage T-cell repertoire may be limited so that it cannot react quickly to a particular antigen. In a sense, as shown here, the T-cell repertoire could not respond in a way that would require the spelling of ZEBRA. Nevertheless, by other processes, it might be able to respond (although more slowly) by recognizing the antigen as "a horse with white and black stripes." Ideas derived from figures and discussions provided by H. Cliff Lane.

Table 11.1 Comparisons of assays for T-cell responses[a]

Feature	ELISPOT	CFC	CD107	MHC-peptide multimers	BrdU or CFSE
0.05% of CD4 or CD8 cells	1:50,000 PBMC	0.05% of CD4 or 0.12% of CD8 T cells	0.2% of CD8 T cells	0.02% of CD8 T cells	0.2% of CD4 or CD8 T cells
Typical background	<1:200,000	0.01% of CD4 cells, 0.03% of CD8 T cells	0.05% of CD8 T cells	0.005% of CD8 cells	0.05% of CD4 or CD8 cells
Detection efficiency	Low	High	High	High	High
Turnaround time	2 days	10 h	10 h	3 h	3–7 days
Information content	Low	High	High	High, but epitope restricted	High, but semiquantitative
Automation potential	Medium	Medium	Medium	High	Low

[a]Enzyme-linked immunospot (ELISPOT) assays detect the secretion of cytokines by cells cultured in filter-bottom wells using enzyme-labeled antibodies and colorimetric substrates. The positive cells are counted under a low-power microscope or with an automated image reader. Cytokine flow cytometry (CFC) uses intracellular staining in the presence of a secretion inhibitor like brefeldin A to detect cytokine production with fluorescently tagged antibodies and multiparameter flow cytometry. CD107 is a constituent protein of cytotoxic granules, which is transiently exported to the cell surface upon CTL degranulation. It can be stained by flow cytometry and thus identifies degranulating cells with cytotoxic activity. CD107 can also be stained in combination with intracellular cytokines and/or MHC-peptide multimers. MHC-peptide multimers include tetramers, pentamers, and dimers of MHC molecules loaded with antigenic peptides and tagged with a fluorescent label. They can be used to directly identify T cells with a given peptide-plus-MHC specificity in flow cytometry assays (e.g., HIV-specific T cells). Bromodeoxyuridine (BrdU) and carboxyfluorescein succinimidyl ester (CFSE) assays are used to measure cellular proliferation by flow cytometry. The assays can be utilized to detect T-cell proliferative responses to HIV antigens. BrdU is a thymidine analog that is incorporated into the DNA of dividing cells and can be detected with a fluorescently labeled antibody. CFSE is a cytophilic dye that labels cellular proteins. With each round of cell division, the level of CFSE in the cells is halved by dilution into daughter cells. The stepwise loss of CFSE is thus a measure of cell division. Reprinted from reference 2755 with permission.

dine) into cells (1472; for a review, see reference 2755). Whether stimulation in vitro provides a true window to the in vivo state is not yet known (3761). Cytotoxic activity can be evaluated by reduction in cell numbers, release of radioactive markers (^{51}Cr) from dying cells (2898), and expression of cell markers of cytotoxicity (2592). A common measure of CTL function is detection of intracellular perforin or expression of CD107, a protein associated with degranulation (i.e., release of cytotoxic peptides) (80, 2592) (Table 11.1). An important consideration is whether the antiviral CTL activity measured has relevance to the autologous virus and to infected primary CD4$^+$ T cells (see Section C.2).

C. CD4$^+$ T Lymphocytes

1. CD4$^+$ HELPER CELL CLASSIFICATION

Similar to the murine system (3135, 3140), human CD4$^+$ T helper (TH) cells can be separated into TH1 and TH2 subsets (813, 814, 3786, 3787, 4091;

for a review, see reference 2688) according to their cytokine production and function (Table 11.2) (see also Chapters 4 and 8). TH1 cells secrete IL-2, IFN-γ, and TNF-α, which are important for strong cell-mediated immunity; TH2 cells produce IL-4, IL-5, IL-6, IL-10, and IL-13, which help increase antibody production. They have characteristics of Tem cells (Table 11.3).

The differential expression of the IL-12β receptor on CD4$^+$ cells has provided another possible means of distinguishing TH1 (present) and TH2 (absent) cells (2837) (Table 11.2). IL-4 can inhibit the expression of this receptor and can thereby induce the development of TH2 cells (2837). IFN-α and IFN-γ can maintain the presence of this IL-12 receptor and restore the ability of the cells to respond to IL-12, which is part of the TH1 pathway (3781, 4354, 4727). Importantly, IL-12 induces IFN-γ production by NK cells (374), and thus the interplay among these different cytokines can be appreciated (Figure 9.6).

Table 11.2 Characterization of CD4+ T helper cell subsets

Characteristic	CD4+ cell subset	
	TH1	TH2
Cytokines	IL-2, IFN-γ, TNF-α	IL-4, IL-5, IL-6, IL-10, IL-13
Cytokines that enhance their development	IL-12	IL-4, IL-13
IL-12Rβ expression	+	−
CCR3 expression	−	+
Sensitivity to apoptosis	+	−
Cytokine effect on apoptosis	Protect	Accelerate
CD95L expression[a]	Normal	Decreased
Relative sensitivity to HIV infection[b]	+	+
CTL activity	+	−
Overall helper function	Increase cell-mediated immunity	Increase antibody production

[a]CD95L is involved in Fas-mediated apoptosis.
[b]Some differences have been reported (see Chapter 4, Section II.C).

The TH subsets are derived from naïve CD4+ T cells. These naïve cells produce IL-2 and express CD45RA, a tyrosine phosphatase that plays a role in TCR-mediated signaling (3761). CCR7, also on these cells, is a chemokine receptor that, as noted above, mediates trafficking to secondary lymphoid tissue (523, 1021). The TH cells appear to represent terminally differentiated CD4+ cells derived from a precursor (or TH0-type) cell capable of expressing many different cytokines, particularly IL-2 and TNF-β (1340) (Figure 11.1). Factors such as antigen dose (4313), the type of APC, and, most importantly, the cytokine milieu determine the type of T helper responses generated. It is important to note that T helper cell differentiation requires a series of extensive cellular and molecular changes that lead to a very heterogeneous response (1340). The induction process cannot change an already committed TH1 or TH2 cell (4376).

IL-12 induces TH1 cell development from naïve cells while down-regulating TH2 cell cytokine expression (e.g., IL-4) (2786, 4023, 4031; for a review of IL-12, see reference 4469) (Figure 11.3). This inhibition of TH2 development by IL-12 may occur indirectly through the stimulation of IFN-γ synthesis (374, 4469). In contrast, IL-4 and, perhaps more so, IL-13 stimulate the development of TH2 cells (2281, 4979), which in turn produce IL-4, which can down-regulate TH1 cytokine expression (817).

These observations indicate that cytokines produced by the TH1 and TH2 subsets can cross-regulate one another (3786, 3787). As other examples, IFN-γ, a product of TH1 cells, can inhibit the generation of TH2 cells (1410), whereas IL-4 (noted above) or IL-10, a product of TH2 cells, can inhibit the generation of TH1 cells and their cytokine production by TH1 cells (817, 1012) (Figure 11.4). The inhibitory effect of IL-10 may be indirect and reflect a block of IL-12 synthesis by macrophages or DCS (938) (see below). Macrophages of HIV-infected symptomatic patients have been found to have increased production of IL-1 and decreased production of IL-12 (766). These findings support an inhibitory effect of IL-4 on type 1 cytokine production (3344).

Because similar cytokines can be produced by other cells in the body, the terminology of type 1 and type 2 responses is preferentially used instead of TH1 and TH2 responses, particularly when the specific cells producing the cytokines are not identified (817, 3786, 3787). It is also important to note that the separation of TH CD4+ cells into TH1 and TH2 cells and the interactions of type 1 and type 2 cytokines (814, 2688, 4023) provide a helpful concept but that the system is more complex. For example, unlike in the murine system, IL-10 can be made by both TH1 and TH2 cell clones (648, 1034, 3786, 3787), although the dominant cell type releasing IL-10 is TH2 (1034, 1739).

In addition, both type 1 and type 2 cytokines can increase immunoglobulin production, although specific differences can be appreciated (e.g., IgE production by type 2 cytokines) (814, 3786). Further-

Table 11.3 Human CD4[+] T-cell subset heterogeneity[a]

Parameter	Naïve	Central memory	TH1[b]	TH2[b]	Terminal effector
CD45 isoform	RA	RO	RO	RO	RA or RO
CCR7	+	+	−	−	−
Chemokine receptors			CXCR3	CRTH2	CX3CR1
HIV coreceptor	CXCR4[d]	CXCR4[d]	CCR5, CXCR4	CCR5, CXCR4	CCR5, CXCR4
CD62L	+	+	+ or −	+ or −	−
CD28/CD27/CD57	+/+/−	+/+/−	+/−/−	+/−/−	−/−/+
Repertoire	Most diverse	Diverse	Intracellular antigens	Extracellular antigens	Oligoclonal
Cytokine receptor	IL-7R	IL-7R	IL-12Rβ1, IL-18R	IL-4R	IL-12Rβ1
Signal transduction	STAT5	STAT5	STAT1/STAT4	STAT6	STAT4?
Transcription factor		?	T-Bet	GATA-3	?
Relative turnover rate	Very low	Low	High	High	Medium, slow accumulation
Proliferative potential	Very high	High	Low	Low	Very low
Response to antigen/ effector function		IL-2	IFN-γ, IL-2, TNF-α	IL-4, IL-5, IL-10, IL-13	Perforin, granzymes, IFN-γ?
Tissue location	Circulation/ lymphoid	Circulation/ lymphoid	Inflammation	Inflammation (allergic)	Circulation, other?
Main interacting cell type(s)	DC[c]	DC?	Monocyte, NK cell, B cell	Mast cell, eosinophil, B cell	Virally infected target cells, especially CMV
Cell function for HIV	No response	IL-2 production	IL-2/IFN-γ production	IL-4/IL-30 production	Cytokine cells

[a]CD4[+] and CD8[+] T cell subsets are defined by their phenotype as noted by cell surface molecules, turnover rates, repertoire, and cytokine production in response to antigen (see also Table 11.4). Differences can be observed depending on initial antigen expression, chronic infection, or treated infection. For example, central (also called resting) and effector memory T cells (Tcm, Tem) are both CD45RO[+] but differ in expression of CCR7 and CD62L (Tcm positive and Tem negative). Effector memory cells have limited proliferative potential but rapid effector function, particularly IFN-γ production (see Table 11.4). They are generally found in non-lymphoid organs and prepared to respond to infection at those sites. Some consider CD4[+] CCR7[−] CD45RO[+] CD57[+] cells to be the principal Tem cells (3394). Central memory CD4[+] T cells have very limited effector function, but share with naïve cells the expression of CCR7 and IL-2 production; they can migrate to lymphoid tissue, with the potential for extensive proliferation and differentiation when exposed to antigens. The Tcm cells are restimulated in response to antigen and then proliferate first before being effective in preventing new infections in the periphery. The difference between resting and activated memory cells appears to be in the expression of activation markers on the cell surface. The terminally differentiated CD28[−] CD57[+] cell population lacks IL-7R but expresses IL-12R. These cells can be distinguished from IL-2-producing proliferating Tcm cells. They have a history of extensive proliferation and lack of telomerase activity and have very limited proliferative potential but often contain cytotoxic granules and perforin consistent with the CTL function.

Essentially, the T cells appear to be in a continuum, with cells going from memory (central or resting memory or effector memory) to activated memory and then to effector cells. Central memory cells can form when effector cells return to a memory state and are not very proliferative. When activated, they express CD38 and become activated effector cells, which may not be distinguishable from newly derived effector cells. Finally, the terminal effector cells appear to be in the final stages in differentiation and do not proliferate very much; they have cytotoxic activity and a short life span. The expression of many of these markers (e.g., chemokines and interleukin receptors) is enriched on several of these subsets and may not be used *exclusively* to identify specific subsets, as there is substantial overlap. For example, CD62L is usually expressed on TH2 cells but can also be present on TH1 cells. TH1 cells bind to CD62L[−] cells (M. Roederer, personal communication). Data obtained from references 134, 768, 1725, 2192, 2590, 2718, 3151, 3152, 3761, 3788, 3896, and 4624. Table adapted from tables provided by J. Zaunders.

[b]T helper type 1 (TH1) and TH2 cells are part of the memory subset of CD4[+] cells. Those, the most common, that lack CCR7 are Tem cells found in nonlymphoid sites; those with CCR7 expression are found in lymphoid tissues and are considered Tcm cells. The majority of HIV-specific CD4[+] cells appear to be of the TH1 type, in which differences can be appreciated among cells that can produce IL-2, IFN-γ, or both cytokines (see Figure 11.1 and text). While TH2 CD4[+] cells producing IL-4 can be detected, the majority of this cell type produce IL-10 and are usually considered to function as T regulatory cells (Section V).

[c]DC, dendritic cell.

[d]When activated they express CCR5 (331).

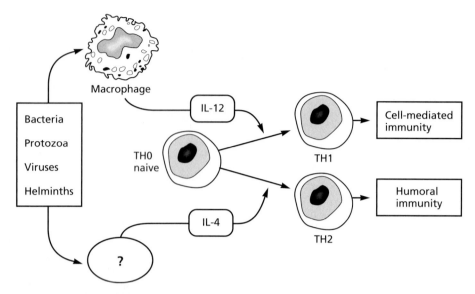

Figure 11.3 Cytokine-driven type 1 cell differentiation. Bacteria, protozoa, probably viruses, and helminths can induce the production of IL-12 by macrophages or other cells. IL-12 then induces differentiation of naïve or TH0 cells into a TH1 subset, which encourages cell-mediated immunity. Other pathogens, particularly helminths, stimulate IL-4 production by cells not yet defined. IL-4 induces TH0 cells toward TH2 cell differentiation. The TH2 cells mediate help for antibody production. What determines the predominant TH1 (type 1) or TH2 (type 2) response in the host is not known. Modified from reference 4023 with permission. Copyright 1993 AAAS.

more, while some type 1 cytokines (e.g., IFN-γ, TNF-α, and IL-2) may increase cellular immune anti-HIV responses, the same cellular factors can augment HIV-1 production (2744, 2871, 3558). In contrast, the type 2 cytokines (e.g., IL-4 and IL-10) suppress HIV expression (2744, 2871, 3558) but reduce CD8+ cell responses (258, 648, 3786, 3787) (see Chapter 8, Table 8.5). The HIV-suppressing effect of IL-10 could be linked to its inhibition of the production of TNF-α, an up-regulator of HIV replication. Because of these dual roles of cytokines (decreasing or increasing CD8+ cell responses and decreasing or increasing HIV production), their clinical use may present problems in terms of the dominant effect observed in the infected person (see Chapter 14).

2. CD4+ HELPER CELL RESPONSES

Early in HIV infection before the occurrence of a substantial decrease in CD4+ cell number (815, 1655, 2398, 3004, 3793, 4079), CD4+ cell responses were reported to be prognostic of the clinical

course (815, 1655, 2398, 3004, 3793, 4079) (see Chapter 8). A poor prognosis correlated with a decrease over time in cell proliferation and IL-2 production after exposure to recall antigens (e.g., tetanus and influenza A), irradiated HLA disparate leukocytes (alloresponse), and phytohemagglutinin (mitogen response) stimulation (Figure 8.2). Approximately one-third of asymptomatic individuals had responses to all three stimuli; those who had no response to the stimuli progressed more rapidly to disease. The decrease in proliferative responses to alloantigens was found in both CD45RA+ naïve and CD45RO+ mature subsets of CD4+ T cells.

Based on studies of HIV-infected individuals over time, a hypothesis was presented that cytokines produced by TH1 and TH2 cells can play an immune regulatory role in HIV infection and affect progression to disease, as has been observed in studies of other infections (814, 1469, 2759, 4079, 4091). The findings suggest that TH1 (or type 1) responses are found primarily in healthy asymptomatic HIV-

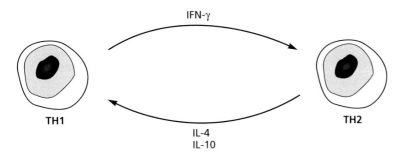

IFN-γ

TH1

IL-4
IL-10

TH2

Figure 11.4 Cross-regulation of the TH1 and TH2 subsets of CD4⁺ cells. The production of certain cytokines by TH1 and TH2 cells can suppress production of cytokines by the corresponding cell subset (3786). From reference 2520 with permission.

infected individuals, whereas a predominance of the TH2 (type 2) responses occurs during the symptomatic stage of disease (805, 814, 4079). These results, observed with purified CD4⁺ cells and confirmed by intracellular staining (2233), indicate a shift from type 1 to type 2 cytokine production with advancement to disease. The data suggest that the type 1 response is protective against disease in an individual (805, 814), whereas progression to disease is associated with a type 2 response (1944, 2010, 3786, 3787). The latter activity may, then, be responsible for suppressing type 1 cytokine production and thereby decreasing the antiviral responses of CD8⁺ effector cells (see above and Section IV.C). Currently, this concept is less popular but does provide a direction for evaluating the immunologic effects of different cytokine expressions.

There is also an IFN-γ-inducible tryptophan-catabolizing enzyme, indoleamine 2,3-dioxygenase (IDO), that can be made in many different cell types, particularly APC. IDO can reduce the function and viability of T cells by depleting tryptophan in the microenvironment (2967). Thus, certain TH1 cells producing IFN-γ may be more susceptible to death by this tryptophan depletion (see Chapter 13).

Another cytokine that can influence TH1 memory CD4⁺ cells is IL-7. It can help form and maintain the memory CD4⁺ T cells (4030) by sustaining their viability, not their proliferative capacity. It can induce naïve CD4⁺ cells to produce IFN-γ (2783). Moreover, CD8⁺ cells have increased survival in the presence of IL-7, but IL-15 is required for their proliferation (Section II.D).

CD4⁺ cell functions that involve anti-HIV responses have been found to be reduced, particularly in terms of cell proliferation (4132) and cytokine production. In general, the TH1 cell responses can be divided into three cell subsets that are primarily Tem cells: those cells secreting IL-2 that is most beneficial to the host defense (Section II.D), those cells that produce IFN-γ and appear to be more differentiated with less proliferative and antigen-responsive activities (3393) (see below), and some CD4⁺ cells that make both cytokines (1724). CMV-specific CD4⁺ cells in the host show equal distribution of these three functionally distinct cell populations. Similar findings are seen with HIV-specific CD4⁺ T cells in subjects with nonprogressive disease. However, solely IFN-γ-secreting cells are primarily observed in HIV-infected individuals with progressive disease and are considered terminal effector cells (Figure 11.1; Table 11.3); they are extremely short-lived and not very functional in antiviral responses. As a corollary, IL-2-secreting and IL-2/IFN-γ-secreting CD4⁺ cells are barely detected in AIDS patients (see below) (1724). The higher frequencies of IL-2- and IL-2/IFN-γ-producing cells in CMV-infected individuals and HIV long-term survivors (see Chapter 13) compared to HIV-infected individuals with progressive disease most likely reflect low levels of viral antigen in the former cases. With high viral loads, a more differentiated type 1 immune response would result consisting mostly of IFN-γ-producing CD4⁺ cells.

HIV infection can cause an alteration in CD4⁺ cell TH1 subsets, with an increase in the IFN-γ-producing poorly replicating cells (e.g., terminal effector cells) versus the IL-2-producing HIV-specific CD4⁺ T cells that have a good proliferative capacity (i.e., Tem versus Tcm cells) (3393, 4888) (Table 11.3). Expression of CD57, a glycosylated member of the N-CAM integrin family, has been used by some investigators to distinguish those cells that produce IFN-γ and have less proliferative capacity from those cells (CD57⁻) that produce IL-2 (3393). Therefore, the IL-2-producing CD4⁺ cells are CCR7⁺ CD45RO⁺ CD57⁻ proliferation-competent cells and classified as Tcm cells (Table 11.3). The IFN-γ-producing cells are of the CCR7⁻ CD45RA⁻ CD57⁺ low proliferating effector Tem phenotype, which is increased with high viral loads (3394) (see above). Nevertheless, the use of CD57 as a marker of different CD4⁺ cell subsets has not been universally accepted. It is more useful with CD8⁺ cell subsets (Section II.D).

Some investigators have demonstrated that CCR7⁻ Tem CD4⁺ cells develop after exposure of naïve CD4⁺ T cells to HIV antigens. As noted above (Section II.A), these cells can then revert to a CCR7⁺ Tcm cell after HIV titers are reduced. If viremia remains high, these cells can instead become a more differentiated (i.e., terminal) Tem cell population (CD4⁺ CCR7⁻ CD45RO⁺ CD57⁺) that produces IFN-γ but not IL-2 (2472, 3394, 4888). Those individuals with low virus levels could have both CD4⁺ memory T-cell types and certainly the IL-2-producing CCR7⁺ CD57⁻ Tcm cells (3393).

In most cases of HIV infection, the HIV-specific CD4⁺ T-cell responses are low (4785). This finding most likely reflects the effect of HIV on the function of these cells (see Chapter 8). The reactive CD4⁺ cells can be targeted for HIV infection because of their proliferative responses (1120). The relative expression of the chemokine coreceptors (CXCR4 on naïve CD4⁺ cells and CCR5 on memory and effector CD4⁺ cells) can also influence these viral effects (Table 11.3) (see Chapter 4) (4919, 4920). In this regard, some studies with acutely infected subjects have suggested that with early HAART, the HIV-specific CD4⁺ T-cell responses can be maintained and are associated with long-term control of HIV infection (3801) (see Chapter 14) (Section II.H). However, the clinical relevance of these initial observations is now not evident since several of these acutely infected subjects off therapy have since progressed to disease (2122).

In this regard, some researchers have questioned the importance of HIV-specific CD4⁺ T-cell responses (2004). They propose that the relative extent of persistent viremia reflecting high immune activation is the most important determinant of the clinical outcome. Low viral loads correlate with an asymptomatic state (see Chapter 13) in which the HIV-specific CD4⁺ T helper cell responses are found (2950, 3802, 4785). Whether this T-cell activity is the cause of the reduction in viremia or a result of the decrease in HIV replication is not resolved. Obviously, further research on the role of HIV-specific CD4⁺ T cells is needed.

In some untreated infected subjects, the CD4⁺ T-cell responses to the HIV-1 Gag protein measured by IL-2 or IFN-γ production have correlated directly with levels of Gag-specific CD8⁺ CTL precursors and particularly with the lowest levels of viremia (2070). These observations most likely reflect the known requirement of CD4⁺ T cells for expansion, function, and memory of CD8⁺ T lymphocytes (2005). Nevertheless, HIV-specific CD8⁺ CTLs can be observed in the absence of substantial numbers of CD4⁺ T cells. In this case, however, the CTLs are tetramer positive and may lack CD8⁺ cell anti-HIV cytotoxic activity (4232) (Section II.D). Others have shown that HIV-specific CD8⁺ CTLs (2231) do not necessarily prevent progression to disease as has been suggested for CD4⁺ cell anti-HIV responses (2004) (noted above). And, in certain studies, HIV-specific CD4⁺ T-cell responses have not consistently correlated with viral load, nor have HIV-specific CD8 T-cell responses (355). Conceivably, the type of CD4⁺ cell present (Tcm or Tem) may determine the CD8⁺ cell function.

3. CYTOTOXIC CD4⁺ CELL ACTIVITY

As noted in Chapter 8 (Section I.C.6), some CD4⁺ T cells can have CTL activity directed either at infected or uninfected CD4⁺ cells or at cells expressing HIV peptides in association with the MHC class II molecule (1035, 1710, 3027, 3279, 3343, 3503). This response is usually found with TH1-type CD4⁺ cells (1035) and is virus strain specific (1710), mediated by perforin (133, 3280, 3281, 3343), or involving Fas/Fas ligand (FasL)-induced apoptosis (3503). Some investigators report that the rapid lysis observed between CD4⁺ CTLs and infected target cells (3343) may be related to cell-to-cell contact and syncytium formation (1788). The level of CD4⁺ cell cytotoxic anti-HIV response is usually low (3279), but a substantial increase in HIV-specific CD4$^+$ CTLs has been reported in primary HIV infection (4920). Some evidence suggests that CD8$^+$ cells play a role in the development of CD4$^+$ cell cytotoxic activity (4777). Moreover, while CD4$^+$ CTLs may help in cell-mediated responses against HIV, they also could have a detrimental effect on uninfected cells (1710, 2796).

D. CD8$^+$ T Lymphocytes

1. SUBSETS OF CD8$^+$ T CELLS

CD8$^+$ T lymphocytes can have cytotoxic (CTL) or noncytotoxic anti-HIV activity (see Section IV). The characterization of CTLs is covered in this section. In terms of CTL response, three major populations of CD8$^+$ T cells, defined by cell surface markers, have been described as naïve, Tcm, and Tem cells. This classification of naïve and memory-type cells resembles that for CD4$^+$ T cells (Tables 11.3 and 11.4) (see Section II.A). Naïve CD8$^+$ cells have not been exposed to antigen. When encountering a microbe like HIV, they can respond quickly and become effector cells. With reduced antigen exposure, they become memory cells. The Tcm cells are CD45RO$^+$ CCR7$^+$ and traffic to lymph nodes, as do naïve CD8$^+$ cells. These Tcm cells have a high proliferative potential but not good cytotoxic activity (perforin low or perforin negative) (see Section II.B), except in the presence of CD4$^+$ cell or DC help (via IL-2, IL-15, or IL-21) (3761). Tcm cells function best at controlling intracellular infections because with their production of IL-2 they can expand into large numbers of effector cells (90, 3761). These cells recognize antigen in lymph nodes and then undergo rapid growth to generate large numbers of Tem cells (Table 11.4). The Tem cells, expressing CD45RO and not CCR7, travel to nonlymphoid tissue (e.g., liver or lung). They become terminal effector cells containing perforin with a very rapid cytotoxic response but do not proliferate well.

For CD8$^+$ T-cell responses to HIV infection, a continuum in a cell-differentiated pattern can be observed beginning with a naïve CD8$^+$ cell that becomes an effector cell when high antigen expression takes place. As the antigen is reduced, Tcm (CCR7$^+$) and Tem (CCR7$^-$) CD8$^+$ cells develop (4741). What influences the formation of Tcm versus Tem cells is not known. When reexposure to antigens occurs, the Tcm and Tem cells both can respond. The Tcm (CCR7$^+$) CD8$^+$ cells, similar to cells with this CD4$^+$ phenotype (see above), persist in vivo primarily in lymphoid tissue, produce IL-2, and are more efficient in proliferation than Tem cells and provide protective immunity. Once activated, the Tcm cells can become Tem cells producing generally IFN-γ. The Tem cells are the immediate responders to the pathogen, becoming T effector cells that go to the nonlymphoid tissue involved and act as terminal effector cells. Once the antigen is cleared, the Tem cells can revert to Tcm cells (Table 11.4) (see also Section II.A).

As with CD4$^+$ T cells, the CD8$^+$ Tcm cells predominate when antigen is cleared or markedly reduced (e.g., with CMV infection); the Tem cell number is greatest when high levels of antigen persist (e.g., with HIV infection). The CD4$^+$ and CD8$^+$ Tcm cells can persist for decades without reexposure to antigen (562, 3760, 3761). As noted above, the CD4$^+$ cells appear to be needed to induce CD8$^+$ cell responses and maintain the CD8$^+$ T-cell memory response (465, 2005, 3761, 4338).

CD28 expression has been used to distinguish between CD8$^+$ cells that have anti-HIV CTL activity (CD8$^+$ CD28$^-$ cells) and those that have a noncytotoxic antiviral response (CD8$^+$ CD28$^+$ cells) (255, 449, 1296, 2396) (Table 11.5) (Section IV). The CD8$^+$ cells lacking CD28 are at an end stage in the replicative cycle and have poor proliferative ability but show cytotoxic activity and secretion of cytokines (for a review, see reference 509). Their stage of senescence is reflected by reduced telomere lengths (1173), and these cells are relatively unresponsive to mitogen and to anti-CD28 antibodies, since they lack the CD28 molecule (449). A possible influence of the aging process on HIV pathogenesis has been considered (953, 1173) (see Chapter 13).

Using other markers (e.g., CD57 and CCR7) along with cytokine production (e.g., IL-2 and IFN-γ), functioning CD8$^+$ cells can be subdivided further in HIV infection (3393). The expression of CD57 reflects chronic immune activation, and this CD8$^+$-cell subset is increased in HIV infection (3419). The CD57 protein is normally found on the effector cytotoxic CD8$^+$ CD28$^-$ cells and is

Table 11.4 Human CD8 T-cell subset heterogeneity

Parameter	Naïve	Central memory	Effector memory	Effector(s)	Terminal effector
CD45	RA	RO	RO	RO	RA
CCR7	+	+	–	–	–
Chemokine receptor(s)			CXCR3, CXCR1, CCR5 +/–	CXCR3, CXCR1, CCR5	CX3CR1
CD38/CD11a (LFA-1)	Low/low	Negative/high	Negative/high	High/high	Negative/high
CD62L addressin	+	+	–	+ or –	–
CD28/CD27/CD57	+/high/–	+/high/–	+/+/–	–/low/–	–/low or –/+
Cytokine receptor(s)	IL-7R (CD127)	IL-7R, IL-2Rβ	IL-7R, IL-2Rβ	IL-12Rβ1, IL-18R, IL-2Rβ	IL-12Rβ1
Turnover	Very low	Low	Intermediate	Very high	Low, with slow accumulation
Repertoire	Most diverse	Diverse	Different from central memory?	Intracellular antigens	Oligoclonal
Response to antigen/effector function	Very high	IL-2	IFN-γ; CAF?	IFN-γ, TNF-α, perforin, granzymes	High perforin, granzymes
Proliferation potential	Very high	High	Low	Very low	Very low
Proportion of tetramer positive for: FLU[b] (cleared virus)		High	Low	Low	Low
CMV (chronic low virus)		Low	Low	Intermediate	High
Untreated HIV (chronic high virus)		Low	Low	Very high	Low
Treated HIV		Low	Intermediate	Intermediate	Low
Location	Circulation/lymphoid	Circulation/lymphoid	Peripheral tissues	Inflammation	Circulation; other?
Cell function	None	IL-2 production	IFN-γ production	IFN-γ production	Cytokine and suppression activity

[a]See Table 11.3, footnote *a*.
[b]FLU, influenza virus antigen.

Table 11.5 Anti-HIV responses by CD8$^+$ T cells

Characteristic	Cytotoxic	Noncytotoxic
MHC restricted	Yes	No
Mechanism	Cell-cell contact, perforin/granzymes, or *fas*-mediated apoptosis	Cell-cell contact and secretion of soluble antiviral protein(s)
Antigen specificity	Fine	Broad?
Cell surface marker	HLA-DR$^+$ CD28$^-$ CD11b$^+$	HLA-DR$^+$ CD28$^+$ CD11b$^-$
Clinical relevance[a]	Develops early after infection but lost with progression to disease	
Vaccine inducible	Yes	nk[b]

[a]Clinical relevance of cytotoxic activity is measured by cell killing or expression of CD107 and perforin (see text).
[b]nk, not known.

usually discordant with CD28 expression. However, its value as a marker of cell function has not been fully assessed. CCR7 expression is absent on the CD28$^-$ CD57$^+$ HIV-specific CD8$^+$ T cells that show reduced proliferative capacity. These cells appear to be terminally differentiated, with a high sensitivity to apoptosis when activated (492). The CD8$^+$ cell effector subsets may therefore be best defined based on their activation status rather than their differentiation phenotype (674) (see below). Recently, the loss of CD127 (IL-7R receptor negative [IL-7R$^-$]) on CD8$^+$ T cells (Table 11.4) has identified another subset of CD8$^+$ cells that is associated with disease progression. These cells produce IFN-γ, but not IL-2, and have decreased proliferative potential, with an increase in susceptibility to apoptosis (3384).

By functional and flow cytometry analysis, the cytotoxic T cells have also been shown to have a CD8$^+$ CD11b$^+$ phenotype, whereas suppressor cells (which can down-modulate immune responses) have a CD8$^+$ CD11b$^-$ phenotype. This phenotype can also distinguish cytotoxic versus noncytotoxic anti-HIV CD8$^+$ cells (2396; S. Killian and J. Levy, unpublished observations) (Table 11.5). In general, the large number of surface markers currently identified on T cells (Tables 11.3 and 11.4) and linked to particular differentiation pathways and functions needs to be better characterized in terms of their clinical relevance.

Finally, the TH classification of CD4$^+$ cells by cytokine production (Table 11.1), discussed above, has also suggested a similar classification for CD8$^+$ cells. In this case, T1 and T2 type cells (or Tc1 and Tc2) could define distinct subsets (3135, 3786, 3787). However, generally the terms type 1 and 2 are used.

Whereas most CD8$^+$ cells appear to secrete IFN-γ, some early studies suggested that type 2 CD8$^+$ cells exist and have decreased CTL activity (2758).

2. ANTI-HIV CYTOTOXIC RESPONSES
a. Overview
The major cell type that can react specifically against virus-infected cells is the cytotoxic subset of CD8$^+$ T lymphocytes described above. Classically, the CD8$^+$ cell cytotoxic response is HLA (MHC) restricted and antigen specific and requires cell-to-cell contact (Table 11.5). It involves both perforin production and Fas/Fas ligand interaction (330, 1964, 2063). The resiliency of the CTL response and its ability to recognize variants appear to be determined by HLA profiles (4783). This finding could explain the protection from infection in some exposed, uninfected individuals (1343) (see Chapter 13). In chronic infection, HIV-1-specific T-cell responses in the blood resemble those in the mucosae (e.g., colon), as observed with Nef as well as Gag (1946). Moreover, HIV-specific cytotoxic T cells can be found in semen and can share epitopes with CTLs from the blood (1922).

Some data have suggested that RANTES production by CTLs enhances their cytotoxicity via an interaction with the chemokine receptor CCR3 (1688). Studies with cell clones following immunization have shown that CD8$^+$ CTLs can be more cross-reactive with divergent HIV-1 strains than CD4$^+$ CTLs (1710). The findings most probably reflect the different epitope presentation mechanisms (MHC class I versus class II) for these two lymphocyte subsets.

Generally, one CD8$^+$ CTL can kill two or three target cells (4751), and this activity can be very important in the control of certain viral infections (576, 1101). In culture, this cellular cytotoxicity is demonstrated by a high input of CD8+ cells, typically a CD8+ cell/target cell (E/T) ratio of 25 to 100:1, and is measured in a 4-h ^{51}Cr release assay (Table 11.1). However, CD8+ CTL clones can show this activity at much lower E/T ratios (e.g., 1:1). Moreover, as expected, the cytotoxicity is observed only with viral protein-expressing cells that have the same MHC class I phenotype as the CD8+ cells. A unique early observation of CTL-mediated lysis on HIV-infected cells was that stimulation of the CTLs with viral antigen before evaluation of their ability to lyse their target is often not necessary. However, the response is generally weaker than that of HIV-stimulated CTLs (2303).

The cytotoxic CD8+ effector cells also have a high expression of CD38 and HLA-DR, indicating their activated state (1858, 2396). Memory CD8+ T cells are primarily CD38− and can expand in the presence of IL-15 (509, 2085). As noted above, current data suggest that HIV-specific cytotoxicity is mediated by a subset of effector CD8+ cells secreting IFN-γ and TNF-α (2590), but particularly expressing perforin and CD107 (1789, 2592, 2593) (Table 11.4) (see below).

In subjects who have control of HIV infection, particularly during treatment of acute infection, mature perforin-expressing CD8+ T cells can be found, indicating that normal cell maturation can take place in the face of HIV infection (1826). In chronic HIV infection, there could be a block in cell maturation so that the CD45RA− CCR7− effector memory cell does not differentiate into a T terminal effector (CD45RA+ CCR7−) cell population (Table 11.4).

b. HIV-specific responses

Studies of the antiviral CTL response have shown that CD8+ lymphocytes can kill cells expressing (via a variety of vector systems) peptides from several different HIV proteins, including reverse transcriptase, envelope, Gag, and some accessory proteins (e.g., Vif and Nef) (1865, 2347a, 3534, 3738, 4656a; for reviews, see references 2943 and 3825). An individual's overall CD8+ T-cell anti-HIV response cannot be fully appreciated by measuring the reaction to single epitopes. For this reason, overlapping peptides need to be used and

a variety of viral proteins should be assessed. Estimates of the frequency of peptide-specific CTL clones range from 0.2 to 1% of T cells (3140). In some cases, the CTL clones persist in vivo for at least 5 years (3140); in others, they are replaced (see below). Most surprising was the finding of anti-HIV Env CTLs in healthy uninfected subjects (1865). This observation has suggested a cross-reactivity of certain viral proteins with cellular proteins (see Chapter 10, Section VI).

In general, CTLs can be found that react with several epitopes on Gag, in particular, three conserved regions of the protein (569). In contrast, CTLs against the HIV envelope protein have been identified for only a limited number of epitopes. Recent evidence suggests that HIV, through its envelope protein, down-modulates the CD40 ligand (CD154) on CD4+ T cells and thus interrupts the interactions that lead to efficient antigen presentation by DCs (4933). This finding in cell culture, if present in vivo, could explain the reduced anti-HIV envelope specific responses of CD8+ CTLs.

Nef proteins generally produce the largest number of CD8+ T-cell responses (1681; for a review, see reference 2589). Nevertheless, with overlapping HIV-1 peptides from autologous viral sequences, an increased detection of Tat-specific CD8+ T cells can be found (83). Cross-reactivity of CTLs to viral antigens from different HIV-1 clades has been observed and depends on the viral protein tested (i.e., Nef or Gag) (887). In this regard, the overlapping peptides for immunodominant regions of various viral proteins such as Gag and Nef can differ among populations (e.g., India versus Africa). Thus, to measure CTL activity, it is optimal to identify conserved regions of the viral antigens (4409) or use autologous virus (see below).

Generally in acute or primary HIV infection, CD8+ T-cell responses are made against the early expressed viral proteins, particularly the accessory proteins: Tat, Nef, and Rev (602). Thus, the kinetics of viral epitope expression is one of the factors involved in the T-cell response. They include antigen processing and presentation as well as expression through certain MHC molecules. Importantly, approaches for a vaccine may need to target virus epitopes that are not frequently recognized by the CD8+ T-cell responses (2589) (see Chapter 15).

Several reports suggest that a strong HIV-specific response of CD8$^+$ cells mirrored by a diverse TCR repertoire pattern and tetramer frequency correlates with a beneficial clinical course (1600, 2189, 3319, 3408, 3409) (see Chapters 8 and 13). As noted in Chapter 13, *HLA-B57* and *HLA-B27* are associated with a slower progression to disease (2114). This protection appears to be associated with an immunodominant HIV-specific CTL response restricted by the HLA allele (82, 1516, 1589, 3006).

A broadly reactive HIV-specific CTL response has been documented in long-term survivors (nonprogressors), suggesting an association with maintenance of an asymptomatic state (1737) (see Chapter 13). Nevertheless, delay in progression to disease was found to be associated with the efficiency of cross-recognition of epitopes by prominent TCRs rather than a broad reaction to HIV-1 epitopes (4507). Moreover, IL-2 therapy can broaden this CD8$^+$ T-cell antiviral response when given in acute infection (B. Walker, unpublished observations). In a well-documented study of infected laboratory workers, group-specific and type-specific anti-Gag CTL responses to the homologous virus proteins were noted initially. These responses appeared to broaden over time (4160). Since the individuals remained asymptomatic, a protective role of the CD8$^+$ cell activity was implied.

HIV-specific CD8$^+$ T cells recognizing consensus viral protein epitopes can remain from earlier responses, but they become less effective in recognizing autologous virus (2466). This finding underlines the necessity of examining the antiviral response against autologous virus and not laboratory strains of virus. Moreover, the use of virus-infected primary CD4$^+$ T cells rather than viral proteins expressed on T cell lines would give more clinically relevant information. Subjects with *HLA-B35* alleles are known to progress more rapidly to AIDS (see Chapter 13). Importantly, those individuals with a particular variant (e.g., *B3501PY* in comparison to *B35-Px*) progress more slowly and have a higher level of virus-specific CTLs as measured with Gag, Nef, and Env epitopes (2031). Again, these findings must reflect the manner by which the viral protein epitopes are expressed by the HLA molecule.

In some cases, the CTL response to some viral peptides (e.g., Gag) may decrease with progression to disease, while this activity against other HIV proteins (e.g., Env) does not (3314, 3737, 4650). Recently, only CTL responses to the Gag protein were found to correlate with low viral loads, whereas anti-envelope CTLs were associated with high viremia (2183a). Part of the reduction in CTL function can be related to aging in which telomeres are shortened, reflecting replicative senescence (953), and the expression of granzyme B and perforin is markedly reduced (117, 4856).

It is noteworthy that a decrease in HIV-specific CTL activity may occur in AIDS patients without a reduction in CD8$^+$ cell cytolytic functions directed at other pathogens (e.g., anti-Epstein-Barr virus activities) (617, 1496, 3407). Similarly, T-cell proliferative responses to HIV proteins can be reduced in HIV-infected patients at the same time that these responses to CMV and herpes simplex virus (HSV) proteins are maintained (674, 4658). In comparison to CMV-specific T cells, the CD8$^+$ T cells from HIV-infected individuals can have lower levels of perforin and have persistent CD27 expression, suggesting impaired maturation and reduction in HIV-specific lytic activity (132). In this regard, strong broadly responsive IFN-γ-producing CD8$^+$ cells directed at autologous viruses are found in the late stages of disease in the absence of mutations in the antigen epitopes of the replicating virus. These observations, reflecting poor control of HIV replication, imply a dysfunction in CD8$^+$ cells not recognized by measuring only IFN-γ production (1127, 2592) (see below).

Some investigators have attempted to determine by mathematical modeling the extent of CTL activity and viral production in HIV infection (2237). CTL response can affect viral loads in the blood by killing virus-infected cells. Considering the turnover rate of infected cells subjected to CTL activity as well as viral cytopathicity, the half-life of an infected CD4$^+$ cell target appears to be about 24 h (3470) (see Chapter 8). The major cytotoxic effect is on productively infected cells; the influence on latently infected cells remains to be determined. This estimate reflects the short-lived nature of most Tem CD4$^+$ cells that are major targets for HIV infection (1120). The Tcm and naïve

CD4[+] T cells are long-lived. Therefore, the overall influence on the half-life of all infected CD4[+] cells (including latent infection) may not be great until the late stages of infection (see Chapters 6 and 8). An escape from CTL activity would subsequently permit renewal of viral production and high levels of circulating virus particles (see below).

3. LACK OF ASSOCIATION OF CD8[+] CTLs WITH THE HIV CLINICAL STATE

In contrast to the above findings, several observations have not indicated a direct correlation of CTLs with control of HIV infection (131, 355, 359, 867, 3733, 4545; for a review, see reference 2232). Progression of the disease can be associated with increasing numbers of HIV-infected cells in the presence of CD8[+] effector cells (1681). In some studies, the number of virus-infected cells in the blood of certain subjects has been found to increase despite a high level of anti-Gag-specific CTLs (2231). These findings could reflect the number of viral epitopes evaluated (for Gag and other HIV proteins) and the CTL assay used (2592). In this regard, recent studies suggest that only Gag-specific CTLs are associated with lower viremia in chronic HIV infection and not responses to the envelope or other viral proteins (2183a). These potentially important findings need to be confirmed.

In some studies, no correlation of CD8[+] cells secreting IFN-γ was found in various stages of disease progression (3472). The breadth and magnitude of the HIV-specific responses also have not correlated consistently with viral load or rate of CD4 cell decline, suggesting some other immune activity responsible for control of HIV (355). Therefore, the strong and broad CTL levels observed in HIV infection with high viremia may be induced by the viral loads and not be responsible for virus control.

Other studies have indicated normal or high levels of CD8[+] T cells in the presence of high-level viremia in progressive disease (1470). Importantly, whereas a CTL phenotype may be present in individuals advancing to disease, the function of the CD8[+] cells may be compromised. These findings indicate that virus-specific CD8[+] cells determined by tetramer staining (87) or cell proliferation do not necessarily indicate cytotoxic function. Several reports show persistence of tetramer-positive T cells at high frequencies despite a loss of IFN-γ-producing cells (2290) and cytotoxic activity (132). This observation can explain the discrepancy in correlating the presence of HIV-specific CTLs as measured by tetramer staining, cell proliferation, or IFN-γ production with cell killing (measured by perforin content and CD107 expression) (2592, 2593) (Table 11.1).

Nevertheless, it is important to note that when autologous HIV-1 Gag-specific CD8[+] CTL clones were expanded in vitro and then transferred back to the HIV-infected individuals, they were found

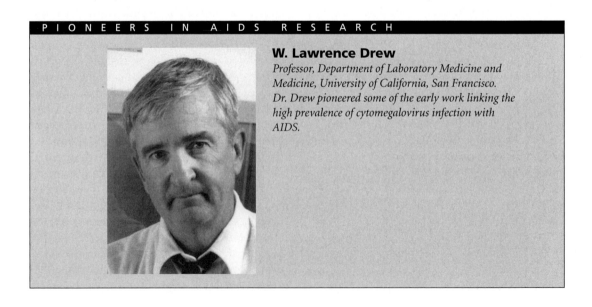

to accumulate near HIV-infected cells and reduce the level of HIV-infected T cells in the blood (518). The results indicated the importance of CD8[+] cells in controlling HIV infection, but could not distinguish between a cytotoxic and a noncytotoxic effect (Section IV). In this regard, studies in primate models using anti-CD8 antibodies have supported a role for CD8[+] cells in controlling HIV infection. With the reduction in CD8[+] cell number, virus replication increased (641, 2869, 3983) (see Chapter 13). Whether CTL activity or the CD8[+] cell noncytotoxic anti-HIV response (CNAR) (2543) is involved needs to be determined (Section IV).

4. CLINICAL RELEVANCE

The above discussion questions the importance of CD8[+] CTLs in controlling HIV infection. Obviously, if these cells function appropriately (i.e., have cytotoxicity) their role could be beneficial. Unfortunately, CTL responses in acute infection are often too late to curtail the extent of the infection (3714). Moreover, HIV-specific CTLs have been found in the gut-associated lymphoid tissue (GALT), even in the absence of CD4[+] T cells (4056), but their function appears to be compromised (1657, 1658). The cells in the GALT expressed granzyme A but not much perforin, although different amounts of perforin RNA were detected in CD8[+] T cells from rectal tissue and PBMC (4057). A lack of strong effector cell function may help maintain the integrity of rectal mucosae but limit the response to HIV. Moreover, the CD8[+] T-cell expression noted after treatment interruption when viremia recurs is mostly due to an increase in preexisting virus-specific CD8[+] cells rather than new immune responses (86). In addition, in chronic HIV infection, CTL activity has been shown to be impaired when the number of CD8[+] cells producing IFN-α, after stimulation with HIV-infected primary CD4[+] T cells, was measured (0.4 to 3%); many more of the CD8[+] cells (25%) were tetramer positive. Importantly, in the subjects studied, the freshly isolated CD8[+] cells also did not kill a peptide-pulsed B cell line or primary HIV-infected CD4[+] T cells (4061a). The results indicate, as noted above, how cytotoxicity using HIV-infected primary CD4[+] T cells as targets may provide a better insight into the effectiveness of this antiviral response.

For the above reasons, it is difficult to assess conclusively the clinical relevance of CTLs in HIV infection. Although this type of antiviral activity has prevented virus spread in some animal model systems (576, 1101), the role of CTLs in HIV infection is not clear. Despite some correlation of CTL activity with a healthy clinical state (617, 3317; for reviews, see references 484, 1573, and 3828), progression of disease with increasing numbers of HIV-infected cells and small numbers of CD4[+] cells occurs in the presence of CD8[+] cells as effector cells (1681). Resistant viruses and dysfunctional CD8[+] cells appear to be involved (Section II.E). Some CTLs could have a detrimental effect on the clinical course (2543, 4971) (Section II.F). It is also conceivable that viruses with lower growth rates may persist because they induce weaker CTLs than more rapidly replicating strains (417).

In summary, measurement of CTL activity against autologous virus in primary CD4[+] cells would appear to provide the best information about the effectiveness of this anti-HIV response. The few studies conducted with autologous virus or its proteins have shown, particularly in advanced-stage disease patients, differences from the antiviral activities observed with HIV consensus peptides (83, 2466, 4061a).

E. HIV Resistance to CTL Activity
1. OVERVIEW

Another property that could differ among HIV isolates is their relative recognition by the cellular immune system, with subsequent killing of the infected cells or suppression of virus replication in the cell. In an early study using PBMC cultures, PCR procedures detected viral genomes from HIV-1 isolates that were not eliminated by antigen-specific CD8[+] CTL, but no consistent isolate of virus could be identified (2988). In another important report, the escape in vivo of a specific virus isolate from the effect of CD8[+] CTLs was described (3499). That finding supported in vitro studies showing that a single amino acid mutation in the viral gp41 protein can eliminate killing of the infected cell by CD8[+] CTLs (956). Several other studies have since described the ability of HIV-1 to avoid CTL activity by selection of escape mutants (4010) (see below). Most recently, viruses that escape CTL activity have been found in individuals with suspected superinfection (84) (see Chapter 4).

Although some mutations are stable, reversions may also reflect a more replication-competent wild-type virus (1374). Moreover, if an HLA type is common in the population, perhaps A2, the mutated virus could be transferred and its resistance to CTLs would remain in the new HLA-A2 individual (1588). However, once an escape mutation takes place, it can revert to the wild type after transmission to an individual with a different HLA allele (2500). In studies of mother-to-child transmission, an escape mutant in the setting of HLA-B27 expression was transferred from the mother to the newborn with a different HLA background, and the CTL escape variant was not effectively targeted by the child's CTLs (1588). Thus, transmission of CTL escape mutants can pose a problem in therapy and vaccine development (see Chapters 14 and 15). A study of two subjects during primary HIV infection identified nonsynonymous nucleotide substitutions in regions of the HIV envelope that were associated with escape from CTL responses. The finding supports further the role of selective pressure in the emergence of CTL-resistant viruses (4213).

2. MECHANISMS FOR HIV RESISTANCE TO CTL ACTIVITIES

a. Escape mutants

In the HIV-infected individual, approximately 14 CD8$^+$ T-cell epitopes at different regions of various viral proteins are presented by different MHC class I molecules (24) and can be targeted by CTLs. Several studies have described the ability of HIV-1 to avoid this CTL activity by selection of escape mutants via mutational events in the recognized epitope (102, 447, 1590, 3603, 4010). These genetic mutations affecting a viral protein occur often and can be influenced by the response of the immune system, particularly CD8$^+$ cytotoxic T cells.

The resistant viruses can be less fit than the wild-type virus (4644). This resistance could occur early in primary infection (447, 3603), reflecting selective pressure by the immune system, and can be associated with progression to disease (1590). However, escape from CTL activity at a limited level seems an unusual reason for a pathogenic course, since CTLs to multiple viral antigens are usually present. For this reason, data on the T-cell repertoire and the

breadth of the CTL response are important in evaluating the effectiveness of this type of antiviral response (see above). In this regard, studies have indicated that CTLs can be generated against the escape virus, thus illustrating the potential breadth of the CD8$^+$ cell anti-HIV activity (68).

Several other mechanisms have been suggested by which HIV-infected cells could escape CTL activity (Table 11.6). For example, R5 virus may be more resistant because macrophages are less sensitive to CTL activity (1731, 4010). HIV infection is also associated with reduced MHC expression on infected cells (1900, 2162, 3962); both the Tat (1900) and Nef (4014) proteins could be involved (see Chapter 7). Several viruses, including herpesviruses, coronaviruses, paramyxoviruses, and adenoviruses, have been shown to decrease both class I and class II antigen expression on cells (for a review, see reference 3732). Nevertheless, some studies suggest that this mechanism is probably not important in affecting CTL activity in HIV infection (4854). Moreover, reduced MHC expression can increase cell susceptibility to lysis by NK cells (see Chapter 9) (540).

Escape mutations in HIV may represent defective antigen processing at presentation in the context

Table 11.6 Possible mechanisms of virus resistance to anti-HIV CTL activity^a

- Mutation in viral peptide recognized by CTLs (102, 447, 1590, 3499, 3603)
- Less sensitivity of R5 viruses growing in macrophages (1731, 4010)
- Down-modulation of MHC expression by viral proteins (e.g., Nef and Tat) (1900, 2162, 3962, 4014)
- Defective antigen presentation by HIV-infected cells (1126, 4881)
- Lack of binding of viral oligopeptide to TAP (2434)
- Abnormal trimming of antigenic peptides (4054)
- Inhibition of virus peptide recognition by small mutant peptides (346)
- Reduced binding of mutant peptides to HLA (102, 3080)
- High levels of circulating free peptides
- Mutant peptide that can inactivate CTLs (i.e., TCR antagonism) (2234, 2960)
- CD8$^+$ cell suppression of HIV antigen expression (2543)
- Association with follicular dendritic cells (4230)

^{a}TAP, transporter associated with antigen processing; TCR, T-cell receptor.

of the HLA molecule (1126, 4881). The resistant viruses may have a mutation in the flanking region of an epitope that leads to an inability of the ERAP1 process (endoplasmic reticulum aminopeptidase 1) to cleave the peptide to the optimal size, particularly at the terminal residues (1126). Processing can involve degradation of viral proteins by cytosolic protease or by peptidases in the cytosol or endoplasmic reticulum. Alternatively, a lack of binding of the oligopeptide to the transporter associated with antigen processing (TAP) and its translocation into the endoplasmic reticulum (2434) could be responsible. In addition, an abnormal trimming of precursors into antigenic peptides that bind to MHC class I molecules may be involved (4054) (see below).

Escape from CTL activity can take place by masking of an epitope recognized by the CTLs through alterations in its peptide structure. Viral resistance to CTL activity occurs if the protein mutation reduces the ability of the HLA molecule to express the epitope or if the mutated protein does not bind well to a CTL (see above). For example, the peptides and assays used can show mutant peptides that are up to 30-fold less efficient in binding to HLA (e.g., HLA-B27) (see Chapter 13) and thus lead to viral escape from CTLs (102, 3080).

In addition, certain class I epitopes in the form of small mutant peptides can inhibit normal lysis of target cells presenting the original epitope (i.e., cells infected with the original virus). These TCR antagonists may induce anergy in CTL clones (346). Thus, HIV could escape the CTL reaction either by replacement of the normal epitope within the HLA class I molecule with a mutant peptide or by the action of the mutant peptide as an antagonist inactivating the CTLs. In support of the latter mechanism, incubation of CTLs with mutant virus-infected cells reduces CTL killing of cells expressing the wild-type virus (346). Moreover, as would be expected, a large variety of circulating free peptides could tie up the CTLs present and prevent them from interacting with the target cell.

Moreover, if the CTL response is to an immunodominant epitope, the development of other CTLs recognizing new epitopes may not occur. The initial CTL reaction to HIV may prevent a new response (2236, 2960) (see Chapter 14). This variation on "original antigenic sin" in comparing CTL responses to a new variant epitope has been well described for murine lymphocytic choriomeningitis virus (2237). Such a T-cell repertoire antagonism has been described in several systems (1998), as well as in HIV infection (for reviews, see references 2235 and 2960). The exact mechanism for the first process is not known but is somewhat reminiscent of the paralysis to B-cell clonal proliferation (see Chapter 10, Section II.G). In the latter case, however, it is the original virus and not the subsequent virus that prevents a sufficient response to a different strain.

Conceivably, suppression of viral antigen expression by the CD8+ cell antiviral factor (Section IV) could lead to the lack of recognition by CTLs (2543) (see below). Alternatively, the ability of CTLs to lyse infected cells may be compromised by the HIV infection (see above). In some cases, both escape from CD8+ T-cell responses and antiretroviral drugs can select for a resistant virus (e.g., protease gene) (2103). Finally, HIV particles bound to follicular dendritic cells may escape CTL lysis because they are not associated with MHC class I molecules.

b. PD-1 expression

The persistence of virus-specific CD8+ T cells lacking effector cell function has sometimes been described as T cell exhaustion (1365a). An explanation for this loss of CD8+ cell activity could be the programmed death 1 (PD-1) protein (CD279). First identified as a protein up-regulated in T-cell hybridomas undergoing apoptotic cell death, it was recently found to be increased on HIV-specific CD8+ T cells (978a, 3490a, 4461a). PD-1 is a known negative regulator of activated T cells, and its presence correlates directly with impaired CD8+ T-cell function and the extent of clinical disease (978a). An up-regulation of PD-1 on CD8+ T cells as well as CD4+ T cells has correlated with increased viral load and low CD4+ T-cell counts (978a; 4461a). Most HIV-specific CD8+ cells express PD-1 (978a; 4461a). PD-1 expression levels on T cells can vary, and thus T-cell function can differ even within the same person (978a; 1252a; 4461a). In one report, the level of PD-1 surface expression correlated with enhanced sensitivity of HIV-specific CD8+ T cells to apoptosis (3490a). In some ways, this mechanism that inhibits the function of cells in which PD-1 is expressed mirrors the activity of T regulatory cells that down-modulate the activity of other activated T cells (Section V).

PD-1 is a member of the CD28 family of co-stimulation molecules that inhibits rather than activates a signal following its interaction with a ligand. It is a transmembrane protein expressed on many activated cells and interacts with two B7-related ligands, PD-L1 (B7-H1; CD274) and PD-L2 (B7-DC; CD273), that are found on a variety of cells, particularly APC and DCs (1252a). Some cytokines, such as the interferons, can up-regulate PD-L1 expression on APCs and endothelial and epithelial cells (1365a). Enhanced expression of PD-L1 has been reported in HIV infection in association with IL-10 production, HIV viremia, and CD4+ T cell loss (4459a). This increase, linked to immune cell activation, could be a marker of disease progression (4459a).

As observed initially with PD-1 expression in mice (243a), the administration of antibodies that block the interaction of this molecule with its ligands, can restore some cell function (978a, 4461a). The reversibility of this inhibition of antigen-specific T cell responses provides promise in therapy for chronic infections but with the understanding that some interactions may cause autoimmune phenomena (1252a, 4461a).

F. Potential Detrimental Effects of CTL Activity

The CTL activity in response to HIV infection may appear to provide a beneficial effect or have no effect in some studies (see above), but some observations suggest that these cells can be part of the pathogenic pathway (2543, 4971) (Table 11.7) (see Chapter 13). In certain infected individuals, CTL have been found that can lyse autologous or heterologous activated uninfected CD4+ lymphocytes (363, 4914). Thus, this non-MHC-restricted cytotoxic activity can contribute to the loss of CD4+ cells in HIV-infected individuals. Antiviral CTL activity has also been found only in infected people who showed clinical symptoms during primary infection (2390). One acutely infected individual who did not have CTL activity maintained high CD4+ cell numbers and an asymptomatic clinical course (1277). The findings are reminiscent of other CTL activities in autoimmune diseases (2657, 4897) and those described in previous work with HIV-infected subjects (4914). A detrimental role of CD8+ cells has been demonstrated with lymphocytic chori-

Table 11.7 Possible evidence for detrimental effects of CD8+ CTL activity in HIV infection[a]

- Lysis of autologous or heterologous activated uninfected CD4+ lymphocytes (363, 4914)
- Lysis of APC (2247, 2985)
- CTL infiltration of lymph nodes (669, 745)
- Continued presence in AIDS patients (1600, 3733)
- Found in the cerebrospinal fluid of symptomatic patients (2011)
- Involved in lung lymphocytic alveolitis (178)
- Absence of CTL responses in disease-free primates naturally infected with simian lentiviruses (2526)
- CTLs are harmful in other viral infections (e.g., lymphocytic choriomeningitis and Theiler's viruses) (445, 3775)

[a]See also references 2543, 3003, and 4971. APC, antigen-presenting cells.

omeningitis virus and Theiler's virus infections in mice (445, 3775). Destruction of virus-infected DC was involved (see Chapter 13, Section II.D) and could occur in HIV infection (2245). The continued presence of CTL in AIDS patients (1600, 3733), and their presence in cerebrospinal fluid (2011), also suggests that they can have a detrimental role. Moreover, the absence of CTL responses in healthy chimpanzees chronically infected with SIV_{cpz} and in other disease-free primates naturally infected with simian lentiviruses has suggested some relationship between this activity and HIV pathogenesis (2526, 2543) (see Chapter 13). Finally, a detrimental role for CD8+ CTLs in HIV-related Sjögren's syndrome (i.e., autoimmune response) and lung lymphocytic alveolitis has been considered (178).

III. Diffuse Infiltrative Lymphocytosis Syndrome

In terms of CD8+ cell responses to HIV infection, the diffuse infiltrative lymphocytosis syndrome (DILS) may reflect some anti-HIV activity of these cells (1966, 2135). DILS has been reported for 0.8 to 7% of HIV-infected individuals (2135, 4775). It appears to have a higher prevalence among African-Americans (4775) and is associated with HLA-DR B1, a subtype of HLA-DR5 (2135).

The syndrome in HIV-infected individuals is defined as bilateral salivary gland enlargement or xerostomia for more than 6 months and salivary or labial gland lymphocyte infiltration with a predominance of CD8+ T cells (1968). In some cases, a neuropathy has been described with a diffuse cellular infiltrative syndrome (1499). The syndrome can include infiltration of the lungs, gastrointestinal tract, and kidneys as well as salivary glands by CD8+ cells.

An increase in the number of circulating CD8+ lymphocytes is also noted and the patients have a delay in CD4+ T-cell loss. The cellular immune response appears to be stimulated by HIV antigens and is found in individuals who have survived a long time with infections. Its occurrence has been associated with expression of EBV and HIV proteins in ductal cells (3736). A similar symptom complex has been described in children who are long-term survivors, particularly those infected around the time of delivery (995). How this syndrome relates to CD8+ cell function is not clear. Nevertheless, the clinical course suggests a beneficial role of these cells perhaps via a noncytotoxic activity (Section IV). DILS patients need to be followed long-term because of the potential development of B-cell lymphoma (1968, 2135).

IV. CD8+ Cell Noncytotoxic Anti-HIV Response

A. General Observations

In addition to having anti-HIV cytotoxic activity associated with CD8+ cells, a subset of these T cells can suppress HIV replication in infected CD4+ cells (Tables 11.5 and 11.8) without killing the cells. Initially, this cellular antiviral activity was recognized by studying individuals who were asymptomatic and did not yield HIV from their cultured PBMC. When their CD8+ cells were removed from the blood sample by panning with monoclonal antibodies to CD8, high levels of virus were released from the CD4+ cells remaining in the culture (4660). The replacement of CD8+ cells in this culture at levels that were far below those used to demonstrate CTL activity (CD8+ cell/CD4+ cell ratio of <1:1) led to complete suppression of virus replication. Subsequent removal of the CD8+ cells again revealed virus-releasing cells. While the effect appears to be most evident when effector and target cells are MHC compatible, non-MHC-restricted suppression can be readily demonstrated (2740, 4658).

This CD8+ cell noncytotoxic anti-HIV response (CNAR) correlates with cell activation (2396, 4763) and the production of a CD8+ cell antiviral factor (CAF) (see below). CNAR has been confirmed by several groups (396, 512, 606, 777, 885, 1554, 2095, 3596, 4444), and all the observations indicate that CD8+ cells suppress HIV production without affecting the proliferation or expression of activation markers on CD4+ cells and without killing the virus-infected cells (2543, 2549, 2735, 4662).

CNAR can be measured with naturally infected CD4+ cells obtained from infected individuals (endogenous assay) as well as with normal CD4+ cells obtained from seronegative individuals and acutely infected in culture with HIV (acute infection assay) (4658) (for a review, see references 2543 and 2549). Suppression of virus replication in both CD4+ lymphocytes and macrophages has been demonstrated (255, 2543, 3108). Moreover, these CD8+ cells show similar responses against many different isolates

Table 11.8 Characteristics of the CD8+ cell noncytotoxic anti-HIV response (CNAR)

- Does not involve cell killing
- Property of CD8+ T cells, not CD4+ cells, NK cells, or macrophages
- Exhibited predominantly by the CD8+ HLA-DR+ CD28+ CD11b− human cell subset
- Associated with VCAM expression on CD8+ cells
- Blocks HIV replication in naturally or acutely infected CD4+ cells
- Can block HIV replication at low CD8+ cell/CD4+ cell ratios (<0.05:1)
- Correlates directly with clinical status and high CD4+ cell counts
- Early response to HIV infection; occurs before seroconversion
- Active against all isolates of HIV-1, HIV-2, and SIV tested
- Dose dependent
- Not MHC restricted
- Blocks HIV at transcription and does not affect earlier steps in virus replication cycle
- Observed with CD8+ cells from infected nonhuman primates
- Mediated (at least in part) by a novel soluble anti-HIV factor (Table 11.12)
- Optimal activity with cell-cell contact
- No effect on activation or proliferation of CD4+ cells

^{a}Measured by in vitro assays. For reviews, see references 2528, 2532, and 2543.

of HIV-1 (including the cytopathic strains), HIV-2, and SIV (Table 11.8) (2745, 4662, 4798).

CD8[+] cell clones with this activity have been described (1911, 4453), and some cell clones may have both CTL and noncytotoxic anti-HIV activities (569, 4855). The latter function may be important in preventing harmful effects of CTLs (2543) (Section II.F and Chapter 13). Cells from infected children show a similar response and a relationship between this antiviral activity and their clinical state (2540, 3531, 3562). Purified CD8[+] CD28[+] CD11b[−] cells show high levels of this anti-HIV response (255, 2396), particularly those cells producing IL-2 (511). Thus, the cellular phenotype of this antiviral CD8[+] cell population differs from that of CD28[−] cytotoxic CD8[+] cells (2543, 2735) (Table 11.5) (Section II.C). In this regard, reduction in antiviral responses correlates with the observed decrease in the CD8[+] CD28[+] cell population associated with disease progression (511, 2396, 3794). DNA microarray studies have in-

dicated that the VCAM gene is up-regulated on CD8[+] cells in association with CNAR and CAF production; therefore, this protein, while not CAF, has proven to be another marker of CD8[+] cells with noncytotoxic anti-HIV activity (1078).

CNAR involving virus suppression takes place after integration, before RNA transcription (713, 885, 2738, 2746, 4444) (Figure 11.5). Naturally infected CD4[+] cells, when mixed with CD8[+] cells, have a marked reduction in viral protein and RNA synthesis but remain viable. Screening assays for detection of CNAR have been developed comparing HIV replication in PBMC from infected subjects and controls (637, 2188, 4011). The approach can be helpful in evaluating vaccine approaches (2038). Finally, unlike CTL function (Section II.C), viral isolates that escape CNAR have not been identified (J. A. Levy, unpublished).

In summary, CNAR can be distinguished from the classical antigen-specific cytotoxic activity of CD8[+] cells (2543, 3267, 3825, 4657, 4662) by the

Figure 11.5 Effect of CD8[+] cells and CD8[+] cell antiviral factor (CAF) on parameters of HIV replication. The CD8[+] cell noncytotoxic antiviral response blocks viral replication, as indicated by decreased reverse transcriptase (RT) activity, viral protein expression measured by immunofluorescent antibody (IFA) techniques, and in situ RNA production. This activity has no effect on the number of infected cells in the culture. The antiviral effect is observed as well in a reduction in unspliced (us), single-spliced (ss), and double-spliced (ds) HIV RNA levels compared to a normal expression of β-actin RNA. Finally, the suppressing effect of CD8[+] cells or CAF does not affect the basal-level expression of HIV LTR-driven transcription but blocks induction of this transcription by HIV, simian virus 40 *tat* expression, or phorbol myristate acetate (PMA) using cells in which the HIV LTR has been linked to a reporter gene (2738).

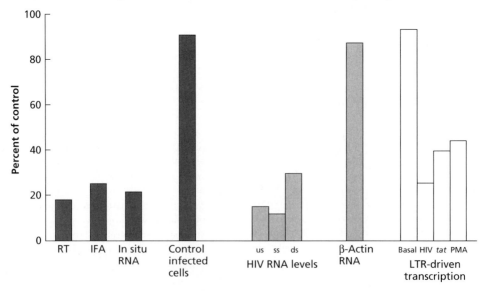

features listed in Tables 11.5 and 11.8. Several of these characteristics have suggested that CNAR is part of the innate immune system (2528, 2549) (Table 11.9) (see also chapter 9).

B. Clinical Relevance

CNAR has been documented in healthy HIV-infected adults as well as children (777, 1554, 2396, 2540, 2543, 2735, 2745, 3562). The CD8+ cell anti-HIV response develops soon after infection (2749) and in combination with the CTL response (446, 2302) can explain the reduction in virus production observed before seroconversion. This CD8+ cell antiviral activity has been shown to diminish over time, concomitant with progression to AIDS (1554, 2396, 2543, 2745). In contrast, in individuals who have been HIV infected for more than 10 years but have resisted development of disease without therapy (i.e., long-term survivors), this anti-HIV response is commonly found at high levels (256, 606, 2520) (see Chapter 13). Thus, CNAR appears to be important in maintaining a healthy clinical state.

In addition, highly exposed uninfected individuals have CNAR without detectable CTL activity (4308) (see Chapter 13). This observation further suggests that this CD8+ cell response resembles a rapid innate immune antiviral activity. Moreover, as noted above (Section II.D.3), temporary depletion of CD8+ cells in chimpanzees chronically infected with HIV-1 and in SIV-infected rhesus monkeys is associated with a return in virus replication (641, 2869, 3983). These findings all indicate that CD8+ cell responses, whether noncytotoxic or cytotoxic, are involved in the control of HIV and SIV infection.

The potential clinical value of CNAR includes as well several features besides its association with long-term survival (Table 11.10). The response

appears to affect both cytopathic and noncytopathic (SI and NSI, X4 and R5) isolates and can reduce virus replication severalfold. By its suppressing activity, it can prevent the emergence of drug-resistant strains, and it does not appear to affect the activation or proliferation of CD4+ cells. Thus, it may in fact restore normal function to infected CD4+ cells. This ability of CD8+ T cells to suppress virus replication has also correlated best with the lack of transmission of virus from infected mothers to newborns (3530). Perhaps importantly, the reduction in expression of viral proteins (e.g., envelope) on cells by this antiviral response could prevent the detrimental effects of CTL activities that might be present in HIV-infected individuals (Section II.F) (Table 11.7) (2543, 4971).

Stimulated CD8+ cells from uninfected subjects have also demonstrated this response (260, 512, 2735, 4660). However, this reactivity is observed more commonly with naturally infected CD4+ cells (214, 3808) and, generally, only at a CD8+ cell/CD4+ cell ratio higher than in HIV-infected individuals (2735, 4660). Moreover, an EBV-specific CTL line from an HIV-seronegative donor has been shown to exhibit CNAR and secrete an antiviral factor (2443). These findings most likely reflect the innate nature of this anti-HIV response (2532), which would be expected in all individuals.

Table 11.9 CD8+ cell noncytotoxic antiviral response is part of the innate immune system

- Not HIV specific; affects several different retroviruses
- Not restricted by MHC class I or class II molecules
- Rapid, early response to HIV infection
- Found in exposed uninfected individuals and decreases after time of exposure—no memory
- Mediated by a secreted cytokine that affects viral transcription

See Section IV and references 2528 and 2532.

Table 11.10 Potential clinical value of CD8+ cell noncytotoxic antiviral activity in HIV infection

- Could ensure long-term survival
- Not affected by viral heterogeneity (HIV-1 and HIV-2); cytopathic and noncytopathic strains are sensitive
- Can prevent several log units of virus replication in vitro (and possibly 3–5 log units in vivo)
- Can prevent emergence of drug-resistant strains and immune escape mutants by blocking virus replication at transcription
- Can prevent dual infection by HIV and recombination
- Does not affect viability, activation, or proliferation of CD4+ cells
- Prevents effects of CTL activities that could be destructive to the host (e.g., death of uninfected as well as infected cells)

For reviews, see references 2543 and 2549.

C. Factors Influencing the CD8+ Cell Noncytotoxic Anti-HIV Response

Why this CD8+ cell noncytotoxic antiviral activity is lost over time is not known, but the phenomenon may reflect the reduction in a particular activated cell subset (e.g., CD8+ HLA-DR+ CD28+ CD11b− cells) (2396) or a loss of its function (Table 11.8). Perhaps the difference in survival of CD8+ cells in culture (3609) and the known presence of apoptosis of CD8+ cells in HIV infection (1581, 2559, 2647, 2984) could help explain this phenomenon. Since apoptosis appears to be related to the cytokines produced (see Chapter 6, Section IV), a shift from type 1 to type 2 cytokines may be partly responsible for this loss in CD8+ cell function (814) (Figure 11.4).

1. ROLE OF CYTOKINES

The possible effect of cytokines on CD8+ cell antiviral activity has been studied in approaches to determine the reason for a reduced CD8+ cell anti-HIV response. As reviewed in Section II.C, it is known that TH1-type CD4+ cells increase cell-mediated immunity, whereas TH2-type CD4+ cells are associated with weak cellular and strong antibody responses. Since cytokines from each cell type can cross-regulate each other (Figure 11.4), whether particular cytokines might influence the CD8+ cell anti-HIV activity has been evaluated. These studies demonstrated that type 1 cytokines (e.g., IL-2) in-crease the CD8+ cell antiviral activity, whereas the type 2 cytokines (e.g., IL-4 and IL-10) reduce the CD8+ cell antiviral activity (258, 2206) (Figure 11.6). IL-12 showed no effect. The results reflect the importance of IL-2 for this response. IL-4 and IL-10 down-modulate IL-2 production (258, 3864). IL-4 can also decrease the expression of the CD28 molecule (2647), which is involved in this response (255) (see below). IL-10 can also decrease B7 expression on APC (4765) and thereby reduce the costimulatory process involved in activating CD8+ cell function (see below). Similar observations have been made with CTL activity: type 1 and not type 2 responses have correlated in vivo with strong CD8+ CTL activity (4687) (Section II.D).

2. CD28 AND CD3 COSTIMULATION

Further studies examining the reduction in CD8+ cell noncytotoxic anti-HIV activity over time indicated the importance of costimulation via the CD28 molecule in maintaining CD8+ cell function. The lymphocyte response is optimal when stimulation occurs both through the TCR (CD3) interaction with antigen within the MHC molecule and through the interaction of the CD8+ cell CD28 molecule with the B7 molecule on APC (e.g., macrophages and DCs) (for review, see references 3698 and 2617). This effect appears to be mediated by increased IL-2 production and ex-

Figure 11.6 Effect of cytokines on the CD8+ cell noncytotoxic anti-HIV response. CD8+ cells were stimulated in the presence of type 1 or type 2 cytokines for 3 days. After being washed, they were tested for their ability to suppress HIV replication in acutely infected CD4+ lymphocytes. From reference 258 with permission.

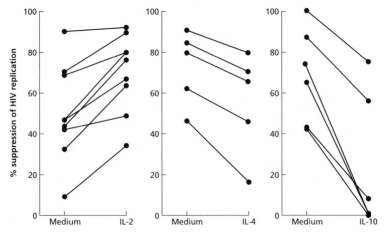

pression of the IL-2R (Figure 11.7) (663, 3282). It involves the transcription of the IL-2 gene through the activation of an enhancer element within the IL-2 promoter (1358, 1727). Cell culture studies demonstrated that anti-CD3 and anti-CD28 antibodies can increase CNAR in both asymptomatic and AIDS patients (Figure 11.8). This costimulation increased IL-2R expression on the cell surface and was mediated by IL-2 (255).

In addition, when CD8$^+$ cells from HIV-infected individuals were stimulated in the presence of macrophages (that express MHC and B7), their noncytotoxic antiviral response was markedly increased, reflecting IL-2 production (255). Moreover, mimicking these beneficial effects of anti-CD3/anti-CD28 antibodies and macrophages on CNAR, the coculture of CD8$^+$ cells with mature DC expressing B7 and MHC restored CNAR in CD8$^+$ cells with diminished anti-HIV activity. The effect was primarily mediated by DC secretion of IL-15 (635). Subsequent studies indicated that besides IL-2, IL-15 alone will enhance CNAR, as will IFN-α. All of these findings place further emphasis on cytokines as immune therapy for enhancing this anti-HIV activity (see Chapter 14).

D. Response to Superinfection

Another finding related to CD8$^+$ cells that potentially affects the clinical outcome is the resistance of cultured PBMC from asymptomatic individuals to superinfection by other strains of HIV-1. Despite the known presence of many uninfected CD4$^+$ cells in their cultured PBMC, no acute infection by X4 or R5 viruses (whether HIV-1 or HIV-2) can take place unless the CD8$^+$ cells are first removed (257, 2095). HIV enters and integrates but is not produced by the infected cells (257). CD8$^+$ cells prevent the superinfected PBMC from releasing virus. With PBMC from symptomatic patients, superinfection can be demonstrated. The replication of both the endogenous and exogenous viruses by these PBMC reflects the absence of a strong CD8$^+$ cell antiviral response (257). These findings are noted in the CNAR screening assay cited above (Section IV.A) (637, 2188).

E. CD8$^+$ Cell Noncytotoxic Responses in Other Virus Infections

CNAR has been demonstrated as well in the SIV system with rhesus macaques (1093, 2094, 3596, 3597), sooty mangabeys (3596), African green monkeys (1208), HIV-infected chimpanzees (641, 1911), and naturally infected chimpanzees (2168). It has also been observed in HIV-2-infected baboons (396) and infected cats (762, 915, 2020). Thus, CNAR appears to be a general immune response to infection by lentiviruses and other retroviruses.

It is noteworthy that a similar type of noncytotoxic suppression of virus expression has been de-

Figure 11.7   Costimulation of CD8$^+$ T cells. The lymphocyte response is optimal following the interaction of the T-cell receptor (TCR) with an MHC class I molecule associated with antigen, together with the interaction of the CD28 molecules on the T cells with the B7 molecules on antigen-presenting cells [APC]) (e.g., macrophages and dendritic cells). The response appears to be mediated by increased IL-2 production and expression of the IL-2 receptor (IL-2R) (663, 3282). A role of IL-15 produced by the APC has also been noted (635).

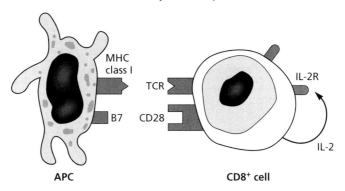

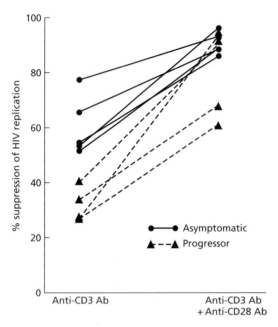

Figure 11.8   When CD8[+] cells are stimulated in the presence of antibodies to the T-cell receptor (TCR) complex (anti-CD3 antibody) together with antibodies to the costimulatory molecule CD28, their ability to suppress HIV replication in infected CD4[+] cells is increased both in asymptomatic individuals and particularly in AIDS patients (progressors). From reference 255 with permission. © 1997 The American Association of Immunologists, Inc.

scribed for hepatitis B virus antigens in transgenic mice and infected chimpanzees. The CD8[+] cells function through secretion of TNF-α and IFN-γ (1662, 1663). Recent evidence suggests that CD8[+] cells also maintain HSV type 1 in a latent stage by production of soluble factors (2178), most probably IFN-γ and TNF-α. Furthermore, human NK cells have been reported to inhibit CMV replica-

tion in infected fibroblasts by a noncytotoxic mechanism involving lymphotoxin-dependent induction of IFN-β (1973).

F. CD8[+] Cell Antiviral Factor (CAF)

A soluble factor secreted by the CD8[+] cells is involved in the CD8[+] cell anti-HIV response (512, 4659). Cell-to-cell contact, however, is the most efficient method for suppressing HIV production. Whether both activities reflect the same antiviral mechanism is not yet clear. The presence of CAF can be shown by adding supernatants from CD8[+] cell cultures directly onto infected CD4[+] cells (2735, 4658). Virus replication is substantially reduced without any effect on cell viability or proliferation. As noted with CNAR, CAF blocks viral transcription (2735) (Figure 11.6), and in some studies, it has reduced reporter gene expression mediated by the LTR from HTLV and Rous sarcoma virus (886). Whether a site in the LTR such as NFAT-2 or NF-κB is affected (885, 886) requires further study. For example, some studies suggest that the anti-HIV activity does not involve NF-κB (2651) or several other domains of the LTR (K. Bonneau, and J. Levy, unpublished observations). The results have suggested that the antiviral effect is upstream from HIV production affecting the transcription/elongation process (e.g. P-TEFb) (C. Mackewicz, M. Peterlin, and J. A. Levy, unpublished observations) (see Chapter 7).

The amount of CAF produced by CD8[+] cells is small; only up to a 25% dilution of culture fluid will still show 50% reduction of HIV replication (Figure 11.9). The level of CAF produced by CD8[+] cells correlates with the clinical state (2735, 4660). The largest production is by CD8[+] cells cultured from healthy individuals with high CD4[+] cell

Figure 11.9   Quantity of CD8[+] cell antiviral factor (CAF) produced by CD8[+] cells. Dilutions of CAF-containing fluid from cultured CD8[+] cells from an asymptomatic individual indicate that a 1:4 dilution will still show a 50% reduction in HIV replication as measured by virus reverse transcriptase (RT) activity in the culture fluid. Fluids from CD8[+] cells of healthy uninfected individuals or those with AIDS do not show evidence of CAF production.

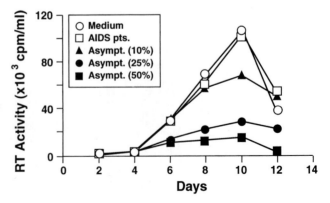

counts. This limited secretion of CAF makes it difficult to identify the anti-HIV protein responsible. It is conceivable that CAF represents a group of factors that are only recognized when used together. Such a situation has been observed, as noted below, with the β-chemokines that are produced by CD8+ cells and block R5 virus infection (822). Nevertheless, the small amount of β-chemokines produced by CD8+ cells in relation to their anti-HIV activity (1609, 2745), the activity of CAF against both X4 and R5 viruses, and the continual ability of CAF fluids to suppress virus replication in the presence of neutralizing antibodies to the β-chemokines support the conclusion that a particular protein, not yet identified, is involved.

CAF was shown to be a protein by its sensitivity to protease and has an estimated size of 10 to 50 kDa (2532). It is resistant to heat (86°C, 10 min) and to low pH (2.0). It can withstand ether extraction and lyophilization (2532, 2543). Whereas most cytokines are made within the first 3 days of stimulation (2744, 2746), CAF is secreted maximally at 5 to 9 days after CD8+ cell activation (2543, 2744). The various characteristics of the factor are listed in Table 11.11. Importantly, it is not found in cellular granules (2747).

Besides the finding of CNAR in SIV-infected rhesus macaques (2094), CD8+ T cells of rhesus macaques infected with attenuated SIV and CD8+

Table 11.11 Characteristics of the CD8+ cell anti-HIV factor[a]

- Produced only by activated CD8+ T cells
- Active against HIV-1, HIV-2, and SIV
- Protease sensitive (e.g., *Staphylococcus* V8 protease)
- Stable at high temperature (86°C, 10 min)
- Stable at low pH (pH 2.0)
- Size of 10–50 kDa
- Resistant to ether and lyophilization
- Lacks identity with other known cytokines
- Blocks HIV replication in naturally and acutely infected CD4+ cells
- Blocks HIV transcription
- Does not affect CD4+ cell activation or proliferation
- Not found in cellular granules
- Precursor protein may be activated by proteolytic cleavage

[a]For a review, see reference 2532.

T cells from a long-term nonprogressing SIV_{mac239}^- infected monkey have been noted to release a soluble factor(s) capable of inhibiting SIV replication in vitro (1464, 4240). Moreover, recent studies with cynomolgus macaques infected with SIV_{mac251}^- indicated that CAF-like activity correlated with plasma viral load and CD4+ T-cell counts (1093). Whether this antiviral response was induced or was associated previously with virus replication remains to be determined. The direct association with CD4+ cell counts suggests a beneficial role for this antiviral factor. In addition, recent studies with CD8+ T cells from HIV-2-infected individuals have shown a greater production of anti-HIV proteins than cells from HIV-1-infected subjects (39). The findings may explain the decreased transmission of HIV-2 and the slower progression to disease in infected individuals (see Chapter 1). Anti-FIV soluble factors are also observed in antigen-stimulated feline CD8+ T lymphocytes, and they suppress viral replication (762) (see below).

As reviewed below, a large number of cytokines have been evaluated, and none has had the characteristics of CAF (Table 11.12).

G. Antiviral Activity of Other Cytokines

1. CD8+ T-CELL-ASSOCIATED FACTORS

Herpesvirus saimiri (HVS)-transformed CD8+ T-cell lines from infected and uninfected children have produced a soluble, heat-stable, pH-stable factor that is less than 10 kDa in size as well as other antiviral factors whose nature has not yet been identified (3136). One low-molecular-weight soluble protein produced by HVS-transformed cells appears to inhibit HIV-1 replication through a STAT1 (signal transducer activator transcription 1)-dependent process (685). The factor activates STAT1, leading to interferon regulatory factor 1 induction with inhibition of gene expression via the HIV-1 LTR. Another protein, prothymosin α, has been found to be associated with the anti-HIV activity in culture fluids of an HVS-transformed CD8+ T-cell line. The activity appears to inhibit HIV-1 LTR transcription (3136a) in macrophages and not in T lymphocytes. Moreover, in a study of an HTLV-1-transformed CD8+ T-cell line, the amino-terminal fragment of a urokinase type plasminogen activator was found in culture fluids

Table 11.12 Proteins lacking identity to the CD8[+] cell antiviral factor (CAF)

- IL-1 to -13, IL-15, IL-18 (2744)
- IL-16 (2742)
- TNF-α, TNF-β (2744)
- IFN-α, IFN-β, IFN-γ (512, 2744)
- TGF-β (2744)
- Granulocyte-macrophage colony-stimulating factor (2744)
- Granuloctye colony-stimulating factor (2744)
- RANTES (407, 2736, 2737, 3108)
- MIP-1α, MIP-1β (2736, 2737, 3108, 3833)
- Monocyte chemoattractant proteins 1, 2, and 3 (1611, 4713)
- Monocyte-derived chemokine (3108)
- SDF-1 (2372)
- Growth-regulated oncogenes α and β (1611)
- Leukemia inhibitory factor (1611)
- Granzymes A and B (2743, 2748)
- IFN-γ-inducible protein 10 (IP-10) (1611)
- Granulolysin (2747)
- Lymphotactin (1611)
- α-Defensins (684, 2750)
- NK cell enhancing factors A and B
- RNase
- Protegrins
- Histatins
- TNF receptors

[a]Those features not referenced are unpublished observations from J. A. Levy et al. (reviewed in references 2532 and 2543).

that inhibited the assembly and binding of HIV-1 (4641a). Production of these two proteins by primary CD8[+] T cells has not been reported, so their clinical relevance is unknown.

Other investigators suggested that α-defensins 1, 2, and 3 represented the anti-HIV activity produced by CD8[+] T cells (4932), but these anti-HIV factors are not made by CD8[+] cells and were found in the non-CD8[+] cells in the irradiated monolayer used to culture the CD8[+] cells (2750). These small innate molecules, both α and β, produced mostly in neutrophils, show anti-HIV activity (2750, 3638, 4676). They are among several natural products aside from CAF that come from various human cells and have anti-HIV activity (Table 11.13).

Other investigators have reported two heat-labile components produced by CD8[+] T-cell lines

that were considered involved in CNAR and CAF activity; one of these bound to heparin and the other did not (1473, 1474). The heparin-binding protein appears to be a modified form of anti-thrombin III (ATIII) that is found in the fetal bovine serum used in CAF assays. These investigators concluded that CAF activates ATIII in the culture medium to give antiviral activity. Nevertheless, this effect was not consistently observed with CAF-containing fluids or in assays conducted without serum proteins (2532).

The observations on ATIII could have relevance to early studies conducted during the evaluation of CAF as a protein. It was found that certain serine protease inhibitors (e.g., leupeptin) used to inactivate the proteases mixed with CAF directly blocked CAF activity and CNAR in up to 70% of cases (2739). Therefore, the anti-HIV activity of CAF could involve a CD8[+] cell protease or a product of CD8[+] cells that binds to a protease inhibitor. The protease could also act on a precursor protein of CAF and cleave it into an active form (2532).

Other natural antiviral factors produced by CD8[+] cells have been identified by gene microarray approaches (1475): NK-enhancing factors A and B. These antioxidant enzymes could inhibit HIV transcription by down-regulation of the NF-κB pathway (2532). Nevertheless, they are made by other cells besides CD8[+] cells and are not present in adequate amounts in CD8[+] cell fluids to represent CAF or have clinical relevance (1475).

2. CHEMOKINES

a. β-Chemokines

In other attempts to define the nature of CAF, several investigators examined cytokines produced by CD8[+] cells. One in vitro study found that three β-chemokines, RANTES, MIP-1α, and MIP-1β, particularly when used together, were anti-HIV factors produced by CD8[+] cells (822). The β-chemokines are found within cytolytic granules of CD8[+] cells and are secreted as sulfated proteoglycans (4642). This association with proteoglycans increases their ability to block HIV infection.

Differences in virus sensitivity to these cytokines are observed. R5 viruses are sensitive, and X4 viruses are not (822, 2009, 2737). The variance can be explained by the fact that only the R5

Table 11.13 Natural human factors with anti-HIV activity

- IFN-α, IFN-β (2744, 4849)
- TGF-β (2744)
- IL-8[a] (2744)
- IL-10 (2744)
- IL-16 (219, 2742)
- IL-18 (761)
- β-Chemokines: RANTES, MIP-1α, MIP-1β (824)
- SDF-1 (409, 3315)
- TNF-α[a] (2744)
- Macrophage-derived chemokine (3385)
- Leukemia inhibitory factor (3440)
- Monocyte chemotactic protein 2 (1611)
- Lymphotactin (1611)
- α-Defensins 1–3 (3205, 4932)
- β-Defensins (3638)
- RNase (3841, 4887)
- Prothymosin α (3136a)
- Secretory leukocyte protease inhibitor (2949)
- α-1-Antitrypsin (4063)
- D-Lactoalbumin (4346)
- CD8+ cell 6-kDa protein (3136)
- 6-kDa protein (3136)
- NK cell enhancing factors A and B (1475)
- CD8+ cell product modifying anti-thrombin III (1473)
- Urokinase-type plasminogen activator[b] (4641a)
- Unidentified CD4+ cell anti-HIV factors (572, 2501, 3871, 4147)
- Factor associated with human chorionic gonadotropin (2697a)
- NK and γδ T-cell anti-HIV factors (1265, 3540)

[a]At high concentrations.
[b]Amino-terminal fragment.

viruses use the β-chemokine receptor CCR5 for virus entry (see Chapter 3). In addition, the R5 isolates can differ in their relative sensitivities to the β-chemokines (i.e., 500 pg to 500 ng) (C. Mackewicz and J. A. Levy, unpublished observations).

Chemokines are a family of structurally related proteins that induce migration of specific subsets of leukocytes to sites in the body and are involved in the generation of cellular inflammation (21, 3340). (For a review on chemokines and their function, see reference 4973; see also Chapter 3, Tables 3.2 and 3.3). These chemoattractant cytokines are also made by a large number of cell types that are sensitive to HIV infection, including CD4+ lymphocytes, NK cells, and macrophages (21, 865, 3340). Thus, both X4 and R5 virus infections can cause the release of chemokines that can recruit cells to lymphoid tissue and increase the spread of HIV (1318, 1610, 4740). This finding has questioned the clinical relevance of these proteins as antiviral factors in HIV infection.

Cell culture studies with the β-chemokines have indicated that in high concentrations, they can act individually in blocking R5 HIV replication, but the presence of all three at amounts ranging from 500 pg to 500 ng is most effective (822); C. Mackewicz and J. A. Levy, unpublished). The block appears to take place at the cell surface by competitive inhibition of the viral envelope protein for the β-chemokine receptor CCR5 and down-regulation of the receptor (see Chapter 3). MIP-1α and other β-chemokines can also inhibit early postentry steps in viral replication by suppressing cell activation (93). Importantly, the chemokines do not block viral LTR transcription (2485), which is suppressed by CAF (2738).

It is noteworthy that β-chemokines, depending on their concentration, can prevent infection via competition at the cell surface (e.g., β-chemokines and SDF-1) or enhance replication through an interaction with cell surface receptors and activation of signal transduction processes. The findings reflect the cell surface and intracellular effects of chemokines (2157). For example, β-chemokines block R5 virus infection of DCs but can enhance X4 virus infection of these cells (4670). They can increase the replication of X4 viruses in CD4+ T cells through signal transduction (2205) probably by up-regulation of CD4 and CXCR4 expression. High concentrations of RANTES oligomers interacting with cell surface glycosaminoglycans can also induce cells to be more permissive to HIV infection (4478).

As noted above, the clinical relevance of the β-chemokines in preventing disease progression has been questioned (2009, 2736), because R5 as well as X4 viruses can be found in individuals progressing to AIDS. Moreover, no significant difference has been noted in levels of chemokine production by activated CD8+ cells from HIV-infected individuals regardless of their clinical state

Murray B. Gardner
Professor Emeritus, University of California, Davis.
Dr. Gardner played an important role in determining
the participation of SIV in immune deficiency and in
defining differences among HIV and SIV strains.

(407, 800, 2736, 3833). In addition, levels of β-chemokines in serum generally do not distinguish patients with AIDS from asymptomatic individuals (2937, 3563, 4868, 4913). The high levels of RANTES (3563) and MIP-1β (4389) that can be found during disease progression most likely reflect immune cell activation.

Some reports indicate that CD8$^+$ T cells from healthy HIV-infected individuals produce high levels of MIP-1α and MIP-1β, but not RANTES, in comparison to the levels produced in uninfected persons or those with progressive disease (824). This association of β-chemokine production by cultured CD8$^+$ cells stimulated by HIV-1 proteins may reflect the overall antiviral responses of CD8$^+$ cells (1275) or reflect the presence of a high number of CD4$^+$ cells in the culture that are major producers of β-chemokines (1610, 4525).

In this regard, studies have found that β-chemokine-producing T-cells are associated with high viremia and chronic T cell activation and not with protection from disease (2022). Importantly, CD4$^+$ cells infected by R5 viruses produce higher levels of β-chemokines than cells infected by X4 viruses (1610). This finding suggests that instead of suppressing virus replication, these cellular products can attract more target cells to the site of infection. Seminal plasma also contains RANTES at levels correlating directly with seminal HIV-1 RNA levels. Whether this β-chemokine recruits more target cells or reduces virus-infected host cells remains to be determined (4301).

CAF lacks identity to the β-chemokines (2736, 2744, 3108). High levels of the β-chemokines do not affect acute infection of CD4$^+$ cells by X4 viruses, but both R5 and X4 strains are sensitive to CAF (2736). Moreover, infection of DCs with X4 or R5 isolates is not inhibited by the β-chemokines (3833). In addition, as noted above (section IV .F), when CD8$^+$ cells are cultured with CD4$^+$ cells infected by either R5 or X4 viruses, neutralizing antibodies to the β-chemokines do not block the suppression of HIV replication (255, 717, 2208, 2736, 3392, 3833). Moreover, neutralizing antibodies to the β-chemokines do not affect the antiviral activity of CAF-containing fluids with HIV-infected CD4$^+$ lymphocytes (2485, 2737) and macrophages (256). Finally, SIV$_{cpz}$, an R5 virus, was suppressed by CD8$^+$ lymphocytes, in a noncytotoxic manner in which the β-chemokines were not involved (3335).

b. Stomal cell-derived factor-1 (SDF-1)
Another chemokine, SDF-1, interacts with CXCR4 and can block X4 virus infection of CD4$^+$ cells (409, 3315) (see Chapter 3). SDF-1 is consistently expressed on mucosal epithelial cells and thus could down-modulate CXCR4 and reduce the efficacy of X4 virus transfer during transmission (28). This chemokine, however, has not been shown to be associated with CD8$^+$ cell suppression (2372). Moreover, high SDF-1 expression in PBMC does not correlate with CD8$^+$ T-cell suppression (3321). In some cases, SDF-1 can increase the ability of Tat to transactivate the HIV-1 LTR

and thus enhance R5 virus replication (2804). It differs from CAF by only inhibiting X4 virus and acting at the cell surface. The X4 virus gp120 can mimic SDF-1 in eliciting chemotactic activity (225).

c. Macrophage-derived chemokine

The macrophage-derived chemokine (MDC) also inhibits HIV replication in primary macrophages but not T lymphocytes, and the function appears to be at a postentry level (906). CAF has been shown not to be MDC (3108). Moreover, the anti-HIV activity of MDC is controversial; suppression of HIV replication can be seen only in some $CD4^+$ lymphocytes, and in certain cases, it enhanced HIV replication in macrophages (3107).

d. IL-16

IL-16 was recognized for its potential role in suppressing SIV replication via $CD8^+$ cells in African green monkeys (219, 1753, 2732). This chemokine-like protein could be a potential anti-HIV factor (219) because of its known interaction with CD4 (928). In some studies, a block of HIV at the cell surface was observed but also at a postentry process (4951), most likely at transcription (96, 4491). Moreover, increased levels of plasma IL-16 have been found during the asymptomatic phase of HIV infection, and a decrease in this cytokine is noted with disease progression (96). However, other studies with purified recombinant IL-16 and antibodies to IL-16 have demonstrated that human $CD8^+$ cells do not make a sufficient amount of this chemokine to block HIV replication. Furthermore, neutralizing antibodies to IL-16 do not affect the antiviral effects of CAF (2742). Finally, levels of IL-16 production by $CD8^+$ cells are not different among HIV-infected individuals in different clinical states (407).

3. OTHER ANTI-HIV CYTOKINES

Various soluble factors, including cytokines not produced only by $CD8^+$ cells, have been found to be associated with anti-HIV activity (Table 11.13). Several have been mentioned above. An unidentified factor that blocks HIV transcription has been reported in $CD4^+$ cell fluids when cocultured with monocytes (572). Its relationship to CAF has not been evaluated. A soluble factor has also been found to be secreted by a transformed $CD4^+$ T-cell line (2501). This HIV-1-resistant factor blocks virus NF-κB activity; thus, it appears to act in a different manner than CAF. Another anti-HIV factor has been found to be secreted by the $CD4^+$ Sup T-1 cell line infected by an NL 4-3 variant virus attenuated with a defect in the *vif* gene. The product blocked HIV at transcription, most likely via an effect on the Tat-mediated LTR during transmission (4147). Further studies on this factor have not been reported. Moreover, soluble factors produced by $CD4^+$ T cells from an HIV-1 long-term survivor appear to block virus after entry and probably after integration (3871). SDF-1 was not responsible, and a factor similar to CAF may be involved. Additional work on this finding has not been published.

Studies examining the noncytotoxic anti-HIV activity resulting from an alloimmune response of PBMC indicated that an RNase was involved (3841). It blocks HIV replication prior to reverse transcription (3521, 4887). Other studies have not shown the presence of mRNA for RNase in $CD8^+$ cells or the presence of this protein in CAF fluids (2532). Another cytokine with antiviral activity is IL-18, which can block early stages of viral infection through the induction of IFN-γ. IL-18 also reduces CD4 expression on the cell surface (761) but is not produced in large amounts by $CD8^+$ cells (unpublished observations). In some studies, a factor found in human chorionic gonadotropin preparations inhibited HIV replication as well as the growth of Kaposi's sarcoma-derived cells (2697a). Its identification has not been reported. Moreover, an antiviral factor has been detected that is produced by placental cells, has a molecular size of less than 50 kDa, and is not one of the known chemokines (4071). It most likely is related to the leukemia inhibitory factor (3440).

Finally, NK cells and γδ T cells have been reported to produce soluble factors that block both R5 and X4 virus infection (1265, 3540). The relationships of these antiviral substances to CAF are not known.

4. SUMMARY

By function and antigenic features, CAF lacks identity to other cytokines, including the interferons, TNF-α, growth factors, defensins, and the chemokines (513, 2737, 2742, 2744) (see above and Tables 9.5, 11.12, and 11.13 for the cytokines evaluated).

V. T Regulatory Cells

Over 10 years ago, the presence of T lymphocytes that regulate the immune response was suggested by studies in mice in which removal of CD4[+] CD25[+] lymphocytes caused a variety of autoimmune diseases (3877). This finding was confirmed by other investigators (for a review, see reference 4096). In mice, four types of regulatory T cells have been identified: antigen-induced CD25[+] type 2-like cells producing IL-4 and IL-10, thereby antagonizing type 2 effector cells; CD4[+] CD25[+] RB[low] TR1 cells that produce IL-10; CD4[+] CD8[+] T cells producing transforming growth factor β (TGF-β); and, most important, naturally occurring CD4[+] CD25[+] regulatory T cells suppressing cell proliferation through cell contact (3877, 4426; for a review, see reference 4096). These observations appeared to revitalize original reports over 30 years ago by Gershon and Kondo (1497) that suppressor T lymphocytes exist that can affect immune activity. In these early studies, however, emphasis was placed on cells that have more of a CD8[+] cell phenotype. These initial studies (1497) could not be pursued further because monoclonal antibodies were not available and cytokines were not well defined (1614).

Importantly, observations from mouse T regulatory cell studies, which have helped to define the field, may not be directly applicable to findings with human T regulatory cells (4096a). In humans, the T regulatory cells have been described by their phenotype (i.e., cellular markers) and function (i.e., suppression of antigen-specific T-cell responses or T-cell activation). In addition, toxic effects (e.g., TGF-β production leading to fibrosis) may also be involved (1226a). Their mechanism(s) of action include cytokine production (e.g., IL-10 or TGF-β), cell-to-cell contact (APC and IDO secretion; see below), and cytotoxic activity (perhaps via perforin or granzymes) (4941a; for reviews, see references 4096 and 4624a) (Table 11.14). The T regulatory cells may differ as well, depending on the location in the body (e.g., lymph node, bowel, thymus, brain, and blood).

Human T regulatory cells were initially defined by CD25 expression on the CD4[+] cell surface but show as well the presence of other molecules such as

Fork-head transcription factor P3 (FoxP3), CTLA-4, the glucocorticoid-induced TNF family-related receptor (GITR) (4096), and, perhaps, PD-1 (D. Nixon, personal communication). Whereas FoxP3 appears to be the most accepted marker of T regulatory cells, some investigators believe that the expression of CD27 and PD-1 are the primary characteristics of human T regulatory cells (766a).

Most current human studies have emphasized the activities of the CD4[+] T regulatory lymphocytes that involve the secretion of TGF-β and IL-10 and cell-to-cell contact (3878, 4096). The findings heralded an appreciation that such T cells could be harmful in HIV infection by down-regulating immune responses to the virus or helpful by depressing the immune activation that is associated with the infection (see below). This immune suppression can be reversible once effector cells are separated from the T regulatory cells (4051a).

Factors that can influence the induction and function of T regulatory cells include cytokines (e.g., IL-4, IL-15, and IL-2), microbes via pattern recognition receptors (e.g., TLR-4, TLR-5, and TLR-8), and an interaction with APC via costimulatory or coinhibitory receptors (e.g., CTLA4, CD28, and GITR) (for reviews, see references 4343a and 4624a). In some cases, T regulatory

Table 11.14 Characteristics of human CD4[+] T regulatory cells[a]

Phenotype markers
CD25[+]
CTLA-4[+]
FoxP3[+]
GITR[+]
PD-1[+b]
CD127 (IL-7R)[−]
CD27[+]

Function
Decrease immune responses
Decrease immune activation

Mechanism of action
Cell-cell contact (e.g., IDO production)
Cytokine production (e.g., IL-10 and TGF-β)
Cell killing

[a]See Section V for details. Evidence for CD8[+] T regulatory cells has also been reported (Section V).
[b]Recently proposed (D. Nixon, unpublished observation).

cells through CTLA-4 can induce the production of the tryptophan-catabolizing enzyme IDO by APC and reduce T effector cell function (3168a) (see Section II.C.2).

TGF-β can promote the conversion of CD4$^+$ cells into T regulatory cells in vitro (716a and 3664a) or following their cocultivation with other T regulatory cells (716a). Most recently, thrombospondin 1, a common extracellular matrix protein, was shown to induce T regulatory cells through an interaction with its receptor, CD47, on naïve or memory CD4$^+$ CD25$^-$ T cells (1631a). CD4$^+$ T regulatory cells express CCR5 and can be infected by HIV (3356a), although no preferential sensitivity to infection has been noted. Moreover, HIV interaction with CD4$^+$ cells can induce increased expression of FoxP3 and enhance the T regulatory cell number. This response is gp120 dependent, and the increased number of T regulatory cells observed appears to be related to a resistance to apoptosis (766a).

HIV infection studies have indicated that human CD4$^+$ T regulatory cells can suppress HIV-specific T-cell responses that are enhanced when CD4$^+$ CD25$^+$ cells are removed from culture (108, 2207). These T regulatory cells that suppressed HIV-specific CD4$^+$ T-cell activity (4711) were reported to be associated in HIV infection with low CD4$^+$ T-cell counts and a type 2 immune response (4499). Lymphoid tissues of HIV-infected subjects with high viral loads have a high concentration of FoxP3 CD4$^+$ CD25$^-$ cells, suggesting a detrimental effect of these cells on anti-HIV responses (118, 3261a). These cells may be different than the T regulatory cell subset in the blood, which is associated with a low viral load (2207). Therefore, T regulatory cells may inhibit immune cell responses in the lymphoid tissue, but in the peripheral blood, they may suppress immune cell activation. The timing of the infection and perhaps different T regulatory cell subsets may be involved. In other studies, the level of CD4$^+$CD25$^+$ T regulatory cells in the gastrointestinal mucosae of untreated HIV-infected subjects was found increased, suggesting a contribution to HIV pathogenesis in this tissue. The number of these cells returned to normal levels after HAART (1212b).

The level of T regulatory cells has been observed to rise with increasing viral load without a direct correlation with immune activation (766a). Some have reported a reduction in T regulatory cells in HIV-infected individuals with T-cell activation (1175a). This finding could reflect a lack of T-regulatory cell response. Moreover, a reduction in T regulatory cells has been noted in long-term survivors (non-progressors) and in subjects receiving HAART (for review, see reference 766a).

Toll-like receptors can be expressed on regulatory T cells (for a review, see reference 4343a). Thus, lipopolysaccharide treatment increases the CD4$^+$ CD25$^+$ cell suppressor function and can also induce this activity in nonsuppressor cell types (609a). Moreover, CD4$^+$ CD25$^-$ T cells can have up-regulated FoxP3 after in vitro activation (4663a), but these cells may not have the function of a conventional T regulatory cell. Moreover, the markers are present for only a short time.

The lack of pathogenicity in SIV-infected mangabeys (2130) or SIV$_{agm}$-infected animals could be associated with an anti-inflammatory response mediated by TGF-β-producing CD4$^+$ CD25$^+$ and CD8$^+$ CD25$^+$ T cells, particularly in the first week after infection (766a, 2286). In this regard, some reports have suggested that the presence of the CD4$^+$ T regulatory cells in HIV infection is associated with a favorable clinical course (2207), perhaps by modulating the effects of a virus-induced hyperactivated state. In other studies, intermittent 5-day cycles of IL-2 used in therapy have been shown to increase CD4$^+$ cells but can lead to the induction of CD4$^+$ CD25$^+$ T regulatory cells (4049). Although showing only weak suppression, these FoxP3$^+$ cells may affect the function of the immune system.

The potential presence of immunoregulatory CD8$^+$ T cells has also been given attention. Treatment of diabetes patients with anti-CD3 antibodies has led to an increase in CD8$^+$ T regulatory cells (CTLA-4$^+$ FoxP3$^+$) that suppressed CD4$^+$ cell proliferation by cell contact (382). Production of TGF-β by some CD8$^+$ cells can reduce the HIV-specific responses of other CD8$^+$ cells (1437). Moreover, TGF-β, IL-10, and IFN-α can induce peripheral CD8$^+$ cells to show T regulatory functions (1517a, 1894, 4698a). These CD8$^+$ T cells mainly regulate the adaptive, secondary, or later phases of immunity and require specific priming. This CD8$^+$ T-cell regulatory pathway differs from this function of NK-T and CD4$^+$ CD25$^+$ regulatory T cells, which act during early and primary immune responses. Finally, CD8^{hi} CD57$^+$ lymphocytes present in chronic infection have been shown to down-modulate the cytotoxic activity of CD8$^+$ cells (2045, 3865, 3866). Further work on this subset, which appears to secrete an inhibitory factor (2045), has not been reported.

■ SALIENT FEATURES • CHAPTER 11

1. The cell-mediated immune response is generally the first immunologic reaction to a viral infection. Innate and adaptive immunity are involved. CD4$^+$ and CD8$^+$ cell anti-HIV-specific activities have been recognized.

2. A variety of assays have been developed to evaluate cellular responses to antigens. The induction of cell proliferation, cytokine production, and cytotoxicity can be measured.

3. The function of both CD4$^+$ and CD8$^+$ T cells has been observed in relationship to specific cell subsets. Essentially, two major functional cells, naïve and memory T cells, are present in the host. The naïve cells have not been exposed to antigen; the memory cells have been exposed to antigen and either respond quickly as effector or terminal effector cells or become memory cells (central and effector).

4. CD4$^+$ cells respond to HIV infection through production of cytokines. These cells can be separated into type 1 and type 2 subsets, depending on the pattern of cytokine release: e.g., IL-2 and IFN-γ for type 1 responses and IL-4 and IL-10 for type 2 responses. Generally, type 1 responses are associated with strong cell-mediated immunity; type 2 responses correlate with humoral immunity.

5. CD4$^+$ cytotoxic cells can also kill virus-infected or uninfected cells through perforin secretion and/or the induction of apoptosis.

6. Cytotoxic CD8$^+$ cell anti-HIV responses are best measured by assays of cell killing or expression of perforin and CD107.

7. The cytotoxic CD8$^+$ cells, similar to CD4$^+$ cells, undergo a differentiation pattern in which naïve cells that encounter antigen either become effector (or terminal effector T cells) with cytotoxic activity or become memory cells that can be restimulated with antigen to respond as effector cells.

8. Cytotoxic CD8$^+$ cells have been identified that react to a variety of viral peptides representing structural or regulatory gene products but primarily to the Gag and Nef proteins. Recognition of Env peptides is low. This response can be mirrored in the diversity of the T-cell population as measured by the T-cell receptor repertoire. Clonal or oligoclonal T-lymphocyte responses may indicate the inability of the host to respond to new foreign antigens.

9. HIV may escape CTL killing by changes within the epitope recognized by CTLs, by masking the epitope through alterations in peptide structure, through down-regulation of MHC expression, or by inducing anergy in the CD8$^+$ cells.

10. The clinical relevance of CD8$^+$ CTLs is not certain. A stable level of CTLs can be found even as individuals progress to disease. Their function in cell killing may be compromised. Some data suggest that CTLs may play a detrimental role in HIV infection.

11. The CD8$^+$ cell noncytotoxic anti-HIV response (CNAR) correlates with the clinical state. It is strong in asymptomatic individuals and is lost with progression to disease. It is active against all types of HIV-1, HIV-2, and SIV isolates.

12. CNAR activity depends on IL-2 production, and its function is associated with production of a CD8$^+$ cell antiviral factor (CAF).

13. Costimulation through CD28 can increase the CD8$^+$ cell noncytotoxic response and CAF production, most likely via induction of IL-2 production.

14. CNAR and CAF act by suppression of HIV transcription.

15. CAF lacks identity to all known cytokines and may be proteolytically cleaved into an active protein during CD8$^+$ cell secretion.

16. Chemokines show anti-HIV activity by blocking virus replication at entry. β-Chemokines suppress R5 HIV isolates. SDF-1 can block X4 virus infection. Their clinical relevance in controlling HIV infection has not been well established.

17. Many natural soluble anti-HIV factors have been identified that may have clinical relevance. None is related to CAF.

18. T regulatory cells have been defined as CD25$^+$ and can suppress immune activation and immune responses through production of a variety of cytokines (e.g., IL-10 and TGF-β), cell-to-cell contact (e.g., antigen-presenting cells), or cell killing. T regulatory cells may have other molecules (e.g., FoxP3) that identify them as playing a role in regulating the immune system. Some evidence for CD8$^+$ cell T regulatory cells has been presented.

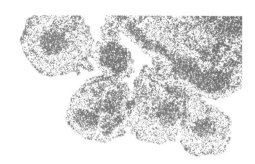

HIV Infection and Development of Cancer

I. Introduction

Cancer will occur in about 40% of individuals with HIV infection (3033). This development of malignancies is not unexpected in association with the immune system disorders caused by HIV infection. However, the finding that certain types of cancer (e.g., Kaposi's sarcoma [KS], B-cell lymphoma, and anal carcinomas) show an important increased prevalence in HIV-infected individuals has led to an emphasis in elucidating their etiology (see below) (for reviews, see references 2714, 3033, and 3646). The first two cancers involve cells of the immune system: endothelial cells and B cells. Endothelial cells have characteristics of immune cells since they express Fc and C3 receptors and can also act as accessory cells in lymphocyte activation (161, 228).

In attempts to find a common link among these malignancies, the possibility of infectious agents can be raised, particularly the herpesviruses and human papillomaviruses (HPV) (Figure 12.1). Human herpesvirus 8 (HHV-8) (also called the KS-associated herpesvirus [KSHV]) has been linked to KS and lymphomas of the peritoneal cavity (see below) (664, 2268). Epstein-Barr virus (EBV) has been found in up to 60% of B-cell lymphomas and in all lymphomas primary to the central nervous system (CNS) (2752, 4117). Nevertheless, although EBV appears to induce B-cell proliferation, it may not play a direct role in transformation (see below). Finally, HPV has been linked to carcinomas in the anus and the cervix.

The development of malignancy in HIV infection could involve three distinct steps: initiation, promotion, and transformation (Figure 12.2). A variety of factors could initiate the malignant process by causing disturbances in the immune or other organ systems. In the case of virus infection, this initiation

293

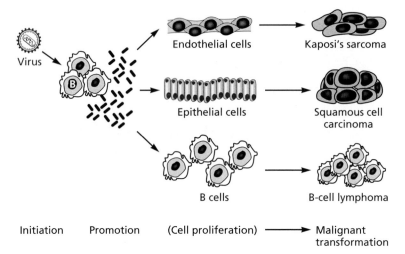

Figure 12.1   Potential role of viruses in induction of malignant disease. Virus can infect host cells, and in the case presented, immune cell cytokine production is induced that promotes proliferation of certain target cells (e.g., endothelial, epithelial, or B cells). With increased replication of cells, other factors can cause chromosomal changes leading to autonomous growth and malignant transformation. Adapted from *The Lancet* (2523), copyright 1995, with permission from Elsevier.

step can be followed by subsequent induction of cytokine (or hormone) production by the immune system that promotes an increased proliferation of the target cell (i.e., endothelium, B cell, or epithelial cell). Finally, a clastogenic event can lead to autonomous cell growth or transformation (2523) (Figure 12.2). Moreover, the host immune system could influence (i.e., promote) the expression of these neoplasms. In some cases, a virus itself could be the direct transforming agent, but most evidence thus far favors a promoter role for viruses.

A leading hypothesis to explain the cancers associated with HIV infection is that immune suppression prevents the proper immune surveillance and inhibition of virus replication or growth of transformed cells. Another possibility linking immune

disorders to cancer is that the malignancies take place secondary to the abnormal secretion of high levels of certain cytokines. These cellular factors would be produced by hyperresponding cells resulting from the disrupted balance in the immune system. They could induce cell proliferation and perhaps virus activation (2523, 2552). Some lymphokines, for example, have angiogenesis-promoting activity and could be linked to KS development (172, 1210).

The cancers in HIV infection could thus result from either depression or enhancement of immune system activity. In any case, a disorder in the immune system is tantamount to the development of certain malignancies found in this infection, as it is for opportunistic infections and other clinical

Figure 12.2   Tumor development appears to be a multistep phenomenon. A variety of agents can initiate the process, which is then promoted often by cellular products such as cytokines or hormones. Finally, a transforming event occurs which generally involves chromosomal changes. This event can be induced directly by virus.

Initiation ⟶ **Promotion** ⟶ **Transformation**

Virus   Cytokines   Chromosomal
Irradiation   Hormones   changes
Chemicals   Virus
Cytokines

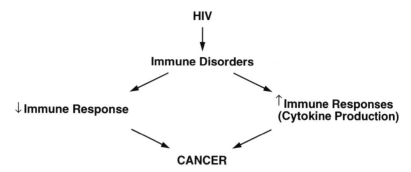

HIV

↓

Immune Disorders

↓**Immune Response**   ↑**Immune Responses (Cytokine Production)**

CANCER

Figure 12.3   HIV infection and cancer development. HIV infection can lead to immune disorders that result in either an increase or a decrease in immune responses. Both processes could be involved in cancer development.

conditions in the host (Figure 12.3). One common observation is that cancers developing in the presence of HIV infection are much more aggressive than those found in noninfected patients (2714). Thus, the immunologic response appears to be important in controlling the progression of cancer.

As individuals are living longer with HIV infection, other malignancies may eventually appear with increased prevalence. In this regard, the incidence of AIDS-associated neoplasms, more so than that of opportunistic infection, appears to increase with age (4595). An increase in other cancers has been suggested, such as Hodgkin's disease, multiple myelomas, and seminomas (1376, 1647, 2714) and leiomyomas and leiomyosarcomas in HIV-infected children (667). In Hodgkin's disease and leiomyosarcomas, EBV may be involved (2890).

Increased rates of cancer of the lips, anus, and lung and of leukemia have also been observed in a large study of people with HIV infection; the highest relative risk from time of HIV diagnosis is associated primarily with Hodgkin's disease and multiple myeloma (1647). People with a mild immune deficiency do not appear to have an increased risk of non-AIDS-defining cancers (1645). Among the nonmelanoma skin cancers increased in HIV infection is Merkel cell carcinoma, which is associated primarily with immune suppression (1206). In Africa, besides KS and non-Hodgkin's lymphoma, squamous cell tumors of the conjunctiva have been frequently observed, most likely resulting from HPV (4052).

Since the introduction of antiretroviral therapy, the incidence of lung cancer in HIV-infected subjects has increased (471). In studies of those lung cancers, no HIV or HPV sequences were detected (4795). The most common finding was widespread genomic instability in the cancer cells. This malignancy could be due to other factors, such as smoking. Penile cancers observed at high frequency could reflect multiple exposures to HPV (1376). The increased incidence of other malignancies, not related to known viruses, may reflect the importance of an immune surveillance system, but also could indicate a microbial etiologic agent yet to be discovered.

This chapter reviews studies of the four cancers frequently associated with HIV infection: KS, B-cell lymphoma, anal carcinoma, and cervical carcinoma. Other tumors that could become more prominent in the HIV-infected host are discussed briefly.

II. Kaposi's Sarcoma

A. Introduction

KS, first reported by the Hungarian physician Moritz Kaposi in 1872 (2100), is a well-demarcated, angioproliferative, often multifocal malignancy that is usually observed in men over the age of 50, particularly those from Eastern Europe and the Mediterranean region (1084, 2333, 4967) (Color Plate 19, following page 366). As the endemic type, it is found frequently in sub-Saharan Africa, at times in an aggressive form, and in men more often than in women, at relatively young ages (2333, 3817, 4967). Unless it is the aggressive form, KS rarely kills the affected person; it remains confined to the skin of the extremities, usually the feet (2333, 4967). For this reason, several groups have considered KS a benign tumor, at least in its initial stages (903, 2552). As noted above, its emergence, usually in cutaneous areas of the body, has been considered a reflection of overall disease expression (i.e., multifocal) and not metastasis (2333, 4967). However, the latter conclusion has been reexamined (Section II.B).

With its increased prevalence in young HIV-infected men, KS received new attention (1373). Moreover, in virus-infected patients, KS can present as an aggressive disease, with both mucocutaneous and visceral involvement (4967).

B. Pathology

The histopathology of KS is complex. The tumor can be divided into four histologic subtypes: nodular, florid, infiltrative, and lymphadenopathic (3868). These subtypes reflect the relative malignancy of the lesion, which appears to have an angiomatous origin. The skin tumors, especially in the early stage, consist of a mixture of cells. The KS lesions often have spaces lined by capillary endothelium, with the cells appearing activated or atypical, not unlike vessels in an inflammatory milieu (Color Plate 20, following page 366). More advanced tumors consist of spindle-shaped cells. The histologic range of endothelial cells, spindle cells, and inflammatory cells within the lesions may account for the controversy surrounding the actual cell of origin (3816, 3817).

Several other cell types besides endothelial cells are prominent in KS lesions, including macrophages, dendritic cells, mast cells, and fibroblasts. Lymph nodes with KS lesions often contain a considerable number of plasma cells (3342). Conceivably, these cells are under cytokine control (e.g., IL-6), as are perhaps the KS cells (2552, 3010) (Sections II.C and II.F).

As noted above, the origin of the cells characterizing the KS lesion is not conclusive. Many researchers linked the endothelial cells to KS (288, 558, 3817, 3847). In some studies, the tumors were considered to be derived from the vascular endothelium (558, 3817) and in others the lymphatic endothelium (288; for reviews, see references 3816 and 3817). Others have suggested that smooth muscle cells (55) and the dermal dendrocytes (3253) are the cells of origin. In the latter case, the properties of the cells could be those shared by macrophages. Early data supported the hypothesis that this neoplasm originated from endothelium and was most probably of vascular origin (3817). More recent studies in the context of KSHV/HHV-8 infection have provided new insight into KS histogenesis (see below).

Genetic analyses of multiple lesions from the same patients have suggested that KS results from the dissemination of monoclonal spindle cells (3644). In this regard, spindle cells can be cultured from the blood of HIV-infected KS patients (535) and have been found to be positive for KSHV/HHV-8 (4162; D. Blackbourn and J. A. Levy, unpublished observations) (Section II.E). The findings on clonality counter previous views that this tumor is multifocal and that different lesions on a patient do not reflect metastases (2333, 4967). This issue has not been resolved.

C. Epidemiology

The geographic distribution of KS varies in parts of the world and even within Africa (4963). It is most prevalent in men in the countries of Eastern Europe and around the Mediterranean basin and sporadically occurs in parts of North America and elsewhere. While present in higher frequency in homosexual men with HIV infection (see below), the overall prevalence in other populations can be equally distributed between men and women (1646). In regions of nonendemicity, KS develops in organ transplant recipients at a rate 400 to 500 times greater than in the general population (3467, 3484).

KS occurs in about 20% of HIV-infected men in the United States (3484) and in approximately 2% of transfusion recipients, hemophiliacs, and women. It declined in prevalence in the cohort of infected homosexual/bisexual men followed in San Francisco, Calif., from 1981 to 1989 (2119) and in other groups studied (315), presumably owing to a change in sexual practices (i.e., transfer of an infectious agent). The incidence has now dropped dramatically with the use of antiretroviral therapy (see Chapter 14).

Transfusion recipients with AIDS are three times more likely to have KS than infected hemophiliacs receiving clotting factor concentrates (3484). Hemophiliacs do not have a high prevalence of this

Table 12.1 Relationship of HIV transmission group and gender to the percentage of adult AIDS patients in the United States with Kaposi's sarcoma[a]

HIV transmission group	Sex	No. of patients/total	% with KS
Homosexual or bisexual	M	23,160/122,170	19.8
Homosexual or bisexual and injecting drug user	M	2,244/13,094	17.1
Born in Caribbean or Africa	M	110/1,849	6.0
	F	27/41	3.6
Heterosexual partner of person born in Caribbean or Africa	M	6/97	6.2
	F	4/78	5.1
Injecting drug user	M	909/33,276	2.7
	F	192/10,608	1.8
Blood transfusion recipient	M	98/2,689	3.6
	F	35/1,647	2.1
Hemophiliac	M	19/1,717	1.1

[a]Data are prior to antiviral therapy. Reprinted from reference 3484 with permission. KS, Kaposi's sarcoma; M, male; F, female.

disease (Table 12.1) (3643), most likely because of the cell association of the causative agent, KSHV/HHV-8, and its inactivation by the clotting factor processes (3484). Transfusions have also been associated with KS development in women, but the risk is much lower than that from sexual contact (Table 12.2).

Cases of children with KS are rare, except in the setting of endemic KS in Africa. It is noteworthy that one infant with this cancer was described in Kaposi's initial report (2100). In general, KS in an HIV-infected child is associated with the mother being in a risk group (3484), again most likely reflecting the presence of KSHV/HHV-8 (Section II.F).

HIV-infected individuals who present with KS as their first manifestation of AIDS generally live longer and have a less compromised immune system at onset than those with opportunistic infections (2333). This finding could even reflect the pathogenesis of this malignancy, which appears when the immune system is not completely suppressed (Section II.D). As noted above, KS could reflect a response to immune enhancement (2552). The disease is characterized by the multifocal appearance of lesions and then spontaneous regressions (3681). This "waxing and waning" of KS lesions supports an influence of the immune system in controlling the emergence and subsequent

Table 12.2 Relation of partner's HIV transmission group to percentage of infected women with Kaposi's sarcoma in the United States[a]

HIV transmission group		No. of women with KS/total	% with KS
Woman	Sexual partner		
Heterosexual	Bisexual man	22/852	2.6
	Injecting drug user	40/4,113	1.0
	Transfusion recipient	1/154	0.7
	Hemophiliac	0/98	0
Injecting drug user	Bisexual man	8/173	4.6
	Injecting drug user	27/1,815	1.5

[a]Reprinted from reference 3484 with permission.

growth of this tumor (285, 3681) or its causative agent (Sections II.D and II.E).

D. Role of the Immune System

The occurrence of both classic KS and HIV-associated KS appears to reflect in part an immune suppression in the host (4649). The presence of high levels of antibodies to known viruses such as EBV and cytomegalovirus (CMV) in HIV-infected KS patients supports the presence of defects in cellular immune regulation. Moreover, in classic Mediterranean KS, this tumor occurs in men with increasing age and has been found to be associated with immune abnormalities (2865). The high prevalence of this cancer in immunosuppressed individuals being treated for kidney transplants (1754, 3466) also supports the importance of immune control in this malignancy (2552, 2865). In addition, if the immunosuppressive therapy is withdrawn, the KS lesions disappear (1754). A direct relationship of KS with immunologic dysfunction, however, is controversial (3816); some patients with endemic KS show no detectable immune disorder (2167). Nevertheless, in several studies, a more rapid loss of CD4+ cells and higher HIV-1 RNA levels were associated with development of KS (1986), supporting the role of immune function in preventing the development of this tumor. Moreover, some individuals may have a genetic susceptibility (e.g., HLA) to KSHV/HHV-8 infection and/or KS development (1468).

The explanations for the potential role of the immune system in KS can be quite diverse. For instance, in the case of transplant recipients, the restoration of immune balance could result in rejection of the tumor by an active immune system. Alternatively, the stimulus (e.g., cytokine production) for endothelial cell growth or "KS cell" replication in the patients could be eliminated once immune equilibrium is reached. The latter possibility is based on the hypothesis that a deficiency in one arm of the immune system may lead to enhancement of the response by another part of the immune system. KS could then be like a hormone-dependent tumor induced through immune enhancement (2552). Upon stimulation by certain angiogenesis-promoting cytokines (172, 3262), the normal endothelial cells (the suspected cells of origin for KS) would replicate continuously. In

support of an immune-based pathology is the observation that KS cells can die by apoptosis, suggesting an effect of cytokines on the tumor. The potential cytolytic effect of a productive virus infection should also be considered (see Section II.E).

KS cells, although perhaps initially benign (903, 2552), if persistently stimulated might undergo karyotypic changes with mutations that establish a stable transformed state. Thus, KS lesions would appear in many parts of the body and, depending on the chromosome changes, could be relatively benign or frankly malignant. In support of this idea, KS lesions at different stages of transformation have been observed in the same HIV-infected individual (4967; J. A. Levy and R. Glogau, unpublished observations). Moreover, the classic Mediterranean form is usually relatively benign (4967). In a sense, the induction of this malignancy by such a process of cytokine production could resemble the role of EBV in some B-cell lymphomas (1215). The virus induces cell proliferation, and in some cases, these replicating activated B cells may evolve into lymphomas (Section III).

In summary, the finding of KS in HIV-infected patients is consistent with the emergence of this cancer in individuals with immune disorders (1373, 1754, 2865, 3466). Moreover, the involvement of other tissues besides the skin (e.g., lungs and lymphoid tissue) reflects the extensive immunocompromised state in AIDS (2333, 4967). However, how the lesions form in response to an infectious agent (e.g., KSHV/HHV-8) and what potential roles the immune system (e.g., lymphatic or vascular endothelium) and secreted cytokines have in KS have not been well defined.

E. Etiology

One of the first suggested causes of KS was the use of an amyl butyl nitrate inhalant (1373, 1764). This drug appears to disturb immune cells, particularly T cells, perhaps through the production of cytokines that was proposed to induce the Kaposi's lesions in the multifocal pattern observed. However, because KS is common in HIV-infected homosexual men (315, 1373), is found on sexual organs (2419), and is prevalent in women with bisexual partners (315, 2419), this tumor was considered a sexually acquired disease (315, 3816, 3817). Supporting this idea is the finding that adoption of "safe sex" guidelines

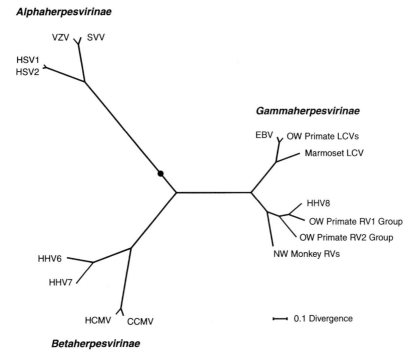

Figure 12.4 A phylogenetic tree for primate herpesvirus lineages. The tree shown is derived from the data set and analyses described in reference 2924. The tree was obtained by a maximum-likelihood method with molecular clock imposed and an input alignment of amino acid sequences for six genes; the species depicted were selected from a total set of 40 species. The root locus is marked with a circle. A divergence scale (substitutions per site) is shown. HSV, herpes simplex virus; VZV, varicella-zoster virus: HCMV, human cytomegalovirus; HVS, herpesvirus saimiri; SVV, simian varicella virus; CCMV, chimpanzee cytomegalovirus; OW, Old World; NW, New World; RV rhadinovirus; LCV, lymphocryptovirus. Figure provided by D. McGeoch.

correlated with a decrease in the incidence of this cancer in HIV-infected individuals (315).

1. DISCOVERY OF KAPOSI'S SARCOMA-ASSOCIATED HERPESVIRUS/HUMAN HERPESVIRUS 8

In 1994, Chang et al. (686) identified unique DNA sequences in KS tumors that were closely related to regions of the genome of EBV and *Herpesvirus saimiri*, members of the gamma herpesvirus subfamily (Figure 12.4). The herpesviruses detected in KS lesions in earlier studies, suspected of being CMV (1523, 1960), could have been this agent, now called KSHV or HHV-8 (for reviews, see references 830 and 3099). For researchers of KS, the term KSHV is the preferred name for this virus; for others, generally HHV-8 is used to designate it as the

eighth human herpesvirus identified and its association with other diseases. In this chapter, these names are combined. Further studies demonstrated the presence of these herpesvirus-like sequences in nearly all forms of KS in both HIV-infected and uninfected people in various parts of the world (for reviews, see references 830 and 3099). They were also noted in B-cell lymphomas found in the peritoneal cavity (664, 2268) and in lymphoid tissue from patients with Castleman's disease (4214) (see below).

The association of these herpesvirus-like sequences with an intact virion was demonstrated by phorbol ester treatment of cultured B lymphoma cells containing this virus (3704). The virus was found in peripheral blood mononuclear cells (PBMC) of KS patients (92, 4742), particularly in CD19+ B cells (92), and detected in peripheral blood cells resembling spindle cells (4162) (D. Blackbourn and J. A. Levy, unpublished observations). The virus has also been found in monocytes in KS tumors (404). The infectivity of KSHV/HHV-8 was demonstrated by taking fluid from either activated peripheral blood B cells, B-cell lymphomas, or KS biopsy specimens in culture and showing replication in CD19$^+$ B cells (391), or in adenovirus-transformed human kidney cells (1328). It appears that DC-SIGN is a virus attachment site for KSHV/HHV-8 infection of myeloid DCs and macrophages (3668).

Herpesviruses are classified into three subfamilies: alpha, beta, and gamma. KSHV/HHV-8 is part of the rhadinovirus genus in the gamma herpesvirus family (Figure 12.4). Phylogenetic analyses of several KSHV/HHV-8 genomes have shown the existence of subtypes A to D as well as N and Q (4978). Distribution studies of this virus, similar to those conducted with HIV, have indicated the predominance of certain subtypes in various parts of the world (subtypes A and C in Europe and subtype B in Africa) (1145). These major subtypes of KSHV/HHV-8 can reflect the spread of human populations over the past 35,000 to 60,000 years (1772, 3716).

2. KSHV/HHV-8 TRANSMISSION

A role for KSHV/HHV-8 in KS has been implicated by the almost universal finding of the virus in KS lesions and within the endothelial cells, spindle cells, and monocytes present in these tumors (404, 451, 2570, 3342). Viral DNA sequences have also been detected in the sensory ganglia of KS patients (891), suggesting a reason for the frequently symmetrical cutaneous distribution of KS lesions in patients. However, the KSHV/HHV-8 sequences have not been detected in tumor-producing cell lines derived from Kaposi's tumors (92, 1307). Thus, whether this virus is a direct cause or a promoter of the malignancy remains to be fully elucidated.

The sexual transmission of KSHV/HHV-8 has been suggested by finding the virus in seminal fluid (1672, 2609, 3057) and the prostate gland (3057) from KS patients and those without KS. KSHV/HHV-8 has also been detected associated with human spermatozoa and within mononuclear cells in semen (213a). However, others have not confirmed the findings in prostate tissue, particularly in relation to healthy virus-infected subjects (92, 890, 1899; for a review, see reference 395).

Besides being detected in seminal fluids from healthy men at low frequency (3057), KSHV/HHV-8 has been found in saliva and nasal secretions of KS patients (393, 427, 488, 633, 4743). The latter fluids would provide a means of transmission aside from the sexual route (2887), particularly since KSHV/HHV-8 in saliva is infectious (4605). The finding of the virus in oral tissues (1071) supports its presence in saliva. Transmission by other routes (e.g., feces/hands) should also be considered. Virus has been found in breast milk of HIV-infected mothers (1024) and occasionally in colostrum (488). In studies of Zimbabwean women, KSHV/HHV-8 was observed in oral, vaginal, and cervical secretions (2392). Thus, sexual transmission of the virus by these routes should be considered (633).

3. KSHV/HHV-8 PATHOGENESIS

Infection with KSHV/HHV-8 has predicted the development of KS up to 21 months before the onset of the tumor in HIV-infected patients (3100). Current understanding of the mechanism behind KSHV/HHV-8 pathogenesis in the context of KS is incomplete. It takes several months to years before KS lesions appear, and the malignant process is influenced by factors associated with immune suppression (Figure 12.5). KSHV/HHV-8 can transform certain endothelial cells, conferring a spindle morphology upon them, reminiscent of that seen in KS lesions (785, 1313, 3021, 3124). The finding suggests that the study of such cells could enlighten our understanding of HHV-8 pathogenesis, and certain viral genes could have transforming capacity (222, 1430, 2462, 3175) (see below). The inability to determine with certainty the histogenesis of the KS spindle cells, whether from blood or lymphatic endothelium (reviewed in reference 3817; also see above), has undoubtedly confounded understanding of the pathogenic process. However, recent studies suggest that KSHV/HHV-8 drives transcriptional reprogramming of infected cells (3218), shifting blood endothelial cells toward a lymphatic phenotype (627, 1886, 4671). Thus, the virus-infected cell of origin of KS could be derived from the blood vasculature, but "reprogrammed" by the virus to a less differentiated or lymphatic state, or vice versa.

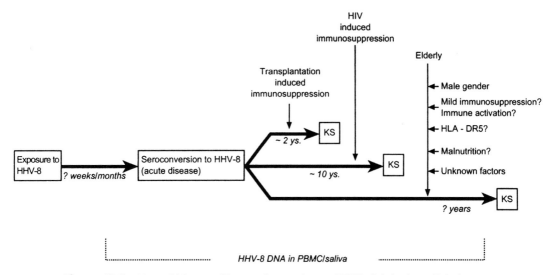

Figure 12.5   Natural history of human herpesvirus 8 (HHV-8) infection: clinical stages and determinants of progression. KS, Kaposi's sarcoma. Reprinted from reference 1145 with permission.

While a transforming role for KSHV/HHV-8 has not been fully demonstrated, its genome does contain sequences that could be responsible for cell transformation (Figure 12.6). These viral regions include the sequence encoding cyclin D (687) (a cell cycle inducer) and a Bcl-2-like sequence that could ensure dominance of a transformed cell by blocking apoptosis (3098, 3848). A potential role for the c-*kit* oncogene in KS tumorigenesis has also been suggested (3125).

Importantly, the gene products most likely to function in cell transformation are associated with lytic cycle replication, when new KSHV/HHV-8 virions are produced, but the virus is predominantly latent in KS. In this regard, the latency-associated nuclear antigen (LANA), found in all KSHV/HHV-8 infections, can inhibit the tumor suppressor proteins p53 and pRB and increase cell proliferation (1370, 3652). A possible explanation for this paradox has been suggested: latent infection permits persistence of the KSHV/HHV-8 genome but is inefficient, and a low level of continuous lytic replication is necessary to maintain the infection and hence the tumor (1650). A hypothesis has been proposed that the KSHV/HHV-8 viral IL-6-related protein, by interacting with its own cell surface receptor (gp130), blocks the activity of IFN-α in inhibiting cell proliferation.

IFN-α through its promoter activates this viral IL-6 production (reviewed in references 698, 3099, and 3251). Cell proliferation results. The virus also encodes certain cytokines and chemokine receptors that could help in resisting host immune responses (3098; for reviews, see references 2527, 3099, 3251, and 3716) (Figure 12.6).

In this regard, immune cell-type-specific influences on KSHV/HHV-8 replication can be observed. Inflammatory cytokines can suppress lytic replication of the virus in endothelial cells, presumably promoting latency (3021). In contrast, in B cells, IFN-γ can reactivate KSHV/HHV-8 into a lytic cycle (392, 682). Moreover, inflammatory cytokines induce phenotypic and functional features in endothelial cells that are consistent with those of KS tumor cells (1295). Thus, inflammatory cytokines, particularly IFN-γ, are proposed to cooperate with KSHV/HHV-8 in promoting its pathogenesis (1211). Furthermore, the mRNAs of some of these contributory cytokines can be stabilized by the KSHV/HHV-8 latent protein, kaposin B (2897).

In further support of the role of KSHV/HHV-8 in KS are studies in transgenic mice in which the constitutively active HHV-8 G-protein coupled receptor (v-GPCR) (159), resembling a cellular chemokine receptor, is expressed (4858). This

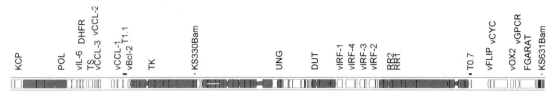

Figure 12.6   Schematic representation of the 137-kb unique region of the Kaposi's sarcoma-associated herpesvirus/human herpesvirus 8 (KSHV/HHV-8) genome, which contains all the known protein-coding regions. The unique region is flanked at each end by multiple copies of a high-GC 801-bp terminal direct repeat (not shown) to give a total genome size of about 170 kbp. The genome termini probably ligate together to circularize the genome during the cellular portion of the viral replicative cycle. The unique region consists of portions containing genes that are widely conserved in other herpesviruses (grey portions) and portions containing genes unique to HHV-8 and, in some cases, its close relatives (white portions). Several genes are regulatory, cytokine, and DNA metabolism genes that are homologous to cellular genes, and many of these are unique to HHV-8. KCP, KSHV complement-binding protein; POL, DNA polymerase; vIL-6, viral IL-6 homolog; DHFR, dihydrofolate reductase; TS, thymidylate synthase; vCCL-1, -2, and -3, viral IL-8-like CC chemokine homologues; vBcl-2, viral Bcl-2 homologues; TK, thymidine kinase; UNG, uracil-DNA glycosylase; DUT, dUTPase; vIRF-1, -2, -3, and -4, viral interferon regulatory factor homologues; RR1 and RR2, subunits of ribonucleotide reductase; vFLIP, viral FLIP-like inhibitor of apoptosis homologue; vCYC, viral D-type cyclin homologue; vOX2, viral OX2 homologue; vGPCR, viral GPCR homologue resembling IL-8Rα; FGARAT, formyl-glycinamide ribotide amidotransferase. Also shown are T1.1 and T0.7, two highly expressed transcripts, and KS330Bam and KS631Bam sequences, originally found by representational difference analysis of an AIDS KS lesion. Provided by A. Davison.

protein induces cell transformation and vascular endothelial growth factor-driven angiogenesis (222, 1431) in KS-like lesions (4858).

4. SEROLOGIC STUDIES

Serologic studies have indicated a close association of KSHV/HHV-8 antibodies with the presence of KS. Assays have included indirect immunofluorescence (2495), immunoblotting (1432, 3015), and use of recombinant viral proteins (974, 2140). Most of these studies show the presence of antibodies in about 1 to 2% of the healthy population, but in these cases, they were measuring primarily the latent or nuclear protein expressed in transformed cells. In other studies (2495), a seroprevalence of about 25% was noted in healthy adults in the United States when antibodies to the cytoplasmic (or viral replicative) antigens were measured. A similar frequency of antibodies to KSHV/HHV-8 in healthy blood donors was noted in serum evaluations by an enzyme-linked immunosorbent assay (ELISA) to a minor viral capsid protein (974). This prevalence seems closer to the occurrence of the virus in the healthy population (rather than 1 to

2%), since the virus has been found in the blood and lymph nodes of healthy individuals without KS or HIV infection and in a healthy blood donor (391). Importantly, the prevalence of antibodies to KSHV/HHV-8 appears to increase at the time of puberty (2495), suggesting transmission primarily through the sexual route, although, as with EBV, saliva seems to be involved (see above). The distribution pattern is similar to that of herpes simplex virus type 2 (for a review, see reference 2527) and EBV (1814).

The reactivity of sera to the KSHV/HHV-8 latent antigen suggests that it represents a tumor-associated protein. Seroconversion to this antigen predicts the development of KS (1432). Moreover, the prevalence of anti-latent-antigen antibodies appears to correlate with the overall incidence of KS in different populations (1429, 2495).

5. THERAPY

Local treatment with cryotherapy, topical retinoic acid, and intralesional chemotherapy as well as local radiation can be used for cosmetic control of tumors. Patients with widespread systematic disease can receive liposomal doxorubicin, which can be highly active and well tolerated. Paclitaxel is another highly effective agent for second-line treatment. IFN-α is also an active agent and when administered with antiretroviral drugs can be used at relatively low and minimally toxic doses (1 million units/day per week). Most recently, thalidomide and Col-3 as well as imatinib have shown some promise in early clinical trials (181, 1066, 2275).

F. Other Human Herpesvirus 8-Associated Cancers

A rare type of HIV-associated lymphoma presents as a primary malignant lymphomatous effusion, called primary effusion lymphoma (PEL) (664, 2268). PEL is generally associated with HHV-8 infection (for reviews, see references 665 and 2268). The virus-encoded vFLIP protein is apparently required for survival of PEL-derived cell lines, suggesting a direct role of HHV-8 in the pathogenesis of this tumor (1660). This tumor can occur late in HIV infection and has a rapid clinical course. In some cases, EBV has been found to be present with HHV-8. Some studies in cell culture have suggested that EBV can enhance the infection of B cells by HHV-8 (394) and may be part of the process involved in this tumor development. As noted in Section II.E, since HHV-8 carries sequences associated with transformation and encodes an IL-6 homolog, its role in inducing these B-cell lymphomas merits further attention. Moreover, LANA has been shown to induce B-cell hyperplasia and lymphoma in

transgenic mice (1243). It is curious that HHV-8 is found predominantly in B-cell lymphomas of the body cavity and not elsewhere. In this regard, it is site specific, as is EBV with brain tumors (see Section IV). Why these B cells carrying particular viruses should proliferate in these locations in the body has yet to be elucidated but could relate to their being immune-privileged sites. The association of HHV-8 with Castleman's disease, a lymphoproliferative disorder, has been described and appears to involve a specific cell subset presenting as plasmablastic lymphoma (1152).

G. Other KSHV/HHV8-Like Viruses

Two different KSHV/HHV-8-related rhadinoviruses are now known to infect nonhuman primates. Those most closely related to KSHV/HHV-8 were identified by molecular probing of retroperitoneal fibromatosis (RF) lesions from two macaque species, the pig-tailed macaque (*Macaca nemestrina*) and the rhesus macaque (*Macaca mulatta*) (3800). RF, a vascular fibroproliferative neoplasm, was initially linked to infection with a type D simian retrovirus (SRV-2), which gives rise to an immunodeficiency syndrome (1508). The rhadinoviruses (RV) were called retroperitoneal fibromatosis herpesviruses Macaca mulatta and Macaca nemestrina, respectively. Although their entire genomes have yet to be sequenced, they have been phylogenetically classified as RV-1 lineage rhadinoviruses, with KSHV/HHV-8 (4007). Another rhadinovirus isolated from rhesus macaques, RRV, is classified according to its genetic sequences as an RV-2 lineage rhadinovirus (1060, 4027) (Figure 12.4). The precise pathogenesis of the rhadinoviruses is unclear and could be strain specific (4813). Inoculation of macaque RRV into monkeys infected with SIV gave rise to B-cell hyperplasia, not unlike that observed in AIDS patients coinfected with KSHV/HHV-8 (4813).

The identification of other nonhuman primate rhadinoviruses supports two major lineages of these viruses (1621, 1622). Primates appear to have both an KSHV/HHV-8-like (RV-1) virus and a separate (RV-2) rhadinovirus (2923). Direct cross-reactivity of antibodies to the primate RV-1 rhadinoviruses with KSHV/HHV-8 has been suggested (1621; for review on serology, see references 697, 1060, 3099, and 3800). However, an RV-2 rhadinovirus subtype in humans has not been identified. In this regard, Kaposi-like tumors occurring in baboons inoculated with HIV-2 (265) were found to have an RV-2-like virus rather than one resembling KSHV/HHV-8 (4743).

H. Conclusions

KSHV/HHV-8 appears to be the proximal agent involved in KS as well as PEL, but it may act to promote the malignant process rather than to transform the cells directly (2523) (Figure 12.1). After stimulation of cell proliferation, transformation may occur by other, non-virus-related, subsequent events, particularly those leading to chromosomal changes, with the emergence of an independently growing cell. For KS development, KSHV/HHV-8 could, through infection of B lymphocytes (92), induce cytokines that enhance proliferation and subsequent transformation of endothelial cells (2552) (Figure 12.2). A similar process can induce B-cell proliferation via IL-6 or IL-10 secretion. Studies of the primate herpesviruses might help elucidate further the pathogenic pathways involved. (For a review of HHV-8 infection and epidemiology, see reference 1145.)

III. B-Cell Lymphomas

A. Introduction

HIV infection is associated with several B-cell abnormalities, including increased B-cell prolifera-

tion, polyclonal hypergammaglobulinemia, and enhanced production of certain B-cell cytokines (see Chapter 8, Table 8.1). These events can be linked to the reactive lymphadenopathy often seen early in HIV infection (12, 1659). The most likely cytokines responsible for B-cell proliferation are IL-6 and IL-10, produced by many cells, particularly monocytes but also B cells, fibroblasts, endothelial cells, and cells in the brain. B-cell proliferation can be demonstrated after incubation with HIV particles (3383) or with the HIV envelope gp41 (749). It may be induced in some B cells via binding of gp120 to a $V_H 3$ immunoglobulin (316) (see Chapter 8).

In one theory, this proliferative state of B cells has been considered a prelude to chromosomal changes that can establish a malignant process (Figures 12.1 and 12.2) (see below). B-cell growth in response to chronic antigenic stimulation (e.g., EBV infection) has been considered the cause of the large number of B-cell lymphomas occurring in immunosuppressed transplant recipients (2203, 2229). Thus, B-cell lymphomas, like KS, are not an entirely unexpected finding in HIV infection. Immunosuppression, as in KS, can play a role in the development of lymphomas through a reduction in appropriate antitumor cell-mediated immunity. Likewise, promotion of cell growth reflecting increased production of cytokines (e.g., IL-6 and IL-10) could be involved (2826), as discussed for KS (Figures 12.1, 12.3, and 12.5). Increased levels of IL-10 reflecting, in some cases, the enhanced activity of the IL-10 promoter have been observed in sera of HIV-infected subjects prior to the development of Hodgkin's B-cell lymphoma (489). The result is usually widespread disease involving sites outside the lymphoid organs (4964; for a review, see reference 1823).

B. Epidemiology and Tumor Characteristics

Although B-cell lymphomas were reported in homosexual men at a time when AIDS was first being recognized (4964, 4965), it was not until 1985 that the Centers for Disease Control revised its guidelines to include lymphoma in the case definition of AIDS (654). B-cell lymphomas are 60 to 100 times more common in AIDS patients than in the general population (314) (Table 12.3).

Table 12.3 Characteristics of B-cell lymphomas in HIV infection[a]

- 60–100 times more common in AIDS patients than in the general population (314)
- Occur more commonly in patients with $CD4^+$ cell counts of <100 cells/µl (360a)
- Up to 30% of AIDS patients are diagnosed with this lymphoma (314)
- Between 5 and 20% of AIDS patients have B-cell lymphoma as their initial or subsequent diagnosis (1823, 3486)
- HIV-infected individuals heterozygous for the CCR5 Δ32 deletion are less likely to develop lymphoma (see Chapter 13)
- HIV-infected subjects with SDF-1 polymorphisms are more likely to develop this cancer (see Chapter 13)
- More common in men than in women (314)
- Twice as common in whites (314)
- Involvement of extranodal sites is common (1823, 2507)
- 40–60% of tumors outside the brain harbor EBV (4099). All CNS lymphomas contain EBV (2752, 2954, 4191).
- Most lymphomas are monoclonal (1823)
- Could reflect increased production of cytokines such as IL-6 and IL-10 (489)

[a]EBV, Epstein-Barr virus; CNS, Central nervous system.

These non-Hodgkin's lymphomas are more likely to occur in patients with a low $CD4^+$ cell count, particularly below 100 (Appendix V). Individuals with $CD4^+$ cell numbers above 350 cells/µl do not have a substantial risk (360a). In an early survey, between 8 and 20% of 36,000 new cases in 1990 were estimated to be in HIV-infected individuals (1407). According to one report, 30% of AIDS patients before 1990 had been diagnosed with lymphoma (314). Furthermore, between 5 and 20% of individuals with AIDS could have B-cell lymphoma as their initial or subsequent diagnosis (1823, 3459). Genetic risk factors have also been described; people heterozygous for the Δ32 deletion of CCR5 are less likely to develop lymphoma, and those with an SDF-1 polymorphism more likely to develop this cancer (see Chapter 13, Table 13.10). Involvement of extranodal sites in the AIDS-associated lymphomas is common, with tumors found in the intestine, CNS, bone marrow, and liver (1823, 2507) (Table 12.3).

The HIV-related B-cell lymphomas are twice as common in whites as in blacks and occur in more men than women (314). All risk groups for HIV infection are susceptible to the development of these lymphomas. These observations contrast with findings in KS, which show that men who have sex with men are at an increased risk for this cancer. This finding suggests that a lymphoma agent (if one exists) is not spread by a sexual route.

The aggressive B-cell lymphomas, commonly seen in HIV disease, have been classified histologically as diffuse large cell (including both large cell and immunoblastic lymphomas) (2364) and Burkitt's lymphoma-like (314, 2954; for reviews, see references 1823 and 2507). The use of two subgroupings represents a simplification of the several subclasses previously used for non-Hodgkin's lymphoma in non-HIV-infected patients (1823, 2507, 4964) (Table 12.4). Small noncleaved lymphomas (Burkitt's or Burkitt-like) associated with HIV infection are at least 1,000 times more common in AIDS patients than in the general U.S. population (314). About 20 to 30% of the lymphomas in HIV-infected patients are of this type, in contrast to B-cell lymphoma in immunosuppressed transplant recipients, among whom approximately 1% have Burkitt's histology (314).

A specific type of B-cell lymphoma termed "primary effusion lymphoma" has been described

Table 12.4 B-cell lymphomas associated with underlying HIV infection[a]

Diffuse large B-cell lymphoma

Large B-cell lymphoma subtypes
- Primary effusion lymphoma
- Plasmablastic lymphoma

Burkitt's lymphoma/leukemia
- Classic Burkitt's lymphoma
- Atypical Burkitt's lymphoma
- Burkitt's lymphoma with plasmacytoid differentiation

Classic Hodgkin's lymphoma
- Nodular sclerosis
- Mixed cellularity
- Lymphocyte-rich classic Hodgkin's lymphoma
- Lymphocyte-depleted Hodgkin's lymphoma

[a]World Health Organization (WHO) classification of lymphoid tumors. Provided by A. Levine.

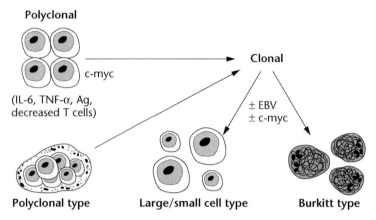

Polyclonal

Clonal

c-myc

(IL-6, TNF-α, Ag,
decreased T cells)

± EBV
± c-myc

Polyclonal type   Large/small cell type   Burkitt type

Figure 12.7 Emergence of B-cell lymphomas in HIV-infected individuals. Polyclonal proliferation of B cells can give rise to monoclonal lymphomas. The factors in parentheses can cause the polyclonal expansion of B cells. The latter type may show evidence of c-*myc* translocation and/or Epstein-Barr virus (EBV) infection. The Burkitt type of lymphoma appears to develop from one malignant cell. EBV and c-*myc* may be detected in polyclonal lymphomas but at a reduced frequency. Figure provided by B. Herndier.

in HIV-infected patients and is associated with HHV-8 infection (see Section II.F). These patients present with malignant infusions (ascites, pleural, and pericardial) often in the absence of any mass lesions. The prognosis is poor. The malignant B cells, as shown by immunoglobulin gene rearrangement studies, usually lack B-cell markers on the cell surface (664, 665).

Lymphomas primary to the brain (e.g., CNS lymphoma) primarily consist of the immunoblastic or large-cell type (not Burkitt's) and occur to the same extent in all ages. It is found in up to 25% of patients with HIV-associated lymphoma (1823) and has been reported for an AIDS patient younger than 1 year old (314). EBV is found in all the AIDS-associated primary lymphomas in the brain (2752, 2954, 4117, 4191). HHV-8 has not been detected (1406). Presenting symptoms in these patients include seizures, headache, focal neurologic abnormalities, cranial nerve palsies, and altered mental state. Although not common, patients have been described as undergoing personality changes (for a review, see reference 2507). Clinically, the patients with primary CNS lymphomas do very poorly, and many are diagnosed only at autopsy (2507, 4194). Generally, the CD4$^+$ cell count at diagnosis is <50/μl (1823).

EBV, often associated with endemic Burkitt's lymphoma (1814), is not required for lymphoma induction in HIV infection; about 40 to 60% of the tumors outside the brain harbor the virus (4099) (Table 12.3). In some reports, the occurrence of EBV-associated diffuse large-cell lymphomas was linked to a loss of anti-EBV cytotoxic T lymphocytes and a rise in the EBV load (2165). EBV, once released from immune control, most probably plays a role in inducing the cell proliferation that can lead in some instances to malignant transformation (see below) (Figures 12.7 and 12.8). With increased cell division, molecular or karyotypic changes can take place, with selection of cells that grow autonomously (Figure 12.2). These events, perhaps directly linked to EBV, may occur preferentially in the brain. In other tumors, cytokine production could be the stimulus for cell proliferation (see below). One immunophenotypic feature of most AIDS lymphomas that could explain the absence of EBV infection is the lack of the viral complement receptor CD21 on the cell surface (4117).

C. Pathogenesis

An increase in B-cell number associated with HIV is mirrored early in infection by the increased size of germinal follicles in the lymph nodes of infected individuals who present clinically with lymphadenopathy (see Chapter 8). This activation of B lymphocytes, observed in other viral infections, can result from HIV itself, a reduction in

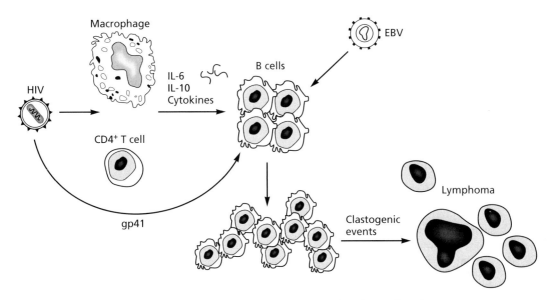

Figure 12.8   Potential mechanisms for transformation of B cells into lymphoma. HIV infection of macrophages or CD4⁺ T cells can result in the production of cytokines that induce the proliferation of B cells. The HIV gp41 envelope protein and EBV can also be involved. The polyclonal activation and chromosomal changes (e.g., c-*myc* translocation) cause the emergence of an autonomously growing malignant cell.

T-cell responses, or a response to cytokines such as IL-4 or IL-6.

The cause of the B-cell lymphomas is not known. As with KS, the cancers could reflect infection by a new agent, spontaneous growth of cells reflecting a lack of T-cell regulation, or a response to cytokines released as a result of HIV infection (Figures 12.7 and 12.8). The last two possibilities most probably overlap, since controls on cytokine production are linked to a normal balance in other arms of the immune system (2523, 2552). The stimulation of B cells, resulting from immune deficiency (see Chapter 10), can cause cell proliferation reflected by high serum immunoglobulin levels, which may predict the onset of non-Hodgkin's lymphomas (1648). Moreover, by CD4:CD40 ligand interaction, vascular cell adhesion molecule expression is induced on the epithelial cell, which permits better attachment of B cells and encourages lymphoma cell growth (3128).

Some investigators believe that these lymphomas occur as a result of germinal-center destruction by a process of follicular lysis (1823). A lack of follicular dendritic cell (FDC) function as antigen-presenting cells renders B cells less sensi-tive to normal apoptotic processes (see Chapter 6), particularly those linked to cytokines. Thus, B cells survive longer and replicate (1823). Perhaps the predominant production of IL-10 by TH2 CD4⁺ cells or B cells or expression of IL-10-like activity by EBV (1908) plays a role in this process (see Chapters 9 and 11). IL-10 prevents the spontaneous death of cultured germinal B cells, most probably by the induction of the antiapoptotic Bcl-2 protein (2554). A similar inhibitory effect on apoptosis by the EBV protein latent membrane protein 1 (LMP-1) has also been described (1808).

One characteristic shared by some HIV-associated lymphomas and lymphomas of patients immunosuppressed for organ transplantation (1720) is the absence of c-*myc* rearrangements (3464, 4099, 4323). This feature, particularly for lymphomas in the brain, distinguishes these tumors from some peripheral lymphomas associated with EBV infection. Small noncleaved lymphomas in AIDS patients (some of the Burkitt's type) often show this c-*myc* genetic abnormality (for a review, see reference 1823) (see also Section III.E). Expression of *ras* and p53 has also been noted (230). The relationship of these genetic changes to the initiation of the cancer is not known. Conceivably, the alterations could have developed as a result of cell proliferation.

While the role of EBV in lymphoma development is unclear, the induction by certain viral proteins (e.g., LMP-1 and BHRF1) of IL-10-like activity and expression of Bcl-2 could be involved in the emergence of the tumor (1808, 1908). The expression of EBV is increased in HIV infection, and the presence of multiple variants in the same host has been reported (Table 12.5) (76, 379). Most EBV-infected tumors are the large-cell type (Table 12.4).

The almost universal finding of EBV in lymphomas occurring in transplant patients has suggested immune suppression as a major factor in the pathogenesis of these tumors (379). Thus, polyclonal B-cell proliferation from EBV activation, decreased apoptosis in association with EBV infection, and/or a lack of cellular immune control could be involved in development of primary CNS lymphomas. Whether karyotypic changes (e.g., translocations) occur before or after polyclonal activation requires further study.

Most of the tumors in AIDS patients are monoclonal, suggesting the outgrowth of one transformation event (1823). In some cases, lymphomas appear to result from the clonal expansion of EBV-transformed B cells (4099). Nevertheless, the possibility that EBV has infected and spread in an already malignant B cell cannot be ruled out.

The existence of polyclonal lymphomas is controversial; if they occur, they may represent B-cell proliferation evolving into a clonal lymphoma (Figure 12.7). Events common to cell transformation could be involved, but a role of cytokines seems to be important. Chronic stimulation by HIV, EBV, HHV-8, or other antigens could cause the proliferative responses observed in HIV-infected patients. Cytokines, including IL-1, IL-2, IL-4, IL-6, IL-7, IL-10, IFN-γ, and TNF-α, have all shown the ability to enhance B-cell proliferation (2017, 2018, 3867) (Figure 12.8). In general, IL-6 and IL-10 seem to be mostly responsible for this proliferation, particularly since they can also be made by B lymphocytes (2862, 4870). Furthermore, reports have shown the induction of high levels of IL-6 production by monocytes in HIV-infected patients (2507, 3202). These cellular factors can maintain the proliferative phase of the lymphoma or B cells through continual growth in an autocrine fashion. Under these conditions, chromosomal changes might not be present and anticytokine approaches might offer effective therapy. This possibility merits further study. In some ways, the polyclonal tumor resembles the murine model of AIDS, in which the proliferating CD4$^+$ cells are persistently stimulated by either viral antigens or superantigens, with cytokines playing a central role (3116).

The duration from initial HIV infection to lymphoma can be about 7 to 8 years, similar to that for opportunistic infections (314). It appears, however, that patients living longer with HIV infection may also have a greater risk of developing this malignancy in time, particularly those with high viremia levels (440, 4595). The introduction of HAART has reduced the incidence of non-Hodgkin's lymphoma dramatically, particularly the primary CNS lymphomas (351; for a review, see reference 4437). Since these tumors are associated with EBV infection, a restored immune response seems to be involved. With HAART as well, a longer survival has been reported in subjects with systemic as well as AIDS-related CNS lymphomas (4163). Moreover, HAART appears to improve substantially the response of non-Hodgkin's and Hodgkin's lymphoma patients to chemotherapy (126), perhaps by reducing the occurrence of opportunistic infections.

Table 12.5 Epstein-Barr virus (EBV) and HIV infection[a]

- Increased levels of EBV in the saliva (10- to 100-fold)
- Increased levels of virus-infected cells in the blood (10-fold)
- Increased EBV replication in the oropharynx
- Can be reinfected with multiple EBV strains
- Multiple EBV genome variants can be found in the same lymphoproliferative lesion
- High titers of antibody to the replicative proteins
- Increased prevalence of brain lymphoma

[a]Data from references 76 and 379 and G. Miller, personal communication.

D. Clinical

Patients with AIDS-related lymphoma may present with the tumor localized to the CNS alone, or with systemic lymphomatous disease. In the latter cir-

Alvin Friedman-Kien

Professor, Departments of Dermatology and Microbiology, New York University Medical Center. Dr. Friedman-Kien was among the first to report the high prevalence of Kaposi's sarcoma in homosexual men, which led to the recognition of AIDS.

cumstance, widespread involvement is expected, with lymphoma present within bone marrow, the gastrointestinal tract, the liver, cerebrospinal fluid, and other sites as well (2507). Patients often seek medical attention because of mass lesions in lymph nodes or extranodal sites, or because of systemic "B" symptoms, which include unexplained fever, drenching night sweats, or weight loss in excess of 10% of normal body weight (2507).

On a population level, the widespread use of HAART, as noted above, has resulted in substantial increases in CD4$^+$ cells and a decrease in the overall incidence of AIDS-related lymphoma (440, 3039). However, whereas the incidence of various opportunistic infections and KS has decreased to a remarkable extent in HIV infection, B-cell lymphoma is now relatively more common as an initial AIDS-defining condition (3037).

Characteristics associated with shorter survival of patients with AIDS lymphoma include stage III or IV disease, elevated lactate dehydrogenase levels, age of >35 years, history of injection drug use, and/or a CD4$^+$ cell level of <100 (4310). The standard or age-adjusted International Prognostic Index has also been validated in patients with AIDS-related lymphoma. Prior to the advent of HAART, the pathological type of lymphoma was not found to be important in terms of prognosis. However, in the HAART era, recent studies have shown that HIV-infected patients with Burkitt's lymphoma, treated with chemotherapy similarly to other patients with AIDS lymphoma, fare statistically less well (2608).

Current therapeutic options include use of standard-dose CHOP (cyclophosphamide, doxorubicin, vincristine, and prednisone) or mBACOD (methotrexate, bleomycin, doxorubicin, cyclophosphamide, vincristine, and dexamethasone), with granulocyte growth factor or infusions of CDE (cyclophosphamide, doxorubicin, and etoposide), which seem to have comparable response rates. Addition of rituximab to CHOP or to the CDE regimen seems to improve both response rates and overall survival (2099, 4236). Care must be taken in using rituximab with chemotherapy in patients with < 50 CD4$^+$ cells/μl since an increased risk of death from infections has been described for this specific subgroup (2099). When combined with HAART, multiagent chemotherapy appears to be well tolerated in terms of hematologic toxicity and results in higher response rates and prolonged survival. Optimal treatment for patients with relapsed or refractory AIDS lymphoma remains undefined at this time. Nonetheless, use of high-dose chemotherapy followed by autologous progenitor cell transplantation appears to be efficacious, with toxicity profiles remarkably similar to those observed in HIV-negative patients with relapsed aggressive lymphoma (2331).

E. Conclusions

In general, the pathogenesis of B-cell lymphomas in HIV infection is considered a result of polyclonal B-cell activation secondary to HIV antigens (e.g., gp41), EBV, HHV-8, or T-cell dysregulation associated with cytokine production

(Figures 12.7 and 12.8). In some cases, a virus (e.g., EBV or HHV-8) may be the direct transforming agent. The induction of B-lymphocyte proliferation by cytokines or other processes can lead to clastogenic events, sometimes including c-*myc* translocation, which is linked to immortalization and outgrowth of clonal transformed B cells (Figures 12.2 and 12.8) (2229, 2764). The concomitant up-regulation of c-*myc* and EBV transcripts has been cited by some to indicate a role for HIV in cell transformation (2427), but this early finding needs further evaluation. The mutations in oncogenes or tumor suppressor genes associated with DNA rearrangements, as noted in Section IV for anal carcinomas, could also be involved in the development of monoclonal B-cell lymphomas (1405). Moreover, normal regulation of B-cell replication may be disturbed by the loss of FDC function in lymphoid tissues (1823). HAART has reduced the incidence of non-Hodgkin's lymphoma (particularly the primary brain lymphomas) (351, 4437) and has provided longer survival in subjects with both systemic and AIDS-related CNS lymphomas (4163).

IV. Anal Carcinoma

A. Introduction

The incidence of anal carcinoma has been estimated to be 7 and 9 per million men and women, respectively, in the general population (3388, 4909). The increased prevalence in women is probably related to receptive anal intercourse as well as exposure to HPV in the nearby vaginal and cervical region (for reviews, see references 3388 and 4985). Nevertheless, there has been a rise in the incidence of anal cancers in both men and women, most probably secondary to the above factors and particularly in association with HIV infection (3388, 3390). In the latter instance, suppression of the immune system may be responsible for the initiation and promotion of the malignant process (see below). Even before the recognition of HIV infection, this cancer was more common among homosexual men; its prevalence was greater than that of cervical cancer in women (961, 3388). For men having sex with men, its incidence is at least twice as high in HIV-infected men.

B. Human Papillomavirus (HPV) Infection

The prevalence of anal cell dysplasia (also known as anal squamous intraepithelial lesions) and HPV infection can be quite high in HIV-infected homosexual men. In one study, 55% of 285 seropositive men versus 23% of 240 seronegative men showed HPV DNA in anal biopsy and cytology studies (2219). The detection of HPV was associated with dysplastic cellular regions. In this study, anal dysplasia was increased more than threefold among HIV-seropositive men with low CD4$^+$ cell counts compared to a seronegative group. Moreover, those with CD4$^+$ cell counts of <500 cells/μl had a sixfold increased risk of dysplasia compared to HIV-infected men with CD4$^+$ cell counts of >500 cells/μl (3388). This direct association suggests that HPV proliferation, dysplasia, and development of carcinoma are linked to the extent of immune compromise. Anal cancer and squamous intraepithelial cell lesions (precursors to anal cancer) have been found as well in HIV-infected subjects who had no history of anal intercourse (3510).

Similarly, the prevalence of cytologic abnormalities and HPV infection of the anus in women confirms the high prevalence of the virus in HIV-infected women (26%) versus uninfected women (7%) (1836). Anal HPV infection is more common than cervical HPV infection in adult HIV-infected and uninfected women at high risk of acquiring HIV infection (3391). Studies of adolescent males and females have shown a similar prevalence of anal HPV infection in HIV-infected and uninfected boys but greater in HIV-infected girls. Virus infection was associated with perianal warts and with a high number of sexual partners (3118, 3391).

Approaches similar to those used in cervical cancer screening (e.g., Pap smear) have been encouraged in screening for dysplasia in the anal canal. Cytology would seem to be important, particularly with individuals at risk, such as HIV-infected men and women (3388). Based on findings thus far, stages in HPV infection can be defined and interpreted for risk of developing carcinoma (Table 12.6).

Table 12.6 Stages in human papillomavirus (HPV) infection[a]

Phase 1: HIV-negative/early infection
Low-level HPV infection
Low prevalence of disease
Low-grade disease

Phase 2: late asymptomatic HIV infection
Active HPV replication
Increasing prevalence of low-grade disease

Phase 3: symptomatic HIV infection
HPV replication
Increasing prevalence of low-grade disease
Increasing prevalence of high-grade disease

[a]From reference 3388.

C. Pathogenesis

Anal cancer, like cervical cancer, often arises in areas of squamous metaplasia near the glandular epithelium. A progressive course can be observed histologically from mild dysplasia to severe dys-

plasia (i.e., carcinoma in situ) (3388) (Figure 12.9). Most cervical and anal cancers develop from intraepithelial neoplasia, called CIN and AIN, respectively (Color Plate 21, following page 366). These lesions appear to be increased in HIV infection (3145, 3646) and have genetic alterations, some of which are found in cervical cancers. This finding, perhaps linked to oncogene expression, suggests a relationship to HPV infection (1690). On cytologic examination, enlarged nuclei and irregular shapes and coarse chromatin are noted (Figure 12.10). HPV has been found to be associated with both cervical and anal cancers, and these malignancies are quite similar histologically (4909, 4985).

The development of cancer in the anal canal (as well as the cervix) is greatly increased in the presence of HPV, particularly the high-risk strains HPV-16 and -18 (4985). A common finding is binding and inactivation of the cellular p53 tumor suppressor protein by HPV proteins (e.g., E6 and

Figure 12.9 Schematic presentation of different grades of anal intraepithelial neoplasia (AIN). AIN grade 1 is characterized by 20 and 25% replacement of the epithelium with immature cells with a high nucleus/cytoplasm ratio. AIN grade 2 has approximately 50% replacement with immature cells, and grade 3 has complete or nearly complete replacement of the normal epithelium with immature cells. Microinvasion, shown at the bottom of the figure, takes place when cells traverse the basement membrane. Microinvasion usually occurs with AIN grades 2 to 3 as indicated. Reprinted from reference 3388 with permission.

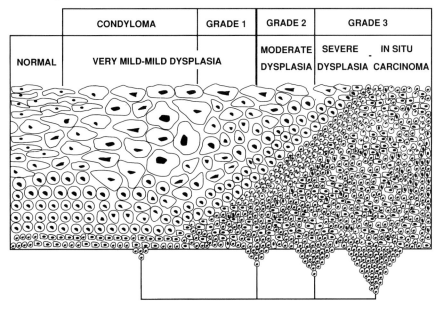

MICROINVASIVE CARCINOMA

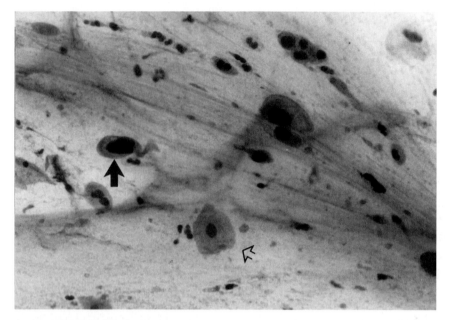

Figure 12.10   Cytologic appearance of AIN grade 2. Note the enlarged nuclei with irregular shape (dark arrow) and cross-chromatin. A normal cell with a small nucleus/cytoplasm ratio is seen nearby (open arrow). Magnification, ×500. Reprinted from reference 3388 with permission.

E7) and, in some cases, mutations in the p53 gene (3960, 4732) (Figure 12.11). This process is more efficient with the high-risk strains of HPV. The HPV early gene product (E7) also inactivates the retinoblastoma (RB) gene product (3959), another tumor suppressor protein that regulates the extent of cell replication. These findings on the effects of E6 and E7 on p53 are mirrored in HPV-negative cervical cancer, in which mutations in p53 have been noted (921). These tumors are usually found in older individuals.

The role of the immune response in HPV expression is reflected in the known appearance in immunosuppressed individuals of warts associated with cancer or organ transplants (3468). Many men who have sex with men have florid condylomata accumulata. The onset of the anal cancer may therefore reflect inadequate cellular immune reactions to HPV or to transformed cell antigens. Alternatively, cytokines produced by HIV replication or immune imbalance (Section I) could influence cell growth and susceptibility to HPV gene transformation.

V. Cervical Carcinoma

A. Epidemiology and Pathology

Several studies (2766) have emphasized that an advanced state of cervical carcinoma can be found in women who are HIV positive. The aggressive tumors are present in those subjects with a poor immune status, as measured by $CD4^+$ cell counts. Variability in response also seems to be directly related to whether women are infected by HIV.

Cervical neoplasia in HIV infection appears to be increasing in prevalence and severity (483, 2863). HIV-infected women have twice the risk of abnormal cytologic results on cervical smears as uninfected women and have a high prevalence of persistent HPV infections (3145). HIV-infected women also have an increased risk of squamous intraepithelial cell lesions, precursors to cervical cancer (1190). Twenty percent of women followed over 3 years developed this lesion. HIV-infected women as well are at an increased risk of developing invasive vulvar carcinoma, indicating that a thorough inspection of the vulva and perianal

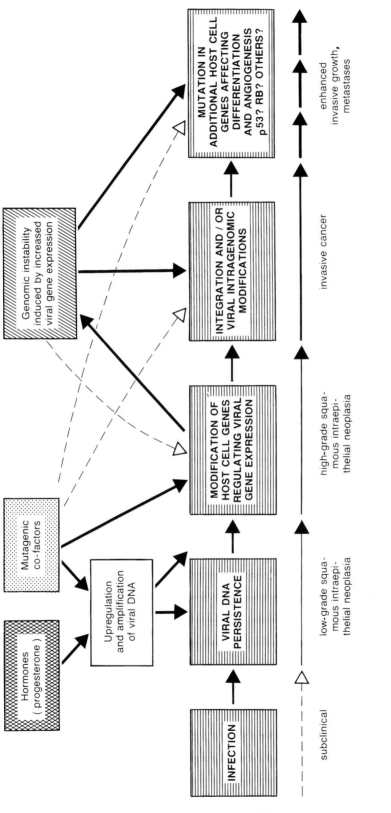

Figure 12.11 Proposed schema of pathogenesis of anal-genital cancer. Subclinical infection with human papillomavirus establishes viral persistence, and various factors interact to lead to a final transformation event. As with other malignancies, chromosomal changes caused by genomic instability would be involved. Control or regression could be mediated by cellular immune responses that are absent in HIV infection. Reprinted from reference 4985 with permission from Elsevier.

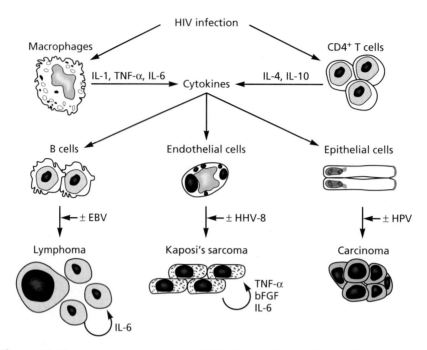

Figure 12.12 Induction of cancers in HIV infection. Virus infection of macrophages, CD4+ cells, or other cells could lead to production of cytokines that enhance the proliferation of certain target cells, such as B cells, endothelial cells, and epithelial cells. The enhanced replication of these cells—either through aprocrine cytokine production or through subsequent viral infection (Epstein-Barr virus [EBV], human papillomavirus [HPV], or human herpesvirus 8 [HHV-8])—could lead to the eventual development of the malignancies noted. In some cases, such as B-cell lymphomas and Kaposi's sarcoma, ongoing cytokine production by the tumor cells maintains the malignant state. (See also Figure 12.8.)

regions is needed for women followed with HIV infection (864).

Whether there is an increased incidence of invasive cervical cancer in HIV-infected women compared to uninfected women remains controversial and may depend upon socioeconomic factors. In certain populations, cervical cancer is one of the most common AIDS-defining illnesses of HIV infection (2766), and its presence, in its invasive form, is now part of the diagnosis of AIDS (643) (see Appendix III). The pathway leading to transformation resembles that of anal carcinoma; likewise, the role of HPV in this tumor is not yet fully defined (Figure 12.11). While the interaction of HPV with tumor suppressor genes seems apparent, why these tumors are more prominent in the immunocompromised individual is not known. Conceivably, as discussed with B-cell lymphomas, cytokines could be produced

that increase the proliferation of epithelial cells and enhance HPV replication (Figure 12.12).

As noted above, HPV may not always be needed for induction of this cancer; on rare occasions, virus-negative cervical carcinomas have been detected (921). These tumors emphasize the molecular aspects of the carcinogenic process, with the viral agents most probably acting as cofactors in the induction of the malignancy (Figures 12.5, 12.7, 12.11, and 12.12). Finally, a possible role in controlling HPV infection has been suggested from studies indicating that women on HAART had reduced progression of HPV disease and tumor regression (3024), including cervical intraepithelial cancers (1782). Nevertheless, HPV infection persisted in the majority of women (1033). Restoration of anti-HPV immune responses could be involved. In this regard, the reduced incidence of cervical carcinoma in women immunized with an

HPV vaccine supports the role of the immune system in preventing this tumor (2306).

B. Conclusions

The findings suggest that HPV infection promotes the development of anal or cervical carcinoma through the suppression of cellular proteins (e.g., p53 and RB) that control cell division. With increased cell replication, chromosome aberrations and transformation can take place. As discussed above, a similar explanation for development of KS and B-cell lymphomas has been considered (Figures 12.1, 12.2, and 12.8). In an immunocompromised host, HPV replication as well as the growth of malignant cells could be enhanced (for reviews, see references 4985 and 4986) (Figure 12.11). It is for this reason that these HPV-associated carcinomas reach much more advanced stages in immunosuppressed hosts (2767). Nevertheless, anal carcinomas and cervical carcinomas can develop, although rarely without evidence of HPV infection (3388). In these cases, the role of cytokines should be further examined (Figures 12. 11 and 12.12). Finally, most reports suggest that HAART has only a limited effect on CIN (1781) and has had no substantial influence on prevalence of or survival from HIV-associated anal cancer (472, 3389).

VI. Summary

HIV infection can set off a chain of events that leads to development of KS, B-cell lymphomas, anal carcinomas, and possibly cervical cancers in the infected individual. Other malignancies may emerge at high frequency in the future. For instance, all of

Table 12.7 Disorders induced by HIV infection that could promote cancer development[a]

- Loss of antibodies to oncogenic virus (e.g., EBV and HPV)
- Loss of cytotoxic CD8[+] T cells (anticancer, antiviral)
- Loss of antibodies to cancer cells
- Loss of NK cell function (anticancer, antiviral)
- Release of cell growth-promoting cytokines (increase cell proliferation)
- Release of cytokines that block apoptosis

[a]EBV, Epstein-Barr virus; HPV, human papillomavirus.

the following have shown an increased incidence in HIV infection: Hodgkin's disease, potentially involving EBV in several cases (1824); multiple myelomas; and seminomas (2714). The mechanisms involved could include either immune suppression or immune enhancement associated with virus infection (Figure 12.3; Table 12.7). A major consideration, because of the potential approaches to therapy, is the role of cytokines in these diseases (Figures 12.1, 12.2, 12.8, and 12.12). B cells, endothelial cells, and epithelial cells could proliferate as a result of cytokine production and could give rise to lymphomas, KS, and anal carcinomas. The chromosomal changes that take place can result from this stimulated growth or directly from an infectious agent, and eventually the malignancy is established. In some cases (e.g., polyclonal B-cell lymphoma), the persistent growth into a cancer could be caused solely by cytokine production. In the presence of immunologic disorders, tumors, such as cervical carcinoma, could spread more readily.

SALIENT FEATURES • CHAPTER 12

1. Malignancies develop in HIV-infected individuals, either through a loss of anticancer immune activity or through hyperactive immune responses that increase proliferation of target cells.

2. The steps involved in transformation could involve increased proliferation of target cells, activation of an oncogenic agent and/or a clastogenic event, and subsequent cell transformation.

3. Kaposi's sarcoma (KS) is the most common malignancy observed in HIV infection and appears to involve endothelial cells, most probably of vascular origin.

4. KS-associated herpesvirus/human herpesvirus 8 (KSHV/HHV-8) appears to be the proximal agent involved in KS and perhaps in body cavity-based lymphomas. It has several genes associated with transforming function, but its direct role in cell transformation has not yet been demonstrated.

5. Serologic studies suggest that KSHV/HHV-8 is present in all KS patients and patients with body cavity-based lymphomas. The virus is found in saliva, nasal secretions, and semen. Antibodies to the virus can be found in up to 25% of the healthy population. Seroconversion occurs primarily around the age of puberty.

6. Diffuse aggressive B-cell lymphomas occur at various sites during HIV infection. The peripheral B-cell lymphomas can have c-*myc* rearrangements. Some peripheral lymphomas and all those primary to the brain contain Epstein-Barr virus (EBV).

7. Lymphomas in the body cavity have either EBV and HHV-8 or HHV-8 alone. Some B-cell lymphomas contain neither HHV-8 nor EBV, indicating that cell transformation does not require infection by these viruses.

8. Despite the use of antiviral therapy, B-cell lymphomas are now more common as an initial AIDS-defining condition.

9. The incidence of anal carcinomas is increased in HIV infection in both men and women. These carcinomas are linked to human papillomavirus (HPV) infections.

10. Anal dysplasia is increased more than threefold in HIV-positive men when they show decreased CD4+ cell counts. This finding suggests a link of HPV activation to dysplasia and the eventual development of cancer.

11. Cervical cancer can be the AIDS-defining illness in some women. It is associated with persistent HPV infection.

12. HPV may promote the development of anal or cervical carcinoma by its suppression of certain cellular proteins (e.g., p53 and RB) that control cell division. With increased cell replication, chromosome aberrations and subsequent cell transformation take place.

13. HPV-associated carcinomas (anal and cervical) reach more advanced stages in immunosuppressed (HIV-infected) hosts.

14. Cervical carcinoma appears to be much more advanced in women who are HIV positive than in those who are not. These women have twice the risk of abnormal cervical smears and a high prevalence of persistent HPV infections.

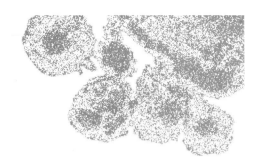

Overall Features of HIV Pathogenesis: Prognosis for Long-Term Survival

HIV PATHOGENESIS REFLECTS the various biologic properties of HIV and the host's immune response to the virus. The differential expression of these two major components of HIV infection determines the final outcome: long-term survival or development of AIDS with its associated opportunistic infections and cancers. How these features of HIV pathogenesis, discussed in the previous chapters, influence survival from HIV infection becomes an important consideration.

I. Cofactors in HIV Infection and Disease Progression

A. General Observations

Whether factors other than HIV itself determine HIV infection and pathogenesis has been an important question (Table 13.1). In terms of HIV transmission (see Chapter 2) it is evident that multiple sexual contacts and sexually transmitted diseases, particularly those leading to genital ulcers, are cofactors in HIV infection of the host and can enhance transmission of the virus. In addition, the use of alcohol and illicit drugs can increase the risk of HIV transmission by compromising mental status.

After infection has occurred, certain factors, in addition to HIV itself, appear to influence progression to disease (Table 13.1). This conclusion is based on the variation in time observed from infection to the development of symptoms and AIDS among different individuals, even those receiving the same contaminated blood. Genetic differences in the host are an obviously important variable (Section III.C). Age has also been recognized as having an influence on progression to disease (Section III.D). In addition, the extent of activation of CD4+ cells needed for effi-

Table 13.1 Potential cofactors in HIV infection and pathogenesis

- Multiple sexual contacts
- Sexually transmitted diseases
- Alcohol and illicit drugs
- Genetic background (Tables 13.9 and 13.10)
- Age
- Immune activation
- Antigenic stimulation (e.g., immunization)
- Other viruses (e.g., herpesvirus and HTLV[a])
- Other infections (e.g., tuberculosis and parasites)
- Immune suppression (e.g., cytokines, drugs, toxins, T regulatory cells)
- Lifestyle (e.g., smoking, depression, and stress)

[a]HTLV, human T-lymphotropic virus.

cient infection and spread of HIV has been considered. Moreover, the consequences of immune activation involving both CD4$^+$ cells and CD8$^+$ cells with the loss of T cells via apoptosis must be appreciated (see Section II.D and Chapter 6). Thus, potential roles in HIV pathogenesis of other viruses (e.g., herpesviruses and papovaviruses), foreign antigens (e.g., vaccinations), and cytokines that increase immune activation have been proposed. Furthermore, additional immune suppression, resulting from other infectious agents, drugs, toxins, or T regulatory cells (Chapter 11), could be a contributing event. Certain potential cofactors are discussed in this section. Other influences on the pathogenic course, including lifestyle, are covered in Section III.

Before the use of HAART, patients with opportunistic diseases had greater declines in CD4$^+$ cell counts and a risk of death (668) independent of initial CD4$^+$ cell count. In most cases, infection by pathogens of both bacterial and viral origin increased plasma viral RNA levels (1113). The enhanced HIV replication during the acute coinfections most likely reflects immune activation with production of TNF-α and interleukin-2 (IL-2) as well as other cytokines (4329). These cellular factors can influence the course of HIV infection (see below). Nevertheless, no specific factor, besides the genetic makeup of the individual, appears to be a consistent determinant of long-term survival versus disease progression.

B. Infection by Other Microbial Organisms

Coinfection of cells with certain viruses, including herpesviruses, papovaviruses, hepatitis viruses, and retroviruses, can increase the expression and production of HIV-1 by other mechanisms besides cytokine production (for a review, see reference 2096) (see Chapter 3). These studies have demonstrated that transactivating factors produced by the infecting virus, usually early gene products, interact directly or via intracellular factors with the HIV long terminal repeat (LTR), usually in the NF-κB region. As examples, cytomegalovirus (CMV), human herpesvirus 6 (HHV-6), and Epstein-Barr virus (EBV) have been shown to activate the HIV LTR, as measured in cell culture by the choramphenicol acetyltransferase assay (977, 1488, 1519, 1893, 2154, 3662, 4129); for a review, see reference 3232) (see Chapter 13). Some experiments, however, indicate that the activation of HIV replication by DNA viruses can involve regions of the viral LTR that are independent of the normal cellular activation pathways (3195, 3362). These studies, showing effects on the HIV LTR by other viruses, have been supported by some observations in vitro with dually infected cells, in which HIV production is increased (629, 1545, 1804, 2705, 4168).

1. HERPESVIRUSES

A possible cofactor in HIV pathogenesis is infection by another virus that could suppress immune responses (3819). Moreover, through genital ulcers, HIV can increase the risk of HIV transmission (589, 1887, 3538) (see Chapter 2). One study suggested that concomitant CMV infection was associated with a more rapid progression toward AIDS in hemophiliacs (4697). In another, acute infection with CMV did not appear to affect substantially the loss of CD4$^+$ cells, but the risk of progression to AIDS in the infected individuals was doubled (3744).

Some investigators have reported enhanced HIV replication following coinfection in cell culture studies with herpesviruses (e.g., CMV, herpes simplex virus [HSV], and HHV-6) (629, 1545, 2705, 3051) (Table 13.2). Some isolates of HHV-6 are reported to induce the CD4 molecule on the surface of CD8$^+$ cells and natural killer (NK) cells

Table 13.2 Herpesviruses as cofactors in HIV infection[a]

- Suppression of immune responses (3819)
- Cause of genital ulcers; enhancement of HIV transmission (589, 1887, 3538)
- Increase progression to disease (e.g., CMV) (3744, 4697)
- Affect HIV replication: enhancement (629, 1545, 2705, 3051, 4934) or inhibition (623, 927, 2313, 2542, 4028)
- Induce CD4 on CD8+ cells and NK cells (2704, 2706)
- Induce β-chemokine receptor (US28) on cells (3537)
- Induction of complement and Fc receptors on infected cells—potential role in antibody-mediated enhancement of infection (2933, 2947)
- Phenotypic mixing (4960)
- Linked to HIV-associated malignancies: KS (i.e., HHV-8) and B-cell lymphoma (i.e., EBV) (686, 1814)
- Induction of hairy leukoplakia (i.e., EBV) (1624)
- Destructive effects on brain and other tissues (e.g., CMV) (4757, 4758)

[a]Includes herpes simplex virus, cytomegalovirus (CMV), Epstein-Barr virus (EBV), human herpesvirus 6 (HHV-6), and HHV-7 KS, Kaposi's sarcoma. See also Table 13.3.

(2704, 2706). Thus, infection by this herpesvirus could permit HIV infection of these cells. Previous EBV transformation of B cells (1804) increases the replication of HIV in these cells (see Chapter 5), and infection of T cells in culture by EBV has enhanced HIV-1 production, possibly via expression of EBNA-2 (954, 3058, 4934). However, other studies have shown that CMV, HHV-6, and EBV suppress HIV replication when cultured cells are coinfected with these viruses (623, 2313, 2542) (see also Chapter 5). The conflicting data could reflect the cell types or the virus isolates used. In addition, HHV-7 utilizes CD4 as its cellular receptor (2707) and could interfere with HIV infection of T cells and macrophages (927). The down-regulation of CXCR4 on CD4+ T cells infected by HHV-6 and HHV-7 has also been reported (4028, 4864). An effect on the viral LTR could be involved (416, 1398).

As discussed in Chapter 3, herpesviruses can also induce the Fc receptor on the surface of cells and may therefore permit HIV infection via antigen:antibody complexes (2933). Since CMV infects

astrocytes and can be found together with HIV in brain cells (3233), such a mechanism could be involved in HIV entry and spread in the brain. The report that CMV can induce a chemokine coreceptor (US28) in infected cells that could be used by HIV for entry (3537) may also have clinical relevance. However, coinfection of lymphocytes by HIV and CMV appears to be very rare in vivo (347).

Clinically, several instances of concomitant infection of the host by different herpesviruses can be cited as evidence for their role as cofactors in HIV infection. Acute HSV infection can cause an increase in HIV viremia (3051), and HSV reactivation can enhance HIV replication in infected subjects. Some other cell culture studies and observations in vivo (see Chapter 5) (1810) suggest that HIV itself might be a cofactor in herpesvirus infections by enhancing or suppressing the replication of these viruses (608, 2542, 4168), possibly through cytokine production. Reactivation of certain herpesviruses has been noted during acute primary HIV infection (2496). These findings could explain the beneficial effect of the use of the antiherpesvirus drug, acyclovir, on survival with HIV infection (3951).

Herpesviruses could also play a role in HIV pathogenesis through their association with Kaposi's sarcoma (KS) (e.g., HHV-8), B-cell lymphomas (e.g., EBV), and hairy leukoplakia (e.g., EBV) (see Chapter 12) (664, 686, 1624, 1814) and their destruction of tissues such as the brain (e.g., CMV) (589, 3538, 4757, 4758).

2. OTHER VIRUSES

HIV replication can also be increased after coinfection of T cells with HTLV-1 (1722) or after their exposure to HTLV antigens in vitro (4904) (Table 13.2). In some cases, these effects of other viruses on HIV were found to be mediated by cytokine production (see Chapters 5 and 9) (1306, 2871). Some investigators have reported an increase in the development of AIDS in HTLV-1-infected subjects (275, 3380), whereas other observations suggest that HTLV-2 infection of CD8+ cells (1700) might delay the course of disease in coinfected subjects (4504, 4614) (Table 13.3).

Hepatitis C virus (HCV) is an RNA virus in the *Flaviviridae* family and is found in about one-third

Table 13.3 Potential effects of infectious agents on HIV replication in culture[a]

Infectious agent(s)	Effect(s)
CMV, HSV, HHV-6, EBV	Increase HIV replication in T cells via LTR activation (1545, 3051, 3232, 4934)
EBV	Enhance replication in B cells (3058)
HHV-6	Induce CD4 expression on CD8[+] lymphocyes and NK cells (2704, 2706)
HTLV and other retroviruses	Increase HIV production (596, 1722)
Influenza virus	Increase CXCR4 expression and X4 virus infection (3624)
Influenza virus	Reduce HIV replication via IFN-α induction (3520)
Measles virus	Suppress HIV replication (1446, 1633)
CMV, HHV-6, HHV-7, and EBV	Inhibit HIV replication (623, 927, 2313, 2542)
HHV-7	Could reduce HIV infection and replication (927, 2707, 4028)
CMV	Induce Fc receptor; permit infection by virus:Ab complex (2933)
	Induce chemokine coreceptor (US28) (3537)
GBV-C	Reduce HIV replication (3221, 4834)
M. tuberculosis	Increase HIV replication (X4) via the LTR or enhanced CCR4 expression on macrophages (1895)
M. tuberculosis and *M. avium*	Increase HIV replication via enhanced CCR5 and CXCR4 expression on T cells and macrophages (2054, 4648)
Neisseria	Increase HIV via LTR (711)
Malaria	Increase HIV replication (4837)

[a]See also Table 13.2. CMV, cytomegalovirus; HSV, herpes simplex virus; HHV-6, human herpesvirus 6; EBV, Epstein-Barr virus; HTLV, human T-lymphotropic virus; GBV-C, GB virus C; LTR, long terminal repeat; IFN-α, alpha interferon; Ab, antibody.

of HIV-infected subjects in the United States (4330). Six different subtypes have been identified. The level of HCV RNA is higher in HIV-coinfected subjects, and there is a more rapid progression to HCV-related liver disease (4330, 4582). Some studies have also suggested that HCV accelerates HIV-related diseases (115, 3524), but others have reported no direct effect of HCV on HIV disease progression (4331, 4989).

Hepatitis B virus (HBV) does not affect the course of HIV infection, but with HIV infection, the extent of inflammatory liver disease due to HBV is reduced (1518). The latter finding might reflect a less aggressive anti-HBV response of an HIV-compromised cellular immune system. In this regard, HIV infection can reduce both HBV- and HCV-specific T-cell responses without affecting the cellular immune activity against EBV (2190, 2416). Recommendations for the care of HBV and HCV coinfection with HIV have been published (2274, 4210).

During acute measles virus infection, HIV replication can be suppressed for short periods, perhaps by the production of type 1 interferon and other virus-inhibitory factors (3141) (see Chapter 11).

Measles virus can also inhibit HIV production in lymphoid tissue culture, particularly by R5 viruses, most likely via the up-regulation of RANTES production (1446, 1633). Influenza virus infection appears to block HIV replication as well by induction of alpha interferon (IFN-α) (3520). Plasmacytoid dendritic cells (PDCs) could be responsible for this cytokine release (see Chapter 9). Nevertheless, some studies suggest that influenza virus can enhance X4 infection via its induction of CXCR4 expression (3624).

GB virus C (GBV-C), another flavivirus, causes no disease in humans but replicates in lymphocytes (4835). Several studies have indicated that HIV-infected subjects with GBV-C viremia live longer, have higher CD4[+] T-cell counts, and have a slower decrease in the number of CD4[+] T cells over time; in some reports, lower plasma viral RNA levels were noted (373, 1820, 4430, 4835). Circulating virus can persist for many years, but in most individuals there is a clearance of GBV-C and a development of antibodies against the viral envelope protein E-2 (4420). Without viremia, the protective effect of this virus on HIV infection appears to be lost (4774). The reason for the observed protection with GBV-C is not known. The virus inhibits HIV replication in peripheral blood mononuclear cells (PBMC) in vitro, perhaps by its induction of a T-cell soluble antiviral factor (2056) or of β-chemokines and the subsequent reduction in CCR5 expression (3221, 4834, 4835). However, in vivo, chemokine (e.g., SDF-1) and cytokine levels in plasma were not found to be increased in GBV-C coinfection (1520).

The preexisting presence of GBV-C viremia does not appear to protect against HIV transmission or affect the viral set point (383). In this regard, in a study of 271 men, GBV-C viremia was significantly associated with prolonged survival 5 to 6 years after HIV infection, but not after 12 to 18 months. Thus, the timing of GBV-C infection may determine the protective effect. The presence of GBV-C viremia could also reflect a nonactivated immune state associated with long-term survival (Section V.C). Alternatively, since GBV-C infects CD4+ cells, some investigators suggest that the GBV-C viremia associated with an asymptomatic state in HIV-infected individuals could merely result from sufficient CD4+ cells being present as target cells for infection (4774).

3. BACTERIA AND PARASITES

It is noteworthy that immune activation from long-term exposure to a variety of antigens or infectious agents can enhance the activation state in individuals and may increase their susceptibility to HIV infection and its spread. Some parasitic diseases, because of a type 2 immune dominant state, may be associated with a poor prognosis for HIV infection (311). Such consideration has been given to HIV-negative Africans who have shown high levels of immune activation markers in their sera (311, 3741; for a review, see reference 310). HIV infection in African subjects appears to be more progressive. In addition, when female sex workers in Kenya were compared with mothers enrolled in HIV vertical-transmission studies, the sex workers had a faster clinical course, most likely reflecting immune activation resulting from concomitant sexually transmitted diseases (574).

In terms of specific bacterial infections, the prevalence of *Mycobacterium tuberculosis* has dramatically increased with the occurrence of the HIV epidemic, reflecting the reduced immune function in infected individuals. Some immunologic studies on HIV-infected individuals with *M. tuberculosis* infection have suggested that the increased immune activation observed with this bacterial infection, most likely via TLR-2, enhances HIV replication and progression to AIDS (208, 4666). Moreover, *M. tuberculosis* can enhance LTR transcription or CXCR4 expression on alveolar macrophages and induce β-chemokine production. This response could help the preferential growth of X4 viruses (1895). In a recent study, *M. tuberculosis* was found to be associated with an increased cellular expression of CCR5 and CXCR4 that could increase HIV infection (3798). Nevertheless, treatment of active tuberculosis for 6 months has not markedly affected HIV viral loads, although the CD4+ cell counts have increased (3113). *Mycobacterium avium* complex as well as *M. tuberculosis* present in HIV-infected people can also increase TNF-α production and the expression of CCR5 and CXCR4, thereby increasing HIV replication (2053, 2054, 4648).

An increase in viral load has been described as well for bacterial pneumonias (570), but no substantial change has been noted in RNA levels with acute respiratory infections most likely caused by viruses (4611). An enhancing effect of *Neisseria gonorrhoeae* on the HIV LTR has also been noted (711). Malarial antigens can enhance HIV replication and the release of cytokines (e.g., TNF-α and IL-6) that are detrimental to the host (4837). Moreover, HIV-1 infection has been associated with increased susceptibility to malarial infections (2084). In Africa, coinfection of HIV-infected individuals with *P. falciparum* leads to severe malaria and increased chance of death (13a, 1631b).

TNF-α, as noted above for *Mycobacterium*, appears to be responsible for the increased HIV replication observed in many cases of this opportunistic infection (4837). Of note, HIV infection has reduced antimalarial antibody responses (3148). *Schistosoma mansoni* coinfection with increased HIV-1 viremia has also been associated with decreased cellular antimicrobial immune responses, including HIV-specific CTL activity, perhaps reflecting an increase in IL-10 production characteristic of a type 2 immune response (2922, 3859). Finally, some studies indicate that acute scrub typhus infection can reduce HIV viral loads (4692). Serum suppressing factors, which have not been identified, could be responsible for this observation.

C. Effect of Vaccinations

Several studies suggest that postinfection immunization procedures will enhance HIV release through antigenic stimulation (1392). An increase in HIV levels in the plasma has been noted after receipt of a pneumococcal vaccine (503). Moreover, both influenza and tetanus immunizations have led to a transient increase in viremia in most studies (3307, 4260, 4262) but not all (1532, 1540). The differences observed may be due to the time of measuring viremia, since the highest increase in viral replication usually occurs in the first few days after immunization. While the above reports have raised the issue of whether infected individuals should be vaccinated, the short duration of the rise in viral load and the importance of protection against several of the infectious agents argue for continuation of immunization in seropositive individuals. In this regard, influenza virus vaccination in HIV-infected individuals often shows a weak antibody response unless the CD4+ cell counts are high (2773). Similar reduced responses to other vaccines (e.g., tetanus and diphtheria toxoids) can be observed in HIV-infected individuals, particularly those with low CD4+ cell counts (2402). Treatment with antiretroviral drugs has restored the antibody response to influenza virus vaccines (2332).

D. Effect of Cytokine Production

The role of TNF-α and other proinflammatory cytokines in increasing HIV viral loads was discussed above and in previous chapters. The ability of certain cytokines to increase and decrease HIV replication could influence the clinical course and has been associated with increased viral loads in coinfections (see above and Chapter 8, Table 8.7). In terms of cytokines affecting an overall immunologic reaction, evidence has suggested that type 2 immune responses (e.g., IL-4 and IL-10 production) can result from infections with helminth or other parasites and exposure to allergens (17, 3787, 3859). Allergy has been associated with enhanced CD4+ cell loss in some infected individuals (1085), perhaps secondary to IL-4 release by mast cells (480). Since type 2 cytokines can suppress the production of type 1 cytokines (see Chapter 11, Section II.C), cell-mediated anti-HIV immune responses could be diminished by these concurrent infections or allergies (17). This possibility is still a hypothesis (311), and further studies need to be conducted to determine whether coinfection by certain pathogens or allergic reactions could influence HIV pathogenesis by production of selective cytokines.

At the cellular level, differences in replication among viruses can certainly result from external stimuli, such as cytokines, acting on intracellular factors that influence the expression of particular HIV isolates (see Chapter 5). For example, TNF-α and IL-1, via protein kinase C activation, appear to enhance the attachment of the NF-κB protein to the promoter region of the viral LTR and increase virus replication (Figure 5.3) (1144, 2317, 2871, 3350). These cytokines are produced by activated macrophages and T cells and by HIV-infected cells.

E. Lifestyle Factors

Certain cell culture and clinical studies have examined the effect of lifestyle conditions on virus expression in peripheral blood (Table 13.1). Morphine and other opiates can increase the production of IFN-γ and IL-2, leading to enhanced virus replication (3301). When methadone was added to cultured human fetal microglia and monocyte-derived macrophages, it increased HIV infection of these cells substantially (2582). This enhancement reflected an up-regulation of CCR5 on the macrophages. When added to latently infected PBMC, methadone increased virus activation and replication (2582). These findings suggest a mechanism by which opioids and other drugs could affect HIV replication and pathogenesis. In this regard, rhesus macaques receiving morphine were shown to have a higher viral set points than control animals (2346).

Some investigators have reported that alcohol can enhance HIV replication (714) in vitro, particularly via an increase in CXCR4 expression (2637). Moreover, alcohol intake was found to increase the sensitivity of a subject's PBMC to HIV infection and growth (209, 212). Alcohol also appeared to have a toxic effect on CD8+ lymphocyte function (209) (Table 13.1). Chronic alcohol consumption in rhesus macaques gave higher SIV levels than in conventional infected animals, most likely related to reduced mucosal T-lymphocyte numbers and function (3573). In other studies, cocaine enhanced HIV replication in cultured PBMC (215, 3489), most probably via TNF-α production (3489). Moreover, morphine sulfate increased SIV replication in T cells (769) and decreased cellular and humoral antiviral immune responses in rhesus monkeys infected with SIV (770). These findings contrast with early observations in vivo that suggested no role for alcohol and other psychoactive drugs in enhancing progression to disease (2111). Smoking has been found to reduce the accessory cell function of alveolar macrophages in HIV-infected individuals (4514). Cigarette smoking also increases the susceptibility of those cells to HIV-1 infection (5). All these factors could influence HIV-related disease (3260, 4514).

Reduced fertility is seen in HIV infection (1607, 3810) secondary to lower rates of conception and increased pregnancy loss. Pregnancy, however, does not appear to influence progression from seroconversion to disease in HIV-infected women (3853).

Acute exercise has induced a transient rise in the number of lymphocytes but not other cells in HIV-positive men (4526). Notably, the association of clinical depression with a decrease in CD4+ cell counts and progression to disease has been reported by some groups (556) but not by others (2711, 3647). Since emotional states, such as stress, can affect hormone (e.g., norepinephrine and cortisol) levels and immunologic functions, a possible increase in HIV replication, which was reported (841, 844, 2179), should be evaluated further. For example, stress may enhance HIV disease progression by increasing viral replication, suppressing immune responses, and inducing harmful behavior patterns (for a review, see reference 3758).

In support of a role for the autonomic nervous system in stimulating HIV replication, recent studies have shown a spatial relationship between catecholaminergic neural fibers and the sites of SIV replication in lymph nodes of SIV-infected rhesus macaques (4173). Active SIV replication was up to fourfold greater in the region of the catecholamine neurotransmitters (e.g., norepinephrine). However, some investigators have reported that norepinephrine, which is increased with exercise and

stress, can inhibit HIV replication in PBMC by inactivating NF-κB (3111). Studies with physiological doses of catecholamines need to be conducted to evaluate these contrasting observations in HIV replication. Finally, rhesus macaques placed under stressful conditions had higher levels of SIV replication and shorter survival, perhaps related to lower concentrations of plasma cortisol (607). In this regard, corticosteroids do not affect HIV growth in vitro (2431), suggesting that short-term treatment with these hormones will not be harmful. Nevertheless, the immune-suppressing effects of steroids need to be considered.

F. Primate Studies of Cofactors in HIV Pathogenesis

In animal studies examining the effect of potential cofactors on the clinical state, HIV-1-infected chimpanzees were inoculated intrarectally with a chimpanzee CMV and monitored for signs of disease. Whereas no evidence of pathology ensued, the chimpanzees began to release HIV-1 in their blood, a characteristic not observed in these animals for over a year previously (641). Whether immune enhancement or suppression brought about this change in viral control is not known. In associated studies, anti-Leu 2a (anti-CD8) antibodies were inoculated into HIV-infected chimpanzees to determine if a reduction in the CD8+ cell count would bring about renewed HIV replication in vivo. Animals treated for 7 to 14 days showed a decrease in their CD8+ cell numbers, and their PBMC released HIV within 2 months (641). No HIV had been recovered from these chimpanzees for 15 to 40 months previously. Subsequent studies with anti-CD8 antibodies in rhesus macaques showed similar results with a reduced control of SIV infection secondary to a decrease in cellular immune function (2869, 3983) (see Chapter 11). These observations in animals indicate that other agents and cytokine effects (e.g., on CD8+ cells by type 2 cytokines) could permit HIV replication from a relatively controlled cellular state (Section II).

G. Conclusions

HIV is the proximal cause of AIDS, but other infectious agents or environmental factors could influence the progression to disease (Tables 13.1,

Table 13.4 Potential effect of microbial infections on HIV pathogenesis

Enhance

HTLV-1[a] (275, 1722)

Hepatitis C[b] (115, 3524)

Parasitic diseases associated with immune activation (311, 3741)

Mycobacterium tuberculosis (208, 2054, 4666)

Mycobacterium avium complex (4648)

Delay

HTLV-2 (4504, 4614)

Measles (3141)

Influenza (3520)

GB virus C (1820, 4430, 4835)

Schistosoma mansoni (2922, 3859)

Scrub typhus (4692)

---

[a]HTLV, human T-lymphotropic virus.

[b]Some studies have not observed an effect (4331, 4989). In terms of hepatitis B, HIV infection has been found to reduce the extent of liver disease (1518) (see text).

13.2, 13.3, and 13.4). How these cofactors could work in the infected individual is not clear. They might induce cytokines or intracellular factors (see Chapter 5) that promote HIV replication or compromise immune responses. They might modify the production of cytokines (type 1 and type 2) that can affect immune function (see Chapters 9 and 11). They could stimulate the immune system abnormally, leading to increased HIV spread, autoimmune responses, or sequelae of immune activation (e.g., apoptosis) (see Chapters 6 and 9 to 11). Alternatively, cofactors might reduce the cellular antiviral activity and permit the escape of HIV from host immunologic control. For this series of events to occur, a continual compromise of the individual's normal immune function would presumably be needed. Clinically, it appears that other factors, including opportunistic infections, can affect the overall health of the infected individual but that the inherited genetic makeup of the host and the nature of the infecting virus are the most important in determining the pathogenic effects of HIV infection. Genetic factors can influence cell susceptibility to HIV infection and host immune antiviral response (see Chapters 3, 4, and 11 and Section III). However, if left unchallenged, HIV is responsible for the disease progression

observed, either by direct infection of cells or by an indirect effect on the immune system and other tissues in the host (see also Section X).

II. Features of HIV Pathogenesis

The pathogenic pathway, after the acute infection period, can be divided into three major phases (Figure 13.1). In the first phase, the reduction in CD4[+] cell number and immune function reflects a common effect of viral infection, but then with HIV these parameters continue to decrease in association with the slow but persistent replication of relatively noncytopathic, usually macrophage-tropic R5 viruses (phase 2). The viruses reduce the CD4[+] cell number either by direct cytotoxicity or, more often, by an indirect means such as apoptosis (3133) (see Chapter 6). This gradual loss of CD4[+] cells is observed in infected individuals from all risk groups, including blood and clotting factor recipients, intravenous drug users, and sexual contacts (1110, 1238, 4041). When the CD4[+] cell number is decreased to a level too low to support strong cell-mediated immunity (e.g., via IL-2 production), CD8[+] cell anti-HIV activity becomes compromised. HIV replication then returns to its high levels, which is the third major phase of pathogenesis (Figure 13.1). At this time, a more virulent X4 cytopathic strain often emerges that is associated with the ultimate demise of the host (see Section II.C).

In the terminal stage, CD8[+] cells, as well as CD4[+] cells, decrease in number, perhaps in part because of the loss of IL-2 production by CD4[+] cells. Apoptosis of both cell types can also be involved (see Chapter 6). Included in this pathogenic pathway is the disruption in the normal immune balance reflected in lymph node structure and bone marrow integrity, often associated with development of severe opportunistic infections and malignancies (see Chapter 12). Moreover, as noted above, the possibility that cytokine production and hyperresponsiveness of the immune system (e.g., autoimmunity and immune activation) also contribute to the final outcome needs to be considered. The reasons for the emergence of the more pathogenic virus are considered in Section VIII.C.

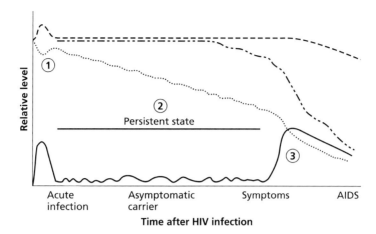

Figure 13.1 Schematic diagram of events occurring after HIV infection. Prior to seroconversion, high levels of virus(—) can be detected in the blood (phase 1). Subsequently, this viremia is reduced to low levels (end of phase 1) and maintained with episodic release of varying amounts of virus over time (phase 2): Months to years later, concurrent with the onset of clinical symptoms, a second high level of viremia occurs and remains raised throughout the terminal period (i.e., development of AIDS) (phase 3). The CD4+ cell number (. . . .) decreases during acute (primary) infection (phase 1) and then returns to a level somewhat below normal. A slow decrease in CD4+ cell count, estimated to be approximately 60 cells/µl per year (2401), occurs over time (the persistent period) (phase 2). Subsequently, in some individuals developing symptoms, a marked decrease in CD4+ cell counts can be observed concomitant with reemergence of high levels of viremia (phase 3). The number of CD8+ cells (- - -) rises during primary infection, as is commonly seen in viral infections. Their number then returns to just above normal and stays elevated until the final stages of disease. In contrast, the CD8+ cell anti-HIV responses (-- — -- —) begin to decrease prior to or around the time of symptoms (late in phase 2) and then to decrease steadily as progression to disease occurs (phase 3). Modified from reference 2516 with permission.

A. Early Period Following Acute Virus Infection (Phase 1)

During sexual transmission, the virus initially enters an individual by infecting "resting" CD4+ cells, activated CD4+ T cells, resident macrophages, dendritic cells (DCs), or mucosal cells lining the rectal or cervicovaginal cavity (1685, 4938) (see Chapter 4). With subsequent transit into the blood, the first cells infected are most probably tissue DCs and macrophages (particularly in lymph nodes or spleen) that are in a differentiated state ready to replicate the virus (see also Chapter 2). These cells then pass virus to T cells after lymphocyte activation. At the time of initial transmission, only a few activated CD4+ lymphocytes are usually circulating in the blood, and peripheral blood monocytes are not very susceptible to infection (see Chapters 3 and 5).

In the initial days following acute infection, virus replication takes place at the site of virus entry, most likely in activated lymphocytes, DCs, and macrophages in the mucosae or the lymphoid tissues (e.g., lamina propria) in the cervicovaginal and gastrointestinal (GI) tracts (1685, 3013) (see Chapters 4 and 9). Sufficient cells must become infected to maintain the infection or it is aborted. This fact can explain the lack of infection in highly exposed individuals (see below) and offers direction for vaccine development. Once the virus infection goes from the initial site to local lymph nodes (within 2 days), the infection has become established (1685, 3013, 4938) (Table 4.4). Viremia results in 5 to 7 days with up to 5,000 infectious particles (IP)/ml, or >10^7 viral RNA molecules per ml of plasma detected (see Chapters 2 and 4). After 10 to 14 days, up to 200 billion CD4+ cells can be infected (1194). The extent of the initial virus production and its subsequent spread reflects the intrinsic susceptibility of the individual mononuclear cells to the entering virus and local immune factors that might limit HIV replication (3013) (see Chapters 3 and 11).

In acute infection, the CD8+ cell numbers rise, as observed in other viral infections (412). Importantly, production of cytokines occurs, primarily of proinflammatory cytokines and chemokines, often causing acute retroviral syndrome (see Chapter 4) and bringing more target cells to the mucosal site of infection. The innate antiviral cytokines (e.g., type 1 interferons) and adaptive CD8+ T cells come too late to prevent the establishment of infection (7, 3714). It is, therefore, during this early period (phase 1), before a sufficient antiviral response develops, that large numbers of cells become infected in lymphoid tissues and other cells in the host (see Chapters 2, 11, and 15). The replicating virus can undergo mutations that increase its virulence (Figure 13.2).

Generally, within weeks after acute infection, viremia is reduced substantially (see Chapter 4), considered by many as a result of the immune response against HIV. Recent studies suggest that this decrease in virus could also reflect a loss of target cells, particularly in the GI tract (i.e., substrate exhaustion) (3494) (see Chapter 8). In the lymph node as well as in the blood at this time, only a small percentage of infected cells (<1%) actively produce virus, most likely reflecting immune cell containment (see Chapters 4 and 11). Cellular immune responses appear to be the first antiviral activity produced; CD8+ cell anti-HIV responses have been noted early and in some cases before seroconversion (446, 804, 2302, 2749) (see Chapters 9 and 11). Virus levels in plasma appear to be reduced before neutralizing antibodies can be detected in recently infected individuals (2302, 2749). However, as observed in the SIV model, the virus-specific CD8+ cells come too late (after 10 to 14 days) to contain the infection (3714). The potential role of innate immune factors (e.g., complement, mannose-binding lectins, interferons, and CD8+ cell antiviral proteins) in suppressing the viremia should also be considered (see Chapters 9 and 11).

Seroconversion takes place within days to weeks after infection but neutralizing antibodies appear to be present only transiently (Figure 13.1) (see Chapters 2, 4, and 10). A virus becomes selected which resists anti-HIV antibodies (see Chapter 10). During the acute or early period, before strong anti-HIV immune responses occur, the viremia reflects replication of a predominant HIV strain detected as a relatively homogeneous virus population (1042, 2104).

B. Persistent Period (Phase 2)

At 3 to 6 months after the primary virus infection, CD4+ cell numbers usually return to near-normal levels (see Chapter 4). They then generally decrease

Figure 13.2 HIV replication permits genetic mutations to the virus. HIV, when replicating through different cells, mutates towards a strain that replicates rapidly, is more cytopathic, and can adapt to grow in various tissues such as the brain. Each replicative cycle can lead to up to 10 mutations (most of them lethal), but the surviving virions generally have a faster replication and a high level of virus replication.

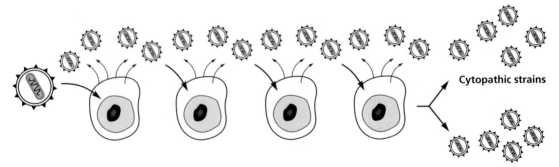

Cytopathic strains

Neuropathic strains

steadily at a rate estimated by some at 25 to 60 cells/μl per year (2401) (Figure 13.1). The reason(s) for this cell loss over time remains one of the unresolved mysteries of this infection (see Chapter 9).

During this asymptomatic period (i.e., phase 2) with virus persistence, HIV replication in the body continues but generally at a low level, particularly in lymph nodes (see Chapter 8). This virus population becomes heterogeneous, probably reflecting the ongoing emergence of virus variants that are selected in the face of anti-HIV immune responses (2915) (see Chapter 4). As discussed in Chapter 4, only 1 in 300 to 400 infected cells in the lymph node may release infectious virus (see Color Plate 9, following page 78) (1194). Peripheral blood contains, in 1 ml, about 1 to 100 IP and 1 to 100,000 infected cells. This continued suppression of HIV replication during the persistent period appears to be mediated by antiviral CD8$^+$ cells (2543, 3827) (see Chapter 11) that help prevent the emergence of a virulent virus.

C. Symptomatic Period (Phase 3)

Within 10 years after infection, many infected individuals develop symptoms, CD4$^+$ cell counts have usually dropped below 350 cells/μl, viral load increases substantially, and a reduction in antiviral CD8$^+$ cell responses can be demonstrated (2396, 2745, 3317) (see Chapter 11) (Figure 13.1). The lack of CD8$^+$ cell suppressing activity is probably reflected in the increased expression of HIV mRNA in CD4$^+$ cells that is detected up to 2 years before the development of disease (3886). In some cases, the CD4$^+$ cell numbers drop precipitously (e.g., up to 200 cells/μl) in just a few months, mirroring a return to high-level virus production (1238, 2516, 3961). This event presages the development of AIDS.

Similar events occur in the lymph node, where virus replication increases concomitant with destruction of the lymphoid tissue, including the follicular dendritic cells (1323) (for reviews, see references 203, 1259, and 3413) and disruption of the normal architecture (see Chapter 4; Chapter 8, Section I.F; and Color Plates 14 and 15, following page 366). The cause of these changes in the lymph nodes is not defined and may represent the effect of the virus or a hyperactivated cellular immune response (see below). The change in the

clinical course appears to be directly related to a reduced cellular immune response, particularly CD8$^+$ cell antiviral activity (484, 2520, 2543, 3827).

During this symptomatic period, and certainly when the individual develops AIDS, the amount of HIV rises to high levels in the blood and lymph node and once again becomes relatively homogeneous. As observed in primary infection, when antiviral immune responses are absent or low, a predominant virus strain emerges. This virus (often with the X4 phenotype) has properties associated with virulence in the host that include an expanded cellular host range, rapid kinetics of replication, and CD4$^+$ cell cytopathicity (Table 13.5) (see Section II.D) (Figures 13.3 and 13.4). The later virus also appears to resist neutralization and can become sensitive to enhancing antibodies (see Chapter 10). This virus is usually related to the early virus at the genomic level (>97%) (731), but certain genetic changes in the regulatory (e.g., *tat*), envelope, and *pol* regions have been found to be associated with these altered in vitro biologic properties (see Chapter 7).

In end-stage disease, CD4$^+$ T cells, rather than macrophages, are still the major source of virus (4546) except perhaps in the GI tract (see Chapter 8). In this regard, lower expression of CXCR4 and higher expression of CCR5 have been found on CD4$^+$ T cells in patients progressing to disease. In these cases, the extent of CD4$^+$ T-cell activation or chemokine receptor expression could not be

Table 13.5 Characteristics of HIV isolates associated with virulence in the host[a]

- Expanded cellular host range
- Rapid kinetics of replication
- High titers of virus production
- Disruption or alteration of cell membrane permeability
- High level of syncytium induction
- Increase in cell killing (cytopathicity)
- Failure to enter a latent state in vitro
- Lack of sensitivity to suppression by the Nef protein[b]
- Sensitivity to antibody-mediated enhancement of infection

[a]Generally observed with X4 viruses but can be noted with R5 viruses isolated in late state disease (2362, 2576).
[b]As assayed with the HIV-1$_{SF2}$ *nef* gene produced in T-cell lines (723).

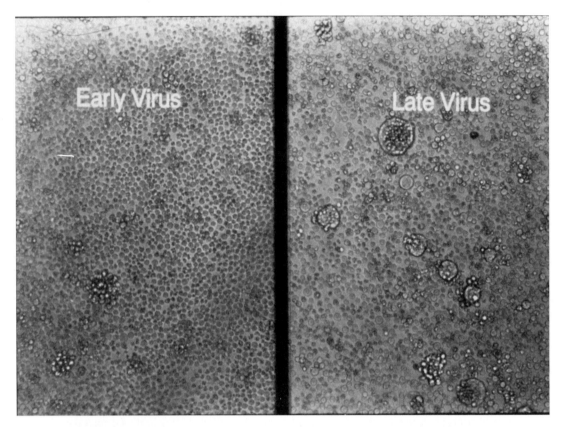

Figure 13.3 HIV-1$_{SF2}$ recovered early during infection from a relatively healthy individual shows very few cytopathic effects when inoculated onto normal peripheral blood mononuclear cells. In contrast, HIV-1$_{SF13}$ isolated later from the same individual when he had AIDS shows the syncytium formation and balloon degeneration characteristic of virulent isolates (Table 13.8). Reprinted from reference 2519 with permission.

distinguished between those individuals infected with X4 versus R5 viruses (3356). Moreover, the R5 isolates in this stage of disease have replicative and cytopathic properties resembling those of X4 viruses (2362, 2576, 4020). In addition, in some cases, the HIV isolates present appear to evolve within the host tissue into neurotropic variants or viruses causing pathology in other organ systems (see Chapter 8).

D. Virologic and Immunologic Factors Responsible for Immune Deficiency

1. POTENTIAL PROCESSES INVOLVED

Several sections of this book have indicated the potential role of R5 versus X4 viruses in the clinical course of HIV infection. Attention, however,

needs to be given to the fact that pathogenesis may be more characteristic of a population of viruses than an individual HIV isolate. Studies with the RNA virus poliovirus have shown that the grouping of viruses with related sequences (i.e., quasispecies) permits greater probability for evolution and adaptation to a new environment (4609). Thus, studies with individual HIV isolates may not provide the correct conclusions relating to in vivo pathogenesis.

The processes leading to a reduction in anti-HIV immune responses, mirrored by the loss of CD4$^+$ cells and CD8$^+$ cell responses, are not yet well defined. Most likely, multiple factors are involved in CD4$^+$ cell loss, and not one factor predominates as the major cause of this decrease (Table 13.6). Some studies suggest that potential

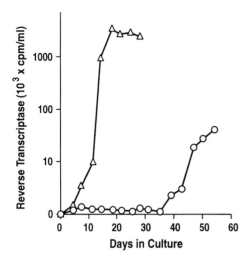

Figure 13.4 Replication of two isolates of HIV-1 recovered from the same individual over time. HIV-1$_{SF2}$ (O), isolated early in the course of infection, replicates slowly and to low titer in the established HUT 78 T-cell line. In contrast, HIV-1$_{SF13}$ (Δ), recovered when the patient had AIDS, grows rapidly and to high titer in the same cells. These and other biologic differences between these two isolates have been used to distinguish viruses in culture as nonvirulent and virulent strains as well as slow/low and rapid/high strains (Table 7.8 and Figure 7.14).

effects of direct infection of CD4$^+$ cells by HIV, an immunologic imbalance, and CD8$^+$ cell cytotoxic responses should be considered (see Chapters 8 and 11). Some early studies established a rapid turnover of the HIV-infected CD4$^+$ cells. This number may not reflect current knowledge, which suggests that these cells could survive longer. However, larger numbers of CD4$^+$ lymphocytes have now been found to be infected than was previously believed, so a direct effect of HIV could explain some loss of CD4$^+$ cells, even though relatively few infected cells show sufficient virus replication that would lead to cell death (see Chapter 4). Moreover, the peripheral blood CD4$^+$ cell level that has been a marker of disease progression may not reflect the large loss of CD4$^+$ cells occurring via HIV infection in the GI tract (493, 2957, 4575) (see Chapter 8) (see below).

Another reason for reduced CD4$^+$ cell function could be the up-regulation of CTLA-4 on CD4$^+$ cells in HIV infection (most likely by immune activation), which can cause a decline in cell number

and anergy (2491). Without dying, the virus-infected cell could still be compromised in its function, including the production of cytokines (e.g., IL-2) necessary for normal immune activity (see Chapters 4 and 11).

Some studies do suggest that a compromise in CD8$^+$ cell anti-HIV function permits a return in high viral replication and immune dysfunction as reflected by a loss in CD4$^+$ cells (Figure 13.5). The relative extent of type 1 and type 2 (4575) cytokine production can influence CD4$^+$ cell numbers, the dominant viral phenotype, and the immune response. The type 1 cytokine pattern has been associated with higher CD4$^+$ cell counts, an R5 virus, and strong CD8$^+$ cell-mediated immunity (see Chapter 11). A high ratio of IL-2 to IL-10 has identified individuals with a good prognosis (799). A dominance of a type 2 immune response is associated with progression to disease (see Chapters 8 and 11). In the case of CD8$^+$ cell noncytotoxic

Table 13.6 Possible causes of reduced CD4$^+$ cell number and function[a]

Direct effects of virus
- Direct infection of CD4$^+$ cells (1736)
- Direct infection of CD4$^+$ cells in the GI tract (493, 2957)
- Infection-mediated death of progenitor cells (e.g., in the thymus) (see Chapter 11)
- Destruction of supporting stromal network required for hematopoiesis (see Chapter 11)
- Up-regulation of CTLA-4 on CD4$^+$ cells (2491)

Indirect effects of HIV infection
- Cytokine imbalance (800, 814, 4575): low IL-2 and IL-10 production (799) (i.e., type 2 response)
- ADCC; killing of CD4$^+$ cells carrying gp120 (see Chapter 10)
- CTL activity against normal CD4$^+$ cells, APC, and B cells (3003, 4914, 4971)
- Autoantibodies (see Chapter 10)
- Immune activation: cell apoptosis (see Chapter 6)
- Opportunistic infection of bone marrow (e.g., by CMV or *Mycobacterium avium-M. intracellulare*)
- Infiltrating malignancies
- Myelotoxic effects of drugs
- Nutritional deficiencies

[a]For other articles, see reference 2901. GI, gastrointestinal; IL-2, interleukin-2; ADCC, antibody-dependent cellular cytotoxicity; CTL, cytotoxic T lymphocyte; APC, antigen-presenting cell; CMV, cytomegalovirus.

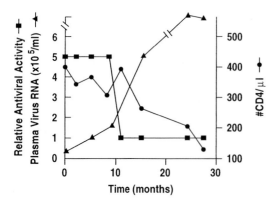

Figure 13.5 CD8+ cell anti-HIV activity in an HIV-infected individual monitored over time. In this subject, the loss of the CD8+ cell response, reflected by the relative ability to suppress virus replication (*y* axis, left) decreases prior to a loss of CD4+ cell number (*y* axis, right). Virus production (▲) resumes at time of reduced CD8+ cell antiviral response. Modified from reference 2520 with permission.

anti-HIV responses, IL-2 production is very important (see Chapter 11) (Figure 13.5). Thus, strengthening of a type 1 response could help in controlling HIV infection.

Normal immune reactions that have gone aberrant and kill CD4+ cells can play a role in an immunopathogenic pathway. These processes, such as apoptosis, ADCC, CTL activity, autoreactive cells, and autoantibodies, reflect a state of immune activation that can be detrimental to the infected individual (see Chapters 6, 10, and 11). Recent data have suggested that a compromise in the gastrointestinal mucosae resulting from the CD4+ cell destruction leads to circulating microbial products such as lipopolysaccharides. They can be a major cause of immune activation and CD4+ cell loss by apoptosis (493a) (see Chapter 6). Hyperactive CTL responses in HIV-infected individuals could also contribute to the immune abnormalities that ultimately lead to AIDS (2543, 3003, 4971). CTL responses could destroy antigen-presenting cells (APC) and prevent the normal cellular immunity needed to maintain an asymptomatic state (2543, 2985). The observed infiltration of lymph nodes by CTLs may reflect destruction of this tissue in vivo (744, 3804) (see Chapter 11). Similar processes, particularly involving bone marrow and thymus, could affect the number and function

of other cells in the immune system (see Chapters 9 and 11).

Finally, with cellular immune responses, some CTLs may react against B cells that produce neutralizing antibodies, as has been reported with lymphocytic choriomeningitis virus (LCMV) in mice. Infection of B cells by a noncytopathic LCMV led to immune destruction of the cells and a persistent infection by these types of viral strains (3533). A similar mechanism might be responsible for the emergence of the R5 viral phenotype. For example, one infected subject had neutralizing antibodies against an X4 virus that was associated with a switch to an R5 virus soon after seroconversion (2420) (see Chapter 10).

2. CONTRIBUTIONS TO HIV PATHOGENESIS

The overall conclusion is that suppression of HIV replication in the host is the most important factor in preventing the progression to disease. Both inhibition of noncytopathic strains (which could cause a slow loss of CD4+ cells by an indirect mechanism) and suppression of more virulent viruses (in which direct cell killing is associated with rapid progression to disease) depend on strong antiviral cell-mediated immune responses. A compromise in this activity appears to be a major determinant for progression to disease (Figure 13.5). Importantly, maintenance of this antiviral activity depends upon cytokines (e.g., IL-2) produced by the very cells that HIV infects, the CD4+ lymphocytes (258, 1259) (see Chapter 11) (Figure 13.6). These features of HIV infection indicate that an immunologic balance reflected by sufficient functioning of both CD4+ and CD8+ cells is needed to control HIV pathogenesis (Figure 13.6). In the case of the CD8+ cell noncytotoxic response (see Chapter 11), the loss of IL-2 or CD8+ cell antiviral factor (CAF) production could lead to the release of virus from its "latent" state and advancement to disease (Figure 13.7). Maintenance of an asymptomatic state appears to depend on an adequate production by CD4+ cells of type 1 cytokines such as IL-2 that are needed for CD8+ cell lymphocyte antiviral activity (258). The CD8+ cells ensure suppression of HIV replication, whether of the nonvirulent or virulent strains, and thus ensure normal CD4+ cell function and a long asymptomatic course. A breakdown in this antiviral activity of CD8+ cells as a result of re-

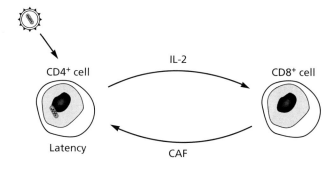

Figure 13.6 Balanced immunogenicity. In this model, sufficient noninfected or non-virus-releasing CD4⁺ cells are present to make interleukin-2 (IL-2), which maintains the production of the CD8⁺ cell antiviral factor (CAF) by CD8⁺ cells. CAF, in turn, suppresses HIV production and prevents the loss of the CD4⁺ cells and their function.

duced type 1 cytokine production could permit the emergence of HIV from a relatively latent state and progression to disease (Section IV).

What causes a decrease in IL-2 production is not known. Since APC, such as DCs, play an important role in inducing and maintaining both CD4⁺ and CD8⁺ cell responses (Figure 13.8), abnormalities in this cell type could be responsible (2247) (see Chapters 8 and 9). Some studies have indicated that CD28:B7 costimulation of CD8⁺ cells or their coculture with mature DCs induces effective CD8⁺ cell antiviral responses (255, 635) (see Chapter 11).

The importance of humoral immune reactions in preventing immune deficiency and disease progression is unclear. HIV infection is associated with a loss of memory B cells (4439a)

(see Chapter 8, Section I.H.). When autologous strains are tested, neutralizing antibodies can be found throughout the course of the infection, albeit generally at low levels and against previous circulating viruses in the host (1881, 3729) (see Chapter 10). The role of these antibodies would appear to be most important during the early phase of HIV infection, when virus neutralization and destruction of virus-infected cells via ADCC could be effective in preventing HIV spread in the host. Later, the humoral immune response does not seem to be involved in defense against HIV and may be detrimental via ADCC or enhancing antibodies (1881) (see Chapter 10).

In summary, the steps involved in HIV infection and progression to disease are multifactorial (Table 13.7). Each has been covered in some detail

Figure 13.7 Immune pathogenesis. CD4⁺ cells produce cytokines such as interleukin-2 (IL-2) that maintain the production of the CD8⁺ cell antiviral factor (CAF). CAF inhibits CD4⁺ cell release of HIV. If an inhibitory event prevents IL-2 production by CD4⁺ cells (pathway 1) or blocks CAF production by CD8⁺ cells (pathway 2), HIV production takes place.

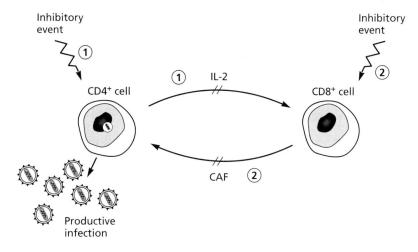

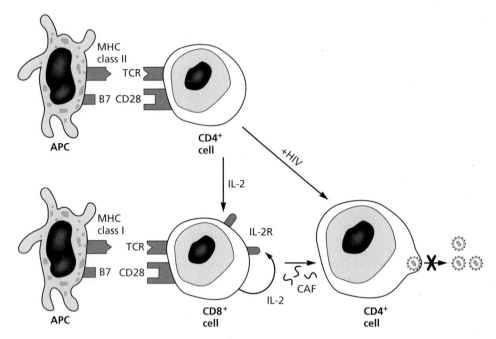

Figure 13.8   Antigen-presenting cells (APC) (e.g., dendritic cells), through their expression of major histocompatibility complex (MHC) molecules and B7 proteins, help in the stimulation of CD4+ and CD8+ cell responses. The ultimate result is an increase in interleukin-2 (IL-2) production and IL-2 receptor (IL-2R) expression. In terms of HIV infection, this costimulation can lead to an increase in the CD8+ cell noncytotoxic antiviral immune response with CAF production and thereby control of virus replication (255).

in this book. The common host factor influencing delay in disease progression is the inherited genetic makeup of the individual, which can determine both the susceptibility of cells to HIV replication (see Chapter 3) and the effectiveness of the antiviral cellular immune response (see Chapters 9 and 11) (Section III). Young age can also have a beneficial influence, most likely reflecting a strong immune response (Section III.D).

III. Prognosis

A. General Observations

Several studies have attempted to define those factors that might be useful in predicting the clinical course (Table 13.8). Obviously, maintaining a normal CD4+ cell level and low virus load are beneficial signs. Those findings often mirror an increased thymus output of T lymphocytes (1248). From the initial recognition of the clinical condition of AIDS,

the most common observation associated with disease progression has been a low circulating CD4+ cell count (1577, 4279). The lowest risk is for subjects with >350 CD4+ cells/μl (1176). Viral RNA levels in the blood are also valuable predictors of clinical progression (2712, 2968, 2969, 4585). Baseline viral loads of >100,000 RNA copies/ml predict clinical progression (1176, 2968, 2969). Furthermore, high-level expression of viral transcripts in PBMC has been useful as a predictor of progression to disease (218, 3886), again most likely reflecting a reduced anti-HIV immune response. In most cases, CD4+ cell counts and viral RNA levels considered together are the most helpful for prognosis (2969). Nevertheless, for decisions on antiviral therapy, the CD4+ cell count has become the most important prognosticator (see Chapter 14). In resource-limited countries, the presence of grey nails may help identify patients with a low CD4+ cell count (3943a).

In this regard, in untreated HIV-infected individuals, the rate of CD4+ T cell decline may not reflect

Table 13.7 Steps involved in HIV infection and pathogenesis

- Virus attachment to cellular receptor(s), fusion and nucleocapsid entry into cells (Figure 3.4)
- Virus replication in cells (influence of intracellular factors)
- Acute virus infection with spread primarily to lymphoid tissues (particularly in the GI tract) and to peripheral blood mononuclear cells
- Virus replication controlled by cellular immunity (CD8$^+$ cell antiviral response) (Figure 13.11)
- Dominant type 1 responses enhancing cell-mediated immunity (Figures 11.6, 11.7)
- Most virus-infected cells placed in a latent state
- Gradual loss of CD4$^+$ cell function and number (role of noncytopathic, macrophage-tropic HIV strains?) (Figure 13.1)
- Switch from type 1 to type 2 cytokine responses (direct role of HIV?)
- Loss of CD8$^+$ cell antiviral responses (Figure 13.5)
- Release of infectious virus and increased numbers of virus-infected cells (lymphoid tissue and peripheral blood)
- Enhanced virus replication
- Emergence of cytopathic isolates (Figures 13.2, 13.3, and 13.4; Table 13.8)
- Further loss of CD4$^+$ cells and function (Figure 13.1)
- Onset of symptoms and progression to AIDS

the HIV RNA levels. Some individuals may have high viral loads without a large decrease in CD4$^+$ cell numbers; others could have low viral loads and low CD4$^+$ cell numbers (3772b). The reasons for this disconnect between viral load and CD4$^+$ cell count are not known, but this observation should be considered in approaches to therapy. Moreover, the process(es) involved need to be understood and may be related to those observed in the nonpathogenic SIV primate models where high levels of virus are found (see Chapter 13, Section VI).

In the case of HIV-infected infants, a rapid rise in plasma viremia soon after infection, without the expected decline in HIV levels within 4 to 6 weeks, gives a poor prognosis (1005). Moreover, as might be expected, severe immune defects in the first year of life in infected children with HIV infection predict rapid progression to disease (750). Furthermore, as noted previously, viral hetero-

geneity correlates with a slower progression to AIDS (1044). This parameter appears to reflect the strength of the immune response shortly after primary infection (1815, 4585) (see above). In resource-poor areas, total lymphocyte count and serum albumin levels can help predict the clinical outcome in children (3044).

Other prognostic factors associated with disease progression (Table 13.8) include elevated levels of p24 antigen or infectious virus in the blood, reflecting again the high viral RNA levels noted above; low titers of antibody against HIV (4585), particularly p24 or p17 Gag proteins (694, 2403) and Tat (3775a); low serum albumin (2959); decreased serum dehydro-3-epiandrosterone levels (1987); high serum urokinase-type plasminogen activation receptor levels (4130); and decreased delayed-type hypersensitivity reactions (4923). In addition, reduced complement receptor 1 (CR-1) expression on erythrocytes (834) and certain major histocompatibility complex (MHC) phenotypes (Table 13.8) are associated with a higher risk of disease progression (626, 1436, 2113, 4735).

A poor prognosis is also associated with features of immune activation such as high levels of β$_2$-microglobulin, soluble IL-2 or TNF receptors, and soluble CD8 in the blood; large amounts of neopterin, TNF-α, and other cytokines in the blood or urine; and increased numbers of activated CD8$^+$ CD38$^+$ cells (1521, 1522, 1654, 2598, 3009, 3038, 3278, 4585). Notably, increased immune activation mirrored by high CD38 expression on CD8$^+$ cells directly correlates with poor prognosis (1521, 1522) (see Chapter 6). Finally, a reduced level of CD8$^+$ cell anti-HIV activity presages development of AIDS (397, 2745, 3317, 3370) (Figure 13.5).

B. Virus Characteristics

As reviewed above, the nature of the infecting virus can have a prognostic value. The cytopathic HIV X4 viruses are more closely associated with a rapid progression to disease than are the R5 viruses (see Chapter 4) (731, 2278, 3792, 4405) (Table 13.5). However, a switch from the R5 to the X4 phenotype is not necessarily observed with progression to disease (1578, 2058). R5 strains are present in up to half of AIDS patients (1578) (see below) and may have greater replicative abilities

Table 13.8 Factors suggesting disease progression in HIV infection[a]

- Low CD4[+] cell number (1015, 1577, 4279)
- Low thymus function (1248)
- High viremia level (2712, 2968, 4585); high cellular viral DNA levels (1669, 4585)
- Cytopathic HIV isolate (731, 2278, 4405) (Table 13.5)
- HIV isolates with high replicative ability (945, 4513)
- High-level expression of viral transcripts in PBMC (3886)
- Plasma p24 antigenemia (2404, 3731, 4033)
- Low lymphocyte count and serum albumin (2959, 3044)
- Low titers of antibody to HIV, particularly p24 or p17 Gag protein (694, 2028, 2403, 4585)
- Decreased serum dehydro-3-epiandrosterone level (1987)
- High serum urokinase type plasminogen activation receptor levels (4130)
- Reduced delayed-type hypersensitivity reactions (4923)
- High serum β_2-microglobulin levels (2598)
- High serum soluble IL-2 receptor levels (3278)
- High serum soluble CD8 levels (3353)
- High serum soluble TNF receptor levels (1537)
- High neopterin levels in blood or urine (3009, 3682)
- High TNF-α levels in blood or urine (1654, 3278, 4585)
- Reduced CR-1 (complement receptor) expression on erythrocytes (834)
- Specific MHC phenotype (1436, 2059, 2113, 4735) (Tables 13.9 and 13.10)
- Increased number of activated CD8[+] CD38[+] cells (1522)
- Reduced CD4[+] and CD8[+] cell antiviral responses (2396, 2745, 3317, 3370)

[a]See Section III for discussion and other references. IL-2, interleukin-2; TNF, tumor necrosis factor; MHC, major histocompatibility complex.

than R5 viruses from HIV-infected asymptomatic individuals (2362, 2576).

An increased replicative ability of a virus determined by the *pol* gene has correlated with CD4[+] T-cell decline and progression to AIDS (945, 4513). Moreover, studies of PBMC infection by viruses from individuals at different clinical states has indicated that the best viral replicative ability (progeny virus production) correlates with progression to disease (3637, 4513). Nevertheless, in some individuals studied over time, a switch from an R5 to an X4 virus did not lead to increased viral RNA levels in the blood (2058, 2120). The findings emphasize the fact that viral load or phenotype alone is not the sole parameter for progression to disease and may not carry the worst prognosis. The overall state of the immune system is the major determinant.

In terms of the virus, deletions in the *nef* gene, particularly in the region of overlap of *nef* with the U3 portion of the LTR, can be associated with slow progression to disease (1016, 1158, 2214). Some of these infected individuals remained healthy for up to 14 years (2447) (see Chapter 7 and Section IV). Delayed progression to disease has also been linked to an R77Q mutation in the viral Vpr gene (2697, 3055).

In evaluating the relationship of different clades to the clinical course, clade D viruses were found to be associated with a lower CD4[+] cell count and a faster progression to death than clade A and B viruses and some recombinant viruses (2072, 4572) (see also Chapter 1). Other studies had noted that people infected with the C, D, or G clade are eight times more likely to develop AIDS than people infected with clade A (2092). The reason for the better prognosis with clade A viruses is not known. Importantly, most evidence does not suggest that individuals in resource-poor countries show a difference in progression to clinical disease, but they do not survive as long with AIDS (1368). This finding most likely reflects the efficacy of clinical care. Some studies suggest that individuals infected early with multiple HIV-1 variants have a faster progression to disease. Such multiple infections appear to be more common in women than in men (3870). These findings probably reflect a poor antiviral immune response of the woman at the time of infection.

C. Cellular Genes

1. RECEPTOR EXPRESSION

Several cellular genes, particularly ones encoding cell surface receptors, have been identified that can affect the clinical course of HIV infection (Table 13.9) (see also http://www.hiv-pharmacogenomics. org) (2829). Although not studied extensively, African populations may have fewer genetic polymorphisms that could provide resistance to HIV

Table 13.9 Cellular genes that affect HIV-1 infection and AIDS progression[a]

Gene	Genotype	Effect	Reference(s)
Cell surface			
CCR5	+/Δ32	Delay AIDS	1003, 1017, 2994, 3028, 4970
CCR5	+/Δ32	↓Risk of lymphoma	1018, 3645
CCR5	+/Δ32	↑Response to antiviral therapy	4533
CCR5	A303/Δ32	Prevent infection	3634
CCR5P	P1/P1	Accelerate AIDS	2830, 2912
CCR2b	+/64I	Delay AIDS	1164, 2292, 2457
HLA (Table 13.10)			
HLA	HLA-A, -B, -C homozygosity	Accelerate AIDS	626, 4379
HLA	HLA-Bw homozygosity	Delay AIDS	1315
HLA	B35Px	Accelerate AIDS	1314, 1436, 4460
HLA	B57, B27, C-14	Delay AIDS	1314, 1435, 2112, 3006, 4460
HLA	A1-B8-DR3, C-D4, C-16, A-29	Accelerate AIDS	2059, 4460
KIR/HLA	KIR3DL1/HLA-B57	Delay AIDS	2667
KIR/HLA	KIR3DS1/HLA-Bw4-80Ile	Delay AIDS	1463, 2831
CX3CR1	249I/M280	Accelerate or delay AIDS; CNS disorders	1260, 1261, 1803, 2360, 2911, 4157, 4600
CCL3L1	Low copy number	Enhance HIV/AIDS susceptibility	1561
CXCR6	E3K	Accelerate PCP pathogenesis	1143
DC-SIGN	−336C	Increased susceptibility to infection	2832
Cytokines			
SDF-1	3'A/3'A	?Delay AIDS	482, 1802, 3164, 4557, 4790
IL-10	−592A	Accelerate AIDS	4110
IFN-γ	−179G/T	Accelerate AIDS	106
TNF-α	−308A/−308A	?Delay AIDS	2248
TNF-β	TNF c2	Delay AIDS	2180
IL-4	IL-41-589T	Delay AIDS	3206, 4750
RANTES	In 1.1C haplotype	Accelerate AIDS	105
RANTES	−403A/−28G	Delay AIDS	2629, 2911
MCP-1Eotaxin	Hap7	Enhance infection	3041
Others			
MBL	Homozygosity for variant alleles; Lower MBL levels	?Accelerate AIDS; enhance infection	1452, 3434, 4337
APOBEC3G	186R	Accelerate AIDS	104
TSG101	HapC	Accelerate AIDS	278
TSG101	HapB	Delay AIDS	278

[a]For more details on genetic determinants influencing HIV pathogenesis, see http://www.hav-pharmacogenomics.org. CNS, central nervous system. PCP, *Pneumocystis jiroveci (carinii)* pneumonia. Table prepared with help from M. Carrington.

infection and disease progression than other populations (4779; for a review, see reference 3303). Besides the HLA phenotype (Section III.C.3), a variety of differences in the CCR5 gene can affect HIV disease progression depending on the nature of the alleles (2912, 3634). As described in Chapter 2, an absence in expression of CCR5 can reduce the risk of infection substantially, and individuals with one allele ($CCR5^{-/+}$) show a decreased progression to AIDS (3159, 4184). Polymorphisms in the CCR5 promoter have been identified that can affect CCR5 mRNA production and reduce the risk of infection, particularly by R5 viruses, and disease progression (2912, 4421a). In addition, *CCR5 Δ32* heterozygosity combined with a CCR5 promoter polymorphism (*−2459 A/G*) is associated with resistance to HIV-1 transmission (1849).

CCR2b is a chemokine receptor that has a minor role as an HIV-1 coreceptor. A G-to-A mutation at position 190 changes the CCR2b codon 64 from valine to isoleucine, affecting the first transmembrane domain of CCR2. The *CCR2b-64I* locus is associated with a 2- to 4-year delay in progression to AIDS (2457, 4184). The mutant protein does not show any difference in its role as a coreceptor, but its effect may reflect a reduced expression of other cell surface proteins. However, a down-modulation of CCR5 was not observed in these studies (2457). Nevertheless, in another study, CCR2b-64I was found to bind to CCR5 in the cytoplasm and reduce its expression (3209). Thus, it is not surprising that a slow progression to disease was observed particularly in individuals with an R5 virus infection. Moreover, an R5-to-X4 conversion appears to take place more commonly in CCR2b-64I+ subjects, again supporting a CCR5-mediated event (4558). This association of the *CCR2b-64I* locus with slow disease progression, however, has not been universally observed (1227). The conflicting reports could again be explained by the fact that the protection provided by the *CCR5 Δ32* genotype appears to be continuous during the course of infection, perhaps because it affects primarily R5 viruses; the *CCR2-64I* genotype shows most of its effect early in infection (3159).

Recently, certain single-nucleotide polymorphisms (e.g., *CCR2-V64I*, *CCR5-2459*, *MIP-1 A+954*, and *IL-2+3896*) and some specific haplotypes in the IL-2 and CCR2/CCR5 regions were found to be associated with increased susceptibility to HIV infection (4122). In addition, HIV-infected individuals homozygous for a variant *CX3CR* haplotype have also shown a rapid progression to AIDS (Table 13.9) (1260). However, this correlation between a CX3CR polymorphism and progression to disease has not been observed in other studies (2360). Moreover, perhaps related to HIV transmission by DCs (see Chapters 4 and 9), certain DC-SIGN (2832) and DC-SIGNR (2628) polymorphisms have been found to be linked to an increase or decrease in susceptibility to HIV infection (2628). Recently, polymorphisms in human TRIMα (see Chapter 5) have been associated with increased susceptibility to HIV infection (2013a). In addition, progression of HIV infection was found associated with TLR9 polymorphisms (417a). This observation places further emphasis on the importance of innate immunity in controlling HIV infection (see Chapter 9).

2. CYTOKINES

Several other genes associated with either chemokine coreceptor expression or the chemokines themselves (e.g., SDF-1) can affect disease progression (Table 13.9) (see below). The *SDF-1 −3′A/3′A* genotype has been associated with a faster progression to late-stage HIV infection, most likely due to a reduced protection of CD4+ lymphocytes by SDF-1 (482). Certain studies in HIV-infected children borne of seropositive mothers have also shown that the presence of *SDF-1 3′A* is associated with accelerated disease progression (4467). However, the homozygous state was found to delay the onset of AIDS in a study of five large AIDS cohorts (4790). The polymorphism was reported to be associated with an increased production of SDF-1 that presumably prevented the emergence of X4 viruses. Nevertheless, these observations were not confirmed in over 1,000 subjects evaluated in the United States, Amsterdam, and Spain (4557, 4599). The conflicting findings could reflect the low frequency of this mutation in various cohorts (4 to 5%) (482, 4790).

Beside the observations on SDF-1 noted above, the relative expression of other cytokines can affect the HIV clinical course. A single-nucleotide polymorphic variation in the IL-10 promoter appears to be present in those individuals progressing more rapidly to AIDS (4110). In addition, a variant of the promoter region of IFN-γ, associated with inducing TNF-α, is associated with accelerated CD4$^+$ T-cell loss most likely via apoptosis (106). Mutations in the TNF-α and TNF-β genes can delay the progression of disease (2180, 2248).

IL-4 can play a role in down-regulation of CCR5 and up-regulation of CXCR4. Thus, a homozygous polymorphism in the IL-4 promoter region (*IL-4-589T*) leading to decreased levels of IL-4 has correlated with increased rates of X4 versus R5 infection in subjects in Japan (3206). This mutation may accelerate the phenotypic switch from R5 to X4 virus infection and could possibly increase disease progression. However, other findings have suggested that this single nucleotide change at position 589 (*589T*) in the IL-4 promoter gene can protect against HIV disease progression, most likely by reducing viral load (3207, 4750). In other studies, some HIV-infected individuals with the *IL-4-589T* promoter polymorphism showed progression to AIDS and survival levels comparable to others but had delayed acquisition of X4 HIV-1 variants (2361). Thus, the conclusive effect of IL-4 polymorphism on HIV infection needs further study.

Diminished transcription of RANTES, which can occur with a mutation in the 1.1c allele, is also associated with progression to AIDS (105). Other mutations in the RANTES gene appear to delay AIDS (2629). Some studies suggest that genetic mutations leading to increased MCP-1 expression can contribute to an accelerated disease progression and increased risk of dementia (1562). Again, these conflicting reports with different cytokines need further evaluation.

3. HLA

Notable attention has been given to the possible relationship of certain MHC human leukocyte antigen (HLA) class I or class II phenotypes (e.g., *HLA-B35*, *HLA-B27*, *HLA-AI*, and *HLA-DR5*) with either delay or enhancement of disease progression (1967, 1968, 2112, 2113, 2793, 4269) (Tables 13.9 and 13.10) (for a review, see reference 4286). The effect of HLA polymorphisms on HIV infection and clinical disease depends on the individual clades involved (4381) and the full genetic makeup of the person infected (4381) (for a review, see reference 4286).

Table 13.10 HLA association with HIV disease progression^a

Fast progressors
HLA class I homozygosity, ancestral haplotypes *8.1, 35.1, 44.2, A23*, supertype *B7, B*08*, haplotype *A*01-B*08-DR3, B22, B35Px, DR3, DR11*

Slow progressors/long-term survivors
Supertype *A2, B27, B51, B57, B1503*, supertype *DR-13*, haplotype *DRB1*13-DQB1*06*

High-risk exposed HIV-seronegative individuals
A2, DR13

^{a}Provided by M. Carrington. For citations see references 499, 626, 1114, 1314, 1347, 1436, 1801, 1967, 1968, 2060, 2112, 2627, 2726, 2777, 4021, 4269, 4381, and 4460.

In studies of clade B infection, in primarily U.S. and Northern European populations, the *HLA-B57* and *HLA-B27* specificities are strongly associated with long-term survival (2112, 3006) defined as infected subjects without therapy, with stable CD4$^+$ T-cell counts and <50 copies of viral RNA/ml for more than 10 years (see Section IV.B and V). Moreover, these infected subjects also present less frequently with the symptomatic acute retroviral syndrome than expected (3.4%); the *HLA-B57* frequency in chronically infected individuals is 9.6% (82, 1435). *HLA-B57* is associated with an early response to the virus leading to rapid HIV control, with reduced viral replication and maintenance of CD4$^+$ cell numbers (1435). In contrast, *HLA-B27* is not linked with a strong CD8$^+$ cell antiviral response and its genetic effect is observed only late in the clinical course (1435) (Tables 13.9 and 13.10). The latter may reflect selection of resistant virus with less replicative ability (102). Some studies suggest that a single amino acid change in an HLA class I molecule, such as *HLA-B35*, can increase the rate of the progression to AIDS (1436) (Tables 13.9 and 13.10).

This predominant role of *HLA-B* alleles rather than *HLA-A* alleles in the control of HIV has also been noted in a study of CD8$^+$ T-cell responses to clade C virus in an African population (2183). The results could reflect a greater diversity of peptides that can be expressed via *HLA-B* (1435). Moreover, *HLA-Bw4* homozygosity has been linked to protection from AIDS (1315). This finding is most likely related to enhanced NK cell function (see below and Chapter 9). In contrast, *HLA-Bw6* homozygosity has been found to be associated with accelerated disease progression (3631).

The delay in disease could result from the effective presentation of antigen in the context of MHC molecules. Thus, a strong CTL or cell-mediated immune response is generated. An alternative reason for the association of the HIV clinical course with certain *HLA* alleles could be immune protection induced by frequent sexual exposures to HLA proteins that are present on the surface of virions or on cells that carry the infectious virus (see Chapter 3, Table 3.10; Chapter 15; and Section VII). Finally, in studies of Zimbabwean women, *HLA-E* and *HLA-G* gene variants independently and synergistically appeared to reduce susceptibility to heterosexual HIV infection (2383) (see Chapter 2). (For other discussions on HLA and protection from infection, see Section VII.C.)

4. KIR PROTEINS

NK cells function through recognition via their KIR proteins of HLA class I molecules on target cells (see Chapter 9). KIR proteins can both stimulate and inhibit NK activity (2408, 2660). In one study, *KIR 3DL1* with *HLA-B57* was associated with delayed progression to disease (2667). As noted above, homozygosity of *HLA-Bw4*, a ligand for an NK cell KIR, was also found to be associated with protection from disease (1315). Moreover, an activating KIR allele, *KIR3DS1*, together with *HLA-B* alleles that encode molecules of isoleucine in posi-

tion 80 (*HLA-Bw4-80I*), appears to be linked to an antiviral affect (Table 13.9). In the absence of this *HLA-B* allele, two copies of *KIR3DS1* are associated with more rapid progression to AIDS (2831). The data suggest an early NK cell response in HIV infection. The mechanism could reflect selective killing of *HLA-Bw4*-infected cells. Thus, HLA class I molecules render protection against HIV by their involvement in both the innate (ligands for NK cell receptors) and the adaptive (presentation of viral antigens to CTLs) immune responses (see Chapters 9 and 11). Nevertheless, a recent observation that HIV infection reduces HLA-Bw4 expression on infected cells (E. Barker, personal communication) questions this conclusion about an in vivo protective effect of this HLA haplotype.

D. Age, Gender, Race, and Ethnicity

Age is an important factor determining the risk for development of AIDS (849) (Table 13.1). Older age (>25 years), particularly in hemophiliacs, has been associated with faster progression to disease (287, 621, 1176, 1238, 4579). Gender does not have a major role in predicting the clinical course (4579; for a review, see reference 3610). Only in the early period after seroconversion is there a difference between men and women in terms of viral load, not later in the course of infection (4287). Viral load can be lower in women (up to 33%) when CD4+ cell counts are comparable to that of men (4287). Importantly, despite the lower viral load in women

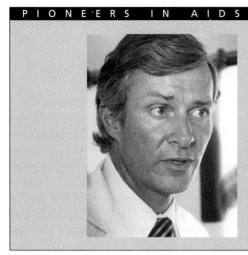

John L. Ziegler

Professor Emeritus, Department of Medicine, University of California, San Francisco (UCSF), and Director, Familial Cancer Risk Core Facility and Cancer Risk Program, UCSF Comprehensive Cancer Center. Dr. Ziegler was among the first to define the cancers (B-cell lymphomas and Kaposi's sarcoma) associated with HIV infection.

having the same CD4+ cell count as men, there is no difference in the gender benefit of antiretroviral therapy (3610). Finally, in the U.S. population, race and ethnicity do not appear to influence viral RNA levels or disease progression (531).

E. Cellular Immune Function

As discussed above and in Chapter 11, another important prognostic factor in HIV pathogenesis is the strength of CD4+ cell proliferative responses to a variety of stimuli. Several studies have indicated that strong HIV-specific CD4+ T-cell and CD8+ cell responses (e.g., CTLs) are associated with slower progression to AIDS (3317, 3370) (see Chapters 9 and 11) (Table 13.8). In a recent study, HIV-specific CD4+ T-cell responses were found to be similar early in infection for infected individuals who went on to become long-term survivors (LTS) or progressors. However, those Gag-specific CD4+ T cells producing IL-2 or IFN-γ were lost in progressors late in infection (2003). Thus, the early presence of the HIV-specific CD4+ cells did not appear to predict the progression to AIDS but rather reflected the extent of viral load and T-cell destruction (see Chapter 11).

In all cases, the cytotoxic function of the HIV-specific CD8+ cells needs to be considered since this activity depends on CD4+ cell function (see below and Chapter 11) and is linked to the HLA phenotypes discussed in Section III.C.3. Importantly, the HIV-specific CD8+ cell responses may not reflect a cytotoxic activity. For example, CD8+ cell HIV-specific responses may be found to be increased with viral load and not show any association with control of HIV infection (867, 4545) (see Chapter 11, Section II.D).

In primary infection, a more diverse CD8+ cell response reflected by a broad T-cell repertoire is associated with a better clinical course, regardless of the initial level or subsequent reduction in viremia (133, 962, 3408). Moreover, as noted earlier in this book (see Chapter 11), a loss of cellular immune responses to recall antigens, alloantigens, and mitogens presages development of disease (814, 815).

Some studies suggest that flow cytometric analyses of CD8+ cell subsets might be useful in defining cellular markers (e.g., activation markers such as CD38) associated with progression to disease (1522, 2396, 2505). The presence of activated CD69+ macrophages in the peripheral blood may also predict neurologic disease (3618) (see Chapter 8). The continual presence of the CD8+ cell antiviral noncytotoxic activity can also be a good marker of resistance to disease progression (2745) (see Chapter 11).

F. Conclusions

Some of the findings on prognosis discussed in this section are controversial, and certain parameters for predicting progression to AIDS (Table 13.8) need further evaluation. Nevertheless, several genetic markers are now well established and helpful in evaluating the risk for infection and disease (Tables 13.9 and 13.10). The use of CD4+ cell counts as a surrogate marker for prognosis is most valuable but can be misleading if the individual is coinfected with HTLV; high CD4+ cell counts can sometimes be observed in advanced HTLV disease (3957). Moreover, as noted above (Section III.A), a disconnect between CD4+ cell number and viral load can be observed (3772b), emphasizing the importance of understanding the processes involved in HIV infection in the individual. Viral RNA levels are a good predictor for clinical progression (2968, 2969), but not necessarily for measuring the effect of therapy (see Chapter 14). A decline in HIV-1 RNA levels during the early period of infection correlates with a better clinical course and is independent of the viral phenotype and CD4+ cell count (2058, 2969) (Figure 13.1). Increased levels of HIV-1 DNA in the PBMC, as well as high numbers of HIV-1-producing CD4+ cells, also correlate with disease progression (1669). These variables most likely reflect the strength of the anti-HIV cellular immune response. In general, most investigators today rely on CD4+ cell numbers combined with viral RNA levels as prognostic markers (2969, 4873). In particular, attention is given to viral RNA levels at the time of seroconversion, when a sharp decrease can portend a long asymptomatic course (Figure 13.1) (2968, 2969).

IV. Differences in Clinical Outcome

A. Overview

1. ADULTS

When evaluating the clinical state of HIV-infected individuals, the stages of infection noted in Section

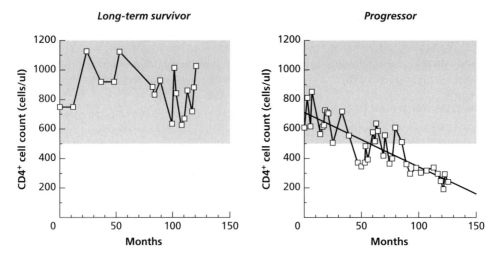

Figure 13.9   CD4$^+$ cell counts in long-term survivors and progressors. Over a 10-year period, CD4$^+$ cell counts remained within the normal range (shaded area) for long-term survivors but persistently decreased in progressors. Figure provided by E. Barker.

II are helpful and certain clinical subgroups can be distinguished (1770). One group of infected individuals consists of typical progressors, whose immune functions appear to be intact early in infection but whose immunologic control weakens within 8 to 10 years, associated with progression to disease. Another clinical group consists of rapid progressors, who show a very quick decline in CD4$^+$ T-cell numbers, usually within 2 to 5 years after primary infection (1770, 4089) (Figure 13.9). They are characterized by low levels of antibodies to HIV proteins and poor HIV-1-neutralizing activity (606, 3416). They may also have enhancing antibodies (1881). Importantly, CTL activity can be present in the rapid progressors (3418, 3733), who may have large numbers of activated CD8$^+$ CD38$^+$ HLA-DR$^+$ cells (1522) (see Chapter 11). This feature underlines the activated immune state associated with a poor prognosis (see above). The role of CTLs in this pathogenic course (4971) is not clear, and their beneficial role may reflect the relative functioning capability of these cells (e.g., perforin expression) (358, 2592, 3005) (see Chapter 11, Section II.D).

The most characteristic feature of rapid progression is a high viral load that does not decrease substantially after primary HIV infection (2058, 2968, 2969). In individuals with this characteristic, homogeneity in HIV isolates is found. In contrast, for typical progressors, a change from viral homogeneity to heterogeneity and back to homogeneity at the time of disease is usually observed (as noted above in Section III.C). Viral homogeneity most probably reflects a poor host antiviral immune response.

A third category of infected individuals consists of the long-term survivors (LTS), also called long-term nonprogressors (LTNP), who have remained asymptomatic with normal CD4$^+$ cell numbers and viral loads for at least 10 years (Figure 13.9) (606, 2520, 3416; for reviews, see references 3352, 3996, and 4040) (see Sections IV.B and V). Some studies have documented that the rate of CD4$^+$ T-cell loss in LTS is markedly reduced (18 cells/μl/year) compared to that in normal progressors (~60 cells/μl/year) (355). Certain groups have predicted that up to 13% of homosexual or bisexual men infected at a young age will remain asymptomatic for more than 20 years (3169). However, the usual percentage of the LTS is 5 to 8% of the total number of infected people (545, 3849) (Figure 13.10) (Section V). These long-term asymptomatic people can be found among infected hemophiliacs, intravenous drug users, sexual contacts, and newborn children (Section IV.B). A subset of the LTS sometimes called "elite controllers" remain healthy for many years with very low or no detectable virus in their blood (358, 1201, 3005) (see below). Strong host anti-HIV immunity appears to be responsible for this control of HIV replication.

Another small group of infected individuals has an unusual clinical presentation. They remain free of illness and AIDS symptoms without therapy for many years after CD4$^+$ cell counts have dropped below 200 cells/μl, some with <100 cells/μl (4215). They have been considered low CD4$^+$ cell LTS (3996). These infected people have a slower decline in CD4$^+$ cell count over time, have less T-cell reactivity than conventional progressors (2146, 3996), and are infected by R5 viruses (3996). The reason for this lack of progression in the absence of treatment has not been explained but could be related to other immune cells (e.g., innate immune activity: NK cells and PDCs) that are active in defense against HIV (1889, 4215) or against opportunistic infections (2549, 4134, 4215) (see Chapters 9 and 11).

2. CHILDREN

In children, a distinction in clinical course similar to that noted in adults can be appreciated (for a review, see reference 4762). Moreover, central nervous system (CNS) disorders in children appear to follow a pattern very comparable to that observed in adults (4762). Very high viral loads in the months soon after infection correlate in newborn children with an increased risk for rapid progression to disease (see Section III). About 10 to 25% of newborn children develop AIDS within the first 2 years of life, whereas the rest have a slow progression to disease, with some remaining healthy for several years (399, 4456). In children with hemophilia, oral candidiasis is the strongest predictor of a poor prognosis (1239). High CD8$^+$ cell counts and high immunoglobulin A (IgA) levels in hemophiliacs in the first years after seroconversion also predict future progression to disease (3496).

Some studies suggested that a rapid progression of HIV infection in the mother correlates with AIDS developing faster in the baby (4455). The data could reflect either transfer of virulent virus strains or increased amounts of virus transmitted to the child. As noted in Chapter 2, the same kind of association has been made for recipients of blood transfusions (3474).

In newborn children, the overall progression to disease is generally more rapid than in adults,

most likely reflecting an immature immune system. Low birth weight, an early decrease in CD4$^+$ cell counts, high viral loads, and clinical symptoms (lymphoadenopathy, splenomegaly, and hepatomegaly) are predictors of this progression (1417, 2882). The symptoms suggest intrauterine infection (see Chapter 2). Progression is also more rapid in infants infected in the perinatal period than in neonates receiving a blood transfusion (544, 1359).

B. Characteristics of Long-Term Survivors (Long-Term Nonprogressors)

The discussion in this chapter underlines an important question about HIV pathogenesis: what is the cause of the wide variations in progression to disease observed among infected individuals? For example, the San Francisco study of HIV infection in a cohort of 622 subjects with well-defined dates of HIV seroconversion (545, 3849) revealed that 87% of the individuals developed AIDS 17 years after HIV seroconversion (545) (S. Buchbinder, personal communication) (Figure 13.10). Importantly, in evaluating the entire cohort with long-term HIV infection at the end of 1995 ($n = 594$; 10 to 15 years after HIV seroconversion), 15% of the cohort remained clinically healthy and 4% of the cohort had normal CD4$^+$ cell counts (Buchbinder, personal communication) (545). These healthy individuals have laboratory markers and clinical histories indicating a slow progression of disease (4090). Although a relatively low percentage of the subjects are in this category, the reasons for their long-term survival could provide insights into possible therapeutic interventions for others. A lack of exposure to sexually transmitted diseases or recreational drugs did not explain the long-term asymptomatic course (545).

This group of asymptomatic HIV-infected individuals, considered LTS or LTNP, maintain a low viral load, both in plasma and in PBMC (606, 2520, 2521, 4597). They usually have in their plasma a less cytopathic (R5) virus, but occasionally an X4 virus is present (3996) (Tables 13.11 and 13.12). In this book this clinical group is called LTS rather than LTNP to give a more positive connotation. Some LTS, as noted above, have little or no detectable virus in their blood and have been considered a separate subset of elite controllers (3005).

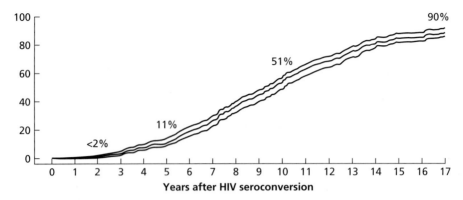

Figure 13.10 Progression to AIDS with time. In the San Francisco city cohort, individuals known to be infected have been monitored since 1978. The results through 1995 show that it takes about 10 years for 50% of the individuals to develop AIDS; 69% of the infected subjects develop the disease within 14 years (545, 2597; S. Buchbinder, personal communication). Figure provided by S. Buchbinder.

LTS have several characteristics, listed in Table 13.11. Some represent very common findings, whereas others relate to features specific for some LTS (Section V). For example, some LTS have anti-CCR5 antibodies associated with a long-lasting down-regulation of CCR5 on the surface of the CD4⁺ T lymphocytes and resistance to R5 virus infection (3435a). Certain early reports indicated that the kinetics of viral replication and progeny production are lower in LTS (606). They can have neutralizing antibodies to the autologous strain but no enhancing antibodies (1881, 2520). Antibodies to the viral envelope V3 region do not correlate with this slow progression to disease (1870). Importantly, HIV-specific CD4⁺ cell and CD8⁺ cell proliferative responses are found in LTS (814, 1737, 3005, 3416, 3794). They can have a high frequency of CTLs (1738, 3416), and the LTS show a strong CD8⁺ cell noncytotoxic antiviral response (259, 2520, 2521).

The structure of the lymph node in LTS is also more intact, and there is a low level of virus replication in PBMC and the lymph nodes; the function of the lymphoid cells is maintained at a high level (397, 3416). A similar finding has been reported for lymphoid tissue from HIV-infected chimpanzees without disease (2276). Finally, as noted above, the diversity of HIV strains in LTS is heterogeneous, in contrast to the homogeneity noted in the rapid progressors. Again, these observations on viral heterogeneity most probably reflect an active anti-HIV immune response in which different escape virus variants can emerge and replicate but are then recognized by the immune system (Section V).

V. Factors Involved in Long-Term Survival

A. Genetic Determinants

People infected with the same or different HIV-1 strains often show similar rates of change in CD4⁺ lymphocyte numbers and viral RNA levels. These findings support the conclusion that host factors, rather than the virus, are most important in determining HIV-1 disease progression (3338) (see above). A report of HIV infection in monozygotic triplets illustrates this importance of the genetic background in host response to the virus. All three children, receiving the same virus through transfusion of a common unit at birth, showed very similar immunologic profiles during several years of infection and developed the same opportunistic infections (3934).

The potential role of multiple genotypes and *HLA* alleles has been evaluated in LTS (see Section III.C) (Table 13.11). These infected individuals have reduced expression of the CCR5 chemokine receptor on CD4⁺ cells (see Chapter 3) as a result of one deleted allele for this coreceptor (1017). This heterozygosity can influence the viral spread and

Table 13.11 Reported characteristics of long-term survivors of HIV infection[a]

- Clinically asymptomatic for ≥10 years*
- Normal CD4+ cell number* (606, 2520, 3416)
- Large number of CD4+ cells in the GI tract* (3915)
- Low virus load (measured by plasma viremia; infected PBMC)* (606, 2520, 3416)
- Low immune activation* (3915)
- CCR2-V64I polymorphism as well as HLA-B54 allele (4183)
- Presence of the HLA-B57 class I allele (3006)
- Viral envelope V2 region is increased in length (2855)
- Virus with deletion in nef region (1016)
- Presence of a predominantly nonvirulent HIV isolate (e.g., R5 virus)* (723)
- Virus with Vpr mutation (2697) or deletion in SP-1 side of the LTR (1246)
- Heterogeneous virus population
- Presence of neutralizing antibodies (606, 1881, 2682)
- Presence of anti-Tat antibodies (1047, 3717)
- Presence of anti-CCR5 antibodies (3435a)
- No enhancing antibodies (1881)
- IgG2 antibodies that react with gp41 together with a CD4+ cell anti-p24 response (2835, 3570)
- Type 1 cytokine production by PBMC* (1159)
- HIV-specific CD4+ T cell and CD8+ T cell responses* (807, 3005, 3416)
- Strong cellular CD8+ cell cytotoxic antiviral response* (256, 357, 1159, 2520)
- Strong NK cell activity (1963)
- Active ADCC (36)
- Lymph node structure is normal* (397, 3406)
- Not on antiretroviral therapy*

[a]Long-term survivors are also called long-term nonprogressors. See Section IV.B. Some of these characteristics have been observed in only a few cases and not generally confirmed. Major factors are noted by an asterisk. GI, gastrointestinal; LTR, long terminal repeat; IgG2, immunoglobulin G2; ADCC, antibody-dependent cellular cytotoxicity.

pathogenicity of R5 strains. In addition, some studies suggest that a mutation in codon 74 of CCR2b (CCR2b-64I) is associated with long-term survival (4184), as is perhaps homozygosity at the SDF-1 locus (Section III.C.2) (Table 13.9). Importantly, long-term survival has been associated with the HLA-B*57O1 class 1 allele (3006). Differences from progressors have been found to be associated particularly with peptides within the Gag regions

that are HLA-B57 restricted (1516). Moreover, the presence of a CCR2-V64I polymorphism as well as the HLA-B54 allele can be associated with long-term survival (4183) (see Section III.C).

These observations on genetic background have indicated that the chance of long-term survival for a subject heterozygous for CCR5 Δ32 can increase 16- and 47-fold when an HLA-B27 allele is present and the HLA-DR6 allele is absent, respectively. A similar increase in survival has been found if at least three of the following alleles were present: HLA-A3, HLA-B14, HLA-B17, and HLA-DR7 (2761). All these HLA genetic differences relate to the effectiveness of the anti-HIV cellular immune response (Section V.C).

B. Virus

As noted earlier, LTS have a low viral load, as reflected by the relatively small number of infected CD4+ cells, as well as low levels of viral RNA, and free infectious virus in the peripheral blood and lymphoid tissues. In LTS, normal CD4+ T-cell numbers and undetectable viral loads in the gut-associated lymphoid tissue have correlated with a control of inflammation and cell activation (3915) (see Chapter 11). Moreover, the viruses recovered from the PBMC are usually R5 strains that are not highly cytopathic. Some studies have indicated that the length of the envelope V2 may be increased by 2 to 13 amino acids in viruses from the LTS (Table 13.11). The findings may reflect the maintenance of an R5 virus in these individuals (2855, 4114).

As noted in Section III.B, some studies indicate that LTS are infected by slowly replicating defective viral mutants, in particular those lacking Nef expression (1016, 2214, 2447, 2993) (see Chapter 8). These studies suggest that Nef could play a role in disease progression. However, this observation is not common. In studies of LTS from Nairobi, Kenya, no sequence change in the virus suggesting attenuation was noted (1247). Other studies characterizing nef sequences in LTS and progressors with HIV infection have not detected deletions or reduced functions of the nef gene that correlate with the rate of disease progression (1923, 2993, 3149). Moreover, defective nef variants have been found in both LTS and those who progress to disease (921a). Obviously, other properties of the

Table 13.12 Factors influencing long-term survival

- Infection with a low replicating virus or an attenuated HIV strain (*nef* mutated) with a reduced replicative ability[a]
- Strong cell-mediated anti-HIV immune response, particularly CD8[+] cell cytotoxic and noncytotoxic antiviral activity: depends on type 1 cytokine production (Section III.E and Chapter 11)
- Genetic background (e.g., receptor polymorphisms— *HLA-B57*, *HLA-B27*, and immune response) (Tables 13.9 and 13.10)
- Young age
- Neutralizing antibody[a]; lack of enhancing antibodies
- Lack of one CCR5 allele[a]
- High levels of plasmacytoid dendritic cells (see Chapter 9)

[a]In some cases.

virus in progressors appear to be responsible for the association with clinical progression (see Section). One potential mechanism for the role of *nef* in HIV attenuation is that a *nef* deletion mutant virus might express its proteins more effectively in vivo, since wild-type Nef has been shown to reduce cellular expression of MHC molecules (4014) (see Chapter 7). The host immune system can therefore recognize the mutant viruses more readily and suppress viral growth. It is noteworthy that the protective effect of a deleted *nef* region can vary, since some of the LTS infected with these attenuated viruses have advanced to disease (371, 921a). Further modifications in other regions of the virus appear to be responsible (371).

A 2-amino-acid insertion into an HIV-1 Vif protein was also found to be associated with a long-term nonprogressor state (59), as was a sequence change that targeted Vif to the nucleus (1253). Conceivably, some interaction with APOBEC3G may be involved (see Chapter 5). Moreover, a deletion in the SP-1 site of the LTR has been linked to an attenuated HIV-1 in an LTS (1246). In addition, the presence of an R77Q mutation in Vpr was found more frequently in LTS than in patients progressing to disease (2697, 3055). The latter virus showed many fewer features associated with the wild-type Vpr, such as induction of apoptosis. However, again, these findings do not account for nonprogression in most LTS. Aside from the

reports cited above, viruses from long-term healthy infected individuals generally do not show other genetic abnormalities such as mutations in the *vif*, *vpr*, or *vpu* sequence (898, 4929).

C. Immune Response

1. HUMORAL IMMUNITY

In terms of the humoral immune responses, no apparent difference can be found between LTS and progressors in immunoglobulin concentrations in the blood (e.g., hypergammaglobulinemia) (9). Certain studies have shown that neutralizing antibodies to autologous and heterologous viral strains correlate with a healthy long-term clinical state (606, 1881, 2678). No enhancing antibodies are detected (1881). This humoral antiviral immune response is not consistently detected in progressors, who, as noted above, can have enhancing antibodies (1881) (see Chapter 10). Some investigators, however, have found that neither neutralizing antibodies nor complement-mediated antibody-dependent enhancement is associated with long-term survival or disease progression (3070). Certain studies suggest that IgG_2 antibodies that react with gp41 are associated with long-term survival, particularly when found together with CD4[+] cell anti-p24 responses (2838, 3246, 3570) (Table 13.11). Moreover, ADCC is found more commonly in LTS (36). Nevertheless, in general, the humoral immune response does not appear to be a major determinant of long-term survival.

2. CELLULAR IMMUNITY

With cellular immune responses, strong anti-HIV CTL activity has been found to be associated with long-term survival (357, 358, 1159) but is not always detected (1159). Moreover, the PBMC from LTS show a type 1 response in cytokine production (i.e., IL-2 and IFN-γ), favoring cellular immune responses (1159) (see Chapter 11). Those LTS with very little, if any, plasma virus (i.e., elite controllers [see above]) have a high frequency of HIV-specific CD8[+] cells with increased proliferative capacity and perforin expression (3005). This CD8[+] cell activity could reflect the high frequency of HIV-specific CD4[+] cells that secrete IL-2 and IFN-α (1201) (see Chapter 11). In this regard, CD8[+] cell function in LTS has recently been shown to be associated with the quality and not the quantity of cell function. Five different activities of CD8+ cells (degranulation and IFN-γ, MIP-1β, TNF-α, and IL-2 production) were all maintained in HIV-specific CD8+ T cells in LTS versus progressors. A possible role of CD4+ T cell help may be involved (358), although some data suggest that IFN-γ-producing CD8+ cells can support independent responses of HIV-specific CD8+ cells (4968).

As noted above, most of these subjects are positive for *HLA-B57* or *HLA-B27*, genetic markers for a healthy clinical state (3005) (Tables 13.9 and 13.10) (Section III.C.3). Because perforin is important in cell killing, the function of the CD8+ cells in LTS appears to be more efficient. Thus, while the frequencies of HIV-specific CD8+ cells can be similar in LTS and progressors (see Section IV.A), the proliferative responses and perforin content can distinguish the CD8+ cells from LTS (358, 3005). Also noteworthy are the findings in LTS of large numbers of CD4+ T cells in the GI tract and mucosal T-cell anti-HIV responses (3915). In most HIV-infected people, marked CD4+ cell depletion occurs in the bowel (see above) (see Chapter 8).

At the time of initial infection, individuals have CD8+ cell antiviral activity, both cytotoxic and noncytotoxic. It can be demonstrated before antibody production and before neutralizing antibodies are seen (446, 2302, 2749) (see Chapters 3 and 11). The CD8+ cell noncytotoxic activity in both PBMC and lymphoid tissue remains strong in LTS (258, 397, 2520, 2745) (Figure 13.11) (see Chapter 11). Both types of CD8+ cell responses are decreased in individuals progressing to disease. Certainly, strong cellular anti-HIV immunity appears to be the major factor in a long-term asymptomatic course (Tables 13.11 and 13.12). Moreover, other innate immune activities may be involved in ensuring long-term survival. Levels of PDCs, major producers of IFN-α, are higher in LTS than in uninfected people (4215). NK cell activity can be strong as well (1963), whereas this function is decreased in many HIV-infected individuals (see Chapter 9). Moreover, as noted above, ADCC, in part mediated by NK and other innate cells, is commonly found in LTS (36) (see Chapters 9 and 10).

These observations on LTS strongly suggest that the low viral load, the noncytopathic nature of the virus, and the absence of viruses sensitive to enhancing antibodies all reflect the anti-HIV ef-

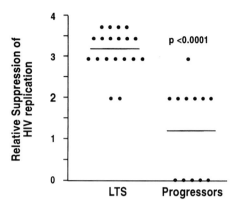

Figure 13.11 Suppression of HIV replication by CD8+ cells. CD8+ cells at different input ratios were added to acutely infected CD4+ cells. The relative extent of suppression was determined. The smallest number of CD8+ cells needed to suppress virus replication by more than 90% was determined. The strength of the CD8+ cell response in long-term survivors was significantly higher than that in progressors ($P = 0.001$). Figure provided by E. Barker.

fect of CD8+ cells, which reduce the ability of HIV strains to replicate and thus to mutate in the host. This response also helps reduce immune cell activation that is found decreased in LTS (3915). As noted above, the CD8+ cell activity depends on strong type 1 cytokine production (see Chapter 11) (Figure 13.6). Whether this protective CD8+ cell antiviral activity is primarily an HIV-specific cytotoxic activity or a noncytotoxic response is not clear. The importance of the latter CD8+ cell noncytotoxic anti-HIV response (CNAR) is reflected in the reduced viral load in asymptomatic individuals and LTS even when X4 strains are present in the blood and lymph nodes (397). In this regard, some studies have suggested that HIV-specific CTLs do not correlate directly with long-term survival (3418) (see Chapter 11). In this case, CNAR may be the most important antiviral response.

VI. Differences in Clinical Course in SIV Infection

Valuable insights into HIV pathogenesis and long-term survival can be gained by observations in primate models having viremia without disease progression (1448, 2526). Notably, uncloned SIV inoculated into sooty mangabeys and rhesus macaques has shown differences in the pathogenic course. Only the macaques had CD4+ T-cell depletion and developed AIDS. The mangabeys showed very little T-cell proliferation but high levels of virus replication. One noteworthy observation is the loss of CD4+ T cells in the bowel of SIV-infected healthy sooty mangabeys similar to that noted in HIV infection (cited in reference 1640). Evidently, this pathological finding occurs even in these presumably asymptomatic animals. Importantly, high-level SIV-specific T-cell responses, immune activation, and immune cell apoptosis are not present in the mangabeys (1150, 4143, 4145). The immunologic control mechanism is therefore unknown and could be related to innate immunity (see Chapter 9). One explanation for the less pathogenic effect of large amounts of SIV in mangabeys is the presence of CD4+ CD25+ regulatory cells and TGFβ production (2286) that could reduce the detrimental effects of immune activation observed in rhesus macaques (2130) (see Chapter 11, Section V). In this regard, CD25 expression was found to be decreased on the CD4+ cells in macaques, but increased in mangabeys. Another explanation is the resistance of central memory SIV-specific CD4+ T cells to anergy (453).

IL-2 and IFN-γ production were also found to be increased in macaques, but IL-10 levels were higher in mangabeys (2130). This cytokine can reduce virus replication and immune activation (see Chapter 11). Moreover, there was a normal T-cell turnover in the healthy SIV-infected mangabeys (2130). In the SIV-infected macaques, this T-cell proliferation is twice that of mangabeys, most likely reflecting early thymic failure (671). Evidently, as noted above, despite high levels of SIV replication in the mangabeys, there is very little bystander death by apoptosis (4144), most likely reflecting less immune activation. Recent studies also suggest that a decreased release of IFN-α by the PDCs from mangabeys could be involved (M. Feinberg, personal communication). This cytokine can induce TRAIL expression on CD4+ cells (1819), making them sensitive to apoptosis (see Chapters 6 and 9). Nevertheless, after 18 years, AIDS did occur in one sooty mangabey with natu-

ral infection (2614). Defining the characteristics of this clinical course could be helpful for HIV studies.

In other SIV studies, naturally infected African green monkeys, which do not develop disease, showed a level of SIV replication even greater than that seen in the naturally infected sooty mangabeys (529, 1551). Thus, again the lack of clinical signs does not reflect host control of viral replication or differences in tissue and cell tropism. Moreover, the same level of diversity was present among viral isolates. The factors involved in this type of nonpathogenic clinical response to infection merit further study. Chimpanzees with a natural infection with a primate lentivirus (SIV_{cpz}) also do not develop disease (3458). One explanation has been the presence of antibody-dependent cytotoxicity in these primates (3982), which is not found in humans. Another explanation could be the high levels of IgA that can be induced in nonhuman primates compared to humans (2323, 2982, 4082). The most common finding in all these primate models is the absence of immune activation (3458, 4145), perhaps reflecting the activity of T regulatory cells and TGFβ production (2130, 2286) (see Chapters 6 and 11). Recently, this lack of immune activation in chimpanzee cells has been related to the presence of sialic acid-recognizing immunoglobulin superfamily lectins (Siglecs) that are associated with down-regulation of immune cell activation (3250). Another explanation could be the Nef alleles from primate lentiviruses (e.g., SIV_{smm}) as well as HIV-2. They appear to down-modulate TCR (CD3) expression, therefore reducing cell activation. Nef alleles from HIV-1 do not participate in this process (3964). Thus, Nef-mediated suppression of T-cell activation may be a characteristic of primate lentiviruses that allows persistence without a great loss of CD4+ cells (3964).

VII. High-Risk HIV-Exposed Seronegative Individuals

A. Overview

Several studies have documented that some individuals who were exposed to infectious virus or viral antigens have not had an established infection.

These high-risk exposed people include sexual partners of infected individuals, intravenous drug users, transfusion recipients, hemophiliacs, children borne of infected mothers, and health care workers with needlestick injuries (317, 745, 804, 807, 2150, 2521, 2540, 3523, 3663, 4684; for reviews, see references 3828 and 4081).

Possible reasons for this resistance to infection have been explored (Table 13.13). These individuals, who do not show evidence of HIV infection (i.e., antibody seroconversion; virus in their blood), have been referred to as exposed seronegative individuals (ESN) or highly exposed uninfected individuals. Since a few of these subjects have later been found to have some evidence of low-level or transient HIV infection (see below) (1189, 4955), it seems best to refer to them as ESN. The characteristics of this group of people are discussed in this section.

B. Genetic Features

ESN can lack CCR5 expression (homozygous for a deletion mutation) (see Chapter 3) (1017, 2635, 3895, 3902). Thus, they are substantially less sensitive to HIV transmission in which R5 viruses dominate. Nevertheless, individuals with this genetic phenotype can be infected by X4 viruses (see Chapter 4). In one large study, only homozygote CCR5 Δ32 subjects (3.2%) were found to be increased among ESN, not individuals with other genetic variants within chemokine receptors or in chemokines (2630). There has been, however, some suggestion that variants of DC-SIGN (2630) and low CCR5 expression in some men with CCR5-Δ32 heterozygosity (4421a) could reduce the risk of HIV infection.

In seronegative sexually exposed adult women and perinatally exposed infants, a decreased risk of HIV infection has been associated with a cluster of closely related *HLA class I A2* alleles and specific viral peptide epitopes (2727). With lack of exposure to the virus, this response decreased (2128, 2726). When some of the women became infected, the CTL response was directed against different viral epitopes (2125, 2726). Thus, both CD4+ and CD8+ cell HIV-specific responses reflecting the inherent strength of cell-mediated immunity appear to be responsible for this protection from HIV infection (see below).

C. Cellular Immune Responses

Some investigators have reported that the resistance to HIV infection in ESN sex workers resides with CTL responses against the virus (3826; for reviews, see references 2406, 3828, and 4081). This prevention of HIV infection correlates with their low level of immune activation (2273). HIV antigen-specific production of IL-2 by PBMC can be demonstrated in some high-risk uninfected subjects (317, 815, 2150). In one study, the pattern of the TCR repertoire appeared to reflect a response to HIV but without infection (354). In other studies, CTL responses to HIV epitopes have been observed in exposed, uninfected adults (354,

Table 13.13 Observations on high-risk seronegative individuals that suggest HIV exposure and protection from infection[a]

Genetic
- Reduced or lack of CCR5 expression (1017, 2630, 3902)
- Genes closely related to *HLA class I A2* alleles (2727)

Immune
- HIV-specific CD4+ T cells (1237, 2137)
- HIV-specific CD8+ CTL (362, 2126, 2769, 3826, 4081)
- CD8+ cell noncytotoxic antiviral response (2520, 2540, 4308)
- Increased NK cell function (4025)
- Increased RANTES levels in the genital tract (2630)
- Reduced susceptibility of PBMC to infection (362, 2038, 4308, 4490)
- Reduced immune activation (2273)
- Serum neutralizing antibodies against cellular components (e.g., HLA and CD4) (317, 2664)[b]
- IgA antibodies react to CCR5 in sera, saliva, and genital fluids (242, 2662, 2664)[b]
- Anti-HIV neutralizing IgA antibodies in serum and vaginal fluids (801, 1065, 2885)[b]
- Cervicovaginal anti-gp41 antibodies that block transcytosis (296)[b]

Other
- Exposure to killed virus or viral antigens
- Low viral load of partner (genital fluid and blood)

[a]CTL, Cytotoxic T lymphocytes; IgA immunoglobulin A.
[b]These observations were made on a small number of exposed seronegative individuals (ESN) and need to be further substantiated.

2406, 3826) and in children born to HIV-1-infected mothers (745, 993, 3826). In one study, a third of ESN subjects who had practiced high-risk sexual activity (13 of 36) had HIV-1-specific CD8$^+$ cell cytotoxicity (1543). Others have noted HIV-specific CD8$^+$ cell T-cell proliferation (807, 3828) in ESN of discordant couples (see Chapter 11). Moreover, CTL against viruses isolated from the infected partner and laboratory isolates were found in 5 of 11 ESN (362).

In other studies, 12 of 18 resistant ESN intravenous drug users had detectable HIV-specific CD8$^+$ cell responses as measured by IFN-γ production after exposure to an HIV peptide (2769). Such HIV-specific CD8$^+$ T-cell responses in 11 of 16 resistant sex workers were also found with cells from the cervix and blood (2126). Overlapping peptides spanning many viral proteins, particularly Vif, have shown this CD8$^+$ cell antiviral response by ESN. The peptides recognized differed from those identified by CTLs from seropositive subjects (2137, 2138). An important study evaluated T-cell responses in two groups of ESN—those who had unprotected sexual contact and those who had shared needles with HIV-infected partners. Similar numbers of uninfected subjects from each group (35 versus 22%) showed a CD8$^+$ cell response to at least one HIV peptide (2768). Thus, this natural HIV resistance was observed in subjects with two different modes of exposure.

CNAR has been noted in 27 of 54 high-risk adults (sexual partners of infected individuals) (4308) (see Chapter 11, Table 11.13) and in 19 of 31 HIV-negative infants born to HIV-positive mothers (2520, 2540). Two of the adult subjects lacked CCR5 expression, suggesting that they were exposed and probably transiently infected by HIV (4308). Very dramatic was the finding of CD8$^+$ cell antiviral responses in an uninfected monozygotic twin whose sister was infected by HIV (2520). Evidently, both twins were exposed to viral antigens and mounted cellular immune responses, but only one twin had established infection. Whether the other twin warded off the infection or was exposed to an amount of infectious virus too small to establish infection is not known.

HIV-1-specific CD4$^+$ T lymphocytes have also been noted in 6 of 8 female ESN sex workers but

at lower numbers than in seropositive individuals (2137, 2138). These cells would be expected to help CD8$^+$ cell anti-HIV CTL activity. HIV-specific CD4$^+$ lymphocyte responses were also detected in 11 of 20 of ESN Nairobi female sex workers (2126, 2129). This resistance of Nairobi prostitutes to HIV infection appears to be associated with HLA-DRB1*0, an anti-HIV-1 class II restricted CD4$^+$ effector cell response (2727). CD8$^+$ lymphocytes responding to HIV epitopes not commonly recognized by seropositive women were also detected (2127). However, in another study, HIV-specific IFN-γ-secreting T cells were not found in male ESN (men having sex with men) (1847).

In other studies, the PBMC from ESN intravenous drug users in Vietnam showed reduced susceptibility to HIV infection in vitro. The presumed CD8$^+$ cell antiviral function appeared to be mediated by a nonchemokine secreted factor (4490). Similar findings in seronegative partners of HIV-infected individuals have been reported (362, 4308). In some cases, the block to HIV infection of the cells appeared to be early in the viral replicative cycle (362). In other studies, PBMC from some ESN were resistant to HIV infection and CD8$^+$ cells were primarily responsible (2038). These findings could reflect the presence of CD8$^+$ cells secreting CAF (see above and Chapter 11). In addition, Gag p24-specific CD4$^+$ T cells that appeared to be somewhat resistant to R5 infection (not mediated by chemokines) have been found in ESN (1237).

In contrast, one study of 80 HIV-exposed Nairobi sex workers who remained uninfected showed that their PBMC were susceptible to both R5 and X4 viruses. Neither chemokine receptor polymorphism nor β-chemokine overproduction by PBMC was found to be responsible for their resistance to HIV infection (1342). Some reports have indicated that enhanced NK cell function in Vietnamese ESN intravenous drug users may contribute to this protection from HIV infection (4025). In another study, elevated RANTES levels in association with increased peripheral blood T-cell counts were found in the genital tracts of uninfected Nairobi sex workers (2630).

All these findings suggest that the ESN were exposed to live virus but have controlled and then, in most cases, eliminated the infection. Effective cellular immune activity (innate and/or adaptive) was induced before antiviral antibodies were elicited. Alternatively, perhaps insufficient viral antigens were presented to the host so that antibodies were not made but cellular immune responses occurred. In this regard, some evidence that previous exposure to low levels of viral antigen induces this immunologic resistance comes from studies of rhesus monkeys receiving small doses of infectious SIV. These animals, which did not seroconvert or have detectable virus, were protected from a low-dose viral challenge that infected the naïve control animals (803). Perhaps related, ESN Nairobi prostitutes were shown to maintain CD8$^+$ CTL responses without seroconversion. Then, after 1 year of reduced sexual exposure, 11 seroconverted in association with a decrease in HIV-specific CD8$^+$ cell responses (2127). The immunologic mechanism for this lack of protection was not known but may reflect loss of adequate innate immune activity that characteristically does not show a memory response (see Chapter 9).

D. Humoral Immune Responses

In some studies, sera from 17 ESN subjects were found to neutralize two different HIV-1 primary isolates (Table 13.13). The antibodies were directed against cellular components (e.g., HLA and CD4) and not viral antigens (2664). In related studies, sera from some ESN reacted with a C-terminal region of HIV gp120 that resembles an HLA class I antigen (533). In some ESN injection drug users, antibodies to HIV-1 envelope epitopes shared with selective HLA class I haplotypes were detected in 7 and envelope-specific CD4$^+$ cellular responses were observed in 16 of 21 subjects (317). All the results indicate some HIV cross-reacting immunity in presumed seronegative highly exposed individuals (317) (see Chapters 10 and 15).

Anti-HIV-1 IgA as well as envelope and Gag-specific IFN-γ-producing CD4$^+$ and CD8$^+$ lymphocytes have also been detected in urine and urethral swabs of ESN (2664; for reviews, see references 2661 and 2886). HIV-1-specific IgA was also noted in sera from 16 of 20 HIV-resistant Nairobi sex workers. Some serum HIV-specific IgA in the ESN has shown anti-HIV neutralizing ability (1065, 2885). The antibodies react with an epitope within gp41 (801). In other studies, antibodies (mostly IgA) reactive with CCR5 have been found in sera, saliva, and genital fluids of ESN (242, 2662, 2664).

Mucosal and plasma IgA from ESN have been shown to inhibit HIV-1 transcytosis across a transmembrane mucosal epithelium culture (1064) (see Chapter 3). Cervicovaginal antibodies reacting to gp41 have blocked transcytosis of cell-associated HIV through a tight epithelial monolayer in vitro (296). A total of 7.5% of 342 ESN female sex workers had these antibodies. This biologic activity could have prevented the transmission of HIV.

Nevertheless, in a study of 31 ESN, serum and cervicovaginal lavage fluids were negative for IgA antibodies against gp120 and did not appear to mediate protection (4778). Moreover, studies of Gambian sex workers who resisted HIV infection found no specific antibodies in genital fluids, and none of the secretions had anti-HIV neutralizing activity (1116). A similar lack of antibodies in vaginal fluids was noted with HIV-discordant couples (4308). In addition, extensive studies examining levels of HIV-specific IgG and IgA antibodies in sera and secretions (saliva, tears, milk, urine, nasal fluids, semen, intestinal washes, and vaginal washes) indicated that if IgA-specific antibodies were present at all, they were at a low level. None was found in vaginal washings obtained from HIV-exposed but uninfected women, thus raising questions about the observations of these antibodies in some cohorts (J. Mestecky, unpublished observations). Finally, whether HIV is present undetected in tissues of ESN requires further study. Thus, whether antiviral antibodies are responsible for protection from HIV infection remains to be determined.

VIII. Diversity of Viruses Involved in Transmission and Infection

A. General Observations

Phylogenetic and molecular analyses of common (signature) sequences in the viral envelope (particularly the V3 loop) have been useful in demonstrating transmission of one HIV-1 isolate to other individuals in the recent past (2946, 4806), and from mothers to infants (2238, 2240, 2389, 4808). In most cases, a selected transfer of one or a limited number of HIV-1 variants was shown

(2240, 4806, 4808) (see Chapter 2). In contrast, for recipients of the same clotting factor preparation, the data from PCR sequencing revealed a lack of substantial differences in the viruses isolated from the individuals involved (781, 2228). This technique was also helpful in demonstrating that a dentist infected five of his patients during surgical procedures (3360). Thus, the route of transmission can greatly influence the virus diversity in the infection.

B. Biologic Properties: the Early Transmitted Virus

A major question still facing the scientific community is why R5 viruses are preferentially expressed after acute and primary infection (Table 13.14). Some investigators believe that these viruses are transmitted predominantly because of their ability to infect mucosal DCs or the presence of high SDF-1 concentrations at mucosal surfaces (28). These explanations are not fully satisfactory since both virus phenotypes have been detected in initial transmission (899, 1294, 1578, 3601). X4 viruses can also infect DCs (2133, 3268), and R5

Table 13.14 Reasons for R5 predominance during acute and primary infection

- R5 viruses have many susceptible CCR5$^+$ CD4$^+$ T-cell targets during immune activation (331, 2363)
- Immune activation up-regulates CCR5 expression (310, 802)
- R5 viruses can more readily infect nonactivated cells (1610, 2650)
- R5 viruses can infect macrophages and dendritic cells (see Chapter 2)
- Higher R5 progeny in infected cells (4018)
- R5 viruses preferentially infect CCR5-expressing CD4$^+$ cells in the gastrointestinal tract (491, 2957, 2972)
- R5 viruses can be passed from CCR5-expressing mucosal cells in the gut to CD4$^+$ T cells (2972)
- R5 virus is less recognized by the immune system (e.g., CTL) (1731, 4010)
- Secreted Tat can inhibit X4 viruses by interacting with CXCR4 (4836)
- The preintegration complex of R5 viruses can more easily enter the nucleus of nonactivated cells (3577)
- CD4$^+$ cell:dendritic cell interaction up-regulates CCR5 expression (4975)

viruses emerge preferentially in primary infection after intravenous drug use, in which circulating CD4$^+$ cells would be the most likely major targets. HIV transmission ability does not seem to determine the result; instead, the environment can influence which virus is found after acute infection. For example, immune activation up-regulates CCR5 expression and can favor R5 virus persistence (310, 802).

The preference in virus phenotype in early infection does not appear to reflect the overall CCR5 and CXCR4 expression levels in peripheral blood CD4$^+$ cells during the initial time of transmission (3088, 4559). Nearly all circulating naïve CD4$^+$ cells express CXCR4 but not CCR5 (389, 410, 3356) and are therefore susceptible to X4 viruses (for a review, see reference 3088) (see Chapter 3). Activated memory T cells express CCR5 (331, 2363). Thus, the immune activation induced by the acute infection could favor R5 virus infection. In addition, a higher progeny production of R5 viruses in PBMC and lymphoid tissue (4018) may be a factor (see Chapter 4). In cell culture, however, X4 viruses can replicate faster, producing more progeny viruses over time than R5 viruses (731, 1122, 2475). Moreover, R5 viruses can replicate in less-activated CD4$^+$ cells (1610, 2650; for a review, see reference 3088). In this regard, inhibitors of costimulation block X4 virus, but not R5 virus, replication, most likely through a reduction in nuclear import of the viral preintegration complex (3578) (see Chapter 5). These findings support the observations that R5 viruses can more readily infect less-activated cells (see Chapter 4).

In addition, CCR5 is expressed on activated CD4$^+$ T cells after interaction with DCs (4975). An effective transfer of R5 viruses from DCs to T cells can also occur via conjugates after R5 virus interaction with the DCs (1596, 2914, 3574; for a review, see reference 1352). Therefore, because of the general state of immune activation, R5 viruses appear in acute infection to have sufficient susceptible targets for their infection and replication.

Importantly, the R5 viruses appear to infect preferentially the CCR5-expressing CD4$^+$ cells in the GI tract (493, 2957, 2971), representing a large reservoir for these cells. Moreover, the R5 viruses can be preferentially transferred to the CCR5$^+$ CD4$^+$ cells by intestinal mucosal cells (see Chapter 4)

(2972). The high viremia observed during acute infection most likely reflects this tissue infection and CD4$^+$ cell loss (see Chapter 8). Studies with rhesus macaques have shown that the R5 SHIVs rather than X4 SHIVs give a great loss of CD4$^+$ intestinal T cells and a later depletion in the peripheral CD4$^+$ cells. In contrast, X4 SHIV infection affected primarily the peripheral CD4$^+$ cells and cells in lymphoid tissue but not a large number of CD4$^+$ cells in the intestine (1733). The host immune system can be involved in this potential distinction in pathogenesis resulting from R5 and X4 virus infections.

The R5 virus may be less recognized by the immune system (e.g., CTLs), particularly because of its presence in macrophages and DCs (1731, 4010). This possibility is suggested by studies in which CD8$^+$ cells were depleted in rhesus macaques coinfected at the same time with R5 and X4 viruses. The X4 virus emerged, suggesting differential control of this virus by CD8$^+$ T cells (1731).

Two noteworthy cases of accidental transmission of HIV provide some insights on the issue. In these cases, nonmucosal transmissions were involved. One resulted from an intravenous inoculation of a small quantity of blood containing predominantly an X4 virus. The other occurred following an intramuscular inoculation of a large quantity of blood containing predominantly an R5 virus. In the first case, persistent X4 virus replication occurred with rapid loss of CD4$^+$ T cells. In the second, receipt of the predominantly R5 virus resulted initially in a selective amplification of the X4 viruses before seroconversion. Then, at seroconversion, R5 viruses emerged and CD4$^+$ T-cell numbers decreased (899). The replacement of an X4 virus with a predominant R5 virus has also been observed by others (2420, 3601) and in one case was associated with the presence of host neutralizing antibodies against the X4 but not the R5 virus (2420). Although the phenomenon of phenotypic switching during primary isolation appears to be rare (1294), it does reflect how the host via target cell or immune response can modify this early infection of the virus and its spread (see Chapter 4).

Finally, some evidence suggests that secreted Tat can inhibit X4 viruses via its interaction with CXCR4 (4836) and could influence the preferential emergence of the R5 viruses. The finding differs from those showing that Tat can up-regulate both the chemokine coreceptors (1920), although, notably, it could induce other cellular factors such as SDF-1 that could block CXCR4 expression (see Chapter 3) (Table 13.14).

C. Switch in HIV Phenotype during the Course of Infection

In half the subjects infected with HIV, an X4 virus emerges after a certain period concomitant with a rapid decline in CD4$^+$ cells and advancement to AIDS (731, 872). The reason for this switch in virus phenotype is not known, and a variety of studies have addressed this issue, with some notable observations (Table 13.15).

One possibility is that a virulent virus present early in infection is suppressed or eliminated by an active antiviral immune system, and a less cytopathic virus dominates. After the reduction in anti-HIV immune response, a virus that has the characteristics of increased virulence reemerges (Table 13.8). Alternatively, the initial transmitted virus is relatively nonpathogenic in the infected individual, but with increased replicative cycles resulting from reduced immune anti-HIV activity, it mutates over time to become a virulent strain (Figures 13.2, 13.3 and 13.4). AIDS can develop

Table 13.15 Potential reasons for a switch from R5 to X4 HIV phenotype during the course of infection[a]

- X4 viruses develop from the early transmitted R5 viruses (4559)
- X4 viruses emerge from low-level replication with the reduction in immune responses (2520)
- Switch from type 1 to type 2 cytokine production (814); IL-4 up-regulates CXCR4 expression (4975)
- X4 viruses have a wide cellular host range (1339)
- X4 viruses show high progeny production within a shorter period (2475)
- Postentry block to R5 HIV replication occurs in memory CD4$^+$ cells (4640)
- X4 viruses can infect both naïve and memory T cells which express CXCR4 (331, 3088)
- Fewer CCR5$^+$ target cells (effector memory CD4$^+$ cells) (3495)

[a]Other citations are given in the text (Section VIII.C). IL-4, interleukin-4.

from either virus biotype (R5 or X4), but the virus involved usually has more cytopathic and greater replicative properties (see Section IV and above) (2362, 2576, 4020).

Emergence of the more virulent viruses appears to depend on an already compromised immune system. This type of virus is not usually found in individuals with CD4+ cell counts above 500 cells/µl. The CD8+ cell noncytotoxic antiviral response is active against all HIV isolates, and this activity decreases with progression to disease (see Chapter 11). A drop in this antiviral response has been observed just before a major reduction in CD4+ cell number (2520) (Figure 13.5). Thus, it would seem that the cytopathic virus strains (either X4 or R5) emerge when sufficient antiviral cellular responses are no longer present in the infected individual.

In several studies, X4 viruses have been found in HIV-infected subjects at all stages of infection (1637, 4004) even though R5 viruses may dominate. In this regard, during HIV infection, the viruses within the CD4+ T cells and macrophages can undergo independent evolution (1388). Other studies suggest that R5 viruses evolve to use CXCR4 as well as CCR5 coreceptors (dual-tropic, R5 or X4) and then eventually become solely X4 virus types (4556). Very few (two or three) amino acid changes in the V3 loop of gp120 can change an R5 virus into an X4 virus (987, 1338, 4112). This V3 loop change may be associated with less replication-competent virus, and additional mutations near V1/V2 may be needed to permit good virus replication. Thus, the time of X4 dominance can be prolonged (3435). The mutations that would occur over time can result from the ongoing production of progeny viruses by the error-prone reverse transcription process (829). Another potential reason for the emergence of the X4 viruses is a switch from type 1 to type 2 cytokine production (812, 814) (see Chapter 11). IL-4 up-regulates CXCR4 expression on DCs and is reduced by IFN-α (4975) (see Chapters 4 and 11).

In any case, whether the two HIV-1 biologic subtypes are transmitted at the same time or the X4 virus evolves from the R5 virus (4565) still remains to be determined. Probably both processes occur. In this regard, a small study in children showed an early emergence of X4 or R5X4 viruses only in immunocompromised children whose mother had an X4 virus detected during pregnancy (632). In other cases, as noted above, an X4 virus was first identified after primary infection but an R5 dominated thereafter (899, 2420, 3601). Thus, both biologic subtypes seemed to be present at transmission.

After an X4 virus emerges, no new X4 variants appear to be generated, suggesting difficulty for other isolates to compete. For those individuals who advance to AIDS with an R5 virus, evidence has been presented, as noted above, that this later virus replicates more quickly and to higher levels than the earlier R5 virus and can be cytopathic (2362, 2576, 4020). The later virus also requires lower CD4/CCR5 expression levels for entrance into cells (1604) and has a decreased sensitivity to RANTES neutralization in comparison with R5 viruses from LTS (2272). Enhanced replication has also been seen with the late versus the early X4 viruses (4565). These later viruses also appear to be less sensitive to CXCR4 antagonists, suggesting a stronger affinity for their receptor (4250).

In summary, the switch from R5 to X4 viruses would appear to reflect, most likely, a change in the immune function of the individual so that X4 viruses already residing in the host emerge (Table 13.15). It could indicate the loss of sufficient target cells (e.g., effector memory CD4+ cells) (1640, 3494) for R5 virus so the more polytropic X4 viruses become dominant. The study in children cited above found that the X4 virus emerged months to years after the CD4+ cell levels began to fall (632). How the X4 viruses compete successfully with R5 viruses is not known, particularly since R5 viruses appear to have progeny that can infect a great number of CD4+ cells and can escape immune surveillance via infection of macrophages and DCs (see above). Conceivably, in the face of reduced immune activity, the ability of X4 viruses to spread to many other cells of the body may be involved, particularly because of the virus' wide cellular host range (1339) and more efficient replicating ability. X4 virus progeny production also usually occurs within a shorter time period than with R5 viruses (1120, 2475). Importantly, R5 and X4 viruses within an individual are usually very similar in the envelope region (see above and

Section II.D) (731), indicating that the viruses are related. Therefore, virus evolution must take place at one time either before or after transmission, depending on the individual infected.

IX. Relationship of HIV Heterogeneity to Pathogenesis in Specific Tissues

In addition to the studies on R5 versus X4 pathogenesis reviewed above and in Section IX.E, several experiments have been initiated to determine if some HIV-1 subtypes distinguished by specific biologic and serologic features are associated with pathology in certain tissues. Viruses appear to evolve independently in different organs and cells of the body (1388). This in vivo compartmentalization can be noted by biologic and genetic differences (see Chapters 4 and 8) (4812). Three major tissues with potential virus subtypes are reviewed below, but others could eventually include HIV-1 isolates isolated from the heart, lung (1969), kidney, and endocrine organs (see Chapter 8).

A. Brain Isolates

Early studies demonstrated that HIV-1 isolates recovered from the brain or cerebrospinal fluid of patients with neurologic symptoms can be distinguished from viruses recovered from the blood of individuals at different clinical states (Table 13.16) (725, 734). In general, the brain-derived isolates are R5 viruses and can grow to high titer in CD4$^+$ lymphocytes. However, they are not cytopathic for these cells and do not down-modulate the CD4 protein on the cell surface (725). These character-

istics could explain in part the finding of CNS disease in some individuals with near-normal CD4$^+$ cell numbers (2535, 3223). These brain-derived isolates grow to higher titer in macrophages than do many blood-derived R5 isolates (2252, 2316, 3487). Moreover, the CNS isolates, reflecting their R5 phenotype, can rarely be propagated in established lines of T cells, B cells, or monocytes (e.g., U937) (734). Finally, brain-derived isolates are not as sensitive to serum neutralization as are the blood isolates (725, 734). In one study, viruses recovered from the brain appeared to be more sensitive to cerebrospinal fluid antibodies than to serum antibodies (4206), but this finding has not been confirmed (4628). These biologic and serologic differences can be appreciated as well when comparing brain and blood isolates from the same individual (734, 748).

Several investigators have shown that only R5 macrophage-tropic HIV-1 isolates (characteristic of brain-derived viruses) grew well in adult microglial cells in culture (4075, 4688). This observation was not unexpected since brain microglia are supposedly derived from macrophage precursor cells. Nevertheless, as noted previously, certain investigators (3493) have challenged the report of infection of microglia, particularly since these cells most likely lack CD4 protein expression. The infected cells could have been peripheral blood macrophages that reside in the brain. In this regard, the CCR5 receptor has been found to be necessary for infection of brain-derived microglia (1777).

When the relative ability of the HIV-1 isolates to replicate in brain-derived cell lines was examined,

Table 13.16 Characteristics of HIV-1 isolates recovered from different tissues[a]

	Source of virus		
Characteristic	Peripheral blood	Brain	Bowel
Growth in CD4$^+$ lymphocytes	++	++	++
Growth in macrophages	± (or ++)*	++	+
Growth in established human T-cell lines	++ (or −)*	−	±
Modulation of CD4 antigen expression	++	−	+
Serum neutralization	++	±	+

[a]Representative of several viral isolates. *, CXCR4 (X4) versus CCR5 (R5) dependent. Relative extent noted by number of plus signs. −, not evident. Modified from reference 2519 with permission.

other noteworthy observations were made that could have relevance to neuropathogenesis (see Chapter 8). In one study, the blood-derived X4 isolates grew better in the human glioma cell lines than did the R5 macrophage-tropic, brain-derived isolates (729). In another, an R5 HIV-1 isolate recovered from the cerebrospinal fluid (and not a brain-derived X4 isolate from the same individual) grew in a glioma explant culture (2316). The relative ability of HIV isolates to infect brain capillary endothelial cells (3123) could determine entry into the CNS and hence selection of a specific isolate. In these studies, X4 and not R5 HIV-1 isolates were infectious for the cells (3123). Therefore, some evolution of the entering virus may take place. Alternatively, damage to the blood-brain barrier by X4 virus infection of endothelial cells and astrocytes could permit entry and the subsequent pathological effects of R5 viruses (see Chapter 8).

The biologic differences between blood and brain isolates have mirrored as well the variations in restriction enzyme sensitivities and viral LTR and envelope V3 loop sequences (Figure 8.9) (2173). Although the HIV-1 isolates from the brain and blood from one individual are related, there are certain genetic differences between them (42, 681, 1213, 4288, 4812). Similar findings have been made with HIV-2 isolates recovered from one individual. The brain virus had an R5 virus phenotype and the blood virus an X4 phenotype (3913). The observations indicate further that distinct but related viral isolates can evolve independently in various tissues in the infected host (2251) (Section IX.B and Chapter 3). This evolution can be responsible for the pathology observed (see Chapter 8).

B. Bowel Isolates

HIV-1 isolates have been detected in the bowel mucosa along the GI tract from the esophagus to the rectum (262, 1515, 1792, 2296, 3234). Studies similar to those described above with brain isolates have indicated some differences between the blood and the bowel viruses (262), but the distinctions were not as great as those defining the brain-derived HIV-1 isolates (Table 13.16). The bowel viruses did show substantial macrophage tropism and were less capable of infecting established

T- and B-cell lines than were blood isolates. This finding is not surprising in consideration of the large number of CCR5-expressing CD4$^+$ cells in the GI tract (see above). In contrast to brain isolates, however, the bowel isolates were sensitive to serum neutralization and were cytopathic for CD4$^+$ cells in culture (262). The existence of subtypes of bowel-tropic R5 HIV-1 isolates is further suggested by the extent of these differences when closely related blood and bowel isolates from the same individual were evaluated (262). This finding is also supported by the enhanced expression of CCR5 on intestinal CD4$^+$ lymphocytes (1733) and intestinal epithelial cells (2972). The latter mucosal lining cells can transfer R5 viruses to T lymphocytes by a process most likely involving endocytosis (2972). Moreover, intestinal epithelial cells can be infected by HIV (262, 3234) (see Chapter 8).

Studies with SIV isolates recovered from different tissues of a monkey have shown sequence changes in the envelope that suggest specific evolution of the virus in the bowel as well as the brain (2251). One tantalizing possibility is that brain and bowel isolates will show an increased ability to enter cells expressing the GalC molecule since cells from both these tissues have this HIV-1 receptor (1730, 4841) (see Chapter 3). The possible role of a bowel HIV isolate in GI disorders is discussed in Chapter 8, Section IV.C.

C. Plasma Virus

Several studies have indicated that most infected individuals have free infectious virus circulating in the blood (875, 1853, 3396) (see Chapter 2). In asymptomatic individuals, it is found in small amounts (1 to 100 infectious particles (IP)/ml); in AIDS patients, it can be detected in larger quantities (100 to 10,000 IP/ml) (Tables 2.2 and 2.3). In most situations, virus has been recovered from both the blood and the cultured PBMC. In others, HIV has been found only in the plasma and not in PBMC (2996). The latter finding may indicate a different source for the plasma virus (e.g., GI tract, lymphoid tissue, and brain).

In this regard, one study has demonstrated that at any one time, the predominant plasma virus variant may be antigenically distinct from the virus in the PBMC (4149). Moreover, in the same individual, only the virus from the plasma, and not viruses obtained from the lymph nodes, was found to be sensitive to serum neutralization (4373). In addition, genetic analyses of HIV-1 isolates grown for a short time in cultured PBMC have revealed some differences between plasma and PBMC isolates (3860). These findings may relate to the escape mutations detected by neutralization assays in individuals over time (see above and Chapter 10).

Finally, during zidovudine (AZT) treatment, plasma virus could be distinguished from viruses represented in cellular proviral DNA (4937) and from viruses (viral sequences) in the lymph node (2376). All these observations suggest that the plasma virus might better represent the actively replicating virus in the host and be a more reliable predictor of clinical state than are isolates from cultured PBMC. The PBMC can contain archival viruses (see Chapter 14). In the same way, the infectious virus in genital fluids better reflects the agent transmitted by sexual contact (see Chapter 2).

D. Thymus

It is noteworthy that protease inhibitor-resistant HIV isolates have shown reduced replication in thymocytes (4297). This resistance correlated with the presence of a large amount of thymus tissue in the infected treated individuals. In other studies, the envelope of an infectious clone of HIV-1 was altered to show either X4 or R5 tropism, and differences in virus replication in the thymus were noted (333). Apparently, X4 viruses can infect nearly all thymocytes and peripheral T cells; the R5 viruses are more limited in the numbers of susceptible target cells (see Chapter 4). As noted above (Section III.B), this difference could help explain the slower progression to disease with R5 viruses (333).

E. Relationship of Changes in HIV Properties over Time to Pathogenesis

1. OVERVIEW

One of the first observations linking biologic heterogeneity to disease was the finding that HIV-1 isolates recovered from AIDS patients differed in biologic properties from those recovered from asymptomatic individuals (165, 731, 1274, 4403, 4405) (Table 13.5). Similarly, viruses obtained from the PBMC of an individual in the early

asymptomatic period were remarkably different from HIV-1 isolated from the same person at later times, when disease had developed (731, 4404). The earlier virus replicated in a limited number of cell types, grew to a relatively low level, and showed slower virus replication than did the later isolate associated with disease in the host (731) (Figure 13.4). Moreover, the early virus or the isolate in asymptomatic individuals, in contrast to the later one, was not very cytopathic for PBMC (Figure 13.3). Other biologic distinctions of HIV-1 isolates probably linked to virulence in the host include lack of induction of latency in established cell lines (C. Cheng-Mayer and J. A. Levy, unpublished observations), resistance to the suppressing effect of Nef as determined in T-cell lines (723), and sensitivity to enhancing and not neutralizing antibodies (1881) (Table 13.5). The possible reasons for the change in biologic characteristics of HIV over time are discussed in Section VIII.C. They appear to be primarily related to a switch from R5 to X4 viruses, although a more highly replicating cytopathic R5 virus can be involved (see above).

2. MOLECULAR DIFFERENCES

Molecular techniques have demonstrated that viruses from the same individual are highly related by restriction enzyme sensitivities and sequence homology (731, 3854). However, at any time, a large number of genetic variants (related but distinguishable) accumulate as a result of the error-prone RT process (829) and can coexist in an individual (1299, 3854). These variants, called quasispecies (2987), appear to be generated more rapidly in vivo than in vitro (3854, 3860), most probably reflecting the selective effect of the immune response on HIV replication and the cell types infected (see below).

The differences among viruses are noted particularly in certain sequences in the envelope region (see below) (731, 732, 1299, 1877) (see Chapter 8). These viral genetic differences, noted over time, have correlated with a wider host range, enhanced cytopathicity, and escape from immune response (731, 732, 2339, 4807) (Section IX.A) (see Chapters 8, 10, and 11). They usually reflect the change from R5 to X4 viruses or to an R5 virus with more virulent-like properties (2362) (Table 13.8).

Many studies of viral sequences have indicated that during acute infection, a homogeneous population of viruses is recovered from the individual. These relatively similar variants are replaced by viral quasispecies with various genetic differences, reflected by high complexity. Finally, during AIDS a more homogeneous population of viruses is again observed (1044). Thus, the initial dominant HIV isolate(s), after infection, appears to change over time, most likely reflecting responses to the antiviral activity of the immune system. This possibility is supported by the finding of greater diversity in HIV isolates in individuals who have been infected and remain asymptomatic for the longest period of time (1044, 2695). The presence of quasispeciess reflects the ongoing conflict between the virus and an effective immune system. Eventually, associated with a demise in the immune system, the viruses acquire properties of virulence in the host (Tables 6.4 and 13.5) (731, 4405). At that time, a dominant isolate again emerges, and the virus population again becomes homogeneous.

3. BIOLOGIC DIFFERENCES

In some studies, this transition in virus phenotype over time seemed evident in the infected individuals, since viruses with different biologic properties (R5 versus X4) could be found in the blood at the same time (1637, 4004) (Section VIII.C). These results mirror those mentioned above for variation in genetic sequences among viral species in one individual (1044). The relevant quantity of each type could influence pathogenesis or be a consequence of immune deficiency.

The association of disease with viruses with more virulent features, as defined in cell culture, is suggestive of causation (Table 13.5). For example, the cytopathic, highly replicative X4 variants appearing 2 years earlier in the blood can predict progression to AIDS (2278). Moreover, individuals showing X4 viruses in primary infection have been reported to advance more rapidly to disease (3257, 3792). Many reports now indicate that the X4 phenotype of HIV leads to a more rapid decline in $CD4^+$ cell counts, which is a major predictor of disease progression (Section II.D). This virus biotype can infect both naïve and memory T cells and readily induces apoptosis (338, 773). Moreover, X4 viruses can induce apoptosis of $CD8^+$ cells, leading to further immune compromise (1816) (see above).

Nevertheless, as noted previously (see Chapter 4), some studies have not shown a direct correlation of X4 isolates with development of disease (2102). Adults or children infected with R5 viruses can also reach the same low $CD4^+$ cell level over time and progress to AIDS (1578, 3727, 4227, 4233). Thus, the virus coreceptor phenotype does not always correlate directly with induction of

AIDS. More importantly, it may be the replicative property and cytopathicity for CD4+ cells that is a common property of R5 virus associated with AIDS (2362, 2576, 4020, 4441, 4892) (see above).

4. RELATIONSHIP TO DEVELOPMENT OF AIDS

How these biologic changes relate to pathogenesis is best evaluated in animal models. In cats, the induction of immune deficiency by the feline leukemia virus has been linked to its envelope region and its ability to cause cytopathic effects in an established feline T-cell line (3364). Similar findings have been reported for the X4 SHIV macaque model (670, 2106). Work in the SIV system has indicated that other portions of the viral genome (e.g., *nef*) could be responsible for its pathogenic characteristics in vivo (2170) (see Chapter 8). Moreover, studies with SCID-hu mice reconstituted with human PBMC have shown that macrophage tropism and not cytopathicity by an HIV isolate correlates best with CD4+ cell loss (3133). The reason for this observation is not known but might involve the relative levels of cytokines produced and their influence on apoptosis (see Chapters 6 and 8). Apoptosis could also be responsible for the loss of thymocytes as shown by HIV infection of fetal liver and thymus implants in SCID-hu mice (441). In this animal model system, in contrast to the SCID-PBMC-hu mouse system (3133), X4 viruses are the most destructive (587). Moreover, a reduction in IL-1 production by R5 HIV-infected macrophages and/or an increased expression of Fas ligand (202) could cause CD4+ cell death by apoptosis (835) (see Chapter 6, Figure 6.4). Thus, the potential role of both biologic virus phenotypes must be considered in CD4+ cell loss and HIV pathogenesis (Section VIII.C).

X. Conclusions: Viral and Immunologic Features of HIV Pathogenesis

Long-term survival (or long-term nonprogression) of HIV infection appears to depend on dominant type 1 immune responses of CD4+ cells (258, 814). The production of type 1 cytokines (e.g., IL-2 and IFN-γ) in LTS helps maintain CD8+ cell anti-HIV activity and other immune functions, including those directed against opportunistic infections and cancer (see Chapters 10 and 11) (Figures 13.6, 13.8, and 13.12). In contrast, in progressors, a shift to type 2 cytokines (e.g., IL-4 and IL-10) (813) suppresses CD8+ cell antiviral responses (see Chapters 9 and 11) (Figure 13.12). The type 2 cytokines can not only turn off the type 1 cytokines needed for strong cell-mediated immune responses but can also directly affect the antiviral responses by CD8+ cells. The emphasis on antibody production can encourage enhancement of virus infection (1881) (see Chapter 10). The reason for this shift in dominant cytokine production is not known but may reflect damage to DCs (2244, 2528, 2543) (see Chapters 9 and 11).

When sufficient numbers of CD4+ cells are lost by direct or indirect mechanisms, the levels of cytokines such as IL-2 that are needed to maintain the functions of CD8+ cells will be reduced (Figure 13.13) (see Chapter 11). The resultant loss of CD8+ cell antiviral activity then leads to the onset of high-level HIV replication from which virulent mutated strains can eventually emerge. A loss of CD8+ cell anti-HIV activity appears to presage the development of disease. This cellular immune response is probably reduced before substantial virus production takes place. A decrease in CD8+ cell noncytotoxic antiviral activity can be demonstrated before a major decrease in CD4+ cell counts occurs and viral RNA production rises (2520) (Figure 13.5).

Progression to disease does not correlate with a reduction in total numbers of CD8+ T cells (2543, 2735). The level of this lymphocyte subset often remains elevated until the late stages of disease (2401) (Figure 13.1). The emergence of a virulent strain that cannot be controlled by CD8+ cells also does not seem to be the major cause. In cell culture, CD8+ cells with CNAR demonstrate high activity against HIV-1 and HIV-2 strains, whether cytopathic or not (257, 2543). Thus, it appears that an intrinsic reduction in CD8+ cell antiviral activity is involved. In the case of CTLs, it could reflect a loss in perforin expression and cytotoxic activity (358, 3005). With CD8+ cell noncytotoxic responses, it could be CAF production (see Chapter 11). Why the antiviral responses are lost over time is an important unanswered question. As with other viruses, one major influence can be the genetic makeup of the individual; protection can

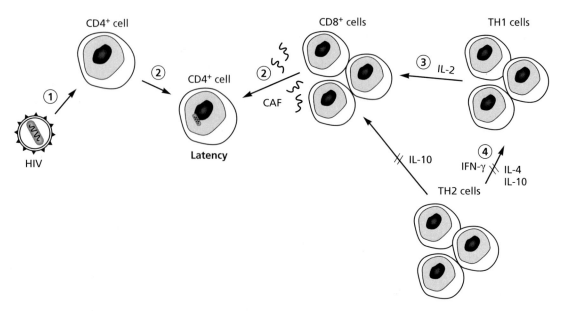

Figure 13.12 Viral and immunologic events in the persistent clinically healthy stage (e.g., in long-term survivors). HIV infection of CD4+ cells (step 1) is placed into a relatively latent state by the action of noncytotoxic CD8+ cells and the CD8+ cell antiviral factor (CAF) (~ ~) (step 2). This CD8+ cell anti-HIV response is increased with the production of type 1 cytokines (e.g., interleukin-2 [IL-2]) secreted by TH1 CD4+ cells (step 3). The type 1 cytokines also suppress the potential inhibitory effects of type 2 cytokines (produced by TH2 CD4+ cells) on this control of HIV infection by CD8+ cells (step 4). Modified from reference 2520 with permission.

come from strong innate and adaptive immune activities, including DC function (635, 2244), appropriate type 1 or type 2 immune responses, and reduced inherent sensitivity of the host cells to virus replication.

Another important factor in HIV pathogenesis is that HIV-infected individuals exhibit alterations in a number of metabolic pathways (1336) and have reduced concentrations in plasma of certain amino acids that could contribute to exacerbation of their disease (1336). In particular, degradation of the essential amino acid tryptophan by indoleamine 2, 3-dioxygenase (IDO) can exert a direct effect on the immune system (2967). IDO catalyzes the rate-limiting step of tryptophan degradation in the kynurenine pathway (2967), which results in downstream products with immunosuppressive (e.g., picolinic acid (2966) and neurotoxic (for example, quinolinic acid (2966, 4300) effects (see Chapter 8). For example, changes in the balance of tryptophan and kynurenine induced by IDO

were reported in Alzheimer's disease (4300) and AIDS dementia (1381). Moreover, inhibition of IDO has facilitated the elimination by the immune system of HIV-1-infected macrophages in an animal model of HIV-1-induced encephalitis (3592).

A reduction in tryptophan associated with a concomitant increase in the catabolites of the kynurenine pathway has been proposed to be responsible for the reduction in T-cell responses against HIV-1 and other pathogens (2966) (Chapter 11, Section V). The ratio between concentrations in plasma of kynurenine and tryptophan is increased in HIV-infected patients in direct correlation with viral load and is reduced by HAART (1381, 4730, 4912). These findings suggest that HIV-1-initiated, IDO-induced changes in tryptophan metabolism can contribute to both the immunologic and neurologic dysfunction seen in HIV-1 disease. Support for this possibility also comes from the observation that HAART partially

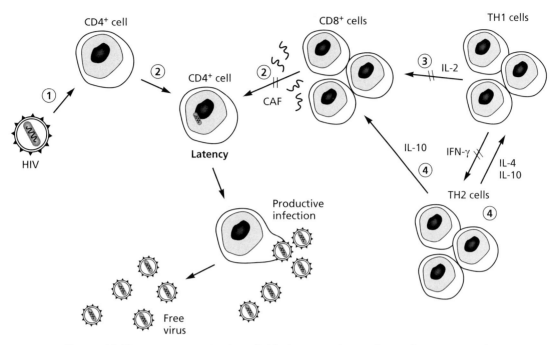

Figure 13.13   Events occurring in individuals progressing to disease (i.e., progressors). The events described in the legend to Figure 13.12 are changed by a predominant expression of the TH2 versus the TH1 cytokine response. Cytokines such as interleukin-4 (IL-4) and IL-10 (step 4) can suppress cytokine production by TH1 cells and thereby affect the CD8⁺ cell antiviral activity. Moreover, these cellular factors can directly inhibit CD8⁺ cell antiviral responses (Figure 13.12). The result of the loss of CD8⁺ cell antiviral activity is release of the HIV from latency and production of virus in lymph nodes and peripheral blood. These events lead to development of disease. Reproduced from reference 2520 with permission.

restores immunity and can reverse some of the neurologic symptoms observed in HIV-1-infected patients (3863). Additional work in this area of metabolic disorders is warranted.

In this consideration of the clinical course in HIV infection, the recognition of ESN offers encouragement that resistance to this infection can occur. While some adaptive immune responses have been found in ESN (e.g., CTLs and mucosal anti-HIV antibodies), they are not universally noted, and it would appear that innate cellular immune responses (DC, NK, and CD8⁺ cell mediated) are very important (see Chapter 9). Nevertheless, the observed cross-reactivity of antibodies with HLA antigens (see Chapter 10, Table 10.6) supports the hypothesis that antialloeneic responses, particularly antibodies, might be helpful in preventing HIV infection (2479) (see Chapter 15). Thus, further work in examining the immuno-

logic and, in some cases, genetic factors that enable some individuals to resist infection, albeit in most cases transiently, is a direction worthy of additional investigation for development of anti-HIV therapies and vaccines. Why this natural resistance is lost when exposure to HIV no longer takes place (e.g., in Nairobi commercial sex workers) (2127) needs to be considered in this pursuit of directions to induce long-standing protection from HIV infection and disease.

If the concept of HIV pathogenesis discussed in this chapter is correct, a major question is, what approaches can be made to maintain the type 1 responses and thus prevent replication of HIV (Figure 13.14)? The possibilities under consideration are the use of type 1 cytokines directly (e.g., IL-2, IL-15, and IL-12) or of neutralizing antibodies to certain type 2 cytokines such as IL-4 and IL-10 (see Chapters 9, 11, and 14) (808, 817). Moreover, the importance of

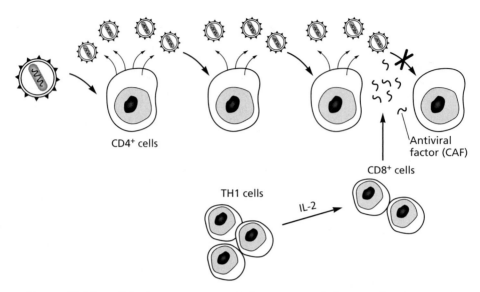

Figure 13.14 Cellular immune responses in long-term survival: approaches for controlling HIV pathogenesis. Methods directed at increasing CD8+ cell anti-HIV activity such as interleukin-2 (IL-2) therapy (e.g., increasing production of CD8+ cell antiviral factor (CAF) or enhancement of type 1 (TH1) cellular responses would suppress HIV infection and maintain a long asymptomatic state. Administration of CAF, once purified, might also be beneficial. Modified from reference 2520 with permission.

CD8+ cells in controlling the infection has been explored through the administration to infected individuals of autologous CD8+ cells previously grown in large quantities ex vivo (1859, 2241) (see Chapter 14). However, this ex vivo culture of T lymphocytes has not been recently utilized. Further approaches to increase CD8+ cell antiviral responses in the host (including CAF production) need to be explored in attempts to bring long-term survival to all HIV-infected individuals.

SALIENT FEATURES • CHAPTER 13

1. Cofactors that might play a role in HIV pathogenesis include the genetic makeup of the host (e.g., *HLA*), infection by other viruses or infectious agents, sexually transmitted diseases, immune-stimulating processes such as allergens, and other factors that influence cytokine production.

2. Lifestyle factors, particularly alcohol, smoking, drugs, and stress, are possible cofactors in HIV pathogenesis, particularly in their effect on mental capacity.

3. HIV pathogenesis involves three major clinical stages of infection: an early period in which high virus production takes place, a persistent period when virus is maintained at a lower threshold primarily by the immune system, and a symptomatic period when viral production has reemerged and presages the development of disease. At these various clinical stages, the virus population shows homogeneity, heterogeneity, and then a return to homogeneity, respectively.

4. Progression to disease is heralded by the emergence of a virus (X4 or R5) with increased replication kinetics and cytopathology and often enhanced progeny production.

5. The factors involved in the decrease in HIV-specific immune function include loss of CD4+ cells by direct killing or by indirect effects such as apoptosis; relative changes in type 1 or type 2 cytokine production that can influence cell-mediated immunity; aberrant immune responses, such as autoreactive T cells; autoantibodies; and an inadequate production of interleukin-2 (IL-2). A possible detrimental role for cytotoxic T lymphocytes should be considered.

6. In the absence of therapy, a delay in progression to disease correlates with low viral RNA levels and high numbers of CD4+ cells in the blood. Several other parameters reflecting immune activation, virus phenotype, and reduced immune function may be predictive of the risk for progression to disease.

7. Three clinical outcomes of HIV infection can be distinguished: a typical progression over 8 to 10 years, a rapid progression within 2 to 5 years, and a long-term survival or nonprogression in which an individual remains healthy without therapy for more than 10 years. Some long-term survivors are elite controllers who can suppress HIV to undetectable levels in the blood. One other noteworthy group, untreated patients with an AIDS diagnosis (<200 CD4+ cells/μl), may not develop terminal disease for several years.

8. HIV pathogenesis reflects a variety of viral and immunologic features. Factors involved in long-term survival can include infection with a virus with reduced cytopathic effects and low replicative ability; an absence of enhancing antibodies; presence of innate immune responses, including a strong CD8+ cell antiviral noncytopathic response; and a dominant type 1 cytokine pattern. Loss of CD8+ cell antiviral activity presages progression to disease.

9. Long-term survival appears to depend on sufficient production of IL-2, which maintains the CD8+ cell anti-HIV response and other immune functions that protect the host from disease. A basic determinant would appear to be normally functioning antigen-presenting cells (e.g., dendritic cells).

10. High-risk exposed seronegative individuals represent a clinical group that has probably been protected from infection by a strong anti-HIV cellular immune response. A role for mucosal anti-HIV antibodies has been suggested.

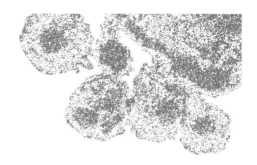

Antiviral Therapies

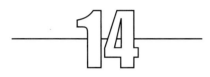

I. Introduction

While this book cannot cover in detail the many therapeutic approaches being evaluated to control HIV infection, some review of work in this field is helpful in the context of HIV pathogenesis. Several steps in the viral infection cycle discussed in the early chapters (Figure 5.1) have been targeted for antiviral action. Many drugs have been evaluated over the past decade, targeting certain features of HIV infection (Table 14.1). Over 20 are now being used (Figure 14.1; Table 14.2) (for reviews, see references 10 and 4318). In addition, certain immune system-based (immune-based) treatments have received increased attention (e.g., interleukin-2 [IL-2]) (2310) (see Section III). The therapies for opportunistic infections among HIV-infected people have greatly improved since the onset of this epidemic (for reviews and treatment recommendations, see references 10, 309, and 4873). Moreover, some clinical symptoms and conditions arising from HIV infection can be improved by restoring normal levels of micronutrients in the body (for a review, see reference 4378) (Section II.D.4).

A brief historic account of anti-HIV therapies is provided in this chapter, followed by an update on present treatment approaches. The current antiviral drugs, when used in combination, now considered a cocktail of highly active antiretroviral therapy (HAART), have shown promise in controlling HIV infection (for a review, see reference 4318). Nevertheless, the need for adherence to treatment and the toxic effects of certain drugs are noteworthy and encourage further studies to improve anti-HIV strategies. The effect of these therapies on neurologic disorders is covered in Chapter 8.

Table 14.1 Potential approaches to therapies for HIV infection[a]

Anti-HIV virions
- sCD4
- Neutralizing antibodies (polyclonal, monoclonal)[b]

Virus entry
- CD4 analogues
- CCR5/CXCR4 analogues or antibodies
- Neutralizing antibodies[b]
- Fusion inhibitor (e.g., T20)
- Saliva glycoproteins
- Sulfated polysaccharides

Early steps prior to integration
- Anti-RT (e.g., nucleoside analogues such as AZT, ddI, ddC, and d4T), nonnucleoside inhibitors (e.g., nevirapine and efavirenz), nucleotide inhibitors (tenofovir)
- Anti-integrase
- Anticapsid
- Antinucleotides (e.g., MPA and HU)
- Interferons
- Intracellular proteins (TRIM5α and APOBEC3G)
- Antiviral accessory proteins (e.g., Tat, Nef, Vif, and Rev)
- Anti-RNA (e.g., hammerhead RNA and siRNA)

Immune cell activation
- Cyclosporine
- Hydroxyurea
- MPA

Postintegration
- Anti-Tat
- Antiprotease
- Antisense nucleotides
- Anti-RNA (ribozymes and siRNA)
- CAF
- Cytokines (immune modulation)

Virus budding
- Glycosylation inhibitors (castanospermine)
- Interferons

Anti-infected cells
- Antiviral antibodies: antibody-dependent cellular cytotoxicity
- rCD4 toxin, rCD25 toxin
- Anti-gp120 toxin
- UV-A plus psoralen
- CD8+ cells

[a]RT, reverse transcriptase; AZT, zidovudine; ddI, didanosine; ddC, zalcitabine; d4T, stavudine; MPA, mycophenolic acid; HU, hydroxyurea; CAF, CD8+ cell antiviral factor; rCD4, recombinant CD4.

[b]By either passive immunotherapy or active immunization.

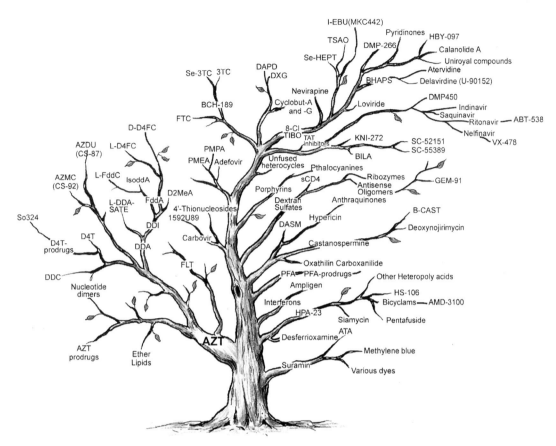

Figure 14.1   Schematic representation of the early development of anti-HIV drugs over time. At the left side are the nucleoside analogues. At the right side are the nonnucleoside drugs. The tree presents several different approaches directed at the replicative cycle of HIV. Modified from reference 3963 with kind permission of Springer Science and Business Media and provided by R. Schinazi.

II. Anti-HIV Therapies

A. Reverse Transcriptase Inhibitors

Recognizing the causative agent of AIDS as a retrovirus led to an immediate emphasis on arresting the replicative cycle of the virus. It is not surprising, therefore, that the first successful drug found was an inhibitor of the required reverse transcription. A compound that had been previously synthesized for potential use against cancer, 3'-azido-3'-deoxythymidine (AZT) (also called zidovudine [Retrovir]), substantially inhibited viral reverse transcriptase (RT) and HIV replication in vitro (3032). Its mechanism of action involved both a termination of viral DNA production and a competition for nucleosides used by the viral

polymerase. Nevertheless, the exact mechanism(s) for AZT activity in vivo is not known.

AZT was soon reported to be effective in preventing the onset of symptoms of HIV infection (1124). At first, large doses of the drug were administered (1,500 mg/day) and were associated with frequent side effects, especially toxicity to the bone marrow (1298). Subsequently, the amount of AZT prescribed was reduced to 500 to 600 mg/day. This level resulted in fewer harmful toxicities (852). Based on the early reports, therapy was recommended for asymptomatic individuals with a CD4$^+$ cell count of <500 cells/μl (4622), but that recommendation was later challenged (4037). Some studies suggested that AZT treatment offered less benefit to asymptomatic subjects than to

Table 14.2 Drugs approved for the treatment of HIV infection[a]

Brand name	Generic name (abbreviation)
NRTIs	
Atripla	Tenofovir, emtricitabine, and efavirenz
Combivir	Lamivudine and zidovudine
Emtriva	Emtricitabine (FTC)
Epivir	Lamivudine (3TC)
Epzicom	Abacavir and lamivudine
Hivid	Zalcitabine; dideoxycytidine (ddC)
Retrovir	Zidovudine; azidothymidine (AZT)
Trizivir	Abacavir, zidovudine, and lamivudine
Truvada	Tenofovir disoproxil and emtricitabine
Videx EC	Enteric coated didanosine
Videx	Didanosine (ddI), dideoxyinosine
Viread[b]	Tenofovir disoproxil fumarate
Zerit	Stavudine (d4T)
Ziagen	Abacavir
NNRTIs	
Rescriptor	Delavirdine
Sustiva	Efavirenz
Viramune	Nevirapine
PIs	
Agenerase	Amprenavir
Aptivus	Tipranavir
Crixivan	Indinavir
Fortovase	Saquinavir
Invirase	Saquinavir mesylate
Kaletra	Lopinavir and ritonavir
Lexiva	Fosamprenavir calcium
Norvir	Ritonavir
Prezista	Darunavir
Reyataz	Atazanavir sulfate
Viracept	Nelfinavir mesylate, NFV
Fusion inhibitors	
Fuzeon	Enfuvirtide, T20

[a] Taken from http://www.fda.gov/oashi/aids/virals.html.
[b] Nucleotide reverse transcriptase inhibitor.

symptomatic patients (1961, 4037). The effect of the drug was short-term and appeared to be greatest when used late in the clinical course.

Over the past 20 years, seven nucleoside RT inhibitors (NRTIs) that compete with nucleosides used by the viral RT to produce the DNA provirus have been introduced into treatment (http://www.fda.gov/oashi/aids/virals.html) (Table 14.2). Several are now given in combination. Like AZT, many need to be activated by intracellular phosphorylation. Didanosine (ddI) (2',3'-dideoxyinosine) and zalcitabine (ddC) (2',3'-dideoxycytidine) were found to be effective and less toxic to bone marrow than AZT (3720, 4088, 4863). Nevertheless, their administration has been associated with pancreatitis and peripheral neuropathy (Section V). Another anti-RT drug, stavudine (d4T) (2',3'-didehydro-3'-deoxythymidine) (534), initially showed less toxicity than the other drugs, with some indication of stabilization of CD4+ cells. However, d4T, although effective against HIV, has been associated with noteworthy metabolic problems (Section V.B). The nucleoside analogue lamivudine (3TC) (−)-2',-deoxy-3'-thiothiadine) was found to have activity against HIV-1 strains resistant to AZT. Monotherapy with 3TC soon gives rise to resistant strains, but the common mutation in the HIV-1 polymerase gene at the 184 Met codon conferring resistance to 3TC maintains or restores the sensitivity of the virus to nucleoside inhibitors such as AZT (1219, 4654, 4701). Thus, 3TC or the related compound emtricitabine (FTC) (3822) is usually used in combination with nucleoside RT inhibitors (Section II.C).

A related NRTI utilizes an analogue for a nucleotide that contain a phosphate group and thus is less dependent on cellular kinase activity for activation. The one drug of this type, 9-(2-phosphonomethoxypropyl) adenine (PMPA), showed promising results in preventing disease development in SIV-infected monkeys (4561). If given soon after SIV transmission, this drug was shown to block the establishment of infection (4492). It is now the most commonly prescribed treatment (as tenofovir [Viread]) in Western countries (Table 14.2). A related compound, adefovir dipivoxil, has also shown anti-HIV activity (1027) but because of renal toxicity is no longer used in doses effective against HIV-1. It is prescribed for hepatitis B virus infection.

Three nonnucleoside RT inhibitors (NNRTIs), nevirapine (NVP), delavirdine, and efavirenz, have also been introduced for therapy (http://www.fda.gov/oashi/aids/virals.html) (Table 14.2). They block the hydrophobic pocket within the polymerase domain of the p66 RT subunit. The use of the NNRTI drugs in combination with nucleoside

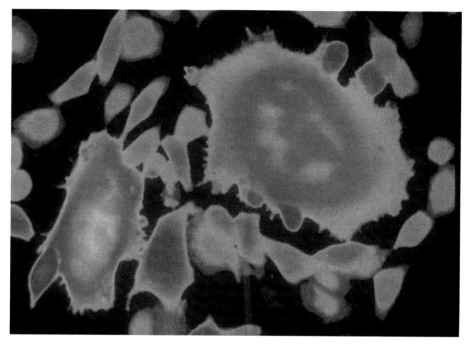

Color Plate 12 The HUT 78 T-cell line (pretreated with dye) was mixed with Chinese hamster ovary (CHO) cells expressing the HIV-1$_{LAI}$ envelope glycoprotein. The resulting fusion between these two cells permitted dye transfer from the T lymphocyte into the CHO cells. Photomicrograph courtesy of C. Weiss. (See page 135.)

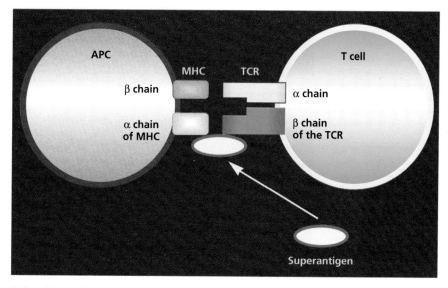

Color Plate 13 A superantigen is not processed by cells but can bind directly to either class II molecules or the Vβ portion of the T-cell receptor (see Color Plate 18). This interaction can lead to a nonspecific activation of T cells. Adapted from reference 900 with permission. (See page 147.)

Color Plate 14 Effects of HIV infection on lymphoid tissue. (A) Early stage. Follicular and paracortical hyperplasia can be seen secondary to an increase in the number of germinal centers associated with B-cell proliferation. Paracortical hyperplasia reflects the increase in the number of CD8+ cells. (B) Follicular lysis stage. In the early advancement to symptomatic infection, germinal centers break down and follicular dendritic cell death occurs. Eventually, an involution of the germinal centers takes place. (C) Terminal stage. At this stage of infection, lymphoid tissue depletion is noted, with an absence of lymphocytes and a complete disruption of normal lymph node architecture. Photomicrographs courtesy of B. Herndier. (See page 175.)

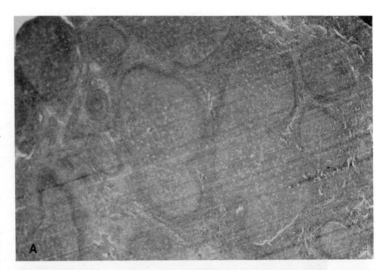

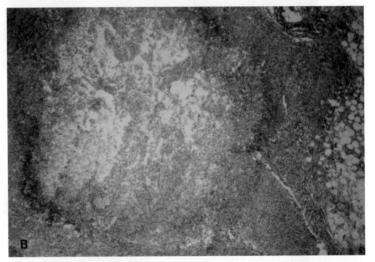

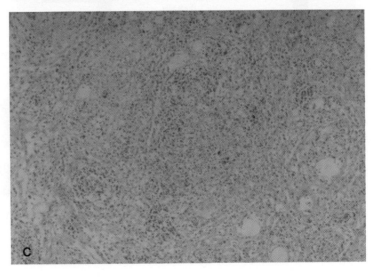

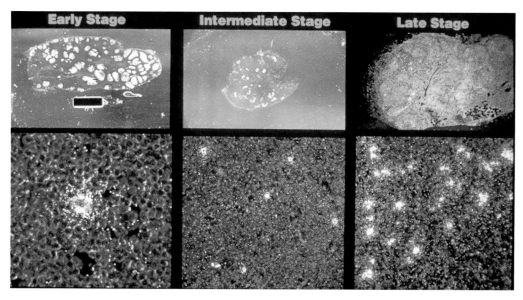

Color Plate 15 Effects of HIV infection on lymphoid tissue. Panels indicate the changes in the lymph node germinal centers as determined by selective staining (top panels) and by the location of virus replication in lymph node tissue (bottom panels). HIV replication was detected by PCR procedures. The events are reflected for the early, intermediate, and late stages of HIV infection. Data provided by the HIV Information Network; figure derived from reference 3414 with permission from Elsevier. (See page 175.)

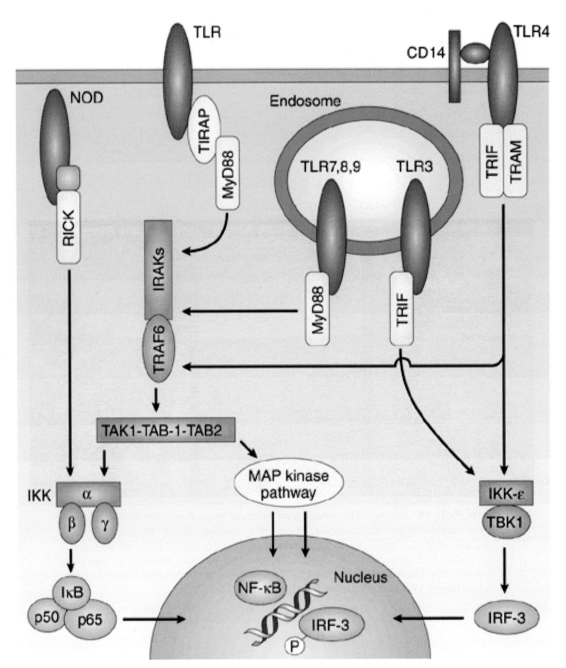

Color Plate 16 Signaling through receptors of the innate immune system. Upon interaction with pathogen-associated molecular patterns (PAMPs), pattern recognition receptors (PRRs) initiate signaling cascades leading to activation of transcription factors (such as NF-kB and IRF3), resulting in expression of inflammatory cytokines and other cellular activation events. A simplified pathway highlighting the main elements is shown, with receptors in green, adaptor proteins in yellow, kinases in purple, and transcription factors in blue. Ligation of different Toll-like receptors (TLRs) may induce distinct gene expression patterns (1086). IKK, IκB kinase complex; IRAK, IL-1 receptor-associated kinase; IRF, interferon regulatory protein; MyD88, myeloid differentiation factor 88; RICK, receptor-interacting serine/threonine kinase; TAB1/2, TAK1 binding protein; TAK1, transforming growth factor β-activated kinase; TBK1, TRAF family member-associated NFkB activator binding kinase 1; TIR, Toll-IL-1 receptor domain; TIRAP, TIR domain-containing adaptive protein; TRAF, TNF receptor-associated factor; TRAM, TRIF-related adaptor molecules; TRIF, TIR domain-containing adaptor protein inducing IFN-β. Reprinted with permission from Macmillan Publishers Ltd.: *Nature Medicine* (3433), © 2005. (See page 211.)

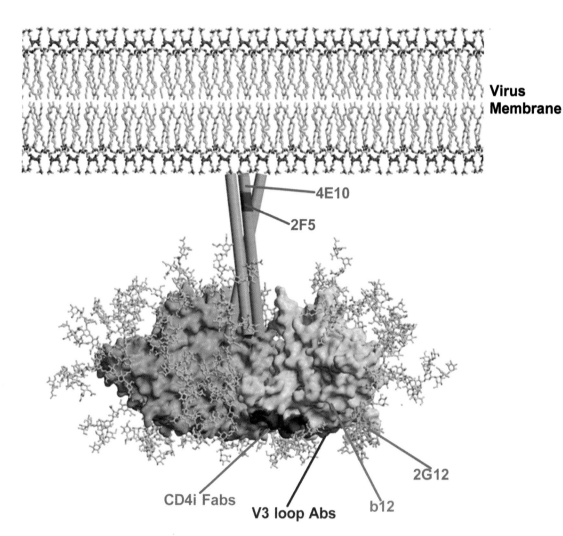

Virus Membrane

4E10

2F5

CD4i Fabs

V3 loop Abs

b12

2G12

Color Plate 17   Neutralizing antibody epitopes on a model of the Env spike of HIV-1 based on the structure of core gp120 (2368, 2369); three gp120 monomers are shown in gray, pale green, and pale blue. gp41 (pink) is shown schematically as three tubes. Carbohydrate chains are shown in yellow, and the oligomannose cluster proposed to interact with monoclonal antibody 2G12 is shown in cyan. Binding sites for other neutralizing monoclonal antibodies are indicated. Figure provided by D. Burton, R. Stanfield, and I. A. Wilson. Reprinted from reference 563 with permission. (See page 241.)

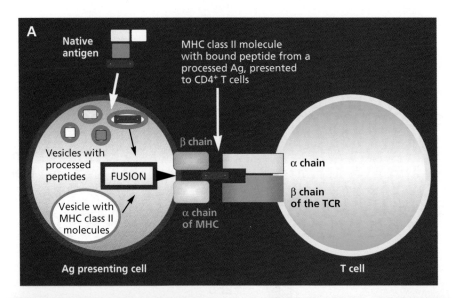

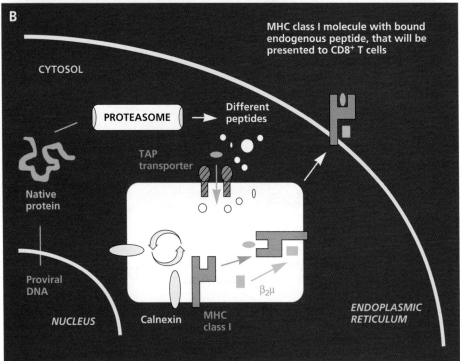

Color Plate 18 (A) Antigen (Ag) presentation to CD4[+] T cells. An exogenous antigen with various epitopes is endocytosed by an antigen-presenting cell and processed in intracellular vesicles such as acidified endosomes. These vesicles then fuse with other vesicles containing major histocompatibility complex (MHC) class II molecules, which transport the peptide to the cell surface. The antigen is subsequently presented to the CD4[+] cells through an interaction with the T-cell receptor (TCR) (generally the alpha and beta chains) and the CD4 molecule. (B) Presentation of antigen to CD8[+] cells. Endogenous antigens expressed by a cell are first processed by proteasomes into small peptides. These molecules are then transported by specific molecules (the TAP transporters) into the endoplasmic reticulum. In this organelle, MHC class I molecules are bound first to calnexin (Csc), a chaperone protein, and then to peptide antigen. Binding of the peptide to the α chain allows for stable interaction with β_2-microglobulin. The peptide bound to the MHC class I complex is transported through the Golgi complex to the cell surface. From this site, it interacts with the TCR and the CD8 molecule on the CD8[+] cell surface TAP, transporter associated with antigen processing. Adapted from reference 900 with permission. (See page 261.)

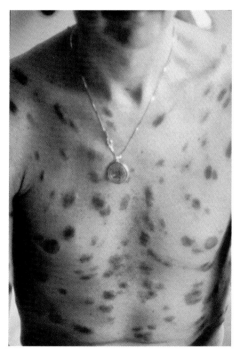

Color Plate 19 Kaposi's sarcoma in a young HIV-infected man. Note the distribution of the lesions suggesting lymphatic involvement. Figure courtesy of P. Volberding. (See page 295.)

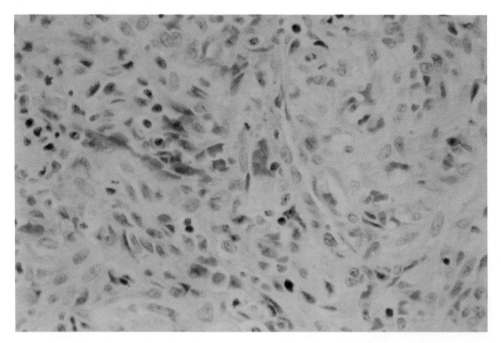

Color Plate 20 Histologic picture of Kaposi's sarcoma. Magnification, ×100. Photomicrograph courtesy of B. Herndier. (See page 296.)

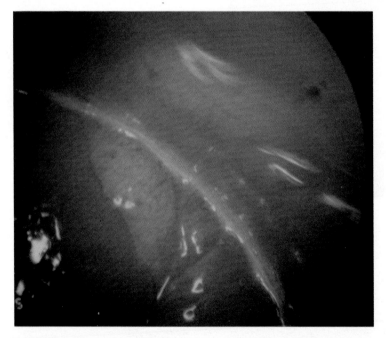

Color Plate 21 AIN grade 2 lesion observed at analscopy. A 3% acidic solution was applied to the surface of the anal canal. A well-circumscribed lesion that has turned white compared to the normal mucosa ("acetowhite") is visualized through an anal scope at ×160 magnification. The lesion is smooth and has prominent vacuolization. Reprinted from reference 3388 with permission. (See page 311.)

analogues has provided dramatic antiviral effects (1025). A hypersensitivity rash can result with administration of the three NNRTIs. Hepatitis occurs with the use of the NVP in patients with a higher baseline CD4+ T-cell count (4552) and most likely reflects a hyperresponse of the immune system (Section II.E). Once these symptoms appear, the drugs cannot be used. Efavirenz also is associated with central nervous system (CNS) effects that resolve within the first weeks of therapy in most patients (2854).

Compounds that prevent the incorporation of the nucleotides into DNA during reverse transcription and act on autoreactive immune cells have also been evaluated. Mycophenolic acid (MPA), at nontoxic concentrations that can be reached in the blood, inhibited HIV-1 and HIV-2 replication in cultured CD4+ lymphocytes and macrophages (1948). It blocks the incorporation of guanidine into proviral DNA (1948) and has shown some promise when used in combination therapy (particularly with abacavir) for HIV infection (692, 2808). Hydroxyurea (HU) also reduces the formation of deoxynucleoside triphosphate substrates

(1434; for a review, see reference 2668). Both MPA and HU may also have value by reducing immune activation (Sections II.D and VII). The addition of HU to RT inhibitors has shown synergistic effects in inhibiting HIV replication in culture (2781) and a moderate effect in vivo (3062). However, its enhancement of peripheral neurotoxicity when used with ddI and d4T has limited its clinical usefulness (2668). Another nucleic acid inhibitor and immune modulator is leflunomide, which blocks pyrimidine (uridine) synthesis (3967). Its antiviral effect is similar to that of HU and appears to be more effective than MPA.

B. Protease Inhibitors

The protease inhibitors (PIs) block the action of another HIV enzyme, which is also encoded by the *pol* gene. Protease autocatalyzes its own precursor protein and then cleaves other polypeptides to bring viral proteins into functional units, particularly the viral core (see Chapter 1). In general, this activity occurs within the virion during or after budding from the cell surface and is blocked by PIs (Figures 1.3 and 14.2). Similar to

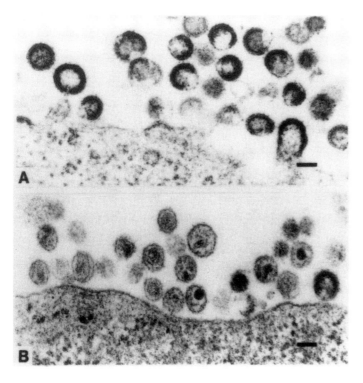

Figure 14.2 (A) Doughnut-shaped HIV-1 particles from a T-cell line infected with a protease-deficient virus (2078). The morphology of the particles resembles that of viruses released from protease inhibitor-treated cells. (B) For comparison, the wild-type virus released from the T-cell line is presented. Bar, 100 nm. Figure provided by K. Ikuta.

the advancement made with crystallization of RT (2256), the crystal structure of the protease enzyme (3224, 4799) helped in the development of these other antiviral drugs. Computer modeling was able to identify compounds that could fit into the active site at the base of a cleft present in the dimeric form of the functional HIV-1 protease (1217, 3754).

Thus far, the U.S. Food and Drug Administration has approved 10 PIs for treatment of HIV infection (http://www.fda.gov/oashi/aids/virals.html) (Table 14.2). These drugs have provided a major boost in the management of HIV infection and have influenced the concepts of treatment along the lines of those used in anticancer therapies (for reviews, see references 1025 and 1031). In essence, the addition of PIs to two drugs with different antiviral effects (e.g., retroviral RT inhibitors, either nucleoside or nonnucleoside) led to the development of HAART.

Each of the PI drugs used, however, can cause substantial adverse effects and can interact with other medications (Section V). For example, several factors need to be considered when prescribing PIs, including their interaction with various statins, antibiotics, anticoagulants, and other antiretroviral drugs (1031, 3526) as well as food supplements such as garlic (3525). Initially, the PIs needed to be given according to a recommended timing (e.g., indinavir [Crixivan] every 8 h); otherwise viral resistance could quickly occur and show cross-reactivity with other PIs (Section III). The recent PI drug formulations do not have that time or food restriction (238, 1031). Tipranavir plus ritanovir has shown a very strong antiviral activity compared to other PIs in subjects with multidrug-resistant HIV infection (577a). Moreover, darunavir (Prezista) is a recently approved PI that works against HIV isolates that have reduced susceptibility to other PIs.

The PI ritonavir is a strong inhibitor of cytochrome P-450, which is involved in the metabolism of PIs by the liver. When it was used along with saquinavir, toxic levels of saquinavir resulted (2979). However, since saquinavir has poor oral bioavailability, ritonavir can increase its therapeutic potential. Thus, lower doses of PIs can be used with ritonavir (for reviews, see references 1031 and 3526). Saquinavir, therefore, is generally used in combination with ritonavir (Table 14.2)

and other PIs (http://www.fda.gov/oashi/aids/virals.html).

A notable concern is the oral bioavailability of certain PIs (especially saquinavir) and their capacity to cross the blood-brain barrier to enter other reservoirs for the virus in the body. For example, none of the PI drugs thus far has shown efficient passage into the cerebrospinal fluid (CSF) (because of the high degree of protein binding), and the development of drug-resistant strains in these sanctuaries must be considered (see Chapter 8 and see below).

C. Combination Therapy

Because the antiviral effects of the RT inhibitor monotherapies were limited, the use of two- or three-drug therapies was begun, and the results were very encouraging (Table 14.2). Initially, AZT, ddI, ddC, and combinations of these drugs were attempted in two-drug therapy trials (1708, 2064, 3921). In general, adding another nucleoside analogue increased the efficacy of the treatment, but often resistance resulted and persistent control of virus replication was not achieved.

As noted above, the most dramatic effect on viral RNA levels has come with triple-drug therapy. R5 and X4 viruses are equally affected (539). This introduction of combination antiretroviral therapy, now known as HAART, has greatly diminished the death rate from AIDS and has reduced clinical symptoms of HIV infection (678, 1062, 1872), including cardiovascular disease (4452). The decline in death rate from AIDS in individuals with >100 $CD4^+$ cells/µl can be credited to the use of such antiretroviral drugs in combination (1872).

PIs taken alone give rise quickly to resistant strains, some of which become cross-resistant to other PIs. However, in combination with other anti-HIV drugs, they add an antiviral effect that can lead to undetectable levels of virus in the plasma, lymphoid tissues, and CSF (1439) for months to years. Pathogenic changes in the follicular dendritic cell (FDC) network of lymphoid tissues can be favorably reversed with HAART (4941) (Section II.G). Moreover, a repopulation of lymphoid tissue with $CD4^+$ cells can take place (4939) (Section II.G). Initially, two anti-RT drugs were combined with a PI (1031). However, because of the toxicities of PIs, two NRTIs and one NNRTI have more recently been recommended (4265)

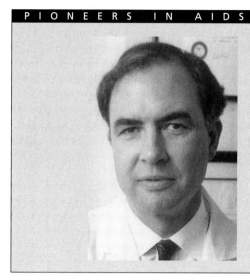

Paul Volberding

Chief of Medical Service, San Francisco Veterans Affairs Medical Center; Professor; Vice-Chair, Department of Medicine; and Co-Director, Center for AIDS Research, University of California, San Francisco. Dr. Volberding was among the first to define the clinical syndromes associated with AIDS and established the first ward (at San Francisco General Hospital) dedicated solely to the care of AIDS patients.

(Section V). In short-term therapy, however, there does not appear to be substantial toxicity from PIs (symptoms can be fatigue, diarrhea, and nausea) (853). In evaluating the effect of HAART, two phases in the loss of HIV-infected cells have been recognized: rapid (2 days) and prolonged (half-life of up to 2 weeks) (3470, 3471) (Table 8.5). HAART is also valuable in reducing immune activation with its associated production of toxic inflammatory cytokines that can give clinical symptoms and cause CD4+ cell loss (119, 1439) (see Chapter 6).

D. Other Antiviral Approaches (Table 14.1)

1. VIRAL PROTEIN TARGETS

Integrase, a third viral enzyme, is essential for productive virus infection (4794) (see Chapter 1). Several years ago, this enzyme was purified and its crystal structure identified at 2.5 Å (1157). Like protease, it has a dimeric form. In general, without the function of integrase, HIV is not infectious. Inhibitors of HIV-1 integrase are being developed that have recently shown effectiveness in rhesus macaque studies (1776).

Attention has also been given to blocking some of the intracellular enzymatic properties that are needed for maturation of the virus. Such anti-HIV compounds, considered maturation inhibitors, can block steps in the processing of Gag (2567). Analogues of myristic acid, which is necessary for the myristoylation of the Gag and Nef proteins, have reduced HIV replication (541). However, the potential effect of these treatments on normal cellular function involving these enzymes needs to be considered.

The recognition of the three-dimensional structures of the HIV MA protein (2864) and the ectodomain portion of gp41 (676, 4718) may permit the development of effective therapies against these molecules. In addition, drugs against glycosylation have been considered (1653, 3672). For example, castanospermine disrupts the glycosylation of the viral envelope and makes the virus noninfectious (504). In addition, drugs that block the zinc finger motif of the HIV NC protein have been reported (3721, 4503). Other therapies under evaluation have been directed at viral accessory proteins or genetic regions (e.g., Tat and the long terminal repeat [LTR]) (1910, 2566) as well as the viral envelope proteins (1011, 4756) (see below). In this regard, the internal fragment of a heterogeneous nuclear ribonuclear protein U has been found to target the 3' LTR in viral mRNA and block HIV transcription (4533a). While not a secreted protein, this nuclear protein may be induced by other factors with antiviral activity (1889a) (e.g., CD8+ cells) (see Chapter 11). Moreover, some studies have shown that the granulin/epithelin precursor can inhibit P-TEFb function and thus block HIV-1 transcription via Tat. This finding also suggests approaches by which selective inhibitors of P-TEFb could provide an antiviral drug (1889a) (see Chapter 5).

2. CELL SURFACE AND ENTRY INHIBITORS

Other directions for antiviral therapy have included blocking HIV attachment to the viral cellular receptor by using recombinant CD4 (see Chapter 3) or compounds to interrupt the interaction of gp120 with CD4 (1667, 4125) (Table 14.1). Early trials with CD4 analogues were not successful because the affinity of HIV for the natural CD4 receptor was stronger than for the analogue (3089). However, a new class of entry inhibitors preventing the interaction of gp120 with CD4 has been reported that can act directly on both R5 and X4 viruses (4942). Blocking virus attachment with sulfated polysaccharides has also been tried (190, 2894).

Importantly, the development of small molecules to prevent HIV attachment to the HIV coreceptors (CCR5 and CXCR4) is under serious consideration (4150; for a review, see reference 31). Some recent results have been encouraging with these chemokine receptor antagonist drugs that by convention will carry the affix *viroc* (1255). The latter approaches offer promise because they do not appear to induce chemotaxic signaling (4150). However, a trial with Aplaviroc, a GlaxoSmithKline drug, was stopped because of potential liver toxicity (1026). Efficacy problems have faced other entry inhibitors, and currently their use only in "salvage" patients is being recommended (1026). Moreover, since HIV can use a variety of different coreceptors (see Chapter 3), decoys for a particular coreceptor may select for viruses that will find other means of cell entry (782) (Section III). The risk of HIV evolving to home out in other cells or tissues must be considered. Another approach has been to induce production of anti-CCR5 antibodies that could block HIV infection (243) (see Chapter 15). Some evidence suggests that such antibodies exist in certain HIV-exposed seronegative individuals (see Chapter 13).

Recently, a concern for anti-CCR5 compounds has arisen. Whereas the absence of CCR5 expression had been considered not to affect immune responses, individuals who lack CCR5 have an increased risk of developing symptomatic West Nile virus infection. *CCR5 Δ32* homozygosity was significantly associated with a fatal outcome (1531).

In studies targeting the cell surface HIV coreceptors, the topical application of an analogue of the β-chemokine RANTES protected rhesus macaques from vaginal challenge with $SHIV_{SF162}$, an R5 virus (2454). In other primate experiments, a small CCR5 inhibitor reduced virus replication in macaques and prevented vaginal transmission of an SHIV-R5 virus (4574). Results from trials in human subjects should be available soon.

Notably, drugs to prevent HIV:cell fusion have also been developed (for a review, see reference 593). Fusion inhibitors such as T20 (enfuvirtide [Fuzeon]) that need to be given by subcutaneous administration have shown effective anti-HIV activity. T20 is a synthetic peptide mimicking a region of the gp41 HIV-1 envelope. It competes with the viral protein and blocks cell fusion and entry (Color Plate 5, following page 78). T20 has been beneficial to individuals who are resistant to many of the antiretroviral drugs (2186, 2441). Sensitivity to T20 is enhanced with less coreceptor expression on the cell surface and less affinity of the virus for coreceptors such as CCR5 (3685). In addition, CD4 binding to gp120 exposes a portion of gp41 (HR1 coiled coil), and this process can be blocked by certain entry inhibitors that bind to gp120. These findings are encouraging the development of other types of fusion inhibitors of HIV entry (for a review, see reference 2185).

3. OTHER STRATEGIES

Ribozymes, antisense molecules, and attempts at gene therapy with intracellular transdominant inhibitors have been proposed after promising results were obtained in vitro (1267, 3465, 3813). Antisense RNAs containing a catalytic domain were targeted to the LTR region of HIV-1 and reduced virus replication in cell culture by >90% (3614). This technology can be used as well to block RNA splicing, and in some studies, the RNA can be introduced into cells via an arginine-rich vehicle (3147). This approach was derived from the observation that the easy entry of Tat appears to be related to its high arginine content (3146).

Another approach, RNA interference, is a post-transcriptional silencing mechanism involving double-stranded RNA. This process uses small interfering RNAs (siRNAs) to target the degradation of mRNAs for HIV proteins or cell surface receptors (1991, 2465) (for a review, see reference 2595). It is an activity found in a variety of organisms and, more recently, in mammalian cells (for a review, see reference 1713). This RNA interference is mediated by siRNAs that are produced from larger RNAs by cleavage via an endonuclease, a ribonuclease III type called Dicer. The 21- to 23-nucleotide siRNAs produced are then placed into a nuclease complex, the RNA-induced silencing complex, that targets and cleaves the mRNA complementary to the siRNA (4911). The siRNA approach has been used in cell culture with HIV to reduce virus replication (609, 3287; for a review, see reference 2595). A major problem is finding ways of avoiding mutant viruses that escape from this interference (969). Many of these theoretical approaches, moreover, need a means of easy delivery to cells.

Other novel strategies may include those that mimic the function of APOBEC3G, counter the effect of Vif, or use the blocking action of TRIM5α, as well as other innate intracellular factors (see Chapter 5) (for a review, see reference 1619). A synthetic HIV-1 Rev inhibitor that interferes with viral mRNA export has also been reported (952).

Some investigators had considered using immunosuppressive drugs such as cyclosporine because of the potential detrimental effects of hyperactive immune responses in HIV pathogenesis (3740, 4017) (see Chapter 11). A randomized controlled trial with cyclosporine did not show any sustained benefit in CD4+ cell number in people with chronic HIV infection, suggesting that the immune activation pathways involved are not sensitive to this drug (2453a). Analogues of cyclosporine lacking immune system-suppressing activity may be useful because they block the association of cyclophilin A with the Gag (p24) protein (478, 1353) (see Chapters 4 and 5). They are believed to prevent the opening of the viral capsid after virus entry and its transport to the nucleus. Thus, infection cannot take place. Murabutide is an immune modulator that down-regulates CD4 and CCR5 expression via an effect on intracellular factors. It reduces virus replication in macrophages and dendritic cells (DCs) (967). Work with other immune modulators is discussed in Section VII.C.

Approaches that destroy the virus-infected cells (380) (Table 14.1) have also been studied. Anti-gp120, CD4 or CD45RO, and CD25 antibodies (2895, 3657) or soluble CD4 linked to ricin or other toxins (e.g., *Pseudomonas* or pokeweed antiviral protein) have been tried in culture alone and in combination with antiviral therapy (162, 2799, 2895). Further work with these approaches has not been reported. More strategies directed at cellular targets are warranted to increase the chance of removing reservoirs of HIV.

4. EFFECT OF NUTRITIONAL SUPPLEMENTS

Besides HAART, some studies have suggested that micronutrients can affect the clinical state of HIV infection (for a review, see reference 4378). For example, trials with multivitamin supplements have reduced pathological conditions such as candidiasis. Moreover, in the absence of HAART, nutritional therapy has helped to raise CD4+ and CD8+ T-cell counts and lower viral loads (1263). In such subjects, it can prolong survival (1263). Vitamin A could be beneficial by preventing R5 replication in macrophages via suppression of the HIV-1 LTR (2731). Vitamin D has been shown to be important for maintaining the function of human macrophages, particularly in response to *Mycobacterium tuberculosis* infection. A deficiency in this vitamin can give higher susceptibility to tuberculosis (2633). However, in some studies, adding vitamin A to a multivitamin supplement can reduce the benefit of the regimen, most likely because of the large amount given (4378).

Multivitamins have helped in long-term survival of children of women with poor nutritional status (1262). Low vitamin A and carotenoid levels have been associated with an increased risk of heterosexual transmission, most likely because of the altered integrity of the genital epithelium or immune dysfunction (2958). However, these nutritional additions can increase HIV transmission, probably by enhancing the differentiation of myeloid cells into macrophages and their expression of CCR5 (2728).

Other studies have suggested that low levels of plasma zinc, particularly in relationship to copper levels, can decrease survival from HIV infection (2382). Selenium deficiency has been associated as well with a higher likelihood of genital mucosal shedding of HIV-infected cells (206).

Finally, the supplementation of micronutrients (vitamins C, A, E, B_{12}, B_1, B_2, B_3, B_6, B_9, selenium, iron, and zinc) given at two to three times the recommended requirement to SIV-infected rhesus macaques led to a higher rate of death (1546). This finding could be related to an increased susceptibility of certain cells (e.g., myeloid cells) to HIV infection after they have undergone differentiation in response to retinoic acid (2728, 4509). The results do suggest that megavitamin supplementations could be dangerous to HIV-infected individuals. From these observations, however, it is evident that additional studies to determine appropriate nutritional therapies are warranted, particularly for resource-poor countries.

E. Genetic Factors

Host *HLA* alleles can determine sensitivity to certain antiretroviral drugs (for a review, see reference 3269). In some cases, polymorphisms in a cytokine receptor (e.g., CX3CR1) (538) or in cytokines (e.g., *TNF-α-308*2*), along with an *HLA-A2 B44* haplotye (3604) can play a role in determining the efficiency of anti-HIV drugs. Polymorphisms in the genes encoding cytochrome P-450 can also affect plasma efavirenz concentrations and perhaps those of other antiretroviral drugs (3776).

Immunologic hypersensitivity to abacavir appears to be associated strongly with *HLA-B57*01* (1829, 2780). NVP hypersensitivity (hepatitis, fever, and rash) has correlated with *HLA-DRBI*0101* in the presence of substantial CD4$^+$ cell numbers (2828). The findings suggest a CD4$^+$ T-cell response to NVP antigens. Some evidence has been shown that MHC class II molecules via cellular immunity may help in HIV control by antiretroviral therapy. In particular, the *DR*13* haplotype was associated with maintenance of virus suppression during treatment (2777). The results do support the importance of coexisting anti-HIV immune responses during antiretroviral therapy.

Some findings also suggest that the presence of a multiple drug resistance (MDR-1) transporter gene which codes for P glycoprotein (particularly the C/T polymorphism) gives better CD4$^+$ cell responses after antiviral therapy (1271). Other studies showed that MDR-1 reduced the uptake of protease inhibitors by CD4$^+$ cells (2047) and can be associated with a lower response to HAART (538).

The results could reflect differential control of drugs (particularly PIs) in various compartments and cells (1271). These observations need further evaluation (for a review, see reference 1934).

F. Virus Selection by Antiretroviral Therapy

There is some suggestion that the use of certain antiretroviral drugs could select for R5 versus X4 viruses (4171, 4945). AZT and d4T need to be phosphorylated by kinases present in activated cells to become effective. In contrast, the phosphorylation/activation processes for ddI, ddC, and 3TC are found in quiescent cells. These differences could explain the selection of R5 viruses with AZT and X4 viruses with ddI (4566). Didanosine (ddI) works well in resting T cells, whereas AZT needs activation within cells (1433, 4118).

Biologic studies mirror the pharmacology findings. R5 viruses can induce activation in resting cells that would permit the antiviral activity of AZT in those cells. X4 viruses would be sensitive to agents that are already activated and therefore respond to ddI (1610, 2650). Thus, in some cases, HAART can lead to a phenotypic switch from X4 to R5 variants that could be resistant to therapy (1216). Again, most results suggest a preferential suppression of X4 viruses by the current anti-HIV drugs (3501, 4171). Finally, approaches to block HIV infection via chemokine receptor analogues carry the risk of selecting for viruses that use a different coreceptor (Sections II.D.2 and III).

G. Effects of Antiretroviral Therapy on HIV in Other Tissues

One of the major challenges of antiretroviral drugs besides plasma bioavailability is their distribution in other tissues, particularly the lymph nodes, brain, and testes (1031). The brain and testes maintain compartments that can be somewhat separated from the blood (see Chapter 2).

Present combination therapies including PIs can markedly decrease the levels of virus and virus-infected cells in both blood and lymphoid tissue (646, 3470). With tonsil tissue as a mirror of the effect of combination therapy on lymph nodes, PCR procedures indicated that productively infected lymphocytes were initially rapidly reduced for a half-life of 1 day and the amount of HIV-1 RNA on FDC decreased at a similar rate (646). After 6 months of combination therapy, both lymphoid mononuclear cell- and FDC-associated virus levels were reduced by several log units. Nevertheless, the established half-life of FDC HIV RNA (1.7 days) indicated that fresh virus is constantly being attached to the FDC (646). HAART has also been shown to decrease substantially the viral RNA in intestinal epithelial cells and to reduce lamina propria CD4$^+$ cell apoptosis (2297).

In the brain, HAART has markedly reduced HIV levels in the CSF (1439) and has been shown to improve neurocognitive function (4459). CSF virus studies have been conducted with subjects receiving HAART by procedures similar to those used to measure plasma virus changes with therapy. They indicated that the reduction in viral RNA in the CSF can be rapid, with a half-life of about 2.6 days, compared to 2.3 days for plasma virus (1177). These times reflect the two phases of virus suppression by therapy (see above). Because the CSF viral load correlated with the CSF cell count, viral production appeared to come primarily from infected lymphocytes (1177) within the CSF. Some of the beneficial effects of therapy may reflect decreased virus replication and immune activation (e.g., cytokine production) in the periphery. Nevertheless, despite success in reducing many clinical disorders with HAART, the CNS, perhaps because of poor blood-brain barrier penetration, continues to show signs and symptoms of HIV infection (2888). Optimal treatment of HIV infection in the CNS appears to be with 3TC and AZT or d4T as well as NVP, since these drugs can penetrate the blood-brain barrier (127; for a review, see reference 1212a).

In terms of viral sanctuaries, several studies indicate that certain antiretroviral drugs such as PIs do not cross the blood-brain and blood-testis barrier very effectively. The concentration of the drugs in seminal fluids can be 10% of that found in blood (4395). However, some studies have shown a reduction in virus shedding during antiviral therapy (1517, 1671) (see Chapter 2). In any case, both resistant and wild-type (not resistant) viruses have been found in these compartments. In contrast, tenofovir is substantially concentrated in seminal fluids, where distinct patterns of drug resistance can be found in comparison to blood (1502). Drug resistance can develop independently in the CNS (935), most likely because of poor penetration of the blood-brain barrier by several drugs (e.g., AZT), except perhaps NVP (127).

In some cases, HAART substantially reduces the viral load in genital fluids (4591), but virus can still be detected in seminal fluid cells in HIV-infected men (4926). In certain studies, HAART effectively reduced virus in plasma and seminal fluids but not in rectal secretions (4983). In others, HIV RNA was reduced in anal/rectal specimens of subjects on therapy, but the number of infected cells was not affected substantially (2391). The relationship of these findings to viral resistance versus viral reservoirs (see below) was not reported. HAART reduces free virus and virus-infected cells in vaginal fluids (1746). However, again, the inability of certain antiviral drugs to penetrate the female genital tract can explain the lack of effectiveness in reducing cell-associated virus and resistant viruses in cervicovaginal fluids (4126). The detection of drug-resistant variants of HIV-1 in genital fluids (2884, 4653) and the association of drug-resistant viruses with sexual transmission (1957) (see above) very much emphasize the potential spread of resistant strains among populations.

H. Therapy for Acute and Primary Infections

The enthusiasm for the great reduction in viral RNA levels by three-drug therapy has led to trials examining the use of these drugs soon after primary infection or early in the symptomatic course. The appropriate time to begin therapy, however, is not yet known, since HAART can affect immune responses to HIV and have toxic side effects (Section V). The toxicity of the drugs versus the emergence of resistant strains should determine how soon an individual is treated. Moreover, beginning antiretroviral therapy before the host immune system has responded to HIV may compromise the ability of the infected individual to control HIV infection after therapy is stopped. The host may have very little defense in warding off an infection that by then has probably spread indolently to many more cells than occurs during acute infection. Such blunting by therapy of an immune response to an acute infection that could establish protective immunity has been reported with rickettsial infections

(4816). Approaches need to be evaluated that may reduce harmful immune activation without compromising the initial immune responses or decrease viral load at the very early stages (before seroconversion) versus later, when the viral set point has been reached. Moreover, physicians need to consider, as noted above, the adverse effects of these drugs, especially PIs, on other medications taken by patients, particularly antibiotics, anticoagulants, and other anti-HIV drugs.

Treatment of acute HIV infection with HAART has suppressed virus replication substantially and appears to protect the HIV-specific CD4$^+$ T helper cell and CD8$^+$ cell responses (77, 3348, 3368, 3801), particularly if used before seroconversion (85). Initiation of HAART within 2 weeks of antibody seroconversion (i.e., acute infection) showed a benefit for up to 24 weeks in viral load and CD4$^+$ cell count after termination of HAART; HAART begun at a later time period (2 weeks to 6 months after infection) gave some benefit, but it was no longer observed after 48 weeks (1785a). The HIV-specific CD8$^+$ T-cell responses were particularly increased if the subjects had brief episodes of viremia (3348). The frequencies of HIV-specific CD8$^+$ T cells observed in subjects treated during acute infection were similar in the blood and in lymphoid tissues. These findings suggested that studies on peripheral blood are appropriate for insight into immune responses in lymphoid organs (3371).

In early infection, HAART has been associated with a return in the number of CD4$^+$ T lymphocytes and a reduced T-cell activation (85, 1774, 3801, 4178), but in some cases, this effect was short-lived (2122). Nevertheless, a short course (~ 3 months) of antiretroviral therapy showed preservation of HIV-specific CD4$^+$ T helper cell responses after a year off therapy (1284). Notably, the decrease in viremia during primary infection is associated with reduced T-cell activation and maturation abnormalities (1774). Treated individuals have also shown a sixfold increase in anti-HIV-1 p24 responses within 3 months (85). HIV-1-specific cytotoxic T lymphocytes (CTLs) remained detectable in most treated patients in this study, but the breadth and magnitude of CTL responses were less than observed in chronic infection (85). Thus, HAART administered for 3 to 4 months after acute infection gave improved CD4$^+$ T-cell memory responses that could help maintain the initial CTL activities and a less diverse HIV population (85).

In primary infection, after 6 to 12 months of HAART, greater candida and tetanus lymphoproliferative responses were noted in treated subjects (2776) than in untreated subjects. Moreover, HAART during primary infection has shown a decreased frequency of minor opportunistic infections, mucocutaneous disorders, and respiratory infections and appeared to reduce the progression to AIDS in 78 weeks of follow-up (342). If HAART is used later, this immune response is lost (77, 3368) and there are less HIV-specific CD4$^+$ T-cell responses. The finding suggests that the drug treatment early in infection can preserve this anti-HIV immunity. In this regard, in animal studies immediate AZT treatment protected newborn monkeys acutely infected with SIV against a rapid clinical course (4562).

Nevertheless, more recent reports suggest that the HAART-mediated control in primary infection can be transient (2122). This finding again raises the question of whether treatment in primary infection is helpful (4178). Antiviral drugs, including AZT, have been shown to decrease PBMC proliferative responses to mitogen (1779) and might blunt the immune response to HIV if used after acute infection (3792, 4433) (Section VI). In this case, a restricted CTL response is maintained without a broadening observed in chronic HIV infection (85). HAART begun during acute or primary infection has reduced the cell-mediated immune responses (963, 2818, 4309) as well as anti-HIV antibody production (2818). In some cases, seroreversion had been observed (1726, 2116). However, over a short period, HAART did not affect the levels of neutralizing antibodies present (3729).

In summary, with the newer drug regimens some clinicians are calling for further evaluation of early treatment of HIV infection (1876; for a review, see reference 2203a). As shown in the SIV model and noted above, early antiviral treatment could block the immune responses needed to establish an anti-HIV state and prevent superinfection (2602, 4816) (see Chapter 4). Maturation of the immune system may be required for the long-term control of HIV; the breadth of the antiviral immune responses may be compromised by early administration of HAART. Thus, the use of intermittent therapy (to permit some virus replication) or therapeutic immunization may be important to induce an HIV-specific immune response in treated individuals (see Section IX). Immune-based therapies can also enhance the effect of HAART in early infection (see Section VIII).

I. Antiretroviral Postexposure and Pre-Exposure Therapy

In connection with exposure to HIV through needlestick injuries, AZT use has reduced the infection rate eightfold (656). The therapy should be initiated preferably within 1 to 2 h after suspected exposure, but the time when it will no longer be useful has not been defined. A 4-week course of therapy should be administered, since this period has been shown to be most effective (658). Additional drugs should be given to increase antiviral activity in the case of suspected resistance (for a review, see reference 1495). Attention has been given as well to post-sexual exposure anti-HIV therapy, and trials on its efficacy are in progress (3785). Most recently, the use of drugs such as tenofovir as preexposure prophylaxis has been advocated, particularly in populations at high risk for infection (1602). This idea requires further evaluation.

J. Immune Restoration Diseases

In some patients receiving HAART, the reconstitution of the immune system has led to clinical syndromes now referred to as immune restoration disease (IRD) (for a review, see reference 1367). This clinical condition includes increased delayed-type hypersensitivity to mycobacteria, an exacerbation of retinitis from CMV, *Cryptococcus neoformans* infection, and various inflammatory skin conditions (468, 1020, 1058, 1644, 2670). Apparently, HAART given soon after the diagnosis of an opportunistic infection carries the highest risk for this syndrome (2670, 4085). Restoration of cellular immune responses to microbial antigens (e.g., *M. tuberculosis*) appears to be involved (464). Treatment of the opportunistic infection should be given first and then HAART, since a return of immune responses with antiretroviral therapy could lead to detrimental antimicrobial responses. Some studies suggest that circulating IL-6 levels prior to HAART may be associated with the development of IRD (4299). Human papillomavirus-associated oral warts are also increased with HAART (1623, 2202), perhaps reflecting immune reconstitution. Most recently, HAART been reported to be associated with an increase in leprosy in people coinfected with the causative mycobacterium. The onset of this disease may reflect a type of immune restoration syndrome in which recovering lymphocytes transmit the organism to various parts of the body, where it induces clinical symptoms.

K. Antiretroviral Therapy: Considerations and Conclusions

1. OVERVIEW

The introduction of HAART has dramatically changed the clinical course and prognosis for HIV-infected individuals. With proper monitoring for drug resistance, the outcome can be very positive, at least for several years. HIV replication in the presence of HAART is much less frequently detected in treatment-naïve subjects than in drug-experienced ones, subjects who change treatment, or those with higher viral loads starting HAART (3040). Moreover, subjects with a more activated immune system show reduced effects of HAART (247). In any case, a low-level HIV viremia (<10,000 copies/ml) does not appear to lead to faster disease progression (3179).

Importantly, as noted above, despite these advances in decreasing the levels of free virus in the blood and lymph nodes, several HIV-infected cells can still remain in lymphoid tissue sites (646, 3406, 3470) (see Section IV). After discontinuation of therapy, high-level HIV replication can return as rapidly as is observed in acute infection (3061) (Section XI). Thus, the reservoir of infected cells that are not directly susceptible to antiviral therapy is a challenge to present treatment approaches.

Currently, several NRTIs and nucleotide and nonnucleotide RT inhibitors as well as PIs are available for anti-HIV therapy (Table 14.2). Of these, tenofovir appears to be the most widely used to date (1027). T20 and entry inhibitors as well as other anti-HIV drugs are also being prescribed or developed. Some studies show a greater susceptibility of group O viruses to antiviral therapies than clade B isolates (1056). Drug combinations are being evaluated in trials similar to those performed with anticancer therapies.

2. RECOMMENDATIONS

For recommended guidelines on treatment, see reference 10, 309, 4873 and http://www.cdc.gov/hiv/topics/treatment/index.htm#treatment (Table 14.3). These reports advise the monitoring of the viral load in plasma and the CD4+ cell count, the use of therapy to prevent the onset of immune deficiency, attempts to sustain undetectable virus levels in the blood, and the selection of new antiviral drugs when viremia returns in the subject (10, 4873). Three-drug therapy is advised for all infected individuals with CD4+ cell counts of <350 cells/μl or with viral loads of >50,000 copies of RNA/ml. HAART is strongly recommended for adults with <200 CD4+ cells/μl (4873). In general, for a newly infected individual in whom genotyping or phenotyping for drug resistance cannot be undertaken, a three-drug combination treatment using NRTIs and nucleotide RT inhibitors is first recommended (e.g., AZT or d4T, or tenofovir or abacavir with 3TC or FTC) (1025) with an NNRTI. Use of AZT is not

Table 14.3 CD4+ cell and virus level considerations for initiating antiretroviral therapy, 2003[a]

Viral load
- Therapy is recommended for all patients with HIV RNA levels above 30,000 copies/ml of plasma.
- Therapy should be considered for all HIV-infected patients with HIV RNA at >10,000 copies/ml in plasma.
- For patients at low risk of progression (low HIV RNA level in plasma and high CD4+ cell count), particularly those whose are not committed to complex antiretroviral regimens, therapy might be safely deferred. These patients should be reevaluated every 3–6 months.

CD4+ cell count
- Therapy is recommended for all patients with CD4+ cell counts of <200 cells/μl.
- Therapy is offered to those HIV-infected subjects with CD4+ cell counts between 200 and 350 cells/μl.
- Therapy is deferred for HIV-infected subjects with CD4+ cell counts of >350 cells/μl if the viral load is <55,000 RNA copies/ml. If the viral load is >55,000 RNA copies/ml, treatment is offered.

[a]From reference 4873 and from the UCSF Center for HIV Information HIV InSite website (http://hivinsite.ucsf.edu/). Three-drug therapy is recommended; monotherapy should not be considered.

usually advised because of its toxicity to the bone marrow, but it is a frequently prescribed drug. For an NNRTI, usually efavirenz is favored (6). The cheapest combination therapy is NVP with 3TC and d4T, but because of the neuropathies from d4T, other NRTIs are recommended. Importantly, as noted above, because of the poor penetration of most antiviral drugs into the brain tissue (127; for a review, see reference 1212a), viral resistance can begin there, and thus neurologic diseases caused by HIV may not be well controlled.

Monotherapy should no longer be considered (Table 14.3). Clinicians are also advised not to add only a single drug to a treatment regimen that is not working, since resistance to the other drugs administered will permit low-level replication of viruses that can eventually become resistant. In resource-limited countries, total lymphocyte count or CDC or WHO clinical classifications can be alternative measures for determining when to begin therapy (162, 1846).

Some evidence has suggested that subjects initiating NNRTI-based regimens rather than PI-based regimens have a more durable treatment and lower rates of virologic failure (2230, 4744). The results may reflect toxicities of the PI drugs. In this regard, reduction in plasma HIV levels to less than 0.72 log unit after 1 week predicts a poor long-term response in most patients (3561). Some explanation for the virologic response to NNRTI-containing salvage regimens may be the hypersusceptibility of some HIV isolates to these drugs (4744). Stress may also affect responses to antiviral therapy. Higher levels of the neurotransmitter norepinephrine enhance replication of HIV-1 in vitro by up-regulating the chemokine receptors (845). Thus, individuals with high levels of autonomic nervous system activity may have increased HIV replication (845) (see Chapter 13).

3. DRUG RESISTANCE ISSUES

Some infected individuals and some clinicians are reluctant to begin early therapy for HIV infection because they fear that resistance will emerge and no further antiviral drugs will be available (see Section III). However, for those needing therapy, new RT inhibitors, PIs, and entry inhibitors are being evaluated, as well as treatments eventually aimed at the other viral enzyme, integrase. In addition, other approaches for limiting viral replication (e.g., the use of Gag antagonists) could provide alternative directions for controlling the virus. Most importantly, the development of medicines that can be taken once a day has made levels of nonadherence, which can lead to virus resistance, much less of a problem (1414) (see Section III.A). Nevertheless, drug resistance can still occur despite high levels of adherence (237). Importantly, patients previously treated for HIV infection and having a partially suppressive drug regimen have an increased risk of resistance mutations, reducing the probability of future drug options (1757a).

The possibility of drug resistance remains a constant challenge. Already some reports are indicating up to a 50% failure in the control of HIV replication in individuals on PI and combination therapy (1025, 2625). Just as we have learned with antibiotic resistance in bacteria (2553), indiscriminate or inappropriate use of antiretroviral drugs can create resistant viruses that will be difficult to control.

4. CONCLUSIONS

The benefits of HAART to people with HIV infection, particularly AIDS, are very encouraging. In 1996, the number of AIDS cases diagnosed in the United States had already decreased after a steady increase over 16 years, and a decrease in deaths from AIDS was noted (1871, 1872). In this regard, with the lack of adequate antiretroviral therapy in most parts of the world, a difference in survival from AIDS around the globe is becoming evident. Eighty percent of people infected with HIV that need therapy do not receive it (UNAIDS 2006 Report [http://www.unaids.org/en/HIVdata]). Whereas initially the times from infection to disease appeared similar in individuals infected in the Western countries and in Africa (see Chapter 13), this pattern will change with the lack of treatment in developing countries. This problem needs to be resolved. In 2000, a global effort was initiated to bring HAART to 3 million people in resource-limited settings by 2005 (the 3×5 Initiative). That goal was not reached, but at the G8 conference that year, the recommendation was made for full global access to drugs by 2010. Fortunately, the development of generic drugs is bringing appropriate benefit to many people in South America (Brazil), India, China, and parts of Africa (Uganda).

One danger is the assumption that therapeutic approaches that mirror the virologic parameter of low viral load in asymptomatic individuals and a normal $CD4^+$ cell count are sufficient to ensure long-term survival. This concept lacks the understanding of the mechanism (i.e., the immune response) by which the untreated healthy individual controls virus replication. Unless the immune system is permitted to return to a normal state, the treated individual retains reservoirs of virus-infected cells that can destroy the immune system further in an indolent fashion and eventually induce a compromised immune state. Even with very good control of viremia and normal $CD4^+$ T-cell levels, symptoms of ongoing infection, particularly inflammation within different tissues, can give rise to clinical conditions involving the brain, lungs, and joints (see Chapter 8). For this reason, in addition to HAART, which can compromise immune cell function (Section VI), approaches to restore the anti-HIV immune response via immune-based therapies must be considered. Particular attention should be given to the control of the reservoir of virus-infected cells (2522) (Sections IV and VII).

III. Drug Resistance

A. Overview

One very important problem with antiviral treatments is the emergence of resistant viruses (1587, 2413; for a review, see reference 4580; for an update on drug resistance mutations, see http://www.iasusa.org/resistance_mutations/index.html). The causes for this selection of resistant viruses appear to be increased transmission, evolution of HIV to avoid the effect of the drugs, and the lack of adherence of subjects taking HAART. In this regard, the availability of three drugs that can be taken orally once daily (1414) should be helpful as well as the development of a one-pill formulation (Atripla) containing tenofovir, FTC, and efavirenz (see http://www.fda.gov/oashi/aids/virals.html).

A recent study has shown that HIV resistance to antiviral drugs increases with duration of therapy and can be found over the past 6 years to be at least 20 to 25% (4523a). Generally, this resistance, if detected in therapy-naïve people, is called primary; in treated individuals it is considered acquired

(4580). This occurrence of drug resistance does not appear to be related to particular HIV-1 subtypes (3513). Importantly, patients previously treated for HIV infection and having a partially suppressive drug regimen have an increased risk of resistance mutations, reducing the probability of future drug options (1757a). In the initial studies of resistance, the most common genetic alteration linked to AZT resistance was a 2-bp modification leading to a change from threonine to tyrosine or phenylalanine at position 215 (2320). At least five genetic alterations associated with AZT resistance were later identified (2151, 2413). Resistances to the other NRTIs (ddC, ddI, and 3TC) and to PIs have also been encountered (see http://www.iasusa .org/resistance_mutations/index.html).

Viral resistance to PIs has been recognized frequently in both in vitro and in vivo studies (863, 1031, 3799). These PI-resistant viruses can be found in untreated individuals (2450) and result from spontaneous mutation or transmission of a resistant virus (see below). The flexibility of structure and function in the protease enzyme may make resistance more easily attainable than with the other viral enzymes. Sustained concentrations of the PIs need to be maintained to avoid the emergence of this resistance (1031), which occurs less frequently when the drugs are used in combination with other antiretroviral therapies. With some of the mutations, cross-resistance to five structurally different protease inhibitors has been found (863). Therapy with two of the PIs (nelfinavir [Viracept] and amprenavir) often results in mutations that do not result in resistance to other antiprotease drugs (3437). Thus, when resistance to nelfinavir or amprenavir occurs, the other PIs may still be effective. However, if therapy with these drugs is continued, mutations occur which result in resistance to the other PIs (see http://www.iasusa.org/resistance_mutations/ index.html). If resistance to other PIs develops first, there is usually also resistance to nelfinavir and amprenavir.

In the laboratory, virus strains with resistance to four different anti-RT drugs have been identified (1974, 2412). Importantly, in one infected patient treated sequentially with five NRTIs and one NNRTI, drug-resistant mutations selected for a strain resistant to all of the dideoxynucleoside analogues tested and many NNRTIs (3978). Thus, this therapy did not prevent the appearance of multidrug-resistant viruses that maintain a stable replication rate. Recently, a multidrug-resistant R5/X4 virus was found to have been transmitted to an infected patient who progressed rapidly to AIDS (2817) (see below).

Viruses resistant to entry inhibitors (e.g., CCR5) have also been reported (4479; for a review, see reference 31). The resistance to CCR5 receptor inhibitors does not appear to modify a virus to use CXCR4, but the exposure selects for a virus with a higher affinity for the receptor (4479). Similar observations were made with CD4 decoys that were not effective in antiviral therapy (see above). However, the important determination is whether, when a mixture of viruses is involved, a CCR5 entry inhibitor would select for an X4 virus. Viruses resistant to T20 are also recognized (3023) but have been associated with reduced replicative ability and more sensitivity to neutralizing antibodies (3687). These findings are a major reason monotherapy with drugs like T20 is not appropriate. Importantly, drug resistance appears to be less prevalent in areas in which adherence to therapy is emphasized (996).

B. Resistant Virus-Infected Cells

In one early study in which wild-type and resistant strains were found in the plasma before therapy, only the resistant virus strain was noted in the plasma after therapy, whereas the PBMC DNA maintained both types of virus (1880). This finding emphasizes the fact that antiretroviral drugs affect only de novo infection and that the majority of circulating virions represent the product of such infection. Cells containing virus before treatment begins can be long-lived and unaffected by the therapy (Sections II.G and IV). In this regard, with HAART, effective elimination of many HIV-infected cells from lymphoid tissues can be achieved (see below) (646, 3470). However, virus-infected cells in several tissues can remain as reservoirs for the virus (see Section IV and Chapter 5). Sometimes cells such as macrophages are refractory to the antiretroviral effects of AZT because of a decreased formation of AZT triphosphate, decreased phosphorylation of thymidine triphosphate, and/or decreased levels of thymidine kinase activity (2951, 3728). These processes can reflect the reduced cell activation noted above.

C. Therapy Options with Drug Resistance

The choice of therapy in drug resistance now depends on examining the various resistance mutations in the RT and protease genes. Such genotyping along with phenotyping can be helpful in finding alternatives to antiretroviral drugs for experienced and newly treated subjects. It can be important in acute infection, in which drug-resistant viruses have been detected (1785, 2625, 2983). Recommended treatments of antiretroviral drug-resistant HIV-1 infections have been published. In general, changes in therapy can be instituted, at least for a while (for a review, see reference 1025). With time, however, even with alternating therapies, resistance to multiple RT inhibitors can occur (1587, 1974) (see above and http://www.iasusa.org/resistance_mutations/index.html). A common therapeutic strategy for initial failure of HAART includes the use of three NRTIs or two NRTIs and an NNRTI. Later, PI are considered (1025) for what has been termed "salvage" therapy in the face of virus resistance.

Subjects with low-level viremia in the presence of HAART appear to still benefit from the treatment. The resistant viruses often have a reduced replicative capability, and certain anti-HIV immune responses are maintained (1028). Mutations in RT can give multiple NRTI drug resistances and a reduced HIV replicative ability (2289). The drug-resistant virus is also not necessarily more virulent (1958). Nevertheless, some drug-resistant viruses have enhanced replicative ability, which is associated with reduced CD4+ T-cell counts (4202). Moreover, a drug-resistant virus variant that grows less well in culture may undergo further mutations (e.g., in the protease gene) in vivo and have increased replicative ability (3261). In this regard, the M184V mutation in the HIV-1 RT associated with 3TC therapy limits the frequency of mutations restoring a virus' replicative ability (4701). Thus, there is a reduced number of HIV-1 variants transmitted with an M184V thymidine analogue mutation (TAM) (4508). Moreover, less immune activation is associated with these drug-resistant viruses, and thus slower CD4+ cell declines are noted (1936).

In some subjects, drug-resistant viruses can be found circulating, but CD4+ cell counts remain relatively high (297). This observation also most likely reflects the reduced replicative ability of resistant viruses (particularly for PIs) (2842, 3708) as well as the observation that protease-resistant strains do not infect the thymus (4297). Nevertheless, further treatment of subjects with high viral loads and moderate CD4+ cell counts can often bring about higher CD4+ cell numbers (1025).

In a noteworthy study, a persistent moderate level of viremia (400 to 20,000 RNA copies/ml) in subjects on HAART was not associated with an increased risk of developing an AIDS-defining illnesses compared to that for treated subjects with viral loads of <400 RNA copies/ml (3653). Thus, the level of virus replication, which could require a change in therapy, needs to be continually evaluated.

D. Effect on Virus Transmission

HAART can also reduce HIV transmission (3582). Nevertheless, drug-resistant viruses are transmitted (see above) (1785, 2625), presumably because antiretroviral therapy does not always reach high enough concentrations and resistant viruses emerge in genital fluids (see Chapter 3). Such viruses are quite frequent (up to 70%) in seminal fluid of treated individuals (1503). The rate of transmission of these resistant viruses by sexual activity, however, appears to be lower than the rate of transmission of wild-type viruses in the HIV-infected population. Their transmission has been estimated to be at about 20% of the frequency expected (2482). These observations may be due to reduced replicative ability of these viruses (see above) or to a reduction in their transmissibility.

As previously noted, some transmissions may give rise to infection by viruses resistant to most of the present antiviral drugs (2817). This observation certainly raises important issues for current prevention trials. Fortunately, infection with drug-resistant viruses does not appear to show a difference in the rate of CD4+ cell decline after seroconversion (360). Moreover, plasma and breast milk from many women given a single dose of nevirapine (NVP) to prevent maternal transmission to newborns also contained NVP-resistant virus (1316, 2459), indicating the concern for the widespread use of this drug.

IV. Cellular Reservoirs of HIV during Antiviral Therapy

A. Presence of Latently Infected Cells

Soon after the introduction of HAART, several studies indicated that despite the absence of detectable circulating HIV, reservoirs of infected CD4+ cells could remain in the infected individual for 4 to 60 years (772, 778, 1292, 1293, 4810). It is still controversial whether new virus infections continue to occur when the antiretroviral therapy-treated subjects show no detectable viremia (778, 4140). In some individuals, viral replication is so suppressed that de novo infection does not appear to take place. That response is represented in individuals in whom the viral envelope sequence does not change, suggesting that the predominant plasma viruses come from cellular reservoirs that are not the circulating CD4+ T cells (221).

Nevertheless, in other studies, changes in the genetic sequence of the suppressed virus over time (1664, 1978) and the reported unintegrated DNA in cells from HAART patients (4068) indicate that some rounds of new infection do take place. The virus present in these different CD4− cells and monocytes can be genetically diverse and vary in replicative ability and drug resistance (1041) (see above). In some cases, the infected cells can continue to produce HIV at high or low levels; in others, a latent infection takes place in which virus production occurs only after its activation (for a discussion of latency, see Chapter 5).

In patients treated for at least 2 years with HAART, HIV RNA and DNA remained detectable in the lymph nodes, but not in genital secretions or CSF (1664). The establishment of long-lived populations of infected CD4− cells (some of which are latently infected) can occur during acute HIV infection (774). Treatment during primary infection therefore may reduce these cellular reservoirs, but not prevent their occurrence (4306; for a review, see reference 403).

These findings should not be so surprising since the nature of retrovirus infection permits an established state without death of the infected cell. Indeed, these cellular reservoirs often show evidence of archival viruses that have previously circulated in the blood of infected individuals (2388, 3056). This finding is particularly true for the presence of drug resistance and wild-type viruses since the drug-resistant viruses often have less efficient replicating ability (see above). The interruption of therapy can give rise to a dominance of the wild-type drug-sensitive viruses. Thus, in some approaches, viruses resistant to the vast majority of antiretroviral drugs may be replaced following cessation of therapy by sensitive viruses (coming from the cellular reservoirs), at least until therapy is

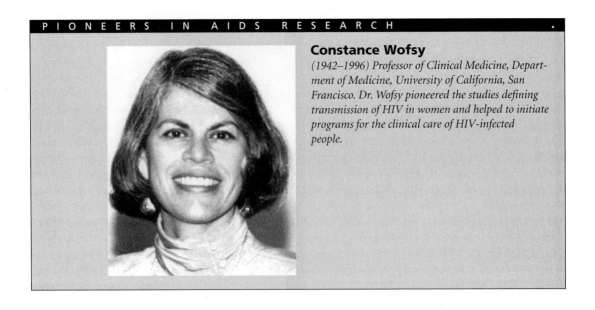

PIONEERS IN AIDS RESEARCH

Constance Wofsy
(1942–1996) Professor of Clinical Medicine, Department of Medicine, University of California, San Francisco. Dr. Wofsy pioneered the studies defining transmission of HIV in women and helped to initiate programs for the clinical care of HIV-infected people.

restored. However, interruption of HAART for subjects with multidrug-resistant HIV in attempts to bring back a sensitive virus have not shown beneficial effects (2437). Reinitiation of therapy usually selects again for resistant virus, which can remain in latent reservoirs (1039) (Section III).

B. Attempts to Eliminate Latently Infected Cells

Several groups have tried to eliminate the HIV latent reservoirs through administration of cytokines or immune-activating agents (775, 2481; for reviews, see references 2342 and 3566). The idea is that inducing virus replication could kill the infected cell or make it susceptible to elimination by the immune system. However, even in subjects treated for 7 years with no detectable viruses, the reservoirs showed a decay in the CD4$^+$ T-cell half-life of 44 months, so eradication seems unlikely (4140). Other studies estimate the half-life of the latent cells to be 20 to 70 weeks (4306), and reestablishment of other latent virus-infected cells occurs. Importantly, several of these cellular reservoirs are not latently infected but can produce HIV without causing cell death (e.g., macrophages and central memory CD4$^+$ cells). Their elimination requires the same approach as latent reservoirs that have been activated to release virus: anticellular therapies.

Most of the approaches to eradicate the virus also emphasize cells of the immune system and do not consider the long-lived viral reservoirs in other organs such as the bowel, brain, and kidney (for a review, see reference 2342) as well as genital tissues and fluids (2517, 3290). All these data strongly suggest that elimination of the virus from an infected individual would not be feasible since leaving even one infected cell can reinitiate the infection when therapy is stopped. In a way, this challenge resembles that of anticancer therapies (see Conclusions, page 429).

In recognizing the fact that the present antiretroviral therapies do not directly attack the virus reservoirs, subjects with viral loads below the level of detection can still show mutations in the polymerase, Nef, and envelope genes of the virus quasispecies (131, 2836). These findings reflect continual HIV replication in the host, even in the face of no detectable plasma viremia. This evidence that current HAART would not be capable of eradicating HIV includes the observation that the virus can persist on FDC in lymphoid tissues for many years despite therapy (1850) (Section XII).

V. Drug Toxicities

A. Overview

While current antiviral drugs have had substantial beneficial effects on HIV infection and development of disease, the side effects can be very harmful to the infected individual (Table 14.4). These include abnormalities in body fat distribution and in lipid and glucose metabolism, cardiac disease, and pancreatic, kidney and liver disorders (for reviews, see references 195, 2585, 3271, and 3869; see also http://www.iasusa.org/resistance_mutations/index.html). (For a review on metabolic complications and HIV therapy in children, see reference 2896.)

B. Lipid Disorders

In the case of lipid abnormalities, a distinction needs to be made between lipoatrophy (i.e., loss of fat in the subcutaneous areas, especially the extremities) and lipohypertrophy (sometimes called lipodystrophy) (i.e., accumulation of lipid deposits in the abdomen and posterior, reflecting increased visceral and upper trunk fat) (195, 2585, 4428). Lipoatrophy affects the lower extremities more than the upper body (195) and involves subcutaneous fat loss. It is not related to the HIV wasting syndrome, which involves a generalized loss of body fat and lean body mass (2585).

There is no linkage between lipoatrophy and lipohypertrophy. In general, those with lipohypertrophy are less likely to have lipoatrophy (195). It is important to note that HIV-infected individuals have more fat loss than uninfected individuals in all peripheral and most central regions of the body (195). With gain of weight, HIV-infected men and women put more fat in the upper trunk and visceral depots than uninfected controls. In comparison to central lipohypertrophy, lipoatrophy has been found more frequently in HIV-infected individuals. Moreover, HIV-infected men with and without lipoatrophy have less subcutaneous adipose tissue than uninfected controls.

Table 14.4 Common side effects of antiretroviral therapy[a]

Side effect(s)	Drug(s)
Allergic rash	Abacavir, nevirapine, efavirenz
Anemia, bone marrow disorder	Zidovudine
Atherosclerosis (accelerated)	Ritonavir, other protease inhibitors
Central nervous system disorders (dizziness, headache, psychiatric effects)	Efavirenz
GI disorders (nausea, vomiting, diarrhea)	All protease inhibitors, zidovudine
Hepatotoxicity, hepatitis	Nevirapine, efavirenz, tipranavir, other protease inhibitors, all NRTIs (uncommon)
Hyperbilirubinemia	Atazanavir, indinavir
Insulin resistance and glucose disorders	Ritonavir, perhaps all protease inhibitors
Injection site reactions	Enfuvirtide
Lactic acidosis and mitochondrial toxicity	All NRTIs (particularly d4T and ddI)
Lipid abnormalities	Protease inhibitors, d4T, efavirenz
Lipoatrophy (fat wasting)	NRTI (particularly d4T and zidovudine), may be enhanced by protease inhibitors
Pancreatitis	ddI, d4T
Peripheral neuropathy	d4T, ddI
Renal disorders	Tenofovir (renal insufficiency), indinavir (nephrolithiasis)
Steven Johnson's syndrome	Nevirapine (women more than men)
Teratogenicity (birth defects)	Efavirenz

[a]The generic names of the most common drugs associated with the disorder are given. For more details, see http://www.aidsmeds.com/lessons/DrugChart.htm and reference 3956. An extensive listing of antiretroviral drug toxicities is maintained by the Department of Health and Human Services (DHHS) (available at http://www.hivatis.org). GI, gastrointestinal; NRTIs, nucleoside reverse transcriptase inhibitors; d4T, stavudine; ddI, didanosine.

The levels of risk of lipoatrophy are similar for men and women, but lipohypertrophy occurs more commonly in women (2585).

Essentially, antiretroviral drugs that are associated with lipoatrophy do not appear to be associated with central lipohypertrophy (195). Lipoatrophy, without necessarily lipohypertrophy, is linked to use of specific antiretroviral drugs using thymidine analogues, especially d4T and, to a lesser extent, AZT and PIs such as indinavir (195). NVP use has been found to be associated with depletion of visceral adipose tissue (195, 819). Lipoatrophy is associated with aging, duration of therapy, and Caucasian background. Mechanisms of lipoatrophy may relate to impairment of adipocyte differentiation, mitochondrial toxicity, and adipocyte apoptosis, perhaps mediated by cytokines such as TNF-α (2585).

Lipohypertrophy is fat accumulation in the abdomen, breast, or dorsal cervical region (e.g., "buffalo hump") and occurs with duration of therapy, older age, disease severity, and use of PIs (2585).

Many of these metabolic problems have been linked to poor function of mitochondria (400; for reviews, see references 901 and 2585), but the evidence is not conclusive. Reductions in mitochondrial DNA occur with HIV infection alone but appear to be most severe with NRTI treatment (907, 2585, 3025, 3270, 4106). In this regard, certain HIV proteins such as Tat, Vpr, and protease can cause mitochondrial damage and induce apoptosis (see Chapter 6) (901). Mitochondrial DNA toxicity has been associated with lactic acidosis, hepatic steatosis, myopathy, cardiomyopathy, peripheral neuropathy, and pancreatitis (907).

The receipt of PIs has become associated with the most serious metabolic side effects of HAART (for reviews, see references 294, 2460). They include increased levels of triglycerides, very low density lipoproteins (VLDL) and cholesterol, as well as deterioration in glucose tolerance. Studies in HIV-seronegative volunteers have shown that some PIs (e.g., indinavir) induce substantial insulin resistance and abnormalities in glucose metabolism (2460), without affecting triglyceride or free fatty acid levels (3273). Other PIs, such as lopinavir and ritonavir, increase triglyceride and free fatty acid levels, with less effect on glucose metabolism (2461). Atazanavir has little effect on either glucose or lipid metabolism (3274). Some investigators have also reported increased levels of adiponectin and TNF-α with PI therapy (4610). Moreover, certain PIs have been noted to have a toxic effect by decreasing adipocyte differentiation (4592). The hyperlipidemia in PI regimens may also reflect the lack of degradation of apolipoprotein B by the proteosome (2583).

Some studies have suggested that gp120 can inhibit growth hormone release (3163) and thus cause depletion of lean body mass. The production of TNF-α associated with immune activation has also been linked to insulin-resistant lipoatrophy (2455, 3190). In addition, a higher level of cortisol in NNRTI-treated subjects may be involved in some of the metabolic disorders (850). These results require further evaluation. Importantly, as noted above, untreated HIV-infected subjects, especially with very low CD4+ cell counts (<100 cells/μl), have abnormal fat loss, particularly in the extremities (195, 2586). Thus, it appears that HAART increases the possibility of lipid disorders associated with HIV infection.

C. Cardiac Disorders

There is debate over the extent to which combination antiretroviral therapy and PI use, in particular, increases the risk of myocardial infarction and other cardiovascular disease (477, 1375, 2853). Given the proatherosclerotic profile of these drugs (increase in VLDL cholesterol and insulin resistance), it is likely that combination therapy with PIs lead to higher rates of cardiovascular disease than combination therapy with NNRTIs (which raise high-density lipoprotein cholesterol, the protective particle). However, drugs in both classes (except atazanavir) usually increase LDL cholesterol. Hence, it is still unknown what treatment per se will enhance the risk of cardiovascular disease.

D. Bone Disorders

Increased prevalence of osteopenia, and to a lesser extent osteoporosis, has been reported in HIV in-

fection, and recent studies suggest an increased risk of fractures (150a). Furthermore, there is no consensus in the field on which factors are associated with osteopenia and osteoporosis. However, some studies have suggested that bone remodeling can take place with HAART (174). Osteonecrosis occurs much more frequently than expected in patients with HIV disease. Prior exposure to glucocorticoids is a major risk factor (for a review, see reference 70).

E. Toxicity in Children

Folic acid antagonists such as trimethoprim can increase the risk of neural tube, cardiovascular, oral, and urinary tract defects in infants whose mothers were exposed to these drugs (1822a). Efaviranz is not allowed to be given to pregnant women because of the risk of teratogenic effects, particularly neural tube defects (1052a; for a review, see reference 4458a).

F. Treatment for Drug Toxicities

Recommendations have been published for the treatment of metabolic complications of HAART, including body fat distribution abnormalities, high cholesterol and triglycerides, lactic acidemia, and bone diseases (see references 2896 and 3956). For example, some studies indicate that replacing a thymidine nucleotide analogue with tenofovir or abacavir can improve lipoatrophy (3153a). A recent report suggests that vitamin E might help prevent the lipid abnormalities associated with PIs (3171). Moreover, some studies suggest that growth hormone therapy (3956) and supervised aerobic and resistance exercise can decrease the symptoms of these lipid disorders (4177, 4312).

VI. Effects of Antiretroviral Therapy on the Immune System

A. Overview

Early studies reported beneficial effects of antiretroviral therapies on immunologic function (806) (Table 14.5), but as noted above (Section II.H), some trials with AZT-treated individuals, particularly in acute infection, suggested that these therapies reduced cell proliferation and would be toxic to the immune system. AZT and 3TC can

Table 14.5 Effects of antiretroviral therapy on the immune system[a]

- Increased CD4[+] cells and naïve CD4[+] lymphocytes (177)
- Increased thymic output of T lymphocytes (1594)
- Improved clonal efficiency of CD4[+] cells (3259)
- Improved T-cell proliferative responses, and antibody production (806, 808, 950, 2153, 4910)[b]
- Improved CTL activity (950)[b]
- Improved CNAR (2741)[b]
- Improved monocyte function (2014)
- Reduced immune system activation (177, 1774)
- Improved responses to other pathogens (Section VI.B).
- Improved delayed-type hypersensitivity and IL-2 production (806, 808, 950, 2153, 4910)
- No immediate repair in T-cell repertoire (873)
- Reduced number of HIV-specific CTLs (3318)[b]
- Reduced HIV-specific CD4[+] T-cell responses (3527)[b]
- Reduced CNAR (4309, 4763)[b]
- Reduced anti-HIV antibodies (369)[b]
- Reduced proliferation of T cells (1779, 2624)

[a]The reduced functions most likely reflect a persistent decrease in viral load resulting from long-term antiviral therapy. CTL, cytotoxic T lymphocyte; CNAR, CD8[+] cell noncytotoxic anti-HIV response; IL-2, interleukin-2.

[b]Improvement or reduction can reflect the length of time the antiviral therapy is received.

interfere with the proliferation of T cells (1779, 2624). Also, HAART can reduce the number of effector CTLs (3318, 4231), HIV-specific CD4[+] T-cell responses (3527), CD8[+] cell noncytotoxic anti-HIV activity (4309, 4763), and anti-HIV antibody production (369, 2116, 2818). In some cases, as noted above, seroreversion has been documented in adults and children (1726, 2116, 2709; for a review, see reference 1697). These findings most likely reflect long-term reduction in viral load by the therapy. Importantly, a recent study of the effect of HAART on the uninfected newborn children of treated mothers showed reduced total lymphocyte counts and reduced CD8[+] cell number until at least 8 years of age (554). These findings merit further evaluation.

In most situations, however, treatment of chronic infection has brought improvement in antibody production (2014, 4910) and cell-mediated immunity, as reflected by delayed-type hypersen-

sitivity skin reaction, IL-2 production, monocyte function (2014), T-cell proliferative responses, CTL activity (806, 950), and CD8[+] cell noncytotoxic anti-HIV responses (2741). HAART also increases thymic output of T lymphocytes (1593). However, in some cases, a low CD4[+] T-cell increase with HAART is observed and considered a result of failure of thymic function (4397). Moreover, a reduction in immune activation takes place (177, 1774). A decrease in activation markers (HLA-DR and CD38 expression) on CD4[+] and CD8[+] T cells and a return in response to recall antigens (e.g., CMV), but not to HIV antigens (177), have been observed. The overall results suggest that the antiviral drugs, either by decreasing virus levels or by acting directly on the immune system, can provide a beneficial response (Table 14.5) (see below).

With PIs, an increase in the number of CD4[+] cells expressing the CD28 molecule has been noted as well as an enhanced proliferation of these cells to mitogens, recall antigens, and HIV core proteins (2153; for a review, see reference 2152). The initial response of lymphocytes to antiretroviral therapies has been primarily an expansion of the existing pool of memory and naïve CD4[+] T cells and not the generation of new naïve cells. The percentage of naïve cells before therapy is the same as that after therapy (873). Thymic output, however, has been observed and can be an important factor, particularly in severely immunodeficient patients (1280). Thus, most studies suggest that prolonged use of HAART increases the number of naïve CD4[+] lymphocytes (177). The clonal efficiency of CD4[+] cells has also been restored, suggesting normal production of T lymphocytes from progenitor cells (3259). Therefore, notable improvement in immune function has been observed, although persistent undetectable viral loads can be associated with reduced anti-HIV responses.

B. Immune Responses to Other Organisms

HAART is particularly helpful in terms of other infectious diseases if the anti-HIV therapy does not lead to IRD (Section II.J). HAART is reported to restore some hepatitis B virus (HBV)-specific CD4[+] and CD8[+] T-cell responses (2416) and can lead to a substantial decrease in CMV viremia in the absence of any specific anti-CMV therapy (3313). HAART has enhanced antibody responses to influenza virus vaccine (2332). Anti-HIV therapy, in most cases, has reduced *Mycobacterium avium* complex and CMV infections via cellular immune responses (252, 1765). HAART has also decreased the incidence of symptomatic visceral leishmaniases (990).

HAART can reduce mortality from HCV or HBV infection, and this effect seems to be much more beneficial than the associated risks of liver toxicity (3641). Nevertheless, some liver abnormalities associated with NNRTI therapy need to be considered (3623) (see above). In addition, HAART also appears to reduce JC virus replication and survival from AIDS-related progressive multifocal leukoencephalopathy (991). Finally, HAART has been shown to improve the response of subjects with non-Hodgkin's lymphoma to chemotherapy (4530), has helped patients live longer with CNS lymphoma (4163), and has been associated with regressions in cervical intraepithelial neoplasias (1782) (see Chapter 12). Improved immune activity appears to be responsible.

C. Function of the Restored Lymphocyte Population

Despite an increase in CD4$^+$ cell numbers during antiviral therapies, the nature and function of these immune cells remain to be elucidated. Based on telomere lengths, the initial return of CD4$^+$ cells most probably results from redistribution of cells from sequestered sites in the body and not from renewal (4809). The slow rise in the CD4$^+$ cell number could be explained by a block in generation of fresh CD4$^+$ cells from the thymus, through infection of stromal cells, events in the microenvironment, or infection of precursor CD4$^+$ cells (4809) (see Chapter 8). The increased turnover of CD8$^+$ T cells in HIV infection (4809) (see Chapter 13) argues against a block in precursor CD8$^+$ cell formation and supports a peripheral expansion in the number of these cells.

Some studies suggest that the replenished CD4$^+$ and CD8$^+$ cells lack the diversity in their repertoire to be effective in immunologic responses to new agents (873, 3417) (see Chapter 11, Figure 11.3). The amount of naïve lymphocytes pro-

duced is limited, usually depending on the number existing before therapy (873). Studies have also demonstrated a reduced function of the restored CD4$^+$ cells (873). For this reason, other strategies need to be taken (see below). Finally, the decision to use HAART must appreciate the possible onset of immune system-related disorders.

D. Conclusions

In summary, with limited increases in the CD4$^+$ cell count to 100 to 150 cells/µl, full improvement of immune function with HAART cannot be expected, at least in the short term. With immune therapeutic approaches, however, some benefit might be achieved, particularly in terms of cell function (for reviews, see references 2152 and 3404) (Section VII). With the increase in CD4$^+$ cell counts resulting from HAART, the use of prophylaxis for *Pneumocystis jiroveci* (*carinii*) pneumonia is no longer recommended in adults and children if the counts are >200 CD4$^+$ cells/µl (3986, 4529). Similarly, with CD4$^+$ cell increases, chemoprophylaxis can be discontinued for cerebral toxoplasmosis and *Mycobacterium avium* complex, CMV retinitis, and other potential opportunistic infections (1187, 2262, 4209). Azithromycin prophylaxis used for *M. avium* is not needed when HAART-treated subjects have CD4$^+$ cell counts that rise to more than 100 cells/µl (1187). All these results reflect most likely improved immune responses against HIV and the resulting recovery of many antimicrobial immune responses. Antiretroviral therapy can also reduce the risk of developing tuberculosis, but other prophylactic approaches are needed to confine this epidemic (1527).

VII. Immune System-Based Therapies

A. Introduction

Direct attempts at restoring immune function affected by HIV infection are being considered (for reviews, see references 505, 2152, 3404, and 4050) (Table 14.6). A return of the CD4$^+$ cell count may be obtained with antiviral therapy, but specific anti-HIV responses, although increased in some cases, do not appear to improve substantially

Table 14.6 Potential immune-based therapies for HIV infection[a]

- IL-2 administration (970, 1983, 2312)
- IL-12 therapy (808, 1989, 2395)
- IL-15 therapy (635, 2085, 3155)
- Antibodies to IL-4 and IL-10 (817, 2395)
- IL-10 therapy (739)
- Type 1 interferons (917, 1198, 1680)
- Granulocyte-macrophage colony-stimulating factor (124, 1051)
- Anti-TNF-α drugs (pentoxifylline [1067], thalidomide [3901], and antibodies [696])
- Passive antibody administration (1200, 4481, 4976)
- Immune modulators (e.g., cyclosporine, hydroxy-urea, and mycophenolic acid) (2373, 2668, 2808, 3404, 3740)
- Thymopentin (2975)
- Thymus replacement (2305, 2814)
- CD8+ cell administration (1859, 2594)

[a]Most of these approaches include the concomitant use of highly active antiretroviral therapy. IL-2, interleukin-2; TNF-α, tumor necrosis factor alpha.

(3404). Moreover, the use of multidrug therapy for several years could be poorly tolerated and compromised by toxicity, nonadherence, and development of drug-resistant virus strains. In addition, the responses against HIV become diminished (Section VI). Thus, immune system-based (or immune-based) therapies need to receive further attention as an approach for controlling HIV. These therapies include the use of cytokines (e.g., IL-2, GM-CSF, G-CSF, interferon-α IL-10, IL-12, IL-15, IL-16, and IL-7) and compounds helpful in decreasing immune activation. Moreover, these immune strategies have involved therapeutic immunizations and adoptive lymphocyte immunotherapy (for a review, see reference 4050).

B. Interleukin-2

With the appreciation that disease progression and HIV infection may be influenced by particular cytokines, some manipulations of these cellular products have been considered. The ability of IL-2 therapy to enhance CD4+ cell numbers in the peripheral blood and lymph nodes has been well established (1811, 2308, 2310, 2312, 2555, 2839, 2840, 4400, 4532). This increase appears to reflect longer survival of naïve and central memory CD4+ cells as well as NK cells but not effector memory T cells (2310) (see Chapters 4 and 9). Therefore, responses to HIV are not improved (see below). Studies have been conducted evaluating IL-2 given subcutaneously either in large doses (7.5 million units twice daily) for 5 days every 2 months or in low doses (1 million units) daily (4374) (see below). In most cases, naïve T-cell expansion appears to be from existing naïve CD4+ cells rather than fresh thymic output (2675, 3220). The T cells can produce IL-2, IL-4, and IFN-γ (1001). Larger trials of administration of IL-2 in 5-day cycles every 2 months or daily with HAART are under study, based on the early encouraging results noted above.

IL-2 can induce HIV replication (284) and thus needs to be given concomitantly with HAART. Under this condition, 1 year of therapy showed CD4+ cell numbers maintained with no increase in viral RNA levels in the plasma (2312). Recently, subcutaneous IL-2 therapy given in 5-day cycles every 2 months for up to 6 years has given consistent increases in CD4+ cell numbers (1252). In a limited trial, subjects who received IL-2 therapy had fewer clinical events than those receiving HAART alone (2801). One report indicated that IL-2 at low doses (3 million units twice a day subcutaneously every 4 weeks) was better tolerated than higher doses (7.5 million units twice a day for 8 weeks); both gave good CD4+ cell proliferation (4374), but the long-term clinical outcome is not known. Two international studies are currently being undertaken to explore the potential beneficial effect of IL-2 on clinical outcomes (SILCAAT and ESPRIT). Both involve the 5-day subcutaneous IL-2 therapy given every 2 months. The first is for infected subjects with low CD4+ cell counts. The second is in subjects with CD4+ T-cell counts of ≥ 300 cells/μl on HAART. Up to 10 cycles (range, 3 to 29) have been conducted, and substantial increases in CD4+ cell number have been noted (1252).

In most subjects receiving IL-2 therapy with HAART, greater increases in CD4+ cells are seen than in those only receiving HAART (see above). IL-2 has also enhanced the level of NK-T cells in subjects with primary infection (3054). In one study, T-cell responses to recall antigens have improved 8.5-fold in IL-2 recipients, who also had better antibody responses to tetanus vaccination (2555). In another study, however, IL-2 did not enhance responses to tetanus vaccination (4532). Cell culture studies have shown an increase in CD8+ cell antiviral responses (Figure 11.9) (258, 2206), and this result could explain the above clinical observations with this cytokine.

An increase in immunologic control of HIV during IL-2 therapy has been observed in 27 HIV-infected subjects treated for over 3 years. CD4+ cell numbers increased and there was a decrease in proviral DNA in the PBMC (1584). Moreover, IL-2 therapy has also increased the CD8+ cell noncytotoxic anti-HIV response (CNAR) when given after 1 year of HAART in subjects acutely infected with HIV (2840). IL-2 given with HAART at the time of primary infection did not enhance CNAR, perhaps because this response had not yet been fully restored (2839). Other studies with IL-2 have suggested that the cytokine can help reduce substantially the latent reservoirs of HIV-infected cells (771). IL-2 therapy may also increase other cytokines, such as IL-7 and Flt-3 ligand, that can have a beneficial effect on immune responses (312) (see Chapters 8 and 11).

Naïve cells go to the lymph node, where they encounter new antigens and can react. With IL-2 therapy, it is important to know the nature of the CD4+ cells whose numbers are expanded; they appear to be primarily naïve and central memory cells (2310). CD4+ cells that enhance HIV-specific cell-mediated immunity (type 1 response) would be a preferred result. Therefore, approaches have been made to initiate HIV-specific CD4+ T-cell responses via the use of IL-2 therapy with therapeutic immunization and intermittent antiretroviral therapy (4838) (see below).

Besides inducing HIV replication, IL-2 therapy could have a detrimental clinical effect by enhancing the proliferation of CD4+ CD25+ regulatory T cells that reduce the anti-HIV immune response (4051). Nevertheless, the CD4+ CD25+ cells increased are low in FoxP3 and may not have the many characteristics of a T regulatory cell (4049) (see Chapter 11, Section V). They also do not show an increased expression of activation markers or cell proliferation. However, IL-2 administered for 5 days every 2 months over a long period can lead to enhanced apoptosis of both CD4+ and CD8+ T cells. This finding, which requires further evaluation, most likely reflects the induced production of inflammatory cytokines (4048).

Finally, low-dose daily IL-2 therapy has also been associated with improvement in CD4+ cell counts and liver function tests in patients who were coinfected with HIV and HCV and may help in reducing HCV levels in the blood (3966). The relative value of low-dose versus high-dose IL-2 treatment needs to be determined. While symptoms with lose-dose therapy are fewer, the CD4+ T-cell responses are more evident with high-dose therapy.

C. Other Strategies

Other cytokine manipulations in the host have been evaluated in cell culture studies and suggest possible use in therapy (Table 14.6). Cell-mediated immune responses of cultured PBMC, as measured by proliferation to recall and allogeneic antigens and to mitogens, have been restored by the addition of IL-12 to the cells (808, 2395). This cytokine, produced by macrophages and DCs, is known to induce the differentiation of TH0 cells into TH1 cells (see Chapter 11). IL-12 administration could also act to compensate for the inhibitory effects of IL-10 on IL-12 production by macrophages (938, 2395, 4023).

With the known effect of IL-12 on NK cell activity as well (see Chapters 6, 8, and 11), the possible use of this cytokine in therapy for HIV infection is under consideration (1989). Since IL-10 reduces HIV-1 replication in vitro, probably via its anti-TNF-α activity, some clinical trials have also evaluated its potential use for HIV infection (739). Obviously, however, a balance in the beneficial and detrimental effects of these immunologic factors needs to be considered; for example, IL-10 can inhibit CD8+ cell responses (258).

A similar restorative effect on T-cell responses and on PBMC cultures from HIV-infected subjects was observed with antibodies to IL-4 and IL-10 (406, 817) (see Chapter 13). Conceivably, IL-12 or the anti-type 2 cytokine antibodies induced a type 1 response that increased the CD8+ cell antiviral activity. Antibodies to type 2 cytokines can increase type 1 cytokine production (4139) (Table 14.6).

Increased attention is currently being given to the use of IL-15, which can enhance CD8+ cell responses without inducing HIV expression (3439). The potential value of this cytokine for expanding memory CD8+ T cells has been emphasized (2085, 4935). IL-15 also helps in CNAR (635) and NK cell differentiation (for a review, see reference 1264). Moreover, studies have indicated that subjects who do not respond well to HAART may have low levels of circulating IL-15 (941) and not viral resistance. Based on these observations, IL-15, a product of epithelial cells and DCs, is being considered for induction of both innate and adaptive immune responses (3155; for a review, see reference 1264).

Administration of granulocyte-macrophage colony-stimulating factor with HAART has shown a substantial increase in CD4$^+$ cell counts and a decrease in virus breakthroughs (124). It can help in the management of neutropenia and also enhance cellular immune responses against HIV and opportunistic infections (for a review, see reference 1051). Moreover, receipt of GM-CSF in one study appeared to reduce HIV replication following cessation of HAART (1241).

Other immunologic approaches include the use of IFN-α, which has an anti-HIV effect (2989, 2997, 4849), although resistance to IFN-α has been noted (2352) (Table 14.6). Trials with pegylated IFN-α have been conducted (620, 1198, 1680), as has been described with HCV coinfection, and are currently being continued. Toxic effects of IFN-α, such as neutropenia, anemia, and drug intolerance, may limit the effectiveness of this treatment given with HAART (1680). IFN-β therapy may also be helpful in preventing HIV infection, particularly with R5 viruses; the cytokine down-regulates CCR5 expression (917). In this regard, current studies are using synthetic oligodeoxynucleotides containing immunostimulatory CpG motifs (see Chapters 9 and 15). By the induction of IFN-α, immune improvements were seen in HIV-infected subjects who were hyporesponsive to HBV vaccine (880). IFN-γ might also have some antiviral potential, since it decreases the cell surface expression of the HIV-1 receptor galactosyl ceramide on bowel cells (4843) and increases cell-mediated immunity. However, thus far, clinical trials with this cytokine have not been encouraging.

Using immune-modulating drugs such as thymopentin (2975), cyclosporine (3740), hydroxyurea (2373, 2668), and mycophenolic acid (MPA) (2808, 3404) in combination with HAART may help reduce T-cell activation. MPA blocks guanidine incorporation, as does abacavir, so the use of

these drugs together has been considered (Section II.D).

Pentoxifylline (1067), thalidomide (3901), and anti-TNFα antibodies (696) have been shown to reduce HIV replication and thus disease progression. These approaches might also improve symptoms related to high levels of TNF-α (2871), such as wasting syndrome (3712) (Section V.B) (Chapter 8). Nevertheless, paradoxically, the successful treatment of oral ulcers with thalidomide was associated with increased TNF-α and HIV-1 levels (1985). Moreover, pentoxifylline has increased CMV replication in HIV-infected people (4245). These approaches have not been given much recent attention.

Finally, the administration of antiviral drugs or HIV-specific immune cells along with cytokine therapy (e.g., currently with IL-2) (see above), as is done in some anticancer protocols (3425), should be considered. In the case of HIV infection, cytokine gene-transduced CD8$^+$ cells might also be useful (Section VIII). In summary, a combined approach of antiviral drugs with immune-based therapy would seem to be the most appropriate to regain control of HIV (2555, 3404).

VIII. Immune System Restoration

While immune-based therapies may help with HAART to restore immune cell numbers and some function, the full restoration of the immune system should be an important objective. Thymopoiesis is needed in the regeneration of peripheral T cells and is dependent on both the age and immune status of the host (1466) (see Chapter 13). The thymus directs T-cell repertoire formation during ontogeny. Later, thymus-independent pathways are needed to replenish the turnover of mature T cells (CD45RO$^+$). Aging is characterized by replacement of naïve T cells by memory cells and an accumulation of functional defects within the cells (3020). Expansion of already formed T cells may not always permit a full repertoire of cellular responses. In the absence of the thymus, it is estimated that peripheral T-cell numbers can expand 100,000-fold in vivo (3768) if the right cytokines are available, but new naïve cells are not regenerated. The overall survival of individual cells (and their repertoires) depends on the extent of self-renewal, particularly via the thymus, versus apoptosis associated with immune activation (2071, 3020).

Some results support evidence that an elevated and continually increasing division rate occurs in both T-cell subsets in HIV-infected people (3379) (see Chapters 8 and 13). This mechanism can help explain the rebound of the CD4$^+$ cell number after the use of antiviral drugs, certainly after the first month, when redistribution plays the major role (547).

In terms of T-cell recovery during anti-HIV therapy (Section VI.C), the telomere length in T cells has suggested that the early return of memory or mature cells results primarily from migration of cells from tissue reservoirs (4809). Measuring the loss of telomere length in CD4$^+$ and CD8$^+$ cells from HIV-1-infected people has suggested, in fact, that an enhanced aging process takes place, particularly in CD8$^+$ CD28$^-$ cells (1173). This cellular aging, mirrored by a reduction in telomere length, appears to be limited to CD8$^+$ cells, since CD4$^+$ cells maintain a telomere length expected for healthy populations (4809). Unless these cells have increased telomerase activity, which seems unlikely, the CD4$^+$ cells in infected individuals (even on therapy) appear to be turning over at a normal rate (4397).

This finding on telomere length supports the conclusion that the initial increases in CD4$^+$ cell counts after antiviral therapy result from a redistribution of cells (2548, 2741, 4809) and not from de novo generation of fresh cells. Thus, in HIV infection, the loss in CD4$^+$ cells may reflect not increased destruction of cells but slow ingress of new cells into the circulation. A disorder in CD4$^+$ cell migration from tissue sites could be involved, as could a loss of only short-lived CD4$^+$ cells or a reduction in thymopoiesis (see Chapters 8 and 11). Studies of the Vβ repertoire have also suggested that with treatment there is not a return to heterogeneous CD8$^+$ or CD4$^+$ cell responses with efficient immunologic activity (873).

Whether immune function can be restored in people on antiviral therapy remains to be determined (4050). An important question is how naïve lymphocytes can be generated if a thymus is not present. A functioning thymus can be detected in some adults (2903), and new T cells can come from this tissue as well as other reservoirs in the body (984, 2733, 2900). Thus, T-cell populations can be maintained after thymic atrophy but regeneration depends on some residual thymus-like function (2733). The use of antiretroviral therapy has indicated that those subjects with a large amount of thymic tissue had a greater rise in naïve CD4$^+$ T cells with HAART but also had a greater chance of virologic rebound, perhaps reflecting the larger number of target cells for infection (2903, 4182) (see discussion on thymus, Chapter 13).

In reference to thymus activity, observations with individuals undergoing intensive chemotherapy suggested that thymus-dependent regeneration of CD4$^+$ T lymphocytes can occur in children but that deficiencies are found in young adults lacking a normal functioning thymus. Recovery can be demonstrated by the number of CD45RA$^+$ CD62L$^+$ CD4$^+$ T lymphocytes (naïve cells) and can take a long time (2733). Other studies have shown that T-cell recovery after immune suppression (e.g., for autologous bone marrow transplantation) is due to proliferation of mature T cells and not naïve ones (984). These estimates on the length of time that naïve and memory cells live within a host and cycle between these stages of maturity need to be considered in modeling immune system restoration in HIV-infected individuals.

Most naïve cells in healthy adults appear to come from pools present in lymphoid tissues throughout the body. In HIV-infected individuals, this naïve population becomes greatly reduced secondary to the cytopathicity of HIV and the activation of the immune system against the virus. Thus, if an extrathymic pathway cannot be utilized, approaches at thymus (explant) restoration (2305, 2814) or bone marrow stem cell therapy merit consideration (Table 14.6) (for a review, see reference 1466). In this regard, administration of IL-7, which can induce thymopoiesis, is being considered (313, 3326).

Finally, based on the observation that CD8$^+$ cells can suppress HIV replication or function as CTLs, some groups have evaluated whether CD8$^+$ cells, grown in large quantities in culture, can be administered as therapy to restore immune function (Section X). Studies on ex vivo-cultured autologous CD8$^+$ cells showed no obvious toxicity in patients (1859, 2594). A remission in Kaposi's sarcoma lesions was noted in two patients (2242).

Other approaches to enhance control of HIV infection include adoptive transfer of autologous PBMC, lymph node lymphocytes, and activated CD4+ T cells (2509, 4471, 4612).

The administration of CD8+ cells along with IL-2 and the use of CD8+ cells genetically engineered to produce this cytokine (3425), as well as the eventual administration of the CD8+ cell antiviral factor, can be considered (see Chapter 11). Conceivably, therapies directed at stimulating CD8+ cell anti-HIV responses can be developed (e.g., CD28 engagement) (255). These other cellular approaches to immune system modulation and recovery, in addition to cytokines, anticytokine antibodies, and anticytokine drugs, merit increased attention (Tables 14.1 and 14.6).

IX. Postinfection Immunization

The suggestion that postinfection therapy could involve therapeutic immunization with a viral protein (3893) has been evaluated. This approach toward immune system stimulation should not be considered a vaccination, since this term is properly reserved for prevention strategies (Chapter 15). In early studies, some investigators (3683) immunized HIV-infected individuals with recombinant gp160 produced in the baculovirus system. No obvious toxicity was noted, and T-cell proliferative responses were noted in vaccinees who had stabilized CD4+ cell counts. Higher levels of antibodies to certain HIV envelope peptides were found in the subjects, and neutralizing antibodies measured in a few individuals were increased. In one study, HIV-1 envelope-specific CTL responses were also increased in immunized HIV-seropositive individuals (2347). However, the potential value of therapeutic immunization was questioned after a randomized trial showed no clinical effect (1218). Moreover, immune stimulation under some circumstances might be harmful by increasing the spread of virus in the host (1392, 4262) (see Chapter 13). Obviously, the type of immunization used in approaching this objective can determine the therapeutic outcome.

Following a similar concept, HIV-infected individuals received immunizations with envelope-depleted virus still containing the HIV-1 Gag proteins. One reason for this strategy was to increase levels of p24 antibodies, which are reduced in symptomatic patients (see Chapter 13). After 5 years, no toxicity from the immunizations was noted (2508) and an increase in cell-mediated antiviral immune cell responses, a reduced rate of increase in the viral load, and a reduced rate of CD4+ cell decline were noted (4461). Preliminary studies suggest that only certain infected people respond to this antiviral therapy. In other studies of infected people, immunization with recombinant p17/p24 Ty virus-like particles had no effect on the level of antibodies to the Gag protein (4576). Therapeutic immunization with inactivated envelope-depleted HIV-1 along with HAART increased HIV-specific CD4+ cell responses in subjects (3746).

In primary infection, if antiviral therapy is accompanied by HIV immunization, a beneficial effect on control of virus has been observed after stopping treatment (2204, 2716, 2816) (see below). Moreover, in a pilot study involving HAART plus four vaccinations with a canarypox virus vector (ALVAC-HIV) and a lipopeptide vaccine followed by three cycles of subcutaneous IL-2, HIV-specific CD4+ cell proliferative responses were observed in 19 of 33 subjects, compared to 9 of 36 controls receiving HAART alone. After interruption of antiviral therapy, 24% of the immunized group lowered their viral set point, compared to 5% of the control group (610, 2555b).

A very encouraging enhancement of anti-HIV responses has been reported using a therapeutic DC immunization in untreated people chronically infected with HIV (2677). This inactivated autologous virus-pulsed DC approach induced HIV-specific CD4+ cells and HIV-1 Gag-specific perforin-expressing CD8+ CTLs, as well as marked reductions in plasma viral loads (2677). Similar results with DC loaded with HIV have recently been reported for subjects on HAART (1440).

X. Passive Immunotherapy and Use of Antibody-Based Approaches

Some investigators have considered the possibility that passive immunotherapy with plasma or purified immunoglobulins from HIV-seropositive individuals who are asymptomatic (2107, 3626) would be helpful (Table 14.6). The potential use of human anti-V3 loop monoclonal antibodies received some attention (1200, 4976). Several monoclonal antibodies with different epitopes would be needed, particularly if the noncontiguous viral CD4 binding site is the target (see Chapter 3).

The initial trials with anti-HIV plasma in AIDS patients showed some success, as measured by improvement in clinical status and stabilization of CD4+ cell counts (2107, 4615). The effect could result from HIV neutralization, antibody-dependent cellular cytotoxicity, or nonspecific stimulation of the immune system of the recipient. Other studies did not demonstrate a clinical benefit in AIDS patients (1984). Large doses of monoclonal antibodies directed against HIV antigens appear to be needed to show a substantial increase in neutralizing activity in the host serum. Protection of cats from feline immunodeficiency virus infection by passive antibody administration has been reported (3612), as has protection of chimpanzees (3608). For example, anti-V3 specific antibodies have protected chimpanzees from infection (75 chimpanzee infectious doses) when given 1 day before virus inoculation or within a few minutes after exposure to the virus (1200). However, this protection has not been seen after longer periods of delay before treatment (A.M. Prince, personal communication) (see Chapter 15, Section XIII).

Increased survival of SIV-infected macaques was achieved by passive treatment with antiviral antibodies (1695). Moreover, SIV hyperimmune serum given subcutaneously prior to oral SIV inoculation protected newborn macaques from infection (4560). Recently, an anti-V3 humanized antibody given 24 h before virus challenge protected cynomolgus monkeys from SHIV infection (1169). Notably, delivery of neutralizing antibodies to subjects prior to interruption of HAART has helped to reduce the virus rebound after treatment was stopped (4481).

A major concern is whether the immunoglobulins inoculated into a host will enhance rather than neutralize the HIV strain present in that infected individual. This result was suggested by some SIV studies (1447) (see Chapter 10). Experimentation with the isolated strain before clinical use might be warranted to avoid a potential danger in this therapy. If passive immunization is effective, immunoglobulins can be produced (i.e.,

monoclonal antibodies) to use in individuals after needlestick injuries or in pregnant women around the time of delivery (see Chapter 2). Finally, as noted in Sections II.D.3 and IV, antibodies linked to ricin or other toxins have been suggested for use in killing infected cells (2799, 2895). The viral envelope or cell surface molecules are targeted.

XI. Structured Treatment Interruption

Because HAART can reduce both humoral and cellular immune responses to HIV (see Section VI), approaches have been initiated to maintain or enhance anti-HIV responses during therapy. These include interruption in antiviral treatment (to permit some virus replication) or therapeutic postinfection immunization (Section IX). During HAART, there are periods of intermittent viremia (e.g., blips), which do not appear to affect CD4+ T-cell counts and may maintain the anti-HIV responses (1073). These kinds of observations encourage approaches that systematically interrupt HAART as a kind of "autovaccination" procedure.

The studies, involving weekly structured or strategic treatment interruption (STI) following a week of therapy, did not give favorable results in terms of delaying virus rebound and avoiding resistant viruses (109). Nevertheless, a brief interruption of HAART has shown improvement in cholesterol and triglyceride levels that could be of benefit to the subject (1758). However, drug resistance still can occur despite high levels of adherence during the treatment phase (237, 2841). In this regard, the pharmacogenetics of various drugs are important. For example, NNRTI drugs usually have a long plasma half-life, and thus stopping HAART that includes these therapies may result in monotherapy (i.e., with an NNRTI) that could select for a drug-resistant virus (3718).

In some studies (3349), STI showed an increase in cellular and humoral responses to HIV but very little consistent control of virus. Other investigators have confirmed that despite a long period of time with HAART, one interruption can bring back a viral load set point that is similar to that observed prior to introduction of therapy. The data appear to reflect an intrinsic amount of virus-infected cells within the host as well as a reduced anti-HIV immune response (1759) (Section VI). Favorable results were obtained with subjects whose CD4+ T-cell count had reached >500 cells/μl after remaining on therapy for more than 1 year. They showed a longer period of time off treatment before HAART had to be restored (1959). Subjects showing prolonged reduction in HIV production after STI have strong HIV-1-specific immune responses (3348, 3349). Notably, the type of CD8+ cell responding is important. In one study, an increase in HIV-specific CD8+ cells occurred after STI but with little control of the virus; the CD8+ cells were of the nondifferentiated perforin-low type (942) (see Chapter 11). Moreover, the CD8+ T-cell expansion noted after STI is mostly due to an increase in preexisting virus-specific CD8+ cells rather than new immune responses (86).

In a recent study, therapeutic immunization with lipopeptides and vaccinia virus-based vaccines (see Chapter 15) given with HAART provided an increased time off treatment in which the viral load was lower in association with HIV-specific CD4+ and CD8+ T-cell responses (2555a). A decrease in up to 40% in receipt antiretroviral drugs was noted in 15 months of follow-up. Moreover, a trial of DNA immunization with tenofovir in rhesus macaques showed a decrease in the viral rebound and CD4+ cell decline following STI (1389). Moreover, IL-2 given with HAART followed by STI has shown a continual increase in CD4+ cell counts in some subjects in comparison to those who did not receive IL-2 with HAART (2148). However, in a pilot study evaluating the effect of IL-2 with HAART on viral load and CD4+ cell count after treatment interruption, no benefit of the cytokine therapy was observed (1815a).

With STI, differences have been noted in chronically infected versus acutely infected subjects. In some of the early STI studies in chronically infected subjects (3842) viral load rebounds were observed, but thereafter, the virus could be controlled by resumption of treatment. Very few changes in CD4+ and CD8+ lymphocyte numbers were noted, and no resistance was seen in the viruses detected (3237). In a study of HIV infection chronically suppressed with antiretroviral therapy, intermittent STI showed a longer doubling time for the initial rise in viral load, a lower

medium peak for the viral load, and a greater number of subjects with viral load setpoints of <1000 RNA copies/ml. Immunization with an ALVAC vaccine (vCP1452) did not affect these results (1985a). In some studies of brief interruptions, HIV-specific responses returned to CD4+ and CD8+ T cells (1755). In general, two phases of CD4+ cell response after STI have been observed: an initial rapid decline and then a slow decrease which can bring the cell number to pre-HAART levels or lower (1442, 4796). Some clinical investigators agree, therefore, that STI should be used for infected individuals whose pre-HAART CD4+ cell counts were >250 cells/μl (2760, 4164). Others suggest that high levels of plasma IL-15 can predict a favorable outcome from STI in chronic infection (95). Moreover, some data indicate that a rapid and high antibody response to p24 and gp120 after STI can predict a better control of HIV (4479a).

Several studies now indicate that STI in chronic HIV infection can augment HIV-specific immune responses, but a marked decline in CD4+ T cells occurs with return of viremia (611). No real benefit of STI (with different protocols) has been seen in terms of virus control and CD4+ cell count (150, 1156, 4796). In another study, patients with CD4+ cell counts of >350 cells/μl and viral loads of <50 copies/ml were randomized to continue therapy or receive STI. Over a 22-month period, substantial drug savings were made with the STI group and no increase in viral resistance was observed. However, low CD4+ cell counts and some manifestations of HIV infection were more frequent in the subjects undergoing STI (108a). Importantly, the concept of autoimmunization from a short STI has not shown better control of virus in chronic infection (1242, 3369). Moreover, CTL activity has not predicted viral response in STI (3369). In some cases, interruption of antiretroviral therapy can lead to an acute retroviral syndrome observed during primary infection (857). Thus, this approach in chronic infection has not been recommended (43, 189, 1442).

In the largest randomized trial ever conducted in HIV infection, over 5,000 people were enrolled in a program entitled "Strategies for Management of Anti-HIV Therapy" (SMART) (1186a). Begun in January 2002, the trial followed treatment-experienced HIV-infected volunteers who were randomly assigned to continue to receive HAART under current HIV treatment guidelines (CD4+ cells <350 cells/µl) or a drug conservation strategy that involved starting and stopping antiretroviral therapy depending on the CD4+ cell count. The latter individuals did not take HAART until their CD4+ cell counts dropped below 250 cells/µl, and they were then taken off HAART when their CD4+ cells were above 350 cells/µl. The trial was stopped after 15 months because, contrary to the expectation, the drug conservation strategy group had twice as many subjects who progressed to AIDS or death. They also had more major complications, such as cardiovascular, kidney, and liver diseases, than those maintained on therapy for the entire time period. The study suggested that subjects who started HAART with baseline HIV RNA levels of <400 RNA copies/ml had a threefold-higher risk of progression to disease and death than those who started HAART at >400 RNA copies/ml. It is unknown whether the long periods on HAART also bring more complications to those on continuous therapy. These results with a large clinical trial supported the above observations on the potential detrimental effects of STI in chronic HAART patients (108a).

Treatment interruption may, however, be beneficial for primary infection in which, following STI, viremia has been found to be controlled for several months (176). In that way, total drug exposure toxicity is reduced even if reinitiation of HAART is eventually needed (1526; for a review, see reference 1864). In other STI studies of primary HIV-1 infection, a long-term full control of virus was not observed but some reduction in viremia was noted (1864).

Short-term treatment interruption has also been found to be beneficial for drug-experienced subjects with multidrug-resistant viruses (1699, 2118). This effect, however, appears to be limited, as resistant viruses, present in cell reservoirs in the body, reemerge (309a, 2436a) (Section I). In most cases, the rebounding virus analyzed genetically appears to come from several compartments in the body (1155), and prevention of resistant viruses is difficult to achieve (1504).

Therapeutic immunization with HIV proteins together with HAART has been evaluated with STI (see Chapter 15). While the approach generated more of an HIV-specific cellular immune response, no substantial improvement of virus control after cessation of therapy was observed (2204). The enhanced CD8+ T-cell response appears to reflect primarily an expression of preexisting HIV-specific cells (86). The immunization of subjects on HAART with DCs loaded with heat-inactivated autologous HIV has given a longer period before virus doubling and lower peak viremia after treatment interruptions (1440). Such approaches to enhance the immune response to HIV before STI merit further evaluation.

In brief, STI protocols need to follow a reduction in CD4+ cell counts, as well as a rise in viral loads. Understanding the biology of the events that take place during STI may permit certain strategies that will be of benefit to the patient (108a). Moreover, an appreciation that anti-HIV responses must be present before STI is initiated should place more emphasis on short interruptions and therapeutic immunizations. Thus far, however, STI in chronic infection is not recommended.

XII. Summary

There is no question that combination antiviral therapy or HAART has changed the course of the AIDS epidemic and enabled HIV-infected people to live longer and survive, perhaps to a normal lifetime. After 4 years of HAART, CD4+ cell counts in the treated patients continued to increase (1937), and this increase was most dramatic in the presence of IL-2. Although some studies show a leveling off of CD4+ cell counts after 5 years of HAART (4596), the result may reflect the emergence of resistant viruses. Antiretroviral therapy not only increases CD4+ cell counts but also can increase total white cells and platelets (1921) as well as help reconstitute lymph nodes. Some investigators suggest that in resource-limited settings, an increase in total lymphocyte count can be used as a measure of the effectiveness of HAART (45, 205, 1872). In general, the virus replication capability and affinity for a coreceptor can influence its susceptibility to antiretroviral therapy (248, 4480).

Substantial emphasis has been placed on finding therapeutic modalities for attacking the virus itself or virus-infected cells (Figure 14.1; Table 14.2). HIV infection presents many challenges for effective antiviral therapies (Table 14.7). Information on many different drugs showing anti-HIV activity in vitro appears regularly in the literature, but their clinical efficacy awaits further evaluation (Section II). Unfortunately, many drugs have shown organ system toxicity that cannot be evaluated in the laboratory (Table 14.4). Most clinicians conclude that combination therapy, similar to the approaches taken to the treatment of malignancies, should be universally utilized to avoid drug resistance. Attention must be given to potential toxicities.

Importantly, the present antiretroviral drugs do not directly attack the potential millions of virus-infected cells in the body, some of which are long-living macrophages and DCs and latently infected CD4$^+$ cells that can eventually release virus particles in the host. Therefore, the optimal situation for control of HIV infection would be a combination of immune-based therapies and antiretroviral drugs (Figure 14.3; Tables 14.2 and 14.4).

When to start therapy is still not a resolved issue. Treatment in acute or early infection may preserve HIV-specific CD4$^+$ cell responses and de-crease the risk of transmission, but following cessation of treatment, eventually the subjects appear to lose virus control (for a review, see reference 1876). Nevertheless, STI does reduce cost and drug toxicity. Importantly, other additional strategies to enhance anti-HIV responses such as the use of immune-modulating agents, adoptive transfer of cells, or therapeutic immunization (with DC) may provide a direction that will maintain control of HIV infection after therapy is stopped. A short course of treatment interruptions may be helpful but should be carefully monitored. That approach may be most beneficial in an acute (1284) and not chronic infection.

Because of the toxicity of the drugs, the recommendation for their initiation has included information on specific cell subsets, virus level, and clinical determinants suggesting advancement to disease (Table 14.3). Although sustained responses to therapy are best seen with higher CD4$^+$ cell counts, most evidence does not suggest that early treatment with current therapies will delay the onset of AIDS (2880).

The overall approach of therapy is to bring HIV-infected individuals to a state of being long-term survivors in whom the immune system has control of the virus infection (see Chapter 13). Where appropriate, organ transplantation (e.g., kidney or

Table 14.7 Biologic and molecular features of HIV that affect antiviral therapy

- Infected cells are a major source of HIV transmission and pathogenesis.
- Infected T cells, B cells, and macrophages can be circulating reservoirs for HIV. Tissue macrophages and stromal cells can be resident HIV reservoirs that persistently release virus.
- Integrated virus can be latent and remain unaffected by the immune response and antiviral therapy.
- Virus can spread by cell-to-cell transfer.
- Virus can infect brain cells (astrocytes and oligodendrocytes) and other tissue sites (Table 4.7). Therapeutic agents must be able to pass through the blood-brain barrier and the blood-testis barrier and into the gastrointestinal tract.
- Virus can "escape" neutralizing antibodies; in some cases, virus infection is sensitive to enhancement by antibodies.
- Antigenic variations occur widely among HIV-1 and HIV-2 strains.
- Sequence mutations can occur early in the regions containing the HIV envelope and regulatory genes.

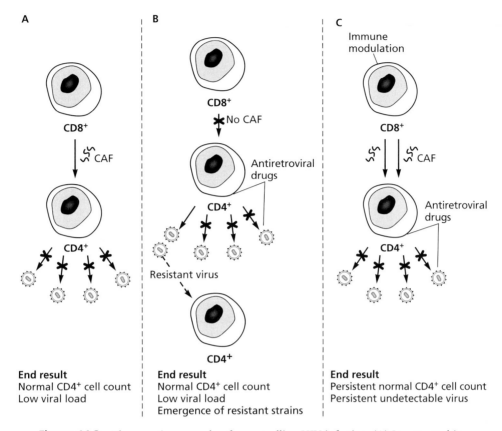

Figure 14.3 Therapeutic approaches for controlling HIV infection. (A) In untreated infected individuals who remain asymptomatic and have normal CD4$^+$ cell counts, control of HIV replication in infected CD4$^+$ cells appears to be mediated by CD8$^+$ cells, particularly noncytotoxic cells that release the CD8$^+$ antiviral factor (CAF). (B) When this cell-mediated immune response decreases (secondary to a variety of factors suggested in the text), HIV is produced. Present combination therapy prevents this released virus from reinfecting fresh cells and can restore CD4$^+$ cell levels. The viral load is reduced. However, resistant strains can emerge if this arrest in virus replication is not complete. (C) The optimal control of HIV infection would come from a dual approach in which immune modulators are used to enhance the CD8$^+$ cell antiviral response and antiretroviral drugs are administered to prevent infection of fresh cells by the free virus remaining in the host.

liver) in HIV-infected individuals should be considered (3784). In all cases, a combination drug regimen and the biologic and molecular features of HIV need to be considered. Eradication of HIV, while a laudable objective, does not currently seem feasible, knowing the biology of retrovirus infections. A recent attempt to achieve this objective in a newborn child given HAART shortly after birth is informative. Whereas plasma virus, proviral DNA, virus culture, and anti-HIV antibodies became negative, HIV replication resumed following therapy interruption 2 years later (4606). Long-term control of the infection appears to be the most achievable goal.

1. Anti-HIV therapies initially began with the use of zidovudine (AZT) and other single reverse transcriptase (RT) inhibitors. Present treatments include three drugs (generally nucleoside or nonnucleoside RT inhibitors). Later, with onset of viral resistance, viral protease inhibitors are added. Monotherapy is not advised.

2. When anti-HIV treatment should begin remains in question, although most physicians recommend administration of drugs if viral loads are above 50,000 RNA copies/ml and CD4$^+$ cell counts are <200 cells/μl.

3. Other antiviral directions under study include integrase inhibitors, drugs against the viral Gag and other proteins, therapy to prevent nucleotide incorporation into viral DNA, and anti-RNA strategies (Tables 14.1 and 14.2).

4. Antiretroviral therapies can reduce the viral load in the lymph nodes, but whether drugs can affect HIV levels in sanctuaries such as the brain or testes remains to be studied.

5. A notable problem encountered with antiviral therapy is drug resistance. Cross-resistance to the protease inhibitors is commonly observed.

6. Importantly, present treatments do not specifically target virus-infected cells, which can remain as reservoirs of HIV production.

7. Antiviral therapies may sometimes compromise the function of the immune system. This effect may reflect direct or indirect (e.g., low viral loads) mechanisms. In most studies, HAART appears to enhance cell-mediated immunity and may be important in helping, either directly or indirectly, the host immune system to function with anti-HIV activity.

8. Immune system-based therapies encourage the use of cytokines (e.g., interleukin-2) that could help restore cell-mediated immunity or approaches that decrease the toxic effects of cellular products, such as tumor necrosis factor alpha.

9. Approaches to restore the function of the immune system in individuals who are receiving antiretroviral therapy are being emphasized. Generating naïve T lymphocytes through thymus-dependent or -independent activities is required.

10. Postinfection immunization studies are being conducted but have not provided initial promising results.

11. Passive immunotherapy and antibody-based antiviral approaches are other directions for treating HIV infection but have not yet shown any consistent beneficial effect.

12. Structured treatment interruption may be helpful in restoring immune function in acute infection but does not appear to be beneficial in chronic infection.

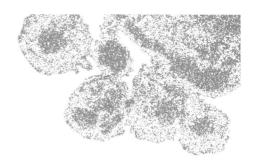

Vaccine Development

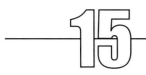

I. Introduction

The previous chapter reviewed the promising results obtained thus far in suppressing virus replication in the infected host with antiviral drugs. Most of the treatments are aimed at the virus and its de novo infection. Controlling or eliminating the reservoirs of virus-infected cells in lymphoid tissue, brain, and other sanctuaries remains the major challenge to obtaining a cure. Some immune system-based therapies have been considered, as well as the need to restore the immune system's anti-HIV responses in individuals in whom virus replication has returned. Nevertheless, despite the promise of effective therapies, the biggest challenge for worldwide control of HIV is preventing HIV infection. The virus continues to spread rapidly, particularly in resource-limited countries (see Preface).

This final chapter reviews the history and recent attempts to develop a vaccine against HIV. Most experimental studies were conducted with SIV or SHIV strains in primates, particularly rhesus macaques, but other animal models have also been evaluated. By assessing past conventional vaccine approaches, a great deal has been learned about what procedures will not work. Now, new directions must be considered that are based on the knowledge that combating HIV infection requires recognition of virus-infected cells, not only free virions.

The discussion in this chapter deals with the true concept of vaccines—prevention of virus infection. Recently, immunogens that may be used in vaccines have been utilized in approaches to boost the immune system of already infected individuals at the same time that antiretroviral drugs are given. This type of therapeutic immunization (which by some is incorrectly called therapeutic vaccination) is covered in Chapter 14. (For overviews on vaccine development in terms of history, future perspectives, and recent challenges, see references 1835, 2942, 3433, and 3761.)

II. Background

In developing a vaccine, several features of HIV infection and transmission must be considered (for reviews, see references 348, 1257, 1592, 1835, 2515, and 3075) (Table 14.7). The approaches for conventional vaccines may not all be relevant for preventing HIV infection (Table 15.1). For example, seropositive individuals who have completely eliminated HIV infection have not been identified, and protection against infection, which is the objective of most vaccines, may not be the appropriate end point for an HIV vaccine. Moreover, previous vaccines have protected against viruses that do not change over time, and they have generally used whole killed or live attenuated viruses. At present, these types of approaches are considered unsafe for an HIV vaccine. Finally, other infectious virions against which effective vaccines have been directed are usually infrequently encountered and have been those that gain entry through mucosal surfaces (e.g., the respiratory and gastrointestinal tracts) aside from the genital tract. The antiviral vaccines presently in use have also been directed against agents that are not passed particularly by certain behavioral patterns (e.g., sexual activity) and are not cell associated (for a review, see reference 1257).

Table 15.1 Features of conventional vaccines[a]

- Establish the state of natural immunity against reinfection similar to that observed in individuals who have recovered from the infection
- Protect against disease and not against infection
- Protect for years against viruses that do not change over time
- Have generally been whole killed or live attenuated
- Protect against infections that occur through mucosal surfaces of the respiratory or gastrointestinal tract, not the genital tract
- Are directed against microbes that are not predominantly related to behavioral patterns
- Are directed at free microbes, not cell-associated pathogens

[a]Adapted from reference 1257.

Table 15.2 Possible correlates of protective immunity against HIV infection[a]

- Innate immune responses (e.g., PDC and CNAR)
- NK cell activity
- CTL activity (CD4+ and CD8+ cells)
- Antibody-dependent cellular cytotoxicity
- Neutralizing antibodies

[a]The presence of these responses at mucosal sites is important. If attenuated virus is used, sufficient replication of the virus must occur to induce protective responses. PDC, plasmacytoid dendritic cells; CNAR, CD8+ cell noncytotoxic anti-HIV response; NK, natural killer; CTL, cytotoxic T lymphocytes (see Chapters 9 and 11).

The initial findings on the serologic cross-reacting region in the V3 loop (i.e., the principal neutralizing domain), the induction of cross-reactive cytotoxic T-lymphocyte (CTL) activity (1710, 2446), and the reported broadening antiviral response in animals immunized with gp120 and the V3 loop (1694, 2012) lent early encouragement to the potential development of a vaccine against HIV (see Chapters 10 and 11). Moreover, the existence of individuals who have been exposed to HIV on many occasions and are not infected (see Chapter 13) indicates that complete protection from HIV infection is possible. Nevertheless, the question of whether the present vaccine directions would protect a host against high doses of the virus (>100 infectious particles) and virus-infected cells (2517, 2522, 2529, 3858) has not been answered.

Importantly, the correlates of protective immunity (Table 15.2) have not been well defined in terms of an HIV vaccine. This vaccine would require longstanding innate immunity that has been shown to be associated with lack of infection in high-risk individuals (see Chapter 13). Approaches are needed to induce this type of immunity without strong immune activation (2533). Essentially, the induction of innate and adaptive immunity as well as mucosal immunity needs to be achieved (2533, 2981, 3011). Similar approaches are being considered in the development of hepatitis C vaccines (1896). Moreover, the most effective immunization strategy involving route of administration and timing needs to be determined (Table 15.3).

Most HIV vaccine approaches are directed at inducing adaptive immune responses, including

Table 15.3 Immunization approaches evaluated for an HIV vaccine[a]

- Parenteral
- Oral administration (adenovirus, poliovirus, salmonella, transgenic plants)
- Intranasal, intravaginal, intrarectal, or intraurethral inoculation
- Use of liposomes, microspheres, microcapsules, immunostimulatory complexes
- DNA immunization
- Use of cytokines (e.g., IL-2 and GM-CSF)

[a]In most cases, adjuvants were used (Section X). IL-2, interleukin-2; GM-CSF, granulocyte-macrophage colony-stimulating factor.

neutralizing antibodies and antigen-specific cellular immune responses. Currently, the requirement for effective innate immune responses has been appreciated (2549, 3433). In this regard, recent studies in rhesus macaques have shown that intravaginal inoculation of SIV leads to a small focus of virus infection (3013). Presumably, if the virus replication at that site is suppressed, the infection cannot be established. The early reaction of innate cells can directly kill incoming virus-infected cells at mucosal surfaces or within lymph nodes (e.g., via NK cells) or suppress virus to prevent its spread (e.g., via interferon release by plasmacytoid dendritic cells or the CD8$^+$ cell antiviral factor (CAF) produced by CD8$^+$ cells) (see Chapters 9 and 11). If, however, the incoming virus cannot be controlled sufficiently, adaptive immune responses will be important with neutralizing antibodies as well as strong CTL activity against virus-infected cells to prevent development of disease. In the SIV intravaginal model, CTLs responded too late (3714). A vaccine needs to elicit a rapid anti-HIV response, and innate immunity can be the means for enhancing both innate and adaptive anti-HIV responses (2533). In this regard, this chapter reviews how the effectiveness of a vaccine may reflect the use of a particular adjuvant containing selected immune potentiators and a delivery vehicle. An ideal adjuvant should induce strong innate immunity.

A major problem in vaccinology is finding an appropriate animal model (Table 15.4) of HIV infection. As noted above, studies of candidate HIV-1 vaccines have relied on primate systems which can mirror to some extent a natural HIV infection. For these studies, infection of macaques with SIV or SIV (HIV-1) (SHIV) chimeric viruses (1449, 2033, 2691, 3692, 4101) has been used and can offer an approach for evaluating HIV-1 vaccines in convenient primate model systems (2502, 2681, 3011, 3013, 3633). Generally, immunogenicity of a potential vaccine is first tested in small animals such as mice, guinea pigs, and rabbits, and then immunogenicity and efficacy are evaluated in primates. If favorable results are obtained, human trials of the vaccine are begun.

For animal studies, chimpanzees, the primate most closely resembling humans, have been used but are expensive and do not generally replicate HIV to high titer or develop disease. Therefore, rhesus macaque studies with SIV have usually been chosen and form the major approach for studying lentivirus vaccines. However, SIV is more virulent than the conventional HIV-1 strains encountered and the results may not be fully applicable to an HIV vaccine. HIV-2 infection of baboons has also been encouraging for vaccine studies (264, 642, 2648), as has been the successful infection of pig-tailed monkeys (*Macaca nemestrina*) with HIV-1 (33) and HIV-2 (4691). Neither of these nonhuman primate models, however, has yet been utilized sufficiently for vaccine studies to permit comparative evaluations.

Nine different types of vaccines for preventing HIV infection are being evaluated or are being considered (Table 15.5) (2515). Each has provided some promise for the development of a vaccine in other viral systems, including the novel use of anti-idiotypes (170, 959). In the future, plants may offer an avenue for vaccine development whereby protection is induced with proteins expressed by plant

Table 15.4 Potential animal models for developing an HIV vaccine

Animal	Virus(es)
Chimpanzee	HIV-1
Rhesus macaque	SIV, SHIV
Baboon	HIV-2
Pig-tailed macaque	HIV-2, SIV
Cynomolgus monkey	HIV-2, SIV
Cat	FIV
Horse	EIAV
Mouse (SCID/hu)	HIV-1, HIV-2

Table 15.5 HIV vaccine approaches[a]

- Whole killed (inactivated) virus: natural or engineered
- Live (attenuated) variants: natural or engineered (e.g., *nef* deleted)
- Subunit vaccine (natural or engineered): envelope glycoproteins (gp120, gp160, gp41); Gag proteins (oligomerization)
- Viral proteins in live vectors (e.g., vaccinia virus, poliovirus, herpes simplex virus, adenovirus, baculovirus, Ty particle, and various bacteria)
- Viral cores with envelope proteins (pseudovirions): virus-like particles
- Sequence-derived peptides of HIV (e.g., V3 epitopes, and CTL/TH epitopes)
- Anti-idiotypes of neutralizing antibodies
- DNA gene transfer
- Plant-derived proteins

[a]Some of these approaches include cytokine enhancement. CTL, cytotoxic T lymphocyte; TH, CD4+ T helper cell.

viruses carrying HIV genes (e.g., alfalfa or cowpea mosaic virus) (4900) or with HIV plant products derived directly through genetic engineering techniques (964) (Table 15.6). Those HIV vaccine approaches that have received the most attention are reviewed below.

For any attempt at vaccine development, the fact must be appreciated that "sterilizing immunity" (i.e., infection is prevented) has never been achieved against other viral infections. Thus, early infection and some replication of HIV would be expected before the subsequent immune responses against the virus could prevent spread in the host (2529). In fact, the realization that HIV itself produces a chronic infection despite strong antiviral immune responses reflects the challenge for an effective AIDS vaccine.

With other conventional vaccines, the virus, when entering the immunized individual, will

Table 15.6 Potential value of transgenic plants in vaccine development

- Economical means for scaling up production of a protein
- Eliminates potential contamination with animal viruses
- Can be delivered either parenterally or as an edible product

replicate for a few cycles and kill the cells infected. Thus, long-term establishment of the infection does not take place and the responding immune system can prevent further virus spread within the host. With HIV, infection of a cell will lead to integration of the viral genome into the chromosome and thus produce an established infection. Unless that cell is killed or sloughed (e.g., in the intestine), the infection will remain in the host (2529). The optimal result of an HIV vaccine, therefore, would be to contain the incoming virus at its site of infection (3013) (see Chapter 9) and arrest its spread. If not eliminated, long-term control of HIV should be maintained and the amount of virus in body fluids would be markedly reduced. In that way, the transmission of HIV would be curtailed. Essentially, the major role of a vaccine is to protect populations from infection, not necessarily the individual (2529). For the individual, protection from disease, but not infection, is a reasonable objective.

In brief, evidence thus far would suggest that approaches which can induce both innate and adaptive immune responses should be incorporated into a vaccine approach. Also very importantly, the first HIV vaccines utilized may show their beneficial effect by preventing the onset of disease rather than preventing infection.

III. Ideal Properties of an Effective Vaccine

The overall aim of any vaccine is to reduce infection in the population (2533). For an AIDS vaccine, prevention of transmission and disease development are the important objectives (Table 15.7). Several challenges to this goal exist (Table 15.8) and are highlighted in this book. Certain properties, in addition to a lack of toxicity, are necessary for a successful vaccine (Table 15.9) (for reviews, see references 18, 1257, 1835, and 2515) (Section II). It should induce strong innate and adaptive humoral and cellular immunity that can respond to HIV and HIV-infected cells (18, 2528, 2533, 4359). Toward this objective, which adjuvants can elicit innate immune reactions and which antigens should be used for adaptive immune responses need to be determined. Both envelope proteins (non-antibody-enhancing regions) and other viral

Table 15.7 Overall objectives of an AIDS vaccine

- Reduce infection in the population
- Reduce virus in body fluids (e.g., genital) and decrease HIV transmission
- Protect the individual from infection
- Protect the individual from development of disease

proteins (e.g., Gag) should be considered. The inclusion of Gag is important since CTL activity against this viral protein seems to correlate with an asymptomatic state (428, 3738, 3827) (see Chapter 11). Moreover, studies show vaccination with the full envelope protein gp160 and the core protein of SIV protected rhesus macaques from challenge with both cloned and uncloned homologous virus (1917) (see below). Cellular immune activity appeared to be the important determinant.

An anti-HIV vaccine should produce long-lasting responses that are present not only in the blood but also in the mucosal linings of the vagina, the rectum, and the oral cavity. This mucosal immunity might require the use of a vaccine administered orally or placed in contact with the mucosal immune system via the vagina, rectum, or nasal/oral passages (2981, 3011) (Table 15.3). In this regard, immunization by the respiratory or gastrointestinal route along with systemic immunization has protected monkeys from HIV challenge via the vagina (2850) (Section IX). However, administering immune potentiators of innate immunity (e.g., CpG) with an SIV vaccine intravaginally has led to marked local inflammation and enhanced SIV infection (4677) (see below).

Side effects such as autoimmune phenomena and enhancing antibodies must be avoided in any

Table 15.8 Challenges of developing an HIV vaccine

- HIV integrates into the cellular genome
- Infected cells transmit the infection
- Cell-to-cell transfer of infection takes place
- Numerous HIV variants
- Virus infects sanctuaries of the body (e.g., brain and testes)
- Virus compromises immune function
- Autoimmune responses may be induced

vaccination procedure (Table 15.9). In this regard, some early studies showed that sera of volunteers immunized with recombinant gp160 had anti-CD4, anti-idiotype antibodies (2136) and anti-HLA class I antibodies (1008) (see below). In this regard, two broadly reactive neutralizing anti-HIV-1 envelope gp41 human monoclonal antibodies, 2F5 and 4E10, were found to be polyspecific autoantibodies reactive with the phospholipid cardiolipin (1768). Thus, as a result of immune tolerance, current HIV-1 vaccines may not induce these types of antibodies because of this autoantigen mimicry (1768) (see Chapter 10).

Several early studies suggested that vaccines that induce a strong cellular immune response rather than a humoral immune response might be most effective in controlling HIV infection (3894) (see Chapters 11 and 13). In this case, the use of selected type 1 cytokines (e.g., interleukin-2 [IL-2]) or antibodies to certain type 2 cytokines along with the vaccine should be considered. Adjuvants that preferentially induce type 1 responses (1649) and a low antigen dose that has been shown to produce a type 1 immune response in murine systems (498, 3428, 4674) have been suggested (Sections VII and IX). Obtaining strong cell-mediated immune responses may require live virus vectors or DNA inoculations so that antigen presentation is optimal for $CD8^+$ cell responses.

Currently, most investigators agree that a vaccine should elicit both humoral and cellular anti-HIV responses. Innate and adaptive immunity should be induced (2533). Finally, as noted above, an ideal HIV vaccine must be safe and preferably would not require multiple booster immunizations (Table 15.9).

IV. Inactivated and Attenuated Viruses

A. Inactivated Whole Virus

The predominant early vaccine studies with lentiviruses used killed SIV in macaques (modeled after the Salk poliovirus vaccine) and showed some prevention from virus infection (1061, 3177, 4248). The approach demonstrated protection against a low-dose challenge with the homologous SIV strain. In general, delays in virus challenge after the

Table 15.9 The ideal HIV vaccine[a]

- Induces local immunity at all entry sites for HIV
- Induces cellular and humoral immune responses against virus-infected cells
- Induces antibodies that neutralize and do not enhance HIV infection
- Induces immune responses that recognize latently infected cells
- Does not induce autoimmune responses
- Safe, with long-lasting effects

[a]Both innate and adaptive immune systems should be induced.

final immunization dose (up to 12 months) gave the best results and formed the basis for further evaluation of these types of vaccines (3177). Nevertheless, other studies soon showed that killed-virus vaccines did not protect against infection or disease when the challenge virus was inoculated onto the genital mucosal lining or when heterologous virus was used (4343). Protection of macaques immunized with killed HIV-2 strains was also reported (3627). Once again, the challenge was a low dose (10 to 40 infectious particles) with a homotypic virus type. Prevention from infection by a heterologous HIV-2 isolate or, more importantly, virus-infected cells was not evaluated.

Very disturbing was the recognition, subsequent to many vaccine studies, that most of the early trials with inactivated SIV strains as immunogens probably measured anticellular and not antiviral responses (913, 2407, 4302). The immunizing and the challenging viruses were grown in the same human cell line. Protection correlated with antibodies against the human cellular proteins (e.g., HLA class I) associated with the virion and not against the viral proteins (156, 679). Thus, protection occurred via anticellular protein responses. The results, however, were impressive in that they suggested complete prevention of SIV transmission. Essentially, sterilizing immunity appeared to be achieved, since any successful infection would have produced progeny viruses lacking the human cell antigens. Thus, they would not be sensitive to that induced immune response. The virus-specific immune activity (e.g., CD8+ cells) responsible for these findings was not defined. However, the potential importance of allostimulation for induction of antiviral immunity is currently receiving attention (Section X.D).

Many of these early SIV studies were reevaluated with appropriate virus preparations. Some did not show protection even with the successful induction of antiviral antibodies (4137). Nevertheless, one study with killed SIV and low-dose homologous SIV challenge did seem to reflect induction of a true antiviral state (1061). Moreover, the vaccination of two rhesus monkeys with whole inactivated HIV-1 protected the animals from an SHIV challenge (2681). Human antigens were not involved, and the results provided further encouragement for using killed virus and the SHIV model to study prevention of HIV infection in nonhuman primates.

Viewing the cat lentivirus as an approach, immunization with inactivated feline immunodeficiency virus (FIV)-infected cells or killed cell-free FIV protected >90% of cats against intraperitoneal infection with small amounts of homologous (2875, 4850) or heterologous (4850) strains. It has also prevented FIV infection in field cats under normal conditions (2876). Neutralizing antibodies were not necessarily present (2875). Moreover, by using a killed-virus vaccine for the equine infectious anemia virus (EIAV), horses were protected against this lentivirus infection by up to 10^5 infectious doses of the homologous virus (1965). The vaccine did not prevent infection by a heterologous virus but protected against disease. These encouraging results did not involve anticellular responses.

Recently, HIV-1, inactivated by low-dose formaldehyde prior to heat treatment, induced antibodies that neutralized homologous and heterologous strains of HIV in mice and nonhuman primates (3572). Other approaches at using inactivated virus include treatment of viruses with psoralen (which causes intercalation of viral nucleic acid) (1031a) and/or aldrithiol-2 (3815). Nevertheless, use of an inactivated HIV vaccine seems remote at this time.

B. Whole Attenuated Virus

1. OBSERVATIONS

Some investigators demonstrated several years ago that immunization of macaques with a live, naturally attenuated SIV strain (SIV$_{mac1A11}$) did not protect against infection but prevented disease in adults and neonates following a subsequent challenge with a virulent virus strain (2827, 3357).

In addition, previous infection of macaques with the SHIV$_{89.6}$ isolate provided protection against vaginal challenge with the pathogenic SIV$_{mac239}$ strain (3633). In this case, cross-reactive cellular responses rather than neutralizing antibodies could be involved. Moreover, macaques immunized orally with two live attenuated SHIV isolates showed protection from disease if the vaccine virus remained active in the animals (2734). Also, preinfection with a weakly pathogenic HIV-2 strain protected one of six macaques from subsequent superinfection with the pathogenic SIV$_{mac251}$ strain given via the rectal route (4655). The protection correlated with high levels of antibodies and cross-reacting neutralizing antibodies. However, the ability to prevent superinfection of the one animal revealed no conclusive information about the correlates of immune protection involved. A similar study suggested protection from SIV infection after an initial HIV-2 infection (3492). Previous infection by one HIV-2 strain has also protected baboons from superinfection by a heterologous HIV-2 strain (2649). In contrast, a prior infection with a nonpathogenic SHIV did not protect against infection by a pathogenic SIV (2502). In the latter case, however, adequate replication of the SHIV may not have taken place.

The common observation from several reports is that a certain threshold of replication of the initiating (attenuated) infectious virus should be reached to induce protective immune responses (425, 4655). These findings on a "threshold effect" (3844, 3845, 4746) (Figure 15.1) could offer insights into the correlates of protection (Table 15.2).

In another approach, a *nef*-deleted attenuated mutant of SIV that does not cause disease in rhesus monkeys (2169, 2170) induced a high titer of antibodies against the virus (965). Results on cellular immune response were not reported. Subsequent challenge of these animals with up to 1,000 rhesus monkey infectious doses of a wild-type virus gave protection from infection (965). Similar findings with *nef*-deleted SIV and SHIV were later reported by other groups (1464, 1949, 3276, 4247). Protection in one case did not correlate with neutralizing antibodies (3276). In another, anti-Env CTLs were considered important (1949). In one report, protection against pathogenic SIV correlated with cytotoxic and noncytotoxic

CD8$^+$ cell responses; the latter was related to nonchemokine, antiviral soluble factors (1464) (see Chapter 11). In one noteworthy study, protection was achieved against challenge with virus-infected cells (71). In other investigations, rhesus macaques previously infected with a *nef*-attenuated SIV strain resisted subsequent exposure to an SHIV strain (425). Since the envelope region differs between these two strains, cell-mediated immune activity rather than neutralizing antibodies must have been involved (2041, 4247). In all these studies, better viral antigen expression may have occurred in the absence of Nef. This viral protein can down-modulate major histocompatibility complex (MHC) class I expression of viral antigens by the infected cell (854, 2444, 4014). Thus, the host CD8$^+$ cell antiviral immune response is reduced (see Chapters 8 and 11).

In other trials, infectious SIVs lacking *nef*, *vpr*, and the upstream sequences in U3 as well as an SIV lacking *nef* were evaluated. Protection was associated with high levels of replication of the vaccine strains in the animals. Some correlation with virus neutralizing and binding antibodies was noted (4828). In addition, using an attenuated SIV strain, three monkeys were protected from disease after inoculation of high-level infectious SHIV. No preexisting neutralizing antibodies were found against the SHIV, nor were they induced after a year of observation following the SHIV challenge. The protection against a totally heterologous envelope must have been related to cell-mediated response (4103), and perhaps involved innate immunity (see Chapters 9 and 11).

Other SIV studies with several independent or combined mutations (e.g., *vpr*, *vpx*, and *vif*) gave similar results (1949; for a review, see reference 1059). In many of these studies, protection correlated with replication of high levels of attenuated virus soon after the initial infection (425, 2502). As suggested by the threshold hypothesis (Figure 15.1), only those attenuated viruses that induced a prolonged sufficiently high viremia provided resistance to challenge by wild-type SIV (2653). A state of protective immunity must be established.

In addition, rhesus macaques sequentially immunized with a SHIV deleted in *vpu* and *nef* followed by one mutant SIV with a deletion in *vpu* had neutralizing antibodies and CTLs that

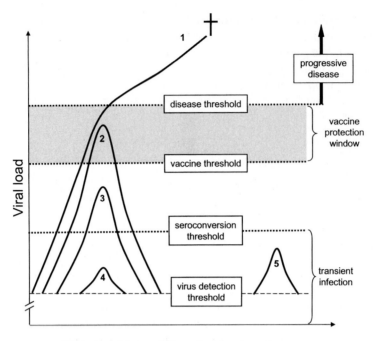

Time post-inoculation (early stage)

Figure 15.1 The threshold hypothesis. After infection with a live attenuated virus, clinical outcomes can vary and depend on multifactorial host-virus dynamics. Persistently high viral loads exceeding the disease threshold result in fatal AIDS (pattern 1); due to high viral replication, more pathogenic viral variants inevitably emerge (pattern 1). If the viral burden exceeds a second putative threshold, the vaccine threshold, but remains below the disease threshold, the host will not develop disease but will instead generate protective responses against subsequent challenge with pathogenic virus (pattern 2, vaccine protection window). If the viral burden remains below the vaccine threshold, as in the case of highly attenuated virus variants, disease will not develop but the host will not be protected against subsequent virus challenge (patterns 3 and 4). If the viral load is so low that the seroconversion threshold is not reached, the host will only be transiently infected (pattern 4). During the chronic phase of infection, occasional blips of viremia can occur, perhaps due to transient disturbances of host control over the vaccine virus (patterns 5). However, live attenuated viruses persist and continue to replicate; with time, aggressive viral escape variants can emerge, causing disease at late stages (not shown). Due to genetic variability in outbred populations, host immune responses may vary considerably, making determination of a discrete vaccine protective window difficult. Adapted from reference 4746 with permission.

recognized both the homologous and the heterologous SHIV and SIV. When challenged via the rectal mucosae, all vaccinated animals were infected but plasma viremia was reduced two- to five-fold and the vaccinated animals maintained CD4$^+$ T-cell levels. Protection from disease appeared to be achieved at least for a short period of time (2343).

This ability of live attenuated SIV to protect against disease may result from the initial induction of strong type 1 type responses and β-chemokine production (1465). In this regard, administration of a live attenuated SIV together with pathogenic virus did not protect against disease (2616). The need for a preexisting immune state for protection against a virulent virus was evident.

2. POTENTIAL PROBLEMS

The use of live attenuated viruses, however, has been challenged by results indicating that inoculation of some of these viruses (e.g., *nef* deleted)

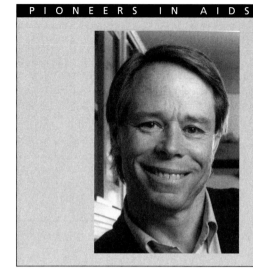

Donald Francis

Executive Director, Global Solutions for Infectious Diseases, a not-for-profit vaccine development company. Dr. Francis led some of the early studies on the epidemiology and etiology of AIDS. He is actively engaged in vaccine research for diseases in less-developed countries.

into neonatal macaques can give rise to AIDS (191). Moreover, some adult animals receiving these attenuated viruses have developed disease several months to years after challenge (1869); in some cases animals receiving the attenuated virus developed disease when the viral deletion was repaired in the animal (3844). This risk of reversion of a deletion mutant to wild-type virus must be appreciated (4247). The *nef*-deleted mutants of SIV may also not prevent infection by heterologous virus strains (2560).

The problem with attenuated viruses could be approached by the use of conditional-live HIV variants whose replication is induced through transient administration of drugs like doxycycline. Withdrawal of the drug arrests virus replication (968, 4188). However, integration of attenuated viruses may lead to other pathogenic processes (e.g., neoplasia) (1134). Acceptance of this approach, therefore, will be difficult unless other vaccine strategies using noninfectious viruses, other viral vectors, or HIV proteins are not successful (see below). Nevertheless, as a model, the attenuated virus comes closest to resembling the relatively persistent replicating virion that would be infecting the host. In this case, an effective antiviral response may be maintained and may control virus pathogenesis. Thus, studies with attenuated viruses are being continued and could indicate what immune responses are needed to induce protective immunity against HIV. For other vaccine studies using live nonpathogenic or less pathogenic SIV, see Section IX.

V. Vaccines Using Purified Proteins: Envelope gp120 or Tat Alone or in Association with an Expression Vector

A. Purified Native or Recombinant Virus Envelope

Some success in inducing anti-HIV immune responses has been achieved with vaccines containing purified envelope glycoproteins expressed in the baculovirus system or in mammalian cells (e.g., Chinese hamster ovary [CHO] cells) in which close to normal glycosylation occurs (158, 335, 1524). In an early trial using chimpanzees, immunization with purified HIV gp120 expressed in CHO cells, but not a variant of gp160 (modified at the cleavage site), prevented infection after a low-dose challenge with homologous HIV (335). Moreover, chimpanzees immunized with multiple booster shots of a recombinant gp120 of HIV-1$_{SF2}$ in the MF59 adjuvant (Section X) resisted challenge with homologous virus (1185). In addition, chimpanzees immunized with the HIV-1$_{MN}$ recombinant gp120 in alum and challenged with the heterologous isolate HIV-1$_{SF2}$ were not infected. Neutralizing antibodies did not correlate with this protection (337). These results encouraged the phase III vaccine trials with gp120 that were recently completed (Section XII). Although certain SIV Env peptide fusion proteins have been reported to show potentially positive results (4060), most studies with native (3178) or recombinant (1506, 1916) envelope proteins have not provided protective efficacy in SIV models. Several early vaccine trials in the SIV system also showed some potentially positive results with native (3178) or recombinant (4060) envelope proteins.

In studies of protection from challenge with infected cells, chimpanzees immunized many times with HIV-1 antigens showed resistance to intravenous injection of infected peripheral blood mononuclear cells (PBMC) (1393). These results provided the first evidence that immunization can induce host responses against HIV-infected cells. Further experiments to confirm these observations are needed, including those using a challenge with infected cells inoculated into the anal and vaginal canals under appropriate physiologic conditions (e.g., in seminal fluid).

In other studies, a recombinant HIV-1 envelope protein derived from a primary R5 isolate was very effective in completely protecting a majority of macaques from SHIV infection delivered by the intravenous route (3078). The adjuvant used, which was known to induce T-cell immunity, was important in eliciting this protection. In later studies with SHIV strains, however, more virulent viruses (growing to higher titer) were less affected by immunization with the R5 recombinant envelope gp120 protein (3077).

Moreover, several experiments have indicated that an oligomer (trimer) structure of gp120 reflecting the native HIV-1 envelope glycoprotein complex can be the best virus envelope immunogen (263, 2696, 4242). In addition, improvement in the ability of the HIV-1 envelope to induce neutralizing antibodies was achieved by preparing a partial deletion of the V2 region (263). In rhesus macaques the resulting recombinant antigen showed induction of some cross-reacting neutralizing antibodies. The approach was based on prior observations that the HIV-1$_{SF162}$ strain lacking the V2 region was neutralized by sera directed against clade B as well as other non-clade B HIV isolates (4253) (see Chapter 10). The potential importance of the neutralizing anti-

bodies in controlling HIV infection was demonstrated by removal of CD8$^+$ cells after immunization with this HIV recombinant envelope protein. All animals challenged intravenously controlled the infection for over 3 years, with the initial immune response being solely neutralizing antibodies (546).

Some investigators have suggested that immunization with a soluble CD4:gp120 complex will best induce neutralizing antibodies to a conformation-dependent epitope on gp120 (2087). These types of studies using a gp140:CD4 or a gp120:CD4 cross-linked complex in rhesus macaques have generated antibodies that neutralized a wide range of primary HIV isolates (both X4 and R5). Thus, a response may be induced against a novel epitope on the HIV envelope revealed by CD4 binding (1341, 4243).

B. Tat Protein

In studies of other viral proteins, vaccination of cynomolgus monkeys with a biologically active Tat protein elicited both humoral and cellular immune responses and reduced infection of macaques with the pathogenic SHIV$_{89.6P}$ virus. The protein was delivered with RIBI or alum as adjuvants (Section X). Protection of animals correlated with low-level CTL activity and the presence of anti-Tat neutralizing antibodies as assessed on acutely infected cells (577). One common cellular immune response in the protected animals was the presence of CD8$^+$ cell noncytotoxic antiviral responses (B. Ensoli, personal communication), (see Chapter 11). In other studies, rhesus macaques immunized with chemically inactivated Tat showed reduced disease and lower viral RNA levels when challenged by the intrarectal route (3449). Nevertheless, in studies with an SIV Tat DNA prime-vaccinia virus Ankara boost vaccination protocol, a substantial anti-Tat CTL response was induced but the macaques did not resist intrarectal challenge with SIV$_{mac239}$ (67). Virus escape mutants with changes in the Tat epitope were found. These studies, however, could reflect the pathogenic nature of SIV$_{mac239}$ (67).

C. Recombinant Envelope Proteins Expressed by Live Vectors

As noted above, studies with live attenuated SIV strains have shown that some can evolve into virulent viruses over time. Therefore, a current emphasis in vaccines has been to attempt to mimic the natural

Table 15.10 Vectors evaluated for HIV vaccines

Viruses

Adenovirus

Bluetongue

Rabies

Canarypox

Equine encephalitis

Hepatitis B

Herpes simplex

Epstein-Barr

Influenza

Poliovirus

Rhinovirus

Semliki Forest

Vaccinia

Ty particle

Potato virus

Bacteria

Mycobacterium (BCG)

Listeria

Salmonella

virus infection with vectors that are not derived directly from a lentivirus (Table 15.10). These live attenuated virus vectors offer a potential vaccine approach. In particular, targeting a vaccine vector to infect dendritic cells (DCs) could elicit strong CD4$^+$ and CD8$^+$ cell anti-HIV responses (1205).

1. POXVIRUSES: PRIME-BOOST APPROACHES

Some promising results in vaccine development have come from studies using poxvirus vectors. The viral proteins are produced in cells of the host in association with vaccinia or canarypox (avipox: ALVAC) virus infection (120, 879, 4905). This approach, which has been helpful in vaccine studies for *Mycobacterium tuberculosis* and malaria, can elicit good humoral and cellular (i.e., CTL) immune anti-HIV responses in animals (for a review, see reference 3761). In many studies, a prime-boost approach has been considered. By this strategy, also used with the Tat vaccine discussed in Section V.B and other vaccine studies discussed below, one method of immunization is followed some months later by a different immunization approach (Table 15.11). The objective is to induce both humoral and cellular anti-HIV immune responses.

In some early vaccine experiments, vaccinia virus vector vaccination expressing HIV gp120 protected chimpanzees from a low-dose HIV challenge (10 to 40 infectious doses), but only after subsequent booster immunizations with a purified baculovirus-derived gp160 and particularly a V3-keyhole limpet hemocyanin (KLH) conjugate (1524). Protection could have come from the anti-V3-specific neutralizing antibodies elicited. Moreover, chimpanzees immunized several times with a live vaccinia virus expressing a recombinant gp160 MN protein or the V3 MN peptide were also protected from intravenous infection with a heterologous HIV-1 strain (1525) (Table 15.12).

Other investigators obtained variable results with a similar prime-boost regimen. When macaques were immunized with a recombinant canarypox vaccine and boosted with subunit HIV-1 proteins, partial protection was observed against infection by a divergent but nonpathogenic HIV-2 (11). Macaques immunized with a modified vaccinia virus Ankara (MVA) expressing multiple SIV antigens followed with inactivated SIV showed no protection against infection from a pathogenic challenge virus. The regimen reduced the virus load, resulting in prolonged disease-free survival (1844). Only reduction of the viral load in a minority of animals challenged with a highly pathogenic virus, SIV$_{mac251}$, was observed, with no apparent benefit in disease outcome (966, 1506). It is possible that immune responses elicited by these early attempts at virus vector priming and protein boosting were suboptimal. They were sufficient to protect against challenge with a virus of low pathogenicity but failed to contain more robust ones.

Table 15.11 Effective HIV immunization[a]

Prime	Boost
Live virus vector (e.g., vaccinia and avipox)	Envelope subunit
DNA vaccines	Pseudovirions
Killed virus	
Pseudovirions	
Envelope subunit	Live virus vector

[a]The first immunization method serves to prime the immune system to respond to an antigen; the second, a boost some months later, usually utilizes a different approach to present antigen(s). Examples are given.

Table 15.12 Vaccination procedures involving the prime-boost approach[a]

Prime	Boost	Primate	Challenge virus	Reference	Protection[b]
Canarypox ($gp160_{MN}$)	V3$_{MN}$ peptides, gp160	Chimpanzee	HIV-1$_{SF2}$	1525	+[c]
Vaccinia ($gp130$)	gp130	Rhesus macaque	SIV$_{mac32H}$	2696	±
Vaccinia ($gp160$)	gp160	Cynomolgus monkey	SIV$_{mne}$ E11S	1914	+
Vaccinia ($gp160$)	gp160	Pig-tailed macaque	SHIV$_{IIIB}$	1917	+[d]
Vaccinia ($gp160$)	gp160	Cynomolgus macaque	Uncloned SIV$_{mne}$ and SIV$_{mne}$ EllS	3550	+
Vaccinia ($gp130$)	gp130				
Vaccinia (*Gag- Pol*)	Gag-Pol				
Canarypox ($gp125$)	gp125, V3 peptides	Cynomolgus monkey	HIV-2	120	±
Vaccinia or canarypox (*gag, pol, env*)	gp160	Rhesus macaque	SIV	1349	+
DNA (CTL epitopes; *tat, rev, nef*)	Vaccinia (rMVA) CTL *gag* epitopes and *tat, rev, nef*	Rhesus macaque	SIV$_{mac239}$	4618	−
DNA (*gag, pol, env, rev, tat, nef*)	Vaccinia (*gag, pol, env, rev, tat, nef, env*)	Rhesus macaque	SIV$_{mac251}$	1794	−
DNA (HIV-1 *env* and *gag*)	gp120	Rhesus macaque	SHIV$_{Ba-L}$	3386	+

[a]Examples of prime-boost vaccine trials. For more examples, see reference 1916. In all cases the prime-boost immunogen used HIV or SIV antigens that matched a challenge virus. Protection from virus infection was observed in some animals but primarily to the homologous virus. In most studies, the challenge virus was given intravenously, except for the intrarectal route used in some animals (1794, 1917, 3386, 4618).

[b]+, protection from virus infection was observed in some animals; ±, limited protection but reduction in viral load set point after challenge was noted; −, no protection, but reduced viremia was observed after challenge.

[c]The two protected animals were immunized with gp160 and the V3 peptide, whereas the two chimpanzees primed with canarypox virus alone were infected. Virus was recovered from peripheral blood mononuclear cells in the acute phase from the latter animals.

[d]Four of six animals were protected, one had a reduced viral load, and one animal showed the presence of virus at 6 months after challenge.

In other experiments, a vaccinia virus vector expressing gp130 of SIV$_{mac}$ followed by a booster of gp130 oligomers elicited protection in some rhesus macaques from challenge with the homologous SIV strain (2696), without a substantial antibody response. Protection against a moderately pathogenic homologous SIV$_{mne}$ clone was achieved in some cynomolgus monkeys after immunization with a vaccinia virus recombinant and a booster with SIV$_{mne}$ gp160 produced in baculovirus or vaccinia virus-infected cells (1914, 1915, 3550). CTL responses sometimes protected animals, suggesting that the challenge virus replicated in the host but was then effectively eliminated (2161). A similar observation was made in vaccination of rhesus macaques with an attenuated poxvirus SIV vaccine expressing virus structural genes. SIV-specific CD4$^+$ and CD8$^+$ cell responses were induced, and six of eight vaccinated animals during primary infection appeared to control virus challenge after interruption of therapy (1795). A poxvirus and protein prime-boost regimen also protected against SHIV$_{IIIB}$ challenge in pig-tailed macaques (for a review, see reference 1916).

In addition, this "prime-boost" vaccine strategy protected rhesus macaques against intraveneously administered homologous virus that represented the majority of the uncloned challenge virus (3550). When the same approach was used with an intrarectal challenge, a more effective protection was achieved against both the cloned and the uncloned virus, most likely because of a selective

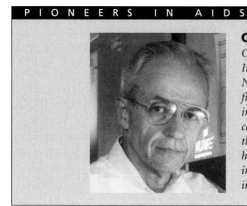

Gene M. Shearer

Chief, Cell-Mediated Immunity Section, Experimental Immunology Branch, National Cancer Institute, National Institutes of Health. Dr. Shearer is one of the first immunologists to approach the challenge of defining the immunologic abnormalities in AIDS. His early concepts dealt with possible activation events within the immune system. With his colleague, Mario Clerici, he pioneered the potential role of a TH1-to-TH2 shift in cytokine production as being responsible in HIV infection for the progression to disease.

transmission of the virus containing the homologous envelope region (3551). Prime-boost immunization with core (Gag-Pol) antigens alone did not achieve protection from infection by the homologus cloned virus but resulted in transient and low viremia in infected animals (3552). Inclusion of both envelope and core antigens in the vaccine design increased the breadth of the response, resulting in protection against both cloned and uncloned SIV_{mne} challenge by the intravenous route (3552).

In related cynomolgus monkey studies with HIV-2, a recombinant canarypox virus was used expressing the HIV-2 envelope gp125 or the V3 synthetic peptide. High antibody titers, some of which were neutralizing, were induced, as were HIV-2-specific CTLs. Despite booster immunizations with gp125, only 4 of 10 animals showed full protection from HIV-2 challenge. There was no correlation between immunologic response and protection (120). In other vaccine experiments, naturally attenuated vaccinia virus or a nonreplicating canarypox virus vector expressing HIV-2 envelope and subunit boosts were used to immunize 18 juvenile rhesus macaques. Despite several boosters and the presence of neutralizing antibodies, none of the animals was protected from HIV-2 challenge (3184). Thus, with HIV-2, this immunization procedure was not sufficient to give protective immunity. Nevertheless, in other earlier studies, protection from SIV infection was achieved with an attenuated HIV-2 envelope recombinant poxvirus in the SIV model (1349). Cross-reactivity must have been involved. However, the general lack of

wide cross-reactivity after vaccination underlines problems faced in developing an effective anti-HIV vaccine based solely on the viral envelope (Section VIII).

Promising studies in rhesus monkeys showed that immunization with recombinant modified vaccinia virus Ankara (MVA) vectors expressing the SIV_{mac239} Gag-Pol and $HIV-1_{89.6}$ Env elicited strong Gag-specific CTL but no envelope neutralizing antibody responses. CTL responses against the $SHIV_{89.6P}$ virus observed prior to challenge correlated with control of viremia and prevention of disease (270).

One caveat to the use of vaccinia virus-based vaccines in humans is the reduced response observed in subjects who have previously been vaccinated for smallpox (879). Repeated boosting with gp160 overcame this problem in the SIV model (1915), and that approach or the use of canarypox virus vectors might avoid this problem in humans.

2. ADENOVIRUS

An adenovirus-based vaccine regimen is currently being emphasized (for a review, see reference 269) and has been effective in protecting chimpanzees from HIV-1 infection (2687). In this regard, a replication-incompetent adenovirus 5 vector containing SIV Gag, Env, or Tat DNA, followed by a booster with the DNA vector, has been evaluated in macaques. The animals immunized with SIV Gag and Env, but not Tat, were able to control the intravenous challenge with $SHIV_{89.6P}$ after immunization. A cellular anti-Gag response seems to have been involved (2584). In other studies, rhesus macaques were immunized with Gag DNA and adenovirus 5 vaccine constructs expressing SIV Gag. They were then challenged with SIV_{mac239} intrarectally. The reduction in viral load after SIV inoculation was observed with the DNA prime-adenovirus 5 boost protocol and not adenovirus 5 immunizations alone (631). However, virus escape was noted within 6 months after challenge. A lack of persistent control of SIV_{mac239} could not be explained by escape from the dominant Gag response (2910). Other mechanisms must be involved (see Chapter 11). In other studies, nearly 40% of the rhesus macaques receiving a prime with a replicating adenovirus-SIV multigene vaccine and a boost with SIV envelope subunits showed strong protection from intrarectal SIV_{mac259} challenge (3442a). Many of these same animals had similar protection during rechallenge one year later. Cellular immunity appeared to be the major factor determining this protection (2778a).

These results have led to the use of adenovirus 5 vector studies in human trials (see Section XII). A concern is that the widespread presence of antibodies to adenovirus 5 in human populations can compromise vaccine efficacy (4119, 4336). Nevertheless, in studies comparing a replication-defective adenovirus serotype 5 vector to MVA, as well as certain DNA vaccine formulations for Gag, the adenovirus vector was the most effective in eliciting anti-Gag CTL response. If rhesus macaques were preexposed to adenovirus subtype 5, the immune responses were reduced but not eliminated. Priming with different DNA vaccine formulations followed by a boost of adenovirus vector has also been found to be most effective and gave promising results for a vaccine that could overcome the existing immunity against adenoviruses (630). Some investigators are also experimenting with a chimpanzee adenovirus to avoid this problem (1302).

Currently, an efficacy vaccine trial sponsored by Merck Pharmaceuticals is in progress involving 3,000 HIV-negative volunteers with or without persistent adenovirus 5 infection. The approach uses nonreplicating adenovirus 5 expressing Gag for priming and a boost with HIV envelope gp120 (VaxGen). If substantial immune responses are elicited, a full experimental human trial will be initiated (see Section XII).

3. OTHER VIRUSES

To have the best expression of an antigen, live virus vectors should infect DCs and express viral proteins after one or two cycles of replication. In this regard, using a Venezuelan equine encephalitis and Sindbis virus chimera vector (VEE/SIN) has offered promising results (1673). Moreover, a recombinant Semliki Forest virus vaccine expressing the SIV_{snm} PBJ14 envelope gp160 given with a recombinant gp120 subunit indicated that the immunized animals, after challenge with SIV, were protected from lethal disease though they became infected with the virus (3142).

The expression of HIV envelope proteins in association with other replicating or nonreplicating viruses has been reported (e.g., Ty, bluetongue virus, hepatitis B virus, adenovirus, Semliki Forest virus, rabies virus, rhinovirus, herpes simplex virus, Epstein-Barr virus, influenza virus, equine encephalitis virus, and polioviruses), as well as with bacteria (*Mycobacterium* [bacillus Calmette Guérin]) (57, 122, 585, 693, 1229, 1629, 2414, 2477, 2577, 2999, 3446, 3709, 3968, 4866) (Table 15.10). Work continues with these approaches, and some have been evaluated in nonhuman primates. A rabies virus vaccine has been derived containing a chimeric HIV-1 Env protein with covalently linked gp140 fused with the cytoplasmic domain of the rabies virus glycoprotein (2936). It is immunogenetic as assessed in murine studies. Moreover, the highly conserved ELDKWA epitope of gp41 has been expressed in the potato virus Xco protein and used to immunize mice intraperineally or intranasally. High levels of anti-HIV-1 antibodies were made which could neutralize HIV (2848).

Some systems, like the approaches using hepatitis B virus, are limited, since only small portions of the viral envelope can be inserted into the viral genome. However, observations on induction of anti-HIV responses with poliovirus chimeras, particularly those involving the replacement of the VP2 and VP3 genes with HIV-1 proteins (122, 3586), have provided encouraging results. In such studies, poliovirus vectors containing SIV *gag, pol, env, nef,* and *tat* in overlapping fragments (cocktails of 20 transgenic polioviruses) were inoculated into seven cynomolgus macaques. All the animals had anti-SIV antibodies, and some had CTL responses. After challenge intravaginally with a pathogenic SIV$_{mac251}$ isolate, 4 of the 7 vaccinated animals showed substantial protection, whereas all 12 control animals became SIV infected (922). Two of the seven vaccinated animals appeared to be completely protected from virus, and two had substantially reduced virus replication. All seven immunized animals remained healthy after challenge.

Another vector being explored is *Listeria monocytogenes* (1951). This gram-positive intracellular bacterium, through the nature of its replicative cycle, can present antigens through either class I or class II MHC molecules (Figure 15.2). Cell-mediated immune responses have been induced in mice by the use of this bacterium as a live vaccine vector for the HIV-1 Gag protein (1356). Other chromosomally modified strains of *L. monocytogenes* may prove useful. In contrast, oral immunization with recombinants from *Salmonella* expressing HIV-2 Gag and gp120 did not induce protection in an SIV model (1349).

4. SUMMARY

Most vaccine studies now suggest that priming with a vector-based vaccine (e.g., vaccinia or canarypox virus or adenovirus) followed by a protein subunit booster offers an excellent chance for induction of protection against virus challenge (Table 15.11). The time of virus challenge is important. At least 6 months appears to be required to establish protective immunity, and longer periods may work better. In studies with HIV-2-expressing recombinant poxviruses, long-lasting protection from SIV infection, even to a second challenge, was achieved in rhesus macaques (1349). A major question is whether promising results in the HIV-2/SIV model can be extrapolated to HIV-1. Currently, as noted above, a pilot adenovirus-based HIV Gag vaccine trial with an envelope gp120 boost is being conducted in humans (Section XII).

Using viral proteins (and not complete virus) as immunogens eliminates the possibility of viral nucleic acids becoming transcribed or undergoing cellular integration even if HIV-1 has been inactivated. Moreover, a killed HIV-1 preparation cannot guarantee antigenic stability of the viral proteins or the lack of residual infectivity. Nevertheless, as with other agents, these vaccine procedures with purified proteins, either alone or with a replicating vector, need to protect against high-dose virus challenge, transmission by infected cells, and mucosal inoculation. Whether their structure will mimic the viral protein associated in a virion is a major concern (Section VI).

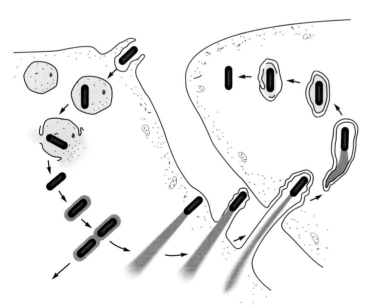

Figure 15.2 Stages in the entry, growth, movement, and spread of *L. monocytogenes*. The bacteria are endocytosed, fused with intracellular vesicles, and digested, and their antigens can be expressed with class II molecules. Alternatively, they can replicate out of the vesicles, become digested, and subsequently be expressed with class I molecules. Because of the value in expressing antigens by these two processes, this bacterium is being evaluated for use in HIV vaccine development. From reference 4431, with permission.

VI. Viral Cores as Vaccines

In a related approach to vaccine development, viral cores containing HIV envelope proteins are produced through the use of HIV or other retrovirus *gag* genetic regions (1931, 4175, 4643). These virus-like particles (VLPs) offer the advantage of a close similarity to HIV without the potential danger of an infectious virion. Thus, they could provide an immunogen that might induce an immune response best suited to recognizing the invading organism. Infection of cells with vaccinia virus constructs containing the core and envelope regions of HIV gives rise to VLPs that express gp120 on the surface and lack the HIV genome (1689, 1931, 4115, 4175) (Figure 15.3). These released retroviral-like structures can be purified in sucrose density gradients and potentially used for immunization (1689, 4087). Moreover, HIV-1-like particles can be produced with unprocessed gp160 glycoproteins that can elicit neutralizing antibodies on immunization of guinea pigs. They represent alternative immunogens for a particle-based AIDS vaccine (3824).

In another approach, the DNA for a replication-defective SIV mutant virus lacking the nucleocapsid was used in which a single infectious cycle takes place (1567) (see Section VII for DNA vaccine studies). Particles were produced that were RNA deficient but contained all the processed viral proteins. The immunized animals after SIV challenge showed decreased peak plasma viral loads and no CD4+ T-cell depletion or clinical disease after 2 years. A boost with an SIV protein did not change these results. The use of these replication-defective structurally complete virions offers another promising approach for an HIV vaccine (1567).

In a prime-boost study, an envelope and Gag DNA immunization was followed by a boost with p55 Gag VLPs and an envelope protein (2504). The booster immunization with the oligomeric envelope protein in MF59 gave strong antibodies and antigen-specific lymphoproliferative responses. The VLPs were effective in enhancing both cellular and humoral immune responses in baboons.

Vaccines with viral cores have also utilized the genetic sequences of other retroviruses or retrovirus-like agents. VLPs expressing the HIV-1 V3 loop have been made with the HIV-2 Gag protein (2701). Moreover, the yeast Ty retrotransposon was manipulated to produce VLPs expressing HIV-1 envelope epitopes (1629, 2440). The induction of mucosal immunity (i.e., anti-SIV antibodies) in primates after vaginal or rectal immunization with a Ty VLP expressing an SIV protein offered some hope for the successful induction of local immune responses (2477, 2478). In other studies, recombinant SIV gp120 and core p27 were inoculated into the iliac lymph nodes draining the genital-rectal region. Infection by the rectal route in four of seven macaques was prevented in association with an increase in immunoglobulin G (IgG) antibody-secreting cells (2480). In addition, VLPs have been derived using baculovirus recombinants containing the HIV-1 envelope (1048). Nevertheless, the potential problem of envelope glycosylation differences between vaccines grown in yeasts and those grown in mammalian cells must be considered. Importantly, for this approach, a major problem is producing sufficient amounts of the viral cores to use in vaccine trials.

VII. Viral DNA Inoculation

Another approach that has received attention during the past decade is the injection of DNA constructs directly into the host (for reviews, see references 3759 and 3761). For effectiveness, certain issues must be considered (Table 15.13). By this procedure, the antigenic epitopes of the immunizing proteins are expressed in a form that would be naturally recognized in the recipient. This procedure is especially helpful in inducing cell-mediated immunity. It was demonstrated as a method of gene therapy for cancer (4805) and for expression of cytokines (3192).

To obtain the most effective anti-HIV response via DNA vaccines, procedures for optimization of the construct for protein expression in human cells have been developed (3632, 4987). One of them involves eliminating the INS element (inhibitory sequences) in the structural genes (*gag*, *pol*, and *env*), thereby giving Rev/RRE-independent and species-independent expression (3987). The uptake of DNA is also important, and a variety of approaches have been used, including direct injection, gene guns, and lipid particles (2648). Electroporation

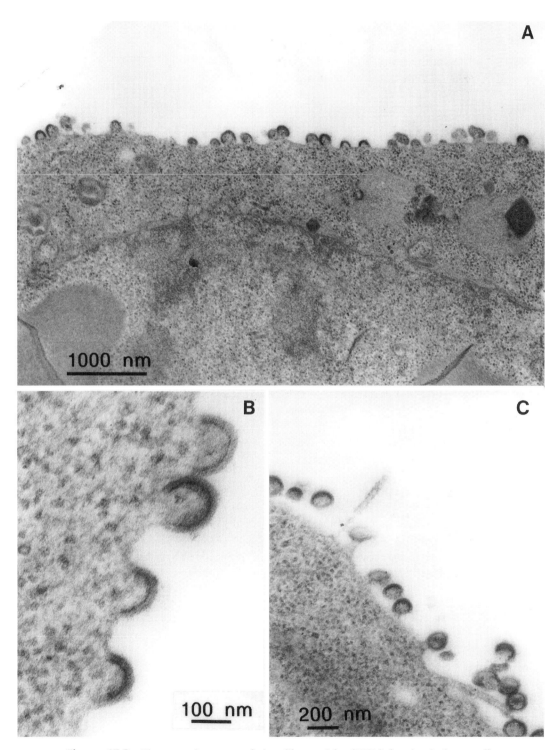

Figure 15.3 Electron microscopy of virus-like particles (VLPs) forming in insect cells transfected with a baculovirus construct expressing Gag/Pol. (A) VLPs budding from the plasma membrane. (B) A high magnification showing several intermediate stages in the budding process. (C) Extracellular VLPs. Reprinted from reference 1933 with permission.

Table 15.13 Important issues with DNA vaccines

- Should deliver to antigen-presenting cells
- Potential integration of plasmid DNA in the host genome must be avoided
- Generation of anti-DNA antibodies must be avoided

can enhance DNA uptake but might not be feasible for human trials (4752). Essentially, delivery to DCs for maximal antigen presentation is the goal (2358).

In studies involving nonhuman primates, inoculation and boosting of chimpanzees with a DNA HIV gp160 plasmid expression vector produced neutralizing and T-cell proliferative responses in all inoculated animals (4668). An HIV-1 envelope DNA vaccine given to rhesus monkeys elicited a type 1-like immune response (2486). Similarly, a plasmid DNA encoding the SIV envelope and Gag proteins induced CTL responses in rhesus macaques (4867). Chimpanzees have been protected against HIV-1 challenge by DNA immunizations with gp160 and *rev* as well as *gag* and *pol* sequences (474). This approach provided encouragement for obtaining protective immunity in humans. Moreover, macaques were primed with an HIV-1 envelope DNA (multiple doses) followed by boosting with the envelope DNA plus the HIV-1 envelope protein itself. An immune response was induced which protected the monkeys from infection with the HIV-1 chimeric SHIV virus. Thus, DNA priming followed by boost with both the DNA and envelope protein showed promise as an effective vaccine strategy (2503).

In this regard, DNA priming followed by a recombinant modified vaccinia virus (MVA) boost induced control of a highly pathogenic SIV in rhesus macaques. Priming with DNA was at 0 and 8 weeks and the boost with the MVA was at 24 weeks. The DNA was given by the intradermal (i.d.) or intramuscular (i.m.) route using a needleless jet injection device (Biojet). The MVA was injected with a needle i.d. and i.m. The DNA and MVA expressed multiple SIV proteins, and the immunization effectively limited virus replication following intrarectal challenge 7 months after the booster (91).

Another vaccine strategy in macaques evaluated DNA constructs encoding CTL epitopes and full-length proteins (Tat, Rev, and Nef) used in a DNA prime-recombinant modified MVA boost regimen. Both virus-specific CTL and CD4+ helper T-cell responses were observed. Intrarectal challenge with SIV_{mac239} controlled the virus in the acute phase but not in the chronic phase. The lack of a long-term effect was attributed to the absence of neutralizing antibodies (4618).

Recent studies in rhesus macaques evaluated a DNA prime-poxvirus boost regimen in which animals were given (i) a chimeric Rev/Tat/Nef protein alone; (ii) a combination of Gag, Pol, and Env proteins; or (iii) a combination of all six antigens (Table 15.12). While a reduction in CD8+ T-cell responses to the individual antigens was noted when all six were given, the vaccination showed a marked delay in the onset and a decrease in the viremia after intrarectal challenge with SIV_{mac251} (1794). The route of DNA administration only affected the humoral responses; intradermal delivery of DNA was 10 times better for antibodies to Gag. However, neither route of DNA delivery gave protection from infection (1794).

Very recently, rhesus macaques immunized with a DNA vaccine coding for four HIV envelope antigens and a Gag antigen from one subtype neutralized the homologous and, to some extent, heterologous HIV isolates. Four of six immunized animals were completely protected following intrarectal challenge with $SHIV_{BAL}$; the other animals had reduced viral loads (3386).

In other experiments, an HIV-2 DNA vaccine was evaluated in baboons in which optimized DNAs coding for the Gag, Pol, Tat, and Nef proteins were used. After four immunizations by the intranasal i.m., and i.d. routes, the baboons were challenged intravaginally with a pathogenic HIV-2 strain. The results indicated that DNA alone can induce both CD8+ and CD4+ cell cytotoxic anti-HIV responses and can dampen the viremia after virus challenge (2648). A surprising observation was that the control vector-immunized animals, after showing an initial burst of viremia, also controlled the HIV-2 challenge, whereas intravaginal titration of this same virus stock in normal baboons showed persistent viremia. The observation could indicate a role for innate immunity since certain motifs on the vector (e.g., CpG) (see Chapter 9) could have elicited an antiviral response (2648).

HIV-1 DNA immunization of human subjects has been conducted and has induced some antiviral immune responses (583, 2195). However, several negative results with DNA vaccines have also been reported. An experimental vaccine containing five DNA plasmids expressing different combinations and forms of the SIV_{mac251} proteins was used for multiple inoculations of rhesus macaques. Some were inoculated intravenously, some i.m., and others by gene gun procedures. CTLs were induced and neutralizing antibodies appeared in all the vaccinated animals but were transient. Some attenuation of the acute phase of infection was noted, but no protection from infection was achieved (2676). These results with DNA alone, as with the HIV-2 DNA vaccine studies (2648), suggested that a prime-boost approach using virus envelope protein as a boost may be the best strategy. In this regard, a DNA prime using a polyvalent HIV *env* vaccine formulation plus a protein boost induced in rabbits broadly reacting anti-HIV neutralizing antibodies (4674a). Nevertheless, most recently, DNA vaccines, because they elicit only limited and short-term cellular immune responses without humoral immunity, have not been highly recommended for a vaccine strategy, particularly when used alone (1112, 3761).

VIII. Other Vaccine Strategies

A. Cytokine Enhancement

Some studies have explored the possibility that immunization of animals with virus or viral proteins together with the administration of cytokines might increase the immune response and enhance protection from virus challenge. For example, vaccination of mice with leishmanial antigens and IL-12 promoted the development of type 1 cells and resistance to subsequent infection (27). Moreover, plasmids encoding the HIV-1 envelope and IL-12, when inoculated into mice, enhanced CTL activity (4497). This type 1 immune response appeared to be mediated by gamma interferon (IFN-γ). The use of IL-1α, IL-12, and IL-18 to replace cholera toxin as an adjuvant for intranasal immunization (to induce mucosal immunity) has also shown promise (481) (Section IX). Work in other infectious disease systems has also suggested that an IL-2-based vaccine might enhance the type 1 responses needed for good cell-mediated immunity (4832).

In experiments with primates, rhesus macaques were vaccinated with an SIV attenuated (*nef* deletion) mutant that expressed IFN-γ. Although the animals became infected on challenge, they had a less pathogenic course and remained healthy for a longer period than did the naïve controls (1505). Other vaccine studies using IL-2 and vaccinia virus constructs in rhesus macaques gave promising results (270, 271). In one study, the immunized animals had good CD4+ and CD8+ cell anti-HIV responses and after challenge had low viral loads, high antibody levels, and no clinical signs (271). In another study, the rhesus macaques were immunized with a DNA vaccine expressing the SIV_{mac239} Gag and the $SHIV_{89.6P}$ envelope or a vaccinia virus fusion protein with or without an IL-2 immunoglobulin plasmid (270). All animals receiving the cytokine-augmented DNA vaccine developed potent virus-specific CD4+ cell proliferation and CTL responses as well as antiviral antibodies. They maintained control of the intravenous $SHIV_{89.6P}$ challenge infection without disease for almost 5 months. However, one animal later showed a single nucleotide mutation within the immunodominant CTL Gag epitope, resulting in virus escape and a return of viral replication and clinical disease (267). These results indicate that solely one or a dominant CTL response against the virus may not be effective for an HIV-1 vaccine (see reference 268 for a review on cytokines as vaccine adjuvants).

If DCs can be brought to the site of immunization through plasmids encoding chemokines or DC-inducing factors (e.g., Flt-3 ligand), the vaccine efficacy can also be improved (4335). The availability of mature DCs at the site of inoculation can be an important rate-limiting factor for DNA vaccine immunogenicity. Giving plasmid MIP-1α and Flt-3 ligands with DNA vaccines has yielded a dramatic increase in DCs at the site of antigen production and augmented the efficacy of a DNA vaccine (4335). Finally, approaches to enhance mucosal immunity have also used selected cytokines (Section IX).

B. Other Approaches

Another strategy could be to generate anti-CCR5 antibodies in the genital mucosa that can be achieved through systemic and mucosal routes (243). Recently, a synthetic form of the HIV-1 coreceptor CCR5 was used to immunize cynomolgus macaques. The antiserum produced reacted with both human and macaque CCR5 and suppressed infection of HIV-1 (R5) in vitro. There was a significantly reduced plasma viral load at 1 week post-intravaginal challenge (3029). This approach may also add to the antiviral responses of other vaccines. In other studies, monocyte-derived dendritic cells pulsed with HIV p24 and other antigens were shown to enhance the recall proliferative responses of CD4$^+$ T cells (3245). The results place further emphasis on DCs as an approach in immunization to enhance HIV-specific responses. Their role in postinfection immunization is discussed in Chapter 14.

IX. Induction of Mucosal Immunity

Mucosal immunity against HIV, particularly in relationship to vaccines, is certainly important (2981) and merits serious consideration. Selective immunization at easily targeted mucosal sites (e.g., the nasal canal) might bring effective responses, since the mucosal immune system appears to be interconnected throughout the body (for reviews, see references 2925 and 2981) (Figure 15.4). Moreover, such approaches should elicit responses of innate immune cells present at the mucosal locations.

One of the first indications that antiviral responses could be present in the vaginal canal came from studies of CTLs in SIV infection (2655). SIV-specific precursor CTLs from chronically infected monkeys and from acutely infected animals were found at a higher frequency at this site. Likewise, virus-specific CTLs have been recovered from the small intestines of SIV-infected macaques. Similar studies of HIV have not been as comprehensive, but the results indicate that infected women (3180) as well as men (1922) have CTL activity in the genital tract (see Chapters 2 and 11). Evidence of humoral responses has also been found in the cervicovaginal region. IgG and IgA antibodies to the envelope protein for both HIV-1 and HIV-2 have

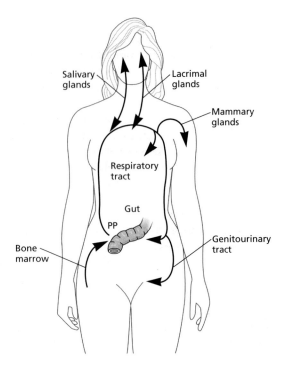

Figure 15.4 Interconnections of the mucosal immune system that involve the oral, nasal, urethral, vaginal, and rectal cavities. PP, Peyer's patches. Provided by J. Mestecky.

been detected. IgA was more prominent in cervical secretions than in the blood and had high specific activity, suggesting local synthesis of antibodies to HIV (317). Antibodies have also been found in nasal (154) and rectal (3046) washes.

In terms of an HIV vaccine, the mucosal immune system of the female genital tract has been well characterized (486) and consists of a variety of secreted factors, including chemokines, defensins, and complement. Cellular components include NK cells, plasmacytoid dendritic cells, γδ T cells, and plasma cells secreting IgA. Studies of the mucosal immune system in female rhesus macaques have indicated the presence of monocytes/macrophages as well as T and B lymphocytes in the lamina propria of the vagina just beneath the vaginal epithelium (2717). A large number of CD8$^+$ T cells are found within the vaginal epithelium and can consist of SIV-specific cytotoxic T cells (2655). These CD8$^+$ cells can also constitute the antiviral response associated with innate immunity. As noted above, anti-HIV CTLs have been found in genital fluids.

Both male and female genital tract tissues lack inductive mucosal sites analogous to the Peyer's patches in the gastrointestional system (2981). Therefore, local immune responses are usually low (see Chapters 10 and 11). It would appear that induction of innate immunity in the mucosae (see Chapter 9) as well as neutralizing antibodies (see Chapter 10) would be important for protection from infection. In attempting to induce immune responses in the mucosae, a variety of techniques using animal models have been evaluated (for reviews, see references 2981 and 3846) (Section III). They consider the fact that the mucosal immune system seems to be interconnected (Figure 15.4) and that immunization by one mucosal route could elicit immune responses in other mucosal sites.

Most vaccines against mucosal infections are given orally (1878). In one series of experiments, young mice were immunized orally with peptides of HIV-1 strains, after stomach acidity was neutralized. A high-titer secretory neutralizing antibody of IgA type was found in the bowel (550). In another group of studies using intranasal administration to mice, a DNA HIV vaccine, combined with liposomes and IL-12 and granulocyte-macrophage colony-stimulating factor (GM-CSF)-expressing plasmids, induced strong levels of both humoral and cellular immune responses (3324). Anti-HIV neutralizing antibodies were found in both feces and serum. As noted in Section VIII, IL-1α, IL-12, and IL-18 have been used as adjuvants to induce mucosal immunity (481). Intranasal immunization of mice with HIV-1 Gag and CpG also gave protection against intravaginal challenge with a vaccinia virus expressing HIV-1 Gag (1148). Intranasal immunization can give protection as well in the upper respiratory tract and the genital region (1878). For example, cold-adapted influenza virus is given via a nasal spray (Flumist). Moreover, studies in humans using the cholera toxin B subunit protein as an immunogen indicated that immunization via the nasal route was optimal for inducing anti-cholera toxin immunoglobulins in nasal secretions as well as vaginal secretions. Oral administration induced antibodies in the vagina but not in the nasal cavity (3837).

In early studies, vaginal, followed by oral, administration of a recombinant, particulate SIV antigen elicited three types of immunity: (i) Gag p27-specific, secretory IgA and IgG in the vaginal fluid, (ii) specific CD4$^+$ T-cell proliferation and helper function in B-cell p27-specific IgA synthesis in the genital lymph nodes, and (iii) specific serum IgA and IgG, with CD4$^+$ T-cell proliferative and helper functions in the circulating blood (2477). In other experiments, direct inoculation of live attenuated SIV into the vaginas of macaques generated IgM and IgA antibodies against the virus in serum and vaginal secretions and viral-specific CTLs in the peripheral blood (2654). Likewise, in an attenuated SIV$_{mac\ 1A11}$ infection of fetal or neonatal rhesus macaques, transient viremia, anti-SIV responses, and weak or no CTL activity were observed. Some of the animals were protected from a subsequent oral challenge with pathogenic SIV$_{mac251}$ shortly after birth. The results showed that protection by the mucosal route can be achieved early in development and confirmed that the virus can be transmitted to newborn monkeys by the oral route (191, 3357).

In another study, nontraumatic inoculation of the vaginas of rhesus macaques was performed with a nonpathogenic SHIV 89.6 chimera that can establish a systemic infection (2680, 2681). Once this infection was controlled in the host, the monkeys were superinfected intravaginally with pathogenic SIV$_{mac239}$, and protection from the second infection was achieved (2680, 2681). In similar studies using the rectal route for HIV-2 administration, monkeys were not protected from subsequent SIV challenge (4655). The result may reflect the low-level replication of the HIV-2 strain (Figure 15.1; Section II and Chapter 1). Nevertheless, macaques infected with a *nef*-deleted SIV were protected against superinfection (via the rectal mucosa) of a pathogenic strain of SIV or a SHIV isolate composed of the envelope of the cytopathic HIV-1$_{SF33}$ strain (914). Moreover, baboons, immunized in part by the intranasal route with viral DNA, appeared to control an intravaginal HIV-2 challenge (2648).

Encouraging results were also obtained when three pregnant macaques were vaccinated with either modified vaccinia virus Ankara (MVA) expressing SIV Gag, Pol, and Env or live attenuated SIV$_{mac1A11}$ against the SIV$_{mac}$ strain. The newborns were challenged with virus via the oral or conjunctival route. Two of the animals were protected against SIV infection at birth. Thus, the immunization and receipt of immunoglobulin from the mother may decrease the rate of perinatal transmission by the mucosal route (4563).

Furthermore, in attempts to generate immune responses at mucosal surfaces, macaques were immunized intranasally, i.m., or intrarectally using a highly attenuated poxvirus, NYVAC SIV$_{gpe}$ vaccine. All animals showed antigen-specific CD8$^+$ T cells in mucosal tissues irrespective of the immunization route (4289). In all cases, following mucosal SIV$_{mac}$ challenge, antigen-specific responses were detected in the mucosal tissues. Thus, a live vector vaccine may elicit a good mucosal response whether administered by the mucosal or parenteral route (4289). In another study, an intrarectal peptide prime-poxvirus boost vaccine in macaques elicited a strong antiviral mucosal CD8$^+$ CTL response and prevented infection or reduced virus spread after a SHIV intrarectal challenge (301). Other encouraging studies have shown that protection from mucosal infection can be achieved by solely parenteral immunization (3551). Thus, with strategies using HIV, mucosal immunity could be elicited by either mucosal or parenteral administration of the vaccine.

Finally, rhesus macaques immunized by the intranasal route with an HIV-1 envelope peptide immunogen showed no anti-HIV antibody responses in nasal or genital mucosal sites, but a limited response was induced when the peptide was used with recombinant IL-1α and GM-CSF. In contrast, the antibody responses at both sites were high in animals immunized parenterally with the peptide and an adjuvant. The results suggested that parenteral vaccine administration with an appropriate adjuvant can elicit human humoral responses in the blood and at mucosal locations (1174).

X. Adjuvants

A. Overview

Immune stimulatory compounds that can enhance vaccines through innate immune responses deserve increased attention (3433). The approach considers the appropriate adjuvants (i.e., immune potentiators and delivery vehicle) for the optimal induction of immune responses against viral antigens (Table 15.14). The delivery system (cationic microparticles or liposomes) can concentrate and present antigens along with immune potentiators in a manner best recognized by antigen-presenting cells. Most current adjuvants are delivery vehicles (e.g., ammonium sulfate [alum] and oil-water emulsions), and immune potentiators need to be included. The strategy can involve cytokines (Section VIII.A), hormones, and nucleic acids, as well as small molecules (3433) (see below).

B. Synthetic

In addition to using the appropriate antigen in a vaccine, an adjuvant containing the immune potentiator in a delivery vehicle is very important for inducing the innate immune system to respond against the virus (for reviews, see references 69 and 3433). This approach aims to elicit both innate and adaptive antiviral activities (2529, 2533). The adjuvant should not produce unacceptable reactions at the injection sites and should have low systemic toxicity. Formulations and delivery systems can be developed to limit systemic distribution of the adjuvant from the injection site.

Table 15.14 Adjuvants to augment cell-mediated and humoral immune responses[a]

Adjuvant	Vehicle
Muramyl dipeptide analogues (e.g., N-acetylmuramyl-t-threonyl-D-isoglutamine)	Squalene L121 emulsion
Muramyl tripeptide phosphatidylethanolamine	Squalene emulsion
Monophosphoryl lipid A (RIBI)	Squalene emulsion liposomes
Saponin (e.g., QS21)	Immune-stimulating complexes

[a]See Section X.B. In addition, the surfactants Tween 80 and Span 85 are used to replace Ariacel A found in Freund's complete adjuvant. The use of cytokines (e.g., interleukin-2 and granulocyte-macrophage colony-stimulating factor) or cell surface ligands as adjuvants is discussed in Sections VIII.A and X.C.

This approach minimizes systemic toxicity and possibly allows higher doses of adjuvant or the use of the adjuvants that would otherwise be too toxic given systemically. The adjuvant should lead to cell-mediated immune responses, including CTL and CNAR (see Chapter 11), as well as antibodies with high affinity for the HIV antigens (see Chapter 10). Antibodies with protective isotypes can also activate complement and function synergistically with effector cells in ADCC processes (see Chapter 10).

The only adjuvants now approved for general human use are aluminum sulfate and aluminum phosphate (alum). Alum augments antibody formation by using most, but not all, antigens; it is ineffective with influenza virus hemagglutinin. Moreover, alum-precipitated antigens do not consistently elicit cell-mediated immunity. Hence, there is a need for adjuvants that have the potency of Freund's complete adjuvant (FCA) in eliciting a cellular immune response but do not induce granulomas at injection sites or produce other unacceptable side effects.

In some new adjuvant formulations, the mycobacterial cell wall component of FCA has been replaced by a synthetic muramyl dipeptide (MDP) or tripeptide (MTP), or by adjuvant-active analogues that are nonpyrogenic and have fewer other side effects, e.g., N-acetylmuramyl-l-threonyl-d-isoglutamine (Table 15.14). FCA is a water-in-mineral oil emulsion. The bulk oil phase remains at the injection site and is infiltrated by macrophages, which is why it produces granulomas. In other adjuvants, the mineral oil in FCA has been replaced by the naturally occurring lipid squalene or squalene in the form of a 5% microfluidized oil-in-water emulsion. The lipids can thus be metabolized by the body. In addition, more-defined surfactants such as Tween 80 and Span 85 are used instead of the Ariacel A surfactant in FCA. Some studies indicate that large animal species (e.g., primates), in contrast to rodents and rabbits, respond best to small-droplet stable emulsions (4554). Thus, this type of adjuvant formulation is recommended for inoculation in humans.

A microfluidized formulation, MF59, consists of an oil-in-water emulsion containing squalene, and surfactants. In addition, it has a phospholipid tail that facilitates association with the lipid phases. MF59 has been demonstrated to be an effective vehicle for influenza virus, herpes simplex virus, and HIV antigens in animal models, and as an adjuvant has been used in clinical trials with these virus vaccines (2065, 2066, 3543). The mechanism of action of MF59 remains to be determined.

With the RIBI adjuvant, the toxicity of the lipid A component of gram-negative bacterial lipopolysaccharide is decreased by removal of a labile phosphate group. The resulting monophosphoryl-lipid A (MPL) is added to squalene emulsions alone or in combination with trehalose dimycolate and/or cell wall skeleton from *Mycobacterium phlei* (3836). One form of the RIBI adjuvant ("Detox") has been used in clinical trials for melanoma and malaria vaccines (3730). MPL has also been combined with liposomes, augmenting their efficacy as adjuvants (3723), and these formulations have also been used in clinical trials with a malaria vaccine (1565). They interact with Toll-like receptor 2 (TLR-2) and TLR-4 (Section X.C). For cell-mediated immunity, liposomes have the potential to carry antigens to antigen-presenting cells such as macrophages, DC, and Langerhans cells in the skin. They can also concentrate the proteins at the site of inoculation and release them gradually, thus maintaining a constant antigenic stimulation.

Yet another group of adjuvants is based on saponins, glycosylated triterpenes derived from plants, usually *Quillaia saponaria*. Saponins are highly surface active and cytolytic, so they can produce tissue damage at injection sites. Such damage is reduced by using purified fractions (e.g., QS21) (2158). This adjuvant has been added to SIV Gag and envelope proteins and has induced CTL responses (3243), but no protection from challenge. Studies using this adjuvant with HIV-1 lipopeptides showed an effect on B-cell and CD4$^+$ cell responses (1404) (see below).

Toxic effects of adjuvants can be avoided as well by decreasing the amount of residual saponin in the vaccine through the formation of immune-stimulating complexes (ISCOMs) (1013, 3101). These are regular, cage-like structures containing saponin and virus envelope glycoproteins. ISCOMs containing gp120 of HIV elicit neutralizing antibodies and CD8$^+$ CTLs in mice (4361). SIV envelope and Gag proteins incorporated into ISCOMs were used to immunize monkeys. Despite CTL and neutralizing antibodies, no protection was achieved (1935). Highly purified saponin has also enhanced cell-mediated immune responses to HIV when used as a component in an experimental gp160 vaccine with alum (4823).

The above adjuvant formulations have been shown to induce protective responses against HIV and perhaps SIV, although in the latter case, cellular antigens could be involved (616, 1061, 3177). Some adjuvants have demonstrated effectiveness in inducing immunogenicity to the vaccine in chimpanzees and humans, e.g., in eliciting anti-HIV responses, with an encouraging safety profile (1524, 2065).

Another approach has been developed that adds a single palmitoyl chain to an HIV-specific peptide and gives the mixture as a lipopeptide vaccine. Promising results with both antibody and cellular anti-HIV immune responses were seen (1403). The use of lipopeptide adjuvants with Tat has been reported (448, 1404) (see above). Phase II clinical trials with such an approach, however, have been associated with cases of neurologic disease, and further studies have not been conducted.

C. Cell Surface Ligands

Agonists to TLR-7 (e.g., imiquimod) and TLR-9 (CpG) induce antiviral cytokines that could enhance innate and adaptive immune responses (880, 1711) (see Chapter 9). However, direct inoculation of innate molecules into the vaginas of rhesus macaques led to inflammation and a subsequent increased risk of SIV transmission (4677).

Immunization of an HIV Gag protein conjugated to a TLR-7/-8 agonist or TLR-9 ligand (CpG) has significantly increased Gag-specific CD4+ T-cell and antibody responses in rhesus macaques (4764). In other studies using a hepatitis B virus antigen vaccine, CpG appeared to be superior to a TLR-7/-8 agonist in inducing humoral and cell-mediated immune responses (4698).

Genetic immune potentiators derived from small DNA sequences (with CpG motifs) have been found to increase immune reactivity, particularly type 1 responses (2328, 4226). CpG oligodeoxynucleotides, by interacting and activating TLR-9, were shown to improve the response of hepatitis B immunization in both healthy and SIV-infected macaques (4593) and in HIV-infected subjects (880). CpG as an efficient vaccine immune potentiator also elicited strong antigen-specific T-cell responses against melanoma antigens (4226), most particularly by inhibition of IFN-α and IL-12 (2328). CpG combined with a Gag-Env pseudovirus induced high levels of anti-gp120 antibodies (1711) (see Chapter 11). Other approaches for eliciting mucosal immunity need to be explored (Section IX). For example, the coadministration of a B7-2 expression plasmid with a DNA vaccine has enhanced the cell-mediated immune response to HIV in mice (4498).

D. Alloimmunogens

Some early work suggested that HLA alloantigens could be used for enhancing immune responses to an antigen, e.g., influenza virus A (816). Since alloimmunization elicits a strong cell-mediated immune response as well as cytokines that can induce both innate and adaptive immune responses, some level of protection might be obtained through this type of approach (2479). The cytokine production could be particularly effective in eliciting innate immunity at mucosal sites to prevent infection by all HIV strains (3485).

Encouragement for this strategy came from the experience with SIV grown in human cells (4302) and other studies with SIV (157) (see Section IV). Moreover, chemokines and CD8+ cell antiviral factors were found to be produced by CD8+ cells from women following alloimmunization (4679). Heterosexual activity elicited mucosal alloimmunization in the partners, leading to reduced susceptibility of their PBMC to HIV infection (3485). Alloresponses can also elicit IFN-α production (3522). Finally, the observation that HLA concordance increases perinatal HIV transmission supports a role of alloresponses in protection from HIV infection (2725). For such alloimmunization, infected human PBMC, cell hybrids, or HLA antigens could be used as immune potentiators in a vaccine (1627, 2479).

XI. Potential Problems Involved in Vaccination

Three major potential risks resulting from vaccination need to be considered.

A. Antibody-Dependent Enhancement

Antibody-dependent enhancement (ADE), discussed in Chapter 10, can result from antiviral antibodies with lower affinity and avidity for the viral proteins (2239). In some vaccine experiments, monkeys immunized with an SIV variable (V2) domain produced neutralizing antibodies to the homologous virus but were not protected from infection. In certain cases, the viral loads were higher in the vaccinated animals than controls, suggesting ADE of virus infection (3968). In other vaccine studies, monkeys immunized against the region in the SIV gp41 transmembrane glycoprotein that is associated with ADE had enhancing antibodies and showed a more rapid progression to disease (3031).

Similar observations were noted with EIAV vaccine studies using a baculovirus-derived virus envelope (1965), which lacks the normal host cell-derived glycosylation pattern. In other studies, horses were protected from infection from a high-dose challenge of homologous but not heterologous EIAV (1965). In these experiments, however, an increase in disease was observed in some immunized animals, suggesting the induction of detrimental immune enhancement responses.

In addition, cats immunized with three different recombinant FIV candidate vaccines, including vaccinia virus-based vectors, showed higher viral loads after challenge. Antibodies produced during the recombinant vaccinia virus immunization were transferred to naïve cats, and enhanced virus infection and replication were noted (4131). Thus, ADE appeared to be a detrimental result of ineffective vaccination. Concern about the possibility of ADE as a result of HIV immunization led to recommendations to evaluate this phenomenon in vaccine trials (2859). Fortunately, some studies have indicated that as titers of neutralizing antibodies increase, the effect of enhancing antibodies can be prevented (3071). The findings suggest that booster immunizations that increase antibody production could elicit more high-affinity neutralizing antibodies.

In vaccine studies with rhesus macaques using an attenuated recombinant herpes zoster virus vaccine expressing the SIV envelope, nonneutralizing envelope antibodies were made and very little CTL activity was observed. After SIV challenge, there was an enhancement of virus replication (4261). The reason for this enhancement was not determined, but one explanation was lymphocyte activation enhancement (2101, 3726); another possibility, not considered, was Fc-mediated antibody enhancement (see Chapter 10). These observations again underline the challenging problem of developing a vaccine that does not enhance the risk of infection.

Finally, most recently, polymorphisms in the genes encoding Fcγ RIIa and RIIIa were found to influence possibly the efficacy of vaccination with recombinant rgp120. In the VaxGen trials (Section XII), individuals who were homozygous for both the high-affinity V allele of Fcγ RIIIa and the high-affinity H allele of FCγ RIIa were more likely to be infected with HIV if they were vaccinated than if they received a placebo (1330). This finding, which needs confirmation, suggests that Fcγ R-mediated antibody enhancement of HIV infection may occur in vivo.

B. Clonal Dominance

Some investigators warn that priming of B cells for an immunologic response may induce a clonal dominant reaction and prevent the response of other B cells to new antigens (2254) (see Chapter 10, Section II.C). This possibility of "original antigenic sin" (1351) has been observed in studies in mice receiving polyvalent mixtures of HIV immunogens (2254). In one model, adult mice were immunized with recombinant gp120 before mating. The 3-week-old offspring were subsequently immunized with the same vaccine, and an inhibition of the IgG response was noted (2019). However, various procedures for changing the sequence of administration or the administration of many components together can overcome some of this suppression (1769). Moreover, masking of the antigenic domain through the addition of carbohydrates and a reduction in net positive charge has been evaluated in animals to counter the suppressive effects of immunodominant epitopes in a primary immune response to HIV. A qualitative shift in antibody production was noted (1454). This approach might be helpful in eliciting a more broadly reactive response from HIV vaccines.

C. T-Cell Receptor Antagonism

In other studies suggesting immune competition, a vaccinated human volunteer who subsequently became infected by HIV showed the presence only of a CTL clone that was able to recognize the vaccine strain. When the CD8+ cells were exposed to a peptide derived from the epitope sequence of the infecting isolate, the CTL activity against the vaccine strain was inhibited (2160). This finding appeared to present the first evidence in vivo of the T-cell receptor antagonism that had been demonstrated by previous in vitro studies (346, 2234).

XII. Human Vaccine Trials

A. Approaches to Clinical Trials

Various steps are involved in conducting vaccine trials. They can be summarized into three phases:

(i) **Phase I**. This trial takes about 12 to 18 months and involves a small group of HIV-seronegative individuals who are tested for the safety of the vaccine candidate and early immunogenicity.

(ii) **Phase II**. This trial with a prospective vaccine involves several hundred individuals and tests safety, dose optimization, and immunogenicity. It can take about 1 to 2 years.

(iii) **Phase III**. This final trial involves several thousand individuals and tests the efficacy of the vaccine approach. Essentially, one group of individuals receives the vaccine and the other gets a placebo control. The extent of HIV transmission is measured as well as the effect of the vaccine on virus replication if transmission takes place. Everyone receives risk reduction counseling and other prevention messages. Phase III trials can take several years (see below).

Recently, a decision was made by developers of HIV vaccine trials to have a limited or "test of concept" efficacy trial in which a smaller number of individuals (about 3,000) than used in a licensure efficacy trial will receive either vaccine or placebo. While efficacy for protection from infection may not be measurable unless a dramatic reduction in transmission occurs, a reduction of 0.5 log unit (threefold or greater) in viral load will be considered effective, as it has been associated with a slower progression to AIDS (see Chapter 13).

There are over 100 phase I trials and 20 phase II vaccine trials completed, on study, or undertaken or being considered in human volunteers. Only two phase III trials are completed; a third is in progress (see the International AIDS Vaccine Initiative website [http://www.iavi.org/] and the (UCSF Center for HIV Information InSite website [http://hivinsite.ucsf.edu/]. Two efficacy trials are also being conducted (see below). The first phase I trial of a human candidate HIV vaccine was done in 1987 based on a recombinant envelope gp120 or gp160 (see below). (1104; for a review, see reference 2052).

B. Viral Proteins and Poxvirus Vectors

Phase I to phase III vaccine trials have been conducted in humans with purified HIV envelope glycoprotein gp160 and gp120 or vaccinia virus-expressed HIV proteins. Moreover, a phase I trial of a Tat vaccine is being evaluated (1209a) (see also Section V). These studies, involving over 10,000 volunteers, have revealed no untoward clinical effects. In early studies the induction of low-level neutralizing antibodies and some cellular immune responses were demonstrated using purified viral envelope proteins (13, 430, 879, 1104, 1175, 1186, 1592, 1595, 1710, 2065, 2066, 2311, 3068, 3343, 4012). CTL responses and possibly CD8+ cell antiviral factor production were induced in seronegative volunteers by a recombinant HIV-1$_{SF2}$ gp160 vaccine (430). A low dose of nonreplicating canarypox virus vector expressing the HIV-1$_{MN}$ envelope-like protein induced CTL activity in seronegative volunteers (1175). Moreover, studies with a vaccine based on muramyl-tripeptide phosphatidylethanolamine (Table 15.14) containing the glycosylated gp120 from the HIV-1$_{SF2}$ strain gave relatively high levels of neutralizing antibodies and cellular immune responses in human volunteers (2065, 2066). Finally, promising results were obtained with HIV-infected subjects immunized with antigens linked to DCs for delivery as has been described in animal systems (528). Mature DCs infected with canarypox virus vector gave strong CD4+ and CD8+ T-cell responses (1205). The approach recently used in therapy (2677) (see Chapter 14) may be effective in prevention strategies and merits further evaluation in human clinical trials.

Importantly, in the past 20 years only two phase III vaccine trials (VAX003 and VAX004) have been completed. A third one, evaluating a canarypox vaccine with a clade B HIV gp120 boost, is currently being evaluated in Thailand (see below) (3706). Moreover, an HVTN/Merck test of concept efficacy trial is underway using an adenovirus vaccine with about the same number of endpoints projected as the Thailand trial (see section XII.C). The length of time required to develop an effective vaccine reflects this low number of trials (Table 15.15). The VaxGen studies (VAX003 and VAX004) were based on encouraging observations made in chimpanzees in which immunization with recombinant gp120 protected the animals from HIV-1 infection (335) (see Section V.A). The factors involved in the initiation and completion of these trials indicate the current requirements for vaccine development (Table 15.16) (1350).

The first phase III trial, begun in June 1998 (using about 5,000 volunteers in the United States) (3717a), did not show protection using the envelope protein from two different HIV-1 clade B strains (an X4 laboratory strain and an R5 clinical isolate). Despite the presence of neutralizing antibodies induced in the individuals in this placebo-controlled phase III trial, there was no overall protective effect noted (1350, 1514, 3717a). The vaccine did not prevent infection, which occurred in 6.7% of the vaccinees and 7% of the placebo recipients. There was no difference in viral load or the genetic characteristics of the infecting HIV-1 strains between the two groups. A second phase III begun in March 1999 in Thailand with 2,500 volunteers used a bivalent gp120 (from clades B and E). These results also showed no protective effect for HIV infection (1350, 1513). Moreover,

Table 15.15 What is the shortest time that an effective vaccine could be developed?[a]

- Perform phase I studies (1–2 yrs)
- Perform phase II studies (1–2 yrs)
- Perform phase III studies (3–4 yrs)
- License, produce, and distribute (1–2 yrs?)
- Best case scenario: 6–10 yrs from the time a vaccine is ready for phase I testing to distribution

[a]From S. Buchbinder and J. Fuchs.

Table 15.16 Factors involved in the completion of two phase III vaccine trials[a]

Number	Factor
2	Trials (3 yrs each)
4	Countries
78	Clinics
895	Employees
12,114	Volunteers screened
7,963	Volunteers enrolled
135,371	Clinic visits
55,741	Injections
71,667	Blood draws
1,005,000	Case report forms

[a]In the United States, Canada, The Netherlands, and Thailand. Reprinted from reference 1350 with permission.

after 3 years of observation, no effect of the vaccine on the clinical course of the infected subjects has been noted. No evidence of ADE was found (1513, 1514). Nevertheless, these first phase III trials have provided valuable information on the strategies needed to complete an HIV vaccine efficacy study (1350) (Table 15.16; Figure 15.5).

By another approach, a phase II trial with the canarypox virus vector (vCP205) expressing gp120, p55, and protease was conducted with 435 volunteers receiving or not receiving an MN virus recombinant gp120 boost. These studies were conducted after early trials with this protocol showed the induction of cross-reacting CTL activity (1283, 1710). The majority of volunteers given the vaccine (94%) had neutralizing antibodies to the MN strain, whereas 56% given the vector alone showed this humoral response. About one-third of the volunteers had anti-HIV CTLs whether receiving gp120 or not (299). These encouraging results led to a phase III trial that began in Kenya in 2001 and involved another poxvirus vector, MVA, and the *gag* gene as well as multiple CTL epitopes from the HIV-1 clade A subtype (4704). That trial was stopped in 2005 when no substantial immune response was noted (356).

Finally, as noted above, a prime-boost phase III vaccine trial (vCP1521) is in progress in Thailand using a recombinant canarypox vector (ALVAC) engineered to express antigens of HIV-1 gp120 (clade E) linked to the transmembrane-anchoring portion of gp41 (clade B) as well as of HIV-1 *gag* and protease (from clade B). The boost is the AIDSVAX

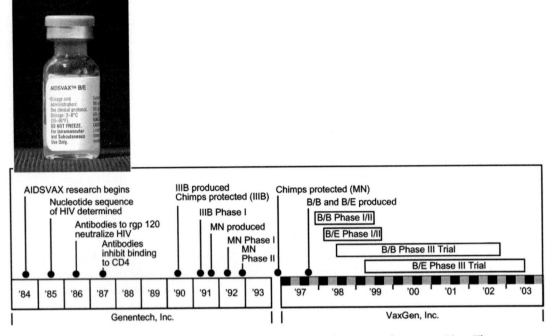

Figure 15.5 Timeline for phase III vaccine trials held in Canada, Puerto Rico, The Netherlands, and the United States. Reprinted from reference 1350 with permission.

gp120 B/E (VaxGen) bivalent HIV-1 gp120 envelope glycoprotein vaccine containing recombinant gp120 from clades B and E (3706).

C. Adenovirus Trial

The Merck pharmaceutical company is currently sponsoring an efficacy vaccine trial with a recombinant adenovirus 5 (rAd5) vector vaccine. It uses three separate clade B Gag, Pol, and Nef vectors for both priming and boosting the immune response in a three-dose regimen (4119a). About 3,000 subjects will be tested, of which some will have pre-existing adenovirus immunity. Protection of infection will be measurable, but only substantial reductions (~45%) in infection rate will be detectable. A threefold reduction in viral load can be assessed for those that get infection despite full counseling. The results of this current trial should be known in the next 2 to 3 years.

In addition, a phase II trial is being conducted through the Vaccine Research Center (VRC) at the NIH, in which a DNA vaccine consisting of clade B Gag, Pol, Nef, and Env plus clade A and C Env DNA are given as a prime, followed by a boost with an rAd5 vector that expresses a clade B Gag/Pol fusion protein and the clade A, B, and C envelope glycoproteins. Volunteers are also evaluated for pre-existing immunity to the adenovirus to evaluate the effect of pre-existing immunity on the immune response (for review, see reference 3761a).

XIII. Other HIV Prevention Approaches

Some investigators have explored the possibility that passive immunotherapy with antibodies or serum from HIV-positive individuals would be helpful in preventing infection. This approach for already-infected individuals is discussed in Chapter 14 (Section X). Animal studies using chimpanzees at first showed no protection from HIV after the administration of anti-HIV antibodies followed by a high-dose virus challenge (100 chimpanzee-infectious doses for a 50% infection rate [CID_{50}]) (3607). Nevertheless, a subsequent study with 10 CID_{50} prevented infection (3608). In one animal in the first experiment, enhancement of HIV infection was suspected (3607).

In another study, an anti-V3 loop monoclonal antibody was found to protect chimpanzees from infection with 75 CID given 24 h after the antibodies (1200). Moreover, when 75 CID was first inoculated into chimpanzees and followed 10 min later by the antiviral antibodies, protection from infection was also observed (1200). A similar finding on protection by passive immunization has been made with HIV and SIV in macaques (3626). However, the efficacy of this approach appears to be limited to just a few minutes after virus inoculation (A.M. Prince, personal communication). Passive immunization of macaques with immune sera or a pool of neutralizing monoclonal antibodies did not protect against an SIV challenge (72, 2159). This finding counters the results of the earlier study (3626), but the viruses in that earlier study were grown in human PBMC and not monkey PBMC. Moreover, macaques have been protected against vaginal transmission of pathogenic SHIV by passive infusion of anti-HIV monoclonal antibodies and immunoglobulins (2860). The application of passive immunization to prevention of infection, particularly after needlestick injuries or during childbirth, requires much further study, including the use of selected (even monoclonal) antibodies (4976).

XIV. Summary and Conclusions

Despite over two decades of research, work on an HIV vaccine remains a challenge. A great deal of information on why vaccines will not work has been accumulated. Very few experiments, primarily in nonhuman primates, have been conclusive in showing protection from virus infection (i.e., SIV). Some observations, however, have provided encouragement for the eventual development of an effective AIDS vaccine (Table 15.17). Nevertheless, the challenges for a rapid development of a vaccine are notable (Tables 15.6, 15.8, 15.15, and 15.16). Unfortunately, many of the animal (i.e., SIV) studies were done with so few animals that conclusions on efficacy are not possible. A full review of SIV trials is needed to determine what vaccine strategy does or does not show promise. Moreover, animal models can give us a direction, but human efficacy trials need to be conducted for definitive results.

Table 15.17 Examples of presumed protection against HIV or SIV infection

- Chimpanzees immunized with recombinant gp120 and challenged with primary or laboratory HIV-1 isolates
- Macaques protected against HIV-2 or SIV following various vaccine approaches
- Macaques vaccinated with live attenuated (*nef*-deleted) SIV
- Macaques exposed to low-dose rectal inoculation of SIV
- Macaques and baboons infected with attenuated SIV or HIV-2 protected from superinfection by pathogenic strains
- Seronegative individuals with multiple exposures to HIV (see Chapter 13)

An effective HIV vaccine will induce acute-phase innate immune responses that along with subsequent activated adaptive innate activity (Table 15.2) (3761) can prevent HIV infection (2533). Some investigators have emphasized the importance of T-cell memory in achieving protective immunity with vaccination (for review, see reference 4912a). Low antigen doses that can elicit T-cell help without overt inflammation are prerequisites for this induction of memory T-cells. In this regard, naïve CD8+ cells after initial exposure to antigen divide 7 to 10 times and differentiate into effector CTLs and long-lived functional memory CD8 T cells (for review, see reference 4912a) (see Chapter 11). The establishment of these central memory cells depends on the initial immune responses to vaccination, which involve the activity of the innate immune system (for review, see reference 3615a). Certainly elucidating the mechanisms by which innate immunity can affect the quantity and quality of long-term T- and B-cell memory can influence the effectiveness of immune responses to pathogens, as observed with some of the conventional vaccines (for review, see reference 3615a).

New approaches to elicit very early immune responses are needed, particularly those that consider innate immunity (2533, 3615a). Importantly, for a vaccine, the choice of an epitope should be based on its immunogenicity as well as whether an escape mutant would be less replication competent (see Chapter 9). In all these discussions is the recognition that HIV-1 transmission by the virus-infected cell can occur readily and that identifying and destroying this cell before transmission takes place will require new strategies in vaccine development (2522, 2529) (Tables 15.8 and 15.9).

The DNA vaccine approaches, through inoculation of specific viral genes, had offered encouraging results for clinical trials because the viral proteins can be expressed with MHC molecules on the surface of the host cells (3759) (Section VII). These vaccines are safe but unfortunately appear to be weakly immunogenic (3761). Nevertheless, a recent Vaccine Research Center DNA vaccine appears to be immunogenic, particularly for Env (3194). Adenovirus 5 vaccines offer a direction but can show reduced immunogenicity if antiadenovirus immunity is preexisting.

Unfortunately, the two phase III trials with an HIV-1 envelope vaccine alone were not successful. The best promise thus far has come from heterologous prime-boost combinations in which priming is performed with a live vector, attenuated strain, or DNA and the boost is done with a subunit viral protein alone or with a virus vector (Tables 15.11 and 15.12). More insight into vaccine approaches will come from present trials. Currently, however, only infection after homologous virus challenge in animal trials has been consistently prevented.

It appears that, in general, a type 1 immune response is the most effective in protecting against infection, although neutralizing antibodies that can block incoming free virus are important. Broadly cross-reacting neutralizing antibodies have been described (see Chapter 10). New information has been provided on mechanisms for inducing mucosal immunity, and new animal models have been described that could facilitate evaluation of vaccine strategies. These approaches include the other SHIV models and HIV-2 infection of pig-tailed macaques and baboons. In these studies, it is necessary to define the correlates of protective immunity that can be addressed in human trials (Table 15.2).

Because of the wide variety of HIV-1 and HIV-2 types, whether a vaccine directed at the envelope and other proteins of one particular virus will be effective is not known. Most investigators would agree that a shared viral region (e.g., certain domains of gp41) would be very important in vaccine development. However, it is also conceivable

that if an innate immune response can be induced, it would have a more general anti-HIV effect and could control infection by all types of HIV-1 strains (see Chapter 9). Innate immune responses appear to be responsible for protection against infection in highly exposed uninfected individuals (see Chapter 13).

Despite the lack of convincing evidence that an effective vaccine for HIV is available, many phase I and II human trials are being conducted in the United States, Thailand, and parts of Africa. Currently, 30 vaccine candidates are in human trials in 19 countries on five continents (http://www.iavi.org/). What perhaps needs continual consideration is the use of whole killed virus. While this technique carries a risk of live-virus survival, this risk should be controllable (e.g., by multiple inactivation steps and the use of killed attenuated HIV strains). This method, which has not received sufficient attention, offers the advantage of presenting a similar viral structure that would be encountered by the infected host. Importantly, studies of high-risk uninfected people suggest that frequent exposure to HIV antigens is important to maintain a viral defense (see Chapter 13). Thus, although certainly difficult to achieve, yearly booster shots or a persistent virus vector, perhaps controlled by inducible genes (e.g., tetracycline) may be needed. Furthermore, protein subunit vaccines should be delivered as oligomers of viral envelope (2696) or polymers containing mixtures of viral proteins, as has been used in malaria (3436).

One concern is whether weak vaccines will induce enhancing antibodies that will increase the chance of infection in some individuals. Moreover, through the induction of clonal dominance (2254), a limited immune response to one vaccine might prevent induction of a better antiviral response with a subsequent, more effective vaccine. For this reason, those conducting large-scale vaccine trials should consider not only the correlates of immunity that might be induced but also the parameters that might be detrimental to the immunized host (Section XI) and that might prevent an effective immune response when a more successful vaccine is developed. In this regard, the VaxGen trials did not show evidence of immune enhancement (1514).

Vaccine development could be targeted to mimic the immune responses that prevent establishment of HIV infection (e.g., in high-risk seronegative individuals). While some adaptive immune responses have been noted (CTL anti-HIV antibodies), they are not universally found, and it would appear that innate immune activity (DC and CD8$^+$ cell mediated) would be the most important (for review, see references 2533 and 3615a) (see Chapter 9). The cross-reactivity with HLA antigens does support the hypothesis of some that anti-allo responses might be helpful in preventing HIV infection (2479) (see Chapter 10). Thus, further work in examining the immunologic and, in some cases, genetic factors that enable some individuals to resist infection, albeit in most cases transiently, may be a direction worthy of additional investigation both for vaccine development and therapeutic strategies. Why this resistance is lost when exposure to HIV no longer takes place (e.g., in Nairobi sex workers) (see Chapter 13) needs to be considered in terms of vaccine development and approaches to induce longstanding protection from HIV infection and disease. One should not be discouraged. It took a long time to develop several conventional vaccines (Table 15.18). Compare these times to the length of time and the factors required for the ultimate licensing of an HIV vaccine (Tables 15.15 and 15.16).

This urgent need to develop an HIV vaccine has fortunately brought forward new funding programs for support of research and development (http://www.niaid.nih.gov/daids/vaccine/funding

.htm). These sources include the Global HIV/AIDS Vaccine Enterprise, which is funded in part by the Gates Foundation and the National Institutes of Health (NIH) (884, 2226). Part of this enterprise is the newly created Center for HIV/AIDS Vaccine Initiative; established by the U.S. government, it funds a virtual HIV/AIDS Vaccine Institute in the United States that resembles the Vaccine Center at NIH. Moreover, initiatives have been funded by the Gates Foundation that focus on neutralizing antibodies, T-cell-mediated immunity, and programs to develop methods for detection of immune correlates in resource-poor countries. It is hoped that this increased attention to vaccine development will bring success in the very near future.

Table 15.18 Development of licensed vaccines[a]

Vaccine	Discovery of etiologic agent	Vaccine developed or licensed in the United States	Years elapsed
Typhoid	1884	1896	12
Pertussis	1906	1926	20
Polio	1908	1955	47
Measles	1953	1983	30
Hepatitis B	1965	1981	16
Rotavirus	1970	1998	28
Hepatitis A	1973	1995	22
Lyme disease	1982	1998	16
HIV	1983	?	>20

[a]Provided by S. Buchbinder and J. Fuchs.

SALIENT FEATURES • CHAPTER 15

1. Development of a vaccine for prevention of HIV infection has included approaches with inactivated virus, attenuated viruses, viral cores, and purified envelope gp120, alone or in association with live expression vectors (virus or bacteria).

2. DNA inoculation offers a direction for a vaccine but has not recently given promising results.

3. The ideal vaccine is one that is safe and long lasting. It will induce local immunity with cellular and humoral immune responses of both innate and adaptive type, as well as antibodies that neutralize and do not enhance the infection.

4. Inoculation of attenuated virus has induced the best protection in animal studies but is not acceptable for human trials.

5. Thus far, the most safe and effective procedure for immunization has been to prime the host with a live vector (i.e., vaccinia, adenovirus) expressing HIV proteins, followed by a boost with a subunit protein or a live virus vector.

6. The success of vaccination may be increased through the coadministration of cytokines or Toll-like receptor agonists that can enhance the immune response.

7. Attention to mucosal immunity requires induction of both innate and adapative immune responses. Immunization via mucosal routes (e.g., intranasal and oral) is being explored.

8. All vaccine approaches require appropriate adjuvants that may selectively enhance innate and adaptive cell-mediated and humoral immunity.

9. Trials involving several human subjects have been conducted that have used subunit envelope vaccines. They did not show any efficacy.

10. Human trials involving a prime with poxvirus-based vaccine and an envelope boost have been conducted or are under study.

11. Prime-boost vaccine efficacy trials are being conducted with an adenovirus prime and an HIV envelope boost or a DNA prime with an adenovirus boost.

12. Potential problems involved in vaccination include autoimmunity, induction of enhancing antibody, clonal dominance, and T-cell receptor antagonism.

13. Passive immunotherapy to prevent HIV transmission is successful in animals when antibodies are administered within a few minutes after infection. This procedure for protection from infection requires more study.

14. Because of the intracellular nature of HIV, cell-mediated immune responses appear to be the most important mechanism for controlling or preventing HIV infection in the host.

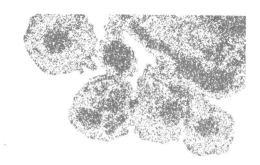

Conclusions

ENCOURAGING PROGRESS HAS BEEN made in understanding the pathogenesis of HIV infection, from the initial isolation of representative viruses in 1983 to the more recent development of effective antiviral drugs. Nevertheless, the path toward the eventual control of HIV still requires major efforts toward immune restoration and the development of an effective vaccine. While the direction appears to be more focused today, many avenues of study still need to be explored. Great advances continue to come from the treatment of opportunistic infections (for a review, see reference 1414). Importantly, HIV represents a new type of organism arising in human populations in epidemic proportions. Its characteristics define the challenges posed for its eventual control (Table A). Notably, whereas some reports of HIV replication in vitro suggested a recent attenuation of the virus (146), other studies examining the clinical course of HIV-1 infection over two decades do not suggest this result (3162). The virus, in several genetic diversities, maintains its pathogenic course. Obviously, virus virulence or "fitness" in vivo is the most important determinant of its clinical pathway.

The exact mechanisms for CD4$^+$ cell depletion and immune deficiency are not yet well defined, and its cellular latency, as well as several other features of HIV infection, remain mysterious. Moreover, whether recombinant viruses and more virulent and drug-resistant viruses are emerging in human populations as a result of continual transmission merits attention. Most importantly, how the advancements made in detection and, particularly, treatment of HIV infection in this country can be shared with less economically developed countries is a vital question.

New therapeutic avenues should now consider some of the approaches described in Chapter 14, such as targeting viral integrase and other HIV proteins. Harnessing the innate and adaptive

Table A How does HIV differ from other epidemic pathogens?

- Directly attacks the immune system
- Involves virus incorporation into the cellular genome
- Establishes a chronic infection before becoming pathogenic
- Involves an agent that frequently changes or modulates itself within the host
- Can recruit other cells by direct infection or cell-to-cell transfer

immune responses against HIV is an important direction. Can a further intracellular factor(s) that influences the relative replicating abilities of HIV be identified, and can the knowledge gained be used therapeutically? Certainly the advancement of our understanding of how the APOBEC3G and TRIM5α proteins can affect HIV infection are encouraging examples of the progress made in this field. Can the virulence gene(s) of HIV (already identified and others to be defined) be countered by direct approaches? What action can be taken to increase all effective immune responses against the virus in the already infected and even the treated host? Many of the experimental procedures proposed can be studied in animal model systems such as SIV and FIV. These systems provide an excellent means for evaluation, since the disease in these animal species also involves lentiviruses that replicate well in CD4$^+$ lymphocytes (Table 1.1).

In all studies, therapeutic and vaccine strategies must consider the potential danger of detrimentally affecting the immune system. For example, attempts to increase CD8$^+$ cell activity (via PD-L antibodies or a reduction in T regulatory cells) may result in immune activation leading to enhanced virus replication and progression to disease. The effects could reflect the loss in balance of CD8$^+$ cell function, cytokine induction, cellular toxicity, autoimmune responses, or production of enhancing antibodies. Immunologic approaches involving specific cytokines or anti-cytokine therapies require the same consideration in approaches to prevent HIV pathogenesis. The ability to control HIV infection clearly requires a full understanding of the virus in all its heterogeneous forms, its genetic differences, its capacity for molecular

mimicry, and its dramatic mechanisms for evolving to become more virulent and to escape immune responses.

Most importantly, the diverse effects of HIV on the immune system must be appreciated. In other viral infections, antiviral approaches were successfully directed at cell-free agents passed through blood or body fluids. With HIV, transmission through *virus-infected* cells presents a major challenge to both anti-HIV therapies and vaccine development. In this regard, the directions taken can resemble those used to attack the cancer cell (Table B). Treatment of HIV infection resembles that of malignancies in that the initial therapies can give excellent control and then subsequent treatments, because of drug resistance of the cancer cell or the virus, show limited efficacy. Furthermore, in an analogy to cancer, the number of virus-infected cells may be sufficiently reduced that many infected cells surviving the therapy will die by normal processes. However, like single cancer cells remaining after chemotherapy, the long-lived HIV-infected lymphocytes, macrophages, or other cells in the body (e.g., brain) can be the source from which resistant or wild-type strains can emerge and spread.

Eventually, viruses within the persistently infected cells can reset the biologic clock to the time (during primary infection) when virus replication

Table B Common features of cancer and AIDS that should be considered for development of effective vaccines

- Both involve an abnormal cell.
- The abnormal cell can exist in a latent state.
- Both can recruit other cells into the process.
- Both involve modulation of antigens on the abnormal cell surface.
- Both can have compromising antibody production: blocking antibodies in cancer and enhancing antibodies in HIV infection.
- Both produce cellular products (cytokines) that can suppress the host immune response.
- Both are affected by cytokines (direct or indirect).
- Both can be associated with apoptosis (direct or indirect).
- Both can be associated with autoimmunity.
- Both require strong cell-mediated immunity (i.e., type 1 response).

took place unchallenged. In this regard, the acute retroviral syndrome has been noted in some HIV-infected subjects after cessation of HAART (857). However, importantly, now the replicating virus may be more pathogenic since it is less well handled by the host; the immune system has been compromised by previous antiviral therapies.

All approaches to the control of HIV continue to require cooperation from various sectors of the population, including government officials and political activists advocating the support needed to continue adequate financial backing for research and care. Along the way, new features of virology and cell biology will be uncovered. Already, the recognition and function of HIV accessory genes, particularly *rev, tat, vif, nef,* and their respective targets, offer insights into potential eukaryotic processes that could have widespread application. Transactivation, RNA binding proteins, and modification in RNA splicing are just a few examples of the biologic processes that have been learned from molecular studies of HIV.

Several challenges remain as we approach future attempts to control HIV infection (Table C). Understanding further how the virus can enter a cell via its variety of receptors can be valuable, and how it can remain latent in cells can shed light on mechanisms by which the host carries a variety of viruses for a lifetime. How the immune system, both innate and adaptive components, reacts to

Table C Future directions

- Understanding HIV latency
- Appreciating the role of innate immunity
- Targeting the virus-infected cell
- Recognizing the emergence of recombinant viruses
- Instituting immune-based therapies
- Developing an effective vaccine

HIV can also help in approaches to control autoimmune disease and infections by other intracellular pathogens, such as those causing malaria and tuberculosis. Importantly, as noted above, the biologic and immunologic challenges of HIV infection mimic those of cancer (Table B). Eliminating the HIV-infected cell and preventing virus replication in the host have parallels in cancer, in which the transformed cell is also the most important culprit. Thus, approaches at solving either pathogenic process through therapy (particularly immune system based) or vaccines could have relevance to both diseases. In addition, knowledge about variations in HIV and recombinant viruses and how they form will be very helpful in vaccine development. Finally, knowing how the host responds to changes in an infectious agent can help further our understanding of viral pathogenesis in general and, in particular, of the diseases caused by human retroviruses.

1993 Revised Classification System for HIV Infection and Expanded AIDS Surveillance Case Definition for Adolescents and Adults[†]

| CD4+ T-cell categories[a] | Clinical categories[b,c] | | |
	A Asymptomatic, acute (primary) HIV or PGL[d]	B Symptomatic, not (A) or (C) conditions	C AIDS-indicator conditions[e]
1. ≥ 500/μl	A1	B1	C1
2. 200–499/μl	A2	B2	C2
3. 200/μl AIDS-indicator T-cell count	A3	B3	C3

[a]See Appendix IV.

[b]See Appendix II.

[c]The shaded areas illustrate the expanded AIDS surveillance case definition. Persons with AIDS-indicator conditions (category C) as well as those with CD4+ T-lymphocyte counts of <200/μl (categories A3 or B3) were reportable as AIDS cases in the United States and territories effective January 1, 1993.

[d]PGL, persistent generalized lymphadenopathy. Clinical category A includes acute (primary) HIV infection (Chapter 4).

[e]See Appendix III.

†Reprinted from reference 643.

APPENDIX II
Clinical Categories†

Category A

Category A consists of one or more of the conditions listed below in an adolescent or adult (≥13 years) with documented HIV infection. Conditions listed in categories B and C must not have occurred.

- Asymptomatic HIV infection
- Persistent generalized lymphadenopathy
- Acute (primary) HIV infection with accompanying illness or history of acute HIV infection

Category B

Category B consists of symptomatic conditions in an HIV-infected adolescent or adult that are not included among conditions listed in clinical category C and that meet at least one of the following criteria: (i) the conditions are attributed to HIV infection or are indicative of a defect in cell-mediated immunity, or (ii) the conditions are considered by physicians to have a clinical course or to require management that is complicated by HIV infection. Examples of conditions in clinical category B include, but are not limited to,

- Bacillary angiomatosis
- Candidiasis, oropharyngeal (thrush)
- Candidiasis, vulvovaginal; persistent, frequent, or poorly responsive to therapy

- Cervical dysplasia (moderate or severe)/ cervical carcinoma in situ
- Constitutional symptoms, such as fever (38.5°C) or diarrhea lasting >1 month
- Hairy leukoplakia, oral
- Herpes zoster (shingles), involving at least two distinct episodes or more than one dermatome
- Idiopathic thrombocytopenic purpura
- Listeriosis
- Pelvic inflammatory disease, particularly if complicated by tubo-ovarian abscess
- Peripheral neuropathy

For classification purposes, category B conditions take precedence over those in category A. For example, someone previously treated for oral or persistent vaginal candidiasis (and who has not developed a category C disease) but who is now asymptomatic should be classified in clinical category B.

Category C

Category C includes the clinical conditions listed in the AIDS surveillance case definition (Appendix III). For classification purposes, once a category C condition has occurred, the person will remain in category C.

†Reprinted from reference 643.

Conditions Included in the 1993 AIDS Surveillance Case Definition[†]

- Candidiasis of bronchi, trachea, or lungs
- Candidiasis, esophageal
- Cervical cancer, invasive[a]
- Coccidioidomycosis, disseminated or extra-pulmonary
- Cryptococcosis, extrapulmonary
- Cryptosporidiosis, chronic intestinal (>1 month's duration)
- Cytomegalovirus disease (other than liver, spleen, or nodes)
- Cytomegalovirus retinitis (with loss of vision)
- Encephalopathy, HIV-related
- Herpes simplex: chronic ulcer(s) (>1 month's duration); or bronchitis, pneumonitis, or esophagitis
- Histoplasmosis, disseminated or extrapulmonary
- Isosporiasis, chronic intestinal (>1 month's duration)
- Kaposi's sarcoma
- Lymphoma, Burkitt's (or equivalent term)
- Lymphoma, immunoblastic (or equivalent term)
- Lymphoma, primary, of brain
- *Mycobacterium avium* complex or *Mycobacterium kansasii*, disseminated or extra-pulmonary
- *Mycobacterium tuberculosis*, any site (pul-monary[a] or extrapulmonary)
- *Mycobacterium*, other species or unidentified species, disseminated or extrapulmonary
- *Pneumocystis carinii* pneumonia
- Pneumonia, recurrent[a]
- Progressive multifocal leukoencephalopathy
- *Salmonella* septicemia, recurrent
- Toxoplasmosis of brain
- Wasting syndrome due to HIV

[†]Reprinted from reference 643.
[a]Added in the 1993 expansion of the AIDS surveillance case definition.

Other Definitions in HIV Infection: CD4$^+$ T-Lymphocyte Categories[†]

CD4$^+$ category	CD4$^+$ cells/μl	CD4$^+$ cell percentage
1	≥500	≥29
2	200–400	14–28
3[a]	<200	<14

[a]Diagnosis of AIDS.

[†]Reprinted from reference 643.

Relationship of CD4$^+$ Cell Count to the Risk of Developing Opportunistic Infections and Cancer

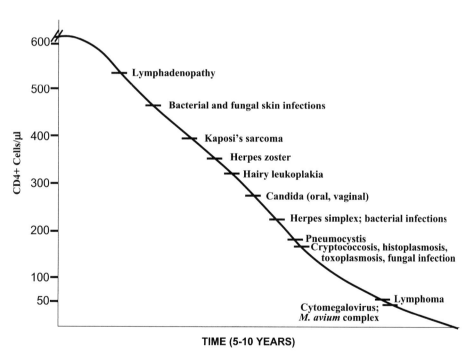

HIV disease progression. High risk of various clinical conditions at the most commonly observed CD4$^+$ T lymphocyte counts. Tuberculosis, Kaposi's sarcoma, and non-Hodgkin's lymphoma can occur any time, but particularly when CD4$^+$ cell counts drop below 400 cells/μl for tuberculosis and Kaposi's sarcoma and 50 cells/μl for non-Hodgkin's lymphoma.

References

1. Aarons, E., M. Fernandez, A. Rees, M. McClure, and J. Weber. 1997. CC-chemokine receptor 5 genotypes and *in vitro* susceptibility to HIV-1 of a cohort of British HIV-exposed uninfected homosexual men. *AIDS* 11:688–689.

2. Aasa-Chapman, M. M. I., S. Holuigue, K. Aubin, M. Wong, N. A. Jones, D. Cornforth, P. Pellegrino, P. Newton, I. Williams, P. Borrow, and A. McKnight. 2005. Detection of antibody-dependent complement-mediated inactivation of both autologous and heterologous virus in primary human immunodeficiency virus type 1 infection. *J. Virol.* 79:2823–2830.

3. Abada, P., B. Noble, and P. M. Cannon. 2005. Functional domains within the human immunodeficiency virus type 2 envelope protein required to enhance virus production. *J. Virol.* 79:3627–3638.

4. Abbas, A. K., and A. H. Sharpe. 1999. T-cell stimulation: an abundance of B7s. *Nat. Med.* 5:1345–1346.

5. Abbud, R. A., C. K. Finegan, L. A. Guay, and E. A. Rich. 1995. Enhanced production of human immunodeficiency virus type 1 by *in vitro*-infected alveolar macrophages from otherwise healthy cigarette smokers. *J. Infect. Dis.* 172:859–863.

6. Abdala, N., P. C. Stephens, B. P. Griffith, and R. Heimer. 1999. Survival of HIV-1 in syringes. *J. Acquir. Immune Defic. Syndr. Hum. Retrovirol.* 20:73–80.

7. Abel, K., D. M. Rocke, B. Chohan, L. Fritts, and C. J. Miller. 2005. Temporal and anatomic relationship between virus replication and cytokine gene expression after vaginal simian immunodeficiency virus infection. *J. Virol.* 79:12164–12172.

8. Abel, S., R. Cesaire, D. Cales-Quist, O. Bera, G. Sobesky, and A. Cabie. 2000. Occupational transmission of human immunodeficiency virus and hepatitis C virus after a punch. *Clin. Infect. Dis.* 31:1494–1495.

9. Abelian, A., K. Burling, P. Easterbrook, and G. Winter. 2004. Hyperimmunoglobulinemia and rate of HIV type 1 infection progression. *AIDS Res. Hum. Retrovir.* 20:127–128.

10. Aberg, J. A., J. E. Gallant, J. Anderson, J. M. Oleske, H. Libman, J. S. Currier, V. E. Stone, and J. E. Kaplan. 2004. Primary care guidelines for the management of persons infected with human immunodeficiency virus: recommendations of the HIV Medicine Association of the Infectious Diseases Society of America. *Clin. Infect. Dis.* 39:609–629.

10a. Abgrall, S. 2006. Initial strategy for antiretroviral-naive patients. *Lancet* 368:2107–2109.

11. Abimiku, A. G., G. Franchini, J. Tartaglia, K. Aldrich, M. Myagkikh, P. D. Markham, P. Chong, M. Klein, M. P. Kieny, E. Paoletti, et al. 1995. HIV-1 recombinant poxvirus vaccine induces cross-protection against HIV-2 challenge in rhesus macaques. *Nat. Med.* 1:321–329.

12. Abrams, D. I., B. J. Lewis, J. H. Beckstead, C. A. Casavant, and W. L. Drew. 1984. Persistent diffuse lymphadenopathy in homosexual men: endpoint or prodrome? *Ann. Intern. Med.* 100:801–808.

13. Abrignani, S., D. Montagna, M. Jeannet, J. Wintsch, N. L. Haigwood, J. R. Shuster, K. S. Steimer, A. Cruchaud, and T. Staehelin. 1990. Priming of CD4+ T cells specific for conserved regions of human immunodeficiency virus glycoprotein gp120 in humans immunized with a recombinant envelope protein. *Proc. Natl. Acad. Sci. USA* 87:6136–6140.

13a. Abu-Raddad, L. J., P. Patnaik, and J. G. Kublin. 2006. Dual infection with HIV and malaria fuels the spread of both diseases in sub-Saharan Africa. *Science* 314:1603–1606.

14. Accola, M. A., S. Hoglund, and H. G. Gottlinger. 1998. A putative α-helical structure which overlaps the capsid-p2 boundary in the human immunodeficiency virus type 1 Gag precursor is crucial for viral particle assembly. *J. Virol.* 72:2072–2078.

15. Accornero, P., M. Radrizzani, D. Delia, F. Gerosa, R. Kurrle, and M. P. Colombo. 1997. Differential susceptibility to HIV-gp120-sensitized apoptosis in CD4+ T-cell clones with different T-helper phenotypes: role of CD95/CD95L interactions. *Blood* 89:558–569.

16. Achim, C. L., M. P. Heyes, and C. A. Wiley. 1993. Quantitation of human immunodeficiency virus, immune activation factors, and quinolinic acid in AIDS brains. *J. Clin. Investig.* 91:2769–2775.

17. Actor, J. K., M. Shirai, M. C. Kullberg, M. L. Buller, A. Sher, and J. A. Berzofsky. 1993. Helminth infection results in

443

decreased virus-specific CD8+ cytotoxic T-cell and Th1 cytokine responses as well as delayed virus clearance. *Proc. Natl. Acad. Sci. USA* **90**:948–952.

18. Ada, G. L., and M. J. McElrath. 1997. HIV type 1 vaccine-induced cytotoxic T cell responses: potential role in vaccine efficacy. *AIDS Res. Hum. Retrovir.* **13**:205–210.

19. Adachi, A., S. Koenig, H. E. Gendelman, D. Daugherty, S. Gattoni-Celli, A. S. Fauci, and M. A. Martin. 1987. Productive, persistent infection of human colorectal cell lines with human immunodeficiency virus. *J. Virol.* **61**:209–213.

20. Adachi, Y., N. Oyaizu, S. Than, T. W. McCloskey, and S. Pahwa. 1996. IL-2 rescues *in vitro* lymphocyte apoptosis in patients with HIV infection. *J. Immunol.* **157**:4184–4193.

21. Adams, D. H., and A. R. Lloyd. 1997. Chemokines: leucocyte recruitment and activation cytokines. *Lancet* **349**:490–495.

22. Adams, L. E., R. Donovan-Brand, A. Friedman-Kien, K. el Ramahi, and E. V. Hess. 1988. Sperm and seminal plasma antibodies in acquired immune deficiency (AIDS) and other associated syndromes. *Clin. Immunol. Immunopathol.* **46**:442–449.

23. Adamson, D. C., B. Wildemann, M. Sasaki, J. D. Glass, J. C. McArthur, V. I. Christov, T. M. Dawson, and V. L. Dawson. 1996. Immunologic NO synthase: elevation in severe AIDS dementia and induction by HIV-1 gp41. *Science* **274**:1917–1921.

24. Addo, M. D., X. G. Yu, A. Rathod, D. Cohen, R. L. Eldridge, D. Strick, M. N. Johnston, C. Corcoran, A. G. Wurcel, C. A. Fitzpatrick, M. E. Feeney, W. R. Rodriguez, N. Basgoz, R. Draenert, D. R. Stone, C. Brander, P. J. Goulder, E. S. Rosenberg, M. Altfeld, and B. D. Walker. 2003. Comprehensive epitope analysis of human immunodeficiency virus type 1 (HIV-1)-specific T-cell responses directed against the entire expressed HIV-1 genome demonstrate broadly directed responses, but no correlation to viral load. *J. Virol.* **77**:2081–2092.

25. Ades, A. E., M. L. Newell, and C. S. Peckham. 1991. Children born to women with HIV-1 infection: natural history and risk of transmission. *Lancet* **337**:253–260.

26. Adleman, L. M., and D. Wofsy. 1993. T-cell homeostasis: implications in HIV infection. *J. Acquir. Immune Defic. Syndr.* **6**:144–152.

27. Afonso, L. C. C., T. M. Scharton, L. Q. Vieira, M. Wysocka, G. Trinchieri, and P. Scott. 1994. The adjuvant effect of interleukin-12 in a vaccine against *Leishmania major*. *Science* **263**:235–237.

28. Agace, W. W., A. Amara, A. I. Roberts, J. L. Pablos, S. Thelen, M. Uguccioni, X. Y. Li, J. Marsal, F. Arenzana-Seisdedos, T. Delaunay, E. C. Ebert, B. Moser, and C. M. Parker. 2000. Constitutive expression of stromal derived factor-1 by mucosal epithelia and its role in HIV transmission and propagation. *Curr. Biol.* **10**:325–328.

29. Aghokeng, A. F., W. Liu, F. Bibollet-Ruche, S. Loul, E. Mpoudi-Ngole, C. Laurent, J. M. Mwenda, D. K. Langat, G. K. Chege, H. M. McClure, E. Delaporte, G. M. Shaw, B. H. Hahn, and M. Peeters. 2006. Widely varying SIV prevalence rates in naturally infected primate species from Cameroon. *Virology* **345**:174–189.

30. Agostini, C., L. Trentin, R. Sancetta, M. Facco, C. Tassinari, A. Cerutti, M. Bortolin, A. Milani, M. Siviero, R. Zambello, and G. Semenzato. 1997. Interleukin-15 triggers activation and growth of the CD8 T-cell pool in extravascular tissues of patients with acquired immunodeficiency syndrome. *Blood* **90**:1115–1123.

31. Agrawal, L., G. Alkhatib, and L. Agrawal. 2001. Chemokine receptors: emerging opportunities for new anti-HIV therapies. *Expert Opin. Ther. Targets* **5**:303–326.

32. Agrawal, L., X. Lu, J. Qingwen, Z. VanHorn-Ali, I. V. Nicoloescu, D. H. McDermott, P. M. Murphy, and G. Alkhatib. 2004. Role for CCR5Δ32 protein in resistance to R5, R5X4, and X4 human immunodeficiency virus type 1 in primary CD4+ cells. *J. Virol.* **78**:2277–2287.

33. Agy, M. B., L. R. Frumkin, L. Corey, R. W. Coombs, S. M. Wolinsky, J. Koehler, W. R. Morton, and M. G. Katze. 1992. Infection of *Macaca nemestrina* by human immunodeficiency virus type-1. *Science* **257**:103–106.

34. Agy, M. B., M. Wambach, K. Foy, and M. G. Katze. 1990. Expression of cellular genes in CD4 positive lymphoid cells infected by the human immunodeficiency virus, HIV-1: evidence for a host protein synthesis shut-off induced by cellular mRNA degradation. *Virology* **177**:251–258.

35. Ahmad, A., and J. Menezes. 1996. Antibody dependent cellular cytotoxicity in HIV infections. *FASEB J.* **10**:258–266.

36. Ahmad, A., R. Morisset, R. Thomas, and J. Menezes. 1994. Evidence for a defect of antibody-dependent cellular cytotoxic (ADCC) effector function and anti-HIV gp120/41-specific ADCC-mediating antibody titres in HIV-infected individuals. *J. Acquir. Immune Defic. Syndr.* **7**:428–437.

37. Ahmad, N., and S. Venkatesan. 1988. Nef protein of HIV-1 is a transcriptional repressor of HIV-1 LTR. *Science* **241**:1481–1485.

38. Ahmad, R., S. T. Sindhu, E. Toma, R. Morisset, J. Vincelette, J. Menezes, and A. Ahmad. 2001. Evidence for a correlation between antibody-dependent cellular cytotoxicity-mediating anti-HIV-1 antibodies and prognostic predictors of HIV infection. *J. Clin. Immunol.* **21**:227–233.

39. Ahmed, R. K., H. Norrgren, Z. da Silva, A. Blaxhult, E. L. Fredriksson, G. Biberfeld, S. Andersson, and R. Thorstensson. 2005. Antigen-specific b-chemokine production and CD8 T-cell noncytotoxic antiviral activity in HIV-2-infected individuals. *Scand. J. Immunol.* **61**:63–71.

40. Aiken, C., and D. Trono. 1995. Nef stimulates human immunodeficiency virus type 1 proviral DNA synthesis. *J. Virol.* **69**:5048–5056.

41. Aikhionbare, F. O., T. Hodge, L. Kuhn, M. Bulterys, E. J. Abrams, and V. C. Bond. 2001. Mother-to-child discordance in HLA-G exon 2 is associated with a reduced risk of perinatal HIV-1. *AIDS* **15**:2196–2198.

42. Ait-Khaled, M., J. E. McLaughlin, M. A. Johnson, and V. C. Emery. 1995. Distinct HIV-1 long terminal repeat quasispecies present in nervous tissues compared to that in lung, blood and lymphoid tissues of an AIDS patient. *AIDS* **9**:675–683.

43. Aiuti, F., and A. Giovannetti. 2003. Structured interruptions of therapy: looking for the best protocol. *AIDS* **17**:2257–2258.

44. Akari, H., S. Bour, S. Kao, A. Adachi, and K. Strebel. 2001. The human immunodeficiency virus type 1 accessory protein Vpu induces apoptosis by suppressing the nuclear factor kappaB-dependent expression of antiapoptotic factors. *J. Exp. Med.* **194**:1299–1311.

45. Akinola, N. O., O. Olasode, I. A. Adediran, O. Onayemi, A. Murainah, O. Irinoye, A. A. Elujoba, and M. A. Durosinmi. 2004. The search for a predictor of CD4 cell count continues: total lymphocyte count is not a substitute for CD4 cell count in the management of HIV-infected individuals in a resource-limited setting. *Clin. Infect. Dis.* **39**:579–581.

46. Akira, S., and K. Takeda. 2004. Toll-like receptor signalling. *Nat. Rev. Immunol.* **4**:499–511.

46a. Akira, S., S. Uematsu, and O. Takeuchi. 2006. Pathogen recognition and innate immunity. *Cell* **124**:783–801.

47. Akridge, R. E., and S. G. Reed. 1996. Interleukin-12 decreases human immunodeficiency virus type 1 replication in human macrophage cultures reconstituted with autologous peripheral blood mononuclear cells. *J. Infect. Dis.* **173**:559–564.

48. Al-Harthi, L., L. J. Guilbert, J. A. Hoxie, and A. Landay. 2002. Trophoblasts are productively infected by CD4-independent isolate of HIV type 1. *AIDS Res. Hum. Retroviruses* **18**:13–17.

49. Al-Harthi, L., A. Kovacs, R. W. Coombs, P. S. Reichelderfer, D. J. Wright, M. H. Cohen, J. Cohn, S. Cu-Uvin, H. Watts, S. Lewis, S. Beckner, and A. Landay. 2001. A menstrual cycle pattern for cytokine levels exists in HIV-positive women: implication for HIV vaginal and plasma shedding. *AIDS* **15**:1535–1543.

50. Alabi, A. S., S. Jaffar, K. Ariyoshi, T. Blanchard, M. van der Loeff, A. Awasana, T. Corrah, S. Sabally, R. Sarge-Njie, F. Cham-Jallow, A. Jaye, N. Berry, and H. Whittle. 2003. Plasma viral load, CD4 cell percentage, HLA and survival of HIV-1, HIV-2, and dually infected Gambian patients. *AIDS* **17**:1513–1520.

51. Albert, J., B. Abrahamsson, K. Nagy, E. Aurelius, H. Gaines, G. Nystrom, and E. M. Fenyo. 1990. Rapid development of isolate-specific neutralizing antibodies after primary HIV-1 infection and consequent emergence of virus variants which resist neutralization by autologous sera. *AIDS* **4**:107–112.

52. Albert, J., U. Bredberg, F. Chiodi, B. Bottiger, E. M. Fenyo, E. Norrby, and G. Biberfeld. 1987. A new human retrovirus isolate of West African origin (SBL-6669) and its relationship to HTLV-IV, LAV-II, and HTLV-IIIB. *AIDS Res. Hum. Retrovir.* **3**:3–10.

53. Albert, J., P. Stalhandske, S. Marquina, J. Karis, R. A. M. Fouchier, E. Norrby, and F. Chiodi. 1996. Biological phenotype of HIV type 2 isolates correlates with V3 genotype. *AIDS Res. Hum. Retrovir.* **12**:821–828.

54. Albini, A., R. Benelli, D. Giunciuglio, T. Cai, G. Mariani, S. Ferrini, and D. M. Noonan. 1998. Identification of a novel domain of HIV Tat involved in monocyte chemotaxis. *J. Biol. Chem.* **273**:15895–15900.

55. Albini, A., C. D. Mitchell, and E. W. Thompson. 1988. Invasive activity and chemotactic response to growth factors by Kaposi's sarcoma cells. *J. Cell. Biochem.* **36**:369–376.

56. Albright, A. V., J. Strizki, J. M. Harouse, E. Lavi, M. O'Connor, and F. Gonzalez-Scarano. 1996. HIV-1 infection of cultured human adult oligodendrocytes. *Virology* **217**:211–219.

57. Aldovini, A., and R. A. Young. 1991. Humoral and cell-mediated immune responses to live recombinant BCG-HIV vaccines. *Nature* **351**:479–482.

58. Aldrovandi, G. M., G. Feuer, L. Gao, B. Jamieson, M. Kristeva, I. S. Y. Chen, and J. A. Zack. 1993. The SCID-hu mouse as a model for HIV-1 infection. *Nature* **363**:732–736.

59. Alexander, L., M. J. Aquino-DeJesus, M. Chan, and W. A. Andiman. 2002. Inhibition of human immunodeficiency virus type 1 (HIV-1) replication by a two-amino-acid insertion in HIV-1 Vif from a nonprogressing mother and child. *J. Virol.* **76**:10533–10539.

60. Alexander, M., Y. Bor, K. S. Ravichandran, M. Hammarskjold, and D. Rekosh. 2004. Human immunodeficiency virus type 1 nef associates with lipid rafts to downmodulate cell surface CD4 and class I major histocompatibility complex expression and to increase viral infectivity. *J. Virol.* **78**:1685–1696.

61. Alexander, S., and J. H. Elder. 1994. Carbohydrate dramatically influences immune reactivity of antisera to viral glycoprotein antigens. *Science* **226**:1328–1330.

62. Alizon, M., P. Sonigo, F. Barre-Sinoussi, J.-C. Chermann, P. Tiollais, L. Montagnier, and S. Wain-Hobson. 1984. Molecular cloning of lymphadenopathy-associated virus. *Nature* **312**:757–760.

63. Alizon, M., S. Wain-Hobson, L. Montagnier, and P. Sonigo. 1986. Genetic variability of the AIDS virus: nucleotide sequence analysis of two isolates from African patients. *Cell* **46**:63–74.

64. Alkhatib, G., C. Combadiere, C. C. Broder, Y. Feng, P. E. Kennedy, P. M. Murphy, and E. A. Berger. 1996. CC-CKR-5: a RANTES, MIP-1α, MIP-1β receptor as a fusion cofactor for macrophage-tropic HIV-1. *Science* **272**:1955–1958.

65. Allain, J. P., C. Bianco, M. A. Blajchman, M. E. Brecher, M. Busch, D. Leiby, L. Lin, and S. Stramer. 2005. Protecting the blood supply from emerging pathogens: the role of pathogen inactivation. *Transfus. Med. Rev.* **19**:110–126.

66. Allan, J. S., J. Strauss, and D. W. Buck. 1990. Enhancement of SIV infection with soluble receptor molecules. *Science* **247**:1084–1088.

67. Allen, T. M., L. Mortara, B. R. Mothe, M. Liebl, P. Jing, B. Calore, M. Piekarczyk, R. Ruddersdorf, D. H. O'Connor, X. Wang, C. Wang, D. B. Allison, J. D. Altman, A. Sette, R. C. Desrosiers, G. Sutter, and D. I. Watkins. 2002. Tat-vaccinated macaques do not control simian immunodeficiency virus SIV-mac239 replication. *J. Virol.* **76**:4108–4112.

68. Allen, T. M., X. G. Yu, E. T. Kalife, L. L. Reyor, M. Lichterfeld, M. John, M. Cheng, R. L. Allgaier, S. Mui, N. Frahm, G. Alter, N. V. Brown, M. N. Johnston, E. S. Rosenberg, S. A. Mallal, C. Brander, B. D. Walker, and M. Altfeld. 2005. De novo generation of escape variant-specific CD8+ T-cell responses following cytotoxic T-lymphocyte escape in chronic human immunodeficiency virus type 1 infection. *J. Virol.* **79**:12952–12960.

69. Allison, A. C., and N. E. Byars. 1992. Adjuvants for new generation vaccines, p. 133–141. *In* R. W. Ellis (ed.), *Vaccines: New Approaches to Immunological Problems.* Butterworths, Stoneham, Mass.

70. Allison, G. T., M. P. Bostrom, and M. J. Glesby. 2003. Osteonecrosis in HIV disease: epidemiology, etiologies, and clinical management. *AIDS* **17**:1–9.

71. Almond, N., K. Kent, M. Cranage, E. Rud, B. Clarke, and E. J. Stott. 1995. Protection by attenuated simian immunodeficiency virus in macaques against challenge with virus-infected cells. *Lancet* **345**:1342–1344.

72. Almond, N., J. Rose, R. Sangster, P. Silvera, B. Stebbings, B. Walker, and E. J. Stott. 1997. Mechanisms of protection induced by attenuated simian immunodeficiency virus. I. Protection cannot be transferred with immune serum. *J. Gen. Virol.* **78**:1919–1922.

73. Aloia, R. C., H. Tian, and F. C. Jensen. 1993. Lipid composition and fluidity of the human immunodeficiency virus envelope and host cell plasma membranes. *Proc. Natl. Acad. Sci. USA* **90**:5181–5185.

74. Aloisi, F., F. Ria, G. Penna, and L. Adorini. 1998. Microglia are more efficient than astrocytes in antigen processing and in Th1 but not Th2 cell activation. *J. Immunol.* **160**:4671–4680.

75. Alonso, A., D. Derse, and B. M. Peterlin. 1992. Human chromosome 12 is required for optimal interactions between

Tat and TAR of human immunodeficiency virus type 1 in rodent cells. *J. Virol.* **66**:4617–4621.

76. **Alsip, G. R., Y. Ench, C. V. Sumaya, and R. N. Boswell.** 1988. Increased Epstein-Barr virus DNA in oropharyngeal secretions from patients with AIDS, AIDS-related complex, or asymptomatic human immunodeficiency virus infections. *J. Infect. Dis.* **157**:1072–1076.

77. **Alter, G., G. Hatzakis, C. M. Tsoukas, K. Pelley, D. Rouleu, R. LeBlanc, J.-G. Baril, H. Dion, E. Lefebvre, R. Thomas, P. Coté, N. Lapointe, J.-P. Routy, R.-P. Sékaly, B. Conway, and N. F. Bernard.** 2003. Longitudinal assessment of changes in HIV-specific effector activity in HIV-infected patients starting highly active antiretroviral therapy in primary infection. *J. Immunol.* **171**:477–488.

78. **Alter, G., J. M. Malenfant, R. M. Delabre, N. D. Burgett, X. G. Yu, M. Lichterfeld, J. Zaunders, and M. Altfeld.** 2004. Increased natural killer cell activity in viremic HIV-1 infection. *J. Immunol.* **173**:5305–5311.

79. **Alter, G., A. Merchant, C. M. Tsoukas, D. Rouleau, R. P. LeBlanc, P. Cote, J. G. Baril, R. Thomas, V. K. Nguyen, R. P. Sekaly, J. P. Routy, and N. F. Bernard.** 2002. Human immunodeficiency virus (HIV)-specific effector CD8 T cell activity in patients with primary HIV infection. *J. Infect. Dis.* **185**:755–765.

79a. **Alter, G., T. J. Suscovich, M. Kleyman, N. Teigen, H. Streeck, M. T. Zaman, A. Meier, and M. Altfeld.** 2006. Low perforin and elevated SHIP-1 expression is associated with functional anergy of natural killer cells in chronic HIV-1 infection. *AIDS* **20**:1549–1551.

80. **Alter, G., N. Teigen, B. T. Davis, M. M. Addo, T. J. Suscovich, M. T. Waring, H. Streeck, M. N. Johnston, K. D. Staller, M. T. Zaman, X. G. Yu, M. Lichterfeld, N. Basgoz, E. S. Rosenberg, and M. Altfeld.** 2005. Sequential deregulation of NK cell subset distribution and function starting in acute HIV-1 infection. *Blood* **106**:3366–3369.

81. **Alter, G., C. M. Tsoukas, D. Rouleau, P. Cote, J.-P. Routy, R.-P. Sekaly, and N. F. Bernard.** 2004. Assessment of longitudinal changes in HIV-specific effector activity in subjects undergoing untreated primary HIV infection. *AIDS* **18**:1979–1989.

82. **Altfeld, M., M. M. Addo, E. S. Rosenberg, F. M. Hecht, P. K. Lee, M. Vogel, X. G. Yu, R. Draenert, M. N. Johnston, D. Strick, T. M. Allen, M. E. Feeney, J. O. Kahn, R. P. Sekaly, J. A. Levy, J. K. Rockstroh, P. J. Goulder, and B. D. Walker.** 2003. Influence of HLA-B57 on clinical presentation and viral control during acute HIV-1 infection. *AIDS* **17**:2581–2591.

83. **Altfeld, M., M. M. Addo, R. Shankarappa, P. K. Lee, T. M. Allen, X. G. Yu, A. Rathod, J. Harlow, K. O'Sullivan, M. N. Johnston, P. J. Goulder, J. I. Mullins, E. S. Rosenberg, C. Brander, B. Korber, and B. D. Walker.** 2003. Enhanced detection of human immunodeficiency virus type 1-specific T-cell responses to highly variable regions by using peptides based on autologous virus sequences. *J. Virol.* **77**:7330–7340.

84. **Altfeld, M., T. M. Allen, X. G. Yu, M. N. Johnston, D. Agrawal, B. T. Korber, D. C. Montefiori, D. H. O'Connor, B. T. Davis, P. K. Lee, E. L. Maler, J. Harlow, P. J. R. Goulder, C. Brander, E. S. Rosenberg, and B. D. Walker.** 2002. HIV-1 superinfection despite broad CD8+ T-cell responses containing replication of the primary virus. *Nature* **420**:434–439.

85. **Altfeld, M., E. S. Rosenberg, R. Shankarappa, J. S. Mukherjee, F. M. Hecht, R. L. Eldridge, M. M. Addo, S. H. Poon, M. N. Phillips, G. K. Robbins, P. E. Sax, S. Boswell, J. O. Kahn, C. Brander, P. J. Goulder, J. A. Levy, J. I. Mullins, and B. D. Walker.** 2001. Cellular immune responses and viral diversity in individuals treated during acute and early HIV-1 infection. *J. Exp. Med.* **193**:169–180.

86. **Altfeld, M., J. van Lunzen, N. Frahm, X. G. Yu, C. Schneider, R. L. Eldridge, M. E. Feeney, D. Meyer-Olson, H. J. Stellbrink, and B. D. Walker.** 2002. Expansion of pre-existing, lymph node-localized CD8+ T cells during supervised treatment interruptions in chronic HIV-1 infection. *J. Clin. Investig.* **109**:837–843.

87. **Altman, J. D., P. A. Moss, P. J. Goulder, D. H. Barouch, M. G. McHeyzer-Williams, J. I. Bell, A. J. McMichael, and M. M. Davis.** 1996. Phenotypic analysis of antigen-specific T lymphocytes. *Science* **274**:94–96.

88. **Amadori, A., G. de Silvestro, R. Zamarchi, M. L. Veronese, M. R. Mazza, G. Schiavo, M. Panozzo, A. de Rossi, L. Ometto, J. Mous, A. Barelli, A. Borri, L. Salmaso, and L. Chieco-Bianchi.** 1992. CD4 epitope masking by gp120/anti-gp120 antibody complexes. *J. Immunol.* **148**:2709–2716.

89. **Amadori, A., R. Zamarchi, V. Ciminale, A. Del Mistro, S. Siervo, A. Alberti, M. Colombatti, and L. Chieco-Bianchi.** 1989. HIV-1 specific B cell activation: a major constituent of spontaneous B cell activation during HIV-1 infection. *J. Immunol.* **143**:2146–2152.

90. **Amadori, A., R. Zamarchi, M. L. Veronese, M. Panozzo, A. Barelli, A. Borri, M. Sironi, F. Colotta, A. Mantovani, and L. Chieco-Bianchi.** 1991. B cell activation during HIV-1 infection. II. Cell-to-cell interactions and cytokine requirement. *J. Immunol.* **146**:57–62.

91. **Amara, R. R., F. Villinger, J. D. Altman, S. L. Lydy, S. P. O'Neil, S. I. Staprans, D. C. Montefiori, Y. Xu, J. G. Herndon, L. S. Wyatt, M. A. Candido, N. L. Kozyr, P. L. Earl, J. M. Smith, H. L. Ma, B. D. Grimm, M. L. Hulsey, J. Miller, H. M. McClure, J. M. McNicholl, B. Moss, and H. L. Robinson.** 2001. Control of a mucosal challenge and prevention of AIDS by a multiprotein DNA/MVA vaccine. *Science* **292**:69–74.

92. **Ambroziak, J. A., D. J. Blackbourn, B. G. Herndier, R. G. Glogau, J. H. Gullett, A. R. McDonald, E. T. Lennette, and J. A. Levy.** 1995. Herpes-like sequences in HIV-infected and uninfected Kaposi's sarcoma patients. *Science* **268**:582–583.

93. **Amella, C.-A., B. Sherry, D. H. Shepp, and H. Schmidt-mayerova.** 2005. Macrophage inflammatory protein 1α inhibits postentry steps of human immunodeficiency virus type 1 infection via suppression of intracellular cyclic AMP. *J. Virol.* **79**:5625–5631.

94. **Amerongen, H. M., R. Weltzin, C. M. Farnet, P. Michetti, W. A. Haseltine, and M. R. Neutra.** 1991. Transepithelial transport of HIV-1 by intestinal M cells: a mechanism for transmission of AIDS. *J. Acquir. Immune Defic. Syndr.* **4**:760–765.

95. **Amicosante, M., F. Poccia, C. Gioia, C. Montesano, S. Topino, F. Martini, P. Narciso, L. P. Pucillo, and G. D'Offizi.** 2003. Levels of interleukin-15 in plasma may predict a favorable outcome of structured treatment interruption in patients with chronic human immunodeficiency virus infection. *J. Infect. Dis.* **188**:661–665.

96. **Amiel, C., E. Darcissac, M. Troung, J. Dewulf, M. Loyens, Y. Mouton, A. Capron, and G. Bahr.** 1999. Interleukin-16 (IL-16) inhibits human immunodeficiency virus replication in cells from infected subjects, and serum IL-16 levels drop with disease progression. *J. Infect. Dis.* **179**:83–91.

97. **Amirhessami-Aghili, N., and S. A. Spector.** 1991. Human immunodeficiency virus type 1 infection of human placenta: potential route for fetal infection. *J. Virol.* **65**:2231–2236.

98. Ammann, A. J., and J. A. Levy. 1986. Laboratory investigation of pediatric acquired immunodeficiency syndrome. *Clin. Immunol. Immunopathol.* **40:**122–127.

99. Ammann, A. J., M. J. Cowan, D. W. Wara, P. Weintrub, S. Dritz, H. Goldman, and H. A. Perkins. 1983. Acquired immunodeficiency in an infant: possible transmission by means of blood products. *Lancet* i:956–958.

100. Ammann, A. J., G. Schiffman, D. Abrams, P. Volberding, J. Ziegler, and M. Conant. 1984. B cell immunodeficiency in acquired immune deficiency syndrome. *JAMA* **251:**1447–1449.

101. Ammar, A., C. Cibert, A. M. Bertoli, V. Tsilivakos, C. Jasmin, and V. Georgoulias. 1991. Biological and biochemical characterization of a factor produced spontaneously by adherent cells of human immunodeficiency virus-infected patients inhibiting interleukin-2 receptor alpha chain (Tac) expression on normal T cells. *J. Clin. Investig.* **87:**2048–2055.

102. Ammaranond, P., J. Zaunders, C. Satchell, D. van Bockel, D. A. Cooper, and A. D. Kelleher. 2005. A new variant cytotoxic T lymphocyte escape mutation in HLA-B27-positive individuals infected with HIV type 1. *AIDS Res. Hum. Retrovir.* **21:**395–397.

103. Amory, J., N. Martin, J. A. Levy, and D. W. Wara. 1992. The large molecular weight glycoprotein MG1, a component of human saliva, inhibits HIV-1 infectivity. *Clin. Res.* **40:**51A. (Abstract.)

104. An, P., G. Beliber, P. Duggal, G. Nelson, M. May, B. Mangeat, I. Alobwede, D. Trono, D. Vlahov, S. Donfield, J. J. Goedert, J. Phair, S. Buchbinder, S. J. O'Brien, A. Telenti, and C. A. Winkler. 2004. APOBEC3G genetic variants and their influence on the progression to AIDS. *J. Virol.* **78:**11070–11076.

105. An, P., G. N. Nelson, L. Wang, S. Donfield, J. J. Goedert, J. Phair, D. Vlahov, S. Buchbinder, W. L. Farrar, W. Modi, S. J. O'Brien, and C. A. Winkler. 2002. Modulating influence on HIV/AIDS by interacting RANTES gene variants. *Proc. Natl. Acad. Sci. USA* **99:**10002–10007.

106. An, P., D. Vlahov, J. B. Margolick, J. Phair, T. R. O'Brien, J. Lautenberger, S. J. O'Brien, and C. A. Winkler. 2003. A tumor necrosis factor-alpha-inducible promoter variant of interferon-gamma accelerates CD4+ T cell depletion in human immunodeficiency virus-1-infected individuals. *J. Infect. Dis.* **188:**228–231.

107. Anand, R., F. Siegal, C. Reed, T. Cheung, S. Forlenza, and J. Moore. 1987. Non-cytocidal natural variants of human immunodeficiency virus isolated from AIDS patients with neurological disorders. *Lancet* ii:234–238.

108. Anandahl, E. M., J. Michaelsson, W. J. Moretto, F. M. Hecht, and D. F. Nixon. 2004. Human CD4+ CD25+ regulatory T cells control T-cell responses to human immunodeficiency virus and cytomegalovirus antigens. *J. Virol.* **78:**2454–2459.

108a. Ananworanich, J., A. Gayet-Ageron, M. Le Braz, W. Prasithsirikul, P. Chetchotisakd, S. Kiertiburanakul, W. Munsakul, P. Raksakulkarn, S. Tansuphasawasdikul, S. Sirivichayakul, M. Cavassini, U. Karrer, D. Genne, R. Nuesch, P. Vernazza, E. Bernasconi, D. Leduc, C. Satchell, S. Yerly, L. Perrin, A. Hill, T. Perneger, P. Phanuphak, H. Furrer, D. Cooper, K. Ruxrungtham, and B. Hirschel. 2006. CD4-guided scheduled treatment interruptions compared with continuous therapy for patients infected with HIV-1: results of the Staccato randomised trial. *Lancet* **368:**459–465.

109. Ananworanich, J., R. Nuesch, M. Le Braz, P. Chetchotisakd, A. Vibhagool, S. Wicharuk, K. Ruxrungtham, H. Furrer, D. Cooper, B. Hirschel, et al. 2003. Failures of 1 week on, 1 week off antiretroviral therapies in a randomized trial. *AIDS* **17:**F33-F37.

110. Andersen, J. L., E. S. Zimmerman, J. L. DeHart, S. Murala, O. Ardon, J. Blackett, J. Chen, and V. Planelles. 2005. ATR and GADD45alpha mediate HIV-1 Vpr-induced apoptosis. *Cell Death Differ.* **12:**326–334.

111. Anderson, D. J., and J. A. Hill. 1987. CD4 (T4+) lymphocytes in semen of healthy heterosexual men: implications for the transmission of AIDS. *Fertil. Steril.* **48:**703–704.

112. Anderson, D. J., T. R. O'Brien, J. A. Politch, A. Martinez, G. R. Deage III, N. Padian, C. R. Horsburgh, and K. H. Mayer. 1992. Effects of disease stage and zidovudine therapy on the detection of human immunodeficiency virus type 1 in semen. *JAMA* **267:**2769–2774.

113. Anderson, D. J., J. A. Politch, A. Martinez, B. J. Van Voorhis, N. S. Padian, and T. R. O'Brien. 1991. White blood cells and HIV-1 in semen from vasectomised seropositive men. *Lancet* **338:**573–574.

114. Anderson, J. P., A. G. Rodrigo, G. H. Learn, A. Madan, C. Delahunty, M. Coon, M. Girard, S. Osmanov, L. Hood, and J. I. Mullins. 2000. Testing the hypothesis of a recombinant origin of human immunodeficiency virus type 1 subtype E. *J. Virol.* **74:**10752–10765.

115. Anderson, K. B., J. L. Guest, and D. Rimland. 2004. Hepatitis C virus coinfection increases mortality in HIV-infected patients in the highly active antiretroviral therapy era: data from the HIV Atlanta VA cohort study. *Clin. Infect. Dis.* **39:**1507–1513.

116. Anderson, S. J., M. Lenburg, N. R. Landau, and J. V. Garcia. 1994. The cytoplasmic domain of CD4 is sufficient for its down-regulation from the cell surface by human immunodeficiency virus type 1 Nef. *J. Virol.* **68:**3092–3101.

117. Andersson, J., H. Behbahani, J. Lieberman, E. Connick, A. Landay, B. Patterson, A. Sonnerborg, K. Lore, S. Uccini, and T. E. Fehniger. 1999. Perforin is not co-expressed with granzyme A within cytotoxic granules in CD8 T lymphocytes present in lymphoid tissue during chronic HIV infection. *AIDS* **13:**1295–1303.

118. Andersson, J., A. Boasso, J. Nilsson, R. Zhang, N. J. Shire, S. Lindback, G. M. Shearer, and C. A. Chougnet. 2005. The prevalence of regulatory T cells in lymphoid tissue is correlated with viral load in HIV-infected patients. *J. Immunol.* **174:** 3143–3147.

119. Andersson, J., T. E. Fehniger, B. K. Patterson, J. Pottage, M. Agnoli, P. Jones, H. Behbahani, and A. Landay. 1998. Early reduction of immune activation in lymphoid tissue following highly active HIV therapy. *AIDS* **12:**F123-F129.

120. Andersson, S., B. Makitalo, R. Thorstensson, G. Franchini, J. Tartaglia, K. Limbach, E. Paoletti, P. Putkonen, and G. Biberfeld. 1996. Immunogenicity and protective efficacy of a human immunodeficiency virus type 2 recombinant canarypox (ALVAC) vaccine candidate in cynomolgus monkeys. *J. Infect. Dis.* **174:**977–985.

121. Andeweg, A. C., P. Leeflang, A. D. M. E. Osterhaus, and M. L. Bosch. 1993. Both the V2 and V3 regions of the human immunodeficiency virus type 1 surface glycoprotein functionally interact with other envelope regions in syncytium formation. *J. Virol.* **67:**3232–3239.

122. Andino, R., D. Silvera, S. D. Suggett, P. L. Achacoso, C. J. Miller, D. Baltimore, and M. B. Feinberg. 1994. Engineering

poliovirus as a vaccine vector for the expression of diverse antigens. *Science* 265:1448–1451.

123. Andreo, S. S., L. C. Barra, L. J. Costa, M. A. Sucupira, I. L. Souza, and R. Diaz. 2004. HIV type 1 transmission by human bite. *AIDS Res. Hum. Retrovir.* 20:349–350.

124. Angel, J. B., K. High, F. Rhame, D. Brand, J. B. Whitmore, J. M. Agosti, M. J. Gilbert, S. Deresinskic, et al. 2000. Phase III study of granulocyte-macrophage colony-stimulating factor in advanced HIV disease: effect on infections, CD4 cell counts and HIV suppression. *AIDS* 14:387–395.

125. Annunziata, P., C. Cioni, S. Toneatto, and E. Paccagnini. 1998. HIV-1 gp120 increases the permeability of rat brain endothelium cultures by a mechanism involving substance P. *AIDS* 12:2377–2385.

126. Antinori, A., A. Cingolani, L. Alba, A. Ammassari, D. Serraino, B. C. Ciancio, F. Palmieri, A. De Luca, L. M. Larocca, L. Ruco, G. Ippolito, and R. Cauda. 2001. Better response to chemotherapy and prolonged survival in AIDS-related lymphomas responding to highly active antiretroviral therapy. *AIDS* 15:1483–1491.

127. Antinori, A., C. F. Perno, M. L. Giancola, F. Forbici, G. Ippolito, R. M. Hoetelmans, and S. C. Piscitelli. 2005. Efficacy of cerebrospinal fluid (CSF)-penetrating antiretroviral drugs against HIV in the neurological compartment: different patterns of phenotypic resistance in CSF and plasma. *Clin. Infect. Dis.* 41:1787–1793.

128. Anton, P. A., R. T. Mitsuyasu, S. G. Deeks, D. T. Scadden, B. Wagner, C. Huang, C. Macken, D. D. Richman, C. Christopherson, F. Borellini, R. Lazar, and K. M. Hege. 2003. Multiple measures of HIV burden in blood and tissue are correlated with each other but not with clinical parameters in aviremic subjects. *AIDS* 17:53–63.

129. Antoni, B. A., P. Sabbatini, A. B. Rabson, and E. White. 1995. Inhibition of apoptosis in human immunodeficiency virus-infected cells enhances virus production and facilitates persistent infection. *J. Virol.* 69:2384–2392.

130. Apetrei, C., P. A. Marx, and S. M. Smith. 2004. The evolution of HIV and its consequences. *Infect. Dis. Clin. N. Am.* 18:369–394.

131. Appay, V., P. Hansasuta, J. Sutton, R. D. Schrier, J. K. Wong, M. Furtado, D. V. Havlir, S. M. Wolinsky, A. J. McMichael, D. D. Richman, S. L. Rowland-Jones, and C. A. Spina. 2002. Persistent HIV-1-specific cellular responses despite prolonged therapeutic viral suppression. *AIDS* 16:161–170.

132. Appay, V., D. F. Nixon, S. M. Donahoe, G. M. A. Gillespie, T. Dong, A. King, G. S. Ogg, H. M. L. Spiegel, C. Conlon, C. A. Spina, D. V. Havlir, D. D. Richman, A. Waters, P. Easterbrook, A. J. McMichael, and S. L. Rowland-Jones. 2000. HIV-specific CD8+ T cells produce antiviral cytokines but are impaired in cytolytic function. *J. Exp. Med.* 192:63–75.

133. Appay, V., L. Papagno, C. A. Spina, P. Hansasuta, A. King, L. Jones, G. S. Ogg, S. Little, A. J. McMichael, D. D. Richman, and S. L. Rowland-Jones. 2002. Dynamics of T cell responses in HIV infection. *J. Immunol.* 168:3660–3666.

134. Appay, V., and S. L. Rowland-Jones. 2004. Lessons from the study of T-cell differentiation in persistent human virus infection. *Semin. Immunol.* 16:205–212.

135. Aranda-Anzaldo, A., and D. Viza. 1992. Human immunodeficiency virus type 1 productive infection in staurosporine-blocked quiescent cells. *FEBS Lett.* 308:170–174.

136. Arase, H., N. Arase, Y. Kobayashi, Y. Nishimura, S. Yonehara, and K. Onoe. 1994. Cytotoxicity of fresh NK1.1+ T cell receptor alpha/beta+ thymocytes against a CD4+8+ thymocyte population associated with intact Fas antigen expression on the target. *J. Exp. Med.* 180:423–432.

137. Archibald, D. W., and G. A. Cole. 1990. *In vitro* inhibition of HIV-1 infectivity by human salivas. *AIDS Res. Hum. Retrovir.* 6:1425–1432.

138. Arden, B., S. P. Clark, D. Kabelitz, and T. W. Mak. 1995. Human T-cell receptor variable gene segment families. *Immunogenetics* 42:455–500.

139. Ardman, B., M. A. Sikorski, M. Settles, and D. E. Staunton. 1990. Human immunodeficiency virus type 1-infected individuals make autoantibodies that bind to CD43 on normal thymic lymphocytes. *J. Exp. Med.* 172:1151–1158.

140. Arendrup, M., J. E. Hansen, H. Clausen, C. Nielsen, L. R. Mathiesen, and J. O. Nielsen. 1991. Antibody to histo-blood group A antigen neutralizes HIV produced by lymphocytes from blood group A donors but not from blood group B or O donors. *AIDS* 5:441–444.

141. Arendrup, M., C. Nielsen, J.-E. S. Hansen, C. Pedersen, L. Mathiesen, and J. O. Nielsen. 1992. Autologous HIV-1 neutralizing antibodies: emergence of neutralization-resistant escape virus and subsequent development of escape virus neutralizing antibodies. *J. Acquir. Immune Defic. Syndr.* 5:303–307.

142. Arese, M., C. Ferrandi, L. Primo, G. Camussi, and F. Bussolino. 2001. HIV-1 Tat protein stimulates in vivo vascular permeability and lymphomononuclear cell recruitment. *J. Immunol.* 166:1380–1388.

143. Arias, R. A., L. D. Muñoz, M. Angeles, and A. Muñoz-Fernandez. 2003. Transmission of HIV-1 infection between trophoblast placental cells and T-cells take place via an LFA-1-mediated cell to cell contact. *Virology* 307:266–277.

144. Arien, K. K., A. Abraha, M. E. Quinones-Mateu, L. Kestens, G. Vanham, and E. J. Arts. 2005. The replicative fitness of primary human immunodeficiency virus type 1 (HIV-1) group M, HIV-1 group O, and HIV-2 isolates. *J. Virol.* 79:8979–8990.

145. Arien, K. K., Y. Gali, A. El-Abdellati, L. Heyndrickx, W. Janssens, and G. Vanham. 2006. Replicative fitness of CCR5-using and CXCR4-using human immunodeficiency virus type 1 biological clones. *Virology* 347:65–74.

146. Arien, K. K., R. M. Troyer, Y. Gali, R. L. Colebunders, E. J. Arts, and G. Vanham. 2005. Replicative fitness of historical and recent HIV-1 isolates suggests HIV-1 attenuation over time. *AIDS* 19:1555–1564.

147. Ariyoshi, K., S. Jaffar, A. S. Alabi, N. Berry, M. S. van der Loeff, S. Sabally, P. T. N'Gom, T. Corrah, R. Tedder, and H. Whittle. 2000. Plasma RNA viral load predicts the rate of CD4 T cell decline and death in HIV-2-infected patients in West Africa. *AIDS* 14:339–344.

148. Ariyoshi, K., M. Schim, M. van der Loeff, S. Sabally, F. Cham, T. Corrah, and H. Whittle. 1997. Does HIV-2 infection provide cross-protection against HIV-1 infection? *AIDS* 11:1053–1054.

149. Armstrong, J. A., and R. Horne. 1984. Follicular dendritic cells and virus-like particles in AIDS related lymphadenopathy. *Lancet* ii:370–372.

150. Arnedo-Valero, M., M. Plana, A. Mas, M. Guila, C. Gil, P. Castro, F. Garcia, E. Domingo, J. M. Gatell, and T. Pumarola. 2004. Similar HIV-1 evolution and immunological responses at

10 years despite several therapeutic strategies and host HLA Types. *J. Med. Virol.* **73:**495–501.

150a. Arnsten, J. H., R. Freeman, A. A. Howard, M. Floris-Moore, Y. Lo, and R. S. Klein. Decreased bone mineral density and increased fracture risk in aging men with or at risk for HIV infection. *AIDS,* in press.

151. Arold, S. T., and A. S. Baur. 2001. Dynamic nef and nef dynamics: how structure could explain the complex activities of this small HIV protein. *Trends Biochem. Sci.* **26:**356–363.

152. Arron, S. T., R. M. Ribeiro, A. Gettie, R. Bohm, J. Blanchard, J. Yu, A. S. Perelson, D. D. Ho, and L. Zhang. 2005. Impact of thymectomy on the peripheral T cell pool in rhesus macaques before and after infection with simian immunodeficiency virus. *Eur. J. Immunol.* **35:**46–55.

153. Artenstein, A. W., T. C. VanCott, J. R. Mascola, J. K. Carr, P. A. Hegerich, J. Gaywee, E. Sanders-Buell, M. L. Robb, D. E. Dayhoff, S. Thitivichianlert, S. Nitayaphan, J. G. McNeil, D. L. Birx, R. A. Michael, D. S. Burke, and F. E. McCutchan. 1995. Dual infection with human immunodeficiency virus type 1 of distinct envelope subtypes in humans. *J. Infect. Dis.* **171:**805–810.

154. Artenstein, A. W., T. C. VanCott, K. V. Sitz, M. L. Robb, K. F. Wagner, S. C. D. Veit, A. F. Rogers, R. P. Garner, J. W. Byron, P. R. Burnett, and D. L. Birx. 1997. Mucosal immune responses in four distinct compartments of women infected with human immunodeficiency virus type 1: a comparison by site and correlation with clinical information. *J. Infect. Dis.* **175:**265–271.

155. Arthos, J., K. C. Deen, M. A. Chaikin, J. A. Fornwald, G. Sathe, Q. J. Sattentau, P. R. Clapham, R. A. Weiss, J. S. McDougal, C. Pietropaolo, R. Axel, A. Truneh, P. J. Maddon, and R. W. Sweet. 1989. Identification of the residues in human CD4 critical for the binding of HIV. *Cell* **57:**469–481.

156. Arthur, L. O., J. W. Bess, Jr., R. C. Sowder II, R. E. Benveniste, D. L. Mann, J. C. Chermann, and L. E. Henderson. 1992. Cellular proteins bound to immunodeficiency viruses: implications for pathogenesis and vaccines. *Science* **258:**1935–1938.

157. Arthur, L. O., J. W. Bess, Jr., R. G. Urban, J. L. Strominger, W. R. Morton, D. L. Mann, L. E. Henderson, and R. E. Benveniste. 1995. Macaques immunized with HLA-DR are protected from challenge with simian immunodeficiency virus. *J. Virol.* **69:**3117–3124.

158. Arthur, L. O., J. W. Bess, Jr., D. J. Waters, S. W. Pyle, J. C. Kelliher, P. L. Nara, K. Krohn, W. G. Robey, A. J. Langlois, R. C. Gallo, and P. J. Fischinger. 1989. Challenge of chimpanzees (*Pan troglodytes*) immunized with human immunodeficiency virus envelope glycoprotein gp120. *J. Virol.* **63:**5046–5053.

159. Arvanitakis, L., E. Geras-Raaka, A. Varma, M. C. Gershengorn, and E. Cesarman. 1997. Human herpesvirus KSHV encodes a constitutively active G-protein-coupled receptor linked to cell proliferation. *Nature* **385:**347–350.

160. Ascher, M. S., and H. W. Sheppard. 1990. AIDS as immune system activation. II. The panergic imnesia hypothesis. *J. Acquir. Immune Defic. Syndr.* **3:**177–191.

161. Ashida, E. R., A. R. Johnson, and P. E. Lipsky. 1981. Human endothelial cell-lymphocyte interaction. *J. Clin. Investig.* **67:**1490–1499.

162. Ashorn, P., B. Moss, J. N. Weinstein, V. K. Chaudhary, D. J. FitzGerald, I. Pastan, and E. A. Berger. 1990. Elimination of infectious human immunodeficiency virus from human T-cell cultures by synergistic action of CD4-*Pseudomonas* exotoxin and reverse transcriptase inhibitors. *Proc. Natl. Acad. Sci. USA* **87:**8889–8893.

163. Asin, S. N., M. W. Fanger, D. Wildt-Perinic, P. L. Ware, C. R. Wira, and A. L. Howell. 2004. Transmission of HIV-1 by primary human uterine epithelial cells and stromal fibroblasts. *J. Infect. Dis.* **190:**236–245.

164. Asjo, B., J. Albert, F. Chiodi, and E. M. Fenyo. 1988. Improved tissue culture technique for production of poorly replicating human immunodeficiency virus strains. *J. Virol. Methods* **19:**191–196.

165. Asjo, B., J. Albert, A. Karlsson, L. Morfeldt-Mamson, G. Biberfeld, K. Lidman, and E. M. Fenyo. 1986. Replicative properties of human immunodeficiency virus from patients with varying severity of HIV infection. *Lancet* **ii:**660–662.

166. Asmuth, D. M., S. M. Hammer, and C. A. Wanke. 1994. Physiological effects of HIV infection on human intestinal epithelial cells: an in vitro model for HIV enteropathy. *AIDS* **8:**205–211.

167. Asselin-Paturel, C., A. Boonstra, M. Dalod, I. Durand, N. Yessaad, C. Dezutter-Dambuyant, A. Vicari, A. O'Garra, C. Biron, F. Briere, and G. Trinchieri. 2001. Mouse type I IFN-producing cells are immature APCs with plasmacytoid morphology. *Nat. Immunol.* **2:**1144–1150.

168. Atchison, R. E., J. Gosling, F. S. Monteclaro, C. Franci, L. Digilio, I. F. Charo, and M. A. Goldsmith. 1996. Multiple extracellular elements of CCR5 and HIV-1 entry: dissociation from response to chemokines. *Science* **274:**1924–1926.

169. Atkins, M. C., E. M. Carlin, V. C. Emery, P. D. Griffiths, and F. Boag. 1996. Fluctuations of HIV load in semen of HIV positive patients with newly acquired sexually transmitted diseases. *Br. Med. J.* **313:**341–342.

170. Attanasio, R., and R. C. Kennedy. 1990. Idiotypic cascades associated with the CD4-HIV gp120 interaction: principles for idiotype-based vaccines. *Int. Rev. Immunol.* **7:**109–119.

171. Aucouturier, P., L. J. Couderc, D. Gouet, F. Danon, J. Gombert, S. Matheron, A. G. Saimot, J. P. Clauvel, and J. L. Preud'homme. 1986. Serum immunoglobulin G subclass dysbalances in the lymphadenopathy syndrome and acquired immune deficiency syndrome. *Clin. Exp. Immunol.* **63:**234–240.

172. Auerbach, R., and Y. A. Sidky. 1979. Nature of the stimulus leading to lymphocyte-induced angiogenesis. *J. Immunol.* **123:**751–754.

173. Auewarakul, P., S. Louisirirotchanakul, R. Sutthent, T. Taechowisan, C. Kanoksinsombat, and C. Wasi. 1996. Analysis of neutralizing and enhancing antibodies to human immunodeficiency virus type 1 primary isolates in plasma of individuals infected with env Genetic subtype B and E viruses in Thailand. *Viral Immunol.* **9:**175–185.

174. Aukrust, P., C. J. Haug, T. Ueland, E. Lien, F. Muller, T. Espevik, J. Bollerslev, and S. S. Froland. 1999. Decreased bone formative and enhanced resorptive markers in human immunodeficiency virus infection: indication of normalization of the bone-remodeling process during highly active antiretroviral therapy. *J. Clin. Endocrinol. Metab.* **84:**145–150.

175. Aukrust, P., N.-B. Liabakk, F. Muller, E. Lien, T. Espevik, and S. S. Freland. 1994. Serum levels of tumor necrosis factor-α (TNFα) and soluble TNF receptors in human immunodeficiency virus type 1 infection-correlations to clinical, immunologic, and virologic parameters. *J. Infect. Dis.* **169:**420–424.

176. Autran, B., G. Carcelain, and P. Debre. 2001. Immune reconstitution after highly active anti-retroviral treatment of HIV infection. *Adv. Exp. Med. Biol.* **495:**205–212.

177. Autran, B., G. Carcelain, T. S. Li, C. Blanc, D. Mathez, R. Tubiana, C. Katlama, P. Debre, and J. Liebowitch. 1997. Positive effects of combined antiretroviral therapy on CD4+ T cell homeostasis and function in advanced HIV disease. *Science* 277:112–116.

178. Autran, B., C. M. Mayaud, M. Raphael, F. Plata, M. Denis, A. Bourguin, J. M. Guillon, P. Debre, and G. Akoun. 1988. Evidence for a cytotoxic T-lymphocyte alveolitis in human immunodeficiency virus-infected patients. *AIDS* 2:179–183.

179. Autran, B., F. Triebel, C. Katlama, W. Rozenbaum, T. Hercend, and P. Debre. 1989. T cell receptor γ/δ+ lymphocyte subsets during HIV infection. *Clin. Exp. Immunol.* 75:206–210.

180. Auvert, B., D. Taljaard, E. Lagarde, J. Sobngwi-Tambekou, R. Sitta, and A. Puren. 2005. Randomized, controlled intervention trial of male circumcision for reduction of HIV infection risk: the ANRS 1265 Trial. *PLOS Med.* 2:e298.

181. Aversa, S. M., A. M. Cattelan, L. Salvagno, G. Crivellari, G. Banna, M. Trevenzoli, V. Chiarion-Sileni, and S. Monfardini. 2005. Treatments of AIDS-related Kaposi's sarcoma. *Crit. Rev. Oncol. Hematol.* 53:253–265.

182. Ayehunie, S., E. A. Garcia-Zepeda, J. A. Hoxie, R. Horuk, T. S. Kupper, A. D. Luster, and R. M. Ruprecht. 1997. Human immunodeficiency virus-1 entry into purified blood dendritic cells through CC and CXC chemokine coreceptors. *Blood* 90:1397.

183. Ayouba, A., P. Mauclere, P. M. Martin, P. Cunin, J. Mfoupouendoun, B. Njinku, S. Souquieres, and F. Simon. 2001. HIV-1 group O infection in Cameroon, 1986 to 1998. *Emerg. Infect. Dis.* 7:466–467.

184. Ayouba, A., S. Souquieres, B. Njinku, P. M. V. Martin, M. C. Muller-Trutwin, P. Roques, F. Barre-Sinoussi, P. Mauclere, F. Simon, and E. Nerrienet. 2000. HIV-1 group N among HIV-1-seropositive individuals in Cameroon. *AIDS* 14:2623–2625.

185. Ayouba, A., G. Tene, P. Cunin, Y. Foupouapouognigni, E. Menu, A. Kfutwah, J. Thonnon, G. Scarlatti, M. Monney-Lobe, N. Eteki, C. Kouanfack, M. Tardy, R. Leke, M. Nkam, A. E. Nlend, F. Barre-Sinoussi, P. M. V. Martin, E. Nerrienet, and The Yaounde European Network for the Study of in Utero Transmission of HIV-1. 2003. Low rate of mother-to-child transmission of HIV-1 after Nevirapine intervention in a pilot public health program in Yaounde, Cameroon. *J. Acquir. Immune Defic. Syndr.* 34:274–280.

186. Ayyavoo, V., A. Mahboubi, S. Mahalingam, R. Ramalingam, S. Kudchodkar, W. V. Williams, D. R. Green, and D. B. Weiner. 1997. HIV-1 vpr suppresses immune activation and apoptosis through regulation of nuclear factor κB. *Nat. Med.* 3:1117–1123.

187. Aziz, S., O. T. Fackler, A. Meyerhans, N. Muller-Lantzsch, M. Zeitz, and T. Schneider. 2005. Replication of M-tropic HIV-1 in activated human intestinal lamina propria lymphocytes is the main reason for increased virus load in the intestinal mucosa. *J. Acquir. Immune Defic. Syndr.* 68:23–30.

188. Azzoni, L., E. Papasavvas, J. Chehimi, J. R. Kostman, K. Mouner, J. Ondercin, B. Perussia, and L. J. Montaner. 2002. Sustained impairment of IFN-γ secretion in suppressed HIV-infected patients despite mature NK cell recovery: evidence for a defective reconstitution of innate immunity. *J. Immunol.* 168:5764–5770.

189. Azzoni, L., E. Papasavvas, and L. J. Montaner. 2003. Lessons learned from HIV treatment interruption: safety, cor-relates of immune control, and drug sparing. *Curr. HIV Res.* 1:329–342.

190. Baba, M., R. Pauwels, J. Balzarini, J. Arnout, J. Desmyter, and E. DeClerq. 1988. Mechanism of inhibitory effect of dextran sulfate and heparin on replication of human immunodeficiency virus *in vitro*. *Proc. Natl. Acad. Sci. USA* 85:6132–6136.

191. Baba, T. W., Y. S. Jeong, D. Pennick, R. Bronson, M. F. Greene, and R. M. Ruprecht. 1995. Pathogenicity of live, attenuated SIV after mucosal infection of neonatal macaques. *Science* 267:1820–1825.

192. Baba, T. W., A. M. Trichel, L. An, V. Liska, L. N. Martin, M. Murphey-Corb, and R. M. Ruprecht. 1996. Infection and AIDS in adult macaques after nontraumatic oral exposure to cell-free SIV. *Science* 272:1486–1489.

193. Babas, T., J. B. Dewitt, J. L. Mankowski, P. M. Tarwater, J. E. Clements, and M. C. Zink. 2006. Progressive selection for neurovirulent genotypes in the brain of SIV-infected macaques. *AIDS* 20:197–205.

194. Babas, T., D. Munoz, J. L. Mankowski, P. M. Tarwater, J. E. Clements, and M. C. Zink. 2003. Role of microglial cells in selective replication of simian immunodeficiency virus genotypes in the brain. *J. Virol.* 77:208–216.

195. Bacchetti, P., B. Gripshover, C. Grunfeld, S. Heymsfield, H. McCreath, D. Osmond, M. Saag, R. Scherzer, M. Shlipak, and P. Tien. 2005. Fat distribution in men with HIV infection. *J. Acquir. Immune Defic. Syndr.* 40:121–131.

196. Bachelder, R. E., J. Bilancieri, W. Lin, and N. L. Letvin. 1995. A human recombinant Fab identifies a human immunodeficiency virus type 1-induced conformational change in cell surface-expressed CD4. *J. Virol.* 69:5734–5742.

197. Bachelerie, F., J. Alcami, U. Hazan, N. Israel, B. Goud, F. Arenzana-Seisdedos, and J.-L. Virelizier. 1990. Constitutive expression of human immunodeficiency virus (HIV) *nef* protein in human astrocytes does not influence basal or induced HIV long terminal repeat activity. *J. Virol.* 64:3059–3062.

198. Bachrach, E., H. Dreja, Y.-L. Lin, C. Mettling, V. Pinet, P. Corbeau, and M. Piechaczyk. 2005. Effects of virion surface gp120 density on infection by HIV-1 and viral production by infected cells. *Virology* 332:418–429.

199. Back, N. K. T., L. Smit, M. Schutten, P. L. Nara, M. Tersmette, and J. Goudsmit. 1993. Mutations in human immunodeficiency virus type 1 gp41 affect sensitivity to neutralization by gp120 antibodies. *J. Virol.* 67:6897–6902.

200. Back, N. T., L. Smit, J.-J. De Jong, W. Keulen, M. Schutten, J. Goudsmit, and M. Tersmette. 1994. An N-glycan within the human immunodeficiency virus type 1 gp120 V3 loop affects virus neutralization. *Virology* 199:431–438.

201. Badley, A. D., D. Dockrell, M. Simpson, R. Schut, D. H. Lynch, P. Leibson, and C. V. Paya. 1997. Macrophage-dependent apoptosis of CD4+ T lymphocytes from HIV-infected individuals is mediated by FasL and tumor necrosis factor. *J. Exp. Med.* 185:55–64.

202. Badley, A. D., J. A. McElhinny, P. J. Leibson, D. H. Lynch, M. R. Alderson, and C. V. Paya. 1996. Upregulation of Fas ligand expression by human immunodeficiency virus in human macrophages mediates apoptosis of uninfected T lymphocytes. *J. Virol.* 70:199–206.

203. Badley, A. D., A. A. Pilon, A. Landay, and D. H. Lynch. 2000. Mechanisms of HIV-associated lymphocyte apoptosis. *Blood* 96:2951–2964.

204. Badou, A., Y. Bennasser, M. Moreau, C. Leclerc, M. Benki-rane, and E. Bahraoui. 2000. Tat protein of human immunodeficiency virus type 1 induces interleukin-10 in human peripheral blood monocytes: implication of protein kinase C-dependent pathway. *J. Virol.* 74:10551–10562.

205. Badri, M., and R. Wood. 2003. Usefulness of total lymphocyte count in monitoring highly active antiretroviral therapy in resource-limited settings. *AIDS* 17:541–545.

206. Baeten, J. M., S. B. Mostad, M. P. Hughes, J. Overbaugh, D. D. Bankson, K. Mandaliya, J. O. Ndinya-Achola, J. J. Bwayo, and J. K. Kreiss. 2001. Selenium deficiency is associated with shedding of HIV-1-infected cells in the female genital tract. *J. Acquir. Immune Defic. Syndr.* 26:360–364.

207. Baeten, J. M., B. A. Richardson, L. Lavreys, J. P. Rakwar, K. Mandaliya, J. J. Bwayo, and J. K. Kreiss. 2005. Female-to-male infectivity of HIV-1 among circumcised and uncircumcised Kenyan men. *J. Infect. Dis.* 191:546–553.

208. Bafica, A., C. A. Scanga, M. L. Schito, S. Hieny, and A. Sher. 2003. In vivo induction of integrated HIV-1 expression by mycobacteria is critically dependent on toll-like receptor 2. *J. Immunol.* 171:1123–1127.

209. Bagasra, O., S. E. Bachman, L. Jew, R. Tawadros, J. Cater, G. Boden, I. Ryan, and R. J. Pomerantz. 1996. Increased human immunodeficiency virus type 1 replication in human peripheral blood mononuclear cells induced by ethanol: potential immunopathogenic mechanisms. *J. Infect. Dis.* 173:550–558.

210. Bagasra, O., H. Farzadegan, T. Seshamma, J. W. Oakes, A. Saah, and R. J. Pomerantz. 1994. Detection of HIV-1 proviral DNA in sperm from HIV-1-infected men. *AIDS* 8:1669–1674.

211. Bagasra, O., S. P. Hauptman, H. W. Lischner, M. Sachs, and R. J. Pomerantz. 1992. Detection of human immunodeficiency virus type 1 provirus in mononuclear cells by *in situ* polymerase chain reaction. *N. Engl. J. Med.* 326:1385–1391.

212. Bagasra, O., A. Kajdacsy-Balla, H. W. Lischner, and R. J. Pomerantz. 1993. Alcohol intake increases human immunodeficiency virus type 1 replication in human peripheral blood mononuclear cells. *J. Infect. Dis.* 167:789–797.

213. Bagasra, O., E. Lavi, L. Bobroski, K. Khalili, J. P. Pestaner, R. Tawadros, and R. J. Pomerantz. 1996. Cellular reservoirs of HIV-1 in the central nervous system of infected individuals: identification by the combination of *in situ* polymerase chain reaction and immunohistochemistry. *AIDS* 10:573–585.

213a. Bagasra, O., D. Patel, L. Bobroski, J. A. Abbasi, A. U. Bagasra, H. Baidouri, T. Harris, A. El-Roeiy, Z. Lengvarszky, H. Farzadegan, and C. Wood. 2005. Locatization of human herpesvirus type 8 in human sperms by in situ PCR. *J. Mol. Histol.* 36:401–412.

214. Bagasra, O., and R. J. Pomerantz. 1993. Human immunodeficiency virus type 1 provirus is demonstrated in peripheral blood monocytes *in vivo:* a study utilizing an *in situ* polymerase chain reaction. *AIDS Res. Hum. Retrovir.* 9:69–76.

215. Bagasra, O., and R. J. Pomerantz. 1993. Human immunodeficiency virus type 1 replication in peripheral blood mononuclear cells in the presence of cocaine. *J. Infect. Dis.* 168:1157–1164.

216. Bagasra, O., T. Seshamma, J. W. Oakes, and R. J. Pomerantz. 1993. High percentages of CD4-positive lymphocytes harbor the HIV-1 provirus in the blood of certain infected individuals. *AIDS* 7:1419–1425.

217. Bagetta, G., M. T. Corasaniti, L. Aloe, L. Berliocchi, N. Costa, A. Finazzi-Agro, and G. Nistico. 1996. Intracerebral injection of human immunodeficiency virus type 1 coat protein gp120 differentially affects the expression of nerve growth factor and nitric oxide synthase in the hippocampus of rat. *Proc. Natl. Acad. Sci. USA* 93:928–933.

218. Bagnarelli, P., A. Valenza, S. Menzo, A. Manzin, G. Scalise, P. E. Varaldo, and M. Clementi. 1994. Dynamics of molecular parameters of human immunodeficiency virus type 1 activity in vivo. *J. Virol.* 68:2495–2502.

219. Baier, M., A. Werner, N. Bannert, K. Metzner, and R. Kurth. 1995. HIV suppression by interleukin-16. *Nature* 378:563.

220. Bailes, E., F. Gao, F. Bibollet-Ruche, V. Courgnaud, M. Peeters, P. A. Marx, B. H. Hahn, and P. M. Sharp. 2003. Hybrid origin of SIV in chimpanzees. *Science* 300:1713.

221. Bailey, J. R., A. R. Sedaghat, T. Kieffer, T. Brennan, P. K. Lee, M. Wind-Rotolo, C. M. Haggerty, A. R. Kamireddi, Y. Liu, J. Lee, D. Persaud, J. E. Gallant, J. Cofrancesco, Jr., T. C. Quinn, C. O. Wilke, S. C. Ray, J. D. Siliciano, R. E. Nettles, and R. F. Siliciano. 2006. Residual human immunodeficiency virus type 1 viremia in some patients on antiretroviral therapy is dominated by a small number of invariant clones rarely found in circulating CD4$^+$ T cells. *J. Virol.* 80:6441–6457.

222. Bais, C., B. Santomasso, O. Coso, L. Arvanitakis, E. G. Raaka, J. S. Gutkind, A. S. Asch, E. Cesarman, M. C. Gerhengorn, and E. A. Mesr. 1998. G-protein-coupled receptor of Kaposi's sarcoma-associated herpesvirus is a viral oncogene and angiogenesis activator. *Nature* 391:86–87.

223. Bakri, Y., A. Mannioui, L. Ylisastigui, F. Sanchez, J. C. Gluckman, and A. Benjouad. 2002. CD40-activated macrophages become highly susceptible to X4 strains of human immunodeficiency virus type 1. *AIDS Res. Hum. Retrovir.* 18:103–113.

224. Bakri, Y., C. Schiffer, V. Zennou, P. Charneau, E. Kahn, A. Benjouad, J. C. Gluckman, and B. Canque. 2001. The maturation of dendritic cells results in postintegration inhibition of HIV-1 replication. *J. Immunol.* 166:3780–3788.

225. Balabanian, K., J. Harriague, C. Decrion, B. Lagane, S. Shorte, F. Baleux, J.-L. Virelizier, F. Arenzana-Seisdedos, and L. A. Chakrabarti. 2004. CXCR4-tropic HIV-1 envelope glycoprotein functions as a viral chemokine in unstimulated primary CD4+ T lymphocytes. *J. Immunol.* 173:7150–7160.

226. Balachandran, R., P. Thampatty, A. Enrico, C. Rinaldo, and P. Gupta. 1991. Human immunodeficiency virus isolates from asymptomatic homosexual men and from AIDS patients have distinct biologic and genetic properties. *Virology* 180:229–238.

227. Baldeweg, T., J. Catalan, E. Lovett, J. Gruzelier, M. Riccio, and D. Hawkins. 1995. Long-term zidovudine reduces neurocognitive deficits in HIV-1 infection. *AIDS* 9:589–596.

228. Baldwin, W. M. I. 1982. The symbiosis of immunocompetent and endothelial cells. *Immunol. Today* 3:267–269.

229. Ball, S. C., A. Abraha, K. R. Collins, A. J. Marozsan, H. Baird, M. E. Quinones-Mateu, A. Penn-Nicholson, M. Murray, N. Richard, M. Lobritz, P. A. Zimmerman, T. Kawamura, A. Blauvelt, and E. J. Arts. 2003. Comparing the ex vivo fitness of CCR5-tropic human immunodeficiency virus type 1 isolates of subtypes B and C. *J. Virol.* 77:1021–1038.

230. Ballerini, P., G. Gianluca, J. Z. Gong, V. Tassi, G. Saglio, D. M. Knowles, and R. Dalla-Favera. 1993. Multiple genetic

lesions in acquired immunodeficiency syndrome-related non-Hodgkin's lymphoma. *Blood* 81:166–176.

231. **Balliet, J. W., D. L. Kolson, G. Eiger, F. M. Kim, K. A. McGann, A. Srinivasan, and R. Collman.** 1994. Distinct effects in primary macrophages and lymphocytes of the human immunodeficiency virus type 1 accessory genes *vpr, vpu,* and *nef:* mutational analysis of a primary HIV-1 isolate. *Virology* 200:623–631.

232. **Balzarini, J., K. Van Laethem, S. Hatse, K. Vermeire, E. De Clercq, W. Peumans, E. Van Damme, A. Vandamme, A. Bohlmstedt, and D. Schols.** 2004. Profile of resistance of human immunodeficiency virus to mannose-specific plant lectins. *J. Virol.* 78:10617–10627.

233. **Banchereau, J., F. Briere, C. Caux, J. Davoust, S. Lebecque, Y.-J. Liu, B. Pulendran, and K. Palucka.** 2000. Immunobiology of dendritic cells. *Annu. Rev. Immunol.* 18:767–811.

234. **Banchereau, J., and R. M. Steinman.** 1998. Dendritic cells and the control of immunity. *Nature* 392:245–252.

235. **Banda, N. K., J. Bernier, D. K. Kurahara, R. Kurrle, N. Haigwood, R.-P. Sekaly, and T. H. Finkel.** 1992. Crosslinking CD4 by HIV gp120 primes T cells for activation-induced apoptosis. *J. Exp. Med.* 176:1099–1106.

236. **Bandres, J. C., J. Trial, D. M. Musher, and R. D. Rossen.** 1993. Increased phagocytosis and generation of reactive oxygen products by neutrophils and monocytes of men with stage 1 human immunodeficiency virus infection. *J. Infect. Dis.* 168:75–83.

236a. **Bangs, S. C., A. J. McMichael, and X. N. Xu.** 2006. Bystander T cell activation—implications for HIV infection and other diseases. Trends Immunol. 27:518–524.

237. **Bangsberg, D. R., E. D. Charlebois, R. M. Grant, M. Holodniy, S. G. Deeks, S. Perry, K. N. Conroy, R. Clark, D. Guzman, A. Zolopa, and A. Moss.** 2003. High levels of adherence do not prevent accumulation of HIV drug resistance mutations. *AIDS* 17:1925–1932.

238. **Bangsberg, D. R., A. R. Moss, and S. G. Deeks.** 2004. Paradoxes of adherence and drug resistance to HIV antiretroviral therapy. *J. Antimicrob. Chemother.* 53:696–699.

239. **Banki, Z., L. Kacani, P. Rusert, M. Pruenster, D. Wilflingseder, B. Falkensammer, H. Stellbrink, J. van Lunzen, A. Trkola, M. P. Dierich, and H. Stoiber.** 2005. Complement dependent trapping of infectious HIV in human lymphoid tissues. *AIDS* 19:481–486.

240. **Banks, W. A., E. O. Freed, K. M. Wolf, S. M. Robinson, M. Franko, and V. B. Kumar.** 2001. Transport of human immunodeficiency virus type 1 pseudoviruses across the blood-brain barrier: role of envelope proteins and adsorptive endocytosis. *J. Virol.* 75:4681–4691.

241. **Bannert, N., M. Farzan, D. S. Friend, H. Ochi, K. S. Price, J. Sodroski, and J. A. Boyce.** 2001. Human mast cell progenitors can be infected by macrophagetropic human immunodeficiency virus type 1 and retain virus with maturation in vitro. *J. Virol.* 75:10808–10814.

242. **Barassi, C., A. Lazzarin, and L. Lopalco.** 2004. CCR5-specific mucosal IgA in saliva and genital fluids of HIV-exposed seronegative subjects. *Blood* 104:2205–2206.

243. **Barassi, C., E. Soprana, C. Pastori, R. Longhi, E. Burati, F. Lillo, C. Marenzi, A. Lazzarin, A. G. Siccardi, and L. Lopalco.** 2005. Induction of murine mucosal CCR5-reactive antibodies as an anti-human immunodeficiency virus strategy. *J. Virol.* 79:6848–6858.

243a. **Barber, D. L., E. J. Wherry, D. Masopust, B. Zhu, J. P. Allison, A. H. Sharpe, G. J. Freeman, and R. Ahmed.** 2006. Restoring function in exhausted CD8 T cells during chronic viral infection. *Nature* 439:682–687.

244. **Barber, S. A., L. Gama, J. M. Dudaronek, T. Voelker, P. M. Tarwater, and J. E. Clements.** 2006. Mechanism for the establishment of transcriptional HIV latency in the brain in a simian immunodeficiency virus-macaque model. *J. Infect. Dis.* 193:963–970.

245. **Barbiano di Belgiojoso, G., A. Genderini, L. Vago, C. Parravicini, S. Bertoli, and N. Landriani.** 1990. Absence of HIV antigens in renal tissue from patients with HIV-associated nephropathy. *Nephrol. Dial. Transplant.* 5:489–492.

246. **Barboric, M., J. Kohoutek, J. P. Price, D. Blazek, D. H. Price, and B. M. Peterlin.** 2005. Interplay between 7SK snRNA and oppositely charged regions in HEXIM1 direct the inhibition of P-TEFb. *EMBO J.* 24:4291–4303.

247. **Barbour, J. D., F. M. Hecht, T. Wrin, M. R. Segal, C. A. Ramstead, T. J. Liegler, M. P. Busch, C. J. Petropoulos, N. S. Hellman, J. O. Kahn, and R. M. Grant.** 2004. Higher CD4+ T cell counts associated with low viral pol replication capacity among treatment-naive adults in early HIV-1 infection. *J. Infect. Dis.* 190:251–256.

248. **Barbour, J. D., T. Wrin, R. M. Grant, J. N. Martin, M. R. Segal, C. J. Petropoulos, and S. G. Deeks.** 2002. Evolution of phenotypic drug susceptibility and viral replication capacity during long-term virologic failure of protease inhibitor therapy in human immunodeficiency virus-infected adults. *J. Virol.* 76:11104–11112.

249. **Barboza, A., B. A. Castro, M. Whalen, C. C. D. Moore, J. S. Parkin, W. L. Miller, F. Gonzalez-Scarano, and J. A. Levy.** 1992. Infection of cultured adrenal cells by different strains of human immunodeficiency virus, types 1 and 2. *AIDS* 6:1437–1444.

250. **Barcova, M., L. Kacani, C. Speth, and M. P. Dierich.** 1998. gp41 envelope protein of human immunodeficiency virus induces interleukin (IL)-10 in monocytes, but not in B, T, or NK cells, leading to reduced IL-2 and interferon-gamma production. *J. Infect. Dis.* 177:905–913.

251. **Baribaud, F., and R. W. Doms.** 2001. The impact of chemokine receptor conformational heterogeneity on HIV infection. *Cell. Mol. Biol.* (Noisy-le-grand) 47:653–660.

252. **Baril, L., M. Jouan, R. Agher, E. Cambau, E. Caumes, F. Bricaire, and C. Katlama.** 2000. Impact of highly active antiretroviral therapy on onset of Mycobacterium avium complex infection and cytomegalovirus disease in patients with AIDS. *AIDS* 14:2593–2596.

253. **Barker, C. F., and R. E. Billingham.** 1997. Immunologically privileged sites. *Adv. Immunol.* 25:1–54.

254. **Barker, E., S. W. Barnett, L. Stamatatos, and J. A. Levy.** 1995. The human immunodeficiency viruses, p. 1–96. *In* J. A. Levy (ed.), *The Retroviridae*, vol. 4. Plenum Press, New York, N.Y.

255. **Barker, E., K. N. Bossart, S. H. Fujimura, and J. A. Levy.** 1997. CD28-costimulation increases CD8+ cell suppression of HIV replication. *J. Immunol.* 159:5123–5131.

256. **Barker, E., K. N. Bossart, and J. A. Levy.** 1998. Primary CD8+ cells from HIV-infected individuals can suppress

productive infection of macrophages independent of β-chemokines. *Proc. Natl. Acad. Sci. USA* 95:1725–1729.

257. Barker, E., K. N. Bossart, C. P. Locher, B. K. Patterson, and J. A. Levy. 1996. CD8+ cells from asymptomatic human immunodeficiency virus-infected individuals suppress superinfection of their peripheral blood mononuclear cells. *J. Gen. Virol.* 77:2953–2962.

258. Barker, E., C. E. Mackewicz, and J. A. Levy. 1995. Effects of TH1 and TH2 cytokines on CD8+ cell response against human immunodeficiency virus: implications for long-term survival. *Proc. Natl. Acad. Sci. USA* 92:11135–11139.

259. Barker, E., C. E. Mackewicz, G. Reyes-Teran, A. Sato, S. A. Stranford, S. H. Fujimura, C. Christopherson, S. Y. Chang, and J. A. Levy. 1998. Virological and immunological features of long-term human immunodeficiency virus-infected individuals who have remained asymptomatic compared to those who have progressed to acquired immunodeficiency syndrome. *Blood* 92:3105–3114.

260. Barker, T. D., D. Weissman, J. A. Daucher, K. M. Roche, and A. S. Fauci. 1996. Identification of multiple and distinct CD8+ T cell suppressor activities: dichotomy between infected and uninfected individuals, evolution with progression of disease, and sensitivity to gamma irradiation. *J. Immunol.* 156:4476–4483.

261. Barnes, P. J., and M. Karin. 1997. Nuclear factor-κB: a pivotal transcription factor in chronic inflammatory diseases. *N. Engl. J. Med.* 336:1066–1071.

262. Barnett, S., A. Barboza, C. M. Wilcox, C. E. Forsmark, and J. A. Levy. 1991. Characterization of human immunodeficiency virus type 1 strains recovered from the bowel of infected individuals. *Virology* 182:802–809.

263. Barnett, S. W., S. Lu, I. Srivastava, S. Cherpelis, A. Gettie, J. Blanchard, S. Wang, I. Mboudjeka, L. Leung, Y. Lian, A. Fong, C. Buckner, A. Ly, S. Hilt, J. Ulmer, C. T. Wild, J. R. Mascola, and L. Stamatatos. 2001. The ability of an oligomeric human immunodeficiency virus type 1 (HIV-1) envelope antigen to elicit neutralizing antibodies against primary HIV-1 isolates is improved following partial deletion of the second hypervariable region. *J. Virol.* 75:5526–5540.

264. Reference deleted.

265. Barnett, S. W., K. K. Murthy, B. G. Herndier, and J. A. Levy. 1994. An AIDS-like condition induced in baboons by HIV-2. *Science* 266:642–646.

266. Barnett, S. W., M. Quiroga, A. Werner, D. Dina, and J. A. Levy. 1993. Distinguishing features of an infectious molecular clone of the highly divergent and non-cytopathic HIV-2$_{UC1}$ strain. *J. Virol.* 67:1006–1014.

267. Barouch, D. H., J. Kunstman, M. J. Kuroda, J. E. Schmitz, S. Santra, F. W. Peyerl, G. R. Krivulka, K. Beaudry, M. A. Lifton, D. A. Gorgone, D. C. Montefiori, M. G. Lewis, S. M. Wolinsky, and N. L. Letvin. 2002. Eventual AIDS vaccine failure in a rhesus monkey by viral escape from noncytotoxic T lymphocytes. *Nature* 415:335–338.

268. Barouch, D. H., N. L. Letvin, and R. A. Seder. 2004. The role of cytokine DNAs as vaccine adjuvants for optimizing cellular immune responses. *Immunol. Rev.* 202:266–274.

269. Barouch, D. H., and G. J. Nabel. 2005. Adenovirus vector-based vaccines for human immunodeficiency virus type 1. *Hum. Gene Ther.* 16:149–156.

270. Barouch, D. H., S. Santra, M. J. Kuroda, J. E. Schmitz, R. Plishka, A. Buckler-White, A. E. Gaitan, R. Zin, J. H. Nam, L. S. Wyatt, M. A. Lifton, C. E. Nickerson, B. Moss, D. C. Montefiori, V. M. Hirsch, and N. L. Letvin. 2001. Reduction of simian-human immunodeficiency virus 89.6p viremia in rhesus monkeys by recombinant modified vaccinia virus Ankara vaccination. *J. Virol.* 75:5151–5158.

271. Barouch, D. H., S. Santra, J. E. Schmitz, M. J. Kuroda, T.-M. Fu, W. Wagner, M. Bilska, A. Craiu, X. X. Zheng, G. R. Krivulka, K. Beaudry, M. A. Lifton, C. E. Nickerson, W. L. Trigona, K. Punt, D. C. Freed, L. Guan, S. Dubey, D. Casimiro, A. Simon, M.-E. Davies, M. Chastain, T. B. Strom, R. S. Gelman, D. C. Montefiori, M. G. Lewis, E. A. Emini, J. W. Shiver, and N. L. Letvin. 2000. Control of viremia and prevention of clinical AIDS in rhesus monkeys by cytokine-augmented DNA vaccination. *Science* 290:463–465.

272. Barre-Sinoussi, F., J.-C. Chermann, F. Rey, M. T. Nugeyre, S. Chamaret, J. Gruest, C. Dauguet, C. Axler-Blin, F. Vezinet-Brun, C. Rouzioux, W. Rozenbaum, and L. Montagnier. 1983. Isolation of a T-lymphotropic retrovirus from a patient at risk for acquired immune deficiency syndrome (AIDS). *Science* 220:868–871.

273. Barrett, A. D. T., and E. A. Gould. 1986. Antibody-mediated early death *in vivo* after infection with yellow fever virus. *J. Gen. Virol.* 67:2539–2542.

274. Barron, M. A., N. Blyveis, B. E. Palmer, S. MaWhinney, and C. C. Wilson. 2003. Influence of plasma viremia on defects in number and immunophenotype of blood dendritic cell subsets in human immunodeficiency virus 1-infected individuals. *J. Infect. Dis.* 187:26–37.

275. Bartholomew, C., W. Blattner, and F. Cleghorn. 1987. Progression to AIDS in homosexual men co-infected with HIV-1 and HTLV-1 in Trinidad. *Lancet* ii:1469.

276. Bartholomew, C. F., and A. M. Jones. 2006. Human bites: a rare risk factor for HIV transmission. *AIDS* 20:631–632.

277. Bartz, S. R., and M. Emerman. 1999. Human immunodeficiency virus type 1 Tat induces apoptosis and increases sensitivity to apoptotic signals by up-regulating FLICE/caspase-8. *J. Virol.* 73:1956–1963.

278. Bashirova, A., G. Bleiber, Y. Qi, H. Hutcheson, T. Yamashita, R. C. Johnson, J. Cheng, G. Alter, J. Goedert, S. Buchbinder, K. Hoots, D. Vlahov, M. May, F. Maldarelli, L. Jacobson, S. J. O'Brien, A. Telenti, and M. Carrington. 2006. Consistent effects of TSG101 genetic variability on multiple outcomes of exposure to human immunodeficiency virus type 1. *J. Virol.* 80:6757–6763.

279. Batman, P. A., S. C. Fleming, P. M. Sedgwick, T. T. MacDonald, and G. E. Griffin. 1994. HIV infection of human fetal intestinal explant cultures induces epithelial cell proliferation. *AIDS* 8:161–167.

280. Baucke, R. B., and P. B. Spear. 1979. Membrane proteins specified by herpes simplex viruses. V. Identification of an Fc-binding glycoprotein. *J. Virol.* 32:779–789.

281. Baum, L. L., K. J. Cassutt, K. Knigge, R. Khattri, J. Margolick, C. Rinaldo, C. A. Kleeberger, P. Nishanian, D. R. Henrard, and J. Phair. 1996. HIV-1 gp120-specific antibody-dependent cell-mediated cytotoxicity correlates with rate of disease progression. *J. Immunol.* 157:2168–2173.

282. Baum, M. K., G. Shor-Posner, Y. Lu, B. Rosner, H. E. Sauberlich, M. A. Fletcher, J. Szapocznik, C. Eisdorfer, J. E. Buring, and C. H. Hennekens. 1995. Micronutrients and HIV-1 disease progression. *AIDS* 9:1051–1056.

283. Baur, A. S., E. T. Sawai, P. Dazin, W. J. Fantl, C. Cheng-Mayer, and B. M. Peterlin. 1994. HIV-1 Nef leads to inhibition or activation of T cells depending on its intracellular localization. *Immunity* 1:373–384.

284. Bayard-McNeeley, M., H. Doo, S. He, A. Hafner, W. D. Johnson, Jr., and J. L. Ho. 1996. Differential effects of interleukin-12, interleukin-15, and interleukin-2 on human immunodeficiency virus type 1 replication in vitro. *Clin. Diagn. Lab. Immunol.* 3:547–553.

285. Bayley, A. C. 1991. Occurrence, clinical behavior and management of Kaposi's sarcoma. *Cancer Surv.* 10:53–71.

286. Beausejour, Y., and M. J. Tremblay. 2004. Interaction between the cytoplasmic domain of ICAM-1 and pr55^{Gag} leads to acquisition of host ICAM-1 by human immunodeficiency virus type 1. *J. Virol.* 78:11916–11925.

287. Becherer, P. R., M. L. Smiley, T. J. Matthews, K. J. Weinhold, C. W. McMillan, and G. C. White II. 1990. Human immunodeficiency virus-1 disease progression in hemophiliacs. *Am. J. Hematol.* 34:204–209.

288. Beckstead, J. H., G. S. Wood, and V. Fletcher. 1985. Evidence for the origin of Kaposi's sarcoma from lymphatic endothelium. *Am. J. Pathol.* 119:294–300.

289. Becquart, P., N. Chomont, P. Roques, A. Ayouba, M. D. Kazatchkine, L. Belec, and H. Hocini. 2002. Compartmentalization of HIV-1 between breast milk and blood of HIV-infected mothers. *Virology* 300:109–117.

290. Becquart, P., H. Hocini, M. Levy, A. Sepou, M. D. Kazatchkine, and L. Belec. 2000. Secretory anti-human immunodeficiency virus (HIV) antibodies in colostrum and breast milk are not a major determinant of the protection of early postnatal transmission of HIV. *J. Infect. Dis.* 181:532–539.

291. Becquart, P., G. Petitjean, Y. A. Tabaa, D. Valea, M. F. Huguet, E. Tuaillon, N. Meda, J. P. Vendrell, and P. Van de Perre. 2006. Detection of a large T-cell reservoir able to replicate HIV-1 actively in breast milk. *AIDS* 20:1453–1455.

292. Bednarik, D. P., J. D. Mosca, and N. B. Raj. 1987. Methylation as a modulator of expression of human immunodeficiency virus. *J. Virol.* 61:1253–1257.

293. Behets, F., M. Kashamuka, M. Pappaioanou, T. A. Green, R. W. Ryder, V. Batter, J. R. George, W. H. Hannon, and T. C. Quinn. 1992. Stability of human immunodeficiency virus type 1 antibodies in whole blood dried on filter paper and stored under various tropical conditions in Kinshasa. *J. Clin. Microbiol.* 30:1179–1182.

294. Behrens, G. M., A. R. Boerner, K. Weber, J. van den Hoff, J. Ockenga, G. Brabant, and R. E. Schmidt. 2002. Impaired glucose phosphorylation and transport in skeletal muscle cause insulin resistance in HIV-1-infected patients with lipodystrophy. *J. Clin. Investig.* 110:1319–1327.

295. Beignon, A. S., K. McKenna, M. Skoberne, O. Manches, I. DaSilva, D. G. Kavanagh, M. Larsson, R. J. Gorelick, J. D. Lifson, and N. Bhardwaj. 2005. Endocytosis of HIV-1 activates plasmacytoid dendritic cells via Toll-like receptor-viral RNA interactions. *J. Clin. Investig.* 115:3265–3275.

296. Belec, L., P. D. Ghys, H. Hocini, J. N. Nkengasong, J. Tranchot-Diallo, M. O. Diallo, V. Ettiegne-Traore, C. Maurice, P. Becquart, M. Matta, A. Si-Mohamed, N. Chomont, I. M. Coulibaly, S. Z. Wiktor, and M. D. Kazatchkine. 2001. Cervicovaginal secretory antibodies to human immunodeficiency virus type 1 (HIV-1) that block viral transcytosis through tight ep-

ithelial barriers in highly exposed HIV-1-seronegative African women. *J. Infect. Dis.* 184:1412–1422.

297. Belec, L., C. Piketty, A. Si-Mohamed, C. Goujon, M.-C. Hallouin, S. Cotigny, L. Weiss, and M. D. Kazatchkine. 2000. High levels of drug-resistant human immunodeficiency virus variants in patients exhibiting increasing CD4+ T cell counts despite virologic failure of protease inhibitor-containing antiretroviral combination therapy. *J. Infect. Dis.* 181:1808–1812.

298. Bell, I., C. Ashman, J. Maughan, E. Hooker, F. Cook, and T. A. Reinhart. 1998. Association of simian immunodeficiency virus Nef with the T-cell receptor (TCR) ζchain leads to TCR down-modulation. *J. Gen. Virol.* 79:2717–2727.

299. Belshe, R. B., C. Stevens, G. J. Gorse, S. Buchbinder, K. Weinhold, H. Sheppard, D. Stablein, S. Self, J. McNamara, S. Frey, J. Flores, J. L. Excler, M. Klein, R. E. Habib, A. M. Duliege, C. Harro, L. Corey, M. Keefer, M. Mulligan, P. Wright, C. Celum, F. Judson, K. Mayer, D. McKirnan, M. Marmor, and G. Woody. 2001. Safety and immunogenicity of a canarypox-vectored human immunodeficiency virus Type 1 vaccine with or without gp120: a phase 2 study in higher- and lower-risk volunteers. *J. Infect. Dis.* 183:1343–1352.

300. Belsito, D. V., M. R. Sanchez, R. L. Baer, F. Valentine, and G. J. Thorbecke. 1984. Reduced Langerhans' cell Ia antigen and ATPase activity in patients with the acquired immunodeficiency syndrome. *N. Engl. J. Med.* 310:1279–1282.

301. Belyakov, I. M., V. A. Kuznetsov, B. Kelsall, D. Klinman, M. Moniuszko, M. Lemon, P. D. Markham, R. Pal, J. D. Clements, M. G. Lewis, W. Strober, G. Franchini, and J. A. Berzofsky. 2006. Impact of vaccine-induced mucosal high avidity CD8+ CTL in delay of AIDS-viral dissemination from mucosa. *Blood* 107:3258–3264.

302. Benedict, C. A., P. S. Norris, and C. F. Ware. 2002. To kill or be killed: viral evasion of apoptosis. *Nat. Immunol.* 3:1013–1018.

303. Benito, J. M., J. M. Zabay, J. Gil, M. Bermejo, A. Escudero, E. Sanchez, and E. Fernandez-Cruz. 1997. Quantitative alterations of the functionally distinct subsets of CD4 and CD8 T lymphocytes in asymptomatic HIV infection: changes in the expression of CD45RO, CD45RA, CD11b, CD38, HLA-DR, and CD25 antigens. *J. Acquir. Immune Defic. Syndr. Hum. Retrovirol.* 14:128–135.

304. Benjouad, A., J.-C. Gluckman, H. Rochat, L. Montagnier, and E. Bahraoui. 1992. Influence of carbohydrate moieties on the immunogenicity of human immunodeficiency virus type 1 recombinant gp160. *J. Virol.* 66:2473–2483.

305. Benki, S., S. B. Mostad, B. A. Richardson, K. Mandaliya, J. K. Kreiss, and J. Overbaugh. 2004. Cyclic shedding of HIV-1 RNA in cervical secretions during the menstrual cycle. *J. Infect. Dis.* 189:2192–2201.

306. Benn, S., R. Rutledge, T. Folks, J. Gold, L. Baker, J. McCormick, P. Feorino, P. Piot, T. Quinn, and M. Martin. 1985. Genomic heterogeneity of AIDS retroviral isolates from North America and Zaire. *Science* 230:949–951.

307. Bennasser, Y., S.-Y. Le, M. Benkirane, and K.-T. Jeang. 2005. Evidence that HIV-1 encodes an siRNA and a suppressor of RNA silencing. *Immunity* 22:607–619.

308. Benos, D. J., B. H. Hahn, J. K. Bubien, S. K. Ghosh, N. A. Mashburn, M. A. Chaikin, G. M. Shaw, and E. N. Benveniste. 1994. Envelope glycoprotein gp120 of human immunodeficiency virus type 1 alters ion transport in astrocytes:

implications for AIDS dementia complex. *Proc. Natl. Acad. Sci. USA* 91:494–498.

309. Benson, C. A., J. E. Kaplan, H. Masur, A. Pau, and K. K. Holmes. 2005. Treating opportunistic infections among HIV-infected adults and adolescents: recommendations from CDC, the National Institutes of Health, and the HIV Medicine Association/Infectious Diseases Society of America. *Clin. Infect. Dis.* 40:S131.

309a. Benson, C. A., F. Vaida, D. V. Havlir, G. F. Downey, M. M. Lederman, R. M. Gulick, M. J. Glesby, M. Wantman, C. J. Bixby, A. R. Rinehart, S. Snyder, R. Wang, S. Patel, and J. W. Mellors. 2006. A randomized trial of treatment interruption before optimized antiretroviral therapy for persons with drug-resistant HIV: 48-week virologic results of ACTG A5086. *J. Infect. Dis.* 194:1309–1318.

310. Bentwich, Z., G. Maartens, D. Torten, A. A. Lal, and R. B. Lal. 2000. Concurrent infections and HIV pathogenesis. *AIDS* 14:2071–2081.

311. Bentwich, Z., Z. Weisman, C. Moroz, S. Bar-Yehuda, and A. Kalinkovich. 1996. Immune dysregulation in Ethiopian immigrants in Israel: relevance to helminth infections? *Clin. Exp. Immunol.* 103:239–243.

312. Beq, S., A. Fontanet, J. Theze, and J.-H. Colle. 2004. IL-7 and Flt-3L plasma levels are increased during highly active antiretroviral therapy-associated IL-2 therapy. *AIDS* 18:2089–2091.

313. Beq, S., M. T. Nugeyre, R. H. Fang, D. Gautier, R. Legrand, N. Schmitt, J. Estaquier, F. Barre-Sinoussi, B. Hurtrel, R. Cheynier, and N. Israel. 2006. IL-7 induces immunological improvement in SIV-infected rhesus macaques under antiviral therapy. *J. Immunol.* 176:914–922.

314. Beral, V., T. Peterman, R. Berkelman, and H. Jaffe. 1991. AIDS-associated non-Hodgkin lymphoma. *Lancet* 337:805–809.

315. Beral, V., T. A. Peterman, R. L. Berkelman, and H. W. Jaffe. 1990. Kaposi's sarcoma among persons with AIDS: a sexually transmitted infection? *Lancet* 335:123–128.

316. Berberian, L., L. Goodglick, T. J. Kipps, and J. Braun. 1993. Immunoglobulin V_H3 gene products: natural ligands for HIV gp120. *Science* 261:1588–1590.

317. Beretta, A., S. H. Weiss, G. Rappocciolo, R. Mayur, C. De Santis, J. Quirinale, A. Cosma, P. Robbioni, G. M. Shearer, J. A. Berzofsky, et al. 1996. Human immunodeficiency virus type 1 (HIV-1)-seronegative injection drug users at risk for HIV exposure have antibodies to HLA class I antigens and T cells specific for HIV envelope. *J. Infect. Dis.* 173:472–476.

318. Bergamini, A., F. Bolacchi, C. D. Pesce, M. Carbone, F. Cepparulo, F. Demin, and G. Rocchi. 2002. Increased CD4 and CCR5 expression and human immunodeficiency virus type 1 entry in CD40 ligand-stimulated macrophages. *J. Infect. Dis.* 185:1567–1577.

319. Bergamini, A., L. Dini, M. Capozzi, L. Ghibelli, R. Placido, E. Faggioli, A. Salanitro, E. Buonanno, L. Cappannoli, L. Ventura, M. Cepparulo, L. Falasca, and G. Rocchi. 1996. Human immunodeficiency virus-induced cell death in cytokine-treated macrophages can be prevented by compounds that inhibit late stages of viral replication. *J. Infect. Dis.* 173:1367–1378.

320. Berger, E. A. 1997. HIV entry and tropism: the chemokine receptor connection. *AIDS* 11:S3–S16.

321. Berger, E. A., R. W. Doms, E. M. Fenyo, B. T. Korber, D. R. Littman, J. P. Moore, Q. J. Sattentau, H. Schuitemaker, J.

Sodroski, and R. A. Weiss. 1998. A new classification for HIV-1. *Nature* 391:240.

322. Berger, E. A., J. D. Lifson, and L. E. Eiden. 1991. Stimulation of glycoprotein gp120 dissociation from the envelope glycoprotein complex of human immunodeficiency virus type 1 by soluble CD4 and CD4 peptide derivatives: implications for the role of the complementarity-determining region 3-like region in membrane fusion. *Proc. Natl. Acad. Sci. USA* 88:8082–8086.

323. Berger, E. A., P. M. Murphy, and J. M. Farber. 1999. Chemokine receptors as HIV-1 coreceptors: roles in viral entry, tropism, and disease. *Annu. Rev. Immunol.* 17:657–700.

324. Berger, E. A., J. R. Sisler, and P. L. Earl. 1992. Human immunodeficiency virus type 1 envelope glycoprotein molecules containing membrane fusion-impairing mutations in the V3 region efficiently undergo soluble CD4-stimulated gp120 release. *J. Virol.* 66:6208–6212.

325. Berger, J., and J. A. Levy. 1992. The human immunodeficiency virus, type 1: the virus and its role in neurologic disease. *Semin. Neurol.* 12:1–9.

326. Berger, J. R. 2000. Progressive multifocal leukoencephalopathy. *Curr. Treat. Options Neurol.* 2:361–368.

327. Bergeron, L., and J. Sodroski. 1992. Dissociation of unintegrated viral DNA accumulation from single-cell lysis induced by human immunodeficiency virus type 1. *J. Virol.* 66:5777–5787.

328. Bergeron, L., N. Sullivan, and J. Sodroski. 1992. Target cell-specific determinants of membrane fusion within the human immunodeficiency virus type 1 gp120 third variable region and gp41 amino terminus. *J. Virol.* 66:2389–2397.

329. Bergey, E. J., M.-I. Cho, B. M. Blumberg, M.-L. Hammarskjold, D. Rekosh, L. G. Epstein, and M. J. Levine. 1994. Interaction of HIV-1 and human salivary mucins. *J. Acquir. Immune Defic. Syndr.* 7:995–1002.

330. Berke, G. 1991. Lymphocyte-triggered internal target disintegration. *Immunol. Today* 12:396–403.

331. Berkowitz, R., K. P. Beckerman, T. J. Schall, and J. M. McCune. 1998. CXCR4 and CCR5 expression delineates targets for HIV-1 disruption of T cell differentiation. *J. Immunol.* 161:3702–3710.

332. Berkowitz, R. D., S. Alexander, C. Bare, V. Linquits-Stepps, M. Bogan, M. E. Moreno, L. Gibson, E. D. Wieder, J. Kosek, C. A. Stoddart, and J. M. McCune. 1998. CCR5- and CXCR4-utilizing strains of human immunodeficiency virus type 1 exhibit differential tropism and pathogenesis in vivo. *J. Virol.* 72:10108–10117.

333. Berkowitz, R. D., S. Alexander, and J. M. McCune. 2000. Causal relationships between HIV-1 coreceptor utilization, tropism, and pathogenesis in human thymus. *AIDS Res. Hum. Retrovir.* 16:1039–1045.

334. Berkowitz, R. D., A. Ohagen, S. Hoglund, and S. P. Goff. 1995. Retroviral nucleocapsid domains mediate the specific recognition of genomic viral RNAs by chimeric gag polyproteins during packaging in vivo. *J. Virol.* 69:6445–6456.

335. Berman, P. W., T. J. Gregory, L. Riddle, G. R. Nakamura, M. A. Champe, J. P. Porter, F. M. Wurm, R. D. Hershberg, E. K. Cobb, and J. W. Eichberg. 1990. Protection of chimpanzees from infection by HIV-1 after vaccination with recombinant glycoprotein gp120 but not gp160. *Nature* 345:622–625.

336. Berman, P. W., T. J. Matthews, L. Riddle, M. Champe, M. R. Hobbs, G. R. Nakamura, J. Mercer, D. J. Eastman, C. Lucas,

A. J. Langlois, F. M. Wurm, and T. J. Gregory. 1992. Neutralization of multiple laboratory and clinical isolates of human immunodeficiency virus type 1 (HIV-1) by antisera raised against gp120 from the MN isolate of HIV-1. *J. Virol.* **66:**4464–4469.

337. Berman, P. W., K. K. Murthy, T. Wrin, J. C. Vennari, E. K. Cobb, D. J. Eastman, M. Champe, G. R. Nakamura, D. Davison, M. F. Powell, J. Bussiere, D. P. Francis, T. Matthews, T. J. Gregory, and J. F. Obijeski. 1996. Protection of MN-rgp120-immunized chimpanzees from heterologous infection with a primary isolate of human immunodeficiency virus type 1. *J. Infect. Dis.* **173:**52–59.

338. Berndt, C., B. Mopps, S. Angermuller, P. Gierschik, and P. H. Krammer. 1998. CXCR4 and CD4 mediate a rapid CD95-independent cell death in CD4+ T cells. *Proc. Natl. Acad. Sci. USA* **95:**12556–12561.

339. Bernier, R., and M. Tremblay. 1995. Homologous interference resulting from the presence of defective particles of human immunodeficiency virus type 1. *J. Virol.* **69:**291–300.

340. Bernstein, M. S., S. E. Tong-Starksen, and R. M. Locksley. 1991. Activation of human monocyte-derived macrophages with lipopolysaccharide decreases human immunodeficiency virus replication in vitro at the level of gene expression. *J. Clin. Investig.* **88:**540–545.

341. Berrada, F., D. Ma, J. Michaud, G. Doucet, L. Giroux, and A. Kessous-Elbaz. 1995. Neuronal expression of human immunodeficiency virus type 1 env proteins in transgenic mice: distribution in the central nervous system and pathological alterations. *J. Virol.* **69:**6770–6778.

342. Berrey, M. M., T. Schacker, A. C. Collier, T. Shea, S. J. Brodie, D. Mayers, R. Coombs, J. Krieger, T. W. Chun, A. Fauci, S. G. Self, and L. Corey. 2001. Treatment of primary human immunodeficiency virus type 1 infection with potent antiretroviral therapy reduces frequency of rapid progression to AIDS. *J. Infect. Dis.* **183:**1466–1475.

343. Berrios, D. C., A. L. Avins, K. Haynes-Sanstad, R. Eversley, and W. J. Woods. 1995. Screening for human immunodeficiency virus antibody in urine. *Arch. Pathol. Lab. Med.* **119:**139–141.

344. Berson, J. F., D. Long, B. J. Doranz, J. Rucker, F. R. Jirik, and R. W. Doms. 1996. A seven-transmembrane domain receptor involved in fusion and entry of T-cell-tropic human immunodeficiency virus type 1 strains. *J. Virol.* **70:**6288–6295.

345. Berthier, A., S. Chamaret, R. Fauchet, J. Fonlupt, N. Genetet, M. Gueguen, M. Pommereuil, A. Ruffault, and L. Montagnier. 1986. Transmissibility of human immunodeficiency virus in haemophilic and non-haemophilic children living in a private school in France. *Lancet* **ii:**598–601.

346. Bertoletti, A., A. Sette, F. V. Chisari, A. Penna, M. Levrero, M. De Carli, F. Fiaccadori, and C. Ferrari. 1994. Natural variants of cytotoxic epitopes are T-cell receptor antagonists for antiviral cytotoxic T cells. *Nature* **369:**407–410.

347. Bertram, S., F. T. Hufert, J. van Lunzen, and D. von Laer. 1996. Coinfection of individual leukocytes with human cytomegalovirus and human immunodeficiency virus is a rare event *in vivo*. *J. Med. Virol.* **49:**283–288.

348. Berzofsky, J. A., and I. J. Berkower. 1995. Novel approaches to peptide and engineered protein vaccines for HIV using defined epitopes: advances in 1994–1995. *AIDS* **9:**S143-S157.

349. Besansky, N. J., S. T. Butera, S. Sinha, and T. M. Folks. 1991. Unintegrated human immunodeficiency virus type 1 DNA in chronically infected cell lines is not correlated with surface CD4 expression. *J. Virol.* **65:**2695–2698.

350. Besnier, C., Y. Takeuchi, and G. Towers. 2002. Restriction of lentivirus in monkeys. *Proc. Natl. Acad. Sci. USA* **99:**11920–11925.

351. Besson, C., A. Goubar, J. Gabarre, W. Rosenbaum, G. Pialoux, F. P. Chatelet, C. Katlama, F. Charlotte, B. Dupont, N. Brousse, M. Huerre, J. Mikol, P. Camparo, K. Mokhtari, M. Tulliez, D. Salmon-Ceron, F. Boue, D. Costagliola, and M. Raphael. 2001. Changes in AIDS-related lymphoma since the era of highly active antiretroviral therapy. *Blood* **98:**2339–2344.

352. Best, S., P. Le Tissier, G. Towers, and J. P. Stoye. 1996. Positional cloning of the mouse retrovirus restriction gene Fv 1. *Nature* **382:**826–829.

353. Bettaieb, A., P. Fromont, F. Louache, E. Oksenhendler, W. Vainchenker, N. Duedari, and P. Bierling. 1992. Presence of cross-reactive antibody between human immunodeficiency virus (HIV) and platelet glycoproteins in HIV-related immune thrombocytopenic purpura. *Blood* **80:**162–169.

354. Bettinardi, A., L. Imberti, A. Sottini, E. Quiros-Roldan, M. Puoti, F. Castelli, G. P. Cadeo, R. Gorla, and D. Primi. 1997. Detection of clonal T cell populations with closely related T cell receptor junctional sequences in persons at high risk for human immunodeficiency virus (HIV) infection and in patients acutely infected with HIV. *J. Infect. Dis.* **175:**272–282.

355. Betts, M. R., D. R. Ambrozak, D. C. Douek, S. Bonhoeffer, J. M. Brenchley, J. P. Casazza, R. A. Koup, and L. J. Picker. 2001. Analysis of total human immunodeficiency virus (HIV)-specific CD4+ and CD8+ T-cell responses: relationship to viral load in untreated HIV infection. *J. Virol.* **75:**11983–11991.

356. Betts, M. R., B. Exley, D. A. Price, A. Bansal, Z. T. Camacho, V. Teaberry, S. M. West, D. R. Ambrozak, G. Tomaras, M. Roederer, J. M. Kilby, J. Tartaglia, R. Belshe, F. Gao, D. C. Douek, K. J. Weinhold, R. A. Koup, P. Goepfert, and G. Ferrari. 2005. Characterization of functional and phenotypic changes in anti-Gag vaccine-induced T cell responses and their role in protection after HIV-1 infection. *Proc. Natl. Acad. Sci. USA* **102:**4512–4517. (First published 7 March 2005; doi:10.1073/pnas.0408773102).

357. Betts, M. R., J. F. Krowka, T. B. Kepler, M. Davidian, C. Christopherson, S. Kwok, L. Louie, J. Eron, H. Sheppard, and J. A. Frelinger. 1999. Human immunodeficiency virus type 1-specific cytotoxic T lymphocyte activity is inversely correlated with HIV type 1 viral load in HIV type 1-infected long-term survivors. *AIDS Res. Hum. Retrovir.* **15:**1219–1228.

358. Betts, M. R., M. C. Nason, S. M. West, S. C. De Rosa, S. A. Migueles, J. Abraham, M. M. Lederman, J. M. Benito, P. A. Goepfert, M. Connors, M. Roederer, and R. A. Koup. 2006. HIV nonprogressors preferentially maintain highly functional HIV-specific CD8+ T-cells. *Blood* **107:**4781–4789.

359. Bevan, M. J., and T. J. Braciale. 1995. Why can't cytotoxic T cells handle HIV? *Proc. Natl. Acad. Sci. USA* **92:**5765–5767.

360. Bhaskaran, K., D. Pillay, A. S. Walker, M. Fisher, D. Hawkins, R. Gilson, K. McLean, and K. Porter. 2004. Do patients who are infected with drug-resistant HIV have a different CD4 cell decline after seroconversion? An exploratory analysis in the UK Register of HIV seroconverters. *AIDS* **18:**1471–1473.

360a. Bhaskaran, K., R. Brettle, K. Porter, A. S. Walker, and the CASCADE Collaboration. 2004. Systemic non-Hodgkin lymphoma in individuals with known dates of HIV seroconversion: incidence and predictors. *AIDS* **18:**673–681.

361. Bieniasz, P. D. 2004. Intrinsic immunity: a front-line defense against viral attack. *Nat. Immunol.* 5:1109–1115.

362. Bienzle, D., K. S. MacDonald, F. M. Smaill, C. Kovacs, M. Baqi, B. Courssaris, M. A. Luscher, S. L. Walmsley, and K. L. Rosenthal. 2000. Factors contributing to the lack of human immunodeficiency virus type 1 (HIV-1) transmission in HIV-1-discordant partners. *J. Infect. Dis.* 182:123–132.

363. Bienzle, D., F. M. Smaill, and K. L. Rosenthal. 1996. Cytotoxic T-lymphocytes from HIV-infected individuals recognize an activation-dependent, non-polymorphic molecule on uninfected CD4+ lymphocytes. *AIDS* 10:247–254.

364. Biggar, R. J., S. Cassol, N. Kumwenda, V. Lema, M. Janes, R. Pilon, V. Senzani, F. Yellin, T. E. T. Taha, and R. L. Broadhead. 2003. The risk of human immunodeficiency virus-1 infection in twin pairs born to infected mothers in Africa. *J. Infect. Dis.* 188:850–855.

365. Biggar, R. J., M. Janes, R. Pilson, R. Roy, R. Broadhead, N. Kumwenda, T. E. T. Taha, and S. Cassol. 2002. Human immunodeficiency virus type 1 infection in twin pairs infected at birth. *J. Infect. Dis.* 186:281–285.

366. Biggar, R. J., P. G. Miotti, T. E. Taha, L. Mtimavalye, R. Broadhead, A. Justesen, F. Yellin, G. Liomba, W. Miley, D. Waters, J. D. Chiphangwi, and J. J. Goedert. 1996. Perinatal intervention trial in Africa: effect of a birth canal cleansing intervention to prevent HIV transmission. *Lancet* 347:1647–1650.

367. Biggs, B.-A., M. Hewish, S. Kent, K. Hayes, and S. M. Crowe. 1995. HIV-1 infection of human macrophages impairs phagocytosis and killing of Toxoplasma gondii. *J. Immunol.* 154:6132–6139.

368. Biglino, A., A. Sinicco, B. Forno, A. M. Pollono, M. Sciandra, C. Martini, P. Pich, and P. Gioannini. 1996. Serum cytokine profiles in acute primary HIV-1 infection and in infectious mononucleosis. *Clin. Immunol. Immunopathol.* 78:61–69.

369. Binley, J. M., A. Trkola, T. Ketas, D. Schiller, B. Clas, S. Little, D. Richman, A. Hurley, M. Markowitz, and J. P. Moore. 2000. The effect of highly active antiretroviral therapy on binding and neutralizing antibody responses to human immunodeficiency virus type 1 infection. *J. Infect. Dis.* 182:945–949.

370. Binley, J. M., T. Wrin, B. Korber, M. B. Zwick, M. Wang, C. Chappey, G. Stiegler, R. Kunert, S. Zolla-Pazner, H. Katinger, C. J. Petropoulos, and D. R. Burton. 2004. Comprehensive cross-clade neutralization analysis of a panel of anti-human immunodeficiency virus type 1 monoclonal antibodies. *J. Virol.* 78:13232–13252.

371. Birch, M. R., J. C. Learmont, W. B. Dyer, N. J. Deacon, J. J. Zaunders, N. Saksena, A. L. Cunningham, J. Mills, and J. S. Sullivan. 2001. An examination of signs of disease progression in survivors of the Sydney Blood Bank Cohort (SBBC). *J. Clin. Virol.* 22:263–270.

372. Birdsall, H. H., J. Trial, H. J. Lin, D. M. Green, G. W. Sorrentino, E. B. Siwak, A. L. de Jong, and R. D. Rossen. 1997. Transendothelial migration of lymphocytes from HIV-1-infected donors. *J. Immunol.* 158:5968–5977.

373. Birk, M., S. Lindback, and C. Lidman. 2002. No influence of GB virus C replication on the prognosis in a cohort of HIV-1-infected patients. *AIDS* 16:2482–2484.

374. Biron, C. A. 1997. Activation and function of natural killer cell responses during viral infections. *Curr. Opin. Immunol.* 9:24–34.

375. Biron, C. A. 1998. Role of early cytokines, including alpha and beta interferons (IFN-alpha/beta), in innate and adaptive immune responses to viral infections. *Semin. Immunol.* 10:383–390.

376. Biron, C. A. 2001. Interferons alpha and beta as immune regulators—a new look. *Immunity* 14:661–664.

377. Biron, C. A., K. B. Nguyen, G. C. Pien, L. P. Cousens, and T. P. Salazar-Mather. 1999. Natural killer cells in antiviral defense: function and regulation by innate cytokines. *Annu. Rev. Immunol.* 17:189–220.

378. Birx, D. L., M. G. Lewis, M. Vahey, K. Tencer, P. M. Zack, C. R. Brown, P. B. Jahrling, G. Tosato, D. Burke, and R. Redfield. 1993. Association of interleukin-6 in the pathogenesis of acutely fatal SIVsmm/PBj-14 in pigtailed macaques. *AIDS Res. Hum. Retrovir.* 9:1123–1129.

379. Birx, D. L., R. R. Redfield, and G. Tosato. 1986. Defective regulation of Epstein-Barr virus infection in patients with acquired immunodeficiency syndrome (AIDS) or AIDS-related disorders. *N. Engl. J. Med.* 314:874–879.

380. Bisaccia, E., C. Berger, and A. S. Klainer. 1990. Extracorporeal photopheresis in the treatment of AIDS-related complex: a pilot study. *Ann. Intern. Med.* 113:270–275.

380a. Bishop, K. N., R. K. Holmes, and M. H. Malim. 2006. Antiviral potency of APOBEC proteins does not correlate with cytidine deamination. *J. Virol.* 80:8450–8458.

381. Bishop, K. N., R. K. Holmes, A. M. Sheehy, and M. H. Malim. 2004. APOBEC-mediated editing of viral RNA. *Science* 305:645.

382. Bisikirska, B., J. Colgan, J. Luban, J. A. Bluestone, and K. C. Herold. 2005. TCR stimulation with modified anti-CD3 mAb expands CD8+ T cell population and induces CD8+CD25+ Tregs. *J. Clin. Investig.* 115:2904–2913.

383. Bisson, G. P., B. L. Strom, R. Gross, D. Weissman, D. Klinzman, W. T. Hwang, J. R. Kostman, D. Metzger, J. T. Stapleton, and I. Frank. 2005. Effect of GB virus C viremia on HIV acquisition and HIV set-point. *AIDS* 19:1910–1912.

384. Biti, R., R. Ffrench, J. Young, B. Bennetts, G. Stewart, and T. Liang. 1997. HIV-1 infection in an individual homozygous for the CCR5 deletion allele. *Nat. Med.* 3:252–253.

385. Bjorck, P. 2001. Isolation and characterization of plasmacytoid dendritic cells from Flt3 ligand and granulocyte-macrophage colony-stimulating factor-treated mice. *Blood* 98:3520–3526.

386. Bjork, R. L., Jr. 1991. HIV-1: seven facets of functional molecular mimicry. *Immunol. Lett.* 28:91–96.

387. Bjorling, E., K. Broliden, D. Bernardi, G. Utter, R. Thorstensson, F. Chiodi, and E. Norrby. 1991. Hyperimmune antisera against synthetic peptides representing the glycoprotein of human immunodeficiency virus type 2 can mediate neutralization and antibody-dependent cytotoxic activity. *Proc. Natl. Acad. Sci. USA* 88:6082–6086.

388. Bjorling, E., G. Scarlatti, A. Von Gegerfelt, J. Albert, G. Biberfeld, F. Chiodi, E. Norrby, and E. M. Fenyo. 1993. Autologous neutralizing antibodies prevail in HIV-2 but not in HIV-1 infection. *Virology* 193:528–530.

388a. Blaak, H., M. E. van der Ende, P. H. Boers, H. Schuitemaker, and A. D. Osterhaus. 2006. In vitro replication capacity of HIV-2 variants from long-term aviremic individuals. *Virology* 353:144–154.

389. Blaak, H., A. B. van't Wout, M. Brouwer, B. Hooibrink, E. Hovenkamp, and H. Schuitemaker. 2000. In vivo HIV-1 infection of CD45RA(+)CD4(+) T cells is established primarily by syncytium-inducing variants and correlates with the rate of CD4(+) T cell decline. *Proc. Natl. Acad. Sci. USA* 97:1269–1274.

390. Blackard, J. T., D. E. Cohen, and K. H. Mayer. 2002. Human immunodeficiency virus superinfection and recombination: current state of knowledge and potential clinical consequences. *Clin. Infect. Dis.* 34:1108–1114.

390a. Blackard, J. T., B. Renjifo, W. Fawzi, E. Hertzmark, G. Msamanga, D. Mwakagile, D. Hunter, D. Spiegelman, N. Sharghi, C. Kagoma, and M. Essex. 2001. HIV-1 LTR subtype and perinatal transmission. *Virology* 287:261–5.

391. Blackbourn, D. J., J. Ambroziak, E. Lennette, M. Adams, B. Ramachandran, and J. A. Levy. 1997. Infectious HHV-8 in a healthy North American blood donor. *Lancet* 349:609–611.

392. Blackbourn, D. J., S. Fujimura, T. Kutzkey, and J. A. Levy. 2000. Induction of human herpesvirus-8 gene expression by recombinant interferon gamma. *AIDS* 14:98–99.

393. Blackbourn, D. J., E. Lennette, J. Ambroziak, D. V. Mourich, and J. A. Levy. 1998. Human herpesvirus 8 detection in nasal secretions and saliva. *J. Infect. Dis.* 177:213–216.

394. Blackbourn, D. J., E. Lennette, B. Klencke, A. Moses, B. Chandran, M. Weinstien, R. G. Glougau, M. H. Witte, D. L. Way, T. Kutzkey, B. Herndier, and J. A. Levy. 2000. The restricted cellular host range of human herpesvirus 8. *AIDS* 14:1123–1133.

395. Blackbourn, D. J., and J. A. Levy. 1997. Human herpesvirus 8 in semen and prostate. *AIDS* 11:249–250.

396. Blackbourn, D. J., C. P. Locher, B. Ramachandran, S. W. Barnett, K. K. Murthy, K. D. Carey, K. M. Brasky, and J. A. Levy. 1997. CD8+ cells from HIV-2-infected baboons control HIV replication. *AIDS* 11:737–746.

397. Blackbourn, D. J., C. E. Mackewicz, E. Barker, T. K. Hunt, B. Herndier, A. T. Haase, and J. A. Levy. 1996. Suppression of HIV replication by lymphoid tissue CD8+ cells correlates with the clinical state of HIV-infected individuals. *Proc. Natl. Acad. Sci. USA* 93:13125–13130.

398. Blackburn, R., M. Clerici, D. Mann, D. R. Lucey, J. Goedert, B. Golding, G. M. Shearer, and H. Golding. 1991. Common sequence in HIV-1 gp41 and HLA Class II beta chains can generate crossreactive autoantibodies with immunosuppressive potential early in the course of HIV-1 infection, p. 63–69. In M. Z. Atassi (ed.), *Immunobiology of Proteins and Peptides*, vol. VI. Plenum Press, New York, N.Y.

399. Blanche, S., M. Tardieu, A. Duliege, C. Rouzioux, F. Le Deist, K. Fukunaga, M. Caniglia, C. Jacomet, A. Messiah, and C. Griscelli. 1990. Longitudinal study of 94 symptomatic infants with perinatally acquired human immunodeficiency virus infection. *Am. J. Dis. Child.* 144:1210–1215.

400. Blanche, S., M. Tardieu, P. Rustin, A. Slama, B. Barret, G. Firtion, N. Ciraru-Vigneron, C. Lacroix, C. Rouzioux, L. Mandelbrot, I. Desguerre, A. Rotig, M. J. Mayaux, and J. F. Delfraissy. 1999. Persistent mitochondrial dysfunction and perinatal exposure to antiretroviral nucleoside analogues. *Lancet* 354:1084–1089.

401. Blancou, P., J. P. Vartanian, C. Christopherson, N. Chenciner, C. Basilico, S. Kwok, and S. Wain-Hobson. 2001. Polio vaccine samples not linked to AIDS. *Nature* 410:1045–1046.

402. Blander, J. M., and R. Medzhitov. 2006. Toll-dependent selection of microbial antigens for presentation by dendritic cells. *Nature* 440:808–812.

403. Blankson, J. N., J. D. Siliciano, and R. F. Siliciano. 2005. The effect of early treatment on the latent reservoir of HIV-1. *J. Infect. Dis.* 191:1394–1396.

404. Blasig, C., C. Zietz, B. Haar, F. Neipel, S. Esser, N. H. Brockmeyer, E. Tschachler, S. Colombini, B. Ensoli, and M. Sturzl. 1997. Monocytes in Kaposi's sarcoma lesions are productively infected by human herpesvirus 8. *J. Virol.* 71:7963–7968.

405. Blauvelt, A., H. Asada, M. W. Saville, V. Klaus-Kovtun, D. J. Altman, R. Yarchoan, and S. I. Katz. 1997. Productive infection of dendritic cells by HIV-1 and their ability to capture virus are mediated through separate pathways. *J. Clin. Investig.* 100:2043–2053.

406. Blauvelt, A., C. Chougnet, G. M. Shearer, and S. I. Katz. 1996. Modulation of T cell responses to recall antigens presented by Langerhans cells in HIV-discordant identical twins by anti-interleukin (IL)-10 antibodies and IL-12. *J. Clin. Investig.* 97:1550–1555.

407. Blazevic, V., M. Heino, A. Ranki, T. Jussila, and K. J. E. Krohn. 1996. RANTES, MIP and interleukin-16 in HIV infection. *AIDS* 10:1435–1436.

408. Bleijs, D. A., T. B. Geijtenbeek, C. G. Figdor, and Y. van Kooyk. 2001. DC-SIGN and LFA-1: a battle for ligand. *Trends Immunol.* 22:457–463.

409. Bleul, C. C., M. Farzan, H. Choe, C. Parolin, I. Clark-Lewis, J. Sodroski, and T. A. Springer. 1996. The lymphocyte chemoattractant SDF-1 is a ligand for LESTR/fusin and blocks HIV-1 entry. *Nature* 382:829–832.

410. Bleul, C. C., L. Wu, J. A. Hoxie, T. A. Springer, and C. R. Mackay. 1997. The HIV coreceptors CXCR4 and CCR5 are differentially expressed and regulated on human T lymphocytes. *Proc. Natl. Acad. Sci. USA* 94:1925–1930.

411. Blom, B., S. Ho, S. Antonenko, and Y. J. Liu. 2000. Generation of interferon alpha-producing predendritic cell (Pre-DC)2 from human CD34(+) hematopoietic stem cells. *J. Exp. Med.* 192:1785–1796.

412. Blomberg, R. S., and R. T. Schooley. 1985. Lymphocyte markers in infectious diseases. *Semin. Hematol.* 22:81–114.

413. Bloom, E. J., D. I. Abrams, and G. Rodgers. 1986. Lupus anticoagulant in the acquired immunodeficiency syndrome. *JAMA* 256:491–493.

414. Bobardt, M. D., P. Salmon, L. Wang, J. D. Esko, D. Gabuzda, M. Fiala, D. Trono, B. Van der Schueren, G. David, and P. A. Gallay. 2004. Contribution of proteoglycans to human immunodeficiency virus type 1 brain invasion. *J. Virol.* 78:6567–6584.

415. Bobkov, A., R. Cheingsong-Popov, M. Garaev, A. Rzhaninova, P. Kaleebu, S. Beddows, M. H. Bachmann, J. I. Mullins, J. Louwagie, W. Janssens, G. van der Groen, F. McCutchan, and J. Weber. 1994. Identification of an env G subtype and heterogeneity of HIV-1 strains in the Russian Federation and Belarus. *AIDS* 8:1649–1655.

416. Boccuni, M. C., F. Campanini, M. C. Battista, G. Bergamini, P. Dal Monte, A. Ripalti, and M. P. Landini. 1998. Human cytomegalovirus product UL44 downregulates the transactivation of HIV-1 long terminal repeat. *AIDS* 12:365–372.

417. Bocharov, G., B. Ludewig, A. Bertoletti, P. Klenerman, T. Junt, P. Krebs, T. Luzyanina, C. Fraser, and R. M. Anderson.

2004. Underwhelming the immune response: effect of slow virus growth on CD8+-T-lymphocyte responses. *J. Virol.* **78:**2247–2254.

417a. Bochud, P., M. Hersberger, P. Taffe, M. Bochud, C. M. Stein, S. D. Rodrigues, T. Calandra, A. Telenti, R. F. Speck, and A. Aderem. Polymorphism in toll-like receptor 9 influence the clinical course of HIV-1 infection. *AIDS,* in press.

418. Boeri, E., A. Giri, F. Lillo, G. Ferrari, O. E. Varnier, A. Ferro, S. Sabbatani, W. C. Saxinger, and G. Franchini. 1992. In vivo genetic variability of the human immunodeficiency virus type 2 V3 region. *J. Virol.* **66:**4546–4550.

419. Bofill, M., N. J. Borthwick, and H. A. Simmonds. 1999. Novel mechanism for the impairment of cell proliferation in HIV-1 infection. *Immunol. Today* **20:**258–261.

420. Bofill, M., W. Gombert, N. J. Borthwick, A. N. Akbar, J. E. McLaughlin, C. A. Lee, M. A. Johnson, A. J. Pinching, and G. Janossy. 1995. Presence of CD3+CD8+Bcl-2^{low} lymphocytes undergoing apoptosis and activated macrophages in lymph nodes of HIV-1+ patients. *Am. J. Pathol.* **146:**1542–1555.

421. Bofill, M., A. Mocroft, M. Lipman, E. Medina, N. J. Borthwick, C. A. Sabin, A. Timms, M. Winter, L. Baptista, M. A. Jonson, C. A. Lee, A. N. Phillips, and G. Janossy. 1996. Increased numbers of primed activated CD8+CD38+CD45RO+ T cells predict the decline of CD4+ T cells in HIV-1-infected patients. *AIDS* **10:**827–834.

422. Bogdan, C. 2000. The function of type I interferons in antimicrobial immunity. *Curr. Opin. Immunol.* **12:**419–424.

423. Bogerd, H. P., B. P. Doehle, H. L. Wiegand, and B. R. Cullen. 2004. A single amino acid difference in the host APOBEC3G protein controls the primate species specificity of HIV type 1 virion infectivity factor. *Proc. Natl. Acad. Sci. USA* **101:**3770–3774.

424. Bogerd, H. P., H. L. Wiegand, B. P. Doehle, K. K. Lueders, and B. R. Cullen. 2006. APOBEC3A and APOBEC3B are potent inhibitors of LTR-retrotransposon function in human cells. *Nucleic Acids Res.* **34:**89–95.

425. Bogers, W. M., H. Niphuis, P. ten Haaft, J. D. Laman, W. Koornstra, and J. L. Heeney. 1995. Protection from HIV-1 envelope-bearing chimeric simian immunodeficiency virus (SHIV) in rhesus macaques infected with attenuated SIV: consequences of challenge. *AIDS* **9:**F13-F18.

426. Bohler, T., J. Walcher, G. Holzl-Wenig, M. Geiss, B. Buchholz, R. Linde, and K.-M. Debatin. 1999. Early effects of antiretroviral combination therapy on activation, apoptosis and regeneration of T cells in HIV-1-infected children and adolescents. *AIDS* **13:**779–789.

427. Boldogh, I., P. Szaniszlo, W. A. Bresnahan, C. M. Flaitz, M. C. Nichols, and T. Albrecht. 1996. Kaposi's sarcoma herpesvirus-like DNA sequences in the saliva of individuals infected with human immunodeficiency virus. *Clin. Infect. Dis.* **23:**406–407.

428. Bollinger, R. C., M. A. Egan, T.-W. Chun, B. Mathieson, and R. F. Siliciano. 1996. Cellular immune responses to HIV-1 in progressive and non-progressive infections. *AIDS* **10:**S85–S96.

429. Bollinger, R. C., Jr., R. L. Kline, H. L. Francis, M. W. Moss, J. G. Bartlett, and T. C. Quinn. 1992. Acid dissociation increases the sensitivity of p24 antigen detection for the evaluation of antiviral therapy and disease progression in asymptomatic human immunodeficiency virus-infected persons. *J. Infect. Dis.* **165:**913–916.

430. Bollinger, R. C., T. C. Quinn, A. Y. Liu, P. E. Stanhope, S. A. Hammond, R. Viveen, M. L. Clements, and R. F. Siliciano. 1993. Cytokines from vaccine-induced HIV-1 specific cytotoxic T lymphocytes: effects on viral replication. *AIDS Res. Hum. Retrovir.* **9:**1067–1077.

431. Bolton, D. L., B. I. Hahn, E. A. Park, L. L. Lehnhoff, F. Hornung, and M. J. Lenardo. 2002. Death of CD4(+) T-cell lines caused by human immunodeficiency virus type 1 does not depend on caspases or apoptosis. *J. Virol.* **76:**5094–5107.

432. Bomsel, M. 1997. Transcytosis of infectious human immunodeficiency virus across a tight human epithelial cell line barrier. *Nat. Med.* **3:**42–47.

433. Bomsel, M., and V. David. 2002. Mucosal gatekeepers: selecting HIV viruses for early infection. *Nat. Med.* **8:**114–116.

434. Bomsel, M., M. Heyman, H. Hocini, S. Lagaye, L. Belec, C. Dupont, and C. Desgranges. 1998. Intracellular neutralization of HIV transcytosis across tight epithelial barriers by anti-HIV envelope protein dIgA or IgM. *Immunity* **9:**277–287.

435. Bonaparte, M. I., and E. Barker. 2003. Inability of natural killer cells to destroy autologous HIV-infected T lymphocytes. *AIDS* **17:**487–494.

436. Bonaparte, M. I., and E. Barker. 2004. Killing of human immunodeficiency virus-infected primary T-cells by autologous natural killer cells is dependent on the ability of the virus to alter the expression of major histocompatibility complex class I molecules. *Blood* **104:**2087–2094.

437. Bonavida, B., J. Katz, and M. Gottlieb. 1986. Mechanism of defective NK cell activity in patients with acquired immunodeficiency syndrome (AIDS) and AIDS-related complex. I. Defective trigger on NK cells for NKCF production by target cells, and partial restoration by IL-2. *J. Immunol.* **137:**1157–1163.

438. Bonecchi, R., G. Bianchi, P. P. Bordignon, D. D'Ambrosio, R. Lang, A. Borsatti, S. Sozzani, P. Allavena, P. A. Gray, A. Mantovani, and F. Sinigaglia. 1998. Differential expression of chemokine receptors and chemotactic responsiveness of type 1 T helper cells (Th1s) and Th2s. *J. Exp. Med.* **187:**129–134.

439. Boniotto, M., S. Crovella, D. Pirulli, G. Scarlatti, A. Spano, L. Vatta, S. Zezlina, P. A. Tovo, E. Palomba, and A. Amoroso. 2000. Polymorphisms in the MBL2 promoter correlated with risk of HIV-1 vertical transmission and AIDS progression. *Genes Immun.* **1:**346–348.

440. Bonnet, F., E. Balestre, R. Thiebaut, P. Morlat, J. L. Pellegrin, D. Neau, and F. Dabis. 2006. Factors associated with the occurrence of AIDS-related non-Hodgkin lymphoma in the era of highly active antiretroviral therapy: Aquitaine Cohort, France. *Clin. Infect. Dis.* **42:**411–417.

441. Bonyhadi, M. L., L. Rabin, S. Salimi, D. A. Brown, J. Kosek, J. N. McCune, and H. Kaneshima. 1993. HIV induces thymus depletion in vivo. *Nature* **363:**728–736.

442. Bor, Y. C., M. D. Miller, F. D. Bushman, and L. E. Orgel. 1996. Target-sequence preferences of HIV-1 integration complexes *in vitro. Virology* **222:**283–288.

443. Bordon, J., P. S. Evans, N. Propp, C. E. Davis, Jr., R. R. Redfield, and C. D. Pauza. 2004. Association between longer duration of HIV-suppressive therapy and partial recovery of the V gamma 2 T cell receptor repertoire. *J. Infect. Dis.* **189:**1482–1486.

444. Borkowsky, W., and K. Krasinski. 1992. Perinatal human immunodeficiency virus infection: ruminations on mechanisms

of transmission and methods of intervention. *Pediatrics* **90**: 133–136.

445. Borrow, P., C. F. Evans, and M. B. A. Oldstone. 1995. Virus-induced immunosuppression: immune system-mediated destruction of virus-infected dendritic cells results in generalized immune suppression. *J. Virol.* **69**:1059–1070.

446. Borrow, P., H. Lewicki, B. H. Hahn, G. M. Shaw, and M. B. A. Oldstone. 1994. Virus-specific CD8+ cytotoxic T-lymphocyte activity associated with control of viremia in primary human immunodeficiency virus type 1 infection. *J. Virol.* **68**: 6103–6110.

447. Borrow, P., H. Lewicki, X. Wei, M. S. Horwitz, N. Peffer, H. Meyers, J. A. Nelson, J. E. Gairin, B. H. Hahn, M. B. A. Oldstone, and G. M. Shaw. 1997. Antiviral pressure exerted by HIV-1-specific cytotoxic T lymphocytes (CTLs) during primary infection demonstrated by rapid selection of CTL escape virus. *Nat. Med.* **3**:205–211.

448. Reference deleted.

449. Borthwick, N. J., M. Bofill, W. M. Gombert, A. N. Akbar, E. Medina, K. Sagawa, M. C. Lipman, M. A. Johnson, and G. Janossy. 1994. Lymphocyte activation in HIV-1 infection. II. Functional defects of CD28-T cells. *AIDS* **8**:431–441.

450. Bosch, V., and T. Pfeiffer. 1992. HIV-1-induced cytopathogenicity in cell culture despite very decreased amounts of fusion-competent viral glycoprotein. *AIDS Res. Hum. Retrovir.* **8**:1815–1821.

451. Boshoff, C., T. F. Schulz, M. M. Kennedy, A. K. Graham, C. Fisher, A. Thomas, J. O. D. McGee, R. A. Weiss, and J. J. O'Leary. 1995. Kaposi's sarcoma-associated herpesvirus infects endothelial and spindle cells. *Nat. Med.* **1**:1274–1278.

452. Bossi, P., N. Dupin, A. Coutellier, F. Bricaire, C. Lubetzki, C. Katlama, and V. Calvez. 1998. The level of human immunodeficiency virus (HIV) type 1 RNA in cerebrospinal fluid as a marker of HIV encephalitis. *Clin. Infect. Dis.* **26**:1072–1073.

453. Bostik, P., E. S. Noble, A. E. Mayne, L. Gargano, F. Villinger, and A. A. Ansari. 2006. Central memory CD4 T cells are the predominant cell subset resistant to anergy in SIV disease resistant sooty mangabeys. *AIDS* **20**:181–188.

454. Bottiger, B., K. Ljunggren, A. Karlsson, K. Krohn, E. M. Fenyo, and G. Biberfeld. 1988. Neutralizing antibodies in relation to antibody dependent cellular cytotoxicity inducing antibodies against human immunodeficiency virus type 1. *Clin. Exp. Immunol.* **73**:339–342.

455. Boudet, F., H. Lecoeur, and M. L. Gougeon. 1996. Apoptosis associated with ex vivo down-regulation of Bcl-2 and up-regulation of Fas in potential cytotoxic CD8+ T lymphocytes during HIV infection. *J. Immunol.* **156**:2282–2293.

456. Boue, F., C. Wallon, C. Goujard, F. Barre-Sinoussi, P. Galanud, and J.-F. Delfraissy. 1992. HIV induces IL-6 production by human B lymphocytes. *J. Immunol.* **148**:3761–3767.

457. Bouhlal, H., N. Chomont, N. Haeffner-Cavaillon, M. D. Kazatchkine, L. Belec, and H. Hocini. 2002. Opsonization of HIV-1 by semen complement enhances infection of human epithelial cells. *J. Immunol.* **169**:3301–3306.

458. Bouhlal, H., V. Latry, M. Requena, S. Aubry, S. V. Kaveri, M. D. Kazatchkine, L. Belec, and H. Hocini. 2005. Natural antibodies to CCR5 from breast milk block infection of macrophages and dendritic cells with primary R5-tropic HIV-1. *J. Immunol.* **174**:7202–7209.

459. Boullier, S., G. Dadaglio, A. Lafeuillade, T. Debord, and M. L. Gougeon. 1997. V delta 1 T cells expanded in the blood throughout HIV infection display a cytotoxic activity and are primed for TNF-alpha and IFN-gamma production but are not selected in lymph nodes. *J. Immunol.* **159**:3629–3637.

460. Bounou, S., J. E. Leclerc, and M. J. Tremblay. 2002. Presence of host ICAM-1 in laboratory and clinical strains of human immunodeficiency virus type 1 increases virus infectivity and CD4(+)-T- cell depletion in human lymphoid tissue, a major site of replication in vivo. *J. Virol.* **76**:1004–1014.

461. Bour, S., H. Akari, E. Miyagi, and K. Strebel. 2003. Naturally occurring amino acid substitutions in the HIV-2 ROD envelope glycoprotein regulate its ability to augment viral particle release. *Virology* **309**:85–98.

462. Bour, S., C. Perrin, and K. Strebel. 1999. Cell surface CD4 inhibits HIV-1 particle release by interfering with Vpu activity. *J. Biol. Chem.* **274**:33800–33806.

463. Bour, S., U. Schubert, K. Peden, and K. Strebel. 1996. The envelope glycoprotein of human immunodeficiency virus type 2 enhances viral particle release: a VPU-like factor? *J. Virol.* **70**:820–829.

464. Bourgarit, A., G. Carcelain, V. Martinez, C. Lascoux, V. Delcey, B. Gicquel, E. Vicaut, P. H. Lagrange, D. Sereni, and B. Autran. 2006. Explosion of tuberculin-specific Th1-responses induces immune restoration syndrome in tuberculosis and HIV co-infected patients. *AIDS* **20**:F1–F7.

465. Bourgeois, C., B. Rocha, and C. Tanchot. 2002. A role for CD40 expression on CD8+ T cells in the generation of CD8+ T cell memory. *Science* **297**:2060–2063.

466. Bourinbaiar, A. S., and R. Nagorny. 1992. Effect of human chorionic gonadotropin (hCG) on HIV-1 transmission from lymphocytes to trophoblasts. *FEBS Lett.* **309**:82–84.

467. Bourinbaiar, A. S., and D. M. Phillips. 1991. Transmission of human immunodeficiency virus from monocytes to epithelia. *J. Acquir. Immune Defic. Syndr.* **4**:56–63.

468. Bouscarat, F., E. Maubec, S. Matheron, and V. Descamps. 2000. Immune recovery inflammatory folliculitis. *AIDS* **14**: 617–618.

469. Bouyac-Bertoia, M., J. D. Dvorin, R. A. Fouchier, Y. Jenkins, B. E. Meyer, L. I. Wu, M. Emerman, and M. H. Malim. 2001. HIV-1 infection requires a functional integrase NLS. *Mol. Cell* **7**:1025–1035.

470. Boven, L. A., L. Gomes, C. Hery, F. Gray, J. Verhoef, P. Portegies, M. Tardieu, and H. S. Nottet. 1999. Increased peroxynitrite activity in AIDS dementia complex: implications for the neuropathogenesis of HIV-1 infection. *J. Immunol.* **162**: 4319–4327.

471. Bower, M., T. Powles, M. Nelson, P. Shah, S. Cox, S. Mandelia, and B. Gazzard. 2003. HIV-related lung cancer in the era of highly active antiretroviral therapy. *AIDS* **17**:371–375.

472. Bower, M., T. Powles, C. Newsom-Davis, C. Thirlwell, J. Stebbing, S. Mandalia, M. Nelson, and B. Gazzard. 2004. HIV-associated anal cancer: has highly active antiretroviral therapy reduced the incidence or improved the outcome? *J. Acquir. Immune Defic. Syndr.* **37**:1563–1565.

473. Boyer, J., K. Bebenek, and T. A. Kunkel. 1992. Unequal human immunodeficiency virus type 1 reverse transcriptase error rates with RNA and DNA templates. *Proc. Natl. Acad. Sci. USA* **89**:6919–6923.

474. Boyer, J. D., K. E. Ugen, B. Wang, M. Agadjanyan, L. Gilbert, M. L. Bagarazzi, M. Chattergoon, P. Frost, A. Javadian, W. V. Williams, Y. Refaeli, R. B. Ciccarelli, D. McCallus, L. Coney, and D. B. Weiner. 1997. Protection of chimpanzees from high-dose heterologous HIV-1 challenge by DNA vaccination. *Nat. Med.* 3:526–532.

475. Boyer, V., C. Delibrais, N. Noraz, F. Fischer, M. D. Kazatchkine, and C. Desgranges. 1992. Complement receptor type 2 mediates infection of the human CD4-negative Raji B-cell line with opsonized HIV. *Scand. J. Immunol.* 36:879–883.

476. Boyer, V., C. Desgranges, M. A. Trabaud, E. Fischer, and M. Kazatchkine. 1991. Complement mediates human immunodeficiency virus type 1 infection of a human T cell line in a CD4- and antibody-independent fashion. *J. Exp. Med.* 173:1151–1158.

477. Bozzette, S. A., C. F. Ake, H. K. Tam, S. W. Chang, and T. A. Louis. 2003. Cardiovascular and cerebrovascular events in patients treated for human immunodeficiency virus infection. *N. Engl. J. Med.* 348:702–710.

478. Braaten, D., E. K. Franke, and J. Luban. 1996. Cyclophilin A is required for the replication of Group M human immunodeficiency virus type 1 (HIV-1) and simian immunodeficiency virus SIV$_{CPZ}$GAB but not group O HIV-1 or other primate immunodeficiency viruses. *J. Virol.* 70:4220–4227.

479. Brack-Werner, R., A. Kleinschmidt, A. Ludvigsen, W. Mellert, M. Neumann, R. Herrmann, M. C. L. Khim, A. Burny, N. Muller-Lantzsch, D. Stavrou, and V. Erfle. 1992. Infection of human brain cells by HIV-1: restricted virus production in chronically infected human glial cell lines. *AIDS* 6:273–285.

480. Bradding, P., I. H. Feather, P. H. Howarth, R. Mueller, J. A. Roberts, K. Britten, J. P. A. Bews, T. C. Hunt, Y. Okayama, C. H. Heusser, G. R. Bullock, M. K. Church, and S. T. Holgate. 1992. Interleukin 4 is localized to and released by human mast cells. *J. Exp. Med.* 176:1381–1386.

481. Bradney, C. P., G. D. Sempowski, H. X. Liao, B. F. Haynes, and H. F. Staats. 2002. Cytokines as adjuvants for the induction of anti-human immunodeficiency virus peptide immunoglobulin G (IgG) and IgA antibodies in serum and mucosal secretions after nasal immunization. *J. Virol.* 76:517–524.

482. Brambilla, A., C. Villa, G. Rizzardi, F. Veglia, S. Ghezzi, A. Lazzarin, M. Cusini, S. Muratori, E. Santagostino, A. Gringeri, L. G. Louie, H. W. Sheppard, G. Poli, N. L. Michael, G. Pantaleo, and E. Vicenzi. 2000. Shorter survival of SDF1–3'A/3'A homozygotes linked to CD4+ T cell decrease in advanced human immunodeficiency virus type 1 infection. *J. Infect. Dis.* 182: 311–315.

483. Branca, M., G. Migliore, M. L. Giuliani, G. Ippolito, G. Cappiello, A. R. Garbuglia, A. Schiesari, G. Rezza, et al. 2000. Squamous intraepithelial lesions (SILs) and HPV associated changes in HIV infected women or at risk of HIV. *Eur. J. Gynaecol. Oncol.* 21:155–159.

484. Brander, C., and Y. Riviere. 2002. Early and late cytotoxic T lymphocyte responses in HIV infection. *AIDS* 16 (Suppl. 4):S97–S103.

485. Brandes, M., K. Willimann, and B. Moser. 2005. Professional antigen-presentation function by human gammadelta T cells. *Science* 309:264–268.

486. Brandtzaeg, P. 1997. Mucosal immunity in the female genital tract. *J. Reprod. Immunol.* 36:23–50.

487. Bray, M., S. Prasad, J. W. Dubay, E. Hunter, K. T. Jeang, D. Rekosh, and M. L. Hammarskjold. 1994. A small element from the Mason-Pfizer monkey virus genome makes human im-

munodeficiency virus type 1 expression and replication Rev-independent. *Proc. Natl. Acad. Sci. USA* 91:1256–1260.

488. Brayfield, B. P., C. Kankasa, J. T. West, G. Bhat, W. Klaskala, C. D. Mitchell, and C. Wood. 2004. Distribution of Kaposi sarcoma-associated herpesvirus/human herpesvirus 8 in maternal saliva and breast milk in Zambia: implications for transmission. *J. Infect. Dis.* 189:2260–2270.

489. Breen, E. C., W. J. Boscardin, R. Detels, L. P. Jacobson, M. W. Smith, S. J. O'Brien, J. S. Chmiel, C. R. Rinaldo, S. Lai, and O. Martinez-Maza. 2003. Non-Hodgkin's B cell lymphoma in persons with acquired immunodeficiency syndrome is associated with increased serum levels of IL10, or the IL10 promoter -592 C/C genotype. *Clin. Immunol.* 109:119–129.

490. Breen, E. C., A. R. Rezai, K. Nakajima, G. N. Beall, R. T. Mitsuyasu, T. Hirano, T. Kishimoto, and O. Martinez-Maza. 1990. Infection with HIV is associated with elevated IL-6 levels and production. *J. Immunol.* 144:480–484.

491. Brenchley, J. M., B. J. Hill, D. R. Ambrozak, D. A. Price, F. J. Guenaga, J. P. Casazza, J. Kuruppu, J. Yazdani, S. A. Migueles, M. Connors, M. Roederer, D. C. Couek, and R. A. Koup. 2004. T-cell subsets that harbor human immunodeficiency virus (HIV) in vivo: implications for HIV pathogenesis. *J. Virol.* 78:1160–1168.

492. Brenchley, J. M., N. J. Karandikar, M. R. Betts, D. R. Ambrozak, B. J. Hill, L. E. Crotty, J. P. Casazza, J. Kuruppu, S. A. Migueles, M. Connors, M. Roederer, D. C. Douek, and R. A. Koup. 2003. Expression of CD57 defines replicative senescence and antigen-induced apoptotic death of CD8+ T cells. *Blood* 101:2711–2720.

493. Brenchley, J. M., T. W. Schacker, L. E. Ruff, D. A. Price, J. H. Taylor, G. J. Beilman, P. L. Nguyen, A. Khoruts, M. Larson, A. T. Haase, and D. C. Douek. 2004. CD4+ T cell depletion during all stages of HIV disease occurs predominantly in the gastrointestinal tract. *J. Exp. Med.* 200:749–759.

493a. Brenchley, J. M., D. A. Price, T. W. Schacker, T. E. Asher, G. Silvestri, S. Rao, Z. Kazzaz, E. Bornstein, O. Lambotte, D. Altmann, B. R. Blazar, B. Rodriguez, L. Teixeira-Johnson, A. Landay, J. N. Martin, F. M. Hecht, L. J. Picker, M. M. Lederman, S. G. Deeks, and D. C. Douek. 2006. Microbial translocation is a cause of systemic immune activation in chronic HIV infection. *Nat. Med.* 12:1365–1371.

494. Brenneman, D. E., G. L. Westbrook, S. P. Fitzgerald, D. L. Ennist, K. L. Elkins, M. R. Ruff, and C. B. Pert. 1988. Neuronal cell killing by the envelope protein of HIV and its prevention by vasoactive intestinal peptide. *Nature* 335:639–642.

495. Brenner, B., J. Routy, Y. Quan, D. Moisi, M. Oliveira, D. Turner, and M. A. Wainberg. 2004. Persistence of multidrug-resistant HIV-1 in primary infection leading to superinfection. *AIDS* 18:1653–1660.

496. Brenner, B. G., C. Gryllis, and M. A. Wainberg. 1991. Role of antibody-dependent cellular cytotoxicity and lymphokine-activated killer cells in AIDS and related diseases. *J. Leukoc. Biol.* 50:628–640.

497. Bretscher, P. A. 1999. A two-step, two-signal model for the primary activation of precursor helper T cells. *Proc. Natl. Acad. Sci. USA* 96:185–190.

498. Bretscher, P. A., G. Wei, J. N. Menon, and H. Bielefeldt-Ohmann. 1992. Establishment of stable, cell-mediated immunity that makes "susceptible" mice resistant to *Leishmania major*. *Science* 257:539–542.

499. Brettle, R. P., A. J. McNeil, S. Burns, S. M. Gore, A. G. Bird, P. L. Yap, L. MacCallum, C. S. Leen, and A. M. Richardson. 1996. Progression of HIV: follow-up of Edinburgh injecting

drug users with narrow seroconversion intervals in 1983–1985. *AIDS* 10:419–430.

500. Brew, B. J., N. Dunbar, L. Pemberton, and J. Kaldor. 1996. Predictive markers of AIDS dementia complex: CD4 cell count and cerebrospinal fluid concentrations of β_2-microglobulin and neopterin. *J. Infect. Dis.* 174:294–298.

501. Briant, L., C. M. Wade, J. Puel, A. J. Leigh Brown, and M. Guyader. 1995. Analysis of envelope sequence variants suggests multiple mechanisms of mother-to-child transmission of human immunodeficiency virus type 1. *J. Virol.* 69:3778–3788.

502. Briat, A., E. Dulioust, J. Galimand, H. Fontaine, M. L. Chaix, H. Letur-Konirsch, S. Pol, P. Jouannet, C. Rouzioux, and M. Leruez-Ville. 2005. Hepatitis C virus in the semen of men coinfected with HIV-1: prevalence and origin. *AIDS* 19:1827–1835.

503. Brichacek, B., S. Swindells, E. N. Janoff, S. Pirruccello, and M. Stevenson. 1996. Increased plasma human immunodeficiency virus type 1 burden following antigenic challenge with pneumococcal vaccine. *J. Infect. Dis.* 174:1191–1199.

504. Bridges, C. G., T. M. Brennan, D. L. Taylor, M. McPherson, and A. S. Tyms. 1994. The prevention of cell adhesion and the cell-to-cell spread of HIV-1 in vitro by the alpha-glucosidase 1 inhibitor, 6-O-butanoyl castanospermine (MDL 28574). *Antivir. Res.* 25:169–175.

505. Bridges, S. H., and N. Sarver. 1995. Gene therapy and immune restoration for HIV disease. *Lancet* 345:427–432.

506. Briggs, J. A., T. Wilk, R. Welker, H. G. Krausslich, and S. D. Fuller. 2003. Structural organization of authentic, mature HIV-1 virions and cores. *EMBO J.* 22:1707–1715.

507. Brigino, E., S. Haraguchi, A. Koutsonikolis, G. J. Cianciolo, U. Owens, R. A. Good, and N. K. Day. 1997. Interleukin 10 is induced by recombinant HIV-1 Nef protein involving the calcium/calmodulin-dependent phosphodiesterase signal transduction pathway. *Proc. Natl. Acad. Sci. USA* 94:3178–3182.

508. Brigl, M., and M. B. Brenner. 2004. CD1: antigen presentation and T cell function. *Annu. Rev. Immunol.* 22:817–890.

509. Brinchmann, J. E. 2000. Differential responses of T cell subsets: possible role in the immunopathogenesis of AIDS. *AIDS* 14:1689–1700.

510. Brinchmann, J. E., J. Albert, and F. Vartdal. 1991. Few infected CD4+ T cells but a high proportion of replication-competent provirus copies in asymptomatic human immunodeficiency virus type 1 infection. *J. Virol.* 65:2019–2023.

511. Brinchmann, J. E., J. H. Dobloug, B. H. Heger, L. L. Haaheim, M. Sannes, and T. Egeland. 1994. Expression of costimulatory molecule CD28 on T cells in human immunodeficiency virus type 1 infection: functional and clinical correlations. *J. Infect. Dis.* 169:730–738.

512. Brinchmann, J. E., G. Gaudernack, and F. Vartdal. 1990. CD8+ T cells inhibit HIV replication in naturally infected CD4+ T cells: evidence for a soluble inhibitor. *J. Immunol.* 144:2961–2966.

513. Brinchmann, J. E., G. Gaudernack, and F. Vartdal. 1991. *In vitro* replication of HIV-1 in naturally infected CD4+ T cells is inhibited by rIFN alpha2 and by a soluble factor secreted by activated CD8+ T cells, but not by rIFN beta, rIFN gamma, or recombinant tumor necrosis factor-alpha. *J. Acquir. Immune Defic. Syndr.* 4:480–488.

514. Brinkmann, R., A. Schwinn, O. Narayan, C. Zink, H. W. Kreth, W. Roggendorf, R. Dorries, S. Schwender, H. Imrich, and V. ter Meulen. 1992. Human immunodeficiency virus infection in microglia: correlation between cells infected in the brain and cells cultured from infectious brain tissue. *Ann. Neurol.* 31:361–365.

515. Brinkmann, V., T. Geiger, S. Alkan, and C. H. Heusser. 1993. Interferon alpha increases the frequency of interferon gamma-producing human CD4+ T cells. *J. Exp. Med.* 178:1655–1663.

516. Broder, C. C., and E. A. Berger. 1993. CD4 molecules with a diversity of mutations encompassing the CDR3 region efficiently support human immunodeficiency virus type 1 envelope glycoprotein-mediated cell fusion. *J. Virol.* 67:913–926.

517. Broder, C. C., D. S. Dimitrov, R. Blumenthal, and E. A. Berger. 1993. The block to HIV-1 envelope glycoprotein-mediated membrane fusion in animal cells expressing human CD4 can be overcome by a human cell component(s). *Virology* 193:483–491.

518. Brodie, S. J., D. A. Lewinsohn, B. K. Patterson, D. Jiyamapa, J. Krieger, L. Corey, P. D. Greenberg, and S. R. Riddell. 1999. In vivo migration and function of transferred HIV-1-specific cytotoxic T cells. *Nat. Med.* 5:34–41.

519. Brodine, S. K., J. R. Mascola, P. J. Weiss, S. I. Ito, K. R. Porter, A. W. Artenstein, F. C. Garland, F. E. McCutchan, and D. S. Burke. 1995. Detection of diverse HIV-1 genetic subtypes in the USA. *Lancet* 346:1198–1199.

520. Brogi, A., R. Presentini, D. Solazzo, P. Piomboni, and E. Constantino-Ceccarini. 1996. Interaction of human immunodeficiency virus type 1 envelope glycoprotein gp120 with a galactoglycerolipid associated with human sperm. *AIDS Res. Hum. Retrovir.* 12:483–489.

521. Broliden, P.-A., A. von Gegerfelt, P. Clapham, J. Rosen, E.-M. Fenyo, B. Wahren, and K. Broliden. 1992. Identification of human neutralization-inducing regions of the human immunodeficiency virus type 1 envelope glycoproteins. *Proc. Natl. Acad. Sci. USA* 89:461–465.

522. Broliden, P. A., B. Makitalo, L. Akerblom, J. Rosen, K. Broliden, G. Utter, M. Jondal, E. Norrby, and B. Wahren. 1991. Identification of amino acids in the V3 region of gp120 critical for virus neutralization by human HIV-1-specific antibodies. *Immunology* 73:371–376.

523. Bromley, S. K., S. Y. Thomas, and A. D. Luster. 2005. Chemokine receptor CCR7 guides T cell exit from peripheral tissues and entry into afferent lymphatics. *Nat. Immunol.* 6:895–901.

524. Brooke, S., R. Chan, S. Howard, and R. Sapolsky. 1997. Endocrine modulation of the neurotoxicity of gp120: implications for AIDS-related dementia complex. *Proc. Natl. Acad. Sci. USA* 94:9457–9462.

525. Brooks, D. G., S. G. Kitchen, C. M. Kitchen, D. D. Scripture-Adams, and J. A. Zack. 2001. Generation of HIV latency during thymopoiesis. *Nat. Med.* 7:459–464.

526. Brooks, D. G., and J. A. Zack. 2002. Effect of latent human immunodeficiency virus infection on cell surface phenotype. *J. Virol.* 76:1673–1681.

527. Brossard, Y., J. T. Aubin, L. Mandelbrot, C. Bignozzi, D. Brand, A. Chaput, J. Roume, N. Mulliez, F. Mallet, H. Agut, F. Barin, C. Brechot, A. Goudeau, J. M. Huraux, J. Barrat, P. Blot, J. Chavinie, N. Ciraru-Vigneron, P. Engelman, F. Herve,

E. Papiernik, and R. Henrion. 1995. Frequency of early *in utero* HIV-1 infection: a blind DNA polymerase chain reaction study on 100 fetal thymuses. *AIDS* 9:359–366.

528. Brossart, P., A. W. Goldrath, E. A. Butz, S. Martin, and M. J. Bevan. 1997. Virus-mediated delivery of antigenic epitopes into dendritic cells as a means to induce CTL. *J. Immunol.* 158:3270–3276.

529. Broussard, S. R., S. I. Staprans, R. White, E. M. Whitehead, M. B. Feinberg, and J. S. Allan. 2001. Simian immunodeficiency virus replicates to high levels in naturally infected African green monkeys without inducing immunologic or neurologic disease. *J. Virol.* 75:2262–2275.

530. Brouwers, P., M. P. Heyes, H. A. Moss, P. L. Wolters, D. G. Poplack, S. P. Markey, and P. A. Pizzo. 1993. Quinolinic acid in the cerebrospinal fluid of children with symptomatic human immunodeficiency virus type 1 disease: relationships to clinical status and therapeutic response. *J. Infect. Dis.* 168:1380–1386.

531. Brown, A. E., J. D. Malone, S. Y. Zhou, J. R. Lane, and C. A. Hawkes. 1997. Human immunodeficiency virus RNA levels in US adults: a comparison based upon race and ethnicity. *J. Infect. Dis.* 176:794–797.

532. Brown, J. A., T. K. Howcroft, and D. S. Singer. 1998. HIV Tat protein requirements for transactivation and repression of transcription are separable. *J. Acquir. Immune Defic. Syndr. Hum. Retrovirol.* 17:9–16.

533. Brown, L., B. E. Souberbielle, J. B. Marriott, M. Westby, U. Desselberger, T. Kaye, M. L. Gougeon, and A. Dalgleish. 1999. The conserved carboxy terminal region of HIV-1 gp120 is recognized by seronegative HIV-exposed people. *AIDS* 13:2515–2521.

534. Browne, M. J., K. H. Mayer, S. B. D. Chafee, M. N. Dudley, M. R. Posner, S. M. Steinberg, K. K. Graham, S. M. Geletko, S. H. Zinner, S. L. Denman, L. M. Dunkle, S. Kaul, C. McLaren, G. Skowron, N. M. Kouttab, T. A. Kennedy, A. B. Weitberg, and G. A. Curt. 1993. 2',3'-didehydro-3'-deoxythymidine (d4T) in patients with AIDS or AIDS-related complex: a phase I trial. *J. Infect. Dis.* 167:21–29.

535. Browning, P. J., J. M. G. Sechler, M. Kaplan, R. H. Washington, R. Gendelman, R. Yarchoan, B. Ensoli, and R. C. Gallo. 1994. Identification and culture of Kaposi's sarcoma-like spindle cells from the peripheral blood of human immunodeficiency virus-1-infected individuals and normal controls. *Blood* 84:2711–2720.

536. Bruggeman, L. A., S. Dikman, C. Meng, S. E. Quaggin, T. M. Coffman, and P. E. Klotman. 1997. Nephropathy in human immunodeficiency virus-1 transgenic mice is due to renal transgene expression. *J. Clin. Investig.* 100:84–92.

537. Bruggeman, L. A., M. D. Ross, N. Tanji, A. Cara, S. Dikman, R. E. Gordon, G. C. Burns, V. D. D'Agati, J. A. Winston, M. E. Klotman, and P. E. Klotman. 2000. Renal epithelium is a previously unrecognized site of HIV-1 infection. *J. Am. Soc. Nephrol.* 11:2079–2087.

538. Brumme, Z. L., W. W. Y. Dong, K. J. Chan, R. S. Hogg, J. S. G. Montaner, M. V. O'Shaughnessy, and P. R. Harrigan. 2003. Influence of polymorphisms within the CX3CR1 and MDR-1 genes on initial antiretroviral therapy response. *AIDS* 17:201–208.

539. Brumme, Z. L., J. Goodrich, H. B. Mayer, C. J. Brumme, B. M. Henrick, B. Wynhoven, J. J. Asselin, P. K. Cheung, R. S. Hogg, J. S. Montaner, and P. R. Harrigan. 2005. Molecular and clinical epidemiology of CXCR4-using HIV-1 in a large population of antiretroviral-naive individuals. *J. Infect. Dis.* 192:466–474.

540. Brutkiewicz, R. R., and R. M. Welsh. 1995. Major histocompatibility complex class I antigens and the control of viral infections by natural killer cells. *J. Virol.* 69:3967–3971.

541. Bryant, M. L., L. Ratner, R. J. Duronio, N. S. Kishore, B. Devadas, S. P. Adams, and J. I. Gordon. 1991. Incorporation of 12-methoxydodecanoate into the human immunodeficiency virus 1 gag polyprotein precursor inhibits its proteolytic processing and virus production in a chronically infected human lymphoid cell line. *Proc. Natl. Acad. Sci. USA* 88:2055–2059.

542. Bryant, M. L., J. Yamamoto, P. Luciw, R. Munn, P. Marx, J. Higgins, N. Pedersen, A. Levine, and M. B. Gardner. 1985. Molecular comparison of retroviruses associated with human and simian AIDS. *Hematol. Oncol.* 3:187–197.

543. Bryceson, Y. T., M. E. March, H. G. Ljunggren, and E. O. Long. 2006. Synergy among receptors on resting NK cells for the activation of natural cytotoxicity and cytokine secretion. *Blood* 107:159–166.

544. Bryson, Y. J., K. Luzuriaga, J. L. Sullivan, and D. W. Wara. 1992. Proposed definitions for *in utero* versus intrapartum transmission of HIV-1. *N. Engl. J. Med.* 327:1246–1247.

545. Buchbinder, S. P., M. H. Katz, N. A. Hessol, P. M. O'Malley, and S. D. Holmberg. 1994. Long-term HIV-1 infection without immunologic progression. *AIDS* 8:1123–1128.

546. Buckner, C., L. G. Gines, C. J. Saunders, L. Vojtech, I. Srivastava, A. Gettie, R. Bohm, J. Blanchard, S. W. Barnett, J. T. Safrit, and L. Stamatatos. 2004. Priming B cell-mediated anti-HIV envelope responses by vaccination allows for the long-term control of infection in macaques exposed to a R5-tropic SHIV. *Virology* 320:167–180.

547. Bucy, R. P., R. D. Hockett, C. A. Derdeyn, M. S. Saag, K. Squires, M. Sillers, R. T. Mitsuyasu, and J. M. Kilby. 1999. Initial increase in blood CD4+ lymphocytes after HIV antiretroviral therapy reflects redistribution from lymphoid tissues. *J. Clin. Investig.* 103:1391–1398.

548. Budhraja, M., H. Levendoglu, F. Kocka, M. Mangkornkanok, and R. Sherer. 1987. Duodenal mucosal T cell subpopulation and bacterial cultures in acquired immune deficiency syndrome. *Am. J. Gastroenterol.* 82:427–431.

549. Budka, H., C. A. Wiley, P. Kleihues, J. Artigas, A. K. Asbury, E. S. Cho, D. R. Cornblath, M. C. Dal Canto, U. DeGirolami, D. Dickson, L. G. Epstein, M. M. Esiri, F. Giangaspero, G. Gosztonyi, F. Gray, J. W. Griffin, D. Henin, Y. Iwasaki, R. S. Janssen, R. T. Johnson, P. L. Lantos, W. D. Lyman, J. C. McArthur, K. Nagashima, N. Peress, C. K. Petito, R. W. Price, R. H. Rhodes, M. Rosenblum, G. Said, F. Scaravilli, L. R. Sharer, and H. V. Vinters. 1991. HIV-associated disease of the nervous system: review of nomenclature and proposal for neuropathology-based terminology. *Brain Pathol.* 1:143–152.

550. Bukawa, H., J. I. Sekigawa, K. Hamajima, J. Fukushima, Y. Yamada, H. Kiyono, and K. Okuda. 1995. Neutralization of HIV-1 by secretory IgA induced by oral immunization with a new macromolecular multicomponent peptide vaccine candidate. *Nat. Med.* 1:681–685.

551. Bukrinsky, M. I., S. Haggerty, M. P. Dempsey, N. Sharova, A. Adzhubel, L. Spitz, P. Lewis, D. Goldfarb, M. Emerman, and M. Stevenson. 1993. A nuclear localization signal within HIV-1 matrix protein that governs infection of non-dividing cells. *Nature* 365:666–669.

552. Bukrinsky, M. I., N. Sharova, M. P. Dempsey, T. L. Stanwick, A. G. Bukrinskaya, S. Haggerty, and M. Stevenson. 1992.

Active nuclear import of human immunodeficiency virus type 1 preintegration complexes. *Proc. Natl. Acad. Sci. USA* **89**: 6580–6584.

553. Bukrinsky, M. I., T. L. Stanwick, M. P. Dempsey, and M. Stevenson. 1991. Quiescent T lymphocytes as an inducible virus reservoir in HIV-1 infection. *Science* **254**:423–427.

553a. Bulterys, M., D. J. Jamieson, M. J. O'Sullivan, M. H. Cohen, R. Maupin, S. Nesheim, M. P. Webber, R. Van Dyke, J. Wiener, and B. M. Branson. 2004. Rapid HIV-1 testing during labor: a multicenter study. *JAMA* **292**:219–223.

554. Bunders, M., C. Thorne, and M. L. Newell. 2005. Maternal and infant factors and lymphocyte, CD4 and CD8 cell counts in uninfected children of HIV-1-infected mothers. *AIDS* **19**:1071–1079.

555. Buonaguro, L., G. Barillari, H. K. Chang, C. A. Bohan, V. Kao, R. Morgan, R. C. Gallo, and B. Ensoli. 1992. Effects of the human immunodeficiency virus type 1 *tat* protein on the expression of inflammatory cytokines. *J. Virol.* **66**:7159–7167.

556. Burack, J. H., D. C. Barrett, R. D. Stall, M. A. Chesney, M. L. Ekstrand, and T. J. Coates. 1993. Depressive symptoms and CD4 lymphocyte decline among HIV-infected men. *JAMA* **270**:2568–2573.

557. Burgard, M., M. J. Mayaux, S. Blanche, A. Ferroni, M. L. Guihard-Moscato, M. C. Allemon, N. Ciraru-Vigneron, G. Firtion, C. Floch, F. Guillot, E. Lachassine, M. Vial, C. Griscelli, and C. Rouzioux. 1992. The use of viral culture and p24 antigen testing to diagnose human immunodeficiency virus infection in neonates. *N. Engl. J. Med.* **327**:1192–1197.

558. Burgdorf, W. H. C., K. Mukai, and J. Rsai. 1981. Immunohistochemical identification of factor VIII-related antigen in endothelial cells of cutaneous lesions of alleged vascular nature. *Am. J. Clin. Pathol.* **75**:167–171.

559. Burkala, E. J., J. He, J. T. West, C. Wood, and C. K. Petito. 2005. Compartmentalization of HIV-1 in the central nervous system: role of the choroid plexus. *AIDS* **19**:675–684.

560. Burke, A. P., D. Anderson, P. Mannan, J. L. Ribas, Y.-H. Liang, J. Smialek, and R. Virmani. 1994. Systemic lymphadenopathic histology in human immunodeficiency virus-1-seropositive drug addicts without apparent acquired immunodeficiency syndrome. *Hum. Pathol.* **25**:248–256.

561. Burns, B. F., G. S. Wood, and R. F. Dorfman. 1991. The varied histopathology of lymphadenopathy in the homosexual male. *Am. J. Surg. Pathol.* **9**:287–296.

562. Burton, D. R., R. C. Desrosiers, R. W. Doms, W. C. Koff, P. D. Kwong, J. P. Moore, G. J. Nabel, J. Sodroski, I. A. Wilson, and R. T. Wyatt. 2004. HIV vaccine design and the neutralizing antibody protection. *Nat. Immunol.* **5**:233–236.

563. Burton, D. R., R. L. Stanfield, and I. A. Wilson. 2005. Antibody vs. HIV in a clash of evolutionary titans. *Proc. Natl. Acad. Sci. USA* **102**:14943–14948. (First published 11 October 2005; doi:10.1073/pnas.0505126102.)

564. Reference deleted.

565. Busch, M. P., S. A. Glynn, S. L. Stramer, D. M. Strong, S. Caglioti, D. J. Wright, B. Pappalardo, and S. H. Kleinman. 2005. A new strategy for estimating risks of transfusion-transmitted viral infections based on rates of detection of recently infected donors. *Transfusion* (Paris) **45**:254–264.

566. Busch, M. P., L. L. L. Lee, and G. A. Satten. 1995. Time course of detection of viral and serological markers preceding HIV-1 seroconversion; implications for blood and tissue donor screening. *Transfusion* (Paris) **35**:91–97.

567. Busch, M. P., E. A. Operskalski, and J. W. Mosley. 1996. Factors influencing HIV-1 transmission by blood transfusion. *J. Infect. Dis.* **174**:26–33.

568. Busch, M. P., and G. A. Satten. 1997. Time course of viremia and antibody seroconversion following human immunodeficiency virus exposure. *Am. J. Med.* **102**:117–124.

569. Buseyne, F., M. McChesney, F. Porrot, S. Kovarik, B. Guy, and Y. Riviere. 1993. Gag-specific cytotoxic T lymphocytes from human immunodeficiency virus type 1-infected individuals: Gag epitopes are clustered in three regions of the p24 gag protein. *J. Virol.* **67**:694–702.

570. Bush, C. E., R. M. Donovan, N. P. Markowitz, P. Kvale, and L. D. Saravolatz. 1996. A study of HIV RNA viral load in AIDS patients with bacterial pneumonia. *J. Acquir. Immune Defic. Syndr. Hum. Retrovirol.* **13**:23–26.

571. Bushman, F., M. Lewinski, A. Ciuffi, S. Barr, J. Leipzig, S. Hannenhalli, and C. Hoffmann. 2005. Genome-wide analysis of retroviral DNA integration. *Nat. Rev. Microbiol.* **3**:848–858.

572. Butera, S. T., T. L. Pisell, K. Limpakarnjanarat, N. L. Young, T. W. Hodge, T. D. Mastro, and T. M. Folks. 2001. Production of a novel viral suppressive activity associated with resistance to infection among female sex workers exposed to HIV type 1. *AIDS Res. Hum. Retrovir.* **17**:735–744.

573. Buzy, J. M., L. M. Lindstrom, M. C. Zink, and J. E. Clements. 1995. HIV-1 in the developing CNS: developmental differences in gene expression. *Virology* **210**:361–371.

574. Bwayo, J. J., N. J. D. Nagelkerke, S. Moses, J. Embree, E. N. Ngugi, A. Mwatha, J. Kimani, A. Anzala, S. Choudhri, J. O. N. Achola, and F. A. Plummer. 1995. Comparison of the declines in CD4 counts in HIV-1 seropositive female sex workers and women from the general population in Nairobi, Kenya. *J. Acquir. Immune Defic. Syndr. Hum. Retrovirol.* **10**:457–461.

575. Byrn, R. A., and A. A. Kiessling. 1998. Analysis of human immunodeficiency virus in semen: indications of a genetically distinct virus reservoir. *J. Reprod. Immunol.* **41**:161–176.

576. Byrne, J. A., and M. B. A. Oldstone. 1984. Biology of cloned cytotoxic T lymphocytes specific for lymphocytic choriomeningitis virus: clearance of virus in vivo. *J. Virol.* **51**:682–686.

577. Cafaro, A., A. Caputo, C. Fracasso, M. T. Maggiorella, D. Goletti, S. Baroncelli, M. Pace, L. Sernicola, M. L. Koanga-Mogtomo, M. Betti, A. Borsetti, R. Belli, L. Akerblom, F. Corrias, S. Butto, J. Heeney, F. Verani, F. Titti, and B. Ensoli. 1999. Control of SHIV-89.6P-infection of cynomolgus monkeys by HIV-1 Tat protein vaccine. *Nat. Med.* **5**:643–650.

577a. Cahn, P., J. Villacian, A. Lazzarin, C. Katlama, B. Grinsztejn, K. Arasteh, P. Lopez, N. Clumeck, J. Gerstoft, N. Stavrianeas, S. Moreno, F. Antunes, D. Neubacher, and D. Mayers. 2006. Ritonavir-boosted tipranavir demonstrates superior efficacy to ritonavir-boosted protease inhibitors in treatment-experienced HIV-infected patients: 24-week results of the RESIST-2 trial. *Clin. Infect. Dis.* **43**:1347–1356.

578. Cai, Q., X.-L. Huang, G. Rappocciolo, and C. R. Rinaldo, Jr. 1990. Natural killer cell responses in homosexual men with early HIV infection. *J. Acquir. Immune Defic. Syndr.* **3**:669–676.

579. Cai, R., B. Carpick, R. F. Chun, K.-T. Jeang, and B. R. G. Williams. 2000. HIV-1 TAT inhibits PKR activity by both RNA-dependent and RNA-independent mechanisms. *Arch. Biochem. Biophys.* **373**:361–367.

580. Calabrese, L. H., D. M. Kelley, A. Myers, M. O'Connell, and K. Easley. 1991. Rheumatic symptoms and human immunodeficiency virus infection. *Arthritis Rheum.* **34**:257–263.

581. Calabro, M. L., C. Zanotto, F. Calerazzo, C. Crivellaro, A. Del Mistro, A. De Rossi, and L. Chieco-Bianchi. 1995. HIV-1 infection of the thymus: evidence for a cytopathic and thymotropic viral variant *in vivo. AIDS Res. Hum. Retrovir.* **11:**11–19.

582. Calarese, D. A., C. N. Scanlan, M. B. Zwick, S. Deechongkit, Y. Mirmura, R. Kunert, P. Zhu, M. R. Wormald, R. L. Stanfield, K. H. Roux, J. W. Kelly, P. M. Rudd, R. A. Dwek, H. Katinger, D. R. Burton, and I. A. Wilson. 2003. Antibody domain exchange is an immunological solution to carbohydrate cluster recognition. *Science* **300:**2065–2066.

583. Calarota, S. A., A.-C. Leandersson, G. Bratt, J. Hinkula, D. M. Klinman, K. J. Weinhold, E. Sandstrom, and B. Wahren. 1999. Immune responses in asymptomatic HIV-1-infected patients after HIV-DNA immunization followed by highly active antiretroviral treatment. *J. Immunol.* **163:**2330–2338.

584. Caldwell, R. L., B. S. Egan, and V. L. Shepherd. 2000. HIV-1 tat represses transcription from the mannose receptor promoter. *J. Immunol.* **165:**7035–7041.

585. Caley, I. J., M. R. Betts, D. M. Irlbeck, N. L. Davis, R. Swanstrom, J. A. Frelinger, and R. E. Johnston. 1997. Humoral, mucosal, and cellular immunity in response to a human immunodeficiency virus type 1 immunogen expressed by a Venezuelan equine encephalitis virus vaccine vector. *J. Virol.* **71:**3031–3038.

586. Camaur, D., and D. Trono. 1996. Characterization of human immunodeficiency virus type 1 Vif particle incorporation. *J. Virol.* **70:**6106–6111.

587. Camerini, D., B. D. Jamieson, J. A. Zack, and I. S. Y. Chen. 1994. Pathogenesis of syncytium-inducing and non-syncytium inducing HIV-1 isolates and molecular clones in SCID-hu mice. *Keyst. Symp. Mol. Cell. Biol.* **1994** (Suppl. 18B):155.

588. Camerini, D., and B. Seed. 1990. A CD4 domain important for HIV-mediated syncytium formation lies outside the virus binding site. *Cell* **60:**747–754.

589. Cameron, D. W., J. N. Simonsen, L. J. D'Costa, A. R. Ronald, G. M. Maitha, M. N. Gakinya, M. Cheang, J. O. Ndinya-Achola, P. Piot, R. C. Brunham, and F. A. Plummer. 1989. Female to male transmission of human immunodeficiency virus type 1: risk factors for seroconversion in men. *Lancet* **ii:**403–407.

590. Cameron, M. L., D. L. Granger, T. J. Matthews, and J. B. Weinberg. 1994. Human immunodeficiency virus (HIV)-infected human blood monocytes and peritoneal macrophages have reduced anticryptococcal activity whereas HIV-infected alveolar macrophages retain normal activity. *J. Infect. Dis.* **170:**60–67.

591. Cameron, P., M. Pope, A. Granelli-Piperno, and R. M. Steinman. 1996. Dendritic cells and the replication of HIV-1. *J. Leukoc. Biol.* **59:**158–171.

592. Cameron, P. U., P. S. Freudenthal, J. M. Barker, S. Gezelter, K. Inaba, and R. M. Steinman. 1992. Dendritic cells exposed to human immunodeficiency virus type-1 transmit a vigorous cytopathic infection to CD4+ T cells. *Science* **257:**383–387.

593. Cammack, N. 2001. The potential for HIV fusion inhibition. *Curr. Opin. Infect. Dis.* **14:**13–16.

594. Campbell, I. L., C. R. Abraham, E. Masliah, P. Kemper, J. D. Inglis, M. B. A. Oldstone, and L. Mucke. 1993. Neurologic disease induced in transgenic mice by cerebral overexpression of interleukin 6. *Proc. Natl. Acad. Sci. USA* **90:**10061–10065.

595. Campbell, S. M., S. M. Crowe, and J. Mak. 2001. Lipid rafts and HIV-1: from viral entry to assembly of progeny virions. *J. Clin. Virol.* **22:**217–227.

596. Canivet, M., A. D. Hoffman, D. Hardy, J. Sernatinger, and J. A. Levy. 1990. Replication of HIV-1 in a wide variety of animal cells following phenotypic mixing with murine retroviruses. *Virology* **178:**543–551.

597. Canki, M., J. R. Sparrow, W. Chao, M. J. Potash, and D. J. Volsky. 2000. Human immunodeficiency virus type 1 can infect human retinal pigment epithelial cells in culture and alter the ability of the cells to phagocytose rod outer segment membranes. *AIDS Res. Hum. Retrovir.* **16:**453–463.

598. Canque, B., S. Bakri, S. Camus, M. Yagello, A. Benjouad, and J. C. Gluckman. 1999. The susceptibility to X4 and R5 human immunodeficiency virus-1 strains of dendritic cells derived in vitro from CD34+ hematopoietic progenitor cells is primarily determined by their maturation stage. *Blood* **93:**3866–3875.

599. Cantin, R., J.-F. Fortin, G. Lamontagne, and M. Tremblay. 1997. The presence of host-derived HLA-DR1 on human immunodeficiency virus type 1 increases viral infectivity. *J. Virol.* **71:**1922–1930.

600. Cantin, R., J.-F. Fortin, and M. Tremblay. 1996. The amount of host HLA-DR proteins acquired by HIV-1 is virus strain- and cell type-specific. *Virology* **218:**372–381.

601. Cantrill, H. L., K. Henry, B. Jackson, A. Erice, F. M. Ussery, and H. H. Balfour, Jr. 1988. Recovery of human immunodeficiency virus from ocular tissues in patients with acquired immune deficiency syndrome. *Ophthalmology* **95:**1458–1462.

602. Cao, J., J. McNevin, U. Malhotra, and M. J. McElrath. 2003. Evolution of CD8+ T cell immunity and viral escape following acute HIV-1 infection. *J. Immunol.* **171:**3837–3846.

603. Cao, J., I. W. Park, A. Cooper, and J. Sodroski. 1996. Molecular determinants of acute single-cell lysis by human immunodeficiency virus type 1. *J. Virol.* **70:**1340–1354.

604. Cao, Y., D. Dieterich, P. A. Thomas, Y. Huang, M. Mirabile, and D. D. Ho. 1992. Identification and quantitation of HIV-1 in the liver of patients with AIDS. *AIDS* **6:**65–70.

605. Cao, Y., P. Krogstad, B. T. Korber, R. A. Koup, M. Muldoon, C. Macken, J. L. Song, Z. Jin, J. Q. Zhao, S. Clapp, I. S. Chen, D. D. Ho, and A. Ammann. 1990. CD4-independent, productive human immunodeficiency virus type 1 infection of hepatoma cell lines in vitro. *J. Virol.* **64:**2553–2559.

606. Cao, Y., L. Qin, L. Zhang, J. Safrit, and D. D. Ho. 1995. Virologic and immunologic characterization of long-term survivors of human immunodeficiency virus type 1 infection. *N. Engl. J. Med.* **332:**201–208.

607. Capitanio, J. P., S. P. Mendoza, N. W. Lerche, and W. A. Mason. 1998. Social stress results in altered glucocorticoid regulation and shorter survival in simian acquired immune deficiency syndrome. *Proc. Natl. Acad. Sci. USA* **95:**4714–4719.

608. Capobianchi, M. R., C. Barresi, P. Borghi, S. Gessani, L. Fantuzzi, F. Ameglio, F. Belardelli, S. Papadia, and F. Dianzani. 1997. Human immunodeficiency virus type 1 gp120 stimulates cytomegalovirus replication in monocytes: possible role of endogenous interleukin-8. *J. Virol.* **71:**1591–1597.

609. Capodici, J., K. Kariko, and D. Weissman. 2002. Inhibition of HIV-1 infection by small interfering RNA-mediated RNA interference. *J Immunol.* **169:**5196–5201.

609a. Caramalho, I., T. Lopes-Carvalho, D. Ostler, S. Zelenay, M. Haury, and J. Demengeot. 2003. Regulatory T cells selectively express toll-like receptors and are activated by lipopolysaccharide. *J. Exp. Med.* **197:**403–411.

610. Carcelain, G., R. Tubiana, A. Samri, V. Calvez, C. De-laugerre, H. Agut, C. Katlama, and B. Autran. 2001. Transient mobilization of human immunodeficiency virus (HIV)-specific CD4 T-helper cells fails to control virus rebounds during intermittent antiretroviral therapy in chronic HIV type 1 infection. *J. Virol.* 75:234–241.

611. Cardiello, P. G., E. Hassink, J. Ananworanich, P. Srasue-bkul, T. Samor, A. Mahanontharit, K. Ruxrungtham, B. Hirschel, J. Lange, P. Phanuphak, and D. A. Cooper. 2005. A prospective, randomized trial of structured treatment interruption for patients with chronic HIV type 1 infection. *Clin. Infect. Dis.* 40:594–600.

612. Cardo, D. M., D. H. Culver, C. A. Ciesielski, P. U. Srivastava, R. Marcus, D. Abiteboul, J. Heptonstall, G. Ippolito, F. Lot, P. S. McKibben, D. M. Bell, et al. 1997. A case-control study of HIV seroconversion in health care workers after percutaneous exposure. *N. Engl. J. Med.* 337:1485–1490.

613. Cardoso, A. R., C. Goncalves, D. Pascoalinho, C. Gil, A. F. Ferreira, I. Bartolo, and N. Taveira. 2004. Seronegative infection and AIDS caused by an A2 subsubtype HIV-1. *AIDS* 18:1071–1074.

614. Carl, S., T. C. Greenough, M. Krumbiegel, M. Greenberg, J. Skowronski, J. L. Sullivan, and F. Kirchhoff. 2001. Modulation of different human immunodeficiency virus type 1 Nef functions during progression to AIDS. *J. Virol.* 75:3657–3665.

615. Carlson, J. R. 1988. Serological diagnosis of human immunodeficiency virus infection by Western blot testing. *JAMA* 260:674–679.

616. Carlson, J. R., T. P. McGraw, E. Keddie, J. L. Yee, A. Rosenthal, A. J. Langlois, R. Dickover, R. Donovan, P. A. Luciw, M. B. Jennings, and M. B. Gardner. 1990. Vaccine protection of rhesus macaques against simian immunodeficiency virus infection. *AIDS Res. Hum. Retrovir.* 6:1239–1246.

617. Carmichael, A., X. Jin, P. Sissons, and L. Borysiewicz. 1993. Quantitative analysis of the human immunodeficiency virus type (HIV-1)-specific cytotoxic T lymphocytes (CTL) response at different stages of HIV-1 infection: differential CTL responses to HIV-1 and Epstein-Barr virus in late disease. *J. Exp. Med.* 177:249–256.

618. Carne, C. A., R. S. Tedder, A. Smith, S. Sutherland, S. G. Elkington, H. M. Daly, F. E. Preston, and J. Craske. 1985. Acute encephalopathy coincident with seroconversion for anti-HTLV-III. *Lancet* ii:1206–1208.

619. Carr, J. K., M. Avila, M. G. Carrillo, H. Salomon, J. Hierholzer, V. Watanaveeradej, M. A. Pando, M. Negrete, K. L. Russell, J. Sanchez, D. L. Birx, R. Andrade, J. Vinoles, and F. E. McCutchan. 2001. Diverse BF recombinants have spread widely since the introduction of HIV-1 into South America. *AIDS* 15:F41-F46.

620. Carrat, F., F. Bani-Sadr, S. Pol, E. Rosenthal, F. Lunel-Fabiani, A. Benzekri, P. Morand, C. Goujard, G. Pialoux, L. Piroth, D. Salmon-Ceron, C. Degott, P. Cacoub, and C. Perronne. 2004. Pegylated interferon alfa-2b vs standard interferon alfa-2b, plus ribavirin, for chronic hepatitis C in HIV-infected patients: a randomized controlled trial. *JAMA* 292:2839–2848.

621. Carre, N., C. Deveau, F. Belanger, F. Boufassa, A. Persoz, C. Jadand, C. Rouzioux, J.-F. Delfraissy, and D. Bucquet. 1994. Effect of age and exposure group on the onset of AIDS in heterosexual and homosexual HIV-infected patients. *AIDS* 8:797–802.

622. Carreno, M.-P., N. Chomont, M. D. Kazatchkine, T. Irinopoulou, C. Krief, A.-S. Mohamed, L. Andreoletti, M. Matta, and L. Belec. 2002. Binding of the LFA-1 (CD11a) to intracellular adhesion molecule 3 (ICAM-3; CD50) and ICAM-2 (CD102) triggers transmigration of human immunodeficiency virus type 1-infected monocytes through mucosal epithelial cells. *J. Virol.* 76:32–40.

623. Carrigan, D. R., K. K. Knox, and M. A. Tapper. 1990. Suppression of human immunodeficiency virus type 1 replication by human herpesvirus-6. *J. Infect. Dis.* 162:844–851.

624. Carrillo, A., and L. Ratner. 1996. Cooperative effects of the human immunodeficiency virus type 1 envelope variable loops V1 and V3 in mediating infectivity for T cells. *J. Virol.* 70:1310–1316.

625. Carrillo, A., and L. Ratner. 1996. Human immunodeficiency virus type 1 tropism for T-lymphoid cell lines: role of the V3 loop and C4 envelope determinants. *J. Virol.* 70:1301–1309.

626. Carrington, M., G. W. Nelson, M. P. Martin, T. Kissner, D. Vlahov, J. J. Goedert, R. Kaslow, S. Buchbinder, K. Hoots, and S. J. O'Brien. 1999. HLA and HIV-1: heterozygote advantage and B*35-Cw*04 disadvantage. *Science* 283:1748–1752.

627. Carroll, P. A., E. Brazeau, and M. Lagunoff. 2004. Kaposi's sarcoma-associated herpesvirus infection of blood endothelial cells induces lymphatic differentiation. *Virology* 328:7–18.

628. Carroll-Anzinger, D., and L. Al-Harthi. 2006. Gamma interferon primes productive human immunodeficiency virus infection in astrocytes. *J. Virol.* 80:541–544.

629. Casareale, D., M. Fiala, C. M. Chang, L. A. Cone, and E. S. Mocarski. 1989. Cytomegalovirus enhances lysis of HIV-infected T lymphoblasts. *Int. J. Cancer* 44:124–130.

630. Casimiro, D. R., L. Chen, T. Fu, R. K. Evans, M. J. Caulfield, M. Davies, A. Tang, M. Chen, L. Huang, V. Harris, D. C. Freed, K. A. Wilson, S. Dubey, D. Zhu, D. Nawrocki, H. Mach, R. Troutman, L. Isopi, D. Williams, W. Hurni, Z. Xu, J. G. Smith, S. Wang, X. Liu, L. Guan, R. Long, W. Trigona, G. J. Heidecker, H. C. Perry, N. Persaud, T. J. Toner, Q. Su, X. Liang, R. Youil, M. Chastain, A. J. Bett, D. B. Volkin, E. A. Emini, and J. W. Shiver. 2003. Comparative immunogenicity in rhesus monkeys of DNA plasmid, recombinant vaccinia virus, and replication-defective adenovirus vectors expressing a human immunodeficiency virus type 1 *gag* gene. *J. Virol.* 77:6305–6313.

631. Casimiro, D. R., F. Wang, W. A. Schleif, X. Liang, Z. Q. Zhang, T. W. Tobery, M. E. Davies, A. B. McDermott, H. O'-Connor D, A. Fridman, A. Bagchi, L. G. Tussey, A. J. Bett, A. C. Finnefrock, T. M. Fu, A. Tang, K. A. Wilson, M. Chen, H. C. Perry, G. J. Heidecker, D. C. Freed, A. Carella, K. S. Punt, K. J. Sykes, L. Huang, V. I. Ausensi, M. Bachinsky, U. Sadasivan-Nair, D. I. Watkins, E. A. Emini, and J. W. Shiver. 2005. Attenuation of simian immunodeficiency virus SIVmac239 infection by prophylactic immunization with DNA and recombinant adenoviral vaccine vectors expressing Gag. *J. Virol.* 79:15547–15555.

632. Casper, C., L. Naver, P. Clevestig, E. Belfrage, T. Leitner, J. Albert, S. Lindgren, C. Ottenblad, A. B. Bohlin, E. M. Fenyo, and A. Ehrnst. 2002. Coreceptor change appears after immune deficiency is established in children infected with different HIV-1 subtypes. *AIDS Res. Hum. Retrovir.* 18:343–352.

633. Casper, C., M. Redman, M. L. Huang, J. Pauk, T. M. Lampinen, S. E. Hawes, C. W. Critchlow, R. A. Morrow, L. Corey, N. Kiviat, and A. Wald. 2004. HIV infection and

human herpesvirus-8 oral shedding among men who have sex with men. *J. Acquir. Immune Defic. Syndr.* **35**:233–238.

634. Castedo, M., T. Roumier, J. Blanco, K. F. Ferri, J. Baretina, L. A. Tintignac, K. Andreau, J. L. Perfettini, A. Amendola, R. Nardacci, P. Leduc, D. E. Ingber, S. Druillennec, B. Roques, S. A. Leibovitch, M. Vilella-Bach, J. Chen, J. A. Este, N. Modjtahedi, M. Piacentini, and G. Kroemer. 2002. Sequential involvement of Cdk1, mTOR and p53 in apoptosis induced by the HIV-1 envelope. *EMBO J.* **21**:4070–4080.

635. Castelli, J., E. Thomas, Y.-J. Liu, and J. A. Levy. 2004. Mature dendritic cells can enhance CD8+ cell noncytotoxic anti-HIV responses: the role of IL-15. *Blood* **103**:2699–2704.

636. Castilla, J., J. Del Romero, V. Hernando, B. Marincovich, S. Garcia, and C. Rodriguez. 2005. Effectiveness of highly active antiretroviral therapy in reducing heterosexual transmission of HIV. *J. Acquir. Immune Defic. Syndr.* **40**:96–101.

637. Castillo, R. C., S. Arango-Jaramillo, R. John, K. Weinhold, P. Kanki, L. Carruth, and D. H. Schwartz. 2000. Resistance to human immunodeficiency virus type 1 in vitro as a surrogate of vaccine-induced protective immunity. *J. Infect. Dis.* **181**:897–903.

638. Castro, B. A., S. W. Barnett, L. A. Evans, J. Moreau, K. Odehouri, and J. A. Levy. 1990. Biologic heterogeneity of human immunodeficiency virus type 2 (HIV-2). *Virology* **178**:527–534.

639. Castro, B. A., C. Cheng-Mayer, L. A. Evans, and J. A. Levy. 1988. HIV heterogeneity and viral pathogenesis. *AIDS* **2**:S17–S28.

640. Castro, B. A., J. W. Eichberg, N. W. Lerche, and J. A. Levy. 1989. HIV from experimentally infected chimpanzees: isolation and characterization. *J. Med. Primatol.* **18**:337–342.

641. Castro, B. A., J. Homsy, E. Lennette, K. K. Murthy, J. W. Eichberg, and J. A. Levy. 1992. HIV-1 expression in chimpanzees can be activated by CD8+ cell depletion or CMV infection. *Clin. Immunol. Immunopathol.* **65**:227–233.

642. Castro, B. A., M. Nepomuceno, N. W. Lerche, J. W. Eichberg, and J. A. Levy. 1991. Persistent infection of baboons and rhesus monkeys with different strains of HIV-2. *Virology* **184**:219–226.

643. Castro, K. G., J. W. Ward, L. Slutsker, J. W. Buehler, H. W. Jaffe, R. L. Berkelman, and J. W. Curran. 1992. 1993 revised classification system for HIV infection and expanded surveillance case definition for AIDS among adolescents and adults. *Morb. Mortal. Wkly. Rep.* **41**:1–19.

644. Cauda, R., M. Tumbarello, L. Ortona, P. Kanda, R. C. Kennedy, and T. C. Chanh. 1988. Inhibition of normal human natural killer cell activity by human immunodeficiency virus synthetic transmembrane peptides. *Cell. Immunol.* **115**:57–65.

645. Cavard, C., A. Zider, M. Vernet, M. Bennoun, S. Saragosti, G. Grimber, and P. Briand. 1990. *In vivo* activation by ultraviolet rays of the human immunodeficiency virus type 1 long terminal repeat. *J. Clin. Investig.* **86**:1369–1374.

646. Cavert, W., D. W. Notermans, K. Staskus, S. W. Wietgrefe, M. Zupancic, K. Gebhard, K. Henry, Z. Q. Zhang, R. Mills, H. McDade, J. Goudsmit, S. A. Danner, and A. T. Haase. 1997. Kinetics of response in lymphoid tissues to antiretroviral therapy of HIV-1 infection. *Science* **276**:960–964.

647. Cayota, A., F. Vuillier, D. Scott-Algara, V. Feuillie, and G. Dighiero. 1993. Differential requirements for HIV-1 replication in naive and memory CD4 T cells from asymptomatic HIV-1 seropositive carriers and AIDS patients. *Clin. Exp. Immunol.* **91**:241–248.

648. Cease, K. B., and J. A. Berzofsky. 1994. Toward a vaccine for AIDS: the emergence of immunobiology-based vaccine development. *Annu. Rev. Immunol.* **12**:923–989.

649. Celada, F., C. Cambiaggi, J. Maccari, S. Burastero, T. Gregory, E. Patzer, J. Porter, C. McDanal, and T. Matthews. 1990. Antibody raised against soluble CD4-rgp120 complex recognizes the CD4 moiety and blocks membrane fusion without inhibiting CD4-gp120 binding. *J. Exp. Med.* **172**:1143–1150.

650. Cella, M., F. Facchetti, A. Lanzavecchia, and M. Colonna. 2000. Plasmacytoid dendritic cells activated by influenza virus and CD40L drive a potent T_H1 polarization. *Nat. Immunol.* **1**:305–310.

651. Cella, M., D. Jarrossay, F. Facchetti, O. Alebardi, H. Nakajima, A. Lanzavecchia, and M. Colonna. 1999. Plasmacytoid monocytes migrate to inflamed lymph nodes and produce large amounts of type I interferon. *Nat. Med.* **5**:919–923.

652. Centers for Disease Control. 1981. Pneumocystis pneumonia. *Morb. Mortal. Wkly. Rev.* **30**:250–252.

653. Centers for Disease Control. 1982. *Pneumocystis carinii* pneumonia among persons with hemophilia. *Morb. Mortal. Wkly. Rep.* **31**:365–367.

654. Centers for Disease Control. 1985. Revision of the case definition of acquired immunodeficiency syndrome for national reporting—United States. *Ann. Intern. Med.* **103**:402.

655. Centers for Disease Control. 1994. Zidovudine for the prevention of HIV transmission from mother to infant. *Morb. Mortal. Wkly. Rep.* **43**:285–287.

656. Centers for Disease Control. 1995. Case-control of HIV seroconversion in health-care workers after percutaneous exposure to HIV-infected blood—France, United Kingdom, and United States, January 1988–August 1994. *Morb. Mortal. Wkly. Rep.* **44**:929–933.

657. Reference deleted.

658. Centers for Disease Control. 1996. Update: provisional Public Health Service recommendations for chemoprophylaxis after occupational exposure to HIV. *JAMA* **276**:90–92.

659. Centers for Disease Control. 2002. Sexually transmitted diseases treatment guidelines 2002. *Morb. Mortal. Wkly. Rep.* **51**:1–80.

660. Centers for Disease Control and Prevention. 2006. Twenty-five years of HIV/AIDS—United States, 1981–2006. *Morb. Mortal. Wkly. Rep.* **55**:585–589.

661. Centlivre, M., P. Sommer, M. Michel, R. H. T. Fang, S. Gofflo, J. Valladeau, N. Schmitt, F. Thierry, B. Hurtrel, S. Wain-Hobson, and M. Sala. 2005. HIV-1 clade promoters strongly influence spatial and temporal dynamics of viral replication in vivo. *J. Clin. Investig.* **115**:348–358.

662. Centlivre, M., P. Sommer, M. Michel, R. Ho Tsong Fang, S. Gofflo, J. Valladeau, N. Schmitt, S. Wain-Hobson, and M. Sala. 2006. The HIV-1 clade C promoter is particularly well adapted to replication in the gut in primary infection. *AIDS* **20**:657–666.

663. Cerdan, C., Y. Martin, M. Courcoul, H. Brailly, C. Mawas, F. Birg, and D. Olive. 1992. Prolonged IL-2 receptor-alpha/CD25 expression after T cell activation via the adhesion molecule CD2 and CD28. *J. Immunol.* **149**:2255–2261.

664. Cesarman, E., Y. Chang, P. S. Moore, J. W. Said, and D. M. Knowles. 1995. Kaposi's sarcoma-associated herpesvirus-like

DNA sequences in AIDS-related body-cavity-based lymphomas. *N. Engl. J. Med.* 332:1186–1191.

665. Cesarman, E., and D. M. Knowles. 1999. The role of Kaposi's sarcoma-associated herpesvirus (KSHV/HHV-8) in lymphoproliferative diseases. *Semin. Cancer Biol.* 9:165–174.

666. Chad, D. A., T. W. Smith, A. Blumenfeld, P. G. Fairchild, and U. DeGirolami. 1990. Human immunodeficiency virus (HIV)-associated myopathy: immunocytochemical identification of an HIV antigen (gp 41) in muscle macrophages. *Ann. Neurol.* 28:579–582.

667. Chadwick, E. G., E. J. Connor, C. G. Hanson, V. V. Joshi, H. Abu-Farsakh, R. Yogev, G. McSherry, K. McClain, and S. B. Murphy. 1990. Tumors of smooth-muscle origin in HIV-infected children. *JAMA* 263:3182–3184.

668. Chaisson, R. E., J. E. Gallant, J. C. Keruly, and R. D. Moore. 1998. Impact of opportunistic disease on survival in patients with HIV infection. *AIDS* 12:29–33.

669. Chakrabarti, L., V. Baptiste, E. Khatissian, M.-C. Cumont, A.-M. Aubertin, L. Montagnier, and B. Hurtel. 1995. Limited viral spread and rapid immune response in lymph nodes of macaques inoculated with attenuated simian immunodeficiency virus. *Virology* 213:535–548.

670. Chakrabarti, L. A., T. Ivanovic, and C. Cheng-Mayer. 2002. Properties of the surface envelope glycoprotein associated with virulence of simian-human immunodeficiency virus SHIV(SF33A) molecular clones. *J. Virol.* 76:1588–1599.

671. Chakrabarti, L. A., S. R. Lewin, L. Zhang, A. Gettie, A. Luckay, L. N. Martin, E. Skulsky, D. D. Ho, C. Cheng-Mayer, and P. A. Marx. 2000. Normal T-cell turnover in sooty mangabeys harboring active simian immunodeficiency virus infection. *J. Virol.* 74:1209–1223.

672. Chakraborty, B., L. Valer, C. De Mendoza, V. Soriano, and M. E. Quinones-Mateu. 2004. Failure to detect human immunodeficiency virus type 1 superinfection in 28 HIV-seroconcordant individuals with high risk of reexposure to the virus. *AIDS Res. Hum. Retrovir.* 20:1026–1031.

673. Chakraborty, R. 2005. HIV-1 infection in children: a clinical and immunologic overview. *Curr. HIV Res.* 3:31–41.

674. Champagne, P., G. S. Ogg, A. S. King, C. Knabenhans, K. Ellefsen, M. Nobile, V. Appay, G. P. Rizzardi, S. Fleury, M. Lipp, R. Forster, S. Rowland-Jones, R. P. Sekaly, A. J. McMichael, and G. Pantaleo. 2001. Skewed maturation of memory HIV-specific CD8 T lymphocytes. *Nature* 410:106–111.

675. Chams, V., T. Jouault, E. Fenouillet, J.-C. Gluckman, and D. Klatzmann. 1988. Detection of anti-CD4 autoantibodies in the sera of HIV-infected patients using recombinant soluble CD4 molecules. *AIDS* 2:353–361.

676. Chan, D. C., D. Fass, J. M. Berger, and P. S. Kim. 1997. Core structure of gp41 from the HIV envelope glycoprotein. *Cell* 89:263–273.

677. Chan, D. C., and P. S. Kim. 1998. HIV entry and its inhibition. *Cell* 93:681–684.

678. Chan, K. C., B. Yip, R. S. Hogg, J. S. G. Montaner, and M. V. O'Shaughnessy. 2002. Survival rates after initiation of antiretroviral therapy stratified by CD4 cell counts in two cohorts in Canada and the United States. *AIDS* 16:1693–1694.

679. Chan, W. L., A. Rodgers, R. D. Hancock, F. Taffs, P. Kitchin, G. Farrar, and F. Y. Liew. 1992. Protection in simian immunodeficiency virus-vaccinated monkeys correlates with anti-HLA class I antibody response. *J. Exp. Med.* 176:1203–1207.

680. Chandwani, S., M. A. Greco, K. Mittal, C. Antoine, K. Krasinski, and W. Borkowsky. 1991. Pathology and human immunodeficiency virus expression in placentas of seropositive women. *J. Infect. Dis.* 163:1134–1138.

681. Chang, J., R. Jozwiak, B. Wang, T. Ng, Y. C. Ge, W. Bolton, D. E. Dwyer, C. Randle, R. Osborn, A. L. Cunningham, and N. K. Saksena. 1998. Unique HIV type 1 V3 region sequences derived from six different regions of brain: region-specific evolution within host-determined quasispecies. *AIDS Res. Hum. Retrovir.* 14:25–30.

682. Chang, J., R. Renne, D. Dittmer, and D. Ganem. 2000. Inflammatory cytokines and the reactivation of Kaposi's sarcoma-associated herpesvirus lytic replication. *Virology* 266:17–25.

683. Chang, S.-Y. P., B. H. Bowman, J. B. Weiss, R. E. Garcia, and T. J. White. 1993. The origin of HIV-1 isolate HTLV-IIIB. *Nature* 363:466–469.

684. Chang, T. K.-Y., F. Francois, A. Mosoain, and M. E. Klotman. 2003. CAF-mediated HIV-1 transcriptional inhibition is distinct from α-defensin-1 HIV inhibition. *J. Virol.* 77:6777–6784.

685. Chang, T. L., A. Mosoian, R. Pine, M. E. Klotman, and J. P. Moore. 2002. A soluble factor(s) secreted from CD8+ T lymphocytes inhibits human immunodeficiency virus type 1 replication through STAT1 activation. *J. Virol.* 76:569–581.

686. Chang, Y., E. Cesarman, M. S. Pessin, F. Lee, J. Culpepper, D. M. Knowles, and P. S. Moore. 1994. Identification of herpesvirus-like DNA sequences in AIDS-associated Kaposi's sarcoma. *Science* 266:1865–1869.

687. Chang, Y., P. S. Moore, S. J. Talbot, C. H. Boshoff, T. Zarkowska, D. Godden-Kent, H. Paterson, R. A. Weiss, and S. Mittnacht. 1996. Cyclin encoded by KS herpesvirus. *Nature* 382:410.

688. Chanh, T. C., G. R. Dreesman, P. Kanda, G. P. Linette, J. T. Sparrow, D. D. Ho, and R. C. Kennedy. 1986. Induction of anti-HIV neutralizing antibodies by synthetic peptides. *EMBO J.* 5:3065–3071.

689. Chanh, T. C., R. C. Kennedy, and P. Kanda. 1988. Synthetic peptides homologous to HIV transmembrane glycoprotein suppress normal human lymphocyte blastogenic response. *Cell. Immunol.* 111:77–86.

690. Chapel, A., A. Bensussan, E. Vilmer, and D. Dormont. 1992. Differential human immunodeficiency virus expression in CD4+ cloned lymphocytes: from viral latency to replication. *J. Virol.* 66:3966–3970.

691. Chaperot, L., A. Blum, O. Manches, G. Lui, J. Angel, J. P. Molens, and J. Plumas. 2006. Virus or TLR agonists induce TRAIL-mediated cytotoxic activity of plasmacytoid dendritic cells. *J. Immunol.* 176:248–255.

692. Chapuis, A. G., G. Paolo Rizzardi, C. D'Agostino, A. Attinger, C. Knabenhans, S. Fleury, H. Acha-Orbea, and G. Pantaleo. 2000. Effects of mycophenolic acid on human immunodeficiency virus infection in vitro and in vivo. *Nat. Med.* 6:762–768.

693. Charbit, A., A. Molla, J. Ronco, J. M. Clement, V. Favier, E. Bahraoui, L. Montagnier, A. Leguern, and M. Hofnung. 1990. Immunogenicity and antigenicity of conserved peptides from the envelope of HIV-1 expressed at the surface of recombinant bacteria. *AIDS* 4:545–551.

694. Chargelegue, D., C. M. Stanley, C. M. O'Toole, B. T. Colvin, and M. W. Steward. 1995. The affinity of IgG antibod-

ies to gag p24 and p17 in HIV-1-infected patients correlates with disease progression. *Clin. Exp. Immunol.* **99**:175–181.

695. Charman, H. P., S. Bladen, R. V. Gilden, and L. Coggins. 1976. Equine infectious anemia virus: evidence favoring classification as a retrovirus. *J. Virol.* **19**:1073–1079.

696. Charpentier, B., C. Hiesse, O. Lantz, C. Ferran, S. Stephens, D. O'Shaugnessy, M. Bodmer, G. Benoit, J. F. Bach, and L. Chatenoud. 1992. Evidence that antihuman tumor necrosis factor monoclonal antibody prevents OKT3-induced acute syndrome. *Transplantation* **54**:997–1002.

697. Chatlynne, L. G., and D. V. Ablashi. 1999. Seroepidemiology of Kaposi's sarcoma-associated herpesvirus (KSHV). *Semin. Cancer Biol.* **9**:175–185.

698. Chatterjee, M., J. Osborne, G. Bestetti, Y. Chang, and P. S. Moore. 2002. Viral IL-6-induced cell proliferation and immune evasion of interferon activity. *Science* **298**:1432–1435.

699. Chaturvedi, S., P. Frame, and S. L. Newman. 1995. Macrophages from human immunodeficiency virus-positive persons are defective in host defense against *Histoplasma capsulatum*. *J. Infect. Dis.* **171**:320–327.

700. Chavan, S. J., S. L. Tamma, M. Kaplan, M. Gerstein, and S. G. Pahwa. 1999. Reduction in T cell apoptosis in patients with HIV disease following antiretroviral therapy. *Clin. Immunol.* **93**:24–33.

701. Chayt, K. J., M. E. Harper, L. M. Marselle, E. B. Lewin, R. M. Rose, J. M. Oleske, L. G. Epstein, F. Wong-Staal, and R. C. Gallo. 1986. Detection of HTLV-III RNA in lungs of patients with AIDS and pulmonary involvement. *JAMA* **256**:2356–2359.

702. Chazal, N., G. Singer, C. Aiken, M. L. Hammarskjold, and D. Rekosh. 2001. Human immunodeficiency virus type 1 particles pseudotyped with envelope proteins that fuse at low pH no longer require Nef for optimal infectivity. *J. Virol.* **75**:4014–4018.

703. Cheevers, W. P., and T. C. McGuire. 1988. The lentiviruses: maedi/visna, caprine arthritis-encephalitis, and equine infectious anemia. *Adv. Virus Res.* **34**:189–215.

704. Chehimi, J., S. Bandyopadhyay, K. Prakash, B. Perussia, N. F. Hassan, H. Kawashima, D. Campbell, J. Kornbluth, and S. E. Starr. 1991. In vitro infection of natural killer cells with different human immunodeficiency virus type 1 isolates. *J. Virol.* **65**:1812–1822.

705. Chehimi, J., J. D. Marshall, O. Salvucci, I. Frank, S. Chehimi, S. Kawecki, D. Bacheller, S. Rifat, and S. Chouaib. 1997. IL-15 enhances immune functions during HIV infection. *J. Immunol.* **158**:5978–5987.

706. Chehimi, J., K. Prakash, V. Shanmugam, S. J. Jackson, S. Bandypadhyay, and S. E. Starr. 1993. In vitro infection of peripheral blood dendritic cells with human immunodeficiency virus-1 causes impairment of accessory functions. *Adv. Exp. Med. Biol.* **329**:521–526.

707. Chehimi, J., S. E. Starr, I. Frank, A. D'Andrea, X. Ma, R. R. MacGregor, J. Sennelier, and G. Trinchierei. 1994. Impaired interleukin 12 production in human immunodeficiency virus-infected patients. *J. Exp. Med.* **179**:1361–1366.

708. Chehimi, J., S. E. Starr, I. Frank, M. Rengaraju, S. J. Jackson, C. Llanes, M. Kobayashi, B. Perussia, D. Young, E. Nickbarg, S. F. Wolf, and G. Trinchieri. 1992. Natural killer (NK) cell stimulatory factor increases the cytotoxic activity of NK cells from both healthy donors and human immunodeficiency virus-infected patients. *J. Exp. Med.* **175**:789–796.

709. Chelucci, C., M. Federico, R. Guerriero, G. Mattia, I. Casella, E. Pelosi, U. Testa, G. Mariani, H. J. Hassan, and C. Peschle. 1998. Productive human immunodeficiency virus-1 infection of purified megakaryocytic progenitors/precursors and maturing megakaryocytes. *Blood* **91**:1225–1234.

710. Chelucci, C., H. J. Hannsan, C. Locardi, D. Bulgarini, E. Pelosi, G. Mariani, U. Testa, M. Federico, M. Valtieri, and C. Peschle. 1995. In vitro human immunodeficiency virus-1 infection of purified hematopoietic progenitors in single-cell culture. *Blood* **85**:1181–1187.

711. Chen, A., I. C. Boulton, J. Pongoski, A. Cochrane, and S. D. Gray-Owen. 2003. Induction of HIV-1 long terminal repeat-mediated transcription by *Neisseria gonorrhoeae*. *AIDS* **17**:625–636.

712. Chen, B. K., J. T. Gandhi, and D. Baltimore. 1996. CD4 down-modulation during infection of human T cells with human immunodeficiency virus type 1 involves independent activities of *vpu, env,* and *nef. J. Virol.* **70**:6044–6053.

713. Chen, C. H., K. J. Weinhold, J. A. Bartlett, D. P. Bolognesi, and M. L. Greenberg. 1993. CD8+ T lymphocyte-mediated inhibition of HIV-1 long terminal repeat transcription: a novel antiviral mechanism. *AIDS Res. Hum. Retrovir.* **9**:1079–1086.

714. Chen, H., J. Zha, R. E. Gowans, P. Camargo, J. Nishitani, J. L. McQuirter, S. W. Cole, J. A. Zack, and X. Liu. 2004. Alcohol enhances HIV type 1 infection in normal human oral keratinocytes by up-regulating cell-surface CXCR4 coreceptor. *AIDS Res. Hum. Retrovir.* **20**:513–519.

715. Chen, J., L. Wang, J. J. Chen, G. K. Sahu, S. Tyring, K. Ramsey, A. J. Indrikova, J. R. Petersen, D. Paar, and M. W. Cloyd. 2002. Detection of antibodies to human immunodeficiency virus (HIV) that recognize conformational epitope of glycoproteins 160 and 41 often allows for early diagnosis of HIV infection. *J. Infect. Dis.* **186**:321–331.

715a. Chen, K., J. Huang, C. Zhang, S. Huang, G. Nunnari, F. X. Wang, X. Tong, L. Gao, K. Nikisher, and H. Zhang. 2006. Alpha interferon potently enhances the anti-human immunodeficiency virus type 1 activity of APOBEC3G in resting primary CD4 T cells. *J. Virol.* **80**:7645–7657.

716. Chen, W., S. Antonenko, J. M. Sederstrom, X. Liang, A. S. Chan, H. Kanzler, B. Blom, B. R. Blazar, and Y.-J. Liu. 2004. Thrombopoietin cooperates with FLT3-ligand in the generation of plasmacytoid dendritic cell precursors from human hematopoietic progenitors. *Blood* **103**:2547–2553.

716a. Chen, W., W. Jin, N. Hardegen, K. J. Lei, L. Li, N. Marinos, G. McGrady, and S. M. Wahl. 2003. Conversion of peripheral CD4+CD25- naive T cells to CD4+CD25+ regulatory T cells by TGF-beta induction of transcription factor Foxp3. *J. Exp. Med.* **198**:1875–1886.

717. Chen, Y., and P. Gupta. 1996. CD8+ T-cell-mediated suppression of HIV-1 infection may not be due to chemokines RANTES, MIP-1α, and MIP-1β. *AIDS* **10**:1434–1435.

718. Chen, Z., A. Luckay, D. L. Sodora, P. Telfer, P. Reed, A. Gettie, J. M. Kanu, R. F. Sadek, J. Yee, D. D. Ho, L. Zhang, and P. A. Marx. 1997. Human immunodeficiency virus type 2 (HIV-2) seroprevalence and characterization of a distinct HIV-2 genetic subtype from the natural range of simian immunodeficiency virus-infected sooty mangabeys. *J. Virol.* **71**:3953–3960.

719. Chen, Z., P. Telfier, A. Gettie, P. Reed, L. Zhang, D. D. Ho, and P. A. Marx. 1996. Genetic characterization of new West African simian immunodeficiency virus SIVsm: geographic clustering of household-derived SIV strains with human immunodeficiency virus type 2 subtypes and genetically diverse viruses from a single feral sooty mangabey troop. *J. Virol.* 70:3617–3627.

720. Chene, L., M.-T. Nugeyre, E. Guillemard, N. Moulian, F. Barre-Sinoussi, and N. Israel. 1999. Thymocyte-thymic epithelial cell interaction leads to high-level replication of human immunodeficiency virus exclusively in mature CD4⁺ CD8⁻ CD3⁺ thymocytes: a critical role for tumor necrosis factor and interleukin-7. *J. Virol.* 73:7533–7542.

721. Cheng-Mayer, C., A. Brown, J. Harouse, P. A. Luciw, and A. J. Mayer. 1999. Selection for neutralization resistance of the simian/human immunodeficiency virus SHIVSF33A variant in vivo by virtue of sequence changes in the extracellular envelope glycoprotein that modify N-linked glycosylation. *J. Virol.* 73:5294–5300.

722. Cheng-Mayer, C., J. M. Homsy, L. A. Evans, and J. A. Levy. 1988. Identification of HIV subtypes with distinct patterns of sensitivity to serum neutralization. *Proc. Natl. Acad. Sci. USA* 85:2815–2819.

723. Cheng-Mayer, C., P. Ianello, K. Shaw, P. A. Luciw, and J. A. Levy. 1989. Differential effects of *nef* on HIV replication: implications for viral pathogenesis in the host. *Science* 246:1629–1632.

724. Cheng-Mayer, C., and J. A. Levy. 1988. Distinct biologic and serologic properties of HIV isolates from the brain. *Ann. Neurol.* 23:S58–S61.

725. Cheng-Mayer, C., and J. A. Levy. 1990. Human immunodeficiency virus infection of the CNS: characterization of "neurotropic" strains. *Curr. Top. Microbiol. Immunol.* 160:145–156.

726. Cheng-Mayer, C., and J. A. Levy. 1994. The *nef* protein suppresses HIV-1 replication in T-cells at an early stage of infection. *Proc. Natl. Acad. Sci. USA* 91:1539–1543.

727. Cheng-Mayer, C., R. Liu, N. R. Landau, and L. Stamatatos. 1997. Macrophage tropism of human immunodeficiency virus type 1 and utilization of the CC-CCR5 coreceptor. *J. Virol.* 71:1657–1661.

728. Cheng-Mayer, C., M. Quiroga, J. W. Tung, D. Dina, and J. A. Levy. 1990. Viral determinants of HIV-1 T-cell/macrophage tropism, cytopathicity, and CD4 antigen modulation. *J. Virol.* 64:4390–4398.

729. Cheng-Mayer, C., J. T. Rutka, M. L. Rosenblum, T. McHugh, D. P. Stites, and J. A. Levy. 1987. The human immunodeficiency virus (HIV) can productively infect cultured human glial cells. *Proc. Natl. Acad. Sci. USA* 84:3526–3530.

730. Cheng-Mayer, C., D. Seto, and J. A. Levy. 1991. Altered host range of HIV-1 after passage through various human cell types. *Virology* 181:288–294.

731. Cheng-Mayer, C., D. Seto, M. Tateno, and J. A. Levy. 1988. Biologic features of HIV that correlate with virulence in the host. *Science* 240:80–82.

732. Cheng-Mayer, C., T. Shioda, and J. A. Levy. 1991. Host range, replicative, and cytopathic properties of human immunodeficiency virus type 1 are determined by very few amino acid changes in *tat* and gp120. *J. Virol.* 65:6931–6941.

733. Cheng-Mayer, C., T. Shioda, and J. A. Levy. 1992. Small regions of the *env* and *tat* genes control cellular tropism, cytopathology and replicative properties of HIV-1, p. 188–195. *In* G. B. Rossi, E. Beth-Giraldo, L. Chieco-Bianchi, F. Dianzani, G. Giraldo, and P. Verani (ed.), *Science Challenging AIDS.* S. Karger, Basel, Switzerland.

734. Cheng-Mayer, C., C. Weiss, D. Seto, and J. A. Levy. 1989. Isolates of human immunodeficiency virus type 1 from the brain may constitute a special group of the AIDS virus. *Proc. Natl. Acad. Sci. USA* 80:8575–8579.

735. Chenine, A., Q. Sattentau, and M. Moulard. 2000. Selective HIV-1-induced downmodulation of CD4 and coreceptors. *Arch. Virol.* 145:455–471.

736. Chenine, A. L., M. Pion, E. Matouskova, F. Gondois-Rey, R. Vigne, and I. Hirsch. 2002. Adaptation of a CXCR4-using human immunodeficiency type 1 NDK virus in intestinal cells is associated with CD4-independent replication. *Virology* 304:403–414.

737. Cherepanov, P., Z. Y. Sun, S. Rahman, G. Maertens, G. Wagner, and A. Engelman. 2005. Solution structure of the HIV-1 integrase-binding domain in LEDGF/p75. *Nat. Struct. Mol. Biol.* 12:526–532.

738. Chermann, J. C., G. Donker, N. Yahi, D. Salaun, N. Guettari, O. Gayet, and I. Hirsh. 1991. Discrepancies in AIDS virus data. *Nature* 351:277–278.

739. Chernoff, A. E., E. V. Granowitz, L. Shapiro, E. Vannier, G. Lonnemann, J. B. Angel, J. S. Kennedy, A. R. Rabson, S. M. Wolff, and C. A. Dinarello. 1995. A randomized, controlled trial of IL-10 in humans. Inhibition of inflammatory cytokine production and immune responses. *J. Immunol.* 154:5492–5499.

740. Chertova, E., J. W. Bess, Jr., B. J. Crise, I. R. Sowder, T. M. Schaden, J. M. Hilburn, J. A. Hoxie, R. E. Benveniste, J. D. Lifson, L. E. Henderson, and L. O. Arthur. 2002. Envelope glycoprotein incorporation, not shedding of surface envelope glycoprotein (gp120/SU), is the primary determinant of SU content of purified human immunodeficiency virus type 1 and simian immunodeficiency virus. *J. Virol.* 76:5315–5325.

740a. Chertova, E., O. Chertov, L. V. Coren, J. D. Roser, C. M. Trubey, J. W. Bess, Jr., R. C. Sowder, 2nd, E. Barsov, B. L. Hood, R. J. Fisher, K. Nagashima, T. P. Conrads, T. D. Veenstra, J. D. Lifson, and D. E. Ott. 2006. Proteomic and biochemical analysis of purified human immunodeficiency virus type 1 produced from infected monocyte-derived macrophages. *J. Virol.* 80:9039–9052.

741. Chesebro, B., R. Buller, J. Portis, and K. Wehrly. 1990. Failure of human immunodeficiency virus entry and infection in CD4-positive human brain and skin cells. *J. Virol.* 64:215–221.

742. Chesebro, B., J. Nishio, S. Perryman, A. Cann, W. O'Brien, I. S. Y. Chen, and K. Wehrly. 1991. Identification of human immunodeficiency virus envelope gene sequences influencing viral entry into CD4-positive HeLa cells, T-leukemia cells, and macrophages. *J. Virol.* 65:5782–5789.

743. Cheung, L., L. McLain, M. J. Hollier, S. A. Reading, and N. J. Dimmock. 2005. Part of the C-terminal tail of the envelope gp41 transmembrane glycoprotein of human immunodeficiency virus type 1 is exposed on the surface of infected cells and is involved in virus-mediated cell fusion. *J. Gen. Virol.* 86:131–138.

744. Cheynier, R., S. Henrichwark, F. Hadida, E. Pelletier, E. Oksenhendler, B. Autran, and S. Wain-Hobson. 1994. HIV and T cell expansion in splenic white pulps is accompanied by - infiltration of HIV-specific cytotoxic T lymphocytes. *Cell* 78:373–387.

745. Cheynier, R., P. Langlade-Demoyen, M.-R. Marescot, S. Blanche, G. Blondin, S. Wain-Hobson, C. Griscelli, E. Vilmer, and F. Plata. 1992. Cytotoxic T lymphocyte responses in the

peripheral blood of children born to human immunodeficiency virus-1-infected mothers. *Eur. J. Immunol.* **22:**2211–2217.

746. Chiengsong-Popov, R., D. Callow, S. Beddows, S. Shaunak, C. Wasi, P. Kaleebu, C. Gilks, I. V. Petrascu, M. M. Garaev, D. M. Watts, N. T. Constantine, and J. N. Weber. 1992. Geographic diversity of human immunodeficiency virus type 1: serologic reactivity to *env* epitopes and relationship to neutralization. *J. Infect. Dis.* **165:**256–261.

747. Chin, M. P., T. D. Rhodes, J. Chen, W. Fu, and W. S. Hu. 2005. Identification of a major restriction in HIV-1 intersubtype recombination. *Proc. Natl. Acad. Sci. USA* **102:**9002–9007.

748. Chiodi, F., S. Fuerstenberg, M. Gidlund, B. Asjo, and E. M. Fenyo. 1987. Infection of brain-derived cells with the human immunodeficiency virus. *J. Virol.* **61:**1244–1247.

749. Chirmule, N., V. S. Kalyanaraman, C. Saxinger, F. Wong-Staal, J. Ghrayeb, and S. Pahwa. 1990. Localization of B-cell stimulatory activity of HIV-1 to the carboxyl terminus of gp41. *AIDS Res. Hum. Retrovir.* **6:**299–305.

750. Chirmule, N., M. Lesser, A. Gupta, M. Ravipati, N. Kohn, and S. Pahwa. 1995. Immunological characteristics of HIV-infected children: relationship to age, CD4 counts, disease progression, and survival. *AIDS Res. Hum. Retrovir.* **11:**1209–1219.

751. Chirmule, N., T. W. McCloskey, R. Hu, V. S. Kalyanaraman, and S. Pahwa. 1995. HIV gp120 inhibits T cell activation by interfering with expression of costimulatory molecules CD40 ligand and CD80 (B71). *J. Immunol.* **155:**917–924.

752. Chirmule, N., N. Oyaizu, V. S. Kalyanaraman, and S. Pahwa. 1992. Inhibition of normal B-cell function by human immunodeficiency virus envelope glycoprotein, gp120. *Blood* **79:**1245–1254.

753. Chitnis, A., D. Rawls, and J. Moore. 2000. Origin of HIV type 1 in colonial French Equatorial Africa? *AIDS Res. Hum. Retrovir.* **16:**5–8.

754. Chiu, I. M., A. Yaniv, J. E. Dahlberg, A. Gazit, S. F. Skuntz, S. R. Tronick, and S. A. Aaronson. 1985. Nucleotide sequence evidence for relationship of AIDS retrovirus to lentiviruses. *Nature* **317:**366–368.

755. Chiu, Y. L., V. B. Soros, J. F. Kreisberg, K. Stopak, W. Yonemoto, and W. C. Greene. 2005. Cellular APOBEC3G restricts HIV-1 infection in resting CD4+ T cells. *Nature* **435:**108–114.

756. Chlebowski, R. T., M. B. Grosvenor, and N. H. Bernhard. 1989. Nutritional status, gastrointestinal dysfunction, and survival in patients with AIDS. *Am. J. Gastroenterol.* **84:**1288–1293.

757. Cho, S., K. S. Knox, L. M. Kohli, J. J. He, M. A. Exley, S. B. Wilson, and R. R. Brutkiewicz. 2005. Impaired cell surface expression of human CD1d by the formation of an HIV-1 Nef/CD1d complex. *Virology* **337:**242–252.

758. Choe, H., M. Farzan, Y. Sun, N. Sullivan, B. Rollins, P. D. Ponath, L. Wu, C. R. Mackay, G. LaRosa, W. Newman, N. Gerard, C. Gerard, and J. Sodroski. 1996. The beta-chemokine receptors CCR3 and CCR5 facilitate infection by primary HIV-1 isolates. *Cell* **85:**1135–1148.

759. Choe, W., A. Albright, J. Sulcove, S. Jaffer, J. Hesselgesser, E. Lavi, P. Crino, and D. L. Kolson. 2000. Functional expression of the seven-transmembrane HIV-1 co-receptor APJ in neural cells. *J. Neurovirol.* **6:**S61-S69.

760. Choe, W., D. J. Volsky, and M. J. Potash. 2002. Activation of NF-kappaB by R5 and X4 human immunodeficiency virus type 1 induces macrophage inflammatory protein 1alpha and tumor necrosis factor alpha in macrophages. *J. Virol.* **76:**5274–5277.

761. Choi, H. J., C. A. Dinarello, and L. Shapiro. 2001. Interleukin-18 inhibits human immunodeficiency virus type 1 production in peripheral blood mononuclear cells. *J. Infect. Dis.* **184:**560–568.

762. Choi, I. S., R. Hokanson, and E. W. Collisson. 2000. Antifeline immunodeficiency virus (FIV) soluble factor(s) produced from antigen-stimulated feline CD8(+) T lymphocytes suppresses FIV replication. *J. Virol.* **74:**676–683.

763. Chomont, N., H. Hocini, G. Gresenguet, C. Brochier, H. Bouhlal, L. Andreoletti, P. Becquart, C. Charpentier, J. de Dieu Longo, A. Si-Mohamed, M. D. Kazatchkine, and L. Belec. Early archives of genetically-restricted proviral DNA in the female genital tract after heterosexual transmission of HIV-1. *AIDS,* in press.

764. Chong, Y., H. Ikematsu, K. Kikuchi, M. Yamamoto, M. Murata, M. Nishimura, S. Nabeshima, S. Kashiwagi, and J. Hayashi. 2004. Selective CD27+ (memory) B cell reduction and characteristic B cell alteration in drug-naive and HAART-treated HIV type 1-infected patients. *AIDS Res. Hum. Retrovir.* **20:**219–226.

765. Chou, C. S., O. Ramilo, and E. S. Vitetta. 1997. Highly purified CD25- resting T cells cannot be infected *de novo* with HIV-1. *Proc. Natl. Acad. Sci. USA* **94:**1361–1365.

766. Chougnet, C., E. Thomas, A. L. Landay, H. A. Kessler, S. Buchbinder, S. Scheer, and G. M. Shearer. 1998. CD40 ligand and IFN-γ synergistically restore IL-12 production in HIV-infected patients. *Eur. J. Immunol.* **28:**646–656.

766a. Chougnet, C. A., and G. M. Shearer. Regulatory T cells (Treg) and HIV/AIDS: Summary of the September 7–8, 2006 Workshop, in press.

767. Chowers, M. Y., C. A. Spina, T. J. Kwoh, N. J. S. Fitch, D. D. Richman, and J. C. Guitelli. 1994. Optimal infectivity in vitro of human immunodeficiency virus type 1 requires and intact Nef gene. *J. Virol.* **68:**2906–2914.

768. Chtanova, T., S. G. Tangye, R. Newton, N. Frank, M. R. Hodge, M. S. Rolph, and C. R. Mackay. 2004. T follicular helper cells express a distinctive transcriptional profile, reflecting their role as non-Th1/Th2 effector cells that provide help for B cells. *J. Immunol.* **173:**68–78.

769. Chuang, L. F., K. F. Killam, Jr., and R. Y. Chuang. 1993. Increased replication of simian immunodeficiency virus in CEM x174 cells by morphine sulfate. *Biochem. Biophys. Res. Commun.* **195:**1165–1173.

770. Chuang, R. Y., D. J. Blackbourn, L. F. Chuang, Y. Liu, and K. F. Killam, Jr. 1993. Modulation of simian AIDS by opioids. *Adv. Biosci.* **86:**573–583.

771. Chun, T., D. Engel, S. B. Mizell, C. W. Hallahan, M. Fischette, S. Park, J. Davey, R. T. Davey, Jr., M. Dybul, J. A. Kovacs, J. A. Metcalf, J. M. Mican, M. M. Berrey, L. Corey, H. C. Lane, and A. S. Fauci. 1999. Effect of interleukin-2 on the pool of latently infected resting CD4+T cells in HIV-1-infected patients receiving highly active anti-retroviral therapy. *Nat. Med.* **5:**651–655.

772. Chun, T.-W., L. Carruth, D. Finzi, X. Shen, J. A. DiGiuseppe, H. Taylor, M. Hermankova, K. Chadwick, J. Margolick, T. C. Quinn, Y. H. Kuo, R. Brookmeyer, M. A. Zeiger, P. Barditch-Crovo, and R. F. Siliciano. 1997. Quantification of latent tissue reservoirs and total body viral load in HIV-1 infection. *Nature* **387:**183–187.

773. Chun, T.-W., K. Chadwick, J. Margolick, and R. F. Siliciano. 1997. Differential susceptibility of naive and memory CD4+ T cells to the cytopathic effects of infection with human immunodeficiency virus type 1 strain LAI. *J. Virol.* 71:4436–4444.

774. Chun, T. W., D. Engel, M. M. Berrey, T. Shea, L. Corey, and A. S. Fauci. 1998. Early establishment of a pool of latently infected, resting CD4(+) T cells during primary HIV-1 infection. *Proc. Natl. Acad. Sci. USA* 95:8869–8873.

775. Chun, T. W., D. Engel, S. B. Mizell, L. A. Ehler, and A. S. Fauci. 1998. Induction of HIV-1 replication in latently infected CD4+ T cells using a combination of cytokines. *J. Exp. Med.* 188:83–91.

776. Chun, T. W., D. Finzi, J. Margolick, K. Chadwick, D. Schwartz, and R. F. Siliciano. 1995. *In vivo* fate of HIV-1-infected T cells: quantitative analysis of the transition to stable latency. *Nat. Med.* 1:1284–1290.

776a. Chun, T. W., J. S. Justement, C. Sanford, C. W. Hallahan, M. A. Planta, M. Loutfy, S. Kottilil, S. Moir, C. Kovacs, and A. S. Fauci. 2004. Relationship between the frequency of HIV-specific CD8+ T cells and the level of CD38+ CD8+ T cells in untreated HIV-infected individuals. *Proc. Natl. Acad. Sci. USA* 101:2464–2469.

777. Chun, T. W., J. S. Justement, S. Moir, C. W. Hallahan, L. A. Ehler, S. Liu, M. McLaughlin, M. Dybul, J. M. Mican, and A. S. Fauci. 2001. Suppression of HIV replication in the resting CD4+ T cell reservoir by autologous CD8+ T cells: implications for the development of therapeutic strategies. *Proc. Natl. Acad. Sci. USA* 98:253–258.

778. Chun, T. W., D. C. Nickle, J. S. Justement, D. Large, A. Semerjian, M. E. Curlin, A. O'Shea M, C. W. Hallahan, M. Daucher, D. J. Ward, S. Moir, J. I. Mullins, C. Kovacs, and A. S. Fauci. 2005. HIV-infected individuals receiving effective antiviral therapy for extended periods of time continually replenish their viral reservoir. *J. Clin. Investig.* 115:3250–3255.

779. Cianciolo, G. J., T. D. Copeland, S. Oroszlan, and R. Snyderman. 1985. Inhibition of lymphocyte proliferation by a synthetic peptide homologous to retroviral envelope proteins. *Science* 230:453–455.

780. Cicala, C., J. Arthos, A. Rubbert, S. Selig, K. Wildt, O. J. Cohen, and A. S. Fauci. 2000. HIV-1 envelope induces activation of caspase-3 and cleavage of focal adhesion kinase in primary human CD4(+) T cells. *Proc. Natl. Acad. Sci. USA* 97:1178–1183.

781. Cichutek, K., S. Norley, R. Linde, W. Kreuz, M. Gahr, J. Lower, G. Von Wangenheim, and R. Kurth. 1991. Lack of HIV-1 V3 region sequence diversity in two haemophiliac patients infected with a putative biologic clone of HIV-1. *AIDS* 5:1185–1187.

782. Cilliers, T., S. Willey, W. M. Sullivan, T. Patience, P. Pugach, M. Coetzer, M. Papathanasopoulos, J. P. Moore, A. Trkola, P. Clapham, and L. Morris. 2005. Use of alternate coreceptors on primary cells by two HIV-1 isolates. *Virology* 339:136–144.

783. Cimarelli, A., G. Zambruno, A. Marconi, G. Girolomoni, U. Bertazzoni, and A. Giannetti. 1994. Quantitation by competitive PCR of HIV-1 proviral DNA in epidermal Langerhans cells of HIV-infected patients. *J. Acquir. Immune Defic. Syndr.* 7:230–235.

784. Ciuffi, A., M. Llano, E. Poeschla, C. Hoffmann, J. Leipzig, P. Shinn, J. R. Ecker, and F. Bushman. 2005. A role for LEDGF/p75 in targeting HIV DNA integration. *Nat. Med.* 11:1287–1289.

785. Ciufo, D. M., J. S. Cannon, L. J. Poole, F. Y. Wu, P. Murray, R. F. Ambinder, and G. S. Hayward. 2001. Spindle cell conversion by Kaposi's sarcoma-associated herpesvirus: formation of colonies and plaques with mixed lytic and latent gene expression in infected primary dermal microvascular endothelial cell cultures. *J. Virol.* 75:5614–5626.

786. Clapham, P. R., D. Blanc, and R. A. Weiss. 1991. Specific cell surface requirements for the infection of CD4-positive cells by human immunodeficiency virus types 1 and 2 and by simian immunodeficiency virus. *Virology* 181:703–715.

787. Clapham, P. R., A. McKnight, and R. A. Weiss. 1992. Human immunodeficiency virus type 2 infection and fusion of CD4-negative human cell lines: induction and enhancement by soluble CD4. *J. Virol.* 66:3531–3537.

788. Clapham, P. R., J. N. Weber, D. Whitby, K. McIntosh, A. G. Dalgleish, P. J. Maddon, K. C. Deen, R. W. Sweet, and R. A. Weiss. 1989. Soluble CD4 blocks the infectivity of diverse strains of HIV and SIV for T cells and monocytes but not for brain and muscle cells. *Nature* 337:368–370.

789. Clark, R. A., B. Chong, N. Mirchandani, N. K. Brinster, K. Yamanaka, R. K. Dowgiert, and T. S. Kupper. 2006. The vast majority of CLA+ T cells are resident in normal skin. *J. Immunol.* 176:4431–4439.

790. Clark, S. J., M. S. Saag, W. D. Decker, S. Campbell-Hill, J. L. Roberson, P. J. Veldkamp, J. C. Kappes, B. H. Hahn, and G. M. Shaw. 1991. High titers of cytopathic virus in plasma of patients with symptomatic primary HIV-1 infection. *N. Engl. J. Med.* 324:954–960.

791. Clarke, J. N., J. A. Lake, C. J. Burrell, S. L. Wesselingh, P. R. Gorry, and P. Li. 2006. Novel pathway of human immunodeficiency virus type 1 uptake and release in astrocytes. *Virology* 348:141–155.

792. Clavel, F., D. Guetard, F. Brun-Vezinet, S. Chamaret, M.-A. Rey, M. O. Santos-Ferreira, A. G. Laurent, C. Dauguet, C. Katlama, C. Rouzioux, D. Klatzmann, J. L. Champalimaud, and L. Montagnier. 1986. Isolation of a new human retrovirus from West African patients with AIDS. *Science* 233:343–346.

793. Clavel, F., K. Mansinho, S. Chamaret, D. Guetard, V. Favier, J. Nina, M.-O. Santos-Ferreira, J.-L. Champalimaud, and L. Montagnier. 1987. Human immunodeficiency virus type 2 infection associated with AIDS in West Africa. *N. Engl. J. Med.* 316:1180–1185.

794. Clayton, F., S. Kapetanovic, and D. P. Kotler. 2001. Enteric microtubule depolymerization in HIV infection: a possible cause of HIV-associated enteropathy. *AIDS* 15:123–124.

795. Clayton, F., D. P. Kotler, S. K. Kuwada, T. Morgan, C. Stepan, J. Kuang, J. Le, and J. Fantini. 2001. Gp120-induced Bob/GPR15 activation. *Am. J. Pathol.* 159:1933–1939.

796. Clements, G. J., M. J. Price-Jones, P. E. Stephens, C. Sutton, T. F. Schultz, P. R. Clapham, J. A. McKeating, M. O. McClure, S. Thomson, M. Marsh, J. Kay, R. A. Weiss, and J. P. Moore. 1991. The V3 loops of the HIV-1 and HIV-2 surface glycoproteins contain proteolytic cleavage sites: a possible function in viral fusion? *AIDS Res. Hum. Retrovir.* 7:3–16.

797. Clemetson, D. B. A., G. B. Moss, D. M. Willerford, M. Hensel, P. L. Emonyi, S. Hillier, and J. K. Kreiss. 1993. Detection of HIV DNA in cervical and vaginal secretions. *JAMA* 269:2860–2864.

798. Clerici, M., C. Balotta, M. L., E. Ferrario, C. Riva, D. Trabattoni, A. Ridolfo, M. Villa, G. M. Shearer, M. Moroni, and M. Galli. 1996. Type 1 cytokine production and low prevalence of viral isolation correlate with long-term nonprogression in HIV infection. *AIDS Res. Hum. Retrovir.* 12:1053–1061.

799. Clerici, M., C. Balotta, A. Salvaggio, C. Riva, D. Trabattoni, L. Papagno, A. Berlusconi, S. Rusconi, M. L. Villa, M. Moroni, and M. Galli. 1996. Human immunodeficiency virus (HIV) phenotype and interleukin-2/interleukin-10 ratio are associated markers of protection and progression in HIV infection. *Blood* 88:574–579.

800. Clerici, M., C. Balotta, D. Trabattoni, L. Papagno, S. Ruzzante, S. Rusconi, M. L. Fusi, M. C. Colombo, and M. Galli. 1996. Chemokine production in HIV-seropositive long-term asymptomatic individuals. *AIDS* 10:1432–1433.

801. Clerici, M., C. Barassi, C. Devito, C. Pastori, S. Piconi, D. Trabattoni, R. Longhi, J. Hinkula, K. Broliden, and L. Lopalco. 2002. Serum IgA of HIV-exposed uninfected individuals inhibit HIV through recognition of a region within the α-helix of gp41. *AIDS* 16:1731–1741.

802. Clerici, M., S. Butto, M. Lukwiya, M. Saresella, S. Declich, D. Trabattoni, C. Pastori, S. Piconi, C. Fracasso, M. Fabiani, P. Ferrante, G. Rizzardini, and L. Lopalco. 2000. Immune activation in Africa is environmentally-driven and is associated with upregulation of CCR5. Italian-Ugandan AIDS Project. *AIDS* 14:2083–2092.

803. Clerici, M., E. A. Clark, P. Polacino, I. Axberg, L. Kuller, N. I. Casey, W. R. Morton, G. M. Shearer, and R. E. Benveniste. 1994. T-cell proliferation to subinfectious SIV correlates with lack of infection after challenge of macaques. *AIDS* 8:1391–1395.

804. Clerici, M., J. V. Giorgi, C. C. Chou, V. K. Gudeman, J. A. Zack, P. Gupta, H. N. Ho, P. G. Nishanian, J. A. Berzofsky, and G. M. Shearer. 1992. Cell-mediated immune response to human immunodeficiency virus (HIV) type 1 in seronegative homosexual men with recent sexual exposure to HIV-1. *J. Infect. Dis.* 165:1012–1019.

805. Clerici, M., F. T. Hakim, D. J. Venzon, S. Blatt, C. W. Hendrix, T. A. Wynn, and G. M. Shearer. 1993. Changes in interleukin-2 and interleukin-4 production in asymptomatic, human immunodeficiency virus-seropositive individuals. *J. Clin. Investig.* 91:759–765.

806. Clerici, M., A. L. Landay, H. A. Kessler, J. P. Phair, D. J. Venzon, C. W. Hendrix, D. R. Lucey, and G. M. Shearer. 1992. Reconstitution of long-term T helper cell function after zidovudine therapy in human immunodeficiency virus-infected patients. *J. Infect. Dis.* 166:723–730.

807. Clerici, M., J. M. Levin, H. A. Kessler, A. Harris, J. A. Berzofsky, A. L. Landay, and G. M. Shearer. 1994. HIV-specific T-helper activity in seronegative health care workers exposed to contaminated blood. *JAMA* 271:42–46.

808. Clerici, M., D. R. Lucey, J. A. Berzofsky, L. A. Pinto, T. A. Wynn, S. P. Blatt, M. J. Dolan, C. W. Hendrix, S. F. Wolf, and G. M. Shearer. 1993. Restoration of HIV-specific cell-mediated immune responses by interleukin-12 in vitro. *Science* 262:1721–1724.

809. Clerici, M., D. R. Lucey, R. A. Zajac, R. N. Boswell, H. M. Gebel, H. Takahashi, J. A. Berzofsky, and G. M. Shearer. 1991. Detection of cytotoxic T lymphocytes specific for synthetic peptides of gp160 in HIV-seropositive individuals. *J. Immunol.* 146:2214–2219.

810. Clerici, M., E. Roilides, C. S. Via, P. A. Pizzo, and G. M. Shearer. 1992. A factor from CD8 cells of human immunodeficiency virus-infected patients suppresses HLA self-restricted T helper cell responses. *Proc. Natl. Acad. Sci. USA* 89:8424–8428.

811. Clerici, M., A. Sarin, J. A. Berzofsky, A. L. Landay, H. A. Kessler, F. Hashemi, C. W. Hendrix, S. P. Blatt, J. Rusnak, M. J. Dolan, R. L. Coffman, P. A. Henkart, and G. M. Shearer. 1996. Antigen-stimulated apoptotic T-cell death in HIV infection is selective for CD4+ T cells, modulated by cytokines and affected by lymphotoxin. *AIDS* 10:603–611.

812. Clerici, M., A. Sarin, R. L. Coffman, T. A. Wynn, S. P. Blatt, C. W. Hendrix, S. F. Wolf, G. M. Shearer, and P. A. Henkart. 1994. Type 1/type 2 cytokine modulation of T cell programmed cell death as a model for HIV pathogenesis. *Proc. Natl. Acad. Sci. USA* 91:11811–11815.

813. Clerici, M., and G. M. Shearer. 1993. A TH1 to TH2 switch is a critical step in the etiology of HIV infection. *Immunol. Today* 14:107–111.

814. Clerici, M., and G. M. Shearer. 1994. The Th1-Th2 hypothesis of HIV infection: new insights. *Immunol. Today* 15:575–581.

815. Clerici, M., N. I. Stocks, R. A. Zajac, R. N. Boswell, D. R. Lucey, C. S. Via, and G. M. Shearer. 1989. Detection of three distinct patterns of T helper cell dysfunction in asymptomatic, human immunodeficiency virus-positive patients. Independence of CD4+ cell numbers and clinical staging. *J. Clin. Investig.* 84:1892–1899.

816. Clerici, M., N. I. Stocks, R. A. Zajac, R. N. Boswell, C. S. Via, and G. M. Shearer. 1990. Circumvention of defective CD4 T helper cell function in HIV-infected individuals by stimulation with HLA alloantigens. *J. Immunol.* 144:3266–3271.

817. Clerici, M., T. A. Wynn, J. A. Berzofsky, S. P. Blatt, C. W. Hendrix, A. Sher, R. L. Coffman, and G. M. Shearer. 1994. Role of interleukin-10 in T helper cell dysfunction in asymptomatic individuals infected with the human immunodeficiency virus. *J. Clin. Investig.* 93:768–775.

818. Clever, J. L., D. Mirandar, Jr., and T. G. Parslow. 2002. RNA structure and packaging signals in the 5' leader region of the human immunodeficiency virus type 1 genome. *J. Virol.* 76:12381–12387.

819. Clotet, B., M. van der Valk, E. Negredo, and P. Reiss. 2003. Impact of nevirapine on lipid metabolism. *J. Acquir. Immune Defic. Syndr.* 34(Suppl. 1):S79–S84.

820. Cloyd, M. W., and W. S. Lynn. 1991. Perturbation of host-cell membrane is a primary mechanism of HIV cytopathology. *Virology* 181:500–511.

821. Cloyd, M. W., and B. E. Moore. 1990. Spectrum of biological properties of human immunodeficiency virus (HIV-1) isolates. *Virology* 174:103–116.

822. Cocchi, F., A. L. DeVico, A. Garzino-Demo, S. K. Arya, R. C. Gallo, and P. Lusso. 1995. Identification of RANTES, MIP-1alpha, and MIP-1beta as the major HIV-suppressive factors produced by CD8+ T cells. *Science* 270:1811–1815.

823. Cocchi, F., A. L. DeVico, A. Garzino-Demo, A. Cara, R. C. Gallo, and P. Lusso. 1996. The V3 domain of the HIV-1 gp120 envelope glycoprotein is critical for chemokine-mediated blockade of infection. *Nat. Med.* 2:1244–1247.

824. Cocchi, F., A. L. DeVico, R. Yarchoan, R. Redfield, F. Cleghorn, W. A. Blattner, A. Garzino-Demo, S. Colombini-Hatch, D. Margolis, and R. C. Gallo. 2000. Higher macrophage

inflammatory protein (MIP)-1alpha and MIP-1beta levels from CD8+ T cells are associated with asymptomatic HIV-1 infection. *Proc. Natl. Acad. Sci. USA* 97:13812–13817.

825. Cochrane, A., S. Imlach, C. Leen, G. Scott, D. Kennedy, and P. Simmonds. 2004. High levels of human immunodeficiency virus infection of CD8 lymphocytes expressing CD4 in vivo. *J. Virol.* 78:9862–9871.

826. Coffin, J., A. Haase, J. A. Levy, L. Montagnier, S. Oroszlan, N. Teich, H. Temin, K. Toyoshima, H. Varmus, P. Vogt, and R. Weiss. 1986. Human immunodeficiency viruses. (Letter.) *Science* 232:697.

827. Coffin, J. M. 1992. Structure and classification of retroviruses, p. 19–50. *In* J. A. Levy (ed.), *The Retroviridae*, vol. 1. Plenum Press, New York, N.Y.

828. Coffin, J. M. 1992. Superantigens and endogenous retroviruses: a confluence of puzzles. *Science* 255:411–413.

829. Coffin, J. M. 1995. HIV population dynamics *in vivo*: implications for genetic variation, pathogenesis, and therapy. *Science* 267:483–489.

830. Cohen, A., D. G. Wolf, E. Guttman-Yassky, and R. Sarid. 2005. Kaposi's sarcoma-associated herpesvirus: clinical, diagnostic, and epidemiological aspects. *Crit. Rev. Clin. Lab. Sci.* 42:101–153.

831. Cohen, A. H., N. C. J. Sun, P. Shapshak, and D. T. Imagawa. 1989. Demonstration of human immunodeficiency virus in renal epithelium in HIV-associated nephropathy. *Mod. Pathol.* 2:125–128.

832. Cohen, D. I., Y. Tani, H. Tian, E. Boone, L. W. Samelson, and E. C. Lane. 1992. Participation of tyrosine phosphorylation in the cytopathic effect of human immunodeficiency virus-1. *Science* 256:542–545.

833. Cohen, G. B., R. T. Gandhi, D. M. Davis, O. Mandelboim, B. K. Chen, J. L. Strominger, and D. Baltimore. 1999. The selective downregulation of class I major histocompatibility complex proteins by HIV-1 protects HIV-infected cells from NK cells. *Immunity* 10:661–671.

834. Cohen, J. H. M., C. Geffriaud, V. Caudwell, and M. D. Kazatchkine. 1989. Genetic analysis of CR1 (the C3b complement receptor, CD35) expression on erythrocytes of HIV-infected individuals. *AIDS* 3:397–399.

835. Cohen, J. J., R. C. Duke, V. A. Fadok, and K. S. Sellins. 1992. Apoptosis and programmed cell death in immunity. *Annu. Rev. Immunol.* 10:267–293.

836. Cohen, M. S. 2000. Preventing sexual transmission of HIV—new ideas from sub-Saharan Africa. *N. Engl. J. Med.* 342:970–972.

837. Cohen, M. S., and C. D. Pilcher. 2005. Amplified HIV transmission and new approaches to HIV prevention. *J. Infect. Dis.* 191:1391–1393.

838. Cohen, O. J., G. Pantaleo, M. Holodniy, C. H. Fox, J. M. Orenstein, S. Schnittman, M. Niu, C. Graziosi, G. N. Pavlakis, J. Lalezari, J. A. Bartlett, R. T. Steigbigel, J. Cohn, R. Novak, D. McMahon, J. Bilello, and A. S. Fauci. 1996. Antiretroviral monotherapy in early stage human immunodeficiency virus disease has no detectable effect on virus load in peripheral blood and lymph nodes. *J. Infect. Dis.* 173:849–856.

839. Cohen, O. J., G. Pantaleo, D. J. Schwartzentruber, C. Graziosi, M. Vaccarezza, and A. S. Fauci. 1995. Pathogenic insights from studies of lymphoid tissue from HIV-infected

individuals. *J. Acquir. Immune Defic. Syndr. Hum. Retrovirol.* 10:S6–S14.

840. Cohen, P. S., H. Schmidtmayerova, J. Dennis, L. Dubrovsky, B. Sherry, H. Wang, M. Bukrinsky, and K. J. Tracey. 1997. The critical role of p38 MAP kinase in T cell HIV-1 replication. *Mol. Med.* 3:339–346.

841. Cohen, S., and G. M. Williamson. 1991. Stress and infectious disease in humans. *Psychol. Bull.* 109:5–24.

842. Cohen, S. S., C. Li, L. Ding, Y. Cao, A. B. Pardee, E. M. Shevach, and D. I. Cohen. 1999. Pronounced acute immunosuppression *in vivo* mediated by HIV Tat challenge. *Proc. Natl. Acad. Sci. USA* 96:10842–10847.

843. Cole, J. L., U. M. Marzec, C. J. Gunthel, S. Karpatkin, L. Worford, I. B. Sundell, J. L. Lennox, J. L. Nichol, and L. A. Harker. 1998. Ineffective platelet production in thrombocytopenic human immunodeficiency virus-infected patients. *Blood* 91:3239–3246.

844. Cole, S. W., Y. D. Korin, J. L. Fahey, and J. A. Zack. 1998. Norepinephrine accelerates HIV replication via protein kinase A-dependent effects on cytokine production. *J. Immunol.* 161:610–616.

845. Cole, S. W., B. D. Naliboff, M. E. Kemeny, M. P. Griswold, J. L. Fahey, and J. A. Zack. 2001. Impaired response to HAART in HIV-infected individuals with high autonomic nervous system activity. *Proc. Natl. Acad. Sci. USA* 98:12695–12700.

846. Colgan, J., H. E. Yuan, E. K. Franke, and J. Luban. 1996. Binding of human immunodeficiency virus type 1 Gag polyprotein to cyclophilin A is mediated by the central region of capsid and requires Gag dimerization. *J. Virol.* 70:4299–4310.

847. Reference deleted.

848. Reference deleted.

849. Collaborative-Group on AIDS Incubation and HIV Survival including the CASCADE EU Concerted Action. 2000. Time from HIV-1 seroconversion to AIDS and death before widespread use of highly-active antiretroviral therapy: a collaborative re-analysis. *Lancet* 355:1131–1137.

850. Collazos, J., J. Mayo, E. Martinez, and S. Ibarra. 2002. Serum cortisol in HIV-infected patients with and without highly active antiretroviral therapy. *AIDS* 17:123–125.

851. Collette, Y., H.-L. Chang, C. Cerdan, H. Chambost, M. Algarte, C. Mawas, J. Imbert, A. Burny, and D. Olive. 1996. Specific Th1 cytokine down-regulation associated with primary clinically derived human immunodeficiency virus type 1 *nef* gene-induced expression. *J. Immunol.* 156:360–370.

852. Collier, A. C., S. Bozzette, R. W. Coombs, D. M. Causey, D. A. Schoenfeld, S. A. Spector, C. B. Pettinelli, G. Davies, D. D. Richman, J. M. Leedom, P. Kidd, and L. Corey. 1990. A pilot study of low-dose zidovudine in human immunodeficiency virus infection. *N. Engl. J. Med.* 323:1015–1021.

853. Collier, A. C., R. W. Coombs, D. A. Schoenfeld, R. L. Bassett, J. Timpone, A. Baruch, M. Jones, K. Facey, C. Whitacre, V. J. McAuliffe, H. M. Friedman, T. C. Merigan, R. C. Reichman, C. Hooper, and L. Corey. 1996. Treatment of human immunodeficiency virus infection with saquinavir, zidovudine, and zalcitabine. *N. Engl. J. Med.* 334:1011–1018.

854. Collins, K. L., B. K. Chen, S. A. Kalams, B. D. Walker, and D. Baltimore. 1998. HIV-1 Nef protein protects infected primary cells against killing by cytotoxic T lymphocytes. *Nature* 391:397–401.

855. Collman, R., B. Godfrey, J. Cutilli, A. Rhodes, N. F. Hassan, R. Sweet, S. D. Douglas, H. Friedman, N. Nathanson, and F. Gonzalez-Scarano. 1990. Macrophage-tropic strains of human immunodeficiency virus type 1 utilize the CD4 receptor. *J. Virol.* **64:**4468–4476.

856. Colonna, M., G. Trinchieri, and Y. J. Liu. 2004. Plasmacytoid dendritic cells in immunity. *Nat. Immunol.* **5:**1219–1226.

857. Colven, R., R. D. Harrington, D. H. Spach, C. J. Cohen, and T. M. Hooton. 2000. Retroviral rebound syndrome after cessation of suppressive antiretroviral therapy in three patients with chronic HIV infection. *Ann. Intern. Med.* **133:**430–434.

858. Comeau, A. M., J. Pitt, G. V. Hillyer, S. Landesman, J. Bremer, B. H. Chang, J. Lew, J. Moye, G. F. Grady, K. McIntosh, et al. 1996. Early detection of human immunodeficiency virus on dried blood spot specimens: sensitivity across serial specimens. *J. Pediatr.* **129:**111–118.

859. Conaldi, P. G., L. Biancone, A. Bottelli, A. Wade-Evans, L. C. Racusen, M. Boccellino, V. Orlandi, C. Serra, G. Camussi, and A. Toniolo. 1998. HIV-1 kills renal tubular epithelial cells in vitro by triggering an apoptotic pathway involving caspase activation and fas upregulation. *J. Clin. Investig.* **102:**2041–2049.

860. Conaldi, P. G., A. Bottelli, A. Wade-Evans, L. Biancone, A. Baj, V. Cantaluppi, C. Serra, A. Dolei, A. Toniolo, and G. Camussi. 2000. HIV-persistent infection and cytokine induction in mesangial cells: a potential mechanism for HIV-associated glomerulosclerosis. *AIDS* **14:**2045–2047.

861. Conant, K., A. Garzino-Demo, A. Nath, J. C. McArthur, W. Halliday, C. Power, R. C. Gallo, and E. O. Major. 1998. Induction of monocyte chemoattractant protein-1 in HIV-1 Tat-stimulated astrocytes and elevation in AIDS dementia. *Proc. Natl. Acad. Sci. USA* **95:**3117–3121.

862. Conant, M., D. Hardy, J. Sernatinger, D. Spicer, and J. A. Levy. 1986. Condoms prevent transmission of the AIDS-associated retrovirus by oral-genital contact. *JAMA* **225:**1706.

863. Condra, J. H., W. A. Schleif, O. M. Blahy, L. J. Gabryelski, D. J. Graham, J. C. Quintero, A. Rhodes, H. L. Robbins, E. Roth, M. Shivaprakash, D. Titus, T. Yang, H. Teppler, K. E. Squires, P. J. Deutsch, and E. A. Emini. 1995. In vivo emergence of HIV-1 variants resistant to multiple protease inhibitors. *Nature* **374:**569–571.

864. Conley, L. J., T. V. Ellerbrock, T. J. Bush, M. A. Chiasson, D. Sawo, and T. C. Wright. 2002. HIV-1 infection and risk of vulvovaginal and perianal condylomata acuminata and intraepithelial neoplasia: a prospective cohort study. *Lancet* **359:**108–113.

865. Conlon, K., A. Lloyd, U. Chattopadhyay, N. Lukacs, S. Kunkel, T. Schall, D. Taub, C. Morimoto, J. Osborne, J. Oppenheim, H. Young, D. Kelvin, and J. Ortaldo. 1995. CD8+ and CD45RA+ human peripheral blood lymphocytes are potent sources of macrophage inflammatory protein 1α, interleukin-8 and RANTES. *Eur. J. Immunol.* **25:**751–756.

866. Connick, E., S. MaWhinney, C. C. Wilson, and T. B. Campbell. 2005. Challenges in the study of patients with HIV type 1 seroconversion. *Clin. Infect. Dis.* **40:**1355–1357.

867. Connick, E., R. L. Schlichtemeier, M. B. Purner, K. M. Schneider, D. M. Anderson, S. MaWhinney, T. B. Campbell, D. R. Kuritzkes, J. M. Douglas, Jr., F. N. Judson, and R. T. Schooley. 2001. Relationship between human immunodeficiency virus type 1 (HIV-1)-specific memory cytotoxic T lymphocytes and virus load after recent HIV-1 seroconversion. *J. Infect. Dis.* **184:**1465–1469.

868. Connolly, N. C., S. A. Riddler, and C. R. Rinaldo. 2005. Proinflammatory cytokines in HIV disease-a review and rationale for new therapeutic approaches. *AIDS Rev.* **7:**168–180.

869. Connor, R. I., B. K. Chen, S. Choe, and N. R. Landau. 1995. Vpr is required for efficient replication of human immunodeficiency virus type 1 in mononuclear phagocytes. *Virology* **206:**936–944.

870. Connor, R. I., and D. D. Ho. 1994. Human immunodeficiency virus type 1 variants with increased replicative capacity develop during the asymptomatic stage before disease progression. *J. Virol.* **68:**4400–4408.

871. Connor, R. I., W. A. Paxton, K. E. Sheridan, and R. A. Koup. 1996. Macrophages and CD4+ T lymphocytes from two multiply exposed, uninfected individuals resist infection with primary non-syncytium-inducing isolates of human immunodeficiency virus type 1. *J. Virol.* **70:**8758–8764.

872. Connor, R. I., K. E. Sheridan, D. Ceradini, S. Choe, and N. R. Landau. 1997. Change in coreceptor use correlates with disease progression in HIV-1-infected individuals. *J. Exp. Med.* **185:**621–628.

873. Connors, M., J. A. Kovacs, S. Krevat, J. C. Gea-Banacloche, M. C. Sneller, M. Flanigan, J. A. Metcalf, R. E. Walker, J. Falloon, M. Baseler, R. Stevens, I. Feuerstein, H. Masur, and H. C. Lane. 1997. HIV infection induces changes in CD4+ T-cell phenotype and depletions within the CD4+ T-cell repertoire that are not immediately restored by antiviral or immune-based therapies. *Nat. Med.* **3:**533–540.

874. Conti, L., P. Matarrese, B. Varano, M. C. Gauzzi, A. Sato, W. Malorni, F. Belardelli, and S. Gessani. 2000. Dual role of the HIV-1 vpr protein in the modulation of the apoptotic response of T cells. *J. Immunol.* **165:**3293–3003.

875. Coombs, R. W., A. C. Collier, J.-P. Allain, B. Nikora, M. Leuther, G. F. Gjerset, and L. Corey. 1989. Plasma viremia in human immunodeficiency virus infection. *N. Engl. J. Med.* **321:**1626–1631.

876. Coombs, R. W., D. J. Lockhart, S. O. Ross, L. Deutsch, J. Dragavon, K. Diem, T. M. Hooton, A. C. Collier, L. Corey, and J. N. Krieger. 2006. Lower genitourinary tract sources of seminal HIV. *J. Acquir. Immune Defic. Syndr.* **41:**430–438.

877. Coombs, R. W., P. S. Reichelderfer, and A. L. Landay. 2003. Recent observations on HIV type-1 infection in the genital tract of men and women. *AIDS* **17:**455–480.

878. Coombs, R. W., C. E. Speck, J. P. Hughes, W. Lee, R. Sampoleo, S. O. Ross, J. Dragavon, G. Peterson, T. M. Hooton, A. C. Collier, L. Corey, L. Koutsky, and J. N. Krieger. 1998. Association between culturable human immunodeficiency virus type 1 (HIV-1) in semen and HIV-1 RNA levels in semen and blood: evidence for compartmentalization of HIV-1 between semen and blood. *J. Infect. Dis.* **177:**320–330.

879. Cooney, E. L., M. J. McElrath, L. Corey, S.-L. Hu, A. C. Collier, D. Arditti, M. Hoffman, G. E. Smith, and P. D. Greenberg. 1993. Enhanced immunity to human immunodeficiency virus (HIV) envelope elicited by a combined vaccine regimen consisting of priming with a vaccinia recombinant expressing HIV envelope and boosting with gp160 protein. *Proc. Natl. Acad. Sci. USA* **90:**1882–1886.

880. Cooper, C. L., H. L. Davis, J. B. Angel, M. L. Morris, S. M. Elfer, I. Seguin, A. M. Krieg, and D. W. Cameron. 2005. CPG 7909 adjuvant improves hepatitis B virus vaccine seroprotection in antiretroviral-treated HIV-infected adults. *AIDS* **19:**1473–1479.

881. Cooper, D. A., J. Gold, P. Maclean, B. Donovan, R. Finlayson, T. G. Barnes, H. M. Michelmore, P. Brooke, and R. Penny. 1985. Acute AIDS retrovirus infection: definition of a clinical illness associated with seroconversion. *Lancet* i:537–540.

882. Cooper, D. A., B. Tindall, E. J. Wilson, A. A. Imrie, and R. Penny. 1988. Characterization of T lymphocyte responses during primary infection with human immunodeficiency virus. *J. Infect. Dis.* 157:889–896.

883. Cooper, M. A., T. A. Fehniger, and M. A. Caligiuri. 2001. The biology of human natural killer-cell subsets. *Trends Immunol.* 22:633–640.

884. Coordinating Committee of the Global HIV/AIDS Vaccine Enterprise. 2005, posting date. *The Global HIV/AIDS Vaccine Enterprise: Scientific strategic plan.* [Online.] http://medicine .plosjournals.org/perlserv?request=get-document&doi=10.1371/ journal.pmed.0020025.

885. Copeland, K. F. T., P. J. McKay, and K. L. Rosenthal. 1995. Suppression of activation of the human immunodeficiency virus long terminal repeat by CD8+ T cells is not lentivirus specific. *AIDS Res. Hum. Retrovir.* 11:1321–1326.

886. Copeland, K. F. T., P. J. McKay, and K. L. Rosenthal. 1996. Suppression of the human immunodeficiency virus long terminal repeat by CD8+ T cells is dependent on the NFAT-1 element. *AIDS Res. Hum. Retrovir.* 12:143–148.

887. Coplan, P. M., S. B. Gupta, S. A. Dubey, P. Pitisuttithum, A. Nikas, B. Mbewe, E. Vardas, M. Schechter, E. G. Kallas, D. C. Freed, T. M. Fu, C. T. Mast, P. Puthavathana, J. Kublin, K. Brown Collins, J. Chisi, R. Pendame, S. J. Thaler, G. Gray, J. McIntyre, W. L. Straus, J. H. Condra, D. V. Mehrotra, H. A. Guess, E. A. Emini, and J. W. Shiver. 2005. Cross-reactivity of anti-HIV-1 T cell immune responses among the major HIV-1 clades in HIV-1-positive individuals from 4 continents. *J. Infect. Dis.* 191:1427–1434.

888. Coppenhaver, D. H., P. Sriyuktasuth-Woo, S. Baron, C. E. Barr, and M. N. Qureshi. 1994. Correlation of nonspecific antiviral activity with the ability to isolate infectious HIV-1 from saliva. *N. Engl. J. Med.* 330:1314–1315.

889. Corbeil, J., M. Tremblay, and D. D. Richman. 1996. HIV-induced apoptosis requires the CD4 receptor cytoplasmic tail and is accelerated by interaction of CD4 with p56lck. *J. Exp. Med.* 183:39–48.

890. Corbellino, M., G. Bestetti, M. Galli, and C. Parravicini. 1996. Absence of HHV-8 in prostate and semen. *N. Engl. J. Med.* 335:1237–1238.

891. Corbellino, M., C. Parravicini, J. T. Aubin, and E. Berti. 1996. Kaposi's sarcoma and herpesvirus-like DNA sequences in sensory ganglia. *N. Engl. J. Med.* 334:1341–1342.

892. Corbet, S., M. C. Muller-Trutwin, P. Versmisse, S. Delarue, A. Ayouba, J. Lewis, S. Brunak, P. Martin, F. Brun-Vezinet, F. Simon, F. Barre-Sinoussi, and P. Mauclere. 2000. env sequences of simian immunodeficiency viruses from chimpanzees in Cameroon are strongly related to those of human immunodeficiency virus group N from the same geographic area. *J. Virol.* 74:529–534.

893. Corboy, J. R., J. M. Buzy, M. C. Zink, and J. E. Clements. 1992. Expression directed from HIV long terminal repeats in the central nervous system of transgenic mice. *Science* 258:1804–1808.

894. Cordonnier, A., L. Montagnier, and M. Emerman. 1989. Single amino-acid changes in HIV envelope affect viral tropism and receptor binding. *Nature* 340:571–574.

895. Cordonnier, A., Y. Riviere, L. Montagnier, and M. Emerman. 1989. Effects of mutations in hyperconserved regions of the extracellular glycoprotein of human immunodeficiency virus type 1 on receptor binding. *J. Virol.* 63:4464–4468.

896. Corey, L., A. Wald, C. L. Celum, and T. C. Quinn. 2004. The effects of herpes simplex virus-2 on HIV-1 acquisition and transmission: a review of two overlapping epidemics. *J. Acquir. Immune Defic. Syndr.* 35:435–445.

897. Cornelissen, M., G. Kampinga, F. Zorgdrager, and J. Goudsmit. 1996. Human immunodeficiency virus type 1 subtypes defined by env show high frequency of recombinant gag genes. *J. Virol.* 70:8209–8212.

898. Cornelissen, M., C. Kuiken, F. Zorgdrager, S. Hartman, and J. Goudsmit. 1997. Gross defects in the vpr and vpu genes of HIV type 1 cannot explain the differences in RNA copy number between long-term asymptomatics and progressors. *AIDS Res. Hum. Retrovir.* 13:247–252.

899. Cornelissen, M., G. Mulder-Kampinga, J. Veenstra, F. Zorgdrager, C. Kuiken, S. Hartman, J. Dekker, L. Van der Hoek, C. Sol, R. Coutinho, and J. Goudsmit. 1995. Syncytium-inducing (SI) phenotype suppression at seroconversion after intramuscular inoculation of a non-syncytium-inducing/SI phenotypically mixed human immunodeficiency virus population. *J. Virol.* 69:1810–1818.

900. Cossarizza, A. 1997. T cell repertoire and HIV infection: facts and perspectives. *AIDS* 11:1075–1088.

901. Cossarizza, A., and G. Moyle. 2004. Antiretroviral nucleoside and nucleoside analogues and mitochondria. *AIDS* 18:137–151.

902. Cossarizza, A., C. Ortolani, C. Mussini, G. Guaraldi, N. Mongiardo, V. Borghi, D. Barbieri, E. Bellesia, M. G. Franceschini, B. De Rienzo, and C. Franceschi. 1995. Lack of selective Vβ deletion in CD4+ or CD8+ T lymphocytes and functional integrity of T-cell repertoire during acute HIV syndrome. *AIDS* 9:547–553.

903. Costa, J., and A. S. Rabson. 1983. Generalised Kaposi's sarcoma is not a neoplasm. *Lancet* i:58.

904. Costa, L. J., Y. H. Zheng, J. Sabotic, J. Mak, O. T. Fackler, and B. M. Peterlin. 2004. Nef binds p6* in GagPol during replication of human immunodeficiency virus type 1. *J. Virol.* 78:5311–5323.

905. Coste, J., H. W. Reesing, C. P. Engelfriet, S. Laperche, S. J. Brown, M. P. Busch, H. G. Cuijpers, R. Elgin, B. Ekermo, J. S. Epstein, O. Flesland, H. E. Heier, G. Henn, J. M. Hernandez, I. K. Hewlett, C. Hyland, A. J. Keller, T. Krusius, S. Levicnik-Stezina, G. Levy, C. K. Lin, A. R. Margaritis, L. Muylle, C. Neiderhauser, S. Pastila, J. Pillonel, J. Pineau, C. L. van der Poel, C. Politis, W. K. Roth, S. Sauleda, C. R. Seed, D. Sondag-Thull, S. L. Stramer, M. Strong, E. C. Vamvakas, C. Velati, M. A. Vesga, and A. Zanetti. 2005. Implementation of donor screening for infectious agents transmitted by blood by nucleic acid technology: update to 2003. *Vox Sang.* 88:289–303.

906. Cota, M., M. Mengozzi, E. Vicenzi, P. Panina-Bordignon, F. Sinigaglia, P. Transidico, S. Sozzani, A. Mantovani, and G. Poli. 2000. Selective inhibition of HIV replication in primary macrophages but not T lymphocytes by macrophage-derived chemokine. *Proc. Natl. Acad. Sci. USA* 97:9162–9167.

907. Cote, H. C., Z. L. Brumme, K. J. Craib, C. S. Alexander, B. Wynhoven, L. Ting, H. Wong, M. Harris, P. R. Harrigan, M. V. O'Shaughnessy, and J. S. Montaner. 2002. Changes in

mitochondrial DNA as a marker of nucleoside toxicity in HIV-infected patients. *N. Engl. J. Med.* **346**:811–820.

908. **Couedel-Courteille, A., C. Butor, V. Juillard, J.-G. Guillet, and A. Venet.** 1999. Dissemination of SIV after rectal infection preferentially involves paracolic germinal centers. *Virology* **260**:277–294.

909. **Coulomb-L'Hermine, A., D. Emilie, I. Durand-Gasseline, P. Galanaud, and G. Chaouat.** 2000. SDF-1 production by placental cells: a potential mechanism of inhibition of mother-to-fetus HIV transmission. *AIDS* **16**:1097–1098.

910. **Coutsoudis, A., K. Pillay, L. Kuhn, E. Spooner, W. Tsai, and H. M. Coovadia.** 2001. Method of feeding and transmission of HIV-1 from mothers to children by 15 months of age: prospective cohort study from Durban, South Africa. *AIDS* **15**:379–387.

911. **Cowan, S., T. Hatziioannou, T. Cunningham, M. A. Muesing, H. G. Gottlinger, and P. D. Bieniasz.** 2002. Cellular inhibitors with Fv1-like activity restrict human and simian immunodeficiency virus tropism. *Proc. Natl. Acad. Sci. USA* **99**:11914–11919.

912. **Craigo, J. K., B. K. Patterson, S. Paranjpe, K. Kulka, M. Ding, J. Mellors, R. C. Montelaro, and P. Gupta.** 2004. Persistent HIV type 1 infection in semen and blood compartments in patients after long-term potent antiretroviral therapy. *AIDS Res. Hum. Retrovir.* **20**:1196–1209.

913. **Cranage, M. P., N. Polyanskaya, B. McBride, N. Cook, L. A. E. Ashworth, M. Dennis, A. Baskerville, P. J. Greenaway, T. Corcoran, P. Kitchin, J. Rose, M. Murphy-Corb, R. C. Desrosiers, E. J. Stott, and G. H. Farrar.** 1993. Studies on the specificity of the vaccine effect elicited by inactivated simian immunodeficiency virus. *AIDS Res. Hum. Retrovir.* **9**:13–22.

914. **Cranage, M. P., A. M. Whatmore, S. A. Sharpe, N. Polyanskaya, S. Leech, J. D. Smith, E. W. Rud, M. J. Dennis, and G. A. Hall.** 1997. Macaques infected with live attenuated SIVmac are protected against superinfection via the rectal mucosa. *Virology* **229**:143–154.

915. **Crawford, P. C., G. P. Papadi, J. K. Levy, N. A. Benson, A. Mergia, and C. M. Johnson.** 2001. Tissue dynamics of CD8 lymphocytes that suppress viral replication in cats infected neonatally with feline immunodeficiency virus. *J. Infect. Dis.* **184**:671–681.

916. **Crawford, T. B., D. S. Adams, W. P. Cheevers, and L. C. Cork.** 1980. Chronic arthritis in goats caused by a retrovirus. *Science* **207**:997–999.

916a. **Creagh, E. M., and L. A. O'Neill.** 2006. TLRs, NLRs and RLRs: a trinity of pathogen sensors that co-operate in innate immunity. *Trends Immunol.* **27**:352–357.

917. **Cremer, I., V. Vieillard, and E. De Maeyer.** 1999. Interferon-β-induced human immunodeficiency virus resistance to CD34+ human hematopoietic progenitor cells correlation with a down-regulation of CCR-5 expression. *Virology* **253**:241–249.

918. **Crise, B., L. Buonocore, and J. K. Rose.** 1990. CD4 is retained in the endoplasmic reticulum by the human immunodeficiency virus type 1 glycoprotein precursor. *J. Virol.* **64**:5585–5593.

919. **Crise, B., and J. K. Rose.** 1992. Human immunodeficiency virus type 1 glycoprotein precursor retains a CD4-p56^lck complex in the endoplasmic reticulum. *J. Virol.* **66**:2296–2301.

920. **Crombie, R., R. L. Silverstein, C. MacLow, S. Frieda, A. Pearce, R. L. Nachman, and J. Laurence.** 1998. Identification of a CD36-related thrombospondin 1-binding domain in HIV-1 envelope glycoprotein gp120: relationship to HIV-1-specific inhibitory factors in human saliva. *J. Exp. Med.* **187**:25–35.

921. **Crook, T., D. Wrede, J. Tidy, J. Scholefield, L. Crawford, and K. H. Vousden.** 1991. Status of c-myc, p53 and retinoblastoma genes in human papillomavirus positive and negative squamous cell carcinomas of the anus. *Oncogene* **6**:1251–1257.

921a. **Crotti, A., F. Neri, D. Corti, S. Ghezzi, S. Heltai, A. Baur, G. Poli, E. Santagostino, and E. Vicenzi.** 2006. Nef alleles from human immunodeficiency virus type 1-infected long-term-nonprogressor hemophiliacs with or without late disease progression are defective in enhancing virus replication and CD4 down-regulation. *J. Virol.* **80**:10663–10674.

922. **Crotty, S., C. J. Miller, B. L. Lohman, M. R. Neagu, L. Compton, D. Lu, F. X. Lu, L. Fritts, J. D. Lifson, and R. Andino.** 2001. Protection against simian immunodeficiency virus vaginal challenge by using sabin poliovirus vectors. *J. Virol.* **75**:7435–7452.

923. **Crough, T., M. Nieda, and A. J. Nicol.** 2004. Granulocyte colony-stimulating factor modulates α-galactosylceramide-responsive human Vα24+Vβ11+ NKT cells. *J. Immunol.* **173**:4960–4966.

924. **Crowe, S., J. Mills, and M. S. McGrath.** 1987. Quantitative immunocytofluorographic analysis of CD4 surface antigen expression and HIV infection of human peripheral blood monocyte-macrophages. *AIDS Res. Hum. Retrovir.* **3**:135–145.

925. **Crowe, S., T. Zhu, and W. A. Muller.** 2003. The contribution of monocyte infection and trafficking to viral persistence, and maintenance of the viral reservoir in HIV infection. *J. Leukoc. Biol.* **74**:635–641.

926. **Crowe, S. M., J. Mills, T. Elbeik, J. D. Lifson, J. Kosek, J. A. Marshall, E. G. Engleman, and M. S. McGrath.** 1992. Human immunodeficiency virus-infected monocyte-derived macrophages express surface gp120 and fuse with CD4 lymphoid cells in vitro: a possible mechanism of T lymphocyte depletion in vivo. *Clin. Immunol. Immunopathol.* **65**:143–151.

927. **Crowley, R. W., P. Secchiero, D. Zella, A. Cara, R. C. Gallo, and P. Lusso.** 1996. Interference between human herpesvirus 7 and HIV-1 in mononuclear phagocytes. *J. Immunol.* **156**:2004–2008.

928. **Cruikshank, W. W., D. M. Center, N. Nisar, M. Wu, B. Natke, A. C. Theodore, and H. Kornfeld.** 1994. Molecular and functional analysis of a lymphocyte chemoattractant factor: association of biologic function with CD4 expression. *Proc. Natl. Acad. Sci. USA* **91**:5109–5113.

929. **Cu Uvin, S., A. M. Caliendo, S. E. Reinert, K. H. Mayer, T. P. Flanigan, and C. C. J. Carpenter.** 1998. HIV-1 in the female genital tract and the effect of antiretroviral therapy. *AIDS* **12**:826–827.

930. **Cuevas, M. T., I. Ruibal, M. L. Villahermosa, H. Diaz, E. Delgado, E. Vazquez-de-Parga, L. Perez-Alvarez, M. Blanco de Armas, L. Cuevas, L. Medrano, E. Noa, S. Osmanov, R. Najera, and M. M. Thomson.** 2002. High HIV-1 genetic diversity in Cuba. *AIDS* **16**:1643–1653.

931. **Cullen, B. R.** 2001. Journey to the center of the cell. *Cell* **105**:697–700.

932. **Cullen, B. R. C.** 2006. Role and mechanism of action of the APOBEC3 family of antiretroviral resistance factors. *J. Virol.* **80**:1067–1076.

933. Cunningham, A. L., S. Li, J. Juarez, G. Lynch, M. Alali, and H. Naif. 2000. The level of HIV infection of macrophages is determined by interaction of viral and host cell genotypes. *J. Leukoc. Biol.* 68:311–317.

934. Cunningham, A. L., J. Wilkinson, S. Turville, and M. Pope. Binding and uptake of HIV by dendritic cells and transfer to T lymphocytes: implications for pathogenesis. *In* S. Gessani (ed.), *Dendritic Cells in the Pathogenesis and Immunity of HIV Infection*, in press.

935. Cunningham, P. H., D. G. Smith, C. Satchell, D. A. Cooper, and B. Brew. 2000. Evidence for independent development of resistance to HIV-1 reverse transcriptase inhibitors in the cerebrospinal fluid. *AIDS* 14:1949–1954.

936. Curtis, B. M., S. Scharnowske, and A. J. Watson. 1992. Sequence and expression of a membrane-associated C-type lectin that exhibits CD4-independent binding of human immunodeficiency virus envelope glycoprotein gp120. *Proc. Natl. Acad. Sci. USA* 89:8356–8360.

937. Cvetkovich, T. A., E. Lazar, B. M. Blumberg, Y. Saito, T. A. Eskin, R. Reichman, D. A. Baram, C. del Cerro, H. E. Gendelman, M. del Cerro, and L. G. Epstein. 1992. Human immunodeficiency virus type 1 infection of neural xenografts. *Proc. Natl. Acad. Sci. USA* 89:5162–5166.

938. D'Andrea, A., M. Aste-Amezaga, N. M. Valiante, X. Ma, M. Kubin, and G. Trinchieri. 1993. Interleukin 10 (IL-10) inhibits human lymphocyte interferon gamma-production by suppressing natural killer cell stimulatory factor/IL-12 synthesis in accessory cells. *J. Exp. Med.* 178:1041–1048.

939. D'Aquila, R. T., L. Sutton, A. Savara, M. D. Hughes, and V. A. Johnson. 1998. CCR5/delta(ccr5) heterozygosity: a selective pressure for the syncytium-inducing human immunodeficiency virus type 1 phenotype. *J. Infect. Dis.* 177:1549–1553.

940. D'Costa, S., K. S. Slobod, R. G. Webster, S. W. White, and J. L. Hurwitz. 2001. Structural features of HIV envelope defined by antibody escape mutant analysis. *AIDS Res. Hum. Retroviruses* 17:1205–1209.

941. d'Ettorre, G., G. Forcina, M. Lichtner, F. Mengoni, C. D'Agostino, A. P. Massetti, C. M. Mastroianni, and V. Vullo. 2002. Interleukin-15 in HIV infection: immunological and virological interactions in antiretroviral-naive and -treated patients. *AIDS* 16:181–188.

942. D'Offizi, G., C. Montesano, C. Agrati, C. Gioia, M. Amicosante, S. Topino, P. Narciso, L. P. Pucillo, G. Ippolito, and F. Poccia. 2002. Expansion of pre-terminally differential CD8 T cells in chronic HIV-positive patients presenting a rapid viral rebound during structured treatment interruption. *AIDS* 16:2431–2438.

943. D'Souza, M. P., P. Durda, C. V. Hanson, and G. Milman. 1991. Evaluation of monoclonal antibodies to HIV-1 by neutralization and serological assays: an international collaboration. *AIDS* 5:1061–1070.

944. da Silva, M., M. M. Shevchuck, W. J. Cronin, N. A. Armenakas, M. Tannenbaum, J. A. Fracchia, and H. L. Ioachim. 1989. Detection of HIV-related protein in testes and prostates of patients with AIDS. *Am. J. Clin. Pathol.* 93:196–201.

945. Daar, E. S., K. L. Kesler, T. Wrin, C. J. Petropoulo, M. Bates, A. Lail, N. S. Hellmann, E. Gomperts, and S. Donfield. 2005. HIV-1 pol replication capacity predicts disease progression. *AIDS* 19:871–877.

946. Daar, E. S., S. Little, J. Pitt, J. Santangelo, P. Ho, N. Harawa, P. Kerndt, J. V. Glorgi, J. Bai, P. Gaut, D. D. Richman, S. Mandel, S. Nichols, and the Los Angeles County Primary HIV Infection Recruitment Network. 2001. Diagnosis of primary HIV-1 infection. *Ann. Intern. Med.* 134:25–29.

947. Daar, E. S., T. Moudgil, R. D. Meyer, and D. D. Ho. 1991. Transient high levels of viremia in patients with primary human immunodeficiency virus type 1 infection. *N. Engl. J. Med.* 324:961–964.

948. Dabis, F., P. Msellati, N. Meda, C. Welffens-Ekra, B. You, O. Manigart, V. Leroy, A. Simonon, M. Cartoux, P. Combe, A. Ouangre, R. Ramon, O. Ky-Zerbo, C. Montcho, R. Salamon, C. Rouzioux, P. Van de Perre, and L. Mandelbrot. 1999. 6-month efficacy, tolerance, and acceptability of a short regimen of oral zidovudine to reduce vertical transmission of HIV in breastfed children in Cote d'Ivoire and Burkina Faso: a double-blind placebo-controlled multicentre trial. *Lancet* 353:786–792.

949. Dadaglio, G., S. Garcia, L. Montagnier, and M. L. Gougeon. 1994. Selective anergy of V beta 8+ T cells in human immunodeficiency virus-infected individuals. *J. Exp. Med.* 179:413–424.

950. Dadaglio, G., F. Michel, P. Langlade-Demoyen, P. Sansonetti, D. Chevrier, F. Vuillier, F. Plata, and A. Hoffenbach. 1992. Enhancement of HIV-specific cytotoxic T lymphocyte responses by zidovudine (AZT) treatment. *Clin. Exp. Immunol.* 87:7–14.

951. Daefler, S., M. E. Klotman, and F. Wong-Staal. 1990. Trans-activating rev protein of the human immunodeficiency virus 1 interacts directly and specifically with its target RNA. *Proc. Natl. Acad. Sci. USA* 87:4571–4575.

952. Daelemans, D., E. Afonina, J. Nilsson, G. Werner, J. Kjems, E. De Clercq, G. N. Pavlakis, and A. M. Vandamme. 2002. A synthetic HIV-1 Rev inhibitor interfering with the CRM1-mediated nuclear export. *Proc. Natl. Acad. Sci. USA* 99:14440–14445.

953. Dagarag, M., T. Evazyan, N. Rao, and R. B. Effros. 2004. Genetic manipulation of telomerase in HIV-specific CD8+ T cells: enhanced antiviral functions accompany the increased proliferative potential and telomere length stabilization. *J. Immunol.* 173:6303–6311.

954. Dahl, K., K. Martin, and G. Miller. 1987. Differences among human immunodeficiency virus strains in their capacities to induce cytolysis of persistent infection or a lymphoblastoid cell line immortalized by Epstein-Barr virus. *J. Virol.* 61:1602–1608.

955. Dahl, K. E., T. Burrage, F. Jones, and G. Miller. 1990. Persistent nonproductive infection of Epstein-Barr virus-transformed human B lymphocytes by human immunodeficiency virus type 1. *J. Virol.* 64:1771–1783.

956. Dai, L.-C., K. West, R. Littaua, K. Takahashi, and F. A. Ennis. 1992. Mutation of human immunodeficiency virus type 1 at amino acid 585 on gp41 results in loss of killing by CD8+ A24-restricted cytotoxic T lymphocytes. *J. Virol.* 66:3151–3154.

957. Dalgleish, A. G., P. C. Beverley, P. R. Clapham, D. H. Crawford, M. F. Greaves, and R. A. Weiss. 1984. The CD4 (T4) antigen is an essential component of the receptor for the AIDS retrovirus. *Nature* 312:763–767.

958. Dalgleish, A. G., T. C. Chahn, R. C. Kennedy, P. Kanda, P. R. Clapham, and R. A. Weiss. 1988. Neutralization of diverse HIV-1 strains by monoclonal antibodies raised against a gp41 synthetic peptide. *Virology* 165:209–215.

959. Dalgleish, A. G., B. J. Thomson, T. C. Chanh, M. Malkovsky, and R. C. Kennedy. 1987. Neutralisation of HIV

isolates by anti-idiotypic antibodies which mimic the T4 (CD4) epitope: a potential AIDS vaccine. *Lancet* ii:1047–1049.

960. Dalgleish, A. G., S. Wilson, M. Gompels, C. Ludlam, B. Gazzard, A. M. Coates, and J. Habeshaw. 1992. T-cell receptor variable gene products and early HIV-1 infection. *Lancet* 339:824–828.

961. Daling, J. R., N. S. Weiss, L. L. Klopfenstein, L. E. Cochran, W. H. Chow, and R. Daifuku. 1982. Correlates of homosexual behavior and the incidence of anal cancer. *JAMA* 247:1988–1990.

962. Dalod, M., M. Dupuis, J. C. Deschemin, C. Goujard, C. Deveau, L. Meyer, N. Ngo, C. Rouzioux, J. G. Guillet, J. F. Delfraissy, M. Sinet, and A. Venet. 1999. Weak anti-HIV CD8(+) T-cell effector activity in HIV primary infection. *J. Clin. Investig.* 104:1431–1439.

963. Dalod, M., M. Harzic, I. Pellegrin, B. Dumon, B. Hoen, D. Sereni, J.-C. Deschemin, J.-P. Levy, A. Venet, and E. Gomard. 1998. Evolution of cytotoxic T lymphocytes responses to human immunodeficiency virus type 1 in patients with symptomatic primary infection receiving antiretroviral triple therapy. *J. Infect. Dis.* 178:61–69.

964. Dalsgaard, K., A. Uttenthal, T. D. Jones, F. Xu, A. Merryweather, W. D. O. Hamilton, J. P. M. Langeveld, R. S. Boshuizen, S. Kamstrup, G. P. Lomonossoff, C. Porta, C. Vela, J. I. Casal, R. H. Meloen, and P. B. Rodgers. 1997. Plant-derived vaccine protects target animals against a viral disease. *Nat. Biotechnol.* 15:248–252.

964a. Damond, F., M. Worobey, P. Campa, I. Farfara, G. Colin, S. Matheron, F. Brun-Vezinet, D. L. Robertson, and F. Simon. 2004. Identification of a highly divergent HIV type 2 and proposal for a change in HIV type 2 classification. *AIDS Res. Hum. Retroviruses* 20:666–672.

964b. Dang, Y., X. Wang, W. J. Esselman, and Y. H. Zheng. 2006. Identification of APOBEC3DE as another antiretroviral factor from the human APOBEC family. *J. Virol.* 80:10522–10533.

965. Daniel, M. D., F. Kirchhoff, P. K. Czajak, P. K. Sehgal, and R. C. Desrosiers. 1992. Protective effects of a live attenuated SIV vaccine with a deletion in the *nef* gene. *Science* 258:1938–1941.

966. Daniel, M. D., G. P. Mazzara, M. A. Simon, P. K. Sehgal, T. Kodama, D. L. Panicali, and R. C. Desrosiers. 1994. Higher-titer immune responses elicted by recombinant vaccinia virus priming and particle boosting are ineffective in preventing virulent SIV infection. *AIDS Res. Hum. Retrovir.* 10:839–851.

967. Darcissac, E. C. A., M.-J. Trong, J. Dewulf, Y. Mouton, A. Capron, and G. M. Bahr. 2000. The synthetic immunomodulator murabutide controls human immunodeficiency virus type 1 replication at multiple levels in macrophages and dendritic cells. *J. Virol.* 74:7794–7802.

968. Das, A. T., C. E. Baldwin, M. Vink, and B. Berkhout. 2005. Improving the safety of a conditional-live human immunodeficiency virus type 1 vaccine by controlling both gene expression and cell entry. *J. Virol.* 79:3855–3858.

969. Das, A. T., T. R. Brummelkamp, E. M. Westerhout, M. Vink, M. Madiredjo, R. Bernards, and B. Berkhout. 2004. Human immunodeficiency virus type 1 escapes from RNA interference-mediated inhibition. *J. Virol.* 78:2601–2605.

970. Davey, R. T., Jr., D. G. Chaitt, S. C. Piscitelli, M. Wells, J. A. Kovacs, R. E. Walker, J. Falloon, M. A. Polis, J. A. Metcalf, H. Masur, G. Fyfe, and H. C. Lane. 1997. Subcutaneous administration of interleukin-2 in human immunodeficiency virus type 1-infected persons. *J. Infect. Dis.* 175:781–789.

971. David, F. J., B. Autran, H. C. Tran, E. Menu, M. Raphael, P. Debre, B. L. Hsi, T. G. Wegman, F. Barre-Sinoussi, and G. Chaouat. 1992. Human trophoblast cells express CD4 and are permissive for productive infection with HIV-1. *Clin. Exp. Immunol.* 88:10–16.

972. Davis, B. R., D. H. Schwartz, J. C. Marx, C. E. Johnson, J. M. Berry, J. Lyding, T. C. Merigan, and A. Zander. 1991. Absent or rare human immunodeficiency virus infection of bone marrow stem/progenitor cells in vivo. *J. Virol.* 65:1985–1990.

973. Davis, D., D. M. Stephens, C. Willers, and P. J. Lachmann. 1990. Glycosylation governs the binding of antipeptide antibodies to regions of hypervariable amino acid sequence within recombinant gp120 of human immunodeficiency virus type 1. *J. Gen. Virol.* 71:2889–2898.

974. Davis, D. A., R. W. Humphrey, F. M. Newcomb, T. R. O'Brien, J. J. Goedert, S. E. Straus, and R. Yarchoan. 1997. Detection of serum antibodies to a Kaposi's sarcoma-associated herpesvirus-specific peptide. *J. Infect. Dis.* 175:1071–1079.

975. Davis, I. C., M. Girard, and P. N. Fultz. 1998. Loss of CD4$^+$ T cells in human immunodeficiency virus type 1-infected chimpanzees is associated with increased lymphocyte apoptosis. *J. Virol.* 72:4623–4632.

976. Davis, L. E., B. L. Hjelle, V. E. Miller, D. L. Palmer, A. L. Llewellyn, T. L. Merlin, S. A. Young, R. G. Mills, W. Wachsman, and C. A. Wiley. 1992. Early viral brain invasion in iatrogenic human immunodeficiency virus infection. *Neurology* 42:1736–1739.

977. Davis, M. G., S. C. Kenney, J. Kamine, J. S. Pagano, and E.-S. Huang. 1987. Immediate-early gene region of human cytomegalovirus trans-activates the promoter of human immunodeficiency virus. *Proc. Natl. Acad. Sci. USA* 84:8642–8646.

978. Dawson, V. L., T. M. Dawson, G. R. Uhl, and S. H. Snyder. 1993. Human immunodeficiency virus type 1 coat protein neurotoxicity mediated by nitric oxide in primary cortical cultures. *Proc. Natl. Acad. Sci. USA* 90:3256–3259.

978a. Day, C. L., D. E. Kaufmann, P. Kiepiela, J. A. Brown, E. S. Moodley, S. Reddy, E. W. Mackey, J. D. Miller, A. J. Leslie, C. Depierres, Z. Mncube, J. Duraiswamy, B. Zhu, Q. Eichbaum, M. Altfeld, E. J. Wherry, H. M. Coovadia, P. J. Goulder, P. Klenerman, R. Ahmed, G. J. Freeman, and B. D. Walker. PD-1 expression on HIV-specific T cells is associated with T-cell exhaustion and disease progression. *Nature*, in press.

979. Dayanithi, G., N. Yahi, S. Baghdiguian, and J. Fantini. 1995. Intracellular calcium release induced by human immunodeficiency virus type 1 (HIV-1) surface envelope glycoprotein in human intestinal epithelial cells: a putative mechanism for HIV-1 enteropathy. *Cell Calcium* 18:9–18.

980. Dayton, A. I., J. G. Sodroski, and C. A. Rosen. 1986. The *trans*-activator gene of the human T-cell lymphotropic virus type III is required for replication. *Cell* 4:941–947.

981. De Andreis, C., G. Simoni, C. Castagna, L. Sacchi, S. M. Sirchia, I. Garagiola, T. Persico, P. Serafini, G. Pardi, and A. E. Semprini. 1997. Absence of detectable maternal DNA and identification of proviral HIV in the cord blood of two infants who became HIV-infected. *AIDS* 11:840–841.

982. De Andreis, C., G. Simoni, F. Rossella, C. Castagna, E. Pesenti, G. Porta, G. Colucci, S. Giuntelli, G. Pardi, and A. E. Semprini. 1996. HIV-1 proviral DNA polymerase chain reaction detection in chorionic villi after exclusion of maternal

contamination by variable number of tandem repeats analysis. *AIDS* **10**:711–715.

983. De Cock, K. M., G. Adjoriolo, E. Ekpini, T. Sibailly, J. Kouadio, M. Maran, K. Brattegaard, K. M. Vetter, R. Doorly, and H. D. Gayle. 1993. Epidemiology and transmission of HIV-2: why there is no HIV-2 pandemic. *JAMA* **270**:2083–2086.

984. de Gast, G. C., L. F. Verdonck, J. M. Middeldorp, T. H. The, A. Hekker, J. A. van den Linden, H. A. J. G. Kreeft, and B. J. E. G. Bast. 1985. Recovery of T cell subsets after autologous bone marrow transplantation is mainly due to proliferation of mature T cells in the graft. *Blood* **66**:428–431.

985. de Jong, A. L., D. M. Green, J. A. Trial, and H. H. Birdsall. 1996. Focal effects of mononuclear leukocyte transendothelial migration: TNF-α production by migrating monocytes promotes subsequent migration of lymphocytes. *J. Leukoc. Biol.* **60**:129–136.

986. de Jong, J.-J., A. de Ronde, W. Keulen, M. Tersmette, and J. Goudsmit. 1992. Minimal requirements for the human immunodeficiency virus type 1 V3 domain to support the syncytium-inducing phenotype: analysis by single amino acid substitution. *J. Virol.* **66**:6777–6780.

987. de Jong, J.-J., J. Goudsmit, W. Keulen, B. Klaver, W. Krone, M. Tersmette, and A. De Ronde. 1992. Human immunodeficiency virus type 1 clones chimeric for the envelope V3 domain differ in syncytium formation and replication capacity. *J. Virol.* **66**:757–765.

988. de la Monte, S. M., D. H. Gabuzda, D. D. Ho, R. H. Brown, Jr., E. T. Hedley-Whyte, R. T. Schooley, M. S. Hirsch, and A. K. Bhan. 1988. Peripheral neuropathy in the acquired immunodeficiency syndrome. *Ann. Neurol.* **23**:485–492.

989. de la Rosa, R., and M. Leal. 2003. Thymic involvement in recovery of immunity among HIV-infected adults on highly active antiretroviral therapy. *J. Antimicrob. Chemother.* **52**:155–158.

990. de la Rosa, R., J. A. Pineda, J. Delgado, J. Macias, F. Morillas, J. A. Mira, A. Sanchez-Quijano, M. Leal, and E. Lissen. 2002. Incidence of and risk factors for symptomatic visceral leishmaniasis among human immunodeficiency virus type 1-infected patients from Spain in the era of highly active antiretroviral therapy. *J. Clin. Microbiol.* **40**:762–767.

991. De Luca, A., M. L. Giancola, A. Ammassari, S. Grisetti, M. G. Paglia, M. Gentile, A. Cingolani, R. Murri, G. Liuzzi, A. D. Monforte, and A. Antinori. 2000. The effect of potent antiretroviral therapy and JC virus load in cerebrospinal fluid on clinical outcome of patients with AIDS-associated progressive multifocal leukoencephalopathy. *J. Infect. Dis.* **182**:1077–1083.

992. De Luca, A., L. Teofile, A. Antinori, M. S. Iovino, P. Mencarini, E. Visconti, E. Tamburrini, G. Leone, and L. Ortona. 1993. Haemopoietic CD34+ progenitor cells are not infected by HIV-1 *in vivo* but show impaired clonogenesis. *Br. J. Haematol.* **85**:20–24.

993. de Maria, A., C. Cirillo, and L. Moretta. 1994. Occurrence of human immunodeficiency virus type 1 (HIV-1)-specific cytolytic T cell activity in apparently uninfected children born to HIV-1-infected mothers. *J. Infect. Dis.* **170**:1296–1299.

994. De Maria, A., M. Fogli, P. Costa, G. Murdaca, F. Puppo, D. Mavilio, A. Moretta, and L. Moretta. 2003. The impaired NK cell cytolytic function in viremic HIV-1 infection is associated with a reduced surface expression of natural cytotoxicity receptors (NKp46, NKp30 and NKp44). *Eur. J. Immunol.* **33**:2410–2418.

995. de Martino, M., P. A. Tovo, L. Galli, and C. Gabiano. 1994. Features of children perinatally infected with HIV-1 surviving longer than 5 years. *Lancet* **343**:191–195.

996. de Mendoza, C., C. Rodriguez, J. M. Eiros, J. Colomina, F. Garcia, P. Leiva, J. Torre-Cisneros, J. Aguero, J. Pedreira, I. Viciana, A. Corral, J. del Romero, R. Ortiz de Lejarazu, and V. Soriano. 2005. Antiretroviral recommendations may influence the rate of transmission of drug-resistant HIV type 1. *Clin. Infect. Dis.* **41**:227–232.

997. De Milito, A., C. Morch, A. Sonnerborg, and F. Chiodi. 2001. Loss of memory (CD27) B lymphocytes in HIV-1 infection. *AIDS* **15**:957–964.

998. de Noronha, C. M. C., M. P. Sherman, H. W. Lin, M. V. Cavrois, R. D. Moir, R. D. Goldman, and W. C. Greene. 2001. Dynamic disruptions in nuclear envelope architecture and integrity induced by HIV-1 Vpr. *Science* **294**:1105–1108.

999. de Oliveira Pinto, L. M., S. Garcia, H. Lecoeur, C. Rapp, and M. L. Gougeon. 2002. Increased sensitivity of T lymphocytes to tumor necrosis factor receptor 1 (TNFR1)- and TNFR2-mediated apoptosis in HIV infection: relation to expression of Bcl-2 and active caspase-8 and caspase-3. *Blood* **99**:1666–1675.

1000. De Paoli, P., D. Gennari, P. Martelli, G. Basaglia, M. Crovatto, S. Battistin, and G. Santini. 1991. A subset of gamma delta lymphocytes is increased during HIV-1 infection. *Clin. Exp. Immunol.* **83**:187–191.

1001. De Paoli, P., S. Zanussi, C. Simonelli, M. T. Bortolin, M. D'Andrea, C. Crepaldi, R. Talamini, M. Comar, M. Giacca, and U. Tirelli. 1997. Effects of subcutaneous interleukin-2 therapy on CD4 subsets and in vitro cytokine production in HIV+ subjects. *J. Clin. Investig.* **100**:2737–2743.

1002. de Pasquale, M. P., A. J. Leigh Brown, S. C. Uvin, J. Allega-Ingersoll, A. M. Caliendo, L. Sutton, S. Donahue, and R. T. D'Aquila. 2003. Differences in HIV-1 pol sequences from female genital tract and blood during antiretroviral therapy. *J. Acquir. Immune Defic. Syndr.* **34**:37–44.

1003. de Roda Husman, A. M., M. Koot, M. Corneliessen, I. P. Keet, M. Brouwer, S. M. Broersen, M. Bakker, M. T. Roos, M. Prins, F. de Wolf, R. A. Coutinho, F. Miedema, J. Gudsmit, and H. Schuitemaker. 1997. Association between CCR5 genotype and the clinical course of HIV-1 infection. *Ann. Intern. Med.* **127**:882–890.

1004. de Ronde, A., B. Kalver, W. Keulen, L. Smit, and J. Goudsmit. 1992. Natural HIV-1 *nef* accelerates virus replication in primary human lymphocytes. *Virology* **188**:391–395.

1005. De Rossi, A., S. Masiero, C. Giaquinto, E. Ruga, M. Comar, M. Giacca, and L. Chieco-Bianchi. 1996. Dynamics of viral replication in infants with vertically acquired human immunodeficiency virus type 1 infection. *J. Clin. Investig.* **97**:323–330.

1006. De Rossi, A., L. Ometto, F. Mammano, C. Zanotto, C. Giaquinto, and L. Chieco-Bianchi. 1992. Vertical transmission of human immunodeficiency virus type 1 (HIV-1): lack of detectable virus in peripheral blood cells of infected children at birth. *AIDS* **6**:1117–1120.

1007. De Rossi, A., M. Pasti, F. Mammano, L. Ometto, C. Giaquinto, and L. Chieco-Bianchi. 1991. Perinatal infection by human immunodeficiency virus type 1 (HIV-1): relationship between proviral copy number *in vivo*, viral properties *in vitro*, and clinical outcome. *J. Med. Virol.* **35**:283–289.

1008. De Santis, C., P. Robbioni, R. Longhi, L. Lopalco, A. G. Siccardi, A. Beretta, and N. J. Roberts, Jr. 1993. Cross-reactive response to human immunodeficiency virus type 1 (HIV-1) gp120 and HLA class I heavy chains induced by receipt of HIV-1-derived envelope vaccines. *J. Infect. Dis.* 168:1396–1403.

1009. De Vincenzi, I. 1994. A longitudinal study of human immunodeficiency virus transmission by heterosexual partners. *N. Engl. J. Med.* 331:341–346.

1010. de Vincenzi, I., R. A. Ancell-Park, J. B. Brunet, P. Costigliola, E. Ricchi, F. Chiodo, A. Roumeliotou, G. Papaevengelou, R. A. Coutinhi, and H. J. A. van Haastrecht. 1992. Comparison of female to male and male to female transmission of HIV in 563 stable couples. *Br. Med. J.* 304:809–813.

1011. de Vreese, K., V. Kofler-Mongold, C. Leutgeb, V. Weber, K. Vermeire, S. Schacht, J. Anne, E. de Clercq, R. Datema, and G. Werner. 1996. The molecular target of bicyclams, potent inhibitors of human immunodeficiency virus replication. *J. Virol.* 70:689–696.

1012. de Waal Malefyt, R., H. Yssel, M.-G. Roncarolo, H. Spits, and J. E. de Vries. 1992. Interleukin-10. *Curr. Opin. Immunol.* 4:314–320.

1013. de Wit, E., V. J. Munster, M. I. Spronken, T. M. Bestebroer, C. Baas, W. E. Beyer, G. F. Rimmelzwaan, A. D. Osterhaus, and R. A. Fouchier. 2005. Protection of mice against lethal infection with highly pathogenic H7N7 influenza A virus by using a recombinant low-pathogenicity vaccine strain. *J. Virol.* 79:12401–12407.

1014. de Wolf, F., R. H. Meloen, M. Bakker, F. Barin, and J. Goudsmit. 1991. Characterization of human antibody-binding sites on the external envelope of human immunodeficiency virus type 2. *J. Gen. Virol.* 72:1261–1267.

1015. de Wolf, F. J., M. A. Lange, and T. M. Houwleling. 1988. Numbers of CD4+ cells and the levels of core antigens and of antibodies to the human immunodeficiency virus as predictors of AIDS among seropositive homosexual men. *J. Infect. Dis.* 158:615–622.

1016. Deacon, N. J., A. Tsykin, A. Solomon, K. Smith, M. Ludford-Menting, D. J. Hooker, D. A. McPhee, A. L. Greenway, A. Ellett, C. Chatfield, V. A. Lawson, S. Crowe, A. Maerz, S. Sonza, J. Learmont, J. S. Sullivan, A. Cunningham, D. Dwyer, D. Dowton, and J. Mills. 1995. Genomic structure of an attenuated quasi species of HIV-1 from a blood tranfusion donor and recipients. *Science* 270:988–991.

1017. Dean, M., M. Carrington, C. Winkler, G. A. Huttley, M. W. Smith, R. Allikmets, J. J. Goedert, S. P. Buchbinder, E. Vittinghoff, E. Gomperts, S. Donfield, D. Vlahov, R. Kaslow, A. Saah, C. Rinaldo, R. Detels, and S. J. O'Brien. 1996. Genetic restriction of HIV-1 infection and progression to AIDS by a deletion allele of the CCR5 structural gene. *Science* 273:1856–1862.

1018. Dean, M., L. P. Jacobson, G. McFarlane, J. B. Margolick, F. J. Jenkins, O. M. Howard, H. F. Dong, J. J. Goedert, S. Buchbinder, E. Gomperts, D. Vlahov, J. J. Oppenheim, S. J. O'Brien, and M. Carrington. 1999. Reduced risk of AIDS lymphoma in individuals heterozygous for the CCR5-delta32 mutation. *Cancer Res.* 59:3561–3564.

1019. Dean, N. C., J. A. Golden, L. Evans, M. L. Warnock, T. E. Addison, P. C. Hopewell, and J. A. Levy. 1988. Human immunodeficiency virus recovery from bronchoaveolar lavage fluid in patients with AIDS. *Chest* 93:1176–1179.

1020. Deayton, J. R., P. Wilson, C. A. Sabin, C. C. Davey, M. A. Johnson, V. C. Emery, and P. D. Griffiths. 2000. Changes in the natural history of cytomegalovirus retinitis following the introduction of highly active antiretroviral therapy. *AIDS* 14:1163–1170.

1021. Debes, G. F., C. N. Arnold, A. J. Young, S. Krautwald, M. Lipp, J. B. Hay, and E. C. Butcher. 2005. Chemokine receptor CCR7 required for T lymphocyte exit from peripheral tissues. *Nat. Immunol.* 6:889–894.

1022. DeCarli, C., L. Fugate, J. Falloon, J. Eddy, D. A. Katz, R. P. Friedland, S. I. Rapoport, P. Brouwers, and P. A. Pizzo. 1991. Brain growth and cognitive improvement in children with human immunodeficiency virus-induced encephalopathy after 6 months of continuous infusion zidovudine therapy. *J. Acquir. Immune Defic. Syndr.* 4:585–592.

1023. Decker, J. M., F. Bibollet-Ruche, X. Wei, S. Wang, D. N. Levy, W. Wang, E. Delaporte, M. Peeters, C. A. Derdeyn, S. Allen, E. Hunter, M. S. Saag, J. A. Hoxie, B. H. Hahn, P. D. Kwong, J. E. Robinson, and G. M. Shaw. 2005. Antigenic conservation and immunogenicity of the HIV coreceptor binding site. *J. Exp. Med.* 201:1407–1419.

1024. Dedicoat, M., R. Newton, K. R. Alkharsah, J. Sheldon, I. Szabados, B. Ndlovu, T. Page, D. Casabonne, C. F. Gilks, S. A. Cassol, D. Whitby, and T. F. Schulz. 2004. Mother-to-child transmission of human herpesvirus-8 in South Africa. *J. Infect. Dis.* 190:1068–1075.

1025. Deeks, S. G. 2003. Treatment of antiretroviral-drug-resistant HIV-1 infection. *Lancet* 262:2002–2011.

1026. Deeks, S. G. 2006. Challenges of developing R5 inhibitors in antiretroviral naive HIV-infected patients. *Lancet* 367:711–713.

1027. Deeks, S. G., A. Collier, J. Lalezari, A. Pavia, D. Rodrigue, W. L. Drew, J. Toole, H. S. Jaffe, A. S. Mulato, P. D. Lamy, W. Li, J. M. Cherrington, N. Hellmann, and J. Kahn. 1997. The safety and efficacy of adefovir dipivoxil, a novel anti-HIV therapy, in HIV infected adults: a randomized, double-blind, placebo-trial controlled trial. *J. Infect. Dis.* 176:1517–1523.

1028. Deeks, S. G., R. Hoh, R. M. Grant, T. Wrin, J. D. Barbour, A. Narvaez, D. Cesar, K. Abe, M. B. Hanley, N. S. Hellmann, C. J. Petropoulos, J. M. McCune, and M. K. Hellerstein. 2002. CD4+ T cell kinetics and activation in human immunodeficiency virus-infected patients who remain viremic despite long-term treatment with protease inhibitor-based therapy. *J. Infect. Dis.* 185:315–323.

1029. Deeks, S. G., C. M. Kitchen, L. Liu, H. Guo, R. Gascon, A. B. Narvaez, P. Hunt, J. N. Martin, J. O. Kahn, J. Levy, M. S. McGrath, and F. M. Hecht. 2004. Immune activation set point during early HIV infection predicts subsequent CD4+ T-cell changes independent of viral load. *Blood* 104:942–947.

1030. Deeks, S. G., B. Schweighardt, J. Galovich, R. Hoh, E. Sinclair, P. W. Hunt, J. M. McCune, J. N. Martin, C. J. Petropoulos, and F. M. Hecht. 2006. Neutralizing antibody responses against autologous and heterologous viruses in acute versus chronic human immunodeficiency virus (HIV) infection: evidence for a constraint on the ability of HIV to completely evade neutralizing antibody responses. *J. Virol.* 80:6155–6164.

1031. Deeks, S. G., M. Smith, M. Holodniy, and J. O. Kahn. 1997. HIV-1 protease inhibitors. *JAMA* 277:145–153.

1031a. Deichmann, M., G. Sczakiel, and R. Haas. 1997. Disinfection of cell-associated and extracellular HIV-1 by PUVA treatment. *J. Virol. Methods* 68:89–95.

1032. Del Corno, M., M. C. Gauzzi, G. Penna, F. Belardelli, L. Adorini, and S. Gessani. 2005. Human immunodeficiency virus type 1 gp120 and other activation stimuli are highly effective in triggering alpha interferon and CC chemokine production in circulating plasmacytoid but not myeloid dendritic cells. *J. Virol.* **79**:12597–12601.

1033. Del Mistro, A., R. Bertorelle, M. Franzetti, A. Cattelan, A. Torrisi, M. Giordani, R. Sposetti, E. Bonoldi, L. Sasset, L. Bonaldi, D. Minucci, and L. Chieco-Bianchi. 2004. Antiretroviral therapy and the clinical evolution of human papillomavirus-associated genital lesions in HIV-positive women. *Clin. Infect. Dis.* **38**:737–742.

1034. Del Prete, G., M. De Carli, F. Almerigogna, M. G. Giudizi, R. Biagiotti, and S. Romagnani. 1993. Human IL-10 is produced by both type 1 helper (Th1) and type 2 helper (Th2) T cell clones and inhibits their antigen-specific proliferation and cytokine production. *J. Immunol.* **150**:353–360.

1035. Del Prete, G. F., M. De Carli, M. Ricci, and S. Romagnani. 1991. Helper activity for immunoglobulin synthesis of T helper type 1 (Th1) and Th2 human T cell clones: the help of Th1 clones is limited by their cytolytic capacity. *J. Exp. Med.* **174**:809–813.

1036. del Romero, J., B. Marincovich, J. Castilla, S. Garcia, J. Campo, V. Hernando, and C. Rodriguez. 2002. Evaluating the risk of HIV transmission through unprotected orogenital sex. *AIDS* **16**:1296–1297.

1037. Delamare, C., M. Burgard, M. J. Mayaux, S. Blanche, A. Doussin, S. Ivanoff, M. L. Chaix, C. Khan, and C. Rouzioux. 1997. HIV-1 RNA detection in plasma for the diagnosis of infection in neonates. *J. Acquir. Immune Defic. Syndr. Hum. Retrovirol.* **15**:121–125.

1038. Delassus, S., R. Cheynier, and S. Wain-Hobson. 1991. Evolution of human immunodeficiency virus type 1 *nef* and long terminal repeat sequences over 4 years in vivo and in vitro. *J. Virol.* **65**:225–231.

1039. Delaugerre, C., M.-A. Valantin, M. Mouroux, M. Bonmarchand, G. Carcelain, C. Duvivier, R. Tubiana, A. Simon, F. Bricaire, H. Agut, B. Autran, C. Katalama, and V. Calvez. 2001. Re-occurrence of HIV-1 drug mutations after treatment re-initiation following interruption in patients with multiple treatment failure. *AIDS* **15**:2189–2191.

1040. Delezay, O., N. Koch, N. Yahi, D. Hammache, C. Tourres, C. Tamalet, and J. Fantini. 1997. Co-expression of CXCR4/Fusin and galactosyl ceramide in the human intestinal epithelial cell line HT-29. *AIDS* **11**:1311–1318.

1041. Delobel, P., K. Sandres-Saune, M. Cazabat, C. Pasquier, B. Marchou, P. Massip, and J. Izopet. 2005. R5 to X4 switch of the predominant HIV-1 population in cellular reservoirs during effective highly active antiretroviral therapy. *J. Acquir. Immune Defic. Syndr.* **38**:382–392.

1042. Delwart, E., M. Magierowska, M. Royz, B. Foley, L. Peddada, R. Smith, C. Heldebrant, A. Conrad, and M. Busch. 2002. Homogeneous quasispecies in 16 out of 17 individuals during very early HIV-1 primary infection. *AIDS* **16**:189–195.

1043. Delwart, E. L., S. Orton, B. Parekh, T. Dobbs, K. Clark, and M. P. Busch. 2003. Two percent of HIV-positive U.S. blood donors are infected with non-subtype B strains. *AIDS Res. Hum. Retrovir.* **19**:1065–1070.

1044. Delwart, E. L., H. W. Sheppard, B. D. Walker, J. Goudsmit, and J. I. Mullins. 1994. Human immunodeficiency virus type 1 evolution in vivo tracked by DNA heteroduplex mobility assays. *J. Virol.* **68**:6672–6683.

1045. Delwart, E. L., E. G. Shpaer, J. Louwagie, F. E. McCutchan, M. Grez, H. Rubasamen-Waigmann, and J. I. Mullins. 1993. Genetic relationships determined by a DNA heteroduplex mobility assay: analysis of HIV-1 *env* genes. *Science* **262**:1257–1261.

1046. Demarest, J. F., N. Jack, C. Cleghorn, M. L. Greenberg, T. L. Hoffman, J. S. Ottinger, L. Fantry, J. Edwards, T. R. O'Brien, K. Cao, B. Mahabir, W. A. Blattner, C. Bartholomew, and K. J. Weinhold. 2001. Immunologic and virologic analyses of an acutely HIV type 1-infected patient with extremely rapid disease progression. *AIDS Res. Hum. Retrovir.* **17**:1333–1334.

1047. Demirhan, I., A. Chandra, O. Hasselmayer, P. Biberfeld, and P. Chandra. 1999. Detection of distinct patterns of anti-tat antibodies in HIV-infected individuals with or without Kaposi's sarcoma. *J. Acquir. Immune Defic. Syndr.* **22**:364–368.

1048. Deml, H., G. Kratochwil, N. Osterrieder, R. Knuchel, H. Wolf, and R. Wagner. 1997. Increased incorporation of chimeric human immunodeficiency virus type 1 gp 320 proteins into Pr55^{gag} particles by an Epstein-Barr gp220/350-derived transmembrane domain. *Virology* **235**:10–25.

1049. Deng, H., R. Liu, W. Ellmeier, S. Choe, D. Unutmaz, M. Burkhart, P. Di Marzio, S. Marmon, R. E. Sutton, C. M. Hill, C. B. Davis, S. C. Peiper, T. J. Schall, D. R. Littman, and N. R. Landau. 1996. Identification of a major co-receptor for primary isolates of HIV-1. *Nature* **381**:661–666.

1050. Derdeyn, C. A., J. M. Decker, F. Bibollet-Ruche, J. L. Mokili, M. Muldoon, S. A. Denham, M. L. Heil, F. Kasolo, R. Musonda, B. H. Hahn, G. M. Shaw, B. T. Korber, S. Allen, and E. Hunter. 2004. Envelope-constrained neutralization-sensitive HIV-1 after heterosexual transmission. *Science* **303**:2019–2022.

1051. Deresinski, S. C. 1999. Granulocyte-macrophage colony-stimulating factor: potential therapeutic, immunological and antiretroviral effects in HIV infection. *AIDS* **13**:633–643.

1052. Dern, K., H. Rubsamen-Waigmann, and R. E. Unger. 2001. Inhibition of HIV type 1 replication by simultaneous infection of peripheral blood lymphocytes with human immunodeficiency virus types 1 and 2. *AIDS Res. Hum. Retrovir.* **17**:295–309.

1052a. De Santis, M., B. Carducci, L. De Santis, A. F. Cavaliere, and G. Straface. 2002. Periconceptional exposure to efavirenz and neural tube defects. *Arch. Intern. Med.* **162**:355.

1053. Des Jarlais, D. C., S. R. Friedman, and W. Hopkins. 1985. Risk reduction for the acquired immunodeficiency syndrome among intravenous drug users. *Ann. Intern. Med.* **103**:755–759.

1054. Des Jarlais, D. C., M. Marmor, D. Paone, S. Titus, Q. Shi, T. Perlis, B. Jose, and S. R. Friedman. 1996. HIV incidence among injecting drug users in New York City syringe-exchange programmes. *Lancet* **148**:987–991.

1055. Desai, K., P. M. Loewenstein, and M. Green. 1991. Isolation of a cellular protein that binds to the human immunodeficiency virus *tat* protein and can potentiate transactivation of the viral promoter. *Proc. Natl. Acad. Sci. USA* **88**:8875–8879.

1056. Descamps, D., G. Collin, F. Letourneur, C. Apetrei, F. Damond, I. Loussert-Ajaka, F. Simon, S. Saragosti, and F. Brun-Vezinet. 1997. Susceptibility of human immunodeficiency virus type 1 group O isolates to antiretroviral agents: in vitro phenotypic and genotypic analyses. *J. Virol.* 71:8893–8898.

1057. Desfosses, Y., M. Solis, Q. Sun, N. Grandvaux, C. Van Lint, A. Burny, A. Gatignol, M. A. Wainberg, R. Lin, and J. Hiscott. 2005. Regulation of human immunodeficiency virus type 1 gene expression by clade-specific Tat proteins. *J. Virol.* 79: 9180–9191.

1058. DeSimone, J. A., R. J. Pomerantz, and T. J. Babinchak. 2000. Inflammatory reactions in HIV-1-infected persons after initiation of highly active antiretroviral therapy. *Ann. Intern. Med.* 133:447–454.

1059. Desrosiers, R. C. 2004. Prospects for an AIDS vaccine. *Nat. Med.* 10:221–223.

1060. Desrosiers, R. C., V. G. Sasseville, S. C. Czajak, X. Zhang, K. G. Mansfield, A. Kaur, R. P. Johnson, A. A. Lackner, and J. U. Jung. 1997. A herpesvirus of rhesus monkeys related to the human Kaposi's sarcoma-associated herpesvirus. *J. Virol.* 71:9764–9769.

1061. Desrosiers, R. C., M. S. Wyand, T. Kodama, D. J. Ringler, L. O. Arthur, P. K. Sehgal, N. L. Letvin, N. W. King, and M. D. Daniel. 1989. Vaccine protection against simian immunodeficiency virus infection. *Proc. Natl. Acad. Sci. USA* 86:6353–6357.

1062. Detels, R., A. Munoz, G. McFarlane, L. A. Kingsley, J. B. Margolick, J. Giorgi, L. K. Schrager, and J. P. Phair. 1998. Effectiveness of potent antiretroviral therapy on time to AIDS and death in men with known HIV infection duration. *JAMA* 280:1497–1503.

1063. Deville, J., and Y. Bryson. 2001. Perinatal transmission of HIV: recognition and treatment interventions. *Curr. Infect. Dis. Rep.* 3:388–396.

1064. Devito, C., K. Broliden, R. Kaul, L. Svensson, K. Johansen, P. Kiama, J. Kimani, L. Lopalco, S. Piconi, J. J. Bwayo, F. Plummer, M. Clerici, and J. Hinkula. 2000. Mucosal and plasma IgA from HIV-1-exposed uninfected individuals inhibit HIV-1 transcytosis across human epithelial cells. *J. Immunol.* 165:5170–5176.

1065. Devito, C., J. Hinkula, R. Kaul, L. Lopalco, J. J. Bwayo, F. Plummer, M. Clerici, and K. Broliden. 2000. Mucosal and plasma IgA from HIV-exposed seronegative individuals neutralize a primary HIV-1 isolate. *AIDS* 14:1917–1920.

1066. Dezube, B. J., S. E. Krown, J. Y. Lee, K. S. Bauer, and D. M. Aboulafia. 2006. Randomized phase II trial of matrix metalloproteinase inhibitor COL-3 in AIDS-related Kaposi's sarcoma: an AIDS Malignancy Consortium Study. *J. Clin. Oncol.* 24:1389–1394.

1067. Dezube, B. J., A. B. Pardee, B. Chapman, L. A. Beckett, J. A. Korvick, W. J. Novick, J. Chiurco, P. Kasdan, C. M. Ahlers, L. T. Ecto, and C. S. Crumpacker. 1993. Pentoxifylline decreases tumor necrosis factor expression and serum triglycerides in people with AIDS. *J. Acquir. Immune Defic. Syndr.* 6:787–794.

1068. Dezzutti, C. S., P. C. Guenthner, J. E. Cummins, Jr., T. Cabrera, J. H. Marshall, A. Dillberger, and R. B. Lal. 2001. Cervical and prostate primary epithelial cells are not productively infected but sequester human immunodeficiency virus type 1. *J. Infect. Dis.* 183:1204–1213.

1069. Dhawan, D., and K. H. Mayer. 2006. Microbicides to prevent HIV transmission: overcoming obstacles to chemical barrier protection. *J. Infect. Dis.* 193:36–44.

1070. Dhawan, S., R. K. Puri, A. Kumar, H. Duplan, J. M. Masson, and B. B. Aggarwal. 1997. Human immunodeficiency virus-1-tat protein induces the cell surface expression of endothelial leukocyte adhesion molecule-1, vascular cell adhesion molecule-1, and intercellular adhesion molecule-1 in human endothelial cells. *Blood* 90:1535–1544.

1071. Di Alberti, L., S. L. Ngui, S. R. Porter, P. M. Speight, C. M. Scully, J. M. Zakrewska, I. G. Williams, L. Artese, A. Piattelli, and C. G. Teo. 1997. Presence of human herpesvirus 8 variants in the oral tissues of human immunodeficiency virus-infected persons. *J. Infect. Dis.* 175:703–707.

1072. Di Marzio, P., J. Tse, and N. R. Landau. 1998. Chemokine receptor regulation and HIV type 1 tropism in monocyte-macrophages. *AIDS Res. Hum. Retrovir.* 14:129–138.

1073. Di Mascio, M., M. Markowitz, M. Louis, A. Hurley, C. Hogan, V. Simon, D. Follmann, D. D. Ho, and A. S. Perelson. 2004. Dynamics of intermittent viremia during highly active antiretroviral therapy in patients who initiate therapy during chronic versus acute and early human immunodeficiency virus type 1 infection. *J. Virol.* 78:10566–10573.

1074. Di Stefano, M., L. Monno, J. R. Fiore, G. Buccoliero, A. Appice, L. M. Perulli, G. Pastore, and G. Angarano. 1998. Neurological disorders during HIV-1 infection correlate with viral load in cerebrospinal fluid but not with virus phenotype. *AIDS* 12:737–743.

1075. Diamond, D. C., B. P. Sleckman, T. Gregory, L. A. Lasky, J. L. Greenstein, and S. J. Burakoff. 1988. Inhibition of CD4+ T cell function by the HIV envelope protein, gp120. *J. Immunol.* 141:3715–3717.

1076. Dianzani, F., G. Antonelli, E. Riva, O. Turriziani, L. Antonelli, S. Tyring, D. A. Carrasco, H. Lee, D. Nguyen, J. Pan, J. Poast, M. Cloyd, and S. Baron. 2002. Is human immunodeficiency virus RNA load composed of neutralized immune complexes? *J. Infect. Dis.* 185:1051–1054.

1077. Dianzani, U., and F. Malavasi. 1995. Lymphocyte adhesion to endothelial cells. *Crit. Rev. Immunol.* 15:167–200.

1078. Diaz, L. S., H. Foster, M. R. Stone, S. Fujimura, D. A. Relman, and J. A. Levy. 2005. VCAM-1 expression on CD8+ cells correlates with enhanced anti-HIV suppressing activity. *J. Immunol.* 174:1574–1579.

1079. Diaz, R. S., E. C. Sabino, A. Mayer, C. F. deOliveira, J. W. Mosley, and M. P. Busch. 1996. Lack of dual HIV infection in a transfusion recipient exposed to two seropositive blood components. *AIDS Res. Hum. Retrovir.* 12:1291–1295.

1080. Dick, A. D., M. Pell, B. J. Brew, E. Foulcher, and J. D. Sedgwick. 1997. Direct ex vivo flow cytometric analysis of human microglial cell CD4 expression: examination of central nervous system biopsy specimens from HIV-seropositive patients and patients with other neurological disease. *AIDS* 11:1699–1708.

1081. Dickie, P., J. Felser, M. Eckhaus, J. Bryant, J. Silver, N. Marison, and A. L. Notkins. 1991. HIV-associated nephropathy in transgenic mice expressing HIV-1 genes. *Virology* 185: 109–119.

1082. Dickover, R. E., E. M. Garratty, S. A. Herman, M.-S. Sim, S. Plaeger, P. J. Boyer, M. Keller, A. Deveikis, E. R. Stiehm, and Y. J. Bryson. 1996. Identification of levels of maternal HIV-1 RNA associated with risk of perinatal transmission. *JAMA* 275:599–605.

1083. Diegel, M. L., P. A. Moran, L. K. Gilliland, N. K. Damle, M. S. Hayden, J. M. Zarling, and J. A. Ledbetter. 1993. Regulation of HIV production by blood mononuclear cells from HIV-infected donors. II. HIV-1 production depends on T cell-monocyte interaction. *AIDS Res. Hum. Retrovir.* 9:465–473.

1084. Digiovanna, J. J., and B. Safai. 1981. Kaposi's sarcoma. Retrospective study of 90 cases with particular reference to the familial occurrence, ethnic background, and prevalence of other diseases. *Am. J. Med.* 71:779–783.

1085. Dikeacou, T., A. Katsambas, W. Lowenstein, C. Romana, A. Balamotis, P. Tsianakas, A. Carabinis, N. Renieri, N. Metaxotos, E. Fragouli, and J. Stratigos. 1992. Clinical manifestations of allergy and their relation to HIV infection. *Int. Arch. Allergy Immunol.* 102:408–413.

1086. Dillon, S., A. Agrawal, T. Van Dyke, G. Landreth, L. McCauley, A. Koh, C. Maliszewski, S. Akira, and B. Pulendran. 2004. A Toll-like receptor 2 ligand stimulates Th2 responses in vivo, via induction of extracellular signal-regulated kinase mitogen-activated protein kinase and c-Fos in dendritic cells. *J. Immunol.* 172:4733–4743.

1087. Dimitrov, D. S., H. Golding, and R. Blumenthal. 1991. Initial stages of HIV-1 envelope glycoprotein-mediated cell fusion monitored by a new assay based on redistribution of fluorescent dyes. *AIDS Res. Hum. Retrovir.* 7:799–805.

1088. Dimitrov, D. S., R. L. Willey, M. A. Martin, and R. Blumenthal. 1992. Kinetics of HIV-1 interactions with sCD4 and CD4+ cells: implications for inhibition of virus infection and intitial steps of virus entry into cells. *Virology* 187:398–406.

1089. Dimitrov, D. S., R. L. Willey, H. Sato, L.-J. Chang, R. Blumenthal, and M. A. Martin. 1993. Quantitation of human immunodeficiency virus type 1 infection kinetics. *J. Virol.* 67:2182–2190.

1090. Dimmock, N. J. 1982. Initial stages in infection with animal viruses. *J. Gen. Virol.* 59:1–22.

1091. Dimmock, N. J. 1995. Update on the neutralization of animal viruses. *Rev. Med. Virol.* 5:163–179.

1092. Dion, M. L., J. F. Poulin, R. Bordi, M. Sylvestre, R. Corsini, N. Kettaf, A. Dalloul, M. R. Boulassel, P. Debre, J. P. Routy, Z. Grossman, R. P. Sekaly, and R. Cheynier. 2004. HIV infection rapidly induces and maintains a substantial suppression of thymocyte proliferation. *Immunity* 21:757–768.

1093. Dioszeghy, V., K. Benlhassan-Chahour, B. Delache, N. Dereuddre-Bosquet, C. Aubenque, G. Gras, R. Le Grand, and B. Vaslin. 2006. Changes in soluble factor-mediated CD8+ cell-derived antiviral activity in cynomolgus macaques infected with simian immunodeficiency virus SIVmac251: relationship to biological markers of progression. *J. Virol.* 80:236–245.

1094. Dirac, A. M. G., H. Huthoff, J. Kjems, and B. Berkhout. 2002. Requirements for RNA heterodimerization of the human immunodeficiency virus type 1 (HIV-1) and HIV-2 genomes. *J. Gen. Virol.* 83:2533–2542.

1095. Dittmar, M. T., A. McNight, G. Simmons, P. R. Clapham, R. A. Weiss, and P. Simmonds. 1997. HIV-1 tropism and coreceptor use. *Nature* 385:495–496.

1096. Dittmar, M. T., G. Simmons, S. Hibbitts, M. O'Hare, S. Louisirirotchanakul, S. Beddows, J. Weber, P. R. Clapham, and R. A. Weiss. 1997. Langerhans cell tropism of human immunodeficiency virus type 1 subtype A through F isolates derived from different transmission groups. *J. Virol.* 71:8008–8013.

1097. Dobrescu, D., S. Kabak, K. Mehta, C. H. Suh, A. Asch, P. U. Cameron, A. S. Hodtsev, and D. N. Posnett. 1995. Human immunodeficiency virus 1 reservoir in CD4+ T cells is restricted to certain Vβ subsets. *Proc. Natl. Acad. Sci. USA* 92:5563–5567.

1098. Dockrell, D. H., A. D. Badley, A. Algeciras-Schimnich, M. Simpson, R. Schut, D. H. Lynch, and C. V. Paya. 1999. Activation-induced CD4+ T cell death in HIV-positive individuals correlates with Fas susceptibility, CD4+ T cell count, and HIV plasma viral copy number. *AIDS Res. Hum. Retrovir.* 15:1509–1518.

1099. Doehle, B. P., A. Schafer, and B. R. Cullen. 2005. Human APOBEC3B is a potent inhibitor of HIV-1 infectivity and is resistant to HIV-1 Vif. *Virology* 339:281–288.

1100. Doehle, B. P., A. Schafer, H. L. Wiegand, H. P. Bogerd, and B. R. Cullen. 2005. Differential sensitivity of murine leukemia virus to APOBEC3-mediated inhibition is governed by virion exclusion. *J. Virol.* 79:8201–8207.

1101. Doherty, P. C., B. B. Knowles, and P. J. Wettstein. 1984. Immunological surveillance of tumors in the context of major histocompatibility complex restriction of T cell function. *Adv. Cancer Res.* 42:1–65.

1102. Dolei, A., A. Biolchini, C. Serra, S. Curreli, E. Gomes, and F. Dianzani. 1998. Increased replication of T-cell-tropic HIV strains and CXC-chemokine receptor-4 induction in T cells treated with macrophage inflammatory protein (MIP)-1α, MIP-1β and RANTES β-chemokines. *AIDS* 12:183–190.

1103. Dolei, A., C. Serra, M. V. Arca, and A. Toiolo. 1992. Acute HIV-1 infection of CD4+ human lung fibroblasts. *AIDS* 6:232–233.

1104. Dolin, R., B. S. Graham, S. B. Greenberg, C. O. Tacket, R. B. Belshe, K. Midthun, M. L. Clements, G. J. Gorse, B. W. Horgan, R. L. Atmar, D. T. Larzon, W. Bonnez, B. F. Fernie, D. C. Montefiore, D. M. Stablein, G. E. Smith, and W. C. Koff. 1991. The safety and immunogenicity of a human immunodeficiency virus type 1 (HIV-1) recombinant gp160 candidate vaccine in humans. *Ann. Intern. Med.* 114:119–127.

1105. Dominguez, V., G. Gevorkian, T. Govezensky, H. Rodriguez, M. Viveros, G. Cocho, Y. Macotela, F. Masso, M. Pacheco, J. L. Estrada, C. Lavalle, and C. Larralde. 1998. Antigenic homology of HIV-1 GP41 and human platelet glycoprotein GPIIIa (Integrin β3). *J. Acquir. Immune Defic. Syndr. Hum. Retrovirol.* 17:385–390.

1106. Doms, R. W. 2000. Beyond receptor expression: the influence of receptor conformation, density, and affinity in HIV-1 infection. *Virology* 276:229–237.

1107. Doms, R. W. 2004. Unwelcome guests with master keys: how HIV enters cells and how it can be stopped. *Top. HIV Med.* 12:100–103.

1108. Donaghy, H., A. Pozniak, B. Gazzard, N. Qazi, J. Gilmour, F. Gotch, and S. Patterson. 2001. Loss of blood CD11c(+) myeloid and CD11c(-) plasmacytoid dendritic cells in patients with HIV-1 infection correlates with HIV-1 RNA virus load. *Blood* 98:2574–2576.

1109. Donaghy, H., J. Wilkinson, and A. L. Cunningham. 2006. HIV interactions with dendritic cells: has our focus been too narrow? *J. Leukoc. Biol.* 80:1001–1012.

1109a. Dondi, E., G. Roue, V. J. Yuste, S. A. Susin, and S. Pellegrini. 2004. A dual role of IFN-alpha in the balance between proliferation and death of human CD4+ T lymphocytes during primary response. *J. Immunol.* 173:3740–3747.

1110. Donegan, E., M. Stuart, J. C. Niland, H. S. Sacks, S. P. Azen, S. L. Dietrich, C. Faucett, M. A. Fletcher, S. H. Kleinman, and E. A. Operskalski. 1990. Infection with human immunodeficiency virus type 1 (HIV-1) among recipients of antibody-positive blood donations. *Ann. Intern. Med.* **113**: 733–739.

1111. Donnelly, C., W. Leisenring, P. Kanki, T. Awerbuci, and S. Sandberg. 1993. Comparison of transmission rates of HIV-1 and HIV-2 in a cohort of prostitutes in Senegal. *Bull. Math. Biol.* **55**:731–743.

1112. Donnelly, J. J., B. Wahren, and M. A. Liu. 2005. DNA vaccines: progress and challenges. *J. Immunol.* **175**:633–639.

1113. Donovan, R. M., C. E. Bush, N. P. Markowitz, D. M. Baxa, and L. D. Saravolatz. 1996. Changes in virus load markers during AIDS-associated opportunistic diseases in human immunodeficiency virus-infected persons. *J. Infect. Dis.* **174**:401–403.

1114. Dorak, M. T., J. Tang, S. Tang, A. Penman-Aguilar, R. A. Coutinho, J. J. Godert, R. Detels, and R. A. Kaslow. 2003. Influence of human leukocyte antigen-B22 alleles on the course of human immunodeficiency virus type 1 infection in 3 cohorts of white men. *J. Infect. Dis.* **188**:856–863.

1115. Doranz, B. J., J. Rucker, Y. Yi, R. J. Smyth, M. Samsom, S. C. Peiper, M. Parmentier, R. G. Collman, and R. W. Doms. 1996. A dual-tropic primary HIV-1 isolate that uses fusin and the b-chemokine receptors CKR-5, CKR-3, and CKR-2b as fusion cofactors. *Cell* **85**:1149–1158.

1116. Dorell, L., A. J. Hessell, M. Wang, H. Whittle, S. Sabally, S. Rowland-Jones, D. R. Burton, and P. W. H. I. Parren. 2000. Absence of specific mucosal antibody responses in HIV-exposed uninfected sex workers from Gambia. *AIDS* **14**:1117–1122.

1117. Dorenbaum, A., C. K. Cunningham, R. D. Gelber, M. Culnane, L. Mofenson, P. Britto, C. Rekacewicz, M. L. Newell, J. F. Delfraissy, B. Cunningham-Schrader, M. Mirochnick, and J. L. Sullivan. 2002. Two-dose intrapartum/newborn nevirapine and standard antiretroviral therapy to reduce perinatal HIV transmission: a randomized trial. *JAMA* **288**:189–198.

1118. Dorrucci, M., G. Rezza, D. Vlahov, P. Pezzotti, A. Sinicco, A. Nicolosi, A. Lazzarin, N. Galai, S. Gafa, R. Pristera, and G. Angarano. 1995. Clinical characteristics and prognostic value of acute retroviral syndrome among injecting drug users. *AIDS* **9**:597–604.

1119. Dorsett, B. H., W. Cronin, and H. L. Ioachim. 1990. Presence and prognostic significance of antilymphocyte antibodies in symptomatic and asymptomatic human immunodeficiency virus infection. *Arch. Intern. Med.* **150**:1025–1028.

1120. Douek, D. C., J. M. Brenchley, M. R. Betts, D. R. Ambrozak, B. J. Hill, Y. Okamoto, J. P. Casazza, J. Kuruppu, K. Kunstman, S. Wolinsky, Z. Grossman, M. Dybul, A. Oxenius, D. A. Price, M. Connors, and R. A. Koup. 2002. HIV preferentially infects HIV-specific CD4+ T cells. *Nature* **417**:95–96.

1121. Douek, D. C., R. D. McFarland, P. H. Keiser, E. A. Gage, J. M. Massey, B. F. Haynes, M. A. Polis, A. T. Haase, M. B. Feinberg, J. L. Sullivan, B. D. Jamieson, J. A. Zack, L. J. Picker, and R. A. Koup. 1998. Changes in thymic function with age and during the treatment of HIV infection. *Nature* **396**:690–695.

1122. Douek, D. C., L. J. Picker, and R. A. Koup. 2003. T cell dynamics in HIV-1 infection. *Annu. Rev. Immunol.* **21**:265–304.

1123. Douglas, S. D., S. J. Durako, N. B. Tustin, J. Houser, L. Muenz, S. E. Starr, and C. Wilson. 2001. Natural killer cell enumeration and function in HIV-infected and high-risk uninfected adolescents. *AIDS Res. Hum. Retrovir.* **17**:543–552.

1124. Dournon, E., S. Matheron, W. Rozenbaum, S. Gharakhanian, C. Michon, P. M. Girard, C. Perronne, D. Salmon, P. De Truchis, C. Leport, E. Bouvet, M. C. Dazza, M. Levacher, and B. Regnier. 1988. Effects of zidovudine in 365 consecutive patients with AIDS or AIDS-related complex. *Lancet* **ii**:1297–1302.

1125. Downs, A. M., and I. De Vincenzi. 1996. Probability of heterosexual transmission of HIV: relationship to the number of unprotected sexual contacts. *J. Acquir. Immune Defic. Syndr. Hum. Retrovirol.* **11**:388–395.

1126. Draenert, R., S. Le Gall, K. J. Pfafferott, A. J. Leslie, P. Chetty, C. Brander, E. C. Holmes, S. Chang, M. E. Feeney, M. M. Addo, L. Ruis, D. Ramduth, P. Jeena, M. Altfeld, J. G. Prado, P. Kiepiela, J. Martinez-Picado, B. D. Walker, and P. J. R. Goulder. 2004. Immune selection for altered antigen processing leads to cytotoxic T lymphocyte escape in chronic HIV-1 infection. *J. Exp. Med.* **199**:905–915.

1127. Draenert, R., C. L. Verrill, Y. Tang, T. M. Allen, A. G. Wurcel, M. Boczanowski, A. Lechner, A. Y. Kim, T. Suscovich, N. V. Brown, M. M. Addo, and B. D. Walker. 2004. Persistent recognition of autologous virus by high-avidity CD8 T cells in chronic, progressive human immunodeficiency virus type 1 infection. *J. Virol.* **78**:630–641.

1128. Dragic, T. 2001. An overview of the determinants of CCR5 and CXCR4 co-receptor function. *J. Gen. Virol.* **82**: 1807–1814.

1129. Dragic, T., P. Charneau, F. Clavel, and M. Alizon. 1992. Complementation of murine cells for human immunodeficiency virus envelope/CD4-mediated fusion in human/murine heterokaryons. *J. Virol.* **66**:4794–4802.

1130. Dragic, T., V. Litwin, G. P. Allaway, S. R. Martin, Y. Huang, K. A. Nagashima, C. Cayanan, P. J. Maddon, R. A. Koup, J. P. Moore, and W. A. Paxton. 1996. HIV-1 entry into CD4+ cells is mediated by the chemokine receptor CC-CKR-5. *Nature* **381**:667–673.

1131. Dragic, T., L. Picard, and M. Alizon. 1995. Proteinase-resistant factors in human erythrocyte membranes mediate CD4-dependent fusion with cells expressing human immunodeficiency virus type 1 envelope glycoproteins. *J. Virol.* **69**:1013–1018.

1132. Dreesman, G. R., and R. C. Kennedy. 1985. Anti-idiotypic antibodies: implications of internal image-based vaccines for infectious diseases. *J. Infect. Dis.* **151**:761–765.

1133. Dreyer, E. B., P. K. Kaiser, J. T. Offermann, and S. A. Lipton. 1990. HIV-1 coat protein neurotoxicity prevented by calcium channel antagonists. *Science* **248**:364–367.

1134. Dropulic, B. 2005. Genetic modification of hematopoietic cells using retroviral and lentiviral vectors: safety considerations for vector design and delivery into target cells. *Curr. Hematol. Rep.* **4**:300–304.

1135. Drucker, E., P. G. Alcabes, and P. A. Marx. 2001. The infection century: massive unsterile injections and the emergence of human pathogens. *Lancet* **358**:1989–1992.

1136. Drummond, J. E., P. Mounts, R. J. Gorelick, J. R. Casas-Finet, W. J. Bosche, L. E. Henderson, D. J. Waters, and L. O. Arthur. 1997. Wild-type and mutant HIV type 1 nucleocapsid proteins increase the proportion of long cDNA transcripts by viral reverse transcriptase. *AIDS Res. Hum. Retrovir.* **13**:533–543.

1137. Drysdale, C. M., and G. N. Pavlakis. 1991. Rapid activation and subsequent down-regulation of the human immunodeficiency virus type 1 promoter in the presence of *tat*: possible mechanisms contributing to latency. *J. Virol.* 65:3044–3051.

1138. **Du Pont, H. L., and G. D. Marshall.** 1995. HIV-associated diarrhea and wasting. *Lancet* 346:352–356.

1139. **Duan, L., J. W. Oakes, A. Ferraro, O. Bagasra, and R. J. Pomerantz.** 1994. Tat and Rev differentially affect restricted replication of human immunodeficiency virus type 1 in various cells. *Virology* 199:474–478.

1140. **Dudhane, A., B. Conti, T. Orlikowsky, Z. Q. Wang, N. Mangla, A. Gupta, G. P. Wormser, and M. K. Hoffmann.** 1996. Monocytes in HIV type 1-infected individuals lose expression of costimulatory B7 molecules and acquire cytotoxic activity. *AIDS Res. Hum. Retrovir.* 12:885–892.

1141. **Duerr, A., Z. Xia, T. Nagachinta, S. Tovanabutra, A. Tansuhaj, and K. Nelson.** 1996. Probability of male-female HIV transmission among married couples in Chiang Mai, Thailand. *10th International Conference on AIDS*, Yokohama, Japan.

1142. **Dugas, N., N. Dereuddre-Bosquet, C. Goujard, D. Dormont, M. Tardieu, and J. F. Delfraissy.** 2000. Role of nitric oxide in the promoting effect of HIV type 1 infection and of gp120 envelope glycoprotein on interleukin 4-induced IgE production by normal human mononuclear cells. *AIDS Res. Hum. Retrovir.* 10:251–258.

1143. **Duggal, P., P. An, T. H. Beaty, S. A. Strathdee, H. Farzadegan, R. B. Markham, L. Johnson, S. J. O'Brien, D. Vlahov, and C. A. Winkler.** 2003. Genetic influence of CXCR6 chemokine receptor alleles on PCP-mediated AIDS progression among African Americans. *Genes Immun.* 4:245–250.

1144. **Duh, E. J., W. J. Maury, T. M. Folks, A. S. Fauci, and A. B. Rabson.** 1989. Tumor necrosis factor alpha activates human immunodeficiency virus type 1 through induction of nuclear factor binding to the NF-kappa B sites in the long terminal repeat. *Proc. Natl. Acad. Sci. USA* 86:5794–5978.

1145. **Dukers, N. H. T. M., and G. Rezza.** 2003. Human herpesvirus 8 epidemiology: what we do and do not know. *AIDS* 17:1717–1730.

1146. **Dukes, C. S., Y. Yu, E. D. Rivadeneira, D. L. Sauls, H.-X. Liao, B. F. Haynes, and J. B. Weinberg.** 1995. Cellular CD44s as a determinant of human immunodeficiency virus type 1 infection and cellular tropism. *J. Virol.* 69:4000–4005.

1147. **Dumais, N., B. Barbeau, M. Olivier, and M. J. Tremblay.** 1998. Prostaglandin E$_2$ up-regulates HIV-1 long terminal repeat-driven gene activity in T cells via NF-κB-dependent and -independent signaling pathways. *J. Biol. Chem.* 273:27306–27314.

1148. **Dumais, N., A. Patrick, R. B. Moss, H. L. Davis, and K. L. Rosenthal.** 2002. Mucosal immunization with inactivated human immunodeficiency virus plus CpG oligodeoxynucleotides induces genital immune responses and protection against intravaginal challenge. *J. Infect. Dis.* 186:1098–1105.

1149. **Dumitrescu, O., M. Kalish, S. C. Kliks, C. I. Bandea, and J. A. Levy.** 1994. Characterization of HIV-1 strains isolated from children in Romania: identification of a new envelope subtype. *J. Infect. Dis.* 169:281–288.

1150. **Dunham, R., P. Pagliardini, S. Gordon, B. Sumpter, J. Engram, A. Moanna, M. Paiardini, J. N. Mandl, B. Lawson, S. Garg, H. McClure, Y. X. Xu, C. Ibegbu, K. Easley, N. Katz, I. Pandrea, C. Apetrei, D. L. Sodora, S. I. Staprans, M. B. Feinberg, and G. Silvestri.** 2006. The AIDS resistance of naturally SIV-infected sooty mangabeys is independent of cellular immunity to the virus. *Blood* 108: 209–217.

1151. **Dunn, D. T., M. L. Newell, A. E. Ades, and C. S. Peckham.** 1992. Risk of human immunodeficiency virus type 1 transmission through breastfeeding. *Lancet* 340:585–588.

1152. **Dupin, N., T. L. Diss, P. Kellum, M. Tulliez, M. Du, D. Sicard, R. A. Weiss, P. G. Isaacson, and C. Boshoff.** 2000. HHV-8 is associated with a plasmablastic variant of Castleman disease that is linked to HHV8-positive plasmablastic lymphoma. *Blood* 95:1406–1412.

1153. **Durbin, J. E., A. Fernandez-Sesma, C. K. Lee, T. D. Rao, A. B. Frey, T. M. Moran, S. Vukmanovic, A. Garcia-Sastre, and D. E. Levy.** 2000. Type I IFN modulates innate and specific antiviral immunity. *J. Immunol.* 164:4220–4228.

1154. **Duvall, M. G., A. Jaye, T. Dong, J. M. Brenchley, A. S. Alabi, D. J. Jeffries, M. van der Sande, T. O. Togun, S. J. McConkey, D. C. Douek, A. J. McMichael, H. C. Whittle, R. A. Koup, and S. L. Rowland-Jones.** 2006. Maintenance of HIV-specific CD4+ T cell help distinguishes HIV-2 from HIV-1 infection. *J. Immunol.* 176:6973–6981.

1155. **Dybul, M., M. Daucher, M. A. Jensen, C. W. Hallahan, T. W. Chun, M. Belson, B. Hidalgo, D. C. Nickle, C. Yoder, J. A. Metcalf, R. T. Davey, L. Ehler, D. Kress-Rock, E. Nies-Kraske, S. Liu, J. I. Mullins, and A. S. Fauci.** 2003. Genetic characterization of rebounding human immunodeficiency virus type 1 in plasma during multiple interruptions of highly active antiretroviral therapy. *J. Virol.* 77:3229–3237.

1156. **Dybul, M., E. Nies-Kraske, M. Daucher, K. Hertogs, C. W. Hallahan, G. Csako, C. Yoder, L. Ehler, P. A. Sklar, M. Belson, B. Hidalgo, J. A. Metcalf, R. T. Davey, D. M. Rock Kress, A. Powers, and A. S. Fauci.** 2003. Long-cycle structured intermittent versus continuous highly active antiretroviral therapy for the treatment of chronic infection with human immunodeficiency virus: effects on drug toxicity and on immunologic and virologic parameters. *J. Infect. Dis.* 188:388–396.

1157. **Dyda, F., A. B. Hickman, T. M. Jenkins, A. Engelman, R. Craigie, and D. R. Davies.** 1994. Crystal structure of the catalytic domain of HIV-1 integrase: similarity to other polynucleotidyl transferases. *Science* 266:1981–1986.

1158. **Dyer, W. B., A. F. Geczy, S. J. Kent, L. B. McIntyre, S. A. Blasdall, J. C. Learmont, and J. S. Sullivan.** 1997. Lymphoproliferative immune function in the Sydney Blood Bank Cohort, infected with natural nef/long terminal repeat mutants, and in other long-term survivors of transfusion-acquired HIV-1 infection. *AIDS* 11:1565–1574.

1159. **Dyer, W. B., G. S. Ogg, M. A. Demoitie, X. Jin, A. F. Geczy, S. L. Rowland-Jones, A. J. McMichael, D. F. Nixon, and J. S. Sullivan.** 1999. Strong human immunodeficiency virus (HIV)-specific cytotoxic T-lymphocyte activity in Sydney Blood Bank Cohort patients infected with nef-defective HIV type 1. *J. Virol.* 73:436–443.

1160. **Dykes, C., M. Balakrishnan, V. Planelles, Y. Zhu, R. A. Bambara, and L. M. Demeter.** 2004. Identification of a preferred region for recombination and mutation in HIV-1 *gag*. *Virology* 326:262–279.

1161. **Dzionek, A., A. Fuchs, P. Schmidt, S. Cremer, M. Zysk, S. Miltenyi, D. W. Buck, and J. Schmitz.** 2000. BDCA-2, BDCA-3, and BDCA-4: three markers for distinct subsets of dendritic cells in human peripheral blood. *J. Immunol.* 165:6037–6046.

1162. **Earl, P. L., R. W. Doms, and B. Moss.** 1990. Oligomeric structure of the human immunodeficiency virus type 1 envelope glycoprotein. *Proc. Natl. Acad. Sci. USA* 87:648–652.

1163. Earl, P. L., R. W. Doms, and B. Moss. 1992. Multimeric CD4 binding exhibited by human and simian immunodeficiency virus envelope protein dimers. *J. Virol.* **66:**5610–5614.

1164. Easterbrook, P. J., T. Rostron, N. Ives, M. Troop, B. G. Gazzard, and S. L. Rowland-Jones. 1999. Chemokine receptor polymorphisms and human immunodeficiency virus disease progression. *J. Infect. Dis.* 180:1096–1105.

1165. Eaton, A. M., T. Wildes, and J. A. Levy. 1994. An anti-gp41 human monoclonal antibody which enhances HIV-1 infection in the absence of complement. *AIDS Res. Hum. Retrovir.* 10:13–18.

1166. Ebenbichler, C., P. Westervelt, A. Carrillo, T. Henkel, D. Johnson, and L. Ratner. 1993. Structure-function relationships of the HIV-1 envelope V3 loop tropism determinant: evidence for two distinct conformations. *AIDS* 7:639–646.

1167. Ebenbichler, C. F., C. Roder, R. Vornhagen, L. Ratner, and M. P. Dierich. 1993. Cell surface proteins binding to recombinant soluble HIV-1 and HIV-2 transmembrane proteins. *AIDS* 7:489–495.

1168. Ebenbichler, C. F., N. M. Thielens, R. Vornhagen, P. Marschang, G. J. Arlaud, and M. P. Dierich. 1991. Human immunodeficiency virus type 1 activates the classical pathway of complement by direct C1 binding through specific sites in the transmembrane glycoprotein gp41. *J. Exp. Med.* 174:1417–1424.

1169. Eda, Y., T. Murakami, Y. Ami, T. Nakasone, M. Takizawa, K. Someya, M. Kaizu, Y. Izumi, N. Yoshino, S. Matsushita, H. Higuchi, H. Matsui, K. Shinohara, H. Takeuchi, Y. Koyanagi, N. Yamamoto, and M. Honda. 2006. Anti-V3 humanized antibody KD-247 effectively suppresses ex vivo generation of human immunodeficiency virus type 1 and affords sterile protection of monkeys against a heterologous simian/human immunodeficiency virus infection. *J. Virol.* 80:5563–5570.

1170. Edinger, A. L., J. E. Clements, and R. W. Doms. 1999. Chemokine and orphan receptors in HIV-2 and SIV tropism and pathogenesis. *Virology* 260:211–221.

1171. Edinger, A. L., J. L. Mankowski, B. J. Doranz, B. J. Margulies, B. Lee, J. Rucker, M. Sharron, T. L. Hoffman, J. F. Berson, M. C. Zink, V. M. Hirsch, J. E. Clements, and R. W. Doms. 1997. CD4-independent, CCR5-dependent infection of brain capillary endothelial cells by a neurovirulent simian immunodeficiency virus strain. *Proc. Natl. Acad. Sci.* USA 94:14742–14747.

1172. Edwards, T. G., T. L. Hoffman, F. Baribaud, S. Wyss, C. C. LaBranche, J. Romano, J. Adkinson, M. Sharron, J. A. Hoxie, and R. W. Doms. 2001. Relationships between CD4 independence, neutralization sensitivity, and exposure of a CD4-induced epitope in a human immunodeficiency virus type 1 envelope protein. *J. Virol.* 75:5230–5239.

1173. Effros, R. B., R. Allsopp, C. P. Chiu, M. A. Hausner, K. Hirji, L. Wang, C. B. Harley, B. Villeponteau, M. D. West, and J. V. Giorgi. 1996. Shortened telomeres in the expanded CD28-CD8+ cell subset in HIV disease implicate replicative senescence in HIV pathogenesis. *AIDS* 10:F17-F22.

1174. Egan, M. A., S. Y. Chong, M. Hagen, S. Megati, E. B. Schadeck, P. Piacente, B. J. Ma, D. C. Montefiori, B. F. Haynes, Z. R. Israel, J. H. Eldridge, and H. F. Staats. 2004. A comparative evaluation of nasal and parenteral vaccine adjuvants to elicit systemic and mucosal HIV-1 peptide-specific humoral immune responses in cynomolgus macaques. *Vaccine* 22:3774–3788.

1175. Egan, M. A., W. A. Pavlat, J. Tartaglia, E. Paoletti, K. J. Weinhold, M. Clements, and R. F. Siliciano. 1995. Induction of human immunodeficiency virus type 1 (HIV-1)-specific cytolytic T lymphocyte responses in seronegative adults by a nonreplicating, host-range-restricted canarypox vector (ALVAC) carrying the HIV-1$_{MN}$ env gene. *J. Infect. Dis.* 171:1623–1627.

1175a. Eggena, M. P., B. Barugahare, N. Jones, M. Okello, S. Mutalya, C. Kityo, P. Mugyenyi, and H. Cao. 2005. Depletion of regulatory T cells in HIV infection is associated with immune activation. *J. Immunol.* 174:4407–4414.

1176. Egger, M., M. May, G. Chene, A. N. Phillips, B. Ledergerber, F. Dabis, D. Costagliola, A. Monforte, F. de Wolf, P. Reiss, J. D. Kundgren, A. C. Justice, S. Staszewski, C. Leport, R. S. Hogg, C. S. Sabin, N. Gill, B. Salzberger, and J. A. C. Sterne. 2002. Prognosis of HIV-1-infected patients starting highly active antiretroviral therapy: a collaborative analysis of prospective studies. *Lancet* 360:119–129.

1177. Eggers, C. C., J. van Lunzen, T. Buhk, and H. J. Stellbrink. 1999. HIV infection of the central nervous system is characterized by rapid turnover of viral RNA in cerebrospinal fluid. *J. Acquir. Immune Defic. Syndr. Hum. Retrovirol.* 20:259–264.

1178. Ehrenreich, H., P. Rieckmann, F. Sinowatz, K. A. Weih, L. O. Arthur, F. D. Goebel, P. R. Burd, J. E. Coligan, and K. A. Clouse. 1993. Potent stimulation of monocytic endothelin-1 production by HIV-1 glycoprotein 120. *J. Immunol.* 150:4601–4609.

1179. Ehret, A., M. O. Westendorp, I. Herr, K. M. Debatin, J. L. Heeney, R. Frank, and P. H. Krammer. 1996. Resistance of chimpanzee T cells to human immunodeficiency virus type 1 Tat-enhanced oxidative stress and apoptosis. *J. Virol.* 70:6502–6507.

1180. Ehrnst, A., S. Lindgren, M. Dictor, B. Johansson, A. Sonnerborg, J. Czajkowski, G. Sundin, and A.-B. Bohlin. 1991. HIV in pregnant women and their offspring: evidence for late transmission. *Lancet* 338:203–207.

1181. Ehrnst, A., A. Sonnerborg, S. Bergdahl, and O. Strannegard. 1988. Efficient isolation of HIV from plasma during different stages of HIV infection. *J. Med. Virol.* 26:23–32.

1182. Eisert, V., M. Kreutz, K. Becker, C. Konigs, U. Alex, H. Rubsamen-Waigmann, R. Andreesen, and H. von Briesen. 2001. Analysis of cellular factors influencing the replication of human immunodeficiency virus type 1 in human macrophages derived from blood of different healthy donors. *Virology* 286:31–44.

1183. Eitner, F., Y. Cui, K. L. Hudkins, M. B. Stokes, M. Segerer, M. Mack, P. L. Lewis, A. A. Abraham, D. Schlondorff, G. Gallo, P. L. Kimmel, and C. E. Alpers. 2000. Chemokine receptor CCR5 and CXCR4 expression in HIV-associated kidney disease. *J. Am. Soc. Nephrol.* 11:856–867.

1184. El Messaoudi, K., L. F. Thiry, C. Liesnard, N. Van Tieghem, A. Bollen, and N. Moguilevsky. 2000. A human milk factor susceptible to cathepsin D inhibitors enhances human immunodeficiency virus type 1 infectivity and allows virus entry into a mammary epithelial cell line. *J. Virol.* 74:1004–1007.

1185. El-Amad, Z., K. K. Murthy, K. Higgins, E. K. Cobb, N. L. Haigwood, J. A. Levy, and K. S. Steimer. 1995. Resistance of chimpanzees immunized with recombinant gp120$_{SF2}$ to challenge by HIV-1$_{SF2}$. *AIDS* 9:1313–1322.

1186. El-Daher, N., M. C. Keefer, R. C. Reichman, R. Dolin, and N. J. Roberts, Jr. 1993. Persisting human immunodeficiency virus type 1 gp160-specific human T lymphocyte responses including CD8+ cytotoxic activity after receipt of envelope vaccines. *J. Infect. Dis.* 168:306–313.

1186a. El-Sadr, W. M., J. D. Lundgren, J. D. Neaton, F. Gordin, D. Abrams, R. C. Arduino, A. Babiker, W. Burman, N. Clumeck, C. J. Cohen, D. Cohn, D. Cooper, J. Darbyshire, S. Emery, G. Fatkerheuer, B. Gazzard, B. Brund, J. Howy, K. Klingman, M. Losso, N. Markowitz, J. Neuhaus, A. Phillips, C. Rappoport, and for the Strategies for Management of Antiretroviral Therapy (SMART) Study. 2006. CD4+ count-guided interruption of antiretroviral treatment. *N. Engl. J. Med.* 355:2283–2296.

1187. El-Sadr, W. M., W. J. Burman, L. B. Grant, J. P. Matts, R. Hafner, L. Crane, D. Zeh, B. Gallagher, S. B. Mannheimer, A. Martinez, F. Gordin, and theTerry Beirn Community Programs for Clinical Research on AIDS. 2000. Discontinuation of prophylaxis for Mycobacterium avium complex disease in HIV-infected patients who have a response to antiretroviral therapy. *N. Engl. J. Med.* 342:1085–1092.

1188. Elkins, M. K., E. Vittinghoff, W. E. Baranzini, F. M. Hecht, U. Sriram, M. P. Busch, J. A. Levy, and J. R. Oksenberg. 2005. Longitudinal analysis B cell repertoire and antibody gene rearrangements during early HIV infection. *Genes Immun.* 6:66–69.

1189. Ellenberger, D. L., P. S. Sullivan, J. Dorn, C. Schable, T. J. Spira, T. M. Folks, and R. B. Lal. 1999. Viral and immunologic examination of human immunodeficiency virus type 1-infected, persistently seronegative persons. *J. Infect. Dis.* 180:1033–1042.

1190. Ellerbrock, T. V., M. A. Chiasson, T. J. Bush, X.-W. Sun, D. Sawo, K. Brudney, and T. C. Wright. 2000. Incidence of cervical squamous intraepithelial lesions in HIV-infected women. *JAMA* 283:1031–1037.

1191. Ellerbrock, T. V., J. L. Lennox, K. A. Clancy, R. F. Schinazi, T. C. Wright, M. Pratt-Palmore, T. Evans-Strickfaden, C. Schnell, R. Pai, L. J. Conley, E. E. Parrish-Kohler, T. J. Bush, K. Tatti, and C. E. Hart. 2001. Cellular replication of human immunodeficiency virus type 1 occurs in vaginal secretions. *J. Infect. Dis.* 184:28–36.

1192. Emau, P., H. M. McClure, M. Isahakia, J. G. Else, and P. N. Fultz. 1991. Isolation from African Sykes' monkeys *(Cercopithecus mitis)* of a lentivirus related to human and simian immunodeficiency viruses. *J. Virol.* 65:2135–2140.

1193. Embretson, J., M. Zupancic, J. Beneke, M. Till, S. Wolinsky, J. L. Ribas, A. Burke, and A. T. Haase. 1993. Analysis of human immunodeficiency virus-infected tissues by amplification and *in situ* hybridization reveals latent and permissive infections at single-cell resolution. *Proc. Natl. Acad. Sci. USA* 90:357–361.

1194. Embretson, J., M. Zupancic, J. L. Ribas, A. Burke, P. Racz, K. Tenner-Racz, and A. T. Haase. 1993. Massive covert infection of helper T lymphocytes and macrophages by HIV during the incubation period of AIDS. *Nature* 362:359–362.

1195. Emery, S., and H. C. Lane. 1997. Immune reconstitution in HIV infection. *Curr. Opin. Immunol.* 9:549–550.

1196. Emiliani, S., W. Fischle, M. Ott, C. Van Lint, C. A. Amella, and E. Verdin. 1998. Mutations in the *tat* gene are responsible for human immunodeficiency virus type 1 postintegration latency in the U1 cell line. *J. Virol.* 72:1666–1770.

1197. Emiliani, S., C. Van Lint, W. Fischle, P. Paras, Jr., M. Ott, J. Brady, and E. Verdin. 1996. A point mutation in the HIV-1 Tat responsive element is associated with postintegration latency. *Proc. Natl. Acad. Sci. USA* 93:6377–6381.

1198. Emilie, D., M. Burgard, C. Lascoux-Combe, M. Laughlin, R. Krzysiek, C. Pignon, A. Rudent, J. M. Molina, J. M. Livrozet, F. Souala, G. Chene, L. Grangeot-Keros, P. Galanaud, D. Sereni, and C. Rouzioux. 2001. Early control of HIV replication in primary HIV-1 infection treated with antiretroviral drugs and pegylated IFN alpha: results from the Primoferon A (ANRS 086) Study. *AIDS* 15:1435–1437.

1199. Emilie, D., M. Peuchmaur, M. C. Mailott, M. C. Crevon, N. Brousse, J. F. Delfraissy, J. Dormont, and P. Galanaud. 1990. Production of interleukins in human immunodeficiency virus-1-replicating lymph nodes. *J. Clin. Investig.* 86:148–159.

1200. Emini, E. A., W. A. Schleif, J. H. Nunberg, A. J. Conley, Y. Eda, S. Tokiyoshi, S. D. Putney, S. Matsushita, K. E. Cobb, C. M. Jett, J. W. Eichberg, and K. K. Murthy. 1992. Prevention of HIV-1 infection in chimpanzees by gp120 V3 domain-specific monoclonal antibody. *Nature* 355:728–730.

1201. Emu, B., E. Sinclair, D. Favre, W. J. Moretto, P. Hsue, R. Hoh, J. N. Martin, D. F. Nixon, J. M. McCune, and S. G. Deeks. 2005. Phenotypic, functional, and kinetic parameters associated with apparent T-cell control of human immunodeficiency virus replication in individuals with and without antiretroviral treatment. *J. Virol.* 79:14169–14178.

1202. Enders, P. J., C. Yin, F. Martini, P. S. Evans, N. Propp, F. Poccia, and C. D. Pauza. 2003. HIV-mediated gammadelta T cell depletion is specific for Vgamma2+ cells expressing the Jgamma1.2 segment. *AIDS Res. Hum. Retrovir.* 19:21–29.

1203. Endres, M. J., P. R. Clapham, M. Marsh, M. Ahuja, J. D. Turner, A. McKnight, J. F. Thomas, B. Stoebenau-Haggarty, S. Choe, P. J. Vance, T. N. C. Wells, C. A. Power, S. S. Sutterwala, R. W. Doms, N. R. Landau, and J. A. Hoxie. 1996. CD4-independent infection by HIV-2 is mediated by fusin/CXCR4. *Cell* 87:745–756.

1204. Engelman, A., G. Englund, J. M. Orenstein, M. A. Martin, and R. Craigie. 1995. Multiple effects of mutations in human immunodeficiency virus type 1 integrase on viral replication. *J. Virol.* 69:2729–2736.

1205. Engelmayer, J., M. Larsson, A. Lee, M. Lee, W. I. Cox, R. M. Steinman, and N. Bhardwaj. 2001. Mature dendritic cells infected with canarypox virus elicit strong antihuman immunodeficiency virus CD8+ and CD4+ T-cell responses from chronically infected individuals. *J. Virol.* 75:2142–2153.

1206. Engels, E. A., M. Frisch, J. J. Goedert, R. J. Biggar, and R. W. Miller. 2002. Merkel cell carcinoma and HIV infection. *Lancet* 359:497–498.

1207. Engering, A., S. J. van Vliet, T. B. H. Geijtenbeek, and Y. Van Kooyk. 2002. Subset of DC-SIGN(+) dendritic cells in human blood transmits HIV-1 to T lymphocytes. *Blood* 100:1780–1786.

1208. Ennen, J., H. Findeklee, M. T. Dittmar, S. Norley, M. Ernst, and R. Kurth. 1994. CD8+ T lymphocytes of African green monkeys secrete an immunodeficiency virus-suppressing lymphokine. *Proc. Natl. Acad. Sci. USA* 91:7207–7211.

1209. Ennen, J., I. Seipp, S. G. Norley, and R. Kurth. 1990. Decreased accessory cell function of macrophages after infection with human immunodeficiency virus type 1 *in vitro. Eur. J. Immunol.* 20:2451–2456.

1209a. Ensoli, B., V. Fiorelli, F. Ensoli, A. Cafaro, F. Titti, S. Butto, P. Monini, M. Magnani, A. Caputo, and E. Garaci. 2006. Candidate HIV-1 Tat vaccine development: from basic science to clinical trials. *AIDS* 20:2245–2261.

1210. Ensoli, B., R. Gendelman, P. Markham, V. Fiorelli, S. Colombini, M. Raffeld, A. Cafaro, H. K. Chang, J. N. Brady, and R. C. Gallo. 1994. Synergy between basic fibroblast growth factor and HIV-1 Tat protein in induction of Kaposi's sarcoma. *Nature* 371:674–680.

1211. Ensoli, B., C. Sgadari, G. Barillari, M. C. Sirianni, M. Sturzl, and P. Monini. 2001. Biology of Kaposi's sarcoma. *Eur. J. Cancer* 37:1251–1269.

1212. Ensoli, F., V. Fiorelli, M. DeCristofaro, D. Muratori, A. Novi, B. Vannelli, C. Thiele, G. Luzi, and F. Aiuti. 1999. Inflammatory cytokines and HIV-1-associated neurodegeneration: oncostatin-M produced by mononuclear cells from HIV-1-infected individuals induces apoptosis of primary neurons. *J. Immunol.* 162:6268–6277.

1212a. Enting, R. H., R. M. Hoetelmans, J. M. Lange, D. M. Burger, J. H. Beijnen, and P. Portegies. 1998. Antiretroviral drugs and the central nervous system. *AIDS* 12:1941–1955.

1212b. Epple, H. J., C. Loddenkemper, D. Kunkel, H. Troger, J. Maul, V. Moos, E. Berg, R. Ullrich, J. D. Schulzke, H. Stein, R. Duchmann, M. Zeitz, and T. Schneider. 2006. Mucosal but not peripheral FOXP3+ regulatory T cells are highly increased in untreated HIV infection and normalize after suppressive HAART. *Blood* 108:3072–3078.

1213. Epstein, L. G., C. Kuiken, B. M. Blumberg, S. Hartman, L. R. Sharer, M. Clement, and J. Goudsmit. 1991. HIV-1 V3 domain variation in brain and spleen of children with AIDS: tissue-specific evolution within host-determined quasispecies. *Virology* 180:583–590.

1214. Epstein, L. G., and L. R. Sharer. 1988. Neurology of human immunodeficiency virus infection in children, p. 70–101. *In* M. L. Rosenblum, R. M. Levy, and D. E. Bredesen (ed.), *AIDS and the Nervous System.* Raven Press, New York, N.Y.

1215. Epstein, M. A., and B. G. Achong. 1979. The relationship of the virus to Burkitt's lymphoma, p. 321–337. *The Epstein-Barr Virus.* Springer-Verlag, New York, N.Y.

1216. Ercoli, L., L. Sarmati, E. Nicastri, G. Giannini, C. Galluzzo, S. Vella, and M. Andreoni. 1997. HIV phenotype switching during antiretroviral therapy: Emergence of saquinavir-resistant strains with less cytopathogenicity. *AIDS* 11:1121–1217.

1217. Erickson, J., D. J. Neidhart, J. VanDrie, D. J. Kempf, X.-C. Wang, D. W. Norbeck, J. J. Plattner, J. W. Rittenhouse, M. Turon, N. Wideburg, W. E. Kohlbrenner, R. Simmer, R. Helfrich, D. A. Paul, and M. Knigge. 1990. Design, activity, and 2.8 angstrom crystal structure of a C2 symmetric inhibitor complexed to HIV-1 protease. *Science* 249:527–533.

1218. Eron, J. J., M. A. Ashby, M. F. Giordano, M. Chernow, W. M. Reiter, S. G. Deeks, J. P. Lavelle, M. A. Conant, B. G. Yangco, P. G. Pate, R. A. Torres, R. T. Mitsuyasu, and T. Twaddell. 1996. Randomised trial of MNrgp120 HIV-1 vaccine in symptomless HIV-1 infection. *Lancet* 348:1547–1551.

1219. Eron, J. J., S. L. Benoit, J. Jemsek, R. D. MacArthur, J. Santana, J. B. Quinn, D. R. Kuritzkes, M. A. Fallon, and M. Rubin. 1995. Treatment with lamivudine, zidovudine, or both in HIV-positive patients with 200 to 500 CD4+ cells per cubic millimeter. *N. Engl. J. Med.* 333:1662–1669.

1220. Eron, J. J., Jr., L. M. Smeaton, S. A. Fiscus, R. M. Gulick, J. S. Currier, J. L. Lennox, R. T. D'Aquila, M. D. Rogers, R. Tung, and R. L. Murphy. 2000. The effects of protease inhibitor therapy on human immunodeficiency virus type 1 levels in semen (AIDS Clinical trials Protocol 850). *J. Infect. Dis.* 181:1622–1628.

1221. Escaich, S., J. Ritter, P. Rougier, D. Lepot, J.-P. Lamelin, M. Sepetjan, and C. Trepo. 1991. Plasma viraemia as a marker of viral replication in HIV-infected individuals. *AIDS* 5:1189–1194.

1222. Eshleman, S. H., Y. Lie, D. R. Hoover, S. Chen, S. E. Hudelson, S. A. Fiscus, C. J. Petropoulos, N. Kumwenda,

N. Parkin, and T. E. Taha. 2006. Association between the replication capacity and mother-to-child transmission of HIV-1, in antiretroviral drug-naive Malawian women. *J. Infect. Dis.* 193:1512–1515.

1223. Esnault, C., O. Heidmann, F. Delebecque, M. Dewannieux, D. Ribet, A. J. Hance, T. Heidmann, and O. Schwartz. 2005. APOBEC3G cytidine deaminase inhibits retrotransposition of endogenous retroviruses. *Nature* 433:430–433.

1224. Espinoza, L. R., J. L. Aguilar, C. G. Espinoza, A. Berman, F. Gutierrez, F. B. Vasey, and B. F. Germain. 1990. HIV associated arthropathy: HIV antigen demonstration in the synovial membrane. *J. Rheumatol.* 17:1195–1201.

1225. Estaquier, J., T. Idziorek, F. De Bels, F. Barre-Sinoussi, B. Hurtrel, A. M. Aubertin, A. Benet, M. Mehtali, E. Muchmore, P. Michel, Y. Mouton, M. Girard, and J. C. Ameisen. 1994. Programmed cell death and AIDS: significance of T-cell apoptosis in pathogenic and nonpathogenic primate lentiviral infections. *Proc. Natl. Acad. Sci. USA* 91:9431–9435.

1226. Estaquier, J., M. Tanaka, T. Suda, S. Nagata, P. Golstein, and J. C. Ameisen. 1996. Fas-mediated apoptosis of CD4+ and CD8+ T cells from human immunodeficiency virus-infected persons: differential *in vitro* preventive effect of cytokines and protease antagonists. *Blood* 87:4959–4966.

1226a. Estes, J. D., S. Wietgrefe, T. Schacker, P. Southern, G. Beilman, C. Reilly, J. M. Milush, J. D. Lifson, D. L. Sodora, J. V. Carlis, and A. T. Haase. SIV-induced lymphatic tissue fibrosis is mediated by TGFβ1+ T$_{regs}$ and begins in early infection. *J. Infect. Dis.*, in press.

1227. Eugen-Olsen, J., A. K. N. Iversen, T. L. Benfield, U. Koppelhus, and P. Garred. 1998. Chemokine receptor CCR2b 64I polymorphism and its relation to CD4 T-cell counts and disease progression in a Danish cohort of HIV-infected individuals. *J. Acquir. Immune Defic. Syndr. Hum. Retrovirol.* 18:110–116.

1228. European Collaborative Study. 2005. Mother-to-child transmission of HIV infection in the era of highly active antiretroviral therapy. *Clin. Infect. Dis.* 40:458–465.

1228a. European Mode of Delivery Collaboration. 1999. Elective caesarean-section versus vaginal delivery in prevention of vertical HIV-1 transmission: a randomised clinical trial. *Lancet* 353:1035–1039

1229. Evans, D. J., J. McKeating, J. M. Meredith, K. L. Burke, K. Katrak, A. John, M. Ferguson, P. D. Minor, R. A. Weiss, and J. W. Almond. 1989. An engineered poliovirus chimaera elicits broadly reactive HIV-1 neutralizing antibodies. *Nature* 339:385–388.

1230. Evans, L. A., T. M. McHugh, D. P. Stites, and J. A. Levy. 1987. Differential ability of human immunodeficiency virus isolates to productively infect human cells. *J. Immunol.* 138:3415–3418.

1231. Evans, L. A., J. Moreau, K. Odehouri, A. Barboza, C. Cheng-Mayer, and J. A. Levy. 1988. Characterization of a noncytopathic HIV-2 strain with unusual effects on CD4 expression. *Science* 240:1522–1525.

1232. Evans, L. A., J. Moreau, K. Odehouri, D. Seto, G. Thomson-Honnebier, H. Legg, A. Barboza, C. Cheng-Mayer, and J. A. Levy. 1988. Simultaneous isolation of HIV-1 and HIV-2 from an AIDS patient. *Lancet* ii:1389–1391.

1233. Evans, L. A., G. Thomson-Honnebier, K. Steimer, E. Paoletti, M. Perkus, H. Hollander, and J. A. Levy. 1989. Antibody-dependent cellular cytotoxicity is directed against both the gp120 and gp41 envelope proteins of the human immunodeficiency virus. *AIDS* 3:1357–1360.

1234. Evatt, B. L., R. B. Ramsey, D. N. Lawrence, L. D. Zyla, and J. W. Curran. 1984. The acquired immunodeficiency syndrome in patients with hemophilia. *Ann. Intern. Med.* 100:499–504.

1235. Everall, I. P., P. J. Luthert, and P. L. Lantos. 1991. Neuronal loss in the frontal cortex in HIV infection. *Lancet* 337:1119–1121.

1236. Everett, H., and G. McFadden. 2001. Viruses and apoptosis: meddling with mitochondria. *Virology* 288:1–7.

1237. Eyeson, J., D. King, M. J. Boaz, E. Sefia, S. Tomkins, A. Waters, P. J. Easterbrook, and A. Vyakarnam. 2003. Evidence for Gag p24-specific CD4 T cells with reduced susceptibility to R5 HIV-1 infection in a UK cohort of HIV-exposed-seronegative subjects. *AIDS* 17:2299–2311.

1238. Eyster, M. E., M. H. Gail, J. O. Ballard, H. Al-Mondhiry, and J. J. Goedert. 1987. Natural history of human immunodeficiency virus infections in hemophiliacs: effects of T-cell subsets, platelet counts, and age. *Ann. Intern. Med.* 107:1–6.

1239. Eyster, M. E., C. S. Rabkin, M. W. Hilgartner, L. M. Aledort, M. V. Ragni, J. Sprandio, G. C. White, S. Eichinger, P. de Moerloose, W. A. Andes, A. R. Cohen, M. Manco-Johnson, G. L. Bray, W. Schramm, A. Hatzakis, M. M. Lederman, C. M. Kessler, and J. J. Goedert. 1993. Human immunodeficiency virus-related conditions in children and adults with hemophilia: rates, relationship to CD4 counts, and predictive value. *Blood* 81:828–834.

1240. Ezekowitz, A. B., M. Kuhlman, J. E. Groopman, and R. A. Byrn. 1989. A human serum mannose-binding protein inhibits *in vitro* infection by the human immunodeficiency virus. *J. Exp. Med.* 169:185–196.

1240a. Fackler, O. T., A. Moris, N. Tibroni, S. I. Giese, B. Glass, O. Schwartz, and H. G. Krausslich. 2006. Functional characterization of HIV-1 Nef mutants in the context of viral infection. *Virology* 351:322–339.

1241. Fagard, C., M. Le Braz, H. Gunthard, H. D. Hirsch, M. Egger, P. Vernazza, E. Bernasconi, A. Telenti, C. Ebnother, A. Oxenius, T. Perneger, L. Perrin, B. Hirschel, and Swiss HIV Cohort Study. 2003. A controlled trial of granulocyte macrophage-colony stimulating factor during interruption of HAART. *AIDS* 17:1487–1492.

1242. Fagard, C., A. Oxenius, H. Gunthard, F. Garcia, M. Le Braz, G. Mestre, M. Battegay, H. Furrer, P. Vernazza, E. Bernasconi, A. Telenti, R. Weber, D. Leduc, S. Yerly, D. Price, S. J. Dawson, T. Klimkait, T. V. Perneger, A. McLean, B. Clotet, J. M. Gatell, L. Perrin, M. Plana, R. Phillips, and B. Hirschel. 2003. A prospective trial of structured treatment interruptions in human immunodeficiency virus infection. *Arch. Intern. Med.* 163:1220–1226.

1243. Fakhari, F. D., J. H. Jeong, Y. Kanan, and D. P. Dittmer. 2006. The latency-associated nuclear antigen of Kaposi sarcoma-associated herpesvirus induces B cell hyperplasia and lymphoma. *J. Clin. Investig.* 116:735–742.

1244. Falk, L. A., Jr., D. A. Paul, A. Landay, and H. Kessler. 1987. HIV isolation from plasma of HIV-infected persons. *N. Engl. J. Med.* 316:1547–1548.

1245. Fanales-Belasio, E., S. Moretti, F. Nappi, G. Barillari, F. Micheletti, A. Cafaro, and B. Ensoli. 2002. Native HIV-1 Tat protein targets monocyte-derived dendritic cells and enhances their maturation, function, and antigen-specific T cell responses. *J. Immunol.* 168:197–206.

1246. Fang, G., H. Burger, C. Chappey, S. Rowland-Jones, A. Visosky, C. H. Chen, T. Moran, L. Townsend, M. Murray, and B. Weiser. 2001. Analysis of transition from long-term nonprogressive to progressive infection identifies sequences that may attenuate HIV type 1. *AIDS Res. Hum. Retrovir.* 17:1395–1404.

1247. Fang, G., C. Kuiken, B. Weiser, S. Rowland-Jones, F. Plummer, C.-H. Chen, R. Kaul, A. O. Anzala, J. Bwayo, J. Kimani, S. M. Philpott, C. Kitchen, J. S. Sinsheimer, B. Gaschen, D. Lang, B. Shi, K. S. Kemal, T. Rostron, C. Brunner, S. Beddows, Q. Sattenau, E. Paxinos, J. Oyugi, and H. Burger. 2004. Long-term survivors in Nairobi: complete HIV-1 RNA sequences and immunogenetic associations. *J. Infect. Dis.* 190: 697–701.

1248. Fang, R. H., E. Khatissian, V. Monceaux, M. Cumont, S. Beq, J. Ameisen, A. Aubertin, N. Israel, J. Estaquier, and B. Hurtel. 2005. Disease progression in macaques with low SIV replication levels: on the relevance of TREC counts. *AIDS* 19:663–673.

1249. Fantini, J., N. Yahi, S. Baghdiguian, and J.-C. Chermann. 1992. Human colon epithelial cells productively infected with human immunodeficiency virus show impaired differentiation and altered secretion. *J. Virol.* 66:580–585.

1250. Fantini, J., N. Yahi, and J.-C. Chermann. 1991. Human immunodeficiency virus can infect the apical and basolateral surfaces of human colonic epithelial cells. *Proc. Natl. Acad. Sci. USA* 88:9297–9301.

1251. Faraci, F. M. 1989. Effects of endothelin and vasopressin on cerebral blood vessels. *Am. J. Physiol.* 257:H799–H803.

1252. Farel, C. E., D. G. Chaitt, B. K. Hahn, L. A. Tavel, J. A. Kovacs, M. A. Polis, H. Masur, D. A. Follmann, H. C. Lane, and R. T. Davey, Jr. 2004. Induction and maintenance therapy with intermittent interleukin-2 in HIV-1 infection. *Blood* 103:3282–3286.

1252a. Farrell, A. 2006. Defeating T-cell fatigue in HIV. *Nat. Med.* 12:1124–1125.

1253. Farrow, M. A., M. Somasundaran, C. Zhang, D. Gabuzda, J. L. Sullivan, and T. C. Greenough. 2005. Nuclear localization of HIV type 1 Vif isolated from a long-term asymptomatic individual and potential role in virus attenuation. *AIDS Res. Hum. Retrovir.* 21:565–574.

1254. Fassati, A., and S. P. Goff. 2001. Characterization of intracellular reverse transcription complexes of human immunodeficiency virus type 1. *J. Virol.* 75:3626–3635.

1255. Fatkenheuer, G., A. L. Pozniak, M. A. Johnson, A. Plettenberg, S. Staszewski, A. I. Hoepelman, M. S. Saag, F. D. Goebel, J. K. Rockstroh, B. J. Dezube, T. M. Jenkins, C. Medhurst, J. F. Sullivan, C. Ridgway, S. Abel, I. T. James, M. Youle, and E. van der Ryst. 2005. Efficacy of short-term monotherapy with maraviroc, a new CCR5 antagonist, in patients infected with HIV-1. *Nat. Med.* 11:1170–1172.

1256. Fauci, A. S. 1993. Multifactorial nature of human immunodeficiency virus disease: implications for therapy. *Science* 262:1011–1018.

1257. Fauci, A. S. 1996. An HIV vaccine: breaking the paradigms. *Proc. Assoc. Am. Physicians* 108:6–13.

1258. Fauci, A. S., D. Mavilio, and S. Kottilil. 2005. NK cells in HIV infection: paradigm for protection or targets for ambush. *Nat. Rev. Immunol.* 5:835–843.

1259. Fauci, A. S., G. Pantaleo, S. Stanley, and D. Weissman. 1996. Immunopathogenic mechanisms of HIV infection. *Ann. Intern. Med.* 124:654–663.

1260. Faure, S., L. Meyer, D. Costagliola, C. Vaneensberghe, E. Genin, B. Autran, J. F. Delfraissy, D. H. McDermott, P. M. Murphy, P. Debre, I. Theodorou, and C. Combadiere. 2000. Rapid progression to AIDS in HIV+ individuals with a structural variant of the chemokine receptor CX3CR1. *Science* 287:2274–2277.

1261. Faure, S., L. Meyer, E. Genin, P. Pellet, P. Debre, I. Theodorou, and C. Combadiere. 2003. Deleterious genetic influence of CX3CR1 genotypes on HIV-1 disease progression. *J. Acquir. Immune Defic. Syndr.* 32:335–337.

1262. Fawzi, W. W., G. I. Msamanga, D. Hunter, B. Renjifo, G. Antelman, H. Bang, K. Manji, S. Kapiga, D. Mwakagile, M. Essex, and D. Spiegelman. 2002. Randomized trial of vitamin supplements in relation to transmission of HIV-1 through breastfeeding and early child mortality. *AIDS* 16:1935–1944.

1263. Fawzi, W. W., G. I. Msamanga, D. Spiegelman, R. Wei, S. Kapiga, E. Villamor, D. Mwakagile, F. Mugusi, E. Hertzmark, M. Essex, and D. Hunter. 2004. A randomized trial of multivitamin supplements and HIV disease progression and mortality. *N. Engl. J. Med.* 351:20–29.

1264. Fehniger, T. A., and M. A. Caligiuri. 2001. Interleukin 15: biology and relevance to human disease. *Blood* 97:14–32.

1265. Fehniger, T. A., G. Herbein, H. X. Yu, M. I. Para, Z. P. Bernstein, W. A. Obrien, and M. A. Caligiuri. 1998. Natural killer cells from HIV-1(+) patients produce C-C chemokines and inhibit HIV-1 infection. *J. Immunol.* 161:6433–6438.

1266. Feinberg, M. B., R. F. Jarrett, A. Aldovini, R. C. Gallo, and F. Wong-Staal. 1986. HTLV-III expression and production involve complex regulation at the levels of splicing and translation of viral RNA. *Cell* 46:807–817.

1267. Feinberg, M. B., and D. Trono. 1992. Intracellular immunization: trans-dominant mutants of HIV gene products as tools for the study and interruption of viral replication. *AIDS Res. Hum. Retrovir.* 8:1013–1022.

1268. Feizi, T., and M. Larkin. 1990. AIDS and glycosylation. *Glycobiology* 1:17–23.

1269. Feldman, S., D. Stein, S. Amrute, T. Denny, Z. Garcia, P. Kloser, Y. Sun, N. Megjugorac, and P. Fitzgerald-Bocarsly. 2001. Decreased interferon-alpha production in HIV-infected patients correlates with numerical and functional deficiencies in circulating type 2 dendritic cell precursors. *Clin. Immunol.* 101:201–210.

1270. Feldmann, H., H. Bugany, F. Mahner, H. D. Klenk, D. Drenckhahn, and H. J. Schnittler. 1996. Filovirus-induced endothelial leakage triggered by infected monocytes/macrophages. *J. Virol.* 70:2208–2214.

1271. Fellay, J., C. Marzolini, E. R. Meaden, D. J. Back, T. Buclin, J. P. Chave, L. A. Decosterd, H. Furrer, M. Opravil, G. Pantaleo, D. Retelska, L. Ruiz, A. H. Schinkel, P. Vernazza, C. B. Eap, and A. Telenti. 2002. Response to antiretroviral treatment in HIV-1-infected individuals with allelic variants of the multidrug resistance transporter 1: a pharmacogenetics study. *Lancet* 359:30–36.

1272. Feng, Y., C. C. Broder, P. E. Kennedy, and E. A. Berger. 1996. HIV-1 entry cofactor: functional cDNA cloning of a seven-transmembrane, G protein-coupled receptor. *Science* 272:872–877.

1273. Feng, Y. X., T. D. Copeland, L. E. Henderson, R. J. Gorelick, W. J. Bosche, J. G. Levin, and A. Rein. 1997. HIV-1 nucleocapsid protein induces "maturation" of dimeric retroviral RNA *in vitro*. *Proc. Natl. Acad. Sci. USA* 93:7577–7581.

1274. Fenyo, E. M., L. Morfeldt-Manson, F. Chiodi, B. Lind, A. von Gegerfelt, J. Albert, E. Olausson, and B. Asjo. 1988. Distinct replicative and cytopathic characteristics of human immunodeficiency virus isolates. *J. Virol.* 62:4414–4419.

1275. Ferbas, J. 1998. Perspectives on the role of CD8+ cell suppressor factors and cytotoxic T lymphocytes during HIV infection. *AIDS Res. Hum. Retrovir.* 14:S153–S160.

1276. Ferbas, J., E. S. Daar, K. Grovit-Ferbas, W. J. Lech, R. Detels, J. V. Giorgi, and A. H. Kaplan. 1996. Rapid evolution of human immunodeficiency virus strains with increased replicative capacity during the seronegative window of primary infection. *J. Virol.* 70:7285–7289.

1277. Ferbas, J., A. H. Kaplan, M. A. Hausner, L. E. Hultin, J. L. Matud, Z. Liu, D. L. Panicali, H. Nerng-Ho, R. Detels, and J. V. Giorgi. 1995. Virus burden in long-term survivors of human immunodeficiency virus (HIV) infection is a determinant of anti-HIV CD8+ lymphocyte activity. *J. Infect. Dis.* 172:329–339.

1278. Ferlazzo, G., M. Pack, D. Thomas, C. Paludan, D. Schmid, T. Strowig, G. Bougras, W. A. Muller, L. Moretta, and C. Munz. 2004. Distinct roles of IL-12 and IL-15 in human natural killer cell activation by dendritic cells from secondary lymphoid organs. *Proc. Natl. Acad. Sci. USA* 101:16606–16611.

1279. Fermin, C. D., and R. F. Garry. 1992. Membrane alterations linked to early interactions of HIV with the cell surface. *Virology* 191:941–946.

1280. Fernandez, S., R. C. Nolan, P. Price, R. Krueger, C. Wood, D. Cameron, A. Solomon, S. R. Lewin, and M. A. French. 2006. Thymic function in severely immunodeficient HIV type 1-infected patients receiving stable and effective antiretroviral therapy. *AIDS Res. Hum. Retrovir.* 22:163–170.

1281. Fernandez-Larsson, R., K. K. Srivastava, S. Lu, and H. L. Robinson. 1992. Replication of patient isolates of human immunodeficiency virus type 1 in T cells: a spectrum of rates and efficiencies of entry. *Proc. Natl. Acad. Sci. USA* 89:2223–2226.

1282. Ferrantelli, F., R. A. Rasmussen, K. A. Buckley, P. Li, T. Wang, D. C. Montefiori, H. katinger, G. Stiegler, D. C. Anderson, H. M. McClure, and R. M. Ruprecht. 2004. Complete protection of neonatal rhesus macaques against oral exposure to pathogenic simian-human immunodeficiency virus by human anti-HIV monoclonal antibodies. *J. Infect. Dis.* 189:2167–2173.

1283. Ferrari, G., W. Humphrey, M. J. McElrath, J. L. Excler, A. M. Duliege, M. L. Clements, L. C. Corey, D. P. Bolognesi, and K. J. Weinhold. 1997. Clade B-based HIV-1 vaccines elicit cross-clade cytotoxic T lymphocyte reactivities in uninfected volunteers. *Proc. Natl. Acad. Sci. USA* 94:1396–1401.

1284. Fidler, S., A. Oxenius, M. Brady, J. Clarke, A. Cropley, A. Babiker, H.-T. Zhang, D. Price, R. Phillips, and J. Weber. 2002. Virological and immunological effects of short-course antiretroviral therapy in primary HIV infection. *AIDS* 16:2049–2054.

1285. Fiebig, E. W., C. M. Heldebrant, R. I. F. Smith, A. J. Conrad, E. L. Delwart, and M. P. Busch. 2005. Intermittent low-level viremia in early primary HIV-1 infection. *J. Acquir. Immune Defic. Syndr.* 39:133–137.

1286. Fiebig, E. W., D. J. Wright, B. D. Rawal, P. E. Garrett, R. T. Schumacher, L. Peddada, C. Heldebrant, R. Smith, A. Conrad, S. H. Kleinman, and M. P. Busch. 2003. Dynamics of HIV viremia and antibody seroconversion in plasma donors: implications for diagnosis and staging of primary HIV infection. *AIDS* 17:1871–1879.

1287. Fields, A. P., D. P. Bednarik, A. Hess, and W. S. May. 1988. Human immunodeficiency virus induces phosphorylation of its cell surface receptor. *Nature* 333:278–280.

1288. Figdor, C. G., Y. van Kooyk, and G. J. Adema. 2002. C-type lectin receptors on dendritic cells and Langerhans cells. *Nat. Rev. Immunol.* 2:77–84.

1289. Finkel, E. 2001. The mitochondrion: is it central to apoptosis? *Science* 292:624–626.

1290. Finkel, T. H., G. Tudor-Williams, N. K. Banda, M. F. Cotoon, T. Curiel, C. Monks, T. W. Baba, R. M. Ruprecht, and A. Kupfer. 1995. Apoptosis occurs predominantly in bystander cells and not in productively infected cells of HIV- and SIV-infected lymph nodes. *Nat. Med.* 1:129–134.

1291. Finnegan, A., K. A. Roebuck, B. E. Nakai, D. S. Gu, M. F. Rabbi, S. Song, and A. L. Landay. 1996. IL-10 cooperates with TNF-alpha to activate HIV-1 from latently and acutely infected cells of monocyte/macrophage lineage. *J. Immunol.* 156:841–851.

1292. Finzi, D., J. Blankson, J. D. Siliciano, J. B. Margolick, K. Chadwick, T. Pierson, K. Smith, J. Lisziewicz, F. Lori, C. Flexner, T. C. Quinn, R. E. Chaisson, E. Rosenberg, B. Walker, S. Gange, J. Gallant, and R. F. Siliciano. 1999. Latent infection of CD4+ T cells provides a mechanism for lifelong persistence of HIV-1, even in patients on effective combination therapy. *Nat. Med.* 5:512–517.

1293. Finzi, D., M. Hermankova, T. Pierson, L. M. Carruth, C. Buck, R. E. Chaisson, T. C. Quinn, K. Chadwick, J. Margolick, R. Brookmeyer, J. Gallant, M. Markowitz, D. D. Ho, D. D. Richman, and R. F. Siliciano. 1997. Identification of a reservoir for HIV-1 in patients on highly active antiretroviral therapy. *Science* 278:1295–1300.

1294. Fiore, J. R., A. Bjorndal, K. A. Peipke, M. Di Stefano, G. Angarano, G. Pastore, H. Gaines, E. M. Fenyo, and J. Albert. 1994. The biological phenotype of HIV-1 is usually retained during and after sexual transmission. *Virology* 204:297–303.

1295. Fiorelli, V., R. Gendelman, F. Samaniego, P. D. Markham, and B. Ensoli. 1995. Cytokines from activated T cells induce normal endothelial cells to acquire the phenotypic and functional features of AIDS-Kaposi's sarcoma spindle cells. *J. Clin. Investig.* 95:1723–1734.

1296. Fiorentino, S., M. Dalod, D. Olive, J. G. Guillet, and E. Gomard. 1996. Predominant involvement of CD8+CD28- lymphocytes in human immunodeficiency virus-specific cytotoxic activity. *J. Virol.* 70:2022–2026.

1297. Fischer-Smith, T., S. Croul, A. E. Sverstiuk, C. Capini, D. L'Heureux, E. G. Regulier, M. W. Richardson, S. Amini, S. Morgello, K. Khalili, and J. Rappaport. 2001. CNS invasion by CD14+/CD16+ peripheral blood-derived monocytes in HIV dementia: perivascular accumulation and reservoir of HIV infection. *J. Neurovirol.* 7:528–541.

1298. Fischl, M. A., D. D. Richman, M. H. Grieco, M. S. Gottlieb, P. A. Volberding, O. L. Laskin, J. M. Leedom, J. E. Groopman, D. Mildvan, R. T. Schooley, G. G. Jackson, D. T. Durack, and D. King. 1987. The efficacy of azidothymidine (AZT) in the treatment of patients with AIDS and AIDS-related complex. A double blind placebo controlled trial. *N. Engl. J. Med.* 317:185–191.

1299. Fisher, A. G., B. Ensoli, D. Looney, A. Rose, R. C. Gallo, M. S. Saag, G. M. Shaw, B. H. Hahn, and F. Wong-Staal. 1988. Biologically diverse molecular variants within a single HIV-1 isolate. *Nature* 334:444–447.

1300. Fisher, A. G., M. B. Feinberg, and S. F. Josephs. 1986. The *trans*-activator gene of HTLV-III is essential for virus replication. *Nature* 320:2367–2371.

1301. Fisher, A. G., L. Ratner, H. Mitsuya, L. M. Marselle, M. E. Harper, S. Broder, R. C. Gallo, and F. Wong-Staal. 1986. Infectious mutants of HTLV-III with changes in the 3' region and markedly reduced cytopathic effects. *Science* 233:655–659.

1302. Fitzgerald, J. C., G. P. Gao, A. Reyes-Sandoval, G. N. Pavlakis, Z. Q. Xiang, A. P. Wlazlo, W. Giles-Davis, J. M. Wilson, and H. C. Ertl. 2003. A simian replication-defective adenoviral recombinant vaccine to HIV-1 gag. *J. Immunol.* 170:1416–1422.

1303. Fitzgerald-Bocarsly, P. 1993. Human natural interferon-alpha producing cells. *Pharmacol. Ther.* 60:39–62.

1304. Fitzgerald-Bocarsly, P. 2002. Natural interferon-α producing cells: the plasmacytoid dendritic cells. *BioTechniques* 33:16–29.

1305. Flamand, L., R. W. Crowley, P. Lusso, S. Colombini-Hatch, D. M. Margolis, and R. C. Gallo. 1998. Activation of CD8+ T lymphocytes through the T cell receptor turns on CD4 gene expression: implications for HIV pathogenesis. *Proc. Natl. Acad. Sci. USA* 95:3111–3116.

1306. Flamand, L., J. Gosselin, M. D'Addario, J. Hiscott, D. V. Ablashi, R. C. Gallo, and J. Menezes. 1991. Human herpesvirus 6 induces interleukin-1-beta and tumor necrosis factor alpha, but not interleukin-6, in peripheral blood mononuclear cell cultures. *J. Virol.* 65:5105–5110.

1307. Flamand, L., R. A. Zeman, J. L. Bryant, Y. Lunardi-Iskandar, and R. C. Gallo. 1996. Absence of human herpesvirus 8 DNA sequences in neoplastic Kaposi's sarcoma cell lines. *J. Acquir. Immune Defic. Syndr. Hum. Retrovirol.* 13:194–197.

1308. Fleming, S. C., M. S. Kapembwa, T. T. MacDonald, and G. E. Griffin. 1992. Direct *in vitro* infection of human intestine with HIV-1. *AIDS* 6:1099–1104.

1309. Fletcher, T. M., III, B. Brichacek, N. Sharova, M. A. Newman, G. Stivahtis, P. M. Sharp, M. Emerman, B. H. Hahn, and M. Stevenson. 1996. Nuclear import and cell cycle arrest functions of the HIV-1 Vpr protein are encoded by two separate genes in HIV-2/SIV(SM). *EMBO J.* 15:6155–6165.

1310. Fleuridor, R., B. Wilson, R. Hou, A. Landay, H. Kessler, and L. Al-Harthi. 2003. CD1d-restricted natural killer T cells are potent targets for human immunodeficiency virus infection. *Immunology* 108:3–9.

1311. Fleury, S., D. Lamarre, S. Meloche, S. E. Ryu, C. Cantin, W. A. Hendrickson, and R. P. Sekaly. 1991. Mutational analysis of the interaction between CD4 and Class II MHC: Class II antigens contact CD4 on a surface opposite the gp120-binding site. *Cell* 66:1037–1049.

1312. Fleury, S., G. P. Rizzardi, A. Chapuis, G. Tambussi, C. Knabenhans, E. Simeoni, J. Y. Meuwly, J. M. Corpataux, A. Lazzarin, F. Miedema, and G. Pantaleo. 2000. Long-term kinetics of T cell production in HIV-infected subjects treated with highly active antiretroviral therapy. *Proc. Natl. Acad. Sci. USA* 97:5393–5398.

1313. Flore, O., S. Rafii, S. Ely, J. J. Oleary, E. M. Hyjek, and E. Cesarman. 1998. Transformation of primary human endothelial cells by Kaposi's sarcoma-associated herpesvirus. *Nature* 394:588–592.

1314. Flores-Villanueva, P. O., H. Hendel, S. Caillat-Zucman, J. Rappaport, A. Burgos-Tiburcio, S. Bertin-Maghit, S. Ruiz-Morales, M. E. Teran, J. Rodriguez-Tafur, and J.-F. Zagury.

2003. Associations of MHC ancestral haplotypes with resistance/susceptibility to AIDS disease development. *J. Immunol.* 170:1925–1929.

1315. Flores-Villanueva, P. O., E. J. Yunis, J. C. Delgado, E. Vittinghoff, S. Buchbinder, J. Y. Leung, A. M. Uglialoro, O. P. Clavijo, E. S. Rosenberg, S. A. Kalams, J. D. Braun, S. L. Boswell, B. D. Walker, and A. E. Goldfeld. 2001. Control of HIV-1 viremia and protection from AIDS are associated with HLA-Bw4 homozygosity. *Proc. Natl. Acad. Sci. USA* 98:5140–5145.

1315a. Flynn, N. M., D. N. Forthal, C. D. Harro, F. N. Judson, K. H. Mayer, and M. F. Para. 2005. Placebo-controlled phase 3 trial of a recombinant glycoprotein 120 vaccine to prevent HIV-1 infection. *J. Infect. Dis.* 191:654–665.

1316. Flys, T., D. W. Nissley, C. W. Claasen, D. Jones, C. Shi, L. A. Guay, P. Musoke, F. Mmiro, J. N. Strathern, J. B. Jackson, J. R. Eshleman, and S. H. Eshleman. 2005. Sensitive drug-resistance assays reveal long-term persistence of HIV-1 variants with the K103N nevirapine (NVP) resistance mutation in some women and infants after the administration of single-dose NVP: HIVNET 012. *J. Infect. Dis.* 192:24–29.

1317. Foglia, G., G. D. Royster IV, K. M. Wasunna, R. Kibaya, J. A. Malia, E. K. Calero, W. Sateren, P. O. Renzullo, M. L. Robb, D. L. Birx, and N. L. Michael. 2004. Use of rapid and conventional testing technologies for human immunodeficiency virus type 1 serologic screening in a rural Kenyan reference laboratory. *J. Clin. Microbiol.* 42:3850–3852.

1318. Foley, J. F., C. Yu, R. Solow, M. Yacobucci, K. W. C. Peden, and J. M. Farber. 2005. Roles for CXC chemokine ligands 10 and 11 in recruiting CD4+ T cells to HIV-1-infected monocyte-derived macrophages, dendritic cells, and lymph nodes. *J. Immunol.* 174:4892–4900.

1319. Folks, T., D. M. Powell, M. M. Lightfoote, S. Benn, M. A. Martin, and A. S. Fauci. 1986. Induction of HTLV-III/LAV from a nonvirus-producing T-cell line: implications for latency. *Science* 231:600–602.

1320. Folks, T. M., and D. P. Bednarik. 1992. Mechanisms of HIV-1 latency. *AIDS* 6:3–16.

1321. Folks, T. M., J. Justement, A. Kinter, C. A. Dinarello, and A. S. Fauci. 1987. Cytokine-induced expression of HIV-1 in a chronically infected promonocyte cell line. *Science* 238:800–802.

1322. Folks, T. M., S. W. Kessler, J. M. Orenstein, J. S. Justement, E. S. Jaffe, and A. S. Fauci. 1988. Infection and replication of HIV-1 in purified progenitor cells of normal human bone marrow. *Science* 242:919–922.

1323. Folkvord, J. M., C. Armon, and E. Connick. 2005. Lymphoid follicles are sites of heightened human immunodeficiency virus type 1 (HIV-1) replication and reduced antiretroviral effector mechanisms. *AIDS Res. Hum. Retrovir.* 21:363–370.

1324. Fong, L., M. Mengozzi, N. W. Abbey, B. G. Herdier, and E. G. Engleman. 2002. Productive infection of plasmacytoid dendritic cells with human immunodeficiency virus 1 is triggered by CD40 ligation. *J. Virol.* 76:11033–11041.

1325. Fontana, A., W. Fierz, and H. Wekerle. 1984. Astrocytes present myelin basic protein to encephalitogenic T-cell lines. *Nature* 307:273–276.

1326. Fontana, L., M. C. Sirianni, G. De Sanctis, M. Carbonari, B. Ensoli, and F. Aiuti. 1986. Deficiency of natural killer activity, but not of natural killer binding, in patients with lymphadenopathy syndrome positive for antibodies to HTLV-III. *Immunobiology* 171:425–435.

1327. Fonteneau, J. F., M. Larsson, A. S. Beignon, K. McKenna, I. Dasilva, A. Amara, Y. J. Liu, J. D. Lifson, D. R. Littman, and N. Bhardwaj. 2004. Human immunodeficiency virus type 1 activates plasmacytoid dendritic cells and concomitantly induces the bystander maturation of myeloid dendritic cells. *J. Virol.* 78:5223–5232.

1328. Foreman, K. E., J. Friborg, W. P. Kong, C. Woffendin, P. J. Polverini, B. J. Nickoloff, and G. J. Nabel. 1997. Propagation of a human herpesvirus from AIDS-associated Kaposi's sarcoma. *N. Engl. J. Med.* 336:163–171.

1329. Forshey, B. M., and C. Aiken. 2003. Disassembly of human immunodeficiency virus type 1 cores in vitro reveals association of Nef with the subviral ribonucoleoprotein complex. *J. Virol.* 77:4409–4414.

1330. Forthal, D., G. Landucci, T. Phan, R. Higa-Tanner, and P. Gilbert. 2006. FCγ receptor IIa and IIIa polymorphisms are associated with the risk of HIV infection 2006. Presented at the 13th Conference on Retroviruses and Opportunistic Infections, Denver, Colo.

1331. Forthal, D. N., G. Landucci, and B. Keenan. 2001. Relationship between antibody-dependent cellular cytotoxicity, plasma HIV type 1 RNA, and CD4+ lymphocyte count. *AIDS Res. Hum. Retrovir.* 17:553–561.

1332. Forthal, D. N., G. Landucci, T. B. Phan, and J. Becerra. 2005. Interactions between natural killer cells and antibody Fc result in enhanced antibody neutralization of human immunodeficiency virus type 1. *J. Virol.* 79:2042–2049.

1333. Fortin, J., R. Cantin, G. Lamontagne, and M. Tremblay. 1997. Host-derived ICAM-1 glycoproteins incorporated on human immunodeficiency virus type 1 are biologically active and enhance viral infectivity. *J. Virol.* 71:3588–3596.

1334. Fortin, J. F., B. Barbeau, H. Hedman, E. Lundgren, and M. J. Tremblay. 1999. Role of the leukocyte function antigen-1 conformational state in the process of human immunodeficiency virus type 1-mediated syncytium formation and virus infection. *Virology* 257:228–238.

1335. Fortin, J. F., R. Cantin, M. G. Bergeron, and M. J. Tremblay. 2000. Interaction between virion-bound host intercellular adhesion molecule-1 and the high-affinity state of lymphocyte function-associated antigen-1 on target cells renders R5 and X4 isolates of human immunodeficiency virus type 1 more refractory to neutralization. *Virology* 268:493–503.

1336. Foster, H. D. 2004. How HIV-1 causes AIDS: implications for prevention and treatment. *Med. Hypotheses* 62:549–553.

1337. Fotopoulos, G., A. Harari, P. Michetti, G. Pantaleo, and J. Kraehenbuhi. 2002. Transepithelial transport of HIV-1 by M cells is receptor-mediated. *Proc. Natl. Acad. Sci. USA* 99:9410–9414.

1338. Fouchier, R. A. M., M. Groenink, N. A. Koostra, M. Tersmette, H. G. Huisman, F. Miedema, and H. Schuitemaker. 1992. Phenotype-associated sequence variation in the third variable domain of the human immunodeficiency virus type 1 gp120 molecule. *J. Virol.* 66:3183–3187.

1339. Fouchier, R. A. M., L. Meyaard, M. Brouwer, E. Hovenkamp, and H. Schuitemaker. 1996. Broader tropism and higher cytopathicity for CD4+ T cells of a syncytium-inducing compared to a non-syncytium-inducing HIV-1 isolate as a mechanism for accelerated CD4+ T cell decline *in vivo*. *Virology* 219:87–96.

1340. Foulds, K. E., C. Wu, and R. A. Seder. 2006. Th1 memory: implications for vaccine development. *Immunol. Rev.* 211:58–66.

1341. Fouts, T., K. Godfrey, K. Bobb, D. Montefiori, C. V. Hanson, V. S. Kalyanaraman, A. DeVico, and R. Pal. 2002. Crosslinked HIV-1 envelope-CD4 receptor complexes elicit broadly cross-reactive neutralizing antibodies in rhesus macaques. *Proc. Natl. Acad. Sci. USA* 99:11842–11847.

1342. Fowke, K. R., T. Dong, S. L. Rowland-Jones, J. Oyugi, W. J. Rutherford, J. Kimani, P. Krausa, J. Bwayo, J. N. Simonsen, G. M. Shearer, and F. A. Plummer. 1998. HIV type 1 resistance in Kenyan sex workers is not associated with altered cellular susceptibility to HIV type 1 infection or enhanced beta-chemokine production. *AIDS Res. Hum. Retrovir.* 14:1521–1530.

1343. Fowke, K. R., N. J. D. Nagelkerke, J. Kimani, J. N. Simonsen, A. O. Anzala, J. J. Bwayo, K. S. McDonald, E. N. Ngugi, and F. A. Plummer. 1996. Resistance to HIV-1 among persistently seronegative prostitutes in Nairobi, Kenya. *Lancet* 348:1347–1351.

1344. Fox, C. H., D. Kotler, A. Tierney, C. S. Wilson, and A. S. Fauci. 1989. Detection of HIV-1 RNA in the lamina propria of patients with AIDS and gastrointestinal disease. *J. Infect. Dis.* 159:467–471.

1345. Fox, C. H., K. Tenner-Racz, P. Racz, A. Firpo, P. A. Pizzo, and A. S. Fauci. 1991. Lymphoid germinal centers are reservoirs of human immunodeficiency virus type 1 RNA. *J. Infect. Dis.* 164:1051–1057.

1346. Fox, R., L. J. Eldren, E. J. Fuchs, R. A. Kaslow, B. R. Visscher, M. Ho, J. P. Phair, and B. F. Polk. 1987. Clinical manifestations of acute infection with human immunodeficiency virus in a cohort of gay men. *AIDS* 1:35–38.

1347. Frahm, N., P. Kiepiela, S. Adams, C. H. Linde, H. S. Hewitt, K. Sango, M. E. Feeney, M. M. Addo, M. Lichterfeld, M. P. Lahaie, E. Pae, A. G. Wurcel, T. Roach, M. A. St John, M. Altfeld, F. M. Marincola, C. Moore, S. Mallal, M. Carrington, D. Heckerman, T. M. Allen, J. I. Mullins, B. T. Korber, P. J. Goulder, B. D. Walker, and C. Brander. 2006. Control of human immunodeficiency virus replication by cytotoxic T lymphocytes targeting subdominant epitopes. *Nat. Immunol.* 7:173–178.

1348. Franceschi, C., M. G. Franceschini, A. Boschini, T. Trenti, C. Nuzzo, G. Castellani, C. Smacchia, B. De Rienzo, T. Roncaglia, M. Portolani, P. Pietrosemoli, M. Meacci, M. Pecorari, A. Sabbatini, W. Malorni, and A. Cossarizza. 1997. Phenotypic characteristics and tendency to apoptosis of peripheral blood mononuclear cells from HIV+ long term non progressors. *Cell Death Differ.* 4:815–823.

1348a. Franchi, L., C. McDonald, T. D. Kanneganti, A. Amer, and G. Nunez. 2006. Nucleotide-binding oligomerization domain-like receptors: intracellular pattern recognition molecules for pathogen detection and host defense. *J. Immunol.* 177:3507–3513.

1349. Franchini, G., M. Robert-Guroff, J. Tartaglia, A. Aggarwal, A. Abimiku, J. Benson, P. Markham, K. Limbach, G. Hurteau, J. Fullen, K. Aldrich, N. Miller, J. Sadoff, E. Paoletti, and R. C. Gallo. 1995. Highly attenuated HIV type 2 recombinant poxviruses, but not HIV-2 recombinant *Salmonella* vaccines, induce long-lasting protection in rhesus macaques. *AIDS Res. Hum. Retrovir.* 11:909–920.

1350. Francis, D. P., W. L. Heyward, V. Popovic, P. Orozco-Cronin, K. Orelind, C. Gee, A. Hirsch, T. Ippolito, A. Luck, M. Longhi, V. Gulati, N. Winslow, M. Gurwith, F. Sinangil, and P. W. Berman. 2003. Candidate HIV/AIDS vaccines: lessons learned from the world's first phase III efficacy trials. *AIDS* 17:147–156.

1351. Francis, T., Jr. 1953. Influenza: new acquaintance. *Ann. Intern. Med.* 39:203–221.

1352. Frank, I., and M. Pope. 2002. The enigma of dendritic cell-immunodeficiency virus interplay. *Curr. Mol. Med.* 2:229–248.

1353. Franke, E. K., and J. Luban. 1996. Inhibition of HIV-replication by cyclosporine A or related compounds correlates with the ability to disrupt the Gag-cyclophilin A interaction. *Virology* 222:279–282.

1354. Franke, E. K., H. E. Yuan, and J. Luban. 1994. Specific incorporation of cyclosporin A into HIV-1 virions. *Nature* 372:359–362.

1355. Frankel, A. D., and J. A. Young. 1998. HIV-1: fifteen proteins and an RNA. *Annu. Rev. Biochem.* 67:1–25.

1356. Frankel, F. R., S. Hegde, J. Lieberman, and Y. Paterson. 1995. Induction of cell-mediated immune responses to human immunodeficiency virus type 1 gag protein by using *Listeria monocytogenes* as a live vaccine vector. *J. Immunol.* 155:4775–4782.

1357. Frankel, S. S., B. M. Wenig, A. P. Burke, P. Mannan, L. D. Thompson, S. L. Abbondanzo, A. M. Nelson, M. Pope, and R. M. Steinman. 1996. Replication of HIV-1 in dendritic cell-derived syncytia at the mucosal surface of the adenoid. *Science* 272:115–117.

1358. Fraser, J. D., B. A. Irving, G. R. Crabtree, and A. Weiss. 1991. Regulation of interleukin-2 gene enhancer activity by the T cell accessory molecule CD28. *Science* 251:313–316.

1359. Frederick, T., L. Mascola, A. Eller, L. O'Neil, and B. Byers. 1994. Progression of human immunodeficiency virus disease among infants and children infected perinatally with human immunodeficiency virus or through neonatal blood transfusion. *Pediatr. Infect. Dis. J.* 13:1091–1097.

1360. Freed, E. O. 2002. Viral late domains. *J. Virol.* 76:4679–4687.

1361. Freed, E. O., E. L. Delwart, G. L. Buchschacher, Jr., and A. T. Panganiban. 1992. A mutation in the human immunodeficiency virus type 1 transmembrane glycoprotein gp41 dominantly interferes with fusion and infectivity. *Proc. Natl. Acad. Sci. USA* 89:70–74.

1362. Freed, E. O., and M. A. Martin. 1994. Evidence for a functional interaction between the V1/V2 and C4 domains of human immunodeficiency virus type 1 envelope glycoprotein gp120. *J. Virol.* 68:2503–2512.

1363. Freed, E. O., and D. J. Myers. 1992. Identification and characterization of fusion and processing domains of the human immunodeficiency virus type 2 envelope glycoprotein. *J. Virol.* 66:5472–5478.

1364. Freed, E. O., D. J. Myers, and R. Risser. 1991. Identification of the principal neutralizing determinant of human immunodeficiency virus type 1 as a fusion domain. *J. Virol.* 65:190–194.

1365. Freedman, A. R., F. M. Gibson, S. C. Fleming, C. J. Spry, and G. E. Griffin. 1991. Human immunodeficiency virus infection of eosinophils in human bone marrow cultures. *J. Exp. Med.* 174:1661–1664.

1365a. Freeman, G. J., E. J. Wherry, R. Ahmed, and A. H. Sharpe. 2006. Reinvigorating exhausted HIV-specific T cells via PD-1-PD-1 ligand blockade. *J. Exp. Med.* 203:2223–2227.

1366. Freitas, A. A., and B. B. Rocha. 1993. Lymphocyte lifespans: homeostasis, selection and competition. *Immunol. Today* **14**:25–29.

1367. French, M. A., P. Price, and S. F. Stone. 2004. Immune restoration disease after antiretroviral therapy. *AIDS* **18**: 1615–1627.

1368. French, N., A. Mujugira, J. Nakiyingi, D. Mulder, E. N. Janoff, and C. F. Gilks. 1999. Immunologic and clinical stages in HIV-1-infected Ugandan adults are comparable and provide no evidence of rapid progression but poor survival with advanced disease. *J. Acquir. Defic. Syndr.* **22**:509–516.

1369. Frey, S., M. Marsh, S. Gunther, A. Pelchen-Matthews, P. Stephens, S. Ortlepp, and T. Stegmann. 1995. Temperature dependence of cell-cell fusion induced by the envelope glycoprotein of human immunodeficiency virus type 1. *J. Virol.* **69**:1462–1472.

1370. Friborg, J., Jr., W. Kong, M. O. Hottiger, and G. J. Nabel. 1999. p53 inhibition by the LANA protein of KSHV protects against cell death. *Nature* **402**:889–894.

1371. Fridell, R. A., L. S. Harding, H. P. Bogerd, and B. R. Cullen. 1995. Identification of a novel human zinc finger protein that specifically interacts with the activation domain of lentiviral Tat proteins. *Virology* **209**:347–357.

1372. Friedland, G., P. Kahl, B. Saltzman, M. Rogers, C. Feiner, M. Mayers, C. Schable, and R. S. Klein. 1990. Additional evidence for lack of transmission of HIV infection by close interpersonal (casual) contact. *AIDS* **4**:639–644.

1373. Friedman-Kien, A. E., L. J. Laubenstein, P. Rubinstein, E. Buimovici-Klein, M. Marmor, R. Stahl, I. Spigland, K. S. Kim, and S. Zolla-Pazner. 1982. Disseminated Kaposi's sarcoma in homosexual men. *Ann. Intern. Med.* **96**:693–700.

1374. Friedrich, T. C., E. J. Dodds, L. J. Yant, L. Vojnov, R. Rudersdorf, C. Cullen, D. T. Evans, R. C. Desrosiers, B. R. Mothe, J. Sidney, A. Sette, K. Kunstman, S. Wolinsky, M. Piatak, J. Lifson, A. L. Hughes, N. Wilson, D. H. O'Connor, and D. I. Watkins. 2004. Reversion of CTL escape-variant immunodeficiency viruses *in vivo*. *Nat. Med.* **10**:275–281.

1375. Friis-Moller, N., C. A. Sabin, R. Weber, A. d'Arminio Monforte, W. M. El-Sadr, P. Reiss, R. Thiebaut, L. Morfeldt, S. De Wit, C. Pradier, G. Calvo, M. G. Law, O. Kirk, A. N. Phillips, and J. D. Lundgren. 2003. Combination antiretroviral therapy and the risk of myocardial infarction. *N. Engl. J. Med.* **349**:1993–2003.

1376. Frisch, M., R. J. Biggar, E. A. Engels, and J. J. Goedert. 2001. Association of cancer with AIDS-related immunosuppression in adults. *JAMA* **285**:1736–1745.

1377. Froland, S. S., P. Jenum, C. F. Lindboe, K. W. Wefring, P. J. Linnestad, and T. Bohmer. 1988. HIV-1 infection in Norwegian family before 1970. *Lancet* **i**:1344–1345.

1378. Frost, S. D., Y. Liu, S. L. Pond, C. Chappey, T. Wrin, C. J. Petropoulos, S. J. Little, and D. D. Richman. 2005. Characterization of human immunodeficiency virus type 1 (HIV-1) envelope variation and neutralizing antibody responses during transmission of HIV-1 subtype B. *J. Virol.* **79**:6523–6527.

1379. Fry, T. J., M. Moniuszko, S. Creekmore, S. J. Donohue, D. C. Douek, S. Giardina, T. T. Hecht, B. J. Hill, K. Komschlies, J. Tomaszewski, G. Franchini, and C. L. Mackall. 2003. IL-7 therapy dramatically alters peripheral T-cell homeostasis in normal and SIV-infected nonhuman primates. *Blood* **101**:2294–2299.

1380. Fu, Y. K., T. K. Hart, Z. L. Jonak, and P. J. Bugelski. 1993. Physiochemical dissociation of CD4-mediated syncytium formation and shedding of human immunodeficiency virus type 1 gp120. *J. Virol.* **67**:3818–3825.

1381. Fuchs, D., A. Forsman, L. Hagberg, M. Larsson, G. Norkrans, G. Reibnegger, E. R. Werner, and H. Wachter. 1990. Immune activation and decreased tryptophan in patients with HIV-1 infection. *J. Interferon Res.* **10**:599–603.

1382. Fujii, Y., K. Otake, M. Tashiro, and A. Adachi. 1996. In vitro cytocidal effects of human immunodeficiency virus type 1 Nef in unprimed human CD4+ T cells without MHC restriction. *J. Gen. Virol.* **77**:2943–2951.

1383. Fujii, Y., K. Otake, M. Tashiro, and A. Adachi. 1996. Soluble Nef antigen of HIV-1 is cytotoxic for human CD4+ T cells. *FEBS Lett.* **393**:93–96.

1384. Fujikawa, L. S., S. Z. Salahuddin, A. G. Palestine, R. B. Nussenblatt, and R. C. Gallo. 1985. Isolation of human T-lymphotropic virus type III from the tears of a patient with acquired immunodeficiency syndrome. *Lancet* **ii**:529–530.

1385. Fujino, T., T. Fujiyoshi, S. Yashiki, S. Sonoda, H. Otsuka, and Y. Nagata. 1992. HTLV-I transmission from mother to fetus via placenta. *Lancet* **340**:1157.

1386. Fujiwara, M., R. Tsunoda, S. Shigeta, T. Yokota, and M. Baba. 1999. Human follicular dendritic cells remain uninfected and capture human immunodeficiency virus type 1 through CD54-CD11a interaction. *J. Virol.* **73**:3603–3607.

1387. Fukumori, T., H. Akari, S. Iida, S. Hata, S. Kagawa, Y. Aida, A. H. Koyama, and A. Adachi. 1998. The HIV-1 vpr displays strong anti-apoptotic activity. *FEBS Lett.* **432**:17–20.

1388. Fulcher, J. A., Y. Hwangbo, R. Zioni, D. Nickle, X. Lin, L. Heath, J. I. Mullins, L. Corey, and T. Zhu. 2004. Compartmentalization of human immunodeficiency virus type 1 between blood monocytes and CD4+ T cells during infection. *J. Virol.* **78**:7883–7893.

1389. Fuller, D. H., P. A. Rajakumar, M. S. Wu, C. W. McMahon, T. Shipley, J. T. Fuller, A. Bazmi, A. M. Trichel, T. M. Allen, B. Mothe, J. R. Haynes, D. I. Watkins, and M. Murphey-Corb. 2006. DNA immunization in combination with effective antiretroviral drug therapy controls viral rebound and prevents simian AIDS after treatment is discontinued. *Virology* **348**:200–215.

1390. Fultz, P., H. M. McClure, H. Daugharty, A. Brodie, C. R. McGrath, B. Swenson, and D. P. Francis. 1986. Vaginal transmission of human immunodeficiency virus (HIV) to a chimpanzee. *J. Infect. Dis.* **5**:896–900.

1391. Fultz, P. N. 2004. HIV-1 superinfections: omens for vaccine efficacy? *AIDS* **18**:115–119.

1392. Fultz, P. N., J.-C. Gluckman, E. Muchmore, and M. Girard. 1992. Transient increases in numbers of infectious cells in an HIV-infected chimpanzee following immune stimulation. *AIDS Res. Hum. Retrovir.* **8**:313–317.

1393. Fultz, P. N., P. Nara, F. Barre-Sinoussi, A. Chaput, M. L. Greenberg, E. Muchmore, M.-P. Kieny, and M. Girard. 1992. Vaccine protection of chimpanzees against challenge with HIV-1-infected peripheral blood mononuclear cells. *Science* **256**:1687–1690.

1394. Fultz, P. N., A. Srinivasan, C. R. Greene, D. Butler, R. B. Swenson, and H. M. McClure. 1987. Superinfection of a chimpanzee with a second strain of human immunodeficiency virus. *J. Virol.* **61**:4026–4029.

1395. Fung, M. S. C., C. R. Y. Sun, W. L. Gordon, R.-S. Liou, T. W. Chang, W. N. C. Sun, E. S. Daar, and D. D. Ho. 1992. Identification and characterization of a neutralization site within the second variable region of human immunodeficiency virus type 1 gp120. *J. Virol.* 66:848–856.

1396. Funke, I., A. Hahn, E. P. Rieber, E. Weiss, and G. Riethmuller. 1987. The cellular receptor (CD4) of the human immunodeficiency virus is expressed on neurons and glial cells in human brain. *J. Exp. Med.* 165:1230–1235.

1397. Funkhouser, A., M. L. Clements, S. Slome, B. Clayman, and R. Viscidi. 1993. Antibodies to recombinant gp160 in mucosal secretions and sera of persons infected with HIV-1 and seronegative vaccine recipients. *AIDS Res. Hum. Retrovir.* 9:627–632.

1398. Furukawa, M., M. Yasukawa, Y. Yakushijin, and S. Fujita. 1994. Distinct effects of human herpesvirus 6 and human herpesvirus 7 on surface molecule expression and function of CD4+ T cells. *J. Immunol.* 152:5768–5775.

1399. Furuta, Y., K. Eriksson, B. Svennerholm, P. Fredman, P. Horal, S. Jeansson, A. Vahlne, J. Holmgren, and C. Czerkinsky. 1994. Infection of vaginal and colonic epithelial cells by the human immunodeficiency virus type 1 is neutralized by antibodies raised against conserved epitopes in the envelope glycoprotein gp120. *Proc. Natl. Acad. Sci. USA* 91:12559–12563.

1400. Fust, G., E. Ujhelyi, T. Hidvegi, K. Paloczi, R. Mihalik, S. Hollan, K. Nagy, and M. Kirschfink. 1991. The complement system in HIV disease. *Immunol. Investigo.* 20:231–241.

1401. Gabali, A. M., J. J. Anzinger, G. T. Spear, and L. L. Thomas. 2004. Activation by inflammatory stimuli increases neutrophil binding of human immunodeficiency virus type 1 and subsequent infection of lymphoctes. *J. Virol.* 78:10833–10836.

1402. Gabuzda, D. H., A. Lever, E. Terwilliger, and J. Sodroski. 1992. Effects of deletions in the cytoplasmic domain on biological functions of human immunodeficiency virus type 1 envelope glycoproteins. *J. Virol.* 66:3306–3315.

1403. Gahery-Segard, H., G. Pialoux, B. Charmeteau, S. Sermet, H. Poncelet, M. Raux, A. Tartar, J. P. Levy, H. Gras-Masse, and J. G. Guillet. 2000. Multiepitopic B- and T-cell responses induced in humans by a human immunodeficiency virus type 1 lipopeptide vaccine. *J. Virol.* 74:1694–1703.

1404. Gahery-Segard, H., G. Pialoux, S. Figueiredo, C. Igea, M. Surenaud, J. Gaston, H. Gras-Masse, J. P. Levy, and J. G. Guillet. 2003. Long-term specific immune responses induced in humans by a human immunodeficiency virus type 1 lipopeptide vaccine: characterization of CD8+-T-cell epitopes recognized. *J. Virol.* 77:11220–11231.

1405. Gaidano, G., P. Ballerini, J. Z. Gong, G. Inghirami, A. Neri, E. Q. Mewcomb, I. T. Magrath, D. M. Knowles, and R. Dalla-Favera. 1991. p53 mutations in human lymphoid malignancies: association with Burkitt lymphoma and chronic lymphocytic leukemia. *Proc. Natl. Acad. Sci. USA* 88:5413–5417.

1406. Gaidano, G., D. Capello, C. Pastore, A. Antinori, A. Gloghini, A. Carbone, L. M. Larocca, and G. Saglio. 1997. Analysis of human herpesvirus type 8 infection in AIDS-related and AIDS-unrelated primary central nervous system lymphoma. *J. Infect. Dis.* 175:1193–1197.

1407. Gail, M. H., J. M. Pluda, C. S. Rabkin, R. J. Biggar, J. J. Goedert, J. W. Horm, E. J. Sondik, R. Yarchoan, and S. Broder. 1991. Projections of the incidence of non-Hodgkin's lymphoma related to acquired immunodeficiency syndrome. *J. Natl. Cancer Inst.* 83:695–701.

1408. Gaines, H., J. Albert, M. von Sydow, A. Sonnerborg, F. Chiodi, A. Ehrnst, O. Strannegard, and B. Asjo. 1987. HIV antigenaemia and virus isolation from plasma during primary HIV infection. *Lancet* i:1317–1318.

1409. Gaines, H., M. von Sydow, J. V. Parry, M. Forsgren, P. O. Pehrson, A. Sonnerborg, P. P. Mortimer, and O. Strannegard. 1988. Detection of immunoglobulin M antibody in primary human immunodeficiency virus infection. *AIDS* 2:11–15.

1410. Gajewski, T. F., J. Joyce, and F. W. Fitch. 1989. Antiproliferative effect of IFN-gamma in murine regulation. III. Differential selection of TH1 and TH2 murine helper T lymphocyte clones using recombinant IL-2 and recombinant IFN-gamma. *J. Immunol.* 143:15–22.

1411. Gallaher, W. R. 1987. Detection of a fusion peptide sequence in the transmembrane protein of human immunodeficiency virus. *Cell* 50:327–328.

1412. Gallaher, W. R., J. M. Ball, R. F. Garry, M. C. Grinnin, and R. C. Montelaro. 1989. A general model for the transmembrane proteins of HIV and other retroviruses. *AIDS Res. Hum. Retrovir.* 5:431–440.

1413. Gallaher, W. R., C. DiSimone, and M. J. Buchmeier. 2001. The viral transmembrane superfamily: possible divergence of Arenavirus and Filovirus glycoproteins from a common RNA virus ancestor. *BMC Microbiol.* 1:1.

1414. Gallant, J. E., E. DeJesus, J. R. Arribas, A. L. Pozniak, B. Gazzard, R. E. Campo, B. Lu, D. McColl, S. Chuck, J. Enejosa, J. J. Toole, and A. K. Cheng. 2006. Tenofovir DF, emtricitabine, and efavirenz vs. zidovudine, lamivudine, and efavirenz for HIV. *N. Engl. J. Med.* 354:251–260.

1415. Gallay, P., V. Stitt, C. Mundy, M. Oettinger, and D. Trono. 1996. Role of the karyopherin pathway in human immunodeficiency virus type 1 nuclear import. *J. Virol.* 70:1027–1032.

1416. Gallay, P., S. Swingler, J. Song, F. Bushman, and D. Trono. 1995. HIV nuclear import is governed by the phosphotyrosine-mediated binding of matrix to the core domain of integrase. *Cell* 83:569–576.

1417. Galli, L., M. de Martino, P.-A. Tovo, C. Gabiano, M. Zappa, C. Giaquinto, S. Tulisso, A. Vierucci, M. Guerra, P. Marchisio, P. Dallacasa, and M. Stegagno. 1995. Onset of clinical signs in children with HIV-1 perinatal infection. *AIDS* 9:455–461.

1418. Gallo, D., J. R. George, J. H. Fitchen, A. S. Goldstein, and M. S. Hindahl. 1997. Evaluation of a system using oral mucosal transudate for HIV-1 antibody screening and confirmatory testing. *JAMA* 277:254–258.

1419. Gallo, P., K. Frei, C. Rordorf, J. Lazdins, B. Tavolato, and A. Fontana. 1989. Human immunodeficiency virus type 1 (HIV-1) infection of the central nervous system: an evaluation of cytokines in cerebrospinal fluid. *J. Neuroimmunol.* 23:109–116.

1420. Gallo, R. C., S. Z. Salahuddin, M. Popovic, G. M. Shearer, M. Kaplan, B. F. Haynes, T. J. Palker, R. Redfield, J. Oleske, and B. Safai. 1984. Frequent detection and isolation of cytopathic retroviruses (HTLV-III) from patients with AIDS and at risk for AIDS. *Science* 224:500–503.

1421. Gallo, R. C., P. S. Sarin, E. P. Gelmann, M. Robert-Guroff, E. Richardson, V. S. Kalyanaraman, D. Mann, G. D. Sidhu, R. E. Stahl, S. Zolla-Pazner, J. Leibowitch, and M. Popovic. 1983. Isolation of human T-cell leukemia virus in acquired immune deficiency syndrome (AIDS). *Science* 220:865–867.

1422. Gandhi, R. T., B. K. Chen, S. E. Strauss, J. K. Dale, M. J. Lenardo, and D. Baltimore. 1998. HIV-1 directly kills CD4+ T cells by a Fas-independent mechanism. *J. Exp. Med.* 187:1113–1122.

1423. Ganesh, L., E. Burstein, A. Guha-Niyogi, M. K. Louder, J. R. Mascola, L. W. J. Klomp, C. Wijmenga, C. S. Duckett, and G. J. Nabel. 2003. The gene product Murr1 restricts HIV-1 replication in resting CD4+ lymphocytes. *Nature* 426:853–857.

1424. Gao, F., E. Bailes, D. Robertson, Y. Chen, C. Rodenburg, S. Michael, L. Cummins, L. Authur, M. Peeters, B. Shaw, P. Sharp, and B. Hahn. 1999. Origin of HIV-1 in the chimpanzee *Pan troglodytes troglodytes. Nature* 397:436–441.

1425. Gao, F., D. L. Robertson, C. D. Carruthers, Y. Y. Li, E. Bailes, L. G. Kostrikis, M. O. Salminen, F. Bibollet-Ruche, M. Peeters, D. D. Ho, G. M. Shaw, P. M. Sharp, and B. H. Hahn. 1998. An isolate of human immunodeficiency virus type 1 originally classified as subtype I represents a complex mosaic comprising three different group M subtypes (A, G, and I). *J. Virol.* 72:10234–10241.

1426. Gao, F., S. A. Trask, H. Hui, O. Mamaeva, Y. Chen, T. S. Theodore, B. T. Foley, B. T. Korber, G. M. Shaw, and B. H. Hahn. 2001. Molecular characterization of a highly divergent HIV type 1 isolate obtained early in the AIDS epidemic from the Democratic Republic of Congo. *AIDS Res. Hum. Retrovir.* 17:1217–1222.

1427. Gao, F., L. Yue, D. L. Robertson, S. C. Hill, H. Hui, R. J. Biggar, A. E. Neequaye, T. M. Whelan, D. D. Ho, G. M. Shaw, P. M. Sharp, and B. H. Hahn. 1994. Genetic diversity of human immunodeficiency virus type 2: evidence for distinct sequence subtypes with differences in virus biology. *J. Virol.* 68:7433–7447.

1428. Gao, F., L. Yue, A. T. White, P. G. Pappas, J. Barchue, A. P. Hanson, B. M. Greene, P. M. Sharp, G. M. Shaw, and B. H. Hahn. 1992. Genetically-diverse simian-related human immunodeficiency type-2 viruses in West Africa. *J. Cell. Biochem.* Suppl. 16E:4.

1429. Gao, S., L. Kingsley, M. Li, W. Zheng, C. Parravicini, J. Ziegler, R. Newton, C. R. Rinaldo, A. Saah, J. Phair, R. Detels, Y. Chang, and P. S. Moore. 1996. KSHV antibodies among Americans, Italians and Ugandans with and without Kaposi's sarcoma. *Nat. Med.* 2:925–928.

1430. Gao, S. J., C. Boshoff, K. Jayachandra, R. A. Weiss, Y. Chang, and P. S. Moore. 1997. KSHV *ORF K9* (vIRF) is an oncogene which inhibits the interferon signaling pathway. *Oncogene* 15:1979–1985.

1431. Gao, S. J., J. H. Deng, and F. C. Zhou. 2003. Productive lytic replication of a recombinant Kaposi's sarcoma-associated herpesvirus in efficient primary infection of primary human endothelial cells. *J. Virol.* 77:9738–9749.

1432. Gao, S. J., L. Kingsley, D. R. Hoover, T. J. Spira, C. R. Rinaldo, A. Saah, J. Phair, R. Detels, P. Parry, Y. Chang, and P. S. Moore. 1996. Seroconversion to antibodies against Kaposi's sarcoma-associated herpesvirus-related latent nuclear antigens before the development of Kaposi's sarcoma. *N. Engl. J. Med.* 335:233–241.

1433. Gao, W. Y., R. Agbaria, J. S. Driscoll, and H. Mitsuya. 1994. Divergent anti-human immunodeficiency virus activity and anabolic phosphorylation of 2', 3'-dideoxynucleoside analogs in resting and activated human cells. *J. Biol. Chem.* 269:12633–12638.

1434. Gao, W. Y., A. Cara, R. C. Gallo, and F. Lori. 1993. Low levels of deoxynucleotides in peripheral blood lymphocytes: a strategy to inhibit human immunodeficiency virus type 1 replication. *Proc. Natl. Acad. Sci. USA.* 90:8925–8928.

1435. Gao, X., A. Bashirova, A. K. Iversen, J. Phair, J. J. Goedert, S. Buchbinder, K. Hoots, D. Vlahov, M. Altfeld, S. J. O'Brien, and M. Carrington. 2005. AIDS restriction HLA allotypes target distinct intervals of HIV-1 pathogenesis. *Nat. Med.* 11:1290–1292.

1436. Gao, X., G. W. Nelson, P. Karacki, M. P. Martin, J. Phair, R. Kaslow, J. J. Goedert, S. Buchbinder, K. Hoots, D. Vlahov, S. J. O'Brien, and M. Carrington. 2001. Effect of a single amino acid change in MHC class I molecules on the rate of progression to AIDS. *N. Engl. J. Med.* 344:1668–1675.

1437. Garba, M. L., C. D. Pilcher, A. L. Bingham, J. Eron, and J. A. Frelinger. 2002. HIV antigens can induce TGF-β1-producing immunoregulatory CD8+ T cells. 168:2247–2254.

1438. Garber, D. A., G. Silvestri, A. P. Barry, A. Fedanov, N. Kozyr, H. McClure, D. C. Montefiori, C. P. Larsen, J. D. Altman, S. I. Staprans, and M. B. Feinberg. 2004. Blockade of T cell costimulation reveals interrelated actions of CD4+ and CD8+ T cells in control of SIV replication. *J. Clin. Investigo.* 113:836–845.

1439. Garcia, F., M. M. Alonso, J. Romeu, H. Knobel, J. Arrizabalaga, E. Ferrer, D. Dalmau, I. Ruiz, F. Vidal, A. Frances, F. Segura, J. L. Gomez-Sirvent, A. Cruceta, B. Clotet, T. Pumarola, T. Gallart, W. A. O'Brien, J. M. Miro, J. M. Gatell.et al. 2000. Comparison of immunologic restoration and virologic response in plasma, tonsillar tissue, and cerebrospinal fluid in HIV-1-infected patients treated with double versus triple antiretroviral therapy in very early stages: The Spanish EARTH-2 Study. *J. Acquir. Immune Defic. Syndr.* 25:26–35.

1440. Garcia, F., M. Lejeune, N. Climent, C. Gil, J. Alcami, V. Morente, L. Alos, A. Ruiz, J. Setoain, E. Fumero, P. Castro, A. Lopez, A. Cruceta, C. Piera, E. Florence, A. Pereira, A. Libois, N. Gonzalez, M. Guila, M. Caballero, F. Lomena, J. Joseph, J. M. Miro, T. Pumarola, M. Plana, J. M. Gatell, and T. Gallart. 2005. Therapeutic immunization with dendritic cells loaded with heat-inactivated autologous HIV-1 in patients with chronic HIV-1 infection. *J. Infect. Dis.* 191:1680–1685.

1441. Garcia, F., G. Niebla, J. Romeu, C. Vidal, M. Plana, M. Ortega, L. Ruiz, T. Gallart, B. Clotet, J. M. Miro, T. Pumarola, and J. M. Gatell. 1999. Cerebrospinal fluid HIV-1 RNA levels in asymptomatic patients with early stage chronic HIV-1 infection: support for the hypothesis of local virus replication. *AIDS* 13:1491–1496.

1442. Garcia, F., M. Plana, G. M. Ortiz, S. Bonhoeffer, A. Soriano, C. Vidal, A. Cruceta, M. Arnedo, C. Gil, G. Pantaleo, T. Pumarola, T. Gallart, D. F. Nixon, J. M. Miro, and J. M. Gatell. 2001. The virological and immunological consequences of structured treatment interruptions in chronic HIV-1 infection. *AIDS* 15:F29–F40.

1443. Garcia, F., C. Vidal, J. M. Gatell, J. M. Miro, A. Soriano, and T. Pumarola. 1997. Viral load in asymptomatic patients with CD4+ lymphocyte counts above 500×10^6/l. *AIDS* 11: 53–57.

1444. Garcia, J. V., J. Alfano, and A. D. Miller. 1993. The negative effect of human immunodeficiency virus type 1 Nef on cell surface CD4 expression is not species specific and requires the cytoplasmic domain of CD4. *J. Virol.* 67:1511–1516.

1445. Garcia, J. V., and A. D. Miller. 1991. Serine phosphorylation-independent downregulation of cell-surface CD4 by *nef. Nature* 350:508–511.

1446. Garcia, M., X. F. Yu, D. E. Griffin, and W. J. Moss. 2005. In vitro suppression of human immunodeficiency virus type 1 replication by measles virus. *J. Virol.* 79:9197–9205.

1447. Gardner, M., A. Rosenthal, M. Jennings, J. Yee, L. Antipa, and E. Robinson, Jr. 1995. Passive immunization of rhesus macaques against SIV infection and disease. *AIDS Res. Hum. Retrovir.* 11:843–854.

1448. Gardner, M. B. 1996. The history of simian AIDS. *J. Med. Primatol.* 25:148–157.

1449. Gardner, M. B., M. P. Carlos, and P. A. Luciw. 2004. Simian retroviruses. *In* G. P. Wormser (ed.), *AIDS and Other Manifestations of HIV Infection.* Raven Press, New York, N.Y.

1450. Gardner, M. B., M. Endres, and P. Barry. 1994. The simian retroviruses: SIV and SRV, p. 133–276. *In* J. A. Levy (ed.), *The Retroviridae*, vol. 3. Plenum Press, New York, N.Y.

1451. Garg, H., and R. Blumenthal. 2006. HIV gp41-induced apoptosis is mediated by caspase-3-dependent mitochondrial depolarization, which is inhibited by HIV protease inhibitor nelfinavir. *J. Leukoc. Biol.* 79:351–362.

1452. Garred, P., H. O. Madsen, B. Hofmann, and A. Svejgaard. 1995. Increased frequency of homozygosity of abnormal mannan-binding protein alleles in patients with suspected immunodeficiency. *Lancet* 346:941–943.

1453. Garrett, L. 1998. Social, behavioral, and demographic factors in emerging infections. *J. Urban Health* 75:492–500.

1454. Garrity, R. R., G. Rimmelzwaan, A. Minassian, W. P. Tsai, G. Lin, J. J. deJong, J. Goudsmit, and P. L. Nara. 1997. Refocusing neutralizing antibody response by targeted dampening of an immunodominant epitope. *J. Immunol.* 159:279–289.

1454a. Garrus, J. E., U. K. von Schwedler, O. W. Pornillos, S. G. Morham, K. H. Zavitz, H. E. Wang, D. A. Wettstein, K. M. Stray, M. Cote, R. L. Rich, D. G. Myszka, and W. I. Sundquist. 2001. Tsg101 and the vacuolar protein sorting pathway are essential for HIV-1 budding. *Cell* 107:55–65.

1455. Garry, R. F. 1989. Potential mechanisms for the cytopathic properties of HIV. *AIDS* 3:683–694.

1456. Garry, R. F. 1990. Extensive antigenic mimicry by retrovirus capsid proteins. *AIDS Res. Hum. Retrovir.* 6:1361–1362.

1457. Garry, R. F., and G. Koch. 1992. Tat contains a sequence related to snake neurotoxins. *AIDS* 6:1541–1542.

1458. Garry, R. F., J. J. Kort, F. Koch-Nolte, and G. Koch. 1991. Similarities of viral proteins to toxins that interact with monovalent cation channels. *AIDS* 5:1381–1384.

1459. Gartner, S. 2000. HIV infection and dementia. *Science* 287:602–604.

1460. Gartner, S., P. Markovits, D. M. Markovitz, M. H. Kaplan, R. C. Gallo, and M. Popovic. 1986. The role of mononuclear phagocytes in HTLV-III/LAV infection. *Science* 233:215–219.

1461. Gasque, P., Y. D. Dean, E. P. McGreal, J. VanBeek, and B. P. Morgan. 2000. Complement components of the innate immune system in health and disease in the CNS. *Immunopharmacology* 49:171–186.

1462. Gattegno, R., A. Ramdani, and T. Jouault. 1992. Lectin-carbohydrate interactions and infectivity of human immunodeficiency virus type 1 (HIV-1). *AIDS Res. Hum. Retrovir.* 8:27–37.

1463. Gaudieri, S., D. DeSantis, E. McKinnon, C. Moore, D. Nolan, C. S. Witt, S. A. Mallal, and F. T. Christiansen. 2005. Killer immunoglobulin-like receptors and HLA act both independently and synergistically to modify HIV disease progression. *Genes Immun.* 6:683–690.

1464. Gauduin, M.,R. L. Glickman, Means, and R. Johnson. 1998. Inhibition of simian immunodeficiency virus (SIV) replication by CD8+ T lymphocytes from macaques immunized with live attenuated SIV. *J. Virol.* 72:6315–6324.

1465. Gauduin, M. C., R. L. Glickman, S. Ahmad, T. Yilma, and R. P. Johnson. 1999. Immunization with live attenuated simian immunodeficiency virus induces strong type 1 T helper responses and beta-chemokine production. *Proc. Natl. Acad. Sci. USA* 96:14031–14036.

1466. Gaulton, G. N., J. V. Scobie, and M. Rosenzweig. 1997. HIV-1 and the thymus. *AIDS* 11:403–414.

1467. Gavioli, R., E. Gallerani, C. Fortini, M. Fabris, A. Bottoni, A. Canella, A. Bonaccorsi, M. Marastoni, F. Micheletti, Q. Cafaro, P. Rimessi, A. Caputo, and B. Ensoli. 2004. HIV-1 Tat protein modulates the generation of cytotoxic T cell epitopes by modifying proteasome composition and enzymatic activity. *J. Immunol.* 173:3838–3843.

1468. Gaya, A., A. Esteve, J. Casabona, J. J. McCarthy, J. Martorell, T. F. Schulz, and D. Whitby. 2004. Amino acid residue at position 13 in HLA-DR beta chain plays a critical role in the development of Kaposi's sarcoma in AIDS patients. *AIDS* 18:199–204.

1469. Gazzinelli, R. T., M. Makino, S. K. Chattopadhyay, C. M. Snapper, A. Sher, A. W. Hugin, and H. C. Morse III. 1992. CD4+ subset regulation in viral infection. *J. Immunol.* 148:182–188.

1470. Gea-Banacloche, J. C., S. A. Migueles, L. Martino, W. L. Shupert, A. C. McNeil, M. S. Sabbaghian, L. Ehler, C. Prussin, R. Stevens, L. Lambert, J. Altman, C. W. Hallahan, J. C. de Quiros, and M. Connors. 2000. Maintenance of large numbers of virus-specific CD8+ T cells in HIV-infected progressors and long-term nonprogressors. *J. Immunol.* 165:1082–1092.

1471. Gea-Banacloche, J. C., E. E. Wieskopf, C. Hallahan, J. C. Lopez, B. de Quiros, M. Flanigan, J. M. Mican, J. Falloon, M. Baseler, R. Stevens, H. C. Lane, and M. Connors. 1998. Progression of human immunodeficiency virus disease is associated with increasing disruptions within the CD4+ T cell receptor repertoire. *J. Infect. Dis.* 177:579–585.

1472. Gehrz, R. C., and S. O. Knorr. 1979. Characterization of the role of mononuclear cell subpopulations in the in vitro lymphocyte proliferation assay. *Clin. Exp. Immunol.* 37:551–557.

1473. Geiben-Lynn, R., N. Brown, B. D. Walker, and A. D. Luster. 2002. Purification of a modified form of bovine antithrombin III as an HIV-1 CD8+ T-cell antiviral factor. *J. Biol. Chem.* 277:42352–42357.

1474. Geiben-Lynn, R., M. Kursar, N. V. Brown, E. L. Kerr, A. D. Luster, and B. D. Walker. 2001. Noncytolytic inhibition of X4 virus by bulk CD8+ cells from human immunodeficiency virus type 1 (HIV-1)-infected persons and HIV-1 specific cytotoxic T lymphocytes is not mediated by β-chemokines. *J. Virol.* 75:8306–8316.

1475. Geiben-Lynn, R., M. Kursar, N. W. Brown, M. M. Addo, H. Shau, J. Lieberman, A. D. Luster, and B. D. Walker. 2003. HIV-1 antiviral activity of recombinant natural killer cell enhancing factors NKEF-A and NKEF-B, members of the peroxiredoxin family. *J. Biol. Chem.* 278:1569–1574.

1476. Geijtenbeek, T. B., D. S. Kwon, R. Torensma, S. J. van Vliet, G. C. van Duijnhoven, J. Middel, I. L. Cornelissen,

H. S. Nottet, V. N. KewalRamani, D. R. Littman, C. G. Figdor, and Y. van Kooyk. 2000. DC-SIGN, a dendritic cell-specific HIV-1-binding protein that enhances trans-infection of T cells. *Cell* 100:587–597.

1477. Geijtenbeek, T. B., R. Torensma, S. J. van Vliet, G. C. van Duijnhoven, G. J. Adema, Y. van Kooyk, and C. G. Figdor. 2000. Identification of DC-SIGN, a novel dendritic cell-specific ICAM-3 receptor that supports primary immune responses. *Cell* 100:575–585.

1478. Geijtenbeek, T. B., G. C. van Duijnhoven, S. J. van Vliet, E. Krieger, G. Vriend, C. G. Figdor, and Y. van Kooyk. 2002. Identification of different binding sites in the dendritic cell-specific receptor DC-SIGN for intercellular adhesion molecule 3 and HIV- 1. *J. Biol. Chem.* 277:11314–11320.

1479. Geiss, G. K., R. E. Bumgarner, M. C. An, M. B. Agy, A. B. van't Wout, E. Hammersmark, V. S. Carter, D. Upchurch, J. I. Mullins, and M. G. Katze. 2000. Large-scale monitoring of host cell gene expression during HIV-1 infection using cDNA microarrays. *Virology* 266:8–16.

1480. Geissler, R. G., R. Rossol, U. Mentzel, O. G. Ottmann, A. S. Klein, P. Gute, E. B. Helm, D. Hoelzer, and A. Ganser. 1996. Gamma-delta-T-cell-receptor-positive lymphocytes inhibit human hematopoietic progenitor cell growth in HIV Type 1-infected patients. *AIDS Res. Hum. Retrovir.* 12:577–584.

1481. Gelbard, H. A., K. A. Dzenko, D. DiLoreto, C. del Cerro, M. del Cerro, and L. G. Epstein. 1993. Neurotoxic effects of tumor necrosis factor alpha in primary human neuronal cultures are mediated by activation of the glutamate AMPA receptor subtype: implications for AIDS neuropathogenesis. *Dev. Neurosci.* 15:417–422.

1482. Gelbard, H. A., H. S. L. M. Nottet, S. Swindells, M. Jett, K. A. Dzenko, P. Genis, R. White, L. Wang, Y.-B. Choi, D. Zhang, S. A. Lipton, W. W. Tourtellotte, L. G. Epstein, and H. E. Gendelman. 1994. Platelet-activating factor: a candidate human immunodeficiency virus type-1-induced neurotoxin. *J. Virol.* 68:4628–4635.

1483. Gelderblom, H. R., M. Ozel, E. H. S. Hausmann, T. Winkel, G. Pauli, and M. A. Koch. 1988. Fine structure of human immunodeficiency virus (HIV), immunolocalization of structural proteins and virus-cell relation. *Micron Microscopica* 19:41–60.

1484. Gelderblom, H. R., M. Ozel, and G. Pauli. 1989. Morphogenesis and morphology of HIV. Structure-function relations. *Arch. Virol.* 106:1–13.

1485. Geleziunas, R., W. Xu, K. Takeda, H. Ichijo, and W. C. Greene. 2001. HIV-1 Nef inhibits ASK1-dependent death signalling providing a potential mechanism for protecting the infected host cell. *Nature* 410:834–838.

1486. Gendelman, H. E., J. M. Orenstein, L. M. Baca, B. Weiser, H. Burger, D. C. Kalter, and M. S. Meltzer. 1989. The macrophage in the persistence and pathogenesis of HIV infection. *AIDS* 3:475–495.

1487. Gendelman, H. E., J. M. Orenstein, M. A. Martin, C. Ferruca, R. Mitra, T. Phipps, L. A. Wahl, H. C. Lane, A. S. Fauci, and D. S. Burke. 1988. Efficient isolation and propagation of human immunodeficiency virus on recombinant colony-stimulating factor 1-treated monocytes. *J. Exp. Med.* 167:1428–1441.

1488. Gendelman, H. E., W. Phelps, L. Feigenbaum, J. M. Ostrove, A. Adachi, P. M. Howley, G. Khoury, H. S. Ginsberg, and M. A. Martin. 1986. Trans-activation of the human immunodeficiency virus long terminal repeat sequence by DNA viruses. *Proc. Natl. Acad. Sci. USA* 83:9759–9763.

1489. Genis, P., M. Jett, E. W. Bernton, T. Boyle, H. A. Gelbard, K. Dzenko, R. W. Keane, L. Resnick, Y. Mizrachi, D. J. Volsky, L. G. Epstein, and H. E. Gendelman. 1992. Cytokines and arachidonic metabolites produced during human immunodeficiency virus (HIV)-infected macrophage-astroglia interactions: implications for the neuropathogenesis of HIV disease. *J. Exp. Med.* 176:1703–1718.

1490. Gentric, A., M. Blaschek, C. Julien, J. Jouquan, Y. Pennec, J.-M. Berthelot, D. Mottier, R. Casburn-Budd, and P. Youinou. 1991. Nonorgan-specific autoantibodies in individuals infected with type 1 human immunodeficiency virus. *Clin. Immunol. Immunopathol.* 59:487–494.

1491. George, J. R., C. Y. Ou, B. Parekh, K. Brattegaard, V. Brown, E. Boateng, and K. M. De Cock. 1992. Prevalence of HIV-1 and HIV-2 mixed infections in Cote d'Ivoire. *Lancet* 340:337–339.

1492. George, M. D., E. Reay, S. Sankaran, and S. Dandekar. 2005. Early antiretroviral therapy for simian immunodeficiency virus infection leads to mucosal CD4+ T-cell restoration and enhanced gene expression regulating mucosal repair and regeneration. *J. Virol.* 79:2709–2719.

1493. George, M. D., S. Sankaran, E. Reay, A. C. Gelli, and S. Dandekar. 2003. High-throughput gene expression profiling indicates dysregulation of intestinal cell cycle mediators and growth factors during primary simian immunodeficiency virus infection. *Virology* 312:84–94.

1494. Gerberding, J. L. 1995. Management of occupational exposures to blood-borne viruses. *N. Engl. J. Med.* 332:444–451.

1495. Gerberding, J. L. 2003. Occupational exposure to HIV in health care settings. *N. Engl. J. Med.* 348:826–833.

1496. Geretti, A. M., M. E. M. Dings, C. A. C. M. van Els, C. A. van Baalen, F. Wijnholds, J. C. C. Borleffs, and A. D. M. E. Osterhaus. 1996. Human immunodeficiency virus type 1 (HIV-1)- and Epstein-Barr virus-specific cytotoxic T lymphocyte precursors exhibit different kinetics in HIV-1-infected persons. *J. Infect. Dis.* 174:34–45.

1497. Gershon, R. K., and K. Kondo. 1971. Infectious immunological tolerance. *Immunology* 21:903–914.

1498. Gershon, R. R. M., D. Vlahov, and K. E. Nelson. 1990. The risk of transmission of HIV-1 through non-percutaneous, non-sexual modes—a review. *AIDS* 4:645–650.

1499. Gherardi, R. K., F. Chretien, M. H. Delfau-Larue, F. J. Authier, A. Moulignier, D. Roulland-Dussoix, and L. Belec. 1998. Neuropathy in diffuse infiltrative lymphocytosis syndrome: an HIV neuropathy, not a lymphoma. *Neurology* 50:1041–1044.

1500. Ghorpade, A., A. Nukuna, M. Che, S. Haggerty, Y. Perisidsky, E. Carter, L. Carhart, L. Shafer, and H. E. Gendelman. 1998. Human immunodeficiency virus neurotropism: an analysis of viral replication and cytopathicity for divergent strains in monocytes and microglia. *J. Virol.* 72:3340–3350.

1501. Ghosh, D. 1992. Glucocorticoid receptor-binding site in the human immunodeficiency virus long terminal repeat. *J. Virol.* 66:586–590.

1502. Ghosn, J., M. Chaix, G. Peytavin, E. Rey, J. Bresson, C. Goujard, C. Katlama, J. Viard, J. Treluyer, and C. Rouzioux. 2004. Penetration of enfuvirtide, tenofovir, efavirenz, and protease inhibitors in the genital tract of HIV-1 infected men. *AIDS* 18:1958–1961.

1503. Ghosn, J., J. Viard, C. Katlama, L. de Almeida, R. Tubiana, F. Letourneur, L. Aaron, C. Goujard, D. Salmon, M. Lereuz-Ville, C. Rouzioux, and M. Chaix. 2004. Evidence of genotypic resistance diversity of archived and circulating viral strains in blood and semen of pre-treated HIV-infected men. *AIDS* 18:447–457.

1504. Ghosn, J., M. Wirden, N. Ktorza, G. Peytavin, H. Ait-Mohand, L. Schneider, S. Dominguez, F. Bricaire, V. Calvez, D. Costagliola, and C. Katlama. 2005. No benefit of a structured treatment interruption based on genotypic resistance in heavily pretreated HIV-infected patients. *AIDS* 19:1643–1647.

1505. Giavedoni, L., S. Ahmad, L. Jones, and T. Yilma. 1997. Expression of gamma interferon by simian immunodeficiency virus increases attenuation and reduces postchallenge virus load in vaccinated rhesus macaques. *J. Virol.* 71:866–872.

1506. Giavedoni, L. D., V. Planelles, N. L. Haigwood, S. Ahmad, J. D. Kluge, M. L. Marthas, M. B. Gardner, P. A. Luciw, and T. D. Yilma. 1993. Immune response of rhesus macaques to recombinant simian immunodeficiency virus gp130 does not protect from challenge infection. *J. Virol.* 67:577–583.

1507. Gibbs, J. S., A. A. Lackner, S. M. Lang, M. A. Simon, P. K. Sehgal, M. D. Daniel, and R. C. Desrosiers. 1995. Progression to AIDS in the absence of a gene for *vpr* or *vpx*. *J. Virol.* 69:2378–2383.

1508. Giddens, W. E., Jr., C. C. Tsai, W. R. Morton, H. D. Ochs, G. H. Knitter, and G. A. Blakley. 1985. Retroperitoneal fibromatosis and acquired immunodeficiency syndrome in macaques. Pathologic observations and transmission studies. *Am. J. Pathol.* 119:253–263.

1509. Gigliotti, F. 2005. Pneumocystis carinii: has the name really been changed? *Clin. Infect. Dis.* 41:1752–1755.

1510. Giguere, J., S. Bounou, S. Paquette, J. Madrenas, and M. J. Tremblay. 2004. Insertion of host-derived costimulatory molecules CD80 (B7.1) and CD86 (B7.2) into human immunodeficiency virus type 1 affects the virus life cycle. *J. Virol.* 78:6222–6232.

1511. Gilbert, J. M., D. Mason, and J. M. White. 1990. Fusion of Rous sarcoma virus with host cells does not require exposure to low pH. *J. Virol.* 64:5106–5113.

1512. Gilbert, M., J. Kirihara, and J. Mills. 1991. Enzyme-linked immunoassay for human immunodeficiency virus type 1 envelope glycoprotein 120. *J. Clin. Microbiol.* 29:142–147.

1513. Gilbert, P. B., M. L. Ackers, P. W. Berman, D. P. Francis, V. Popovic, D. J. Hu, W. L. Hayward, F. Sinangil, B. E. Shepherd, and M. Gurwith. 2005. HIV-1 virologic and immunologic progression and initiation of antiretroviral therapy among HIV-1-infected subjects in a trial of the efficacy of recombinant glycoprotein 120 vaccine. *J. Infect. Dis.* 192:974–983.

1514. Gilbert, P. B., M. L. Peterson, D. Follmann, M. G. Hudgens, D. P. Francis, M. Gurwith, W. L. Heyward, D. V. Jobes, V. Popovic, S. G. Self, F. Sinangil, D. Burke, and P. W. Berman. 2005. Correlation between immunologic responses to a recombinant glycoprotein 120 vaccine and incidence of HIV-1 infection in a Phase 3 HIV-1 preventive vaccine trial. *J. Infect. Dis.* 191:666–677.

1515. Gill, M. J., L. R. Sutherland, and D. L. Church. 1992. Gastrointestinal tissue cultures for HIV in HIV-infected/AIDS patients. *AIDS* 6:553–556.

1516. Gillespie, G. M., R. Kaul, T. Dong, H. B. Yang, T. Rostron, J. J. Bwayo, P. Kiama, T. Peto, F. A. Plummer, A. J. McMichael, and S. L. Rowland-Jones. 2002. Cross-reactive cy-totoxic T lymphocytes against a HIV-1 p24 epitope in slow progressors with B*57. *AIDS* 16:961–972.

1517. Gilliam, B. L., J. R. Dyer, S. A. Fiscus, C. Marcus, S. Zhou, L. Wathen, W. W. Freimuth, M. S. Cohen, and J. J. Eron, Jr. 1997. Effects of reverse transcriptase inhibitor therapy on the HIV-1 viral burden in semen. *J. Acquir. Immune Defic. Syndr. Hum. Retrovirol.* 15:54–60.

1518. Gilson, R. J. C., A. E. Hawkins, M. R. Beecham, E. Ross, J. Waite, M. Briggs, T. McNally, G. E. Kelly, R. S. Tedder, and I. V. D. Weller. 1997. Interactions between HIV and hepatitis B virus in homosexual men: effects on the natural history of infection. *AIDS* 11:597–606.

1519. Gimble, J. M., E. Duh, J. M. Ostrove, H. E. Gendelman, E. E. Max, and A. B. Rabson. 1988. Activation of the human immunodeficiency virus long terminal repeat by herpes simplex virus type 1 is associated with induction of a nuclear factor that binds to the NF-kappaB/core enhancer sequence. *J. Virol.* 62:4104–4112.

1520. Gimenez-Barcons, M., M. Ribera, A. Llano, B. Clotet, J. A. Este, and M. A. Martinez. 2005. Analysis of chemokine and cytokine expression in patients with HIV and GB virus type C coinfection. *Clin. Infect. Dis.* 40:1342–1349.

1521. Giorgi, J. V., L. E. Hultin, J. A. McKeating, T. D. Johnson, B. Owens, L. P. Jacobson, R. Shih, J. Lewis, D. J. Wiley, J. P. Phair, S. M. Wolinsky, and R. Detels. 1999. Shorter survival in advanced human immunodeficiency virus type 1 infection is more closely associated with T lymphocyte activation than with plasma virus burden or virus chemokine coreceptor usage. *J. Infect. Dis.* 179:859–870.

1522. Giorgi, J. V., Z. Liu, L. E. Hultin, W. G. Cumberland, K. Hennessey, and R. Detels. 1993. Elevated levels of CD38+ CD8+ T cells in HIV infection add to the prognostic value of low CD4+ T cell levels: results of 6 years of follow-up. *J. Acquir. Immune Defic. Syndr.* 6:904–912.

1523. Giraldo, B., E. Beth, and F. Hagnuenau. 1972. Herpes virus particles in tissue culture of Kaposi's sarcoma from different geographic regions. *J. Natl. Cancer Inst.* 49:1509–1526.

1524. Girard, M., M.-P. Kieny, A. Pinter, F. Barre-Sinoussi, P. Nara, H. Kobe, K. Kusumi, A. Chaput, T. Reinhart, E. Muchmore, J. Ronco, M. Kaczonek, E. Garrard, J.-C. Gluckman, and P. N. Fultz. 1991. Immunization of chimpanzees confers protection against challenge with human immunodeficiency virus. *Proc. Natl. Acad. Sci. USA* 88:542–546.

1525. Girard, M., B. Meignier, F. Barre-Sinoussi, M. P. Kieny, T. Matthews, E. Muchmore, P. L. Nara, Q. Wei, L. Rimsky, K. Weinhold, and P. N. Fultz. 1995. Vaccine-induced protection of chimpanzees against infection by a heterologous human immunodeficiency virus type 1. *J. Virol.* 69:6239–6248.

1526. Girard, P. M., V. Schneider, A. Dehee, C. Mariot, C. Jacomet, N. Delphin, F. Damond, G. Carcelain, B. Autran, A. G. Saimot, J. C. Nicolas, and W. Rozenbaum. 2001. Treatment interruption after one year of triple nucleoside analogue therapy for primary HIV infection. *AIDS* 15:275–277.

1527. Girardi, E., C. A. Sabin, A. d'Arminio Monforte, B. Hogg, A. N. Phillips, M. J. Gill, F. Dabis, P. Reiss, O. Kirk, E. Bernasconi, S. Grabar, A. Justice, S. Staszewski, G. Fatkenheuer, and J. A. Sterne. 2005. Incidence of tuberculosis among HIV-infected patients receiving highly active antiretroviral therapy in Europe and North America. *Clin. Infect. Dis.* 41:1772–1782.

1528. Gisselquist, D. 2003. Emergence of the HIV type 1 epidemic in the twentieth century: comparing hypotheses to evidence. *AIDS Res. Hum. Retrovir.* **19**:1071–1078.

1529. Giulian, D., K. Vaca, and C. A. Noonan. 1990. Secretion of neurotoxins by mononuclear phagocytes infected with HIV-1. *Science* **250**:1593–1596.

1530. Giulian, D., E. Wendt, K. Vaca, and C. A. Noonan. 1993. The envelope glycoprotein of human immunodeficiency virus type 1 stimulates release of neurotoxins from monocytes. *Proc. Natl. Acad. Sci. USA* **90**:2769–2773.

1531. Glass, W. G., D. H. McDermott, J. K. Lim, S. Lekhong, S. F. Yu, W. A. Frank, J. Pape, R. C. Cheshier, and P. M. Murphy. 2006. CCR5 deficiency increases risk of symptomatic West Nile virus infection. *J. Exp. Med.* **203**:35–40.

1532. Glesby, M. J., D. R. Hoover, H. Farzadegan, J. B. Margolick, and A. J. Saah. 1996. The effect of influenza vaccination on human immunodeficiency virus type 1 load: a randomized, double-blind, placebo-controlled study. *J. Infect. Dis.* **174**:1332–1336.

1533. Glick, M., M. Trope, O. Bagasra, and M. E. Pliskin. 1991. Human immunodeficiency virus infection of fibroblasts in dental pulp in seropositive patients. *Oral Surg. Oral Med. Oral Pathol.* **71**:733–736.

1534. Gloster, S. E., P. Newton, D. Cornforth, J. D. Lifson, I. Williams, G. M. Shaw, and P. Borrow. 2004. Association of strong virus-specific CD4 T cell responses with efficient natural control of primary HIV-1 infection. *AIDS* **18**:749–755.

1535. Gnann, J. W., Jr., J. B. McCormick, S. Mitchell, J. A. Nelson, and M. B. A. Oldstone. 1987. Synthetic peptide immunoassay distinguishes HIV type 1 and HIV type 2 infections. *Science* **237**:1346–1349.

1536. Godfrey, D. I., and M. Kronenberg. 2004. Going both ways: immune regulation via CD1d-dependent NKT cells. *J. Clin. Investigo* **114**:1379–1388.

1537. Godfried, M. H., T. van der Poll, J. Jansen, J. A. Romijn, J. K. M. E. Schattekerk, E. Endert, S. J. H. van Deventer, and H. P. Sauerwein. 1993. Soluble receptors for tumour necrosis factor: a putative marker of disease progression in HIV infection. *AIDS* **7**:33–36.

1538. Goedert, J. J., A.-M. Duliege, C. I. Amos, S. Felton, and R. J. Biggar. 1991. High risk of HIV-1 infection for first-born twins. *Lancet* **338**:1471–1475.

1539. Goedert, J. J., C. M. Kessler, L. M. Aledort, R. J. Biggar, W. A. Andes, G. C. White, J. E. Drummond, K. Vaidya, D. L. Mann, M. E. Eyster, M. V. Ragni, M. M. Lederman, A. R. Cohen, G. L. Bray, P. S. Rosenberg, R. M. Friedman, M. W. Hilgartner, W. A. Blattner, B. Kroner, and M. Gail. 1989. A prospective study of human immunodeficiency virus type 1 infection and the development of AIDS in subjects with hemophilia. *N. Engl. J. Med.* **321**:1141–1148.

1540. Goetz, M. B., D. R. Feikin, H. L. Lennox, W. A. O'Brien, C. M. Elie, J. C. Butler, and R. F. Breiman. 2002. Viral load response to a pneumococcal conjugate vaccine, polysaccharide vaccine or placebo among HIV-infected patients. *AIDS* **16**:1421–1428.

1541. Goff, S. P. 1996. Operating under a Gag order: a block against incoming virus by the Fv1 gene. *Cell* **86**:691–693.

1542. Goff, S. P. 2004. Retrovirus restriction factors. *Mol. Cell* **16**:849–859.

1543. Goh, W. C., J. Markee, R. E. Akridge, M. Meldorf, L. Musey, T. Karchmer, M. Krone, A. Collier, L. Corey, M. Emerman, and M. J. McElrath. 1999. Protection against human immunodeficiency virus type 1 infection in persons with repeated exposure: evidence for T cell immunity in the absence of inherited CCR5 coreceptor defects. *J. Infect. Dis.* **179**:548–557.

1544. Goh, W. C., M. E. Rogel, C. M. Kinsey, S. F. Michael, P. N. Fultz, M. A. Nowak, H. B. H., and M. Emerman. 1998. HIV-1 Vpr increases viral expression by manipulation of the cell cycle: a mechanism for selection of Vpr in vivo. *Nat. Med.* **4**:65–71.

1545. Golden, M. P., S. Kim, S. M. Hammer, E. Z. Ladd, P. A. Schaffer, N. DeLuca, and M. A. Albrecht. 1992. Activation of human immunodeficiency virus by herpes simplex virus. *J. Infect. Dis.* **166**:494–499.

1546. Goldin, B. R., W. Li, K. Mansfield, M. Woods, C. Wanke, L. Freeman, A. Shevitz, L. Gualtieri, S. Bussell, and S. L. Gorbach. 2005. The effect of micronutrient supplementation on disease progression and death in simian immunodeficiency virus-infected juvenile make rhesus macaques. *J. Infect. Dis.* **192**:311–318.

1547. Golding, H., R. Blumenthal, J. Manischewitz, D. R. Littman, and D. S. Dimitrov. 1993. Cell fusion mediated by interaction of a hybrid CD4.CD8 molecule with the human immunodeficiency virus type 1 envelope glycoprotein does occur after a long lag time. *J. Virol.* **67**:6469–6475.

1548. Golding, H., F. A. Robey, F. T. Gates III, W. Linder, P. R. Beining, T. Hoffman, and B. Golding. 1988. Identification of homologous regions in human immunodeficiency virus I gp41 and human MHC Class II beta 1 domain. I. Monoclonal antibodies against the gp41-derived peptide and patients' sera react with native HLA Class II antigens, suggesting a role for autoimmunity in the pathogenesis of acquired immune deficiency syndrome. *J. Exp. Med.* **167**:914–923.

1549. Goldsmith, M. A., and R. W. Doms. 2002. HIV entry: are all receptors created equal? *Nat. Immunol.* **3**:709–710.

1550. Goldsmith, M. A., M. T. Warmerdam, R. E. Atchison, M. D. Miller, and W. C. Greene. 1995. Dissociation of the CD4 downregulation and viral infectivity enhancement functions of human immunodeficiency virus type 1 Nef. *J. Virol.* **69**:4112–4121.

1551. Goldstein, S., I. Ourmanov, C. R. Brown, B. E. Beer, W. R. Elkins, R. Plishka, A. Buckler-White, and V. M. Hirsch. 2000. Range of viral load in healthy African green monkeys infected with simian immunodeficiency virus. *J. Virol.* **74**:11744–11753.

1552. Goletti, D., S. Carrara, D. Vincenti, E. Giacomini, L. Fattorini, A. R. Garbuglia, M. R. Capobianchi, T. Alonzi, G. M. Fimia, M. Federico, G. Poli, and E. Coccia. 2004. Inhibition of HIV-1 replication in monocyte-derived macrophages by *Mycobacterium tuberculosis*. *J. Infect. Dis.* **189**:624–633.

1553. Gollub, E. L., and Z. A. Stein. 1993. The new female condom—item 1 on a women's AIDS prevention agenda. *Am. J. Public Health* **83**:498–500.

1554. Gomez, A. M., F. M. Smaill, and K. L. Rosenthal. 1994. Inhibition of HIV replication by CD8+ T cells correlates with CD4 counts and clinical stage of disease. *Clin. Exp. Immunol.* **97**:68–75.

1555. Gomez, C., and T. J. Hope. 2005. The ins and outs of HIV replication. *Cell. Microbiol.* **7**:621–626.

1556. Gomez, L. M., E. Pacyniak, M. Flick, D. R. Hout, M. L. Gomez, E. Nerrienet, A. Ayouba, M. L. Santiago, B. H. Hahn, and E. B. Stephens. 2005. Vpu-mediated CD4 down-regulation and degradation is conserved among highly divergent SIVcpz strains. *Virology* **335**:46–60.

1557. Gomez, M. B., and J. E. K. Hildreth. 1995. Antibody to adhesion molecule LFA-1 enhances plasma neutralization of human immunodeficiency virus type 1. *J. Virol.* **69**:4628–4632.

1558. Gomez-Romain, V. R., L. J. Patterson, D. Venson, D. Liewehr, K. Aldrich, R. Florese, and M. Robert-Guroff. 2005. Vaccine-elicited antibodies mediate antibody-dependent cellular cytotoxicity correlated with significantly reduced acute viremia in rhesus macaques challenged with SIVmac251. *J. Immunol.* **174**:2185–2189.

1559. Gonda, M., F. Wong-Staal, R. C. Gallo, J. E. Clements, O. Narayan, and R. V. Gilden. 1985. Sequence homology and morphologic similarity of HTLV-III and visna virus, a pathogenic lentivirus. *Science* **227**:173–177.

1560. Gonzales, M. J., E. Delwart, S.-Y. Rhee, R. Tsui, A. R. Zolopa, J. Taylor, and R. W. Shafer. 2003. Lack of detectable human immunodeficiency virus type-1 superinfection during 1072 person-years of observation. *J. Infect. Dis.* **188**:397–405.

1561. Gonzalez, E., H. Kulkarni, H. Bolivar, A. Mangano, R. Sanchez, G. Catano, R. J. Nibbs, B. I. Freedman, M. P. Quinones, M. J. Bamshad, K. K. Murthy, B. H. Rovin, W. Bradley, R. A. Clark, S. A. Anderson, J. O'Connell, B. K. Agan, S. S. Ahuja, R. Bologna, L. Sen, M. J. Dolan, and S. K. Ahuja. 2005. The influence of CCL3L1 gene-containing segmental duplications on HIV-1/AIDS susceptibility. *Science* **307**:1434–1440.

1562. Gonzalez, E., B. H. Rovin, L. Sen, G. Cooke, R. Dhanda, S. Mummidi, H. Kulkarni, M. J. Bamshad, V. Telles, S. A. Anderson, E. A. Walter, K. T. Stephan, M. Deucher, A. Mangano, R. Bologna, S. S. Ahuja, M. J. Dolan, and S. K. Ahuja. 2002. HIV-1 infection and AIDS dementia are influenced by a mutant MCP-1 allele linked to increased monocyte infiltration of tissues and MCP-1 levels. *Proc. Natl. Acad. Sci. USA* **99**:13795–13800.

1563. Gonzalez-Scarano, F., and J. Martin-Garcia. 2005. The neuropathogenesis of AIDS. *Nat. Rev. Immunol.* **5**:69–81.

1564. Gonzalez-Scarano, F., M. N. Waxham, A. M. Ross, and J. A. Hoxie. 1987. Sequence similarities between human immunodeficiency virus gp41 and paramyxovirus fusion proteins. *AIDS Res. Hum. Retrovir.* **3**:245–252.

1565. Gordon, D. M., T. W. McGovern, U. Krzych, J. C. Cohen, I. Schneider, R. LaChance, D. G. Heppner, G. Yuan, M. Hollingdale, M. Slaoui, et al. 1995. Safety, immunogenicity, and efficacy of a recombinantly produced Plasmodium falciparum circumsporozoite protein-hepatitis B surface antigen subunit vaccine. *J. Infect. Dis.* **171**:1576–1585.

1566. Gordon, S. 2002. Pattern recognition receptors: doubling up for the innate immune response. *Cell* **111**:927–930.

1567. Gorelick, R. J., R. E. Benveniste, J. D. Lifson, J. L. Yovandich, W. R. Morton, L. Kuller, B. M. Flynn, B. A. Fisher, J. L. Rossio, M. Piatak, Jr., J. W. Bess, Jr., L. E. Henderson, and L. O. Arthur. 2000. Protection of *Macaca nemestrina* from disease following pathogenic simian immunodeficiency virus (SIV) challenge: utilization of SIV nucleocapsid mutant DNA vaccines with and without an SIV protein boost. *J. Virol.* **74**:11935–11949.

1568. Gorny, M. K., A. J. Conley, S. Karwowska, A. Buchbinder, J. Y. Xu, E. A. Emini, S. Koenig, and S. Zolla-Pazner. 1992. Neutralization of diverse human immunodeficiency virus type 1 variants by an anti-V3 human monoclonal antibody. *J. Virol.* **66**:7538–7542.

1569. Gorny, M. K., J. P. Moore, A. J. Conley, S. Karwowska, J. Sodroski, C. Williams, S. Burda, L. J. Boots, and S. Zolla-Pazner. 1994. Human anti-V2 monoclonal antibody that neutralizes primary but not laboratory isolates of human immunodeficiency virus type 1. *J. Virol.* **68**:8312–8320.

1570. Gorny, M. K., J. Y. Xu, S. Karwowska, A. Buchbinder, and S. Zolla-Pazner. 1993. Repertoire of neutralizing human monoclonal antibodies specific for the V3 domain of HIV-1 gp120. *J. Immunol.* **150**:635–643.

1571. Gorochov, G., A. U. Neumann, A. Kereveur, C. Parizot, T. Li, C. Katlama, M. Karmochkine, G. Raguin, B. Autran, and P. Debre. 1998. Perturbation of CD4+ and CD8+ T-cell repertoires during progression to AIDS and regulation of the CD4+ repertoire during antiviral therapy. *Nat. Med.* **4**:215–221.

1572. Gosling, J., F. S. Monteclaro, R. E. Atchison, H. Arai, C. L. Tsou, M. A. Goldsmith, and I. F. Charo. 1997. Molecular uncoupling of C-C chemokine receptor 5-induced chemotaxis and signal transduction from HIV-1 coreceptor activity. *Proc. Natl. Acad. Sci. USA* **94**:5061–5066.

1573. Gotch, F., S. Rowland-Jones, and D. Nixon. 1992. Longitudinal study of HIV-*gag* specific cytotoxic T lymphocyte responses over time in several patients, p. 60–65. *In* P. Racz, N. L. Letvin, and J. C. Gluckman (ed.), *Cytotoxic T Cells in HIV and Other Retroviral Infections.* Karger, Basel, Switzerland.

1574. Gottlieb, G., D. C. Nickle, M. A. Jensen, K. G. Wong, J. Grobler, F. Li, S. Liu, C. Rademeyer, G. H. Learn, S. S. Karim, C. Williamson, L. Corey, J. B. Margolick, and J. I. Mullins. 2004. Dual HIV-1 infection associated with rapid disease progression. *Lancet* **363**:619–622.

1575. Gottlieb, G. S., S. E. Hawes, H. D. Agne, J. E. Stern, C. W. Critchlow, N. B. Kiviat, and P. S. Sow. 2006. Lower levels of HIV RNA in semen in HIV-2 compared with HIV-1 infection: implications for differences in transmission. *AIDS* **20**:895–900.

1576. Gottlieb, M. D., R. Schroff, H. M. Schanker, J. D. Weisman, P. T. Fan, R. A. Wolf, and A. Saxon. 1981. Pneumocystis carinii pneumonia and mucosal candidiasis in previously healthy homosexual men. *N. Engl. J. Med.* **305**:1425–1431.

1577. Gottlieb, M. S., J. E. Groopman, W. M. Weinstein, J. L. Fahey, and R. Detels. 1983. The acquired immunodeficiency syndrome. *Ann. Intern. Med.* **99**:208–220.

1578. Goudsmit, J. 1995. The role of viral diversity in HIV pathogenesis. *J. Acquir. Immune Defic. Syndr. Hum. Retrovirol.* **10**:S15–S19.

1579. Goudsmit, J., J. M. A. Lange, D. A. Paul, and G. J. Dawson. 1987. Antigenemia and antibody titers to core and envelope antigens in AIDS, AIDS-related complex and subclinical human immunodeficiency virus infection. *J. Infect. Dis.* **155**:558–560.

1580. Goudsmit, J., and V. V. Lukashov. 1999. Dating the origin of HIV-1 subtypes. *Nature* **400**:325–326.

1581. Gougeon, M.-L., S. Garcia, J. Heeney, R. Tschopp, H. Lecoeur, D. Guetard, V. Rame, C. Dauguet, and L. Montagnier. 1993. Programmed cell death in AIDS-related HIV and SIV infections. *AIDS Res. Hum. Retrovir.* **9**:553–563.

1582. Gougeon, M.-L., H. Lecoeur, F. Boudet, E. Ledru, S. Marzabal, S. Boullier, R. Roue, S. Nagata, and J. Heeney. 1997. Lack of chronic immune activation in HIV-infected chimpanzees correlates with the resistance of T cells to Fas/Apo-1 (CD95)-induced apoptosis and reservation of a T helper 1 phenotype. *J. Immunol.* **158**:2964–2976.

1583. Gougeon, M.-L., H. Lecoeur, A. Dulioust, M.-G. Enouf, M. Crouvoiser, C. Goujard, T. Debord, and L. Montagnier.

1996. Programmed cell death in peripheral lymphocytes from HIV-infected persons. *J. Immunol.* 156:3509–3520.

1584. Gougeon, M.-L., C. Rouzioux, I. Liberman, M. Burgard, Y. Taoufik, J.-P. Viard, K. Bouchenafa, C. Capitant, J.-F. Delfraissy, ANRS 048 Study Group, and Y. Levy. 2001. Immunological and virological effects of long term therapy in HIV-1-infected patients. *AIDS* 15:1729–1744.

1585. Gougeon, M. L. 2003. Apoptosis as an HIV strategy to escape immune attack. *Nat. Rev. Immunol.* 3:392–404.

1586. Gould, S. J., A. M. Booth, and J. E. K. Hildreth. 2003. The Trojan exosome hypothesis. *Proc. Natl. Acad. Sci. USA* 100:10592–10597.

1587. Goulden, M. G., N. Cammack, P. L. Hopewell, C. R. Penn, and J. M. Cameron. 1996. Selection *in vitro* of an HIV-1 variant resistant to both lamivudine (3TC) and zidovudine. *AIDS* 10:101–102.

1588. Goulder, P. J., C. Brander, Y. Tang, C. Tremblay, R. A. Colbert, M. M. Addo, E. S. Rosenberg, T. Nguyen, R. Allen, A. Trocha, M. Altfeld, S. He, M. Bunce, R. Funkhouser, S. I. Pelton, S. K. Burchett, K. McIntosh, B. T. Korber, and B. D. Walker. 2001. Evolution and transmission of stable CTL escape mutations in HIV infection. *Nature* 412:334–338.

1589. Goulder, P. J., M. Bunce, P. Krausa, K. McIntyre, S. Crowley, B. Morgan, A. Edwards, P. Giangrande, R. E. Phillips, and A. J. McMichael. 1996. Novel, cross-restricted, conserved, and immunodominant cytotoxic T lymphocyte epitopes in slow progressors in HIV type 1 infection. *AIDS Res. Hum. Retrovir.* 12:1691–1698.

1590. Goulder, P. J. R., R. E. Phillips, R. A. Colbert, S. McAdam, G. Ogg, M. A. Nowak, P. Giangrande, G. Luzzi, B. Morgan, A. Edwards, A. J. McMichael, and S. Rowland-Jones. 1997. Late escape from an immunodominant cytotoxic T-lymphocyte response associated with progression to AIDS. *Nat. Med.* 3:212–217.

1591. Gowda, S. D., B. S. Stein, N. Mohagheghpour, C. J. Benike, and E. G. Engleman. 1989. Evidence that T cell activation is required for HIV-1 entry in CD4+ lymphocytes. *J. Immunol.* 142:773–780.

1592. Graham, B. S., and P. F. Wright. 1995. Candidate AIDS vaccines. *N. Engl. J. Med.* 333:1331–1339.

1593. Graham, C. S., A. Wells, T. Liu, K. E. Sherman, M. Peters, R. T. Chung, A. K. Bhan, J. Andersen, and M. J. Koziel. 2005. Antigen-specific immune responses and liver histology in HIV and hepatitis C coinfection. *AIDS* 19:767–773.

1594. Graham, D. B., M. P. Bell, C. J. Huntoon, J. G. Weaver, N. Hawley, A. D. Badley, and D. J. McKean. 2005. Increased thymic output in HIV-negative patients after antiretroviral therapy. *AIDS* 19:1467–1472.

1595. Graham, N. M. H., S. L. Zeger, L. P. Park, S. H. Vermund, R. Detels, C. R. Rinaldo, and J. P. Phair. 1992. The effects on survival of early treatment of human immunodeficiency virus infection. *N. Engl. J. Med.* 326:1037–1042.

1596. Granelli-Piperno, A., E. Delgado, V. Finkel, W. Paxton, and R. M. Steinman. 1998. Immature dendritic cells selectively replicate macrophagetropic (M-tropic) human immunodeficiency virus type 1, while mature cells efficiently transmit both M- and T-tropic virus to T cells. *J. Virol.* 72:2733–2737.

1597. Granelli-Piperno, A., A. Pritsker, M. Pack, I. Shimeliovich, J. F. Arrighi, C. G. Park, C. Trumpfheller, V. Piguet, T. M. Moran, and R. M. Steinman. 2005. Dendritic cell-specific intercellular adhesion molecule 3-grabbing nonintegrin/CD209 is abundant on macrophages in the normal human lymph node and is not required for dendritic cell stimulation of the mixed leukocyte reaction. *J. Immunol.* 175:4265–4273.

1598. Granelli-Piperno, A., I. Shimeliovich, M. Pack, C. Trumpfheller, and R. M. Steinman. 2006. HIV-1 selectively infects a subset of nonmaturing BDCA1-positive dendritic cells in human blood. *J. Immunol.* 176:991–998.

1599. Grant, M. D., F. M. Smail, and K. L. Rosenthal. 1994. Cytotoxic T-lymphocytes that kill autologous CD4+ lymphocytes are associated with CD4+ lymphocyte depletion in HIV-1 infection. *J. Acquir. Immune Defic. Syndr.* 7:571–579.

1600. Grant, M. D., F. M. Smaill, K. Laurie, and K. L. Rosenthal. 1993. Changes in the cytotoxic T-cell repertoire of HIV-1-infected individuals: relationship to disease progression. *Viral Immunol.* 6:85–95.

1601. Grant, M. D., M. S. Weaver, C. Tsoukas, and G. W. Hoffmann. 1990. Distribution of antibodies against denatured collagen in AIDS risk groups and homosexual AIDS patients suggests a link between autoimmunity and the immunopathogenesis of AIDS. *J. Immunol.* 144:1241–1250.

1602. Grant, R. M., S. Buchbinder, W. Cates, Jr., E. Clarke, T. Coates, M. S. Cohen, M. Delaney, G. Flores, P. Goicochea, G. Gonsalves, M. Harrington, J. R. Lama, K. M. MacQueen, J. P. Moore, L. Peterson, J. Sanchez, M. Thompson, and M. A. Wainberg. 2005. AIDS. Promote HIV chemoprophylaxis research, don't prevent it. *Science* 309:2170–2171.

1603. Gray, G. E., M. Urban, M. F. Chersich, C. Bolton, R. van Niekerk, A. Violari, W. Stevens, and J. A. McIntyre. 2005. A randomized trial of two postexposure prophylaxis regimens to reduce mother-to-child HIV-1 transmission in infants of untreated mothers. *AIDS* 19:1289–1297.

1604. Gray, L., J. Sterjovski, M. Churchill, P. Ellery, N. Nasr, S. R. Lewin, S. M. Crowe, S. L. Wesselingh, A. L. Cunningham, and P. R. Gorry. 2005. Uncoupling coreceptor usage of human immunodeficiency virus type 1 (HIV-1) from macrophage tropism reveals biological properties of CCR5-restricted HIV-1 isolates from patients with acquired immunodeficiency syndrome. *Virology* 337:384–398.

1605. Gray, R. H., X. Li, G. Kigozi, D. Serwadda, H. Brahmbhatt, F. Wabwire-Mangen, F. Nalugoda, M. Kiddugavu, N. Sewankambo, T. C. Quinn, S. J. Reynolds, and M. J. Wawer. 2005. Increased risk of incident HIV during pregnancy in Rakai, Uganda: a prospective study. *Lancet* 366:1182–1188.

1606. Gray, R. H., M. J. Wawer, R. Brookmeyer, N. K. Sewankambo, D. Serwadda, F. Wabwire-Mangen, T. Lutalo, X. Li, T. vanCott, and T. C. Quinn. 2001. Probability of HIV-1 transmission per coital act in monogamous, heterosexual, HIV-1-discordant couples in Rakai, Uganda. *Lancet* 357:1149–1153.

1607. Gray, R. H., M. J. Wawer, D. Serwadda, N. Sewankambo, C. Li, F. Wabwire-Mangen, L. Paxton, N. Kiwanuka, G. Kigozi, J. Konde-Lule, T. C. Quinn, C. A. Gaydos, and D. McNairn. 1998. Population-based study of fertility in women with HIV-1 infection in Uganda. *Lancet* 351:98–103.

1608. Graziosi, C., K. R. Gantt, M. Vaccarezza, J. F. Demarest, M. Daucher, M. S. Saag, G. M. Shaw, T. C. Quinn, O. J. Cohen, C. C. Welbon, G. Pantaleo, and A. S. Fauci. 1996. Kinetics of cytokine expression during primary human immunodeficiency virus type 1 infection. *Proc. Natl. Acad. Sci. USA* 93:4386–4391.

1609. Greco, G., E. Barker, and J. A. Levy. 1998. Differences in HIV replication in CD4+ lymphocytes are not related to β-chemokine production. *AIDS Res. Hum. Retrovir.* **14**: 1407–1411.

1610. Greco, G., S. H. Fujimura, D. V. Mourich, and J. A. Levy. 1999. Differential effects of human immunodeficiency virus isolates on beta-chemokine and gamma interferon production and on cell proliferation. *J. Virol.* **73**:1528–1534.

1611. Greco, G., C. Mackewicz, and J. A. Levy. 1999. Sensitivity of HIV infection to various α, β, and γ chemokines. *J. Gen. Virol.* **80**:2369–2373.

1612. Green, D. A., E. Masliah, H. V. Vinters, P. Beizai, D. J. Moore, and C. L. Achim. 2005. Brain deposition of beta-amyloid is a common pathologic feature in HIV positive patients. *AIDS* **19**:407–411.

1613. Green, D. F., L. Resnick, and J. J. Bourgoignie. 1992. HIV infects glomerular endothelial and mesangial but not epithelial cells in vitro. *Kidney Int.* **41**:956–960.

1614. Green, D. R., P. M. Flood, and R. K. Gershon. 1983. Immunoregulatory T-cell pathways. *Annu. Rev. Immunol.* **1**: 439–463.

1615. Greenberg, A. E. 2001. Possible protective effect of HIV-2 against incident HIV-1 infection: review of available epidemiological and *in vitro* data. *AIDS* **15**:2319–2321.

1616. Greenblatt, R. M., N. Ameli, R. M. Grant, P. Bacchetti, and R. N. Taylor. 2000. Impact of the ovulatory cycle on virologic and immunologic markers in HIV-infected women. *J. Infect. Dis.* **181**:82–90.

1617. Greene, L. W., W. Cole, J. B. Greene, and B. Levy. 1984. Adrenal insufficiency as a complication of the acquired immunodeficiency syndrome. *Ann. Intern. Med.* **101**:497–498.

1618. Greene, W. 2004. Redistricting the retroviral restriction factors. *Nat. Med.* **10**:778–780.

1619. Greene, W. C. 2004. The brightening future of HIV therapeutics. *Nat. Immunol.* **5**:867–871.

1620. Greene, W. C., and B. M. Peterlin. 2002. Charting HIV's remarkable voyage through the cell: basic science as a passport to future therapy. *Nat. Med.* **8**:673–680.

1621. Greensill, J., J. A. Sheldon, K. K. Murthy, J. S. Bessonette, B. E. Beer, and T. F. Schulz. 2000. A chimpanzee rhadinovirus sequence related to Kaposi's sarcoma-associated herpesvirus/human herpesvirus 8: increased detection after HIV-1 infection in the absence of disease. *AIDS* **14**:F129–F135.

1622. Greensill, J., J. A. Sheldon, N. M. Renwick, B. E. Beer, S. Norley, J. Goudsmit, and T. F. Schulz. 2000. Two distinct gamma-2 herpesviruses in African green monkeys: a second gamma-2 herpesvirus lineage among old world primates? *J. Virol.* **74**:1572–1577.

1623. Greenspan, D., A. J. Canchola, L. A. MacPhail, B. Cheikh, and J. S. Greenspan. 2001. Effect of highly active antiretroviral therapy on frequency of oral warts. *Lancet* **357**:1411–1412.

1624. Greenspan, D., J. S. Greenspan, M. Conant, V. Petersen, S. Silverman, Jr., and Y. deSouza. 1984. Oral "hairy" leucoplakia in male homosexuals: evidence of association with both papillomavirus and a herpes-group virus. *Lancet* **ii**:831–834.

1625. Greenspan, D., J. S. Greenspan, N. G. Hearst, L.-Z. Pan, M. A. Conant, D. I. Abrams, H. Hollander, and J. A. Levy. 1987. Relation of oral hairy leukoplakia to infection with HIV and the risk of developing AIDS. *J. Infect. Dis.* **155**:475–481.

1626. Greenway, A. L., D. A. McPhee, K. Allen, R. Johnstone, G. Holloway, J. Mills, A. Azad, S. Sankovich, and P. Lambert. 2002. Human immunodeficiency virus type 1 Nef binds to tumor suppressor p53 and protects cells against p53-mediated apoptosis. *J. Virol.* **76**:2692–2702.

1627. Grene, E., D. A. Newton, E. A. Brown, J. A. Berzofsky, S. Gattoni-Celli, and G. M. Shearer. 2000. Semi-allogeneic cell hybrids stimulate HIV-1 envelope-specific cytotoxic T lymphocytes. *AIDS* **14**:1497–1506.

1628. Grice, A. L., I. D. Keer, and M. S. P. Sansom. 1997. Ion channels formed by HIV-1 Vpu: a modelling and simulation study. *FEBS Lett.* **405**:299–304.

1629. Griffiths, J. C., E. L. Berrie, L. N. Holdsworth, J. P. Moore, S. J. Harris, J. M. Senior, S. M. Kingsman, A. J. Kingsman, and S. E. Adams. 1991. Induction of high-titer neutralizing antibodies, using hybrid human immunodeficiency virus V3-Ty virus-like particles in a clinically relevant adjuvant. *J. Virol.* **65**:450–456.

1630. Grimaila, R. J., B. A. Fuller, P. D. Rennert, M. B. Nelson, M.-L. Hammarskjold, B. Potts, M. Murray, S. D. Putney, and G. Gray. 1992. Mutations in the principal neutralization determinant of human immunodeficiency virus type 1 affect syncytium formation, virus infectivity, growth kinetics, and neutralization. *J. Virol.* **66**:1875–1883.

1631. Grimaldi, L. M. E., G. V. Martino, D. M. Franciotta, R. Brustia, A. Castagna, R. Pristera, and A. Lazzarin. 1991. Elevated alpha-tumor necrosis factor levels in spinal fluid from HIV-1-infected patients with central nervous system involvement. *Ann. Neurol.* **29**:21–25.

1631a. Grimbert, P., S. Bouguermouh, N. Baba, T. Nakajima, Z. Allakhverdi, D. Braun, H. Saito, M. Rubio, G. Delespesse, and M. Sarfati. 2006. Thrombospondin/CD47 interaction: a pathway to generate regulatory T cells from human CD4+ CD25- T cells in response to inflammation. *J. Immunol.* **177**:3534–3541.

1631b. Grimwade, K., N. French, D. D. Mbatha, D. D. Zungu, M. Dedicoat, and C. F. Gilks. 2004. HIV infection as a cofactor for severe falciparum malaria in adults living in a region of unstable malaria transmission in South Africa. *AIDS* **18**:547–554.

1632. Grinspoon, S. K., and J. P. Bilezikian. 1992. HIV disease and the endocrine system. *N. Engl. J. Med.* **327**:1360–1365.

1633. Grivel, J.-C., M. Garcia, W. J. Moss, and L. V. Margolis. 2005. Inhibition of HIV-1 replication in human lymphoid tissues ex vivo by measles virus. *J. Infect. Dis.* **192**:71–78.

1634. Grody, W. W., L. Cheng, and W. Lewis. 1990. Infection of the heart by the human immunodeficiency virus. *Am. J. Cardiol.* **66**:203–206.

1635. Groenink, M., A. C. Andeweg, R. A. M. Fouchier, S. Broersen, R. C. M. van der Jagt, H. Schuitemaker, R. E. Y. de Goede, M. L. Bosch, H. G. Huisman, and M. Tersmette. 1992. Phenotype-associated *env* gene variation among eight related human immunodeficiency virus type 1 clones: evidence for in vivo recombination and determinants of cytotropism outside the V3 domain. *J. Virol.* **66**:6175–6180.

1636. Groenink, M., R. A. M. Fouchier, S. Broersen, C. H. Baker, M. Koot, A. B. van't Wout, H. G. Huisman, F. Miedema, M. Tersmette, and H. Schuitemaker. 1993. Relation of phenotype evolution of HIV-1 to envelope V2 configuration. *Science* **260**:1513–1516.

1637. Groenink, M., R. A. M. Fouchier, R. E. Y. de Goede, F. de Wolf, R. A. Gruters, H. T. M. Cuypers, H. G. Huisman, and M. Tersmette. 1991. Phenotypical heterogeneity in a panel of infectious molecular human immunodeficiency virus type 1 clones derived from a single individual. *J. Virol.* **65**:1968–1975.

1638. Groenink, M., J. P. Moore, S. Broersen, and H. Schuitemaker. 1995. Equal levels of gp120 retention and neutralization resistance of phenotypically distinct primary human immunodeficiency virus type 1 variants upon soluble CD4 treatment. *J. Virol.* **69**:523–527.

1639. Groopman, J. E., S. Z. Salahuddin, M. G. Sarngadharan, P. D. Markham, M. Gonda, A. Sliski, and R. C. Gallo. 1984. HTLV-III in saliva of people with AIDS-related complex and healthy homosexual men at risk for AIDS. *Science* **226**:447–449.

1640. Grossman, Z., M. Meier-Schellersheim, W. E. Paul, and L. J. Picker. 2006. Pathogenesis of HIV infection: what the virus spares is as important as what it destroys. *Nat. Med.* **12**:289–295.

1641. Grossman, Z., M. Meier-Schellersheim, A. E. Sousa, R. M. Victorino, and W. E. Paul. 2002. CD4+ T-cell depletion in HIV infection: are we closer to understanding the cause? *Nat. Med.* **8**:319–323.

1642. Grouard, G., M. C. Rissoan, L. Filgueira, I. Durand, J. Banchereau, and Y. J. Liu. 1997. The enigmatic plasmacytoid T cells develop into dendritic cells with interleukin (IL)-3 and CD40-ligand. *J. Exp. Med.* **185**:1101–1111.

1643. Groux, H., G. Torpier, D. Monte, Y. Mouton, A. Capron, and J. C. Ameisen. 1992. Activation-induced death by apoptosis in CD4+ T cells from human immunodeficiency virus-infected asymptomatic individuals. *J. Exp. Med.* **175**:331–340.

1644. Grubb, J. R., A. C. Moorman, R. K. Baker, and H. Masur. 2006. The changing spectrum of pulmonary disease in patients with HIV infection on anti-retroviral therapy. *AIDS*, **20**:1095–1097.

1645. Grulich, A., X. Wan, M. Law, M. Coates, and Kaldor. 1999. Risk of cancer in people with AIDS. *AIDS* **13**:839–843.

1646. Grulich, A. E., and J. M. Kaldor. 1996. The sex ratio of AIDS-associated Kaposi's sarcoma does not provide evidence that sex hormones play a role in pathogenesis. *AIDS* **10**:1595–1609.

1647. Grulich, A. E., Y. Li, A. McDonald, P. K. Correll, M. G. Law, and J. M. Kaldor. 2002. Rates of non-AIDS-defining cancers in people with HIV infection before and after AIDS diagnosis. *AIDS* **16**:1155–1161.

1648. Grulich, A. E., X. Wan, M. G. Law, S. T. Milliken, C. R. Lewis, R. J. Garsia, J. Gold, R. J. Finlayson, D. A. Cooper, and J. M. Kaldor. 2000. B-cell stimulation and prolonged immune deficiency are risk factors for non-Hodgkin's lymphoma in people with AIDS. *AIDS* **14**:133–140.

1649. Grun, J. L., and P. H. Maurer. 1989. Different T helper cell subsets elicited in mice utilizing two different adjuvant vehicles: the role of endogenous interleukin 1 in proliferative responses. *Cell. Immunol.* **121**:134–145.

1650. Grundhoff, A., and D. Ganem. 2004. Inefficient establishment of KSHV latency suggests an additional role for continued lytic replication in Kaposi sarcoma pathogenesis. *J. Clin. Investig.* **113**:124–136.

1651. Grunfeld, C., D. P. Kotler, and R. Hamadeh. 1992. Hypertriglyceridemia in the acquired immunodeficiency syndrome. *Am. J. Med.* **86**:27–31.

1652. Grunfeld, C., M. Pang, and W. Doerrier. 1992. Lipids, lipoproteins, triglyceride clearance and cytokines in HIV infection and AIDS. *J. Clin. Endocrinol. Metab.* **74**:1045–1052.

1653. Gruters, R. A., J. J. Neefjes, M. Tersmette, R. E. Y. de Goede, A. Tulp, H. G. Huisman, F. Miedema, and H. L. Ploegh. 1987. Interference with HIV-induced syncytium formation and viral infectivity by inhibitors of trimming glucosidase. *Nature* **330**:74–77.

1654. Gruters, R. A., F. G. Terpstra, R. E. Y. De Goede, J. W. Mulder, F. De Wolf, P. T. A. Schellekens, R. A. W. Van Lier, M. Tersmette, and F. Miedema. 1991. Immunological and virological markers in individuals progressing from seroconversion to AIDS. *AIDS* **5**:837–844.

1655. Gruters, R. A., F. G. Terpstra, R. De Jong, C. J. M. Van Noesel, R. A. W. Van Lier, and F. Miedema. 1990. Selective loss of T cell function in different stages of HIV infection. Early loss of anti-CD3-induced T cell proliferation followed by decreased anti-CD3-induced cytotoxic T lymphocyte generation in AIDS-related complex and AIDS. *Eur. J. Immunol.* **20**:1039–1044.

1656. Gu, R., P. Westervelt, and L. Ratner. 1993. Role of HIV-1 envelope V3 loop cleavage in cell tropism. *AIDS Res. Hum. Retrovir.* **9**:1007–1015.

1657. Guadalupe, M., E. Reay, S. Sankaran, T. Prindiville, J. Flamm, A. McNeil, and S. Dandekar. 2003. Severe CD4+ T-cell depletion in gut lymphoid tissue during primary human immunodeficiency type 1 infection and substantial delay in restoration following highly active antiretroviral therapy. *J. Virol.* **77**:11708–11717.

1658. Guadalupe, M., S. Sankaran, M. D. George, E. Reay, D. Verhoeven, B. L. Shacklett, J. Flamm, J. Wegelin, T. Prindiville, and S. Dandekar. 2006. Viral suppression and immune restoration in the gastrointestinal mucosa of human immunodeficiency virus type 1-infected patients initiating therapy during primary or chronic infection. *J. Virol.* **80**:8236–8247.

1659. Guarda, L. A., J. J. Butler, P. Mansell, E. M. Hersh, J. Reuben, and G. R. Newell. 1983. Lymphadenopathy in homosexual men: morbid anatomy with clinical and immunologic correlations. *Am. J. Clin. Pathol.* **79**:559–568.

1660. Guasparri, I., S. A. Keller, and E. Cesarman. 2004. KSHV vFLIP is essential for the survival of infected lymphoma cells. *J. Exp. Med.* **199**:993–1003.

1661. Guay, L. A., P. Musoke, T. Fleming, D. Bagenda, M. Allen, C. Nakabiito, J. Sherman, P. Bakaki, C. Ducar, M. Deseyve, L. Emel, M. Mirochnick, M. G. Fowler, L. Mofenson, P. Miotti, K. Dransfield, D. Bray, F. Mmiro, and J. B. Jackson. 1999. Intrapartum and neonatal single-dose nevirapine compared with zidovudine for prevention of mother-to-child transmission of HIV-1 in Kampala, Uganda: HIVNET 012 randomised trial. *Lancet* **354**:795–802.

1662. Guidotti, L. G., K. Ando, M. V. Hobbs, T. Ishikawa, L. Runkel, R. D. Schreiber, and F. V. Chisari. 1994. Cytotoxic T lymphocytes inhibit hepatitis B virus gene expression by a noncytolytic mechanism in transgenic mice. *Proc. Natl. Acad. Sci. USA* **91**:3764–3768.

1663. Guidotti, L. G., R. Rochford, J. Chung, M. Shapiro, R. Purcell, and F. V. Chisari. 1999. Viral clearance without destruction of infected cells during acute HBV infection. *Science* **284**:825–829.

1664. Gunthard, H. F., D. V. Havlir, S. Fiscus, Z. Q. Zhang, J. Eron, J. Mellors, R. Gulick, S. D. Frost, A. J. Brown, W. Schleif, F. Valentine, L. Jonas, A. Meibohm, C. C. Ignacio, R. Isaacs, R. Gamagami, E. Emini, A. Haase, D. D. Richman, and J. K. Wong. 2001. Residual human immunodeficiency virus (HIV) Type 1 RNA and DNA in lymph nodes and HIV RNA in genital secretions and in cerebrospinal fluid after suppression of viremia for 2 years. *J. Infect. Dis.* 183:1318–1327.

1665. Guo, H. G., J. C. Chermann, D. Waters, L. Hall, A. Louie, R. C. Gallo, H. Streicher, M. S. Reitz, M. Popovic, and W. Blattner. 1991. Sequence analysis of original HIV-1. *Nature* 349:745–746.

1666. Guo, M. M. L., and J. E. K. Hildreth. 1995. HIV acquires functional adhesion receptors from host cells. *AIDS Res. Hum. Retrovir.* 11:1007–1013.

1667. Guo, Q., H. Ho, I. Dicker, L. Fan, N. Zhou, J. Friborg, T. Wang, B. V. McAuliffe, H. Wang, R. E. Rose, H. Fang, H. T. Scarnati, D. R. Langley, N. A. Meanwell, R. Abraham, E. J. Colonno, and P. Lin. 2003. Biochemical and genetic characterizations of a novel human immunodeficiency virus type 1 inhibitor that blocks gp120-CD4 interactions. *J. Virol.* 77:10528–10536.

1668. Gupta, P., R. Balachandran, M. Ho, A. Enrico, and C. Rinaldo. 1989. Cell-to-cell transmission of human immunodeficiency virus type 1 in the presence of azidothymidine and neutralizing antibody. *J. Virol.* 63:2361–2365.

1669. Gupta, P., L. Kingsley, J. Armstrong, M. Ding, M. Cottrill, and C. Rinaldo. 1993. Enhanced expression of human immunodeficiency virus type 1 correlates with development of AIDS. *Virology* 196:586–595.

1670. Gupta, P., C. Leroux, B. K. Patterson, L. Kingsley, C. Rinaldo, M. Ding, Y. Chen, K. Kulka, W. Buchanan, B. McKeon, and R. Montelaro. 2000. Human immunodeficiency virus type 1 shedding pattern in semen correlates with the compartmentalization of viral Quasi species between blood and semen. *J. Infect. Dis.* 182:79–87.

1671. Gupta, P., J. Mellors, L. Kingsley, S. Riddler, M. K. Singh, S. Schreiber, M. Cronin, and C. R. Rinaldo. 1997. High viral load in semen of human immunodeficiency virus type 1-infected men at all stages of disease and its reduction by therapy with protease and nonnucleoside reverse transcriptase inhibitors. *J. Virol.* 71:6271–6275.

1672. Gupta, P., M. K. Singh, C. Rinaldo, M. Ding, H. Farzadegan, A. Saah, D. Hoover, P. Moore, and L. Kingsley. 1996. Detection of Kaposi's sarcoma herpesvirus DNA in semen of homosexual men with Kaposi's sarcoma. *AIDS* 10:1596–1598.

1673. Gupta, S., R. Janai, Q. Bin, P. Luciw, C. Greer, S. Perri, H. Legg, J. Donnelly, S. Barnett, D. O'Hagan, J. M. Polo, and M. Vajdy. 2005. Characterization of human immunodeficiency virus Gag-specific gamma interferon-expressing cells following protective mucosal immunization with alphavirus replicon particles. *J. Virol.* 79:7135–7145.

1674. Gurer, C., A. Höglund, S. Höglund, and J. Luban. 2005. ATPγS disrupts human immunodeficiency virus type 1 virion core integrity. *J. Virol.* 79:5557–5567.

1675. Gurney, K. G., J. Elliott, H. Nassanian, C. Song, E. Soilleux, I. McGowan, P. A. Anton, and B. Lee. 2005. Binding and transfer of human immunodeficiency virus by DC-SIGN+ cells in human rectal mucosa. *J. Virol.* 79:5762–5773.

1676. Guy, B., M. P. Kieny, Y. Riviere, C. Le Peuch, K. Dott, M. Girard, L. Montagnier, and J. P. Lecocq. 1987. HIV F/3' orf encodes a phosphorylated GTP-binding protein resembling an oncogene product. *Nature* 330:266–269.

1677. Guy, B., Y. Riviere, K. Dott, A. Regnault, and M. P. Kieny. 1990. Mutational analysis of the HIV *nef* protein. *Virology* 176:413–425.

1678. Guyader, M., M. Emerman, P. Sonigo, F. Clavel, L. Montagnier, and M. Alizon. 1987. Genome organization and transactivation of the human immunodeficiency virus type 2. *Nature* 326:662–669.

1679. Gyorkey, F., J. L. Melnick, and P. Gyorkey. 1987. Human immunodeficiency virus in brain biopsies of patients with AIDS and progressive encephalopathy. *J. Infect. Dis.* 155:870–876.

1680. Haas, D. W., J. Lavelle, J. P. Nadler, S. B. Greenberg, P. Frame, N. Mustafa, M. St Clair, R. McKinnis, L. Dix, M. Elkins, and J. Rooney. 2000. A randomized trial of interferon alpha therapy for HIV type 1 infection. *AIDS Res. Hum. Retrovir.* 16:183–190.

1681. Haas, G., U. Plikat, P. Debre, M. Lucchiari, C. Katlama, Y. Dudoit, O. Bonduelle, M. Bauer, H.-G. Ihlenfeldt, G. Jing, B. Maier, A. Meyerhans, and B. Autran. 1996. Dynamics of viral variants in HIV-1 Nef and specific cytotoxic T lymphocytes in vivo. *J. Immunol.* 157:4212–4221.

1682. Haase, A. 1975. The slow infection caused by visna virus. *Curr. Top. Microbiol. Immunol.* 72:101–156.

1683. Haase, A. T. 1986. Pathogenesis of lentivirus infections. *Nature* 322:130–136.

1684. Haase, A. T. 1999. Population biology of HIV-1 infection: viral and CD4+ T cell demographics and dynamics in lymphatic tissues. *Annu. Rev. Immunol.* 17:625–656.

1685. Haase, A. T. 2005. Perils at mucosal front lines for HIV and SIV and their hosts. *Nat. Rev. Immunol.* 5:783–792.

1686. Haase, A. T., K. Henry, M. Zupancic, G. Sedgewick, R. A. Faust, H. Melroe, W. Cavert, K. Gebhard, K. Staskus, Z. Q. Zhang, P. J. Dailey, H. H. Balfour, Jr., A. Erice, and A. S. Perelson. 1996. Quantitative image analysis of HIV-1 infection in lymphoid tissue. *Science* 274:985–989.

1687. Habeshaw, J. A., A. G. Dalgleish, L. Bountiff, A. L. Newell, D. Wilks, L. C. Walker, and F. Manca. 1990. AIDS pathogenesis: HIV envelope and its interaction with cell proteins. *Immunol. Today* 11:418–425.

1688. Hadida, F., V. Vieillard, B. Autran, I. Clark-Lewis, M. Baggiolini, and P. Debr. 1998. HIV-specific T cell cytotoxicity mediated by RANTES via the chemokine receptor CCR3. *J. Exp. Med.* 188:609–614.

1689. Haffar, O., J. Garrigues, B. Travis, P. Moran, J. Zarling, and S.-L. Hu. 1990. Human immunodeficiency virus-like, non-replicating, *gag-env* particles assemble in a recombinant vaccinia virus expression system. *J. Virol.* 64:2653–2659.

1690. Haga, T., S. H. Kim, R. H. Jensen, T. Darragh, and J. M. Palefsky. 2001. Detection of genetic changes in anal intraepithelial neoplasia (AIN) of HIV-positive and HIV-negative men. *J. Acquir. Immune Defic. Syndr.* 26:256–262.

1691. Hahn, B. H., G. M. Shaw, S. K. Arya, M. Popovic, R. C. Gallo, and F. Wong-Staal. 1984. Molecular cloning and characterization of the HTLV-III virus associated with AIDS. *Nature* 312:166–169.

1692. Hahn, B. H., G. M. Shaw, K. M. De Cock, and P. M. Sharp. 2000. AIDS as a zoonosis: scientific and public health implications. *Science* 287:607–614.

1693. Hahn, B. H., G. M. Shaw, M. E. Taylor, R. R. Redfield, P. D. Markham, S. Z. Salahuddin, F. Wong-Staal, R. C. Gallo, E. S. Parks, and W. P. Parks. 1986. Genetic variation in HTLV-III/LAV over time in patients with AIDS or at risk for AIDS. *Science* 232:1548–1553.

1694. Haigwood, N. L., P. L. Nara, E. Brooks, G. A. Van Nest, G. Ott, K. W. Higgins, N. Dunlop, C. J. Scandella, J. W. Eichberg, and K. S. Steimer. 1992. Native but not denatured recombinant human immunodeficiency virus type 1 gp120 generates broad-spectrum neutralizing antibodies in baboons. *J. Virol.* **66**:172–182.

1695. Haigwood, N. L., A. Watson, W. F. Sutton, J. McClure, A. Lewis, J. Ranchalis, B. Travis, G. Voss, N. L. Letvin, S. L. Hu, V. M. Hirsch, and P. R. Johnson. 1996. Passive immune globulin therapy in the SIV/macaque model: early intervention can alter disease profile. *Immunol. Lett.* **51**:107–114.

1696. Haigwood, N. S., J. R. Shuster, G. K. Moore, H. Lee, P. V. Skiles, K. W. Higgins, P. J. Barr, C. George-Nascimento, and K. S. Steimer. 1990. Importance of hypervariable regions of HIV-1 gp120 in the generation of virus-neutralizing antibodies. *AIDS Res. Hum. Retrovir.* **6**:855–869.

1697. Hainaut, M., C. A. Peltier, T. Goetghebuer, D. Van der Linden, D. Marissens, G. Zissis, and J. Levy. 2005. Seroreversion in children infected with HIV type 1 who are treated in the first months of life is not a rare event. *Clin. Infect. Dis.* **41**:1820–1821.

1698. Halapi, E., D. Gigliotti, V. Hodara, G. Scarlatti, P. A. Tovo, A. DeMaria, H. Wigzell, and P. Rossi. 1996. Detection of CD8 T-cell expansions with restricted T-cell receptor V gene usage in infants vertically infected by HIV-1. *AIDS* **10**:1621–1626.

1699. Halfon, P., J. Durant, P. Clevenbergh, H. Carsenti, L. Celis, H. Khiri, K. De Smet, A. De Brauwer, F. Hulstaert, and P. Dellamonica. 2003. Kinetics of disappearance of resistance mutations and reappearance of wild-type during structured treatment interruptions. *AIDS* **17**:1351–1361.

1700. Hall, W. W., T. Kubo, S. Ijichi, H. Takahashi, and S. W. Zhu. 1994. Human T cell leukemia lymphoma virus, type II (HTLV-II): emergence of an important newly recognized pathogen. *Semin. Virol.* **5**:165–178.

1701. Hallenberger, S., V. Bosch, H. Angliker, E. Shaw, H. D. Klenk, and W. Garten. 1992. Inhibition of furin-mediated cleavage activation of HIV-1 glycoprotein gp160. *Nature* **360**:358–361.

1702. Halperin, D. T., and R. C. Bailey. 1999. Male circumcision and HIV infection: 10 years and counting. *Lancet* **354**:1813–1815.

1703. Halstead, S. B. 1979. *In vivo* enhancement of dengue virus infection in rhesus monkeys by passively transferred antibody. *J. Infect. Dis.* **140**:527–533.

1704. Hamed, K. A., M. A. Winters, M. Holodniy, D. A. Katzenstein, and T. C. Merigan. 1993. Detection of human immunodeficiency virus type 1 in semen: effects of disease stage and nucleoside therapy. *J. Infect. Dis.* **167**:798–802.

1705. Hamilton, D. P. 1991. What next in the Gallo case? *Science* **254**:944–945.

1706. Hammarlund, E., M. W. Lewis, S. G. Hansen, L. I. Srelow, J. A. Nelson, G. J. Sexton, J. M. Hanifin, and M. K. Slifka. 2003. Duration of antiviral immunity after smallpox vaccination. *Nat. Med.* **9**:1131–1137.

1707. Hammer, S. M. 1996. Advances in antiretroviral therapy and viral load monitoring. *AIDS* **10**:S1–S11.

1708. Hammer, S. M., D. A. Katzenstein, M. D. Hughes, H. Gundacker, R. T. Schooley, R. H. Haubrich, W. K. Henry, M. M. Lederman, J. P. Phair, M. Niu, M. S. Hirsch, and T. C. Merigan. 1996. A trial comparing nucleoside monotherapy with combination therapy in HIV-infected adults with CD4 cell counts from 200 to 500 per cubic millimeter. *N. Engl. J. Med.* **335**:1081–1090.

1709. Hammes, S. R., E. P. Dixon, M. H. Malim, B. R. Cullen, and W. C. Greene. 1989. *Nef* protein of human immunodeficiency virus type 1: evidence against its role as a transcriptional inhibitor. *Proc. Natl. Acad. Sci. USA* **86**:9549–9553.

1710. Hammond, S. A., R. C. Bollinger, P. E. Stanhope, T. C. Quinn, D. Schwartz, M. L. Clements, and R. F. Siliciano. 1993. Comparative clonal analysis of human immunodeficiency virus type 1 (HIV-1)-specific CD4+ and CD8+ cytolytic T lymphocytes isolated from seronegative humans immunized with candidate HIV-1 vaccines. *J. Exp. Med.* **176**:1531–1542.

1711. Hammonds, J., X. Chen, T. Fouts, A. DeVico, D. Montefiori, and P. Spearman. 2005. Induction of neutralizing antibodies against human immunodeficiency virus type 1 primary isolates by Gag-Env pseudovirion immunization. *J. Virol.* **79**:14804–14814.

1712. Han, X.-M., A. Laras, M. P. Rounseville, A. Kumar, and P. R. Shank. 1992. Human immunodeficiency virus type 1 Tat-mediated *trans* activation correlates with the phosphorylation state of a cellular TAR RNA stem-binding factor. *J. Virol.* **66**:4065–4072.

1713. Hannon, G. J. 2002. RNA interference. *Nature* **418**:244–251.

1714. Hansen, J.-E. S., H. Clausen, C. Nielsen, L. S. Teglbjaerg, L. L. Hansen, C. M. Nielsen, E. Dabelsteen, L. Mathiesen, S.-I. Hakomori, and J. O. Nielsen. 1990. Inhibition of human immunodeficiency virus (HIV) infection in vitro by anticarbohydrate monoclonal antibodies: peripheral glycosylation of HIV envelope glycoprotein gp120 may be a target for virus neutralization. *J. Virol.* **64**:2833–2840.

1715. Hansen, J. E. S., C. Nielsen, M. Arendrup, S. Olofsson, L. Mathiesen, J. O. Nielsen, and H. Clausen. 1991. Broadly neutralizing antibodies targeted to mucin-type carbohydrate epitopes of human immunodeficiency virus. *J. Virol.* **65**:6461–6467.

1716. Hansen, J. E. S., C. Nielsen, L. R. Mathiesen, and J. O. Nielsen. 1991. Involvement of lymphocyte function-associated antigen-1 (LFA-1) in HIV infection: inhibition by monoclonal antibody. *Scand. J. Infect. Dis.* **23**:31–36.

1717. Hansen, J. E. S., C. M. Nielsen, C. Nielsen, P. Heegaard, L. R. Mathiesen, and J. O. Nielsen. 1989. Correlation between carbohydrate structures on the envelope glycoprotein gp120 of HIV-1 and HIV-2 and syncytium inhibition with lectins. *AIDS* **3**:635–641.

1718. Hanson, A., A. D. Sarr, A. Shea, N. Jones, S. Mboup, P. Kanki, and H. Cao. 2005. Distinct profile of T cell activation in HIV type 2 compared to HIV type 1 infection: differential mechanism for immunoprotection. *AIDS Res. Hum. Retrovir.* **21**:791–798.

1719. Hanson, C. V. 1994. Measuring vaccine-induced HIV neutralization: report of a workshop. *AIDS Res. Hum. Retrovir.* **10**:645–648.

1720. Hanto, D. W., K. J. Gajl-Peczalkska, and G. Frizzera. 1983. Epstein-Barr virus induced polyclonal and monoclonal B-cell lymphoproliferative disease occurring after renal transplantation. *Ann. Surg.* **198**:356–369.

1721. Harada, S., Y. Koyanagi, H. Nakashima, N. Kobayashi, and N. Yamamoto. 1986. Tumor promoter, TPA, enhances replication of HTLV-III/LAV. *Virology* **154**:249–258.

1722. Harada, S., Y. Koyanagi, and N. Yamamoto. 1985. Infection of HTLV-III/LAV in HTLV-I-carrying cells MT-2 and MT-4 and application in a plaque assay. *Science* 229:563–566.

1723. Haraguchi, S., G. J. Cianciolo, R. A. Good, M. James-Yarish, E. Brigino, and N. K. Day. 1998. Inhibition of interleukin-2 and interferon-γ by an HIV-1 Nef-encoded synthetic peptide. *AIDS* 12:820–822.

1724. Harari, A., S. Petitpierre, F. Vallelian, and G. Pantaleo. 2004. Skewed representation of functionally distinct populations of virus-specific CD4 T cells in HIV-1-infected subjects with progressive disease: changes after antiretroviral therapy. *Blood* 103:966–972.

1725. Harari, A., F. Vallelian, P. R. Meylan, and G. Pantaleo. 2005. Functional heterogeneity of memory CD4 T cell responses in different conditions of antigen exposure and persistence. *J. Immunol.* 174:1037–1045.

1726. Hare, C. B., B. L. Pappalardo, A. C. Karlsson, B. H. Phelps, S. S. Alexander, C. Bentsen, C. A. Ramstead, D. F. Nixon, J. A. Levy, and F. M. Hecht. 2006. Seroreversion in subjects treated with antiretroviral therapy during primary HIV infection. *Clin. Infect. Dis.* 42:700–708.

1727. Harhaj, E. W., S. B. Maggirwar, L. Good, and S.-C. Sun. 1996. CD28 mediates a potent costimulatory signal for rapid degradtion of IκBβ which is associated with accelerated activation of various NF-κB/Rel heterodimers. *Mol. Cell. Biol.* 16:6736–6743.

1728. Hariharan, D., S. D. Douglas, B. Lee, J. P. Lai, D. E. Campbell, and W. Z. Ho. 1999. Interferon-gamma upregulates CCR5 expression in cord and adult blood mononuclear phagocytes. *Blood* 93:1137–1144.

1729. Hariharan, D., Y. Li, D. E. Campbell, S. D. Douglas, S. E. Starr, and W. Ho. 1999. Human immunodeficiency virus infection of human placental cord blood CD34+AC133+ stem cells and their progeny. *AIDS Res. Hum. Retrovir.* 15:1545–1552.

1730. Harouse, J. M., S. Bhat, S. L. Spitalnik, M. Laughlin, K. Stefano, D. H. Silberberg, and F. Gonzalez-Scarano. 1991. Inhibition of entry of HIV-1 in neural cell lines by antibodies against galactosyl ceramide. *Science* 253:320–323.

1731. Harouse, J. M., C. Buckner, A. Gettie, R. Fuller, R. Bohm, J. Blanchard, and C. Cheng-Mayer. 2003. CD8+ T cell-mediated CXC chemokine receptor 4-simian/human immunodeficiency virus suppression in dually infected rhesus macaques. *Proc. Natl. Acad. Sci. USA* 100:10977–10982.

1732. Harouse, J. M., R. G. Collman, and F. Gonzalez-Scarano. 1995. Human immunodeficiency virus type 1 infection of SK-N-MC cells: domains of gp120 involved in entry into a CD4-negative, galactosyl ceramide/3' sulfo-galactosyl ceramide-positive cell line. *J. Virol.* 69:7383–7390.

1733. Harouse, J. M., A. Gettie, R. C. Tan, J. Blanchard, and C. Cheng-Mayer. 1999. Distinct pathogenic sequela in rhesus macaques infected with CCR5 or CXCR4 utilizing SHIVs. *Science* 284:816–819.

1734. Harouse, J. M., C. Kunsch, H. T. Hartle, M. A. Laughlin, J. A. Hoxie, B. Wigdahl, and F. Gonzalez-Scarano. 1989. CD4-independent infection of human neural cells by human immunodeficiency virus type 1. *J. Virol.* 63:2527–2533.

1735. Harouse, J. M., Z. Wroblewska, M. A. Laughlin, W. F. Hickey, B. S. Schonwetter, and F. Gonzalez-Scarano. 1989. Human choroid plexus cells can be latently infected with human immunodeficiency virus. *Ann. Neurol.* 25:406–411.

1736. Harper, M. E., L. M. Marselle, R. C. Gallo, and F. Wong-Staal. 1986. Detection of lymphocytes expressing human T-lymphotropic virus type III in lymph nodes and peripheral blood from infected individuals by *in situ* hybridization. *Proc. Natl. Acad. Sci. USA* 83:772–776.

1737. Harrer, T., E. Harrer, S. A. Kalams, P. Barbosa, A. Trocha, R. P. Johnson, T. Elbeik, M. B. Feinberg, S. P. Buchbinder, and B. D. Walker. 1996. Cytotoxic T lymphocytes in asymptomatic long-term nonprogressing HIV-1 infection. *J. Immunol.* 156:2616–2623.

1738. Harrer, T., E. Harrer, S. A. Kalams, T. Elbeik, S. I. Staprans, M. B. Feinberg, Y. Cao, D. D. Ho, T. Yilma, A. M. Caliendo, R. P. Johnson, S. P. Buchbinder, and B. D. Walker. 1996. Strong cytotoxic T cell and weak neutralizing antibody responses in a subset of persons with stable nonprogressing HIV type 1 infection. *AIDS Res. Hum. Retrovir.* 12:585–592.

1739. Harrington, L. E., R. D. Hatton, P. R. Mangan, H. Turner, T. L. Murphy, K. M. Murphy, and C. T. Weaver. 2005. Interleukin 17-producing CD4+ effector T cells develop via a lineage distinct from the T helper type 1 and 2 lineages. *Nat. Immunol.* 6:1123–1132.

1740. Harrington, R. D., and A. P. Geballe. 1993. Cofactor requirement for human immunodeficiency virus type 1 entry into a CD4-expressing human cell line. *J. Virol.* 67:5939–5947.

1741. Harris, C., C. B. Small, R. S. Klein, G. H. Friedland, B. Moll, E. E. Emeson, I. Spigland, and N. H. Steigbigel. 1983. Immunodeficiency in female sexual partners of men with the acquired immunodeficiency syndrome. *N. Engl. J. Med.* 308:1181–1184.

1742. Harris, R. S., K. N. Bishop, A. M. Sheehy, H. M. Craig, S. K. Peterson-Mahrt, I. N. Watt, M. S. Neuberger, and M. H. Malim. 2003. DNA deamination mediates innate immunity to retroviral infection. *Cell* 113:803–809.

1743. Harrison, T. S., and S. M. Levitz. 1997. Mechanisms of impaired anticryptococcal activity of monocytes from donors infected with human immunodeficiency virus. *J. Infect. Dis.* 176:537–540.

1744. Harrison, T. S., and S. M. Levitz. 1997. Priming with interferon-gamma restores deficient IL-12 production by PBMC from HIV-seropositive donors. *J. Immunol.* 158:459–463.

1745. Hart, A. R., and M. W. Cloyd. 1990. Interference patterns of human immunodeficiency viruses HIV-1 and HIV-2. *Virology* 177:1–10.

1746. Hart, C. E., J. L. Lennox, M. Pratt-Palmore, T. C. Wright, R. F. Schinazi, T. Evans-Strickfaden, T. J. Bush, C. Schnell, L. J. Conley, K. A. Clancy, and T. V. Ellerbrock. 1999. Correlation of human immunodeficiency virus type 1 RNA levels in blood and the female genital tract. *J. Infect. Dis.* 179:871–882.

1747. Hart, C. E., C.-Y. Ou, J. C. Galphin, J. Moore, L. T. Bacheler, J. J. Wasmuth, S. R. Petteway, Jr., and G. Schochetman. 1989. Human chromosome 12 is required for elevated HIV-1 expression in human-hamster hybrid cells. *Science* 246:488–491.

1748. Hart, C. E., M. J. Salterelli, J. C. Galphin, and G. Schochetman. 1995. A human chromosome 12-associated 83-kilodalton cellular protein specifically binds to the loop region of human immunodeficiency virus type 1 *trans*-activation response element RNA. *J. Virol.* 69:6593–6599.

1749. Hart, M. L., M. Saifuddin, K. Uemura, E. G. Bremer, B. Hooker, T. Kawasaki, and G. T. Spear. 2002. High mannose glycans and siliac acid on gp120 regulate binding of mannose-binding lectin (MBL) to HIV type 1. *AIDS Res. Hum. Retrovir.* 18:1311–1317.

1750. Hart, T. K., R. Kirsh, H. Ellens, R. W. Sweet, D. M. Lambert, S. R. Petteway, Jr., J. Leary, and P. J. Bugelski. 1991. Binding of soluble CD4 proteins to human immunodeficiency virus type 1 and infected cells induces release of envelope glycoprotein gp120. *Proc. Natl. Acad. Sci. USA* 88:2189–2193.

1751. Hartley, C. A., M. J. Gilbert, L. Brigido, T. Elbeik, J. A. Levy, S. M. Crowe, and J. Mills. 1996. Human immunodeficiency virus grown in CD4-expressing cells is associated with CD4. *J. Gen. Virol.* 77:2015–2023.

1752. Hartley, O., P. J. Klasse, Q. J. Sattentau, and J. P. Moore. 2005. V3: HIV's switch-hitter. *AIDS Res. Hum. Retrovir.* 21:71–89.

1753. Hartung, S., S. G. Norley, R. Ennen, K. Cichutek, R. Plesker, and R. Kurth. 1992. Vaccine protection against SIVmac infection by high- but not low-dose whole inactivated virus immunogen. *J. Acquir. Immune Defic. Syndr.* 5:461–468.

1754. Harwood, A. R., D. Osoba, and S. L. Hofstader. 1979. Kaposi's sarcoma in recipients of renal transplants. *Am. J. Med.* 67:759–765.

1755. Haslett, P. A., D. F. Nixon, Z. Shen, M. Larsson, W. I. Cox, R. Manandhar, S. M. Donahoe, and G. Kaplan. 2000. Strong human immunodeficiency virus (HIV)-specific CD4+ T cell responses in a cohort of chronically infected patients are associated with interruptions in anti-HIV chemotherapy. *J. Infect. Dis.* 181:1264–1272.

1756. Hasunuma, T., H. Tsubota, M. Watanabe, Z. W. Chen, C. I. Lord, L. C. Burkly, J. F. Daley, and N. L. Letvin. 1992. Regions of the CD4 molecule not involved in virus binding or syncytia formation are required for HIV-1 infection of lymphocytes. *J. Immunol.* 148:1841–1846.

1757. Hatakeyama, M., T. Koni, N. Kobyashi, A. Kawahara, S. D. Levin, R. M. Perlmuther, and T. Taniguichi. 1991. Interaction of the IL-2 receptor with the src-family kinase p56 lck: identification of novel intermolecular association. *Science* 252:1523–1528.

1757a. Hatano, H., P. Hunt, J. Weidler, E. Coakley, R. Hoh, T. Liegler, J. N. Martin, and S. G. Deeks. 2006. Rate of viral evolution and risk of losing future drug options in heavily pretreated, HIV-infected patients who continue to receive a stable, partially suppressive treatment regimen. *Clin. Infect. Dis.* 43:1329–1336.

1758. Hatano, H., K. D. Miller, C. P. Yoder, J. A. Yanovski, N. G. Sebring, E. C. Jones, and R. T. Davey, Jr. 2000. Metabolic and anthropometric consequences of interruption of highly active antiretroviral therapy. *AIDS* 14:1935–1942.

1759. Hatano, H., S. Vogel, C. Yoder, J. A. Metcalf, R. Dewar, R. T. Davey Jr., and M. A. Polis. 2000. Pre-HAART HIV burden approximates post-HAART viral levels following interruption of therapy in patients with sustained viral suppression. *AIDS* 14:1357–1636.

1760. Hattori, T., A. Koito, K. Takatsuki, H. Kido, and N. Katunuma. 1989. Involvement of tryptase-related cellular protease(s) in human immunodeficiency virus type 1 infection. *FEBS Lett.* 248:48–52.

1761. Hatziioannou, T., S. Cowan, S. P. Goff, P. D. Bieniasz, and G. J. Towers. 2003. Restriction of multiple divergent retroviruses by LV1 and Ref1. *EMBO. J.* 22:385–394.

1762. Hatziioannou, T., D. Perez-Caballero, S. Cowan, and P. D. Bieniasz. 2005. Cyclophilin interactions with incoming human immunodeficiency virus type 1 capsids with opposing effects on infectivity in human cells. *J. Virol.* 79:176–183.

1763. Hatziioannou, T., D. Perez-Caballero, A. Yang, S. Cowan, and P. D. Bieniasz. 2004. Retrovirus resistance factors Ref1 and Lv1 are species-specific variants of TRIM5a. *Proc. Natl. Acad. Sci. USA* 101:10774–10779.

1764. Haverkos, J. W., P. F. Pinsky, D. Drotman, and D. J. Bregman. 1985. Disease manisfestations among homosexual men with acquired immunodeficiency syndrome: a possible role of nitrites in Kaposi's sarcoma. *Sex. Transm. Dis.* 12:203–208.

1765. Havlir, D. V., R. D. Schrier, F. J. Torriani, K. Chervenak, J. Y. Hwang, and W. H. Boom. 2000. Effect of potent antiretroviral therapy on immune responses to Mycobacterium avium in human immunodeficiency virus-infected subjects. *J. Infect. Dis.* 182:1658–1663.

1766. Hayday, A., E. Theodoridis, E. Ramsburg, and J. Shires. 2001. Intraepithelial lymphocytes: exploring the Third Way in immunology. *Nat. Immunol.* 2:997–1003.

1767. Hayes, R. J., K. F. Schulz, and F. A. Plummer. 1995. The cofactor effect of genital ulcers on the per-exposure risk of HIV transmission in sub-Saharan Africa. *J. Trop. Med. Hyg.* 98:1–8.

1768. Haynes, B. F., J. Fleming, E. W. St Clair, H. Katinger, G. Stiegler, R. Kunert, J. Robinson, R. M. Scearce, K. Plonk, H. F. Staats, T. L. Ortel, H. X. Liao, and S. M. Alam. 2005. Cardiolipin polyspecific autoreactivity in two broadly neutralizing HIV-1 antibodies. *Science* 308:1906–1908.

1769. Haynes, B. F., M. A. Moody, C. S. Heinley, B. Korber, W. A. Millard, and R. M. Scearce. 1995. HIV type 1 V3 region primer-induced antibody suppression is overcome by administration of C4-V3 peptides as a polyvalent immunogen. *AIDS Res. Hum. Retrovir.* 11:211–221.

1770. Haynes, B. F., G. Pantaleo, and A. S. Fauci. 1996. Toward an understanding of the correlates of protective immunity to HIV infection. *Science* 271:324–328.

1771. Hays, E. F., C. H. Uittenbogaart, J. C. Brewer, L. W. Vollger, and J. A. Zack. 1991. In vitro studies of HIV-1 expression in thymocytes from infants and children. *AIDS* 6:265–272.

1772. Hayward, G. S. 1999. KSHV strains: the origins and global spread of the virus. *Semin. Cancer Biol.* 9:187–199.

1773. Hazenberg, M. D., D. Hamann, H. Schuitemaker, and F. Miedema. 2000. T cell depletion in HIV-1 infection: how CD4+ T cells go out of stock. *Nat. Immunol.* 1:285–289.

1774. Hazenberg, M. D., J. W. Stuart, S. A. Otto, J. C. Borleffs, C. A. Boucher, R. J. de Boer, F. Miedema, and D. Hamann. 2000. T-cell division in human immunodeficiency virus (HIV)-1 infection is mainly due to immune activation: a longitudinal analysis in patients before and during highly active antiretroviral therapy (HAART). *Blood* 95:249–255.

1775. Hazenberg, M. D., M. C. Verschuren, D. Hamann, F. Miedema, and J. J. van Dongen. 2001. T cell receptor excision circles as markers for recent thymic emigrants: basic aspects, technical approach, and guidelines for interpretation. *J. Mol. Med.* 79:631–640.

1776. Hazuda, D. J., S. D. Young, J. P. Guare, N. J. Anthony, R. P. Gomez, J. S. Wai, J. P. Vacca, L. Handt, S. L. Motzel, H. J. Klein, G. Dornadula, R. M. Danovich, M. V. Witmer, K. A. A. Wilson, L. Tussey, W. A. Schleif, L. S. Gabryelski, L. Jin, M. D. Miller, D. R. Casimiro, E. A. Emini, and J. W. Shiver. 2004. Integrase inhibitors and cellular immunity suppress retroviral replication in rhesus macaques. *Science* 305:528–532.

1777. He, J., Y. Chen, M. Farzan, H. Choe, A. Ohagen, S. Gartner, J. Busciglio, X. Yang, W. Hofmann, W. Newman, C. R. Mackay, J. Sodroski, and D. Gabuzda. 1997. CCR3 and CCR5 are co-receptors for HIV-1 infection of microglia. *Nature* 385:645–649.

1778. He, J., S. Choe, R. Walker, P. De Marzio, D. O. Morgan, and N. R. Landau. 1995. Human immunodeficiency virus type 1 viral protein R (vpr) arrests cells in the G_2 phase of the cell cycle by inhibiting p34^{cdc2} activity. *J. Virol.* 69:6705–6711.

1779. Heagy, W., C. Crumpacker, P. A. Lopez, and R. W. Finberg. 1991. Inhibition of immune functions by antiviral drugs. *J. Clin. Investig.* 87:1916–1924.

1780. Healey, D., L. Dianda, J. P. Moore, J. S. McDougal, M. J. Moore, P. Estess, D. Buck, P. D. Kwong, P. C. L. Beverley, and Q. J. Sattentau. 1990. Novel anti-CD4 monoclonal antibodies separate human immunodeficiency virus infection and fusion of CD4+ cells from virus binding. *J. Exp. Med.* 172:1233–1242.

1781. Heard, I., J. M. Palefsky, and M. D. Kazatchkine. 2004. The impact of HIV antiviral therapy on human papillomavirus (HPV) infections and HPV-related diseases. *Antivir. Ther.* 9:13–22.

1782. Heard, I., J. Tassie, M. D. Kazatchkine, and G. Orth. 2002. Highly active antiretroviral therapy enhances regression of cervical intraepithelial neoplasia in HIV-seropositive women. *AIDS* 16:1799–1802.

1783. Heath, S. L., J. G. Tew, A. K. Szakal, and G. F. Burton. 1995. Follicular dendritic cells and human immunodeficiency virus infectivity. *Nature* 377:740–744.

1784. Hecht, F. M., M. P. Busch, B. Rawal, M. Webb, E. Rosenberg, M. Swanson, M. Chesney, J. Anderson, B. Walker, J. Levy, and J. O. Kahn. 2002. Use of laboratory tests and clinical symptoms for identification of primary HIV infection. *AIDS* 16:1119–1129.

1785. Hecht, F. M., R. M. Grant, C. J. Petropoulos, B. Dillon, M. A. Chesney, H. Tian, N. S. Hellmann, N. I. Bandrapalli, L. Digilio, B. Branson, and J. O. Kahn. 1998. Sexual transmission of an HIV-1 variant resistant to multiple reverse-transcriptase and protease inhibitors. *N. Engl. J. Med.* 339:307–311.

1785a. Hecht, F. M., L. Wang, A. Collier, S. Little, M. Markowitz, J. Margolick, J. M. Kilby, E. Daar, B. Conway, and S. Holte. 2006. A multicenter observational study of the potential benefits of initiating combination antiretroviral therapy during acute HIV infection. *J. Infect. Dis.* 194:725–733.

1786. Heggelund, L., T. E. Mollnes, T. Ueland, B. Christophersen, P. Aukrust, and S. S. Froland. 2003. Mannose-binding lectin in HIV infection: relation to disease progression and highly active antiretroviral therapy. *J. Acquir. Immune Defic. Syndr.* 32:354–361.

1787. Heil, F., H. Hemmi, H. Hochrein, F. Ampenberger, C. Kirschning, S. Akira, G. Lipford, H. Wagner, and S. Bauer. 2004. Species-specific recognition of single-stranded RNA via toll-like receptor 7 and 8. *Science* 303:1526–1529.

1788. Heinkelein, M., S. Sopper, and C. Jassoy. 1995. Contact of human immunodeficiency virus type 1-infected and uninfected CD4+ T lymphocytes is highly cytolytic for both cells. *J. Virol.* 69:6925–6931.

1789. Heintel, T., M. Sester, M. M. B. Rodriguez, C. Krieg, U. Sester, R. Wagner, H. W. Pees, B. Gartner, R. Maier, and A.

Meyerhans. 2002. The fraction of perforin-expressing HIV-specific CD8 T cells is a marker for disease progression in HIV infection. *AIDS* 16:1497–1501.

1790. Heinzinger, N., L. Baca-Regen, M. Stevenson, and H. Gendelman. 1995. Efficient synthesis of viral nucleic acids following monocyte infection by HIV-1. *Virology* 206:731–735.

1791. Heinzinger, N. K., M. I. Bukinsky, S. A. Haggerty, A. M. Ragland, V. Kewalramani, M. A. Lee, H. E. Gendelman, L. Ratner, M. Stevenson, and M. Emerman. 1994. The Vpr protein of human immunodeficiency virus type 1 influences nuclear localization of viral nucleic acids in nondividing host cells. *Proc. Natl. Acad. Sci. USA* 91:7311–7315.

1792. Heise, C., S. Dandekar, P. Kumar, R. Duplantier, R. M. Donovan, and C. H. Halsted. 1991. Human immunodeficiency virus infection of enterocytes and mononuclear cells in human jejunal mucosa. *Gastroenterology* 100:1521–1527.

1793. Heise, C., C. J. Miller, A. Lackner, and S. Dandekar. 1994. Primary acute simian immunodeficiency virus infection of intestinal lymphoid tissue is associated with gastrointestinal dsyfunction. *J. Infect. Dis.* 169:1116–1120.

1794. Hel, Z., W. P. Tsai, E. Tryniszewska, J. Nacsa, P. D. Markham, M. G. Lewis, G. N. Pavlakis, B. K. Felber, J. Tartaglia, and G. Franchini. 2006. Improved vaccine protection from simian AIDS by the addition of nonstructural simian immunodeficiency virus genes. *J. Immunol.* 176:85–96.

1795. Hel, Z., D. Venzon, M. Poudyal, W. P. Tsai, L. Giuliani, R. Woodward, C. Chougnet, G. Shearer, J. D. Altman, D. Watkins, N. Bischofberger, A. Abimiku, P. Markham, J. Tartaglia, and G. Franchini. 2000. Viremia control following antiretroviral treatment and therapeutic immunization during primary SIV251 infection of macaques. *Nat. Med.* 6:1140–1146.

1796. Helbert, M. R., J. L'age-Stehr, and N. A. Mitchison. 1993. Antigen presentation, loss of immunological memory and AIDS. *Immunol. Today* 14:340–344.

1797. Hellerstein, M., M. B. Hanley, D. Cesar, S. Siler, C. Papageorgopoulos, E. Wieder, D. Schmidt, R. Hoh, R. Neese, D. Macallan, S. Deeks, and J. M. McCune. 1999. Directly measured kinetics of circulating T lymphocytes in normal and HIV-1-infected humans. *Nat. Med.* 5:83–89.

1798. Hellerstein, M. K., R. A. Hoh, B. Hanley, D. Cesar, D. Lee, R. A. Neese, and J. M. McCune. 2003. Subpopulations of long-lived and short-lived T cells in advanced HIV-1 infection. *J. Clin. Investig.* 112:956–965.

1799. Helseth, E., U. Olshevsky, C. Furman, and J. Sodroski. 1991. Human immunodeficiency virus type 1 gp120 envelope glycoprotein regions important for association with the gp41 transmembrane glycoprotein. *J. Virol.* 65:2119–2123.

1800. Hemmi, H., T. Kaisho, O. Takeuchi, S. Sato, H. Sanjo, K. Hoshino, T. Horiuchi, H. Tomizawa, K. Takeda, and S. Akira. 2002. Small anti-viral compounds activate immune cells via the TLR7 MyD88-dependent signaling pathway. *Nat. Immunol.* 22:22.

1801. Hendel, H., S. Caillat-Zucman, H. Lebuanec, M. Carrington, S. O'Brien, J. M. Andrieu, F. Schachter, D. Zagury, J. Rappaport, C. Winkler, G. W. Nelson, and J. F. Zagury. 1999. New class I and II HLA alleles strongly associated with opposite patterns of progression to AIDS. *J. Immunol.* 162:6942–6946.

1802. Hendel, H., N. Henon, H. Lebuanec, A. Lachgar, H. Poncelet, S. Caillat-Sucman, C. A. Winkler, M. W. Smith, L. Kenefic, S. O'Brien, W. Lu, J. M. Andrieu, D. Zahury, F.

Schachter, J. Rappaport, and J. F. Zagury. 1998. Distinctive effects of CCR5, CCR2, and SDF1 genetic polymorphisms in AIDS progression. *J. Acquir. Immune Defic. Syndr. Hum. Retrovirol.* **19**:381–386.

1803. Hendel, H., C. Winkler, P. An, E. Roemer-Binns, G. Nelson, P. Haumont, S. O'Brien, K. Khalilli, D. Zagury, J. Rappaport, and J. F. Zagury. 2001. Validation of genetic case-control studies in AIDS and application to the CX3CR1 polymorphism. *J. Acquir. Immune Defic. Syndr.* **26**:507–511.

1804. Henderson, E. E., J.-Y. Yang, R.-D. Zhang, and M. Bealer. 1991. Altered HIV expression and EBV-induced transformation in coinfected PBLs and PBL subpopulations. *Virology* **182**:186–198.

1805. Henderson, G. J., N. G. Hoffman, L. H. Ping, S. A. Fiscus, I. F. Hoffman, K. M. Kitrinos, T. Banda, F. E. A. Martinson, P. N. Kazembe, D. A. Chilongozi, M. S. Cohen, and R. Swanstrom. 2004. HIV-1 populations in blood and breast milk are similar. *Virology* **330**:295–303.

1806. Henderson, L. A., and M. N. Qureshi. 1993. A peptide inhibitor of human immunodeficiency virus infection binds to novel human cell surface polypeptides. *J. Biol. Chem.* **268**: 15291–15297.

1807. Henderson, L. A., N. M. Qureshi, S. Rasheed, and R. Garry. 1988. Human immunodeficiency virus-induced cytotoxicity for CD8 cells from some normal donors and virus-specific induction of a suppressor factor. *Clin. Immunol. Immunopathol.* **48**:174–186.

1808. Henderson, S., M. Rowe, C. Gregory, D. Croom-Carter, F. Wang, R. Longnecker, E. Kieff, and A. Rickinson. 1991. Induction of bcl-2 expression by Epstein-Barr virus latent membrane protein 1 protects infected B cells from programmed cell death. *Cell* **65**:1107–1115.

1809. Henderson, W. W., R. Ruhl, P. Lewis, M. Bentley, J. A. Nelson, and A. V. Moses. 2004. Human immunodeficiency virus (HIV) type 1 Vpu induces the expression of CD40 in endothelial cells and regulates HIV-induced adhesion of B-lymphoma cells. *J. Virol.* **78**:4408–4420.

1810. Heng, M. C. Y., S. Y. Heng, and S. G. Allen. 1994. Co-infection and synergy of human immunodeficiency virus-1 and herpes simplex virus-1. *Lancet* **343**:255–258.

1811. Hengge, U. R., C. Borchard, S. Esser, M. Schroder, A. Mirmohammadsadegh, and M. Goos. 2002. Lymphocytes proliferate in blood and lymph nodes following interleukin-2 therapy in addition to highly active antiretroviral therapy. *AIDS* **16**:151–160.

1812. Hengge, U. R., N. H. Brockmeyer, S. Esser, M. Maschke, and M. Goos. 1998. HIV-1 RNA levels in cerebrospinal fluid and plasma correlate with AIDS dementia. *AIDS* **12**:818–820.

1813. Henin, Y., L. Mandelbrot, R. Henrion, R. Pradinaud, J. P. Coulaud, and L. Montagnier. 1993. Virus excretion in the cervicovaginal secretions of pregnant and nonpregnant HIV-infected women. *J. Acquir. Immune Defic. Syndr.* **6**:72–75.

1814. Henle, G., and W. Henle. 1979. The virus as the etiologic agent of infectious mononucleosis. *In* M. A. Epstein and B. G. Achong (ed.), *The Epstein-Barr Virus.* Springer-Verlag, Berlin, Germany.

1815. Henrard, D. R., J. F. Phillips, L. R. Muenz, W. A. Blattner, D. Wiesner, M. E. Eyster, and J. J. Goedert. 1995. Natural history of HIV-1 cell-free viremia. *JAMA* **274**:554–558.

1815a. Henry, K., D. Katzenstein, D. W. Cherng, H. Valdez, W. Powderly, M. B. Vargas, N. C. Jahed, J. M. Jacobson, L. S. Myers, J. L. Schmitz, M. Winters, and P. Tebas. 2006. A pilot study evaluating time to CD4 T-cell count <350 cells/mm(3) after treatment interruption following antiretroviral therapy +/− interleukin 2: results of ACTG A5102. *J. Acquir. Immune Defic. Syndr.* **42**:140–148.

1816. Herbein, G., U. Mahlknecht, F. Batliwalla, P. Gergersen, T. Pappas, J. Butler, W. A. O'Brien, and E. Verdin. 1998. Apoptosis of CD8+ T cells is mediated by macrophages through interaction of HIV gp120 with chemokine receptor CXCR4. *Nature* **395**:189–194.

1817. Herbein, G., L. J. Montaner, and S. Gordon. 1996. Tumor necrosis factor alpha inhibits entry of human immunodeficiency virus type 1 into primary human macrophages: a selective role for the 75-kilodalton receptor. *J. Virol.* **70**:7388–7397.

1818. Herbein, G., C. van Lint, J. L. Lovett, and E. Verdin. 1998. Distinct mechanisms trigger apoptosis in human immunodeficiency virus type 1-infected and uninfected bystander T lymphocytes. *J. Virol.* **72**:660–670.

1819. Herbeuval, J. P., A. W. Hardy, A. Boasso, S. A. Anderson, M. J. Dolan, M. Dy, and G. M. Shearer. 2005. Regulation of TNF-related apoptosis-inducing ligand on primary CD4+ T cells by HIV-1: role of type I IFN-producing plasmacytoid dendritic cells. *Proc. Natl. Acad. Sci. USA* **102**:13974–13979.

1820. Heringlake, S., J. Ockenga, H. L. Tillmann, C. Trautwein, D. Meissner, M. Stoll, J. Hunt, C. Jou, N. Solomon, R. E. Schmidt, and M. P. Manns. 1998. GB virus C/hepatitis G virus infection: a favorable prognostic factor in human immunodeficiency virus-infected patients? *J. Infect. Dis.* **177**: 1723–1726.

1821. Hermankova, M., S. C. Ray, C. Ruff, M. Powell-Davis, R. Ingersoll, R. T. D'Aquila, T. C. Quinn, J. D. Siliciano, R. F. Siliciano, and D. Persaud. 2001. HIV-1 drug resistance profiles in children and adults with viral load of <50 copies/ml receiving combination therapy. *JAMA* **286**:196–207.

1822. Hermankova, M., J. D. Siliciano, Y. Zhou, D. Monie, K. Chadwick, J. B. Margolick, T. C. Quinn, and R. F. Siliciano. 2003. Analysis of human immunodeficiency virus type 1 gene expression in latently resting CD4+ T lymphocytes in vivo. *J. Virol.* **77**:7383–7392.

1822a. Hernandez-Diaz, S., M. M. Werler, A. M. Walker, and A. A. Mitchell. 2000. Folic acid antagonists during pregnancy and the risk of birth defects. *N. Engl. J. Med.* **343**:1608–1614.

1823. Herndier, B. G., L. Kaplan, and M. McGrath. 1994. Pathogenesis of AIDS lymphomas. *AIDS* **8**:1025–1049.

1824. Herndier, B. G., H. C. Sanchez, K. L. Chang, Y. Y. Chen, and L. M. Weiss. 1993. High prevalence of Epstein-Barr virus in the Reed-Sternberg cells of HIV-associated Hodgkin's disease. *Am. J. Pathol.* **142**:1073–1079.

1825. Herrmann, C. H., and A. P. Rice. 1993. Specific interaction of the human immunodeficiency virus Tat proteins with a cellular protein kinase. *Virology* **197**:601–608.

1826. Hess, C., M. Altfeld, S. Y. Thomas, M. M. Addo, E. S. Rosenberg, T. M. Allen, R. Draenert, R. L. Eldrige, J. van Lunzen, H. Stellbrink, B. D. Walker, and A. D. Luster. 2004. HIV-1 specific CD8+ T cells with an effector phenotype and control of viral replication. *Lancet* **363**:863–866.

1827. Hess, C., T. Klimkait, L. Schlapback, V. Del Zenero, S. Sadallah, G. Balestra, V. Werder, C. Schaefer, M. Battegay, and J.-A. Schifferli. 2002. A pool of HIV-1 is associated with erythrocytes *in vivo. Lancet* **359**:2230–2234.

1828. Hesselgesser, J., D. Taub, P. Baskar, M. Greenberg, J. Hoxie, D. Kolson, and R. Horuk. 1998. Neuronal apoptosis induced by HIV-1 gp120 and the chemokine SDF-1α is mediated by the chemokine receptor CXCR4. *Curr. Biol.* 8:595–598.

1829. Hetherington, S., A. R. Hughes, M. Mosteller, D. Shortino, K. L. Baker, W. Spreen, E. Lai, K. Davies, A. Handley, D. J. Dow, M. E. Fling, M. Stocum, C. Bowman, L. M. Thurmond, and A. D. Roses. 2002. Genetic variations in HLA-B region and hypersensitivity reactions to abacavir. *Lancet* 359:1121–1122.

1830. Heyes, M. P., B. J. Brew, A. Martin, R. W. Price, A. M. Salazar, J. J. Sidfis, J. A. Vergey, M. M. Mouradian, A. E. Sadler, and J. Keilp. 1991. Quinolinic acid in cerebrospinal fluid and serum in HIV-1 infection: relationship to clinical and neurological status. *Ann. Neurol.* 29:202–209.

1831. Hickey, W. F., B. L. Hsu, and H. Kimura. 1991. T-lymphocyte entry into the central nervous system. *J. Neurosci. Res.* 28:254–260.

1832. Hildeman, D. A., Y. Zhu, T. C. Mitchell, P. Bouillet, A. Strasser, J. Kappler, and P. Marrack. 2002. Activated T cell death in vivo mediated by proapoptotic bcl-2 family member bim. *Immunity* 16:759–767.

1833. Hildreth, J. E., and R. J. Orentas. 1989. Involvement of a leukocyte adhesion receptor (LFA-1) in HIV-induced syncytium formation. *Science* 244:1075–1078.

1834. Hill, J. M., R. F. Mervis, R. Avidor, T. W. Moddy, and D. E. Brenneman. 1993. HIV envelope protein-induced neuronal damage and retardation of behavioral development in rat neonates. *Brain Res.* 603:222–233.

1835. Hilleman, M. R. 2003. Overview of vaccinology in historic and future perspective: the whence and whither of a dynamic science with complex dimensions, p. 1–38. *In* C. J. Hildegrund (ed.), *DNA Vaccine.* Plenum Press, New York, N.Y.

1836. Hillemanns, P., T. V. Ellerbrock, S. McPhillips, P. Dole, S. Alperstein, D. Johnson, X. W. Sun, M. A. Chiasson, and T. C. Wright, Jr. 1996. Prevalence of anal human papillomavirus infection and anal cytologic abnormalities in HIV-seropositive women. *AIDS* 10:1641–1647.

1837. Himathongkham, S., and P. A. Luciw. 1996. Restriction of HIV-1 (subtype B) replication at the entry step in rhesus macaque cells. *Virology* 219:485–488.

1838. Hino, S., K. Yamaguchi, S. Katamine, H. Sugiyama, T. Amagasaki, K. Kinoshita, Y. Yoshida, H. Doi, Y. Tsuji, and T. Miyamoto. 1985. Mother-to-child transmission of human T-cell leukemia virus type-I. *Jpn. J. Cancer Res.* 76:474–480.

1839. Hioe, C. E., L. Bastiani, J. E. Hildreth, and S. Zolla-Pazner. 1998. Role of cellular adhesion molecules in HIV type 1 infection and their impact on virus neutralization. *AIDS Res. Hum. Retrovir.* 14:S124–S254.

1840. Hioe, C. E., J. E. K. Hildreth, and S. Zolla-Pazner. 1999. Enhanced HIV type 1 neutralization by human anti-glycoprotein 120 monoclonal antibodies in the presence of monoclonal antibodies to lymphocyte function-associated molecule 1. *AIDS Res. Hum. Retrovir.* 15:523–531.

1841. Hira, S. K., J. Kamanga, R. Macuacua, N. Mwansa, D. F. Cruess, and P. L. Perine. 1990. Genital ulcers and male circumcision as risk factors for acquiring HIV-1 in Zambia. *J. Infect. Dis.* 161:584–585.

1842. Hiroishi, K., T. Tuting, and M. T. Lotze. 2000. IFN-alpha-expressing tumor cells enhance generation and promote survival of tumor-specific CTLs. *J. Immunol.* 164:567–572.

1843. Hirsch, I., J. de Mareuil, D. Salaun, and J.-C. Chermann. 1996. Genetic control of infection of primary macrophages with T-cell-tropic strains of HIV-1. *Virology* 219:257–261.

1844. Hirsch, V. M., T. R. Fuerst, G. Sutter, M. W. Carroll, L. C. Yang, S. Goldstein, M. Piatak, Jr., W. R. Elkins, W. G. Alvord, D. C. Montefiori, B. Moss, and J. D. Lifson. 1996. Patterns of viral replication correlate with outcome in simian immunodeficiency virus (SIV)-infected macaques: effect of prior immunization with a trivalent SIV vaccine in modified vaccinia virus Ankara. *J. Virol.* 70:3741–3752.

1845. Hirsch, V. M., R. A. Olmsted, M. Murphey-Corb, R. H. Purcell, and P. R. Johnson. 1989. An African primate lentivirus (SIVsm) closely related to HIV-2. *Nature* 339:389–392.

1846. HIV Paediatric Prognostic Markers Collaborative Study. 2005. Use of total lymphocyte count for informing when to start antiretroviral therapy in HIV-infected children: a meta-analysis of longitudinal data. *Lancet* 366:1868–1874.

1847. Hladik, F., A. Desbien, J. Lang, L. Wang, Y. Ding, S. Holte, A. Wilson, Y. Xu, M. Moerbe, S. Schmechel, and M. J. McElrath. 2003. Most highly exposed seronegative men lack HIV-1-specific, IFN-γ-secreting T cells. *J. Immunol.* 171:2671–2683.

1848. Hladik, F., G. Lentz, R. E. Akridge, G. Peterson, H. Kelley, A. McElroy, and M. J. McElrath. 1999. Dendritic cell-T-cell interactions support coreceptor-independent human immunodeficiency virus type 1 transmission in the human genital tract. *J. Virol.* 73: 5833–5842.

1849. Hladik, F., H. Liu, E. Speelmon, D. Livingston-Rosanoff, S. Wilson, P. Sakchalathorn, Y. Hwangbo, B. Greene, T. Zhu, and M. J. McElrath. 2005. Combined effect of CCR5-Delta32 heterozygosity and the CCR5 promoter polymorphism −2459 A/G on CCR5 expression and resistance to human immunodeficiency virus type 1 transmission. *J. Virol.* 79:11677–11684.

1850. Hlavacek, W. S., C. Wofsy, and A. S. Perelson. 1999. Dissociation of HIV-1 from follicular dendritic cells during HAART: mathematical analysis. *Proc. Natl. Acad. Sci. USA* 96:14681–14686.

1851. Ho, D. D., R. E. Byington, R. T. Schooley, T. Flynn, T. R. Rota, and M. S. Hirsch. 1985. Infrequency of isolation of HTLV-III virus from saliva in AIDS. *N. Engl. J. Med.* 313:1606.

1852. Ho, D. D., M. S. C. Fung, Y. Cao, X. L. Li, C. Sun, T. W. Chang, and N. C. Sun. 1991. Another discontinuous epitope on gp120 that is important in human immunodeficiency virus type 1 neutralization is identified by a monoclonal antibody. *Proc. Natl. Acad. Sci. USA* 88:8949–8952.

1853. Ho, D. D., T. Moudgil, and M. Alam. 1989. Quantitation of human immunodeficiency virus type 1 in the blood of infected persons. *N. Engl. J. Med.* 321:1621–1625.

1854. Ho, D. D., A. U. Neumann, A. S. Perelson, W. Chen, J. M. Leonard, and M. Markowitz. 1995. Rapid turnover of plasma virions and CD4 lymphocytes in HIV-1 infection. *Nature* 373:123–126.

1855. Ho, D. D., T. R. Rota, R. T. Schooley, J. C. Kaplan, J. D. Allan, J. E. Groopman, L. Resnick, D. Felsenstein, C. A. Andrews, and M. S. Hirsch. 1985. Isolation of HTLV-III from cerebrospinal fluid and neural tissues of patients with neurologic syndromes related to the acquired immunodeficiency syndrome. *N. Engl. J. Med.* 313:1493–1497.

1856. Ho, D. D., M. G. Sarngadharan, M. S. Hirsch, R. T. Schooley, T. R. Rota, R. C. Kennedy, T. C. Chanh, and V. L. Sato. 1987. Human immunodeficiency virus neutralizing antibodies recognize several conserved domains on the envelope glycoproteins. *J. Virol.* **61**:2024–2028.

1857. Ho, D. D., R. T. Schooley, T. R. Rota, J. C. Kaplan, T. Flynn, S. Z. Salahuddin, M. A. Gonda, and M. S. Hirsch. 1984. HTLV-III in the semen and blood of a healthy homosexual man. *Science* **226**:451–453.

1858. Ho, H. N., L. E. Hultin, R. T. Mitsuyasu, J. L. Matud, M. A. Hausner, D. Bockstoce, C. C. Chou, S. O'Rourke, J. M. G. Taylor, and J. V. Giorgi. 1993. Circulating HIV-specific CD8+ cytotoxic T cells express CD38 and HLA-DR antigens. *J. Immunol.* **150**:3070–3079.

1859. Ho, M., J. Armstrong, D. McMahon, G. Pazin, X.-L. Huang, C. Rinaldo, T. Whiteside, T. Tripoli, G. Levine, D. Moody, T. Okarma, E. Elder, P. Gupta, N. Tauxe, D. Torpey, and R. Herberman. 1993. A phase I study of adoptive transfer of autologous CD8+ T lymphocytes in patients with acquired immunodeficiency syndrome (AIDS)-related complex or AIDS. *Blood* **81**:2093–2101.

1860. Ho, S. H., L. Shek, A. Gettie, J. Blanchard, and C. Cheng-Mayer. 2005. V3 loop-determined coreceptor preference dictates the dynamics of CD4+-T-cell loss in simian-human immunodeficiency virus-infected macaques. *J. Virol.* **79**:12296–12303.

1861. Ho, W.-Z., V. Ayyavoo, A. Srinivasan, M. F. Stinski, S. A. Plotkin, and E. Gonczol. 1991. Human immunodeficiency virus type 1 *tat* gene enhances human cytomegalovirus gene expression and viral replication. *AIDS Res. Hum. Retrovir.* **7**:689–695.

1862. Hocini, H., P. Becquart, H. Bouhlal, N. Chomont, P. Ancuta, M. D. Kazatchkine, and L. Belec. 2001. Active and selective transcytosis of cell-free human immunodeficiency virus through a tight polarized monolayer of human endometrial cells. *J. Virol.* **75**:5370–5374.

1863. Hodara, V. L., M. C. Velasquillo, L. M. Parodi, and L. D. Giavedoni. 2005. Expression of CD154 by a simian immunodeficiency virus vector induces only transitory changes in rhesus macaques. *J. Virol.* **79**:4679–4690.

1864. Hoen, B., I. Fournier, C. Lacabaratz, M. Burgard, I. Charreau, M. L. Chaix, J. M. Molina, J. M. Livrozet, A. Venet, F. Raffi, J. P. Aboulker, and C. Rouzioux. 2005. Structured treatment interruptions in primary HIV-1 infection: the ANRS 100 PRIMSTOP trial. *J. Acquir. Immune Defic. Syndr.* **40**:307–316.

1865. Hoffenbach, A., P. Langlade-Demoyen, G. Dadaglio, E. Vilmer, F. Michel, C. Mayaud, B. Autran, and F. Plata. 1989. Unusually high frequencies of HIV-specific cytotoxic T lymphocytes in humans. *J. Immunol.* **142**:452–462.

1866. Hoffman, T. L., C. C. LaBranche, W. Zhang, G. Canziani, J. Robinson, I. Chaiken, J. A. Hoxie, and R. W. Doms. 1999. Stable exposure of the coreceptor-binding site in a CD4-independent HIV-1 envelope protein. *Proc. Natl. Acad. Sci. USA* **96**:6359–6364.

1867. Hofman, F. M., M. M. Dohadwala, A. D. Wright, D. R. Hinton, and S. M. Walker. 1994. Exogenous Tat protein activates central nervous system-derived endothelial cells. *J. Neuroimmunol.* **54**:19–28.

1868. Hofmann, B., P. Nishanian, R. L. Baldwin, P. Insixiengmay, A. Nel, and J. L. Fahey. 1990. HIV inhibits the early steps of lymphocyte activation, including initiation of inositol phospholipid metabolism. *J. Immunol.* **145**:3699–3705.

1869. Hofmann-Lehmann, R., J. Vlasak, A. L. Williams, A.-L. Chenine, H. M. McClure, D. C. Anderson, S. O'Neil, and R. M. Ruprecht. 2003. Live attenuated, nef-deleted SIV is pathogenic

in most adult macaques after prolonged observation. *AIDS* **17**:157–166.

1870. Hogervorst, E., S. Jurriaans, F. de Wolf, A. van Wijk, A. Wiersma, M. Valk, M. Roos, B. van Gemen, R. Coutinho, F. Miedema, and J. Goudsmit. 1995. Predictors for non- and slow progression in human immunodeficiency virus (HIV) type 1 infection: low viral RNA copy numbers in serum and maintenance of high HIV-1 p24-specific but not V3-specific antibody levels. *J. Infect. Dis.* **171**:811–821.

1871. Hogg, R. S., M. V. O'Shaughnessy, N. Gataric, B. Yip, K. Craib, M. T. Schechter, and J. S. G. Montaner. 1997. Decline in deaths from AIDS due to new antiretrovirals. *Lancet* **349**:1294.

1872. Hogg, R. S., B. Yip, K. J. Chan, E. Wood, K. J. Craib, M. V. O'Shaughnessy, and J. S. Montaner. 2001. Rates of disease progression by baseline CD4 cell count and viral load after initiating triple-drug therapy. *JAMA* **286**:2568–2577.

1873. Hohmann, A. W., K. Booth, V. Peters, D. L. Gordon, and R. M. Comacchio. 1993. Common epitope on HIV p24 and human platelets. *Lancet* **342**:1274–1275.

1874. Hollander, H., and J. A. Levy. 1987. Neurologic abnormalities and recovery of human immunodeficiency virus from cerebrospinal fluid. *Ann. Intern. Med.* **106**:692–695.

1875. Holm, G. H., and D. Gabuzda. 2005. Distinct mechanisms of CD4+ and CD8+ T-cell activation and bystander apoptosis induced by human immunodeficiency virus type 1 virions. *J. Virol.* **79**:6299–6311.

1876. Holmberg, S. D., F. J. Palella, K. A. Lichtenstein, and D. V. Havlir. 2004. The case for earlier treatment of HIV infection. *Clin. Infect. Dis.* **39**:1699–1704.

1877. Holmes, E. C., L. Q. Zhang, P. Simmonds, C. A. Lundlam, and A. J. Leigh Brown. 1992. Convergent and divergent sequence evolution in the surface envelope glycoprotein of human immunodeficiency virus type 1 within a single infected patient. *Proc. Natl. Acad. Sci. USA* **89**:4835–4839.

1878. Holmgren, J., and C. Czerkinsky. 2005. Mucosal immunity and vaccines. *Nat. Med.* **11**:S45–S53.

1879. Holodniy, M., D. A. Katzenstein, S. Sengupta, A. M. Wang, C. Casipit, D. H. Schwartz, M. Konrad, E. Groves, and T. C. Merigan. 1991. Detection and quantification of human immunodeficiency virus RNA in patient serum by use of the polymerase chain reaction. *J. Infect. Dis.* **163**:862–866.

1880. Holodniy, M., L. Mole, D. Margolis, J. Moss, H. Dong, E. Boyer, M. Urdea, J. Kolberg, and S. Eastman. 1995. Determination of human immunodeficiency virus RNA in plasma and cellular viral DNA genotypic zidovudine resistance and viral load during zidovudine-didanosine combination therapy. *J. Virol.* **69**:3510–3516.

1881. Homsy, J., M. Meyer, and J. A. Levy. 1990. Serum enhancement of human immunodeficiency virus (HIV) correlates with disease in HIV infected individuals. *J. Virol.* **64**:1437–1440.

1882. Homsy, J., M. Meyer, M. Tateno, S. Clarkson, and J. A. Levy. 1989. The Fc and not the CD4 receptor mediates antibody enhancement of HIV infection in human cells. *Science* **244**:1357–1360.

1883. Homsy, J., M. Tateno, and J. A. Levy. 1988. Antibody-dependent enhancement of HIV infection. *Lancet* **i**:1285–1286.

1884. Honda, K., S. Sakaguchi, C. Nakajima, A. Watanabe, H. Yanai, M. Matsumoto, T. Ohteki, T. Kaisho, A. Takaoka, S. Akira, T. Seya, and T. Taniguchi. 2003. Selective contribution of IFN-alpha/beta signaling to the maturation of dendritic cells induced by double-stranded RNA or viral infection. *Proc. Natl. Acad. Sci. USA* 100:10872–10877.

1885. Honda, Y., L. Rogers, K. Nakata, R. Zhao, R. Pine, Y. Nakai, K. Kurosu, W. M. Rom, and M. Weiden. 1998. Type I interferon induces inhibitory 16-kD CCAAT/ enhancer binding protein (C/EBP) beta, repressing the HIV-1 long terminal repeat in macrophages: pulmonary tuberculosis alters C/EBP expression, enhancing HIV-1 replication. *J. Exp. Med.* 188:1255–1265.

1886. Hong, Y. K., K. Foreman, J. W. Shin, S. Hirakawa, C. L. Curry, D. R. Sage, T. Libermann, B. J. Dezube, J. D. Fingeroth, and M. Detmar. 2004. Lymphatic reprogramming of blood vascular endothelium by Kaposi sarcoma-associated herpesvirus. *Nat. Genet.* 36:683–685.

1887. Hook, E. W., III, R. O. Cannon, A. J. Nahmias, F. F. Lee, C. H. Campbell, Jr., D. Glasser, and T. C. Quinn. 1992. Herpes simplex virus infection as a risk factor for human immunodeficiency virus infection in heterosexuals. *J. Infect. Dis.* 165:251–255.

1888. Hooper, E. 1999. The river: a journey to the source of HIV/AIDS. Little Brown, New York, N.Y.

1889. Hoover, D. R., C. Rinaldo, Y. He, J. Phair, J. Fahey, and N. M. H. Graham. 1995. Long-term survival without clinical AIDS after CD4+ cell counts fall below 200 × 10⁶/l. *AIDS* 9:145–152.

1889a. Hoque, M., B. Tian, M. B. Mathews, and T. Pe'ery. 2005. Granulin and granulin repeats interact with the Tat.P-TEFb complex and inhibit Tat transactivation. *J. Biol. Chem.* 280:13648–13657.

1890. Hornung, V., S. Rothenfusser, S. Britsch, A. Krug, B. Jahrsdorfer, T. Giese, S. Endres, and G. Hartmann. 2002. Quantitative expression of toll-like receptor 1–10 mRNA in cellular subsets of human peripheral blood mononuclear cells and sensitivity to CpG oligodeoxynucleotides. *J. Immunol.* 168:4531–4537.

1891. Hornung, V., J. Schlender, M. Guenthner-Biller, S. Rothenfusser, S. Endres, K. K. Conzelmann, and G. Hartmann. 2004. Replication-dependent potent IFN-alpha induction in human plasmacytoid dendritic cells by a single-stranded RNA virus. *J. Immunol.* 173:5935–5943.

1892. Horsburgh, C. R., Jr., C.-Y. Ou, J. Jason, S. D. Holmberg, I. M. Longini, Jr., C. Schable, K. H. Mayer, A. R. Lifson, G. Schochetman, J. W. Ward, G. W. Rutherford, B. L. Evatt, G. R. Seage III, and H. W. Jaffe. 1989. Duration of human immunodeficiency virus infection before detection of antibody. *Lancet* ii:637–640.

1893. Horvat, R. T., C. Wood, and N. Balachandran. 1989. Transactivation of human immunodeficiency virus promoter by human herpesvirus 6. *J. Virol.* 63:970–973.

1894. Horwitz, D. A., S. G. Zheng, and J. D. Gray. 2003. The role of the combination of IL-2 and TGF-beta or IL-10 in the generation and function of CD4+ CD25+ and CD8+ regulatory T cell subsets. *J. Leukoc. Biol.* 74:471–478.

1895. Hoshino, Y., D. B. Tse, G. Rochford, S. Prabhakar, S. Hoshino, N. Chitkara, K. Kuwabara, E. Ching, B. Raju, J. A. Gold, W. Borkowsky, W. N. Rom, R. Pine, and M. Weiden. 2004. Mycobacterium tuberculosis-induced CXCR4 and chemokine expression leads to preferential X4 HIV-1 replication in human macrophages. *J. Immunol.* 172:6251–6258.

1896. Houghton, M., and S. Abrignani. 2005. Prospects for a vaccine against the hepatitis C virus. *Nature* 436:961–966.

1897. Housset, C., E. Lamas, B. Courgnaud, O. Boucher, P. M. Girard, C. Marche, and C. Brechot. 1993. Presence of HIV-1 in human parenchymal and non-parenchymal liver cells in vivo. *J. Hepatol.* 19:252–258.

1898. Hout, D. R., E. R. Mulcahy, E. Pacyniak, L. M. Gomez, M. L. Gomez, and E. B. Stephens. 2004. Vpu: a multifunctional protein that enhances the pathogenesis of human immunodeficiency virus type 1. *Curr. HIV Res.* 2:255–270.

1899. Howard, M. R., D. Whitby, G. Bahadur, F. Suggett, C. Boshoff, M. Tenant-Flowers, T. F. Schulz, S. Kirk, S. Matthews, I. V. D. Weller, R. S. Tedder, and R. A. Weiss. 1996. Detection of human herpesvirus (8) DNA in semen from HIV-infected individuals but not healthy semen donors. *AIDS* 11:F15–F19.

1900. Howcroft, T. K., K. Strebel, M. A. Martin, and D. S. Singer. 1993. Repression of MHC class I gene promoter activity by two-exon Tat of HIV. *Science* 260:1320–1323.

1901. Howe, A. Y., J. U. Jung, and R. C. Desrosiers. 1998. Zeta chain of the T-cell receptor interacts with *nef* of simian immunodeficiency virus and human immunodeficiency virus type 2. *J. Virol.* 72:9827–9834.

1902. Howell, A. L., R. D. Edkins, S. E. Rier, G. R. Yeaman, J. E. Stern, M. W. Fanger, and C. R. Wira. 1997. Human immunodeficiency virus type 1 infection of cells and tissues from the upper and lower human female reproductive tract. *J. Virol.* 71:3498–3506.

1903. Hoxie, J. A., J. D. Alpers, J. L. Rackowski, K. Huebner, B. S. Haggarty, A. J. Cedarbaum, and J. C. Reed. 1986. Alterations in T4 (CD4) protein and mRNA synthesis in cells infected with HIV. *Science* 234:1123–1127.

1904. Hoxie, J. A., T. P. Fitzharris, P. R. Youngbar, D. M. Matthews, J. L. Rackowski, and S. F. Radka. 1987. Nonrandom association of cellular antigens with HTLV-III virions. *Hum. Immunol.* 18:39–52.

1905. Hoxie, J. A., B. S. Haggarty, J. L. Rackowski, N. Pilsbury, and J. A. Levy. 1985. Persistent noncytopathic infection of human lymphocytes with AIDS associated retrovirus (ARV). *Science* 229:1400–1402.

1906. Hrimech, M., X.-J. Yao, F. Bachand, N. Rougeau, and E. A. Cohen. 1999. Human immunodeficiency virus type 1 (HIV-1) Vpr functions as an immediate-early protein during HIV-1 infection. *J. Virol.* 73:4101–4109.

1907. Hsia, K., and S. A. Spector. 1991. Human immunodeficiency virus DNA is present in a high percentage of CD4+ lymphocytes of seropositive individuals. *J. Infect. Dis.* 164:470–475.

1908. Hsu, D. H., R. de Waal Malefyt, D. F. Fiorentino, M. N. Dang, P. Vieira, J. DeVries, H. Spits, R. T. Mosmann, and K. W. Moore. 1990. Expression of interleukin-10 activity by Epstein-Barr virus protein BCRF1. *Science* 250:830–832.

1909. Hsu, K., J. Seharaseyon, P. Dong, S. Bour, and E. Marban. 2004. Mutual functional destruction of HIV-1 Vpu and host TASK-1 channel. *Mol. Cell* 14:259–267.

1910. Hsu, M.-C., U. Dhingra, J. V. Earley, M. Holly, D. Keith, C. M. Nalin, A. R. Richou, A. D. Schutt, S. Y. Tam, M. J. Potash, D. J. Volsky, and D. D. Richman. 1993. Inhibition of type 1 human immunodeficiency virus replication by a Tat antagonist to which the virus remains sensitive after prolonged exposure in vitro. *Proc. Natl. Acad. Sci. USA* 90:6395–6399.

1910a. Hsue, P. Y., J. C. Lo, A. Franklin, A. F. Bolger, J. N. Martin, S. G. Deeks, and D. D. Waters. 2004. Progression of atherosclerosis as assessed by carotid intima-media thickness in patients with HIV infection. *Circulation* 109:1603–1608.

1911. Hsueh, F. W., C. M. Walker, D. J. Blackbourn, and J. A. Levy. 1994. Suppression of HIV replication by CD8+ cell clones derived from HIV-infected and uninfected individuals. *Cell. Immunol.* 159:271–279.

1912. Hu, D. J., S. Subbarao, S. Vanichseni, P. A. Mock, A. Ramos, S. Nguyen, P. A. Mock, A. Ramos, L. Nguyen, T. Chaowanachan, F. van Griensven, K. Choopanya, T. D. Mastro, and J. W. Tappero. 2005. Frequency of HIV-1 dual subtype infections, including intersubtype superinfections, among injection drug users in Bangkok, Thailand. *AIDS* 19:303–308.

1913. Hu, J., M. B. Gardner, and C. J. Miller. 2000. Simian immunodeficiency virus rapidly penetrates the cervicovaginal mucosa after intravaginal inoculation and infects intraepithelial dendritic cells. *J. Virol.* 74:6087–6095.

1914. Hu, S.-L., K. Abrams, G. N. Barber, P. Moran, J. M. Zarling, A. J. Langlois, L. Kuller, W. R. Morton, and R. E. Benveniste. 1992. Protection of macaques against SIV infection by subunit vaccines of SIV envelope glycoprotein gp160. *Science* 255:456–459.

1915. Hu, S.-L., V. Stallard, K. Abrams, G. N. Barber, L. Kuller, A. J. Langlois, W. R. Morton, and R. E. Benveniste. 1993. Protection of vaccinia-primed macaques against SIVmne infection by combination immunization with recombinant vaccinia virus and SIVmne gp160. *J. Med. Primatol.* 22:92–99.

1916. Hu, S. L. 2005. Non-human primate models for AIDS vaccine research. *Curr. Drug. Targets Infect. Disord.* 5:193–201.

1917. Hu, S. L., P. Polacino, V. Stallard, J. Klaniecki, S. Pennathur, B. M. Travis, L. Misher, H. Kornas, A. J. Langlois, W. R. Morton, and R. E. Benveniste. 1996. Recombinant subunit vaccines as an approach to study correlates of protection against primate lentivirus infection. *Immunol. Lett.* 51:115–119.

1918. Hu, W.-S., and H. M. Temin. 1990. Retroviral recombination and reverse transcription. *Science* 250:1227–1233.

1919. Huang, A. S., E. L. Palma, and N. Hewlett. 1974. Pseudotype formation between enveloped RNA and DNA viruses. *Nature* 252:743–745.

1920. Huang, L., I. Bosch, W. Hofmann, J. Sodroski, and A. B. Pardee. 1998. Tat protein induces human immunodeficiency virus type 1 (HIV-1) coreceptors and promotes infection with both macrophage-tropic and T-lymphotropic HIV-1 strains. *J. Virol.* 72:8952–8960.

1921. Huang, S. S., J. D. Barbour, S. G. Deeks, J. S. Huang, R. M. Grant, V. L. Ng, and J. M. McCune. 2000. Reversal of human immunodeficiency virus type 1-associated hematosuppression by effective antiretroviral therapy. *Clin. Infect. Dis.* 30:504–510.

1922. Huang, X. L., Z. Fan, P. Gupta, and C. R. Rinaldo, Jr. 2006. Activation of HIV type 1 specific cytotoxic T lymphocytes from semen by HIV type 1 antigen-presenting dendritic cells and IL-12. *AIDS Res. Hum. Retrovir.* 22:93–98.

1923. Huang, Y., L. Zhang, and D. D. Ho. 1995. Characterization of *nef* sequences in long-term survivors of human immunodeficiency virus type 1 infection. *J. Virol.* 69:93–100.

1924. Huang, Z. B., M. J. Potash, M. Simm, M. Shahabuddin, W. Chao, H. E. Gendelman, E. Eden, and D. J. Volsky. 1993. Infection of macrophages with lymphotropic human immunodeficiency virus type 1 can be arrested after viral DNA synthesis. *J. Virol.* 67:6893–6896.

1925. Huck, S., and M. P. Lefranc. 1987. Rearrangements to the JP1, JP and JP2 segments in the human T-cell rearranging gamma gene (TRG gamma) locus. *FEBS Lett.* 224:291–296.

1926. Hudson, C. P. 1993. Concurrent partnerships could cause AIDS epidemics. *Int. J. STD AIDS* 4:249–253.

1927. Huet, T., R. Cheynier, A. Meyerhans, G. Roelants, and S. Wain-Hobson. 1990. Genetic organization of a chimpanzee lentivirus related to HIV-1. *Nature* 345:356–359.

1928. Hufert, F. T., J. Schmitz, M. Schrieber, H. Schmitz, P. Racz, and D. D. von Laer. 1993. Human Kupffer cells infected with HIV-1 in vivo. *J. Acquir. Immune Defic. Syndr.* 6:772–777.

1929. Hufert, F. T., J. van Lunzen, G. Janossy, S. Bertram, J. Schmitz, O. Haller, P. Racz, and D. von Laer. 1997. Germinal centre CD4+ T cells are an important site of HIV replication *in vivo*. *AIDS* 11:849–857.

1930. Hug, P., H. Lin, T. Korte, X. Xiao, D. S. Dimitrov, J. Wang, A. Puri, and R. Blumenthal. 2000. Glycosphingolipids promote entry of a broad range of human immunodeficiency virus type 1 isolates into cell lines expressing CD4, CXCR4, and/or CCR5. *J. Virol.* 74:6377–6385.

1931. Hughes, B. P., T. F. Booth, A. S. Belyaev, D. McIlroy, J. Jowett, and P. Roy. 1993. Morphogenic capabilities of human immunodeficiency virus type 1 gag and gag-pol proteins in insect cells. *Virology* 193:242–255.

1932. Hughes, E. S., J. E. Bell, and P. Simmonds. 1997. Investigation of the dynamics of the spread of human immunodeficiency virus to brain and other tissues by evolutionary analysis of sequences from the p17*gag* and *env* genes. *J. Virol.* 71:1272–1280.

1933. Hughes, R. A., S. E. Macatonia, I. F. Rowe, A. C. S. Keat, and S. C. Knight. 1990. The detection of human immunodeficiency virus DNA in dendritic cells from the joints of patients with aseptic arthritis. *Br. J. Rheumatol.* 29:166–170.

1934. Huisman, M. T., J. W. Smit, and A. H. Schinkel. 2000. Significance of P-glycoprotein for the pharmacology and clinical use of HIV protease inhibitors. *AIDS* 14:237–242.

1935. Hulskotte, E. G. J., A. M. Geretti, K. H. J. Siebelink, G. van Amerongen, M. P. Cranage, E. W. Rud, S. G. Norley, P. de Vries, and A. D. M. E. Osterhaus. 1995. Vaccine-induced virus-neutralizing antibodies and cytotoxic T cells do not protect macaques from experimental infection with simian immunodeficiency virus SIVmac32H (J5). *J. Virol.* 69:6289–6296.

1936. Hunt, P. W., S. G. Deeks, D. R. Bangsberg, A. Moss, E. Sinclair, T. Liegler, M. Bates, G. Tsao, H. Lampiris, R. Hoh, and J. N. Martin. 2006. The independent effect of drug resistance on T cell activation in HIV infection. *AIDS* 20:691–699.

1937. Hunt, P. W., J. N. Martin, E. Sinclair, B. Bredt, E. Hagos, H. Lampiris, and S. G. Deeks. 2003. T cell activation is associated with lower CD4+ T cell gains in HIV-infected patients with sustained viral suppression on antiretroviral therapy. *J. Infect. Dis.* 187:1534–1543.

1938. Hunter, D. J., and B. N. Maggwa. 1994. Sexual behavior, sexually transmitted diseases, male circumcision and risk of HIV infection among women in Nairobi, Kenya. *AIDS* 8:93–99.

1939. Hussain, L. A., C. G. Kelly, E.-M. Hecht, R. Fellowes, M. Jourdan, and T. Lehner. 1991. The expression of Fc receptors for immunoglobulin G in human rectal epithelium. *AIDS* 5:1089–1094.

1940. Hussain, L. A., and T. Lehner. 1995. Comparative investigation of Langerhans' cells and potential receptors for HIV in oral, genitourinary and rectal epithelia. *Immunology* 85:475–484.

1941. Huthoff, H., and M. H. Malim. 2005. Cytidine deamination and resistance to retroviral infection: towards a structural understanding of the APOBEC proteins. *Virology* 334:147–153.

1942. Hwang, S. S., T. J. Boyle, H. K. Lyerly, and B. R. Cullen. 1991. Identification of the envelope V3 loop as the primary determinant of cell tropism in HIV-1. *Science* 253:71–74.

1943. Hwang, S. S., T. J. Boyle, H. K. Lyerly, and B. R. Cullen. 1992. Identification of envelope V3 loop as the major determinant of CD4 neutralization sensitivity of HIV-1. *Science* 257:535–537.

1944. Hyjek, E., H. W. Lischner, T. Hyslop, J. Bartkowiak, M. Kubin, G. Trinchieri, and D. Kozbor. 1995. Cytokine patterns during progression to AIDS in children with perinatal HIV infection. *J. Immunol.* 155:4060–4071.

1945. Iafrate, A. J., S. Bronson, and J. Skowronski. 1997. Separable functions of Nef disrupt two aspects of T cell receptor machinery: CD4 expression and CD3 signaling. *EMBO J.* 16:671–684.

1946. Ibarrondo, F. J., P. A. Anton, M. Fuerst, H. L. Ng, J. T. Wong, J. Matud, J. Elliott, R. Shih, M. Hausner, C. Price, L. E. Hultin, P. M. Hultin, B. D. Jamieson, and O. O. Yang. 2005. Parallel human immunodeficiency virus type 1-specific CD8+ T-lymphocyte responses in blood and mucosa during chronic infection. *J. Virol.* 79:4289–4297.

1947. Ichimura, H., S. C. Kliks, S. Visrutaratna, C. Y. Ou, M. L. Kalish, and J. A. Levy. 1994. Biological, serological, and genetic characterization of HIV-1 subtype E isolates from Northern Thailand. *AIDS Res. Hum. Retrovir.* 10:263–269.

1948. Ichimura, H., and J. A. Levy. 1995. Polymerase substrate depletion: a novel strategy for inhibiting the replication of the human immunodeficiency virus. *Virology* 211:554–560.

1949. Igarashi, T., Y. Ami, H. Yamamoto, R. Shibata, T. Kuwata, R. Mukai, K. Shinohara, T. Komatsu, A. Adachi, and M. Hayami. 1997. Protection of monkeys vaccinated with *vpr*- and/or *nef*-defective simian immunodeficiency virus strain mac/human immunodeficiency virus type 1 chimeric viruses: a potential candidate live-attenuated human AIDS vaccine. *J. Gen. Virol.* 78:985–989.

1950. Ikeuchi, K., S. Kim, R. A. Byrn, S. R. Goldring, and J. E. Groopman. 1990. Infection of nonlymphoid cells by human immunodeficiency virus type 1 or type 2. *J. Virol.* 64:4226–4231.

1951. Ikonomidis, G., F. R. Frankel, D. A. Portnoy, and Y. Paterson. 1995. Listeria monocytogenes: *a Novel Live Vaccine Vector, Vaccines 95.* Cold Spring Harbor Laboratory Press, Cold Spring Harbor, N.Y.

1952. Ilaria, G., J. L. Jacobs, B. Polsky, B. Koll, P. Baron, C. MacLow, D. Armstrong, and P. N. Schlegel. 1992. Detection of HIV-1 DNA sequences in pre-ejaculatory fluid. *Lancet* 340:1469.

1953. Iliff, P. J., E. G. Piqoz, N. V. Tavengwa, C. D. Sunguza, E. T. Marinda, K. J. Nathoo, L. H. Moulton, B. J. Ward, J. H. Humphrey, and the ZVITAMBO study group 2005. Early exclusive breastfeeding reduces the risk of postnatal HIV-1 transmission and increases HIV-free survival. *AIDS* 19:699–708.

1954. Ilyinski, P. O., and R. C. Desrosiers. 1996. Efficient transcription and replication of simian immunodeficiency virus in the absence of NF-κB and Sp1 binding elements. *J. Virol.* 70:3118–3126.

1955. Imberti, L., A. Sottini, A. Bettinardi, M. Puoti, and D. Primi. 1991. Selective depletion in HIV infection of T cells that bear specific T cell receptor V-beta sequences. *Science* 254:860–862.

1956. Imlach, S., C. Leen, and P. Simmonds. 2003. Phenotypic analysis of peripheral blood gammadelta T lymphocytes and their targeting by human immunodeficiency virus type 1 in vivo. *Virology* 305:415–427.

1957. Imrie, A., A. Beveridge, W. Genn, J. Vizzard, and D. A. Cooper. 1997. Transmission of human immunodeficiency virus type 1 resistant to nevirapine and zidovudine. *J. Infect. Dis.* 175:1502–1506.

1958. Imrie, A., A. Carr, C. Duncombe, R. Finlayson, J. Vizzard, M. Law, J. Kaldor, R. Penny, and D. A. Cooper. 1996. Primary infection with zidovudine-resistant human immunodeficiency virus type 1 does not adversely affect outcome at 1 year. *J. Infect. Dis.* 174:195–198.

1959. International Study Group on CD4-monitored Treatment Interruptions. 2005. CD4 cell-monitored treatment interruption in patients with a CD4 cell count >500 × 10⁶ cells/l. *AIDS* 19:287–294.

1960. Ioachim, H. L., B. Dorsett, J. Melamed, V. Adsay, and E. A. Santagada. 1992. Cytomegalovirus, angiomatosis, and Kaposi's sarcoma: new observations of a debated relationship. *Mod. Pathol.* 5:169–178.

1961. Ioannidis, J. P. A., J. C. Cappelleri, J. Lau, P. R. Skolnik, B. Melville, T. C. Chalmers, and H. S. Sacks. 1995. Early or deferred zidovudine therapy in HIV-infected patients without an AIDS-defining illness. *Ann. Intern. Med.* 122:856–866.

1962. Iordanskiy, S., Y. Zhao, P. DiMarzio, I. Agostini, L. Dubrovsky, and M. Bukrinsky. 2004. Heat-shock protein 70 exerts opposing effects on Vpr-dependent and Vpr-independent HIV-1 replication in macrophages. *Blood* 104:1867–1872.

1963. Ironson, G., E. Balbin, G. Solomon, J. Fahey, N. Klimas, N. Schneiderman, and M. A. Fletcher. 2001. Relative preservation of natural killer cell cytotoxicity and number in healthy AIDS patients with low CD4 cell counts. *AIDS* 15:2065–2073.

1964. Isaaz, S., K. Baetz, K. Olsen, E. Podack, and G. M. Griffiths. 1995. Serial killing by cytotoxic T lymphocytes: T cell receptor triggers degranulation, re-filling of the lytic granules and secretion of lytic proteins via a non-granule pathway. *Eur. J. Immunol.* 25:1071–1079.

1964a. Ishii, K. J., C. Coban, H. Kato, K. Takahashi, Y. Torii, F. Takeshita, H. Ludwig, G. Sutter, K. Suzuki, H. Hemmi, S. Sato, M. Yamamoto, S. Uematsu, T. Kawai, O. Takeuchi, and S. Akira. 2006. A Toll-like receptor-independent antiviral response induced by double-stranded B-form DNA. *Nat. Immunol.* 7:40–48.

1965. Issel, C. J., D. W. Horohov, D. F. Lea, W. V. Adams, Jr., S. F. Hagius, J. M. McManus, A. C. Allison, and R. C. Montelaro. 1992. Efficacy of inactivated whole-virus and subunit vaccines in preventing infection and disease caused by equine infectious anemia virus. *J. Virol.* 66:3398–3408.

1966. Itescu, S., J. Dalton, H. Z. Zhang, and R. Winchester. 1993. Tissue infiltration in a CD8 lymphocytosis syndrome associated with human immunodeficiency virus-1 infection has the phenotypic appearance of an antigenically driven response. *J. Clin. Investig.* 91:2216–2225.

1967. Itescu, S., U. Mathur-Wagh, M. L. Skovron, L. J. Brancato, M. Marmor, A. Zeleniuch-Jacquotte, and R. Winchester. 1991. HLA-B35 is associated with accelerated progression to AIDS. *J. Acquir. Immune Defic. Syndr.* 5:37–45.

1968. Itescu, S., S. Rose, E. Dwyer, and R. Winchester. 1994. Certain HLA-DR5 and -DR6 major histocompatibility complex class II alleles are associated with a CD8 lymphocytic host response to human immunodeficiency virus type 1 characterized by low lymphocyte viral strain heterogeneity and slow disease progression. *Proc. Natl. Acad. Sci. USA* 91:11472–11476.

1969. Itescu, S., P. F. Simonelli, R. J. Winchester, and H. S. Ginsberg. 1994. Human immunodeficiency virus type 1 strains in the lungs of infected individuals evolve independently from those in peripheral blood and are highly conserved in the C-terminal region of the envelope V3 loop. *Proc. Natl. Acad. Sci. USA* **91**:11378–11382.

1970. Ito, M., T. Ishida, L. M. He, F. Tanabe, Y. Rongge, Y. Miyakawa, and H. Terunuma. 1998. HIV type 1 Tat protein inhibits interleukin 12 production by human peripheral blood mononuclear cells. *AIDS Res. Hum. Retrovir.* **14**:845–849.

1971. Ito, T., R. Amakawa, M. Inaba, T. Hori, M. Ota, K. Nakamura, M. Takebayashi, M. Miyaji, T. Yoshimura, K. Inaba, and S. Fukuhara. 2004. Plasmacytoid dendritic cells regulate Th cell responses through OX40 ligand and type I IFNs. *J. Immunol.* **172**:4253–4259.

1972. Ito, T., H. Kanzler, O. Duramad, W. Cao, and Y. J. Liu. 2006. Specialization, kinetics, and repertoire of type 1 interferon responses by human plasmacytoid predendritic cells. *Blood* **107**:2423–2431.

1973. Iversen, A. C., P. S. Norris, C. F. Ware, and C. A. Benedict. 2005. Human NK cells inhibit cytomegalovirus replication through a noncytolytic mechanism involving lymphotoxin-dependent induction of IFN-beta. *J. Immunol.* **175**:7568–7574.

1974. Iversen, A. K. N., R. W. Shafer, K. Wehrly, M. A. Winters, J. I. Mullins, B. Chesebro, and T. C. Merigan. 1996. Multidrug-resistant human immunodeficiency virus type 1 strains resulting from combination antiretroviral therapy. *J. Virol.* **70**:1086–1090.

1975. Ivey-Hoyle, M., J. S. Culp, M. A. Chaikin, B. D. Hellmig, T. J. Matthews, R. W. Sweet, and M. Rosenberg. 1991. Envelope glycoproteins from biologically diverse isolates of immunodeficiency viruses have widely different affinities for CD4. *Proc. Natl. Acad. Sci. USA* **88**:512–516.

1976. Iwasaki, A., and R. Medzhitov. 2004. Toll-like receptor control of the adaptive immune responses. *Nat. Immunol.* **5**:987–995.

1977. Iwatani, Y., S. K. Song, L. Wang, J. Planas, H. Sakai, A. Ishimoto, and M. W. Cloyd. 1997. Human immunodeficiency virus type 1 Vpu modifies viral cytopathic effect through augmented virus release. *J. Gen. Virol.* **78**:841–846.

1978. Izopet, J., M. Cazabat, C. Pasquier, K. Sandres-Saune, E. Bonnet, B. Marchou, P. Massip, and J. Puel. 2002. Evolution of total and integrated HIV-1 DNA and change in DNA sequences in patients with sustained plasma virus suppression. *Virology* **302**:393–404.

1979. Izzedine, H., F. Damond, I. Brocheriou, J. Ghosn, H. Lassal, and G. Deray. 2006. HIV-2 infection and HIV-associated nephropathy. *AIDS* **20**:949–950.

1980. Jabbar, M. A., and D. P. Nayak. 1990. Intracellular interaction of human immunodeficiency virus type 1 (ARV-2) envelope glycoprotein gp160 with CD4 blocks the movement and maturation of CD4 to the plasma membrane. *J. Virol.* **64**:6297–6304.

1981. Jacobs, R., H. Heiken, and R. E. Schmidt. 2005. Mutual interference of HIV and natural killer cell-mediated immune response. *Mol. Immunol.* **42**:239–249.

1982. Jacobson, D. L., J. A. McCutchan, P. L. Spechko, I. Abramson, R. S. Smith, A. Bartok, G. R. Boss, D. Durand, S. A. Bozzette, S. A. Spector, and D. D. Richman. 1991. The evolution of lymphadenopathy and hypergammaglobulinemia are evidence for early and sustained polyclonal B lymphocyte activation during human immunodeficiency virus infection. *J. Infect. Dis.* **163**:240–246.

1983. Jacobson, E. L., F. Pilaro, and K. A. Smith. 1996. Rational interleukin 2 therapy for HIV positive individuals: daily low doses enhance immune function without toxicity. *Proc. Natl. Acad. Sci. USA* **93**:10405–10410.

1984. Jacobson, J. M., N. Colman, N. A. Ostrow, R. W. Simson, D. Tomesch, L. Marlin, M. Rao, J. L. Mills, J. Clemens, and A. M. Prince. 1993. Passive immunotherapy in the treatment of advanced human immunodeficiency virus infection. *J. Infect. Dis.* **168**:298–305.

1985. Jacobson, J. M., J. S. Greenspan, J. Spritzler, N. Ketter, J. L. Fahey, J. B. Jackson, L. Fox, M. Chernoff, A. W. Wu, L. A. MacPhail, G. J. Vasquez, and D. A. Wohl. 1997. Thalidomide for the treatment of oral aphthous ulcers in patients with human immunodeficiency virus infection. *N. Engl. J. Med.* **336**:1487–1493.

1985a. Jacobson, J. M., R. Pat Bucy, J. Spritzler, M. S. Saag, J. J. Eron, Jr., R. W. Coombs, R. Wang, L. Fox, V. A. Johnson, S. Cu-Uvin, S. E. Cohn, D. Mildvan, D. O'Neill, J. Janik, L. Purdue, D. K. O'Connor, C. D. Vita, and I. Frank. 2006. Evidence that intermittent structured treatment interruption, but not immunization with ALVAC-HIV vCP1452, promotes host control of HIV replication: the results of AIDS Clinical Trials Group 5068. *J. Infect. Dis.* **194**:623–632.

1986. Jacobson, L. P., F. J. Jenkins, G. Springer, A. Munoz, K. V. Shah, J. Phair, Z. Zhang, and H. Armenian. 2000. Interaction of human immunodeficiency virus type 1 and human herpesvirus type 8 infections on the incidence of Kaposi's Sarcoma. *J. Infect. Dis.* **181**:1940–1949.

1987. Jacobson, M. A., R. E. Fusaro, M. Galmarini, and W. Lang. 1991. Decreased serum dehydroepiandrosterone is associated with an increased progression of human immunodeficiency virus infection in men with CD4 cell counts of 200–499. *J. Infect. Dis.* **164**:864–868.

1988. Jacobson, M. A., H. Khayam-Bashi, J. N. Martin, D. Black, and V. Ng. 2002. Effect of long-term highly active antiretroviral therapy in restoring HIV-induced abnormal B-lymphocyte function. *J. Acquir. Immune Defic. Syndr.* **31**:472–477.

1989. Jacobson, M. A., J. Spritzler, A. Landay, E. Chan, D. Katzenstein, B. Schock, L. Fox, J. Roe, S. Kundu, and R. Pollard. 2002. A Phase I, placebo-controlled trial of multi-dose recombinant human interleukin-12 in patients with HIV infection. *AIDS* **16**:1147–1154.

1990. Jacotot, E., L. Ravagnan, M. Loeffler, K. F. Ferri, H. L. A. Vieria, N. Zamzami, P. Costantini, S. Druillennec, J. Hoebeke, J. P. Briand, T. Irinopoulou, E. Daugas, S. A. Susin, D. Cointe, Z. H. Xie, J. C. Reed, B. P. Roques, and G. Kroemer. 2000. The HIV-1 viral protein R induced apoptosis via a direct effect on the mitochondrial permeability transition pore. *J. Exp. Med.* **191**:33–45.

1991. Jacque, J., K. Triques, and M. Stevenson. 2002. Modulation of HIV-1 replication by RNA interference. *Nature* **418**:1–4.

1992. Jacque, J. M., and M. Stevenson. 2006. The inner-nuclear-envelope protein emerin regulates HIV-1 infectivity. *Nature* **441**:641–645.

1993. Jacquez, J. A., J. S. Koopman, C. P. Simon, and I. M. Longini, Jr. 1994. Role of primary infection in epidemics of HIV infection in gay cohorts. *J. Acquir. Immune Defic. Syndr.* **7**:1169–1184.

1994. Jaffe, H. W., D. J. Bregman, and R. M. Selik. 1983. Acquired immune deficiency syndrome in the United States: the first 1,000 cases. *J. Infect. Dis.* **148**:339–345.

1995. Jakubik, J. J., M. Saifuddin, D. M. Takefman, and G. T. Spear. 2000. Immune complexes containing human immunodeficiency virus type 1 primary isolates bind to lymphoid tissue B lymphocytes and are infectious for T lymphocytes. *J. Virol.* 74:552–555.

1996. James, C. O., M.-B. Huang, M. Khan, M. Garcia-Barrio, M. D. Powell, and V. C. Bond. 2004. Extracellular nef protein targets CD4+ T cells for apoptosis by interacting with CXCR4 surface receptors. *J. Virol.* 78:3099–3109.

1997. Jameson, B. A., P. E. Rao, L. I. Kong, B. H. Hahn, G. M. Shaw, L. E. Hood, and S. B. H. Kent. 1988. Location and chemical synthesis of a binding site for HIV-1 on the CD4 protein. *Science* 240:1335–1339.

1998. Jameson, S. C., F. R. Carbone, and M. J. Bevan. 1993. Clone-specific T cell receptor antagonists of major histocompatibility complex class I-restricted cytotoxic T cells. *J. Exp. Med.* 177:1541–1550.

1999. Jamieson, B. D., G. M. Aldrovandi, V. Planelles, J. B. M. Jowett, L. Gao, L. M. Bloch, I. S. Y. Chen, and J. A. Zack. 1994. Requirement of human immunodeficiency virus type 1 *nef* for in vivo replication and pathogenicity. *J. Virol.* 68:3478–3485.

2000. Jamieson, B. D., D. C. Douek, S. Killian, L. E. Hultin, D. D. Scripture-Adams, J. V. Giorgi, D. Marelli, R. A. Koup, and J. A. Zack. 1999. Generation of functional thymocytes in the human adult. *Immunity* 10:569–575.

2001. Janeway, C. A., Jr. 2001. How the immune system works to protect the host from infection: a personal view. *Proc. Natl. Acad. Sci. USA* 98:7461–7468.

2002. Janoff, E. N., S. M. Wahl, K. Thomas, and P. D. Smith. 1995. Modulation of human immunodeficiency virus type 1 infection of human monocytes by IgA. *J. Infect. Dis.* 172:855–858.

2003. Jansen, C. A., I. M. De Cuyper, B. Hooibrink, A. K. van der Bij, D. van Baarle, and F. Miedema. 2006. Prognostic value of HIV-1 Gag-specific CD4+ T-cell responses for progression to AIDS analyzed in a prospective cohort study. *Blood* 107:1427–1433.

2004. Jansen, C. A., D. van Baarle, and F. Miedema. 2006. HIV-specific CD4(+) T cells and viremia: who's in control? *Trends Immunol.* 27:119–124.

2005. Janssen, E. M., E. E. Lemmens, T. Wolfe, U. Christen, M. G. von Herrath, and S. P. Schoenberger. 2003. CD4+ T cells are required for secondary expansion and memory in CD8+ T lymphocytes. *Nature* 421:852–856.

2006. Janssen, R. S., G. A. Satten, S. L. Stramer, B. D. Rawal, T. R. O'Brien, B. J. Weiblen, F. M. Hecht, N. Jack, F. R. Cleghorn, J. O. Kahn, M. A. Chesney, and M. P. Busch. 1998. New testing strategy to detect early HIV-1 infection for use in incidence estimates and for clinical and prevention purposes. *JAMA* 280:42–48.

2007. Janssens, W., L. Heyndrickx, G. Van der Auwera, J. Nkegasong, E. Beirnaert, K. Vereecken, S. Coppens, B. Willems, K. Fransen, M. Peeters, P. Ndumbe, E. Delaporte, and G. van der Groen. 1999. Interpatient genetic variability of HIV-1 group O. *AIDS* 13:41–48.

2008. Jansson, M., E. Backstrom, G. Scarlatti, A. Bjorndal, S. Matsuda, P. Rossi, J. Albert, and H. Wigzell. 2001. Length variation of glycoprotein 120 V2 region in relation to biochemical phenotypes and coreceptor usage of primary HIV type 1 isolates. *AIDS Res. Hum. Retrovir.* 15:1405–1414.

2009. Jansson, M., M. Popovic, A. Karlsson, F. Cocchi, P. Rossi, J. Albert, and H. Wigzell. 1996. Sensitivity to inhibition by beta-

chemokines correlates with biological phenotypes of primary HIV-1 isolates. *Proc. Natl. Acad. Sci. USA* 93:15382–15387.

2009a. Jardetsky, T. S., and R. A. Lamb. 2004. Virology: a class act. *Nature* 427:307–308.

2010. Jason, J., L. A. Sleeper, S. M. Donfield, J. Murphy, I. Warrier, S. Arkin, and B. Evatt. 1995. Evidence for a shift from a type I lymphocyte pattern with HIV disease progression. *J. Acquir. Immune Defic. Syndr. Hum. Retrovirol.* 10:471–476.

2011. Jassoy, C., R. P. Johnson, B. A. Navia, J. Worth, and B. D. Walker. 1992. Detection of a vigorous HIV-1-specific cytotoxic T lymphocyte response in cerebrospinal fluid from infected persons with AIDS dementia complex. *J. Immunol.* 149:3113–3119.

2012. Javaherian, K., A. J. Langlois, G. J. LaRosa, A. T. Profy, D. P. Bolognesi, W. C. Herlihy, S. D. Putney, and T. J. Matthews. 1990. Broadly neutralizing antibodies elicted by the hypervariable neutralizing determinant of HIV-1. *Science* 250:1590–1593.

2013. Javaherian, K., A. J. Langlois, C. McDanal, K. L. Ross, L. I. Eckler, C. L. Jellis, A. T. Profy, J. R. Rusche, D. P. Bolognesi, S. D. Putney, and T. J. Matthews. 1989. Principal neutralizing domain of the human immunodeficiency virus type 1 envelope protein. *Proc. Natl. Acad. Sci. USA* 86:6768–6772.

2013a. Javanbakht, H., P. An, B. Gold, D. C. Petersen, C. O'Huigin, G. W. Nelson, S. J. O'Brien, G. D. Kirk, R. Detels, S. Buchbinder, S. Donfield, S. Shulenin, B. Song, M. J. Perron, M. Stremlau, J. Sodroski, M. Dean, and C. Winkler. 2006. Effects of human TRIM5alpha polymorphisms on antiretroviral function and susceptibility to human immunodeficiency virus infection. *Virology* 354:15–27.

2014. Jaworowski, A., P. Ellery, C. L. Maslin, E. Naim, A. C. Heinlein, C. E. Ryan, G. Paukovics, J. Hocking, S. Sonza, and S. M. Crowe. 2006. Normal CD16 expression and phagocytosis of Mycobacterium avium complex by monocytes from a current cohort of HIV-1-infected patients. *J. Infect. Dis.* 193:693–697.

2015. Jayakumar, P., I. Berger, F. Autschbach, M. Weinstein, B. Funke, E. Verdin, M. A. Goldsmith, and O. T. Keppler. 2005. Tissue-resident macrophages are productively infected ex vivo by primary X4 isolates of human immunodeficiency virus type 1. *J. Virol.* 79:5220–5226.

2016. Jeeninga, R. E., M. Hoogenkamp, M. Armand-Ugon, M. de Baar, K. Verhoef, and B. Berkhout. 2000. Functional differences between the long terminal repeat transcriptional promoters of human immunodeficiency virus type 1 subtypes A through G. *J. Virol.* 74:3740–3751.

2017. Jelinek, D. F., and P. E. Lipsky. 1987. Enhancement of human B cell proliferation and differentiation by tumor necrosis factor-alpha and interleukin 1. *J. Immunol.* 139:2970–2976.

2018. Jelinek, D. F., J. B. Splawski, and P. E. Lipsky. 1986. The roles of interleukin-2 and interferon-gamma in human B cell activation, growth and differentiation. *Eur. J. Immunol.* 16:925–932.

2019. Jelonek, M. T., J. L. Maskrey, K. S. Steimer, B. J. Potts, K. W. Higgins, and M. A. Keller. 1995. Inhibition of the offspring anti-recombinant gp120 antibody response to a human immunodeficiency virus vaccine by maternal immunization in a murine model. *J. Infect. Dis.* 172:539–542.

2020. Jeng, C. R., R. V. English, T. Childers, M. B. Tompkins, and W. A. F. Tompkins. 1996. Evidence for CD8+ antiviral activity in cats infected with feline immunodeficiency virus. *J. Virol.* 70:2474–2480.

2021. Jenkins, M., M. B. Hanley, M. B. Moreno, E. Wieder, and J. M. McCune. 1998. Human immunodeficiency virus-1 infection interrupts thymopoiesis and multilineage hematopoiesis *in vivo*. *Blood* **91**:2672–2678.

2022. Jennes, W., S. Sawadogo, S. Koblavi-Dème, B. Vuylsteke, C. Maurice, T. H. Roels, T. Chorba, J. N. Nkengasong, and L. Kestens. 2002. Positive association between β-chemokine-producing T cells and HIV type 1 viral load in HIV-infected subjects in Abidjan, Côte d'Ivoire. *AIDS Res. Hum. Retrovir.* **18**:171–177.

2023. Jensen, M. A., F. S. Li, A. B. van 't Wout, D. C. Nickle, D. Shriner, H. X. He, S. McLaughlin, R. Shankarappa, J. B. Margolick, and J. I. Mullins. 2003. Improved coreceptor usage prediction and genotypic monitoring of R5-to-X4 transition by motif analysis of human immunodeficiency virus type 1 env V3 loop sequences. *J. Virol.* **77**:13376–13388.

2024. Jetzt, A. E., H. Yu, G. J. Klarmann, Y. Ron, B. D. Preston, and J. P. Dougherty. 2000. High rate of recombination throughout the human immunodeficiency virus type 1 genome. *J. Virol.* **74**:1234–1240.

2025. Jewett, A., and B. Bonavida. 1990. Peripheral blood monocytes derived from HIV+ individuals mediate antibody-dependent cellular cytotoxicity (ADCC). *Clin. Immunol. Immunopathol.* **54**:192–199.

2026. Jewett, A., M. Cavalcanti, J. Giorgi, and B. Bonavida. 1997. Concomitant killing *in vitro* of both gp120-coated CD4+ peripheral T lymphocytes and natural killer cells in the antibody-dependent cellular cytotoxicity (ADCC) system. *J. Immunol.* **158**:5492–5500.

2027. Ji, X., H. Gewurz, and G. T. Spear. 2005. Mannose binding lectin (MBL) and HIV. *Mol. Immunol.* **42**:145–152.

2028. Jiang, J.-D., F.-N. Chu, P. H. Naylor, J. E. Kirkley, J. Mandeli, J. I. Wallace, P. S. Sarin, A. L. Goldstein, J. F. Holland, and J. G. Bekesi. 1992. Specific antibody responses to synthetic peptides of HIV-1 p17 correlate with different stages of HIV-1 infection. *J. Acquir. Immune Defic. Syndr.* **5**:382–390.

2029. Jiang, S., K. Lin, and A. R. Neurath. 1991. Enhancement of human immunodeficiency virus type 1 infection by antisera to peptides from the envelope glycoproteins gp120/gp41. *J. Exp. Med.* **174**:1557–1563.

2030. Jiang, S., and A. R. Neurath. 1992. Potential risks of eliciting antibodies enhancing HIV-1 infection of monocytic cells by vaccination with V3 loops of unmatched HIV-1 isolates. *AIDS* **6**:331–342.

2031. Jin, X., X. Gao, M. Ramanathan, Jr., G. R. Deschenes, G. W. Nelson, S. J. O'Brien, J. J. Goedert, D. D. Ho, T. R. O'Brien, and M. Carrington. 2002. Human immunodeficiency virus type 1 (HIV-1)-specific CD8+-T-cell responses for groups of HIV-1-infected individuals with different HLA- B*35 genotypes. *J. Virol.* **76**:12603–12610.

2032. Jinquan, T., S. Quan, H. H. Jacobi, H. O. Madsen, C. Glue, P. S. Skov, H. J. Malling, and L. K. Poulsen. 2000. CXC chemokine receptor 4 expression and stromal cell-derived factor-1alpha-induced chemotaxis in CD4+ T lymphocytes are regulated by interleukin-4 and interleukin-10. *Immunology* **99**:402–410.

2033. Joag, S. V., Z. Li, L. Foresman, E. B. Stephens, L.-J. Zhao, I. Adany, D. M. Pinson, H. M. McClure, and O. Narayan. 1996. Chimeric simian/human immunodeficiency virus that causes progressive loss of CD4+ T cells and AIDS in pig-tailed macaques. *J. Virol.* **70**:3189–3197.

2034. Joag, S. V., E. B. Stephens, D. Galbreath, G. W. Zhu, Z. Li, L. Foresman, L. J. Zhao, D. M. Pinson, and O. Narayan. 1995.

2035. John, G. C., R. W. Nduati, D. Mbori-Ngacha, J. Overbaugh, M. Welch, B. A. Richardson, J. Ndinya-Achola, J. Bwayo, J. Krieger, F. Onyango, and J. K. Kreiss. 1997. Genital shedding of human immunodeficiency virus type 1 DNA during pregnancy: association with immunosuppression, abnormal cervical or vaginal discharge, and severe vitamin A deficiency. *J. Infect. Dis.* **175**:57–62.

2036. John, G. C., R. W. Nduati, D. A. Mbori-Ngacha, B. A. Richardson, D. Paneleeff, A. Mwatha, J. Overbaugh, J. Bwayo, J. O. Ndinya-Achola, and J. K. Kreiss. 2001. Correlates of mother-to-child human immunodeficiency virus type 1 (HIV-1) transmission: association with maternal plasma HIV-1 RNA load, genital HIV-1 DNA shedding, and breast infection. *J. Infect. Dis.* **183**:206–212.

2037. John, G. C., C. Rousseau, T. Dong, S. Rowland-Jones, R. Nduati, D. Mbori-Ngacha, T. Rostron, J. K. Kreiss, B. A. Richardson, and J. Overbaugh. 2000. Maternal SDF1 3'A polymorphism is associated with increased perinatal human immunodeficiency virus type 1 transmission. *J. Virol.* **74**:5736–5739.

2038. John, R., S. Arango-Jaramillo, S. Self, and D. H. Schwartz. 2004. Modeling partially effective HIV vaccines in vitro. *J. Infect. Dis.* **189**:616–623.

2039. John-Stewart, G. C., R. W. Nduati, C. M. Rousseau, D. A. Mbori-Ngacha, B. A. Richardson, S. Rainwater, D. D. Panteleeff, and J. Overbaugh. 2005. Subtype C is associated with increased vaginal shedding of HIV-1. *J. Infect. Dis.* **192**:492–496.

2040. Johnson, N., and J. M. Parkin. 1998. Anti-retroviral therapy reverses HIV-associated abnormalities in lymphocyte apoptosis. *Clin. Exp. Immunol.* **113**:229–234.

2041. Johnson, R. P., R. L. Glickman, J. Q. Yang, A. Kaur, J. T. Dion, M. J. Mulligan, and R. C. Desrosiers. 1997. Induction of vigorous cytotoxic T-lymphocyte responses by live attenuated simian immunodeficiency virus. *J. Virol.* **71**:7711–7718.

2042. Johnston, E. R., L. S. Zijenah, S. Mutetwa, R. Kantor, C. Kittinunvorakoon, and D. A. Katzenstein. 2003. High frequency of syncytium-inducing and CXCR4-tropic viruses among human immunodeficiency virus type 1 subtype C-infected patients receiving antiretroviral treatment. *J. Virol.* **77**:7682–7688.

2043. Joling, P., L. J. Bakker, J. A. G. Van Strijp, T. Meerloo, L. deGraaf, M. E. M. Dekker, J. Goudsmit, J. Verhoef, and H. J. Schuurman. 1993. Binding of human immunodeficiency virus type-1 to follicular dendritic cells *in vitro* is complement dependent. *J. Immunol.* **150**:1065–1073.

2044. Jolly, C., K. Kashefi, M. Hollinshead, and Q. J. Sattentau. 2004. HIV-1 cell to cell transfer across an Env-induced, actin-dependent synapse. *J. Exp. Med.* **199**:283–293.

2045. Joly, P., J. M. Guillon, C. Mayaud, F. Plata, I. Theodorou, M. Denis, P. Debre, and B. Autran. 1989. Cell mediated suppression of HIV-specific cytotoxic T lymphocytes. *J. Immunol.* **143**:2193–2201.

2046. Jonassen, T. O., K. Stene-Johansen, E. S. Berg, O. Hungnes, C. F. Lindboe, S. S. Froland, and B. Grinde. 1997. Sequence analysis of HIV-1 group O from Norwegian patients infected in the 1960s. *Virology* **231**:43–47.

2047. Jones, K., P. G. Bray, S. H. Khoo, R. A. Davey, E. R. Meaden, S. A. Ward, and D. J. Back. 2001. P-glycoprotein and transporter MRP1 reduce HIV protease inhibitor uptake in

CD4 cells: potential for accelerated viral drug resistance? *AIDS* 15:1353–1358.

2048. Jones, K. A., J. T. Kadonaga, P. A. Luciw, and R. Tijian. 1986. Activation of the AIDS retrovirus promoter by the cellular transcription factor, Sp1. *Science* 232:755–759.

2049. Jones, N. A., X. Wei, D. R. Flower, M. Wong, F. Michor, M. S. Saag, B. H. Hahn, M. A. Nowak, G. M. Shaw, and P. Borrow. 2004. Determinants of human immunodeficiency virus type 1 escape from the primary CD8+ cytotoxic T lymphocyte response. *J. Exp. Med.* 200:1243–1256.

2050. Jordan, A., P. Defechereux, and E. Verdin. 2001. The site of HIV-1 integration in the human genome determines basal transcriptional activity and response to Tat transactivation. *EMBO J.* 20:1726–1738.

2051. Jordan, C. A., B. A. Watkins, C. Kufta, and M. Bubois-Dalcq. 1991. Infection of brain microglial cells by human immunodeficiency virus type 1 is CD4 dependent. *J. Virol.* 65:736–742.

2052. Joseph, J., F. Etcheverry, J. Alcami, and G. J. Maria. 2005. A safe, effective and affordable HIV vaccine–an urgent global need. *AIDS Rev.* 7:131–138.

2053. Juffermans, N. P., W. A. Paxton, P. E. Dekkers, A. Verbon, E. de Jonge, P. Speelman, S. J. van Deventer, and T. van Der Poll. 2000. Up-regulation of HIV coreceptors CXCR4 and CCR5 on CD4(+) T cells during human endotoxemia and after stimulation with (myco)bacterial antigens: the role of cytokines. *Blood* 96:2649–2654.

2054. Juffermans, N. P., P. Speelman, A. Verbon, J. Veenstra, C. Jie, J. H. van Deventer, and T. van der Poll. 2001. Patients with active tuberculosis have increased expression of HIV coreceptors CXCR4 and CCR5 on CD4+ T cells. *Clin. Infect. Dis.* 32:650–652.

2055. Jung, A., R. Maier, J. Vartanian, G. Bocharov, V. Jung, U. Fischer, E. Meese, S. Wain-Hobson, and A. Meyerhans. 2002. Multiply infected spleen cells in HIV patients. *Nature* 418:144.

2056. Jung, S., O. Knauer, N. Donhauser, M. Eichenmuller, M. Helm, B. Fleckenstein, and H. Reil. 2005. Inhibition of HIV strains by GB virus C in cell culture can be mediated by CD4 and CD8 T-lymphocyte derived soluble factors. *AIDS* 19:1267–1272.

2057. Jurriaans, S., J. T. Dekker, and A. de Ronde. 1992. HIV-1 viral DNA load in peripheral blood mononuclear cells from seroconverters and long-term infected individuals. *AIDS* 6:635–641.

2058. Jurriaans, S., B. Van Gemen, G. J. Weverling, D. Van Strijp, P. Nara, R. Coutinho, M. Koot, H. Schuitemaker, and J. Goudsmit. 1994. The natural history of HIV-1 infection: virus load and virus phenotype independent determinants of clinical course? *Virology* 204:223–233.

2059. Just, J. J. 1995. Genetic predisposition to HIV-1 infection and acquired immune deficiency virus syndrome: a review of the literature examining associations with HLA. *Hum. Immunol.* 44:156–169.

2060. Just, J. J., E. Abrams, L. G. Louie, R. Urbano, D. Wara, S. W. Nicholas, Z. Stein, and M. C. King. 1995. Influence of host genotype on progression to acquired immunodeficiency syndrome among children infected with human immunodeficiency virus type 1. *J Pediatr* 127:544–549.

2061. Kabelitz, D., and D. Wesch. 2003. Features and functions of gamma delta T lymphocytes: focus on chemokines and their receptors. *Crit. Rev. Immunol.* 23:339–370.

2062. Kadowaki, N., S. Ho, S. Antonenko, R. W. Malefyt, R. A. Kastelein, F. Bazan, and Y. J. Liu. 2001. Subsets of human dendritic cell precursors express different toll-like receptors and respond to different microbial antigens. *J. Exp. Med.* 194:863–869.

2063. Kagi, S., P. Seiler, J. Pavlovic, B. Ledermann, K. Burki, R. M. Zinkernagel, and H. Hengartner. 1995. The role of perforin- and Fas-dependent cytotoxiciy in protection against cytopathic and noncytopathic viruses. *Eur. J. Immunol.* 25:3256–3262.

2064. Kahn, J. O., S. W. Lagakos, D. D. Richman, A. Cross, C. Pettinelli, S. Liou, M. Brown, P. A. Volberding, C. S. Crumpacker, G. Beall, H. S. Sacks, T. C. Merigan, M. Beltangady, L. Smaldone, and R. Dolin. 1992. A controlled trial comparing continued zidovudine with didanosine in human immunodeficiency virus infection. *N. Engl. J. Med.* 327:583–587.

2065. Kahn, J. O., F. Sinangil, J. Baenziger, N. Murcar, D. Wynne, R. L. Coleman, K. S. Steimer, C. L. Dekker, and D. Chernoff. 1994. Clinical and immunologic responses to human immunodeficiency virus (HIV) type 1$_{SF2}$ gp120 subunit vaccine combined with MF59 adjuvant with or without muramyl tripeptide dipalmitoyl phosphatidylethanolamine in non-HIV-infected human volunteers. *J. Infect. Dis.* 170:1288–1291.

2066. Kahn, J. O., K. S. Steimer, J. Baenziger, A. M. Duliege, M. Feinberg, T. Elbeik, M. Chesney, N. Murcar, D. Chernoff, and F. Sinangil. 1995. Clinical, immunologic, and virologic observations related to human immunodeficiency virus (HIV) type 1 infection in a volunteer in an HIV-1 vaccine clinical trial. *J. Infect. Dis.* 171:1343–1347.

2067. Kahn, J. O., and B. D. Walker. 1998. Acute human immunodeficiency virus type 1 infection. *N. Engl. J. Med.* 339:33–39.

2068. Kaiser, P. K., J. T. Offermann, and S. A. Lipton. 1990. Neuronal injury due to HIV-1 envelope protein is blocked by anti-gp120 antibodies but not by anti-CD4 antibodies. *Neurology* 40:1757–1761.

2069. Kaiser, S. M., and M. Emerman. 2004. Controlling lentiviruses: single amino acid changes can determine specificity. *Proc. Natl. Acad. Sci. USA* 101:3725–3726.

2069a. Kaizu, M., A. M. Weiler, K. L. Weisgrau, K. A. Vielhuber, G. May, S. M. Piaskowski, J. Furlott, N. J. Maness, T. C. Friedrich, J. T. Loffredo, A. Usborne, and E. G. Rakasz. 2006. Repeated intravaginal inoculation with cell-associated simian immunodeficiency virus results in persistent infection of nonhuman primates. *J. Infect. Dis.* 194:912–916.

2070. Kalams, S. A., S. P. Buchbinder, E. S. Rosenberg, J. M. Billingsley, D. S. Colbert, N. G. Jones, A. K. Shea, A. K. Trocha, and B. D. Walker. 1999. Association between virus-specific cytotoxic T-lymphocyte and helper responses in human immunodeficiency virus type 1 infection. *J. Virol.* 73:6715–6720.

2071. Kalayjian, R. C., J. Spritzler, M. Pu, A. Landay, R. B. Pollard, V. Stocker, L. A. Harthi, B. H. Gross, I. R. Francis, S. A. Fiscus, P. Tebas, R. J. Bosch, V. Valcour, and M. M. Lederman. 2005. Distinct mechanisms of T cell reconstitution can be identified by estimating thymic volume in adult HIV-1 disease. *J. Infect. Dis.* 192:1577–1587.

2072. Kaleebu, P., N. French, C. Mahe, D. Yirrell, C. Watera, F. Lyagoba, J. Nakiyingi, A. Rutebemberwa, D. Morgan, J. Weber, C. Gilks, and J. Whitworth. 2002. Effect of human immunodeficiency virus (HIV) type 1 envelope subtypes A and D on disease progression in a large cohort of HIV-1-positive persons in Uganda. *J. Infect. Dis.* 185:1244–1250.

2073. Kalish, L. A., J. Pitt, J. Lew, S. Landesman, C. Diaz, R. Hershow, F. B. Hollinger, M. Pagano, B. Smeriglio, and J. Moye. 1997. Defining the time of fetal or perinatal acquisition of human immunodeficiency virus type 1 infection on the basis of age at first positive culture. *J. Infect. Dis.* **175:**712–715.

2074. Kalish, M. L., K. E. Robbins, D. Pieniazek, A. Schaefer, N. Nzilambi, T. C. Quinn, M. E. St Louis, A. S. Youngpairoj, J. Phillips, H. W. Jaffe, and T. M. Folks. 2004. Recombinant viruses and early global HIV-1 epidemic. *Emerg. Infect. Dis.* **10:**1227–1234.

2075. Kalter, D. C., H. E. Gendelman, and M. S. Meltzer. 1991. Inhibition of human immunodeficiency virus infection in monocytes by monoclonal antibodies against leukocyte adhesion molecules. *Immunol. Lett.* **30:**219–228.

2076. Kamata, M., Y. Nitahara-Kasahar, Y. Miyamoto, Y. Yoneda, and Y. Aida. 2005. Importin-α promotes passage through the nuclear pore complex of human immunodeficiency virus type 1 Vpr. *J. Virol.* **79:**3557–3564.

2076a. Kamath, A. T., C. E. Sheasby, and D. F. Tough. 2005. Dendritic cells and NK cells stimulate bystander T cell activation in response to TLR agonists through secretion of IFN-alpha beta and IFN-gamma. *J. Immunol.* **174:**767–776.

2077. Kamel-Reid, S., and J. E. Dick. 1988. Engraftment of immune-deficient mice with human hematopoietic stem cells. *Science* **242:**1706–1709.

2078. Kameoka, M., T. Kimura, Y.-H. Zheng, S. Suzuki, K. Fujinaga, R. B. Luftig, and K. Ikuta. 1997. Protease-defective, gp120-containing human immunodeficiency virus type 1 particles induce apoptosis more efficiently than does wild-type virus or recombinant gp120 protein in healthy donor-derived peripheral blood T cells. *J. Clin. Microbiol.* **35:**41–47.

2079. Kamin, D. S., and S. K. Grinspoon. 2005. Cardiovascular disease in HIV-positive patients. *AIDS* **19:**641–652.

2080. Kamine, J., B. Elangovan, T. Subramanian, D. Coleman, and G. Chinnadurai. 1996. Identification of a cellular protein that specifically interacts with the essential cysteine region of the HIV-1 Tat transactivator. *Virology* **216:**357–366.

2081. Kaminsky, L. S., T. McHugh, D. Stites, P. Volberding, G. Henle, W. Henle, and J. A. Levy. 1985. High prevalence of antibodies to AIDS-associated retroviruses (ARV) in acquired immune deficiency syndrome and related conditions and not in other disease states. *Proc. Natl. Acad. Sci. USA* **82:**5535–5539.

2082. Kamp, W., M. B. Berk, C. J. Visser, and H. S. Nottet. 2000. Mechanisms of HIV-1 to escape from the host immune surveillance. *Eur. J. Clin. Investig.* **30:**740–746.

2083. Kampinga, G. A., A. Simonon, P. Van de Perre, E. Karita, P. Msellati, and J. Goudsmit. 1997. Primary infections with HIV-1 of women and their offspring in Rwanda: findings of heterogeneity at seroconversion, coinfection, and recombinants of HIV-1 subtypes A and C. *Virology* **227:**63–76.

2084. Kamya, M. R., A. F. Gasasira, A. Yeka, N. Bakyaita, S. L. Nsobya, D. Francis, P. J. Rosenthal, G. Dorsey, and D. Havlir. 2006. Effect of HIV-1 infection on antimalarial treatment outcomes in Uganda: a population-based study. *J. Infect. Dis.* **193:**9–15.

2085. Kanai, T., E. K. Thomas, Y. Yasutomi, and N. L. Letvin. 1996. IL-15 stimulates the expansion of AIDS virus-specific CTL. *J. Immunol.* **157:**3681–3687.

2086. Kanbe, K., N. Shimizu, Y. Soda, K. Takagishi, and H. Hoshino. 1999. A CXC chemokine receptor, CXCR5/BLR1, is a novel and specific coreceptor for human immunodeficiency virus type 2. *Virology* **265:**264–273.

2087. Kang, C.-Y., K. Hariharan, P. L. Nara, J. Sodroski, and J. P. Moore. 1994. Immunization with a soluble CD4-gp120 complex preferentially induces neutralizing anti-human immunodeficiency virus type 1 antibodies directed to conformation-dependent epitopes of gp120. *J. Virol.* **68:**5854–5862.

2088. Kang, C.-Y., K. Hariharan, M. R. Posner, and P. Nara. 1993. Identification of a new neutralizing epitope conformationally affected by the attachment of CD4 to gp120. *J. Immunol.* **151:**449–457.

2089. Kang, C.-Y., P. Nara, S. Chamat, V. Caralli, T. Ryskamp, N. Haigwood, R. Newman, and H. Kohler. 1991. Evidence for non-V3-specific neutralizing antibodies that interfere with gp120/CD4 binding in human immunodeficiency virus-1-infected humans. *Proc. Natl. Acad. Sci. USA* **88:**6171–6175.

2090. Kanitakis, J., C. Marchand, H. Su, J. Thivolet, G. Zambruno, D. Schmitt, and L. Gazzolo. 1989. Immunohistochemical study of normal skin of HIV-1-infected patients shows no evidence of infection of epidermal Langerhans cells by HIV. *AIDS Res. Hum. Retrovir.* **5:**293–302.

2091. Kanki, P., S. M'Boup, and R. Marlink. 1992. Prevalence and risk determinants of human immunodeficiency virus type 2 (HIV-2) and human immunodeficiency virus type 1 (HIV-1) in West African female prostitutes. *Am. J. Epidemiol.* **136:**895–907.

2092. Kanki, P. J., D. J. Hamel, J. L. Sankale, C. Hsieh, I. Thior, F. Barin, S. A. Woodcock, A. Gueye-Ndiaye, E. Zhang, M. Montano, T. Siby, R. Marlink, I. NDoye, M. E. Essex, and S. MBoup. 1999. Human immunodeficiency virus type 1 subtypes differ in disease progression. *J. Infect. Dis.* **179:**68–73.

2093. Kanmogne, G. D., R. C. Kennedy, and P. Grammas. 2001. Analysis of human lung endothelial cells for susceptibility to HIV type 1 infection, coreceptor expression, and cytotoxicity of gp120 protein. *AIDS Res. Hum. Retrovir.* **17:**45–53.

2094. Kannagi, M., L. V. Chalifoux, C. I. Lord, and N. L. Letvin. 1988. Suppression of simian immunodeficiency virus replication *in vitro* by CD8+ lymphocytes. *J. Immunol.* **140:** 2237–2242.

2095. Kannagi, M., T. Masuda, T. Hattori, T. Kanoh, K. Nasu, N. Yamamoto, and S. Harada. 1990. Interference with human immunodeficiency virus (HIV) replication by CD8+ T cells in peripheral blood leukocytes of asymptomatic HIV carriers in vitro. *J. Virol.* **64:**3399–3406.

2096. Kannangara, S., J. A. DeSimone, and R. J. Pomerantz. 2005. Attenuation of HIV-1 infection by other microbial agents. *J. Infect. Dis.* **192:**1003–1009.

2097. Kao, L. R., and C. F. Wilkinson. 1987. Inhibition of cytochrome P-450c-mediated benzo[a]pyrene hydroxylase and ethoxyresorufin O-deethylase by dihydrosafrole. *Xenobiotica* **17:**793–805.

2098. Kaplan, D., and S. Sieg. 1998. Role of the Fas/Fas ligand apoptotic pathway in human immunodeficiency virus type 1 disease. *J. Virol.* **72:**6279–6282.

2099. Kaplan, L. D., J. Y. Lee, R. F. Ambinder, J. A. Sparano, E. Cesarman, A. Chadburn, A. M. Levine, and D. T. Scadden. 2005. Rituximab does not improve clinical outcome in a randomized phase 3 trial of CHOP with or without rituximab in patients with HIV-associated non-Hodgkin lymphoma: AIDS-Malignancies Consortium Trial 010. *Blood* **106:** 1538–1543.

2100. **Kaposi, M.** 1872. Idiopathigches multiples pigment sarcom der Haut. *Arch. Dermatol. Syphilis* 4:265–273.

2101. **Karlas, J. A., K. H. Siebelink, M. A. Peer, W. Huisman, A. M. Cuisinier, G. F. Rimmelzwaan, and A. D. Osterhaus.** 1999. Vaccination with experimental feline immunodeficiency virus vaccines, based on autologous infected cells, elicits enhancement of homologous challenge infection. *J. Gen. Virol.* 80(Pt. 3):761–765.

2102. **Karlsson, A., K. Parsmyr, E. Sandstrom, E. M. Fenyo, and J. Albert.** 1994. MT-2 cell tropism as prognostic marker for disease progression in human immunodeficiency virus type 1 infection. *J. Clin. Microbiol.* 32:364–370.

2103. **Karlsson, A. C., S. G. Deeks, J. D. Barbour, B. D. Heiken, S. R. Younger, R. Hoh, M. Lane, M. Sallberg, B. D. Ortiz, J. F. Demarest, T. Ligler, R. M. Grant, J. N. Martin, and D. F. Nixon.** 2003. Dual pressure from antiretroviral therapy and cell-mediated immune response on the human immunodeficiency virus type 1 protease gene. *J. Virol.* 77:6743–6752.

2104. **Karlsson, A. C., S. Lindback, H. Gaines, and A. Sonnerborg.** 1998. Characterization of the viral population during primary HIV-1 infection. *AIDS* 12:839–847.

2105. **Karlsson, G. B., F. Gao, J. Robinson, B. Hahn, and J. Sodroski.** 1996. Increased envelope spike density and stability are not required for the neutralization resistance of primary human immunodeficiency viruses. *J. Virol.* 70:6136–6142.

2106. **Karlsson, G. B., M. Halloran, D. Schenten, J. Lee, P. Racz, K. Tenner-Racz, J. Manola, R. Gelman, B. Etemad-Moghadam, E. Desjardins, R. Wyatt, N. P. Gerard, L. Marcon, D. Margolin, J. Fanton, M. K. Axthelm, N. L. Letvin, and J. Sodroski.** 1998. The envelope glycoprotein ectodomains determine the efficiency of CD4+ T lymphocyte depletion in simian-human immunodeficiency virus-infected macaques. *J. Exp. Med.* 188:1159–1171.

2107. **Karpas, A., I. K. Hewlett, F. Hill, J. Gray, N. Byron, D. Gilgen, V. Bally, J. K. Oates, B. Gazzard, and J. E. Epstein.** 1990. Polymerase chain reaction evidence of human immunodeficiency virus 1 neutralization by passive immunization in patients with AIDS and AIDS-related complex. *Proc. Natl. Acad. Sci. USA* 87:7613–7617.

2108. **Karpatkin, S., M. A. Nardi, and Y. H. Kouri.** 1992. Internal-image anti-idiotype HIV-1 gp120 antibody in human immunodeficiency virus 1 (HIV-1)-seropositive individuals with thrombocytopenia. *Proc. Natl. Acad. Sci. USA* 89:1487–1491.

2109. **Karray, S., and M. Zouali.** 1997. Identification of the B cell superantigen-binding site of HIV-1 gp120. *Proc. Natl. Acad. Sci. USA* 94:1356–1360.

2110. **Kaser, A., S. Kaser, N. C. Kaneider, B. Enrich, C. J. Wiedermann, and H. Tilg.** 2004. Interleukin-18 attracts plasmacytoid dendritic cells (DC2s) and promotes Th1 induction by DC2s through IL-18 receptor expression. *Blood* 103:648–655.

2111. **Kaslow, R. A., W. C. Blackwelder, D. G. Ostrow, D. Yerg, J. Palenicek, A. H. Coulson, and R. O. Valdiserri.** 1989. No evidence for a role of alcohol or other psychoactive drugs in accelerating immunodeficiency in HIV-1-positive individuals. *JAMA* 261:3424–3429.

2112. **Kaslow, R. A., M. Carrington, R. Apple, L. Park, A. Munoz, A. J. Saah, J. J. Goedert, C. Winkler, S. J. O'Brien, C. Rinaldo, R. Detels, W. Blattner, J. Phair, H. Erlich, and D. L. Mann.** 1996. Influence of combinations of human major histocompatibility complex genes on the course of HIV-1 infection. *Nat. Med.* 2:405–411.

2113. **Kaslow, R. A., R. Duquesnoy, M. VanRaden, L. Kingsley, M. Marrari, H. Friedman, S. Su, A. J. Saah, R. Detels, J. Phair, and C. Rinaldo.** 1990. A1, Cw7, B8, DR3 HLA antigen combination associated with rapid decline of T-helper lymphocytes in HIV-1 infection. *Lancet* 335:927–930.

2114. **Kaslow, R. A., C. Rivers, J. Tang, T. J. Bender, P. A. Goepfert, R. El Habib, K. Weinhold, and M. J. Mulligan.** 2001. Polymorphisms in HLA class I genes associated with both favorable prognosis of human immunodeficiency virus (HIV) type 1 infection and positive cytotoxic T-lymphocyte responses to ALVAC-HIV recombinant canarypox vaccines. *J. Virol.* 75:8681–8689.

2115. **Kaspar, A. A., S. Okada, J. Kumar, F. R. Poulain, K. A. Drouvalakis, A. Kelekar, D. A. Hanson, R. M. Kluck, Y. Hitoshi, D. E. Johnson, C. J. Froelich, C. B. Thompson, D. D. Newmeyer, A. Anel, C. Clayberger, and A. M. Krensky.** 2001. A distinct pathway of cell-mediated apoptosis initiated by granulysin. *J. Immunol.* 167:350–356.

2116. **Kassutto, S., M. N. Johnston, and E. S. Rosenberg.** 2005. Incomplete HIV type 1 antibody evolution and seroreversion in acutely infected individuals treated with early antiretroviral therapy. *Clin. Infect. Dis.* 40:868–873.

2117. **Kassutto, S., and E. S. Rosenberg.** 2004. Primary HIV-1 type 1 infection. *Clin. Infect. Dis.* 38:1447–1453.

2118. **Katlama, C., S. Dominguez, K. Gourlain, C. Duvivier, C. Delaugerre, M. Legrand, R. Tubiana, J. Reynes, J.-M. Molina, G. Peytavin, V. Calvez, and D. Costagliola.** 2004. Benefit of treatment interruption in HIV-infected patients with multiple therapeutic failures: a randomized controlled trial (ANRS 097). *AIDS* 18:217–226.

2119. **Katz, M. H., N. A. Hessol, S. P. Buchbinder, A. Hirozawa, P. O'Malley, and S. D. Holmberg.** 1994. Temporal trends of opportunistic infections and malignancies in homosexual men with AIDS. *J. Infect. Dis.* 170:198–202.

2120. **Katzenstein, T. L., C. Pedersen, C. Nielsen, J. D. Lundgren, P. H. Jakobsen, and J. Gerstoft.** 1996. Longitudinal serum HIV RNA quantification: correlation to viral phenotype at seroconversion and clinical outcome. *AIDS* 10:167–173.

2121. **Katzman, M., and M. M. Lederman.** 1986. Defective postbinding lysis underlies the impaired natural killer activity in Factor VIII-treated, human T lymphotropic virus type III seropositive hemophiliacs. *J. Clin. Investig.* 77:1057–1062.

2122. **Kaufmann, D. E., M. Lichterfeld, M. Altfeld, M. M. Addo, M. N. Johnston, P. K. Lee, B. S. Wagner, E. T. Kalife, D. Strick, E. S. Rosenberg, and B. D. Walker.** 2004. Limited durability of viral control following treated acute HIV infection. *PLoS Med.* 2:137–148.

2123. **Kaufmann, G. R., P. Cunningham, A. D. Kelleher, J. Zaunders, A. Carr, J. Vizzard, M. Law, D. A. Cooper, et al.** 1998. Patterns of viral dynamics during primary human immunodeficiency virus type 1 infection. *J. Infect. Dis.* 178:1812–1815.

2124. **Kaul, M., and S. A. Lipton.** 1999. Chemokines and activated macrophages in HIV gp120-induced neuronal apoptosis. *Proc. Natl. Acad. Sci. USA* 96:8212–8216.

2125. **Kaul, R., T. Dong, F. A. Plummer, J. Kimani, T. Rostron, P. Kiama, E. Njagi, E. Irungu, B. Farah, J. Oyugi, R. Chakraborty, K. S. MacDonald, J. J. Bwayo, A. McMichael, and S. L. Rowland-Jones.** 2001. CD8(+) lymphocytes respond to different HIV epitopes in seronegative and infected subjects. *J. Clin. Investig.* 107:1303–1310.

2126. Kaul, R., F. A. Plummer, J. Kimani, T. Dong, P. Kiama, T. Rostron, E. Njagi, K. S. MacDonald, J. J. Bwayo, A. J. McMichael, and S. L. Rowland-Jones. 2000. HIV-1-specific mucosal CD8+ lymphocyte responses in the cervix of HIV-1-resistant prostitutes in Nairobi. *J. Immunol.* **164**:1602–1611.

2127. Kaul, R., S. L. Rowland-Jones, J. Kimani, T. Dong, H. B. Yang, P. Kiama, T. Rostron, E. Njagi, J. J. Bwayo, K. S. MacDonald, A. J. McMichael, and F. A. Plummer. 2001. Late seroconversion in HIV-resistant Nairobi prostitutes despite pre-existing HIV-specific CD8+ responses. *J. Clin. Investig.* **107**:341–349.

2128. Kaul, R., S. L. Rowland-Jones, J. Kimani, K. Fowke, T. Dong, P. Kiama, J. Rutherford, E. Njagi, F. Mwangi, T. Rostron, J. Onyango, J. Oyugi, K. S. MacDonald, J. J. Bwayo, and F. A. Plummer. 2001. New insights into HIV-1 specific cytotoxic T-lymphocyte responses in exposed, persistently seronegative Kenyan sex workers. *Immunol. Lett.* **79**:3–13.

2129. Kaul, R., D. Trabattoni, J. J. Bwayo, D. Arienti, A. Zagliani, F. Mwangi, C. Kariuki, E. N. Ngugi, K. S. MacDonald, T. B. Ball, C. Mario, and F. A. Plummer. 1999. HIV-1-specific mucosal IgA in a cohort of HIV-1-resistant Kenyan sex workers. *AIDS* **13**:23–29.

2130. Kaur, A., R. M. Grant, R. E. Means, H. McClure, M. Feinberg, and R. P. Johnson. 1998. Diverse host responses and outcomes following simian immunodeficiency virus SIVmac239 infection in sooty mangabeys and rhesus macaques. *J. Virol.* **72**:9597.

2131. Kawai, T., and S. Akira. 2006. Innate immune recognition of viral infection. *Nat. Immunol.* **7**:131–137.

2132. Kawamura, K., N. Kadowaki, T. Kitawaki, and T. Uchiyama. 2006. Virus-stimulated plasmacytoid dendritic cells induce CD4+ cytotoxic regulatory T cells. *Blood* **107**:1031–1038.

2133. Kawamura, T., M. Qualbani, E. K. Thomas, J. M. Orenstein, and A. Blauvelt. 2001. Low levels of productive HIV infection in Langerhans cell-like dendritic cells differentiated in the presence of TGF-beta 1 and increased viral replication with CD40 ligand-induced maturation. *Eur. J. Immunol.* **31**:360–368.

2134. Kawashima, H., S. Bandyopadhyay, R. Rutstein, and S. A. Plotkin. 1991. Excretion of human immunodeficiency type 1 in the throat but not in urine by infected children. *J. Pediatr.* **118**:80–82.

2135. Kazi, S., P. R. Cohen, F. Williams, R. Schempp, and J. D. Reveille. 1996. The diffuse infiltrative lymphocytosis syndrome: clinical and immunogenetic features in 35 patients. *AIDS* **10**:385–391.

2136. Keay, S., C. O. Tacket, J. R. Murphy, and B. S. Handwerger. 1992. Anti-CD4 anti-idiotype antibodies in volunteers immunized with rgp160 of HIV-1 or infected with HIV-1. *AIDS Res. Hum. Retrovir.* **8**:1091–1098.

2137. Kebba, A., P. Kaleebu, J. Serwanga, S. Rowland, D. Yirrell, R. Downing, J. Gilmour, N. Imami, F. Gotch, and J. Whitworth. 2004. HIV type 1 antigen-responsive CD4+ T-lymphocytes in exposed yet HIV type 1 seronegative Ugandans. *AIDS Res. Hum. Retrovir.* **20**:67–75.

2138. Kebba, A., P. Kallebu, S. Rowland, R. Ingram, J. Whitworth, N. Imami, and F. Gotch. 2004. Distinct patterns of peripheral HIV-1-specific interferon-γ responses in exposed HIV-1-seronegative individuals. *J. Infect. Dis.* **189**:1705–1713.

2139. Keckesova, Z., L. M. J. Ylinen, and G. J. Towers. 2004. The human and African green monkey TRIM5a genes encode Ref1 and LV1 retroviral restriction factor activities. *Proc. Natl. Acad. Sci. USA* **101**:10780–10785.

2140. Kedes, D. H., E. Operskalski, M. Busch, R. Kohn, J. Flood, and D. Ganem. 1996. The seroepidemiology of human herpesvirus 8 (Kaposi's sarcoma-associated herpesvirus): distribution of infection in KS risk groups and evidence for sexual transmission. *Nat. Med.* **2**:918–924.

2141. Kedzierska, K., and S. M. Crowe. 2001. Cytokines and HIV-1: interactions and clinical implications. *Antivir. Chem. Chemother.* **12**:133–150.

2142. Kedzierska, K., P. Ellery, J. Mak, S. R. Lewin, S. M. Crowe, and A. Jaworowski. 2002. HIV-1 down-modulates gamma signaling chain of Fc gamma R in human macrophages: a possible mechanism for inhibition of phagocytosis. *J. Immunol.* **168**:2895–2903.

2143. Kedzierska, K., A. Maerz, T. Warby, A. Jaworowski, H. Chan, J. Mak, S. Sonza, A. Lopez, and S. Crowe. 2000. Granulocyte-macrophage colony-stimulating factor inhibits HIV-1 replication in monocyte-derived macrophages. *AIDS* **14**:1739–1748.

2144. Kedzierska, K., J. Mak, A. Jaworowski, A. Greenway, A. C. Violo, D. Hocking, S. Purcell, J. Sullivan, J. Mills, H. Chan, and S. M. Crowe. 2001. *nef*-deleted HIV-1 inhibits phagocytosis by monocyte-derived macrophages in vitro but not by peripheral blood monocytes in vivo. *AIDS* **15**:945–955.

2145. Keele, B. F., F. Van Heuverswyn, Y. Li, E. Balles, J. Takehisa, M. L. Santiago, F. Bibollet-Ruche, Y. Chen, L. V. Waln, F. Liegeols, S. Loul, E. M. Ngole, Y. Blenvenue, E. Delaporte, J. F. Brookfield, P. M. Sharp, G. M. Shaw, M. Peeters, and B. H. Hahn. 2006. Chimpanzee reservoirs of pandemic and nonpandemic HIV-1. *Science* **313**:523–526.

2146. Keet, I. M. P., M. Janssen, P. J. Veugelers, F. Miedema, M. R. Klein, J. Goudsmit, R. A. Coutinho, and F. de Wolf. 1997. Longitudinal analysis of CD4 T cell counts, T cell reactivity, and human immunodeficiency virus type 1 RNA levels in persons remaining AIDS-free despite CD4 cell counts <200 for >5 years. *J. Infect. Dis.* **176**:665–671.

2147. Keet, I. P. M., P. Krijnen, M. Koot, J. M. A. Lange, F. Miedema, J. Goudsmit, and R. A. Coutinho. 1993. Predictors of rapid progression to AIDS in HIV-1 seroconverters. *AIDS* **7**:51–57.

2148. Keh, C. E., J. M. Shen, B. Hahn, C. W. Hallahan, C. A. Rehm, V. Thaker, S. M. Wynne, R. T. Davey, H. C. Lane, and I. Sereti. 2006. Interruption of antiretroviral therapy blunts but does not abrogate CD4 T-cell responses to interleukin-2 administration in HIV infected patients. *AIDS* **20**:361–369.

2149. Kehrl, J. H., M. Alvarez-Mon, G. A. Delsing, and A. S. Fauci. 1987. Lymphotoxin is an important T cell-derived growth factor for human B cells. *Science* **242**:1144–1146.

2150. Kelker, H. C., M. Seidlin, M. Vogler, and F. T. Valentine. 1992. Lymphocytes from some long-term seronegative heterosexual partners of HIV-infected individuals proliferate in response to HIV antigens. *AIDS Res. Hum. Retrovir.* **8**:1355–1359.

2151. Kellam, P., C. A. B. Bouchers, and B. A. Larder. 1992. Fifth mutation in human immunodeficiency virus type 1 reverse transcriptase contributes to the development of high-level resistance to zidovudine. *Proc. Natl. Acad. Sci. USA* **89**:1934–1938.

2152. Kelleher, A. D., L. Al-Harthi, and A. L. Landay. 1997. Immunological effects of antiretroviral and immune therapies of HIV. *AIDS* **11**:S149–S155.

2153. Kelleher, A. D., A. Carr, J. Zaunders, and D. A. Cooper. 1996. Alterations in the immune response of human immunodeficiency virus (HIV)-infected subjects treated with an HIV-specific protease inhibitor, ritonavir. *J. Infect. Dis.* 173:321–329.

2154. Keller, A., E. D. Garrett, and B. R. Cullen. 1992. The Bel-1 protein of human foamy virus activates human immunodeficiency virus type 1 gene expression via a novel DNA target site. *J. Virol.* 66:3946–3949.

2155. Keller, M. J., B. Zerhouni-Layachi, N. Cheshenko, M. John, K. Hogarty, A. Kasowitz, C. L. Goldberg, S. Wallenstein, A. T. Profy, M. E. Klotman, and B. C. Herold. 2006. PRO 2000 gel inhibits HIV and herpes simplex virus infection following vaginal application: a double-blind placebo-controlled trial. *J. Infect. Dis.* 193:27–35.

2156. Keller, R., K. Peden, S. Paulous, L. Montagnier, and A. Cordonnier. 1993. Amino acid changes in the fourth conserved region of human immunodeficiency virus type 2 strain HIV-2ROD envelope glycoprotein modulate fusion. *J. Virol.* 67:6253–6258.

2157. Kelly, M. D., H. M. Naif, S. L. Adams, A. L. Cunningham, and A. R. Lloyd. 1998. Dichotomous effects of β-chemokines on HIV replication in monocytes and monocyte-derived macrophages. *J. Immunol.* 160:3091–3095.

2158. Kensil, C. R., U. Patel, M. Lennick, and D. Marciani. 1991. Separation and characterization of saponins with adjuvant activity from Quillaja saponaria molina cortex. *J. Immunol.* 146:431–437.

2159. Kent, K. A., P. Kitchin, K. H. G. Mills, M. Page, F. Taffs, T. Corcoran, P. Silvera, B. Flanagan, C. Powell, J. Rose, C. Ling, A. M. Aubertin, and E. J. Stott. 1994. Passive immunization of cynomolgus macaques with immune sera or a pool of neutralizing monoclonal antibodies failed to protect against challenge with SIVmac251. *AIDS Res. Hum. Retrovir.* 10:189–194.

2160. Kent, S. J., P. D. Greenberg, M. C. Hoffman, R. E. Akridge, and M. J. McElrath. 1997. Antagonism of vaccine-induced HIV-1-specific CD4+ T cells by primary HIV-1 infection. *J. Immunol.* 158:807–815.

2161. Kent, S. J., S.-L. Hu, L. Corey, W. R. Morton, and P. D. Greenberg. 1996. Detection of simian immunodeficiency virus (SIV)-specific CD8+ T cells in macaques protected from SIV challenge by prior SIV subunit vaccination. *J. Virol.* 70:4941–4947.

2162. Kerkau, T., R. Schmitt-Landgraf, A. Schimpl, and E. Wecker. 1989. Downregulation of HLA class I antigens in HIV-1-infected cells. *AIDS Res. Hum. Retrovir.* 5:613–620.

2163. Kerr, J. F. R., and B. V. Harmon. 1991. Definition and incidence of apoptosis: an historical perspective, p. 5–30. *In* L. D. Tomei and F. O. Cope (ed.), *Apoptosis: The Molecular Basis of Cell Death*, vol. 3. Cold Spring Harbor Laboratory, Cold Spring Harbor, N.Y.

2164. Kerr, J. F. R., A. H. Wyllie, and A. R. Currie. 1972. Apoptosis: a basic biological phenomenon with wide-ranging implications in tissue kinetics. *Br. J. Cancer* 26:239–257.

2165. Kersten, M. J., M. R. Klein, A. M. Holwerda, F. Miedema, and M. H. J. van Oers. 1997. Epstein-Barr virus-specific cytotoxic T cell responses in HIV-1 infection. *J. Clin. Investig.* 99:1525–1533.

2166. Keshet, E., and H. M. Temin. 1979. Cell killing by spleen necrosis virus is correlated with a transient accumulation of spleen necrosis virus DNA. *J. Virol.* 31:376–388.

2167. Kestens, L., M. Melbye, R. J. Biggar, W. J. Stevens, P. Piot, A. De Muynck, H. Taelman, M. De Feyter, L. Paluku, and P. L. Gigase. 1985. Endemic African Kaposi's sarcoma is not associated with immunodeficiency. *Int. J. Cancer* 36:49–54.

2168. Kestens, L., J. Vingerhoets, M. Peeters, G. Vanham, C. Vereecken, G. Penne, H. Niphuis, P. van Eerd, G. van der Groen, P. Gigase, and J. Heeney. 1995. Phenotypic and functional parameters of cellular immunity in a chimpanzee with a naturally acquired simian immunodeficiency virus infection. *J. Infect. Dis.* 172:957–963.

2169. Kestler, H., T. Kodama, D. Ringler, M. Marthas, N. Pedersen, A. Lackner, D. Regier, P. Sehgal, M. Daniel, N. King, and R. Desrosiers. 1990. Induction of AIDS in rhesus monkeys by molecularly cloned simian immunodeficiency virus. *Science* 248:1109–1112.

2170. Kestler, H. W., III, D. J. Ringler, K. Mori, D. L. Panicali, P. K. Sehgal, M. D. Daniel, and R. C. Desrosiers. 1991. Importance of the *nef* gene for maintenance of high virus loads and for development of AIDS. *Cell* 65:651–662.

2171. Keswani, S. C., C. A. Pardo, C. L. Cherry, A. Hoke, and J. C. McArthur. 2002. HIV-associated sensory neuropathies. *AIDS* 16:2105–2117.

2172. Ketzler, S., S. Weis, H. Haug, and H. Budka. 1990. Loss of neurons in the frontal cortex in AIDS brains. *Acta Neuropathol.* (Berlin) 80:92–94.

2173. Keys, B., J. Karis, B. Fadeel, A. Valentin, G. Norkrans, L. Hagberg, and F. Chiodi. 1993. V3 sequences of paired HIV-1 isolates from blood and cerebrospinal fluid cluster according to host and show variation related to the clinical stage of disease. *Virology* 196:475–483.

2174. Khabbaz, R. F., W. Heneine, J. R. George, B. Parekh, T. Rowe, T. Woods, W. M. Switzer, H. M. McClure, M. Murphey-Corb, and T. M. Folks. 1994. Infection of a laboratory worker with simian immunodeficiency virus. *N. Engl. J. Med.* 330:172–177.

2175. Khan, M., L. Jin, M. Huang, L. Miles, V. C. Bond, and M. D. Powell. 2004. Chimeric human immunodeficiency virus type 1 (HIV-1) virions containing HIV-2 or simian immunodeficiency virus *nef* are resistant to cyclosporine treatment. *J. Virol.* 78:1843–1850.

2176. Khan, M. A., C. Aberham, S. Kao, H. Akari, R. Gorelick, S. Bour, and K. Strebel. 2001. Human immunodeficiency virus type 1 Vif protein is packaged into the nucleoprotein complex through an interaction with viral genomic RNA. *J. Virol.* 75:7252–7265.

2177. Khan, M. A., S. Kao, E. Miyagi, H. Takeuchi, R. Goila-Gaur, S. Opi, C. L. Gipson, T. G. Parslow, H. Ly, and K. Strebel. 2005. Viral RNA is required for the association of APOBEC3G with human immunodeficiency virus type 1 nucleoprotein complexes. *J. Virol.* 79:5870–5874.

2178. Khana, K. M., A. J. Lepisto, and R. L. Hendricks. 2004. Immunity to latent viral infection: many skirmishes but few fatalities. *Trends Immunol.* 25:230–234.

2179. Khansari, D. N., A. J. Murgo, and R. E. Faith. 1990. Effects of stress on the immune system. *Immunol. Today* 11:170–175.

2180. Khoo, S. H., L. Pepper, N. Snowden, A. H. Hajeer, P. Vallely, E. G. Wilins, B. K. Mandal, and W. E. Ollier. 1997. Tumor necrosis factor c2 microsatellite allele is associated with the rate of HIV disease progression. *AIDS* 11:423–428.

2181. Kido, H., A. Fukutomi, and N. Katunuma. 1990. A novel membrane-bound serine esterase in human T4+ lymphocytes immunologically reactive with antibody inhibiting syncytia induced by HIV-1. Purification and characterization. *J. Biol. Chem.* 265:21979–21985.

2182. Kido, H., A. Fukutomi, and N. Katunuma. 1991. Tryptase TL$_2$ in the membrane of human T4+ lymphocytes is a novel binding protein of the V3 domain of HIV-1 envelope glycoprotein gp120. *FEBS J.* **286**:233–236.

2183. Kiepiela, P., A. J. Leslie, I. Honeyborne, D. Ramduth, C. Thobakgale, S. Chetty, P. Rathnavalu, C. Moore, K. J. Pfafferott, L. Hilton, P. Zimbwa, S. Moore, T. Allen, C. Brander, M. M. Addo, M. Altfeld, I. James, S. Mallal, M. Bunce, L. D. Barber, J. Szinger, C. Day, P. Klenerman, J. Mullins, B. Korber, H. M. Coovadia, B. D. Walker, and P. J. Goulder. 2004. Dominant influence of HLA-B in mediating the potential co-evolution of HIV and HLA. *Nature* **432**:769–775.

2183a. Kiepiela, P., K. Ngumbela, C. Thobakgale, D. Ramduth, I. Honeyborne, E. Moodley, S. Reddy, C. de Pierres, Z. Mncube, N. Mkhwanazi, K. Bishop, M. van der Stok, K. Nair, N. Khan, H. Crawford, R. Payne, A. Leslie, J. Prado, A. Prendergast, J. Frater, N. McCarthy, C. Brander, G. H. Learn, D. Nickle, C. Rousseau, H. Coovadia, J. I. Mullins, D. Heckerman, B. D. Walker, and P. Goulder. 2007. CD8(+) T-cell responses to different HIV proteins have discordant associations with viral load. *Nat. Med.* **13**:46–53.

2184. Kikukawa, R., Y. Koyanagi, S. Harada, N. Kobayashi, M. Hatanaka, and N. Yamamoto. 1986. Differential susceptibility to the acquired immunodeficiency syndrome retrovirus in cloned cells of human leukemic T cell line Molt-4. *J. Virol.* **57**:1159–1162.

2185. Kilby, J. M., and J. J. Eron. 2003. Novel therapies based on mechanisms of HIV-1 cell entry. *N. Engl. J. Med.* **348**:2228–2238.

2186. Kilby, J. M., S. Hopkins, T. M. Venetta, B. DiMassimo, G. A. Cloud, J. Y. Lee, L. Alldredge, E. Hunter, D. Lambert, D. Bolognesi, T. Matthews, M. R. Johnson, M. A. Nowak, G. M. Shaw, and M. S. Saag. 1998. Potent suppression of HIV-1 replication in humans by T-20, a peptide inhibitor of gp41-mediated virus entry. *Nat. Med.* **4**:1302–1307.

2187. Killian, M. S., S. Fujimura, F. M. Hecht, and J. A. Levy. 2006. Similar changes in plasmacytoid dendritic cell and CD4+ T cell counts during primary HIV-1 infection and treatment. *AIDS* **20**:1247–1252.

2188. Killian, M. S., S. Ng, C. E. Mackewicz, and J. A. Levy. 2005. A screening assay for detecting CD8(+) cell non-cytotoxic anti-HIV responses. *J. Immunol. Methods* **304**:137–150.

2189. Killian, M. S., R. L. Sabado, S. Kilpatrick, M. A. Hausner, B. D. Jamieson, and O. O. Yang. 2005. Clonal breadth of the HIV-1-specific T-cell receptor repertoire in vivo as determined by subtractive analysis. *AIDS* **19**:887–896.

2190. Kim, A. Y., G. M. Lauer, K. Ouchi, M. M. Addo, M. Lucas, J. Schullze zur Wiesch, J. Timm, M. Boczanowski, J. E. Duncan, A. G. Wurchel, D. Casson, R. T. Chung, R. Draenert, P. Klenerman, and B. D. Walker. 2005. The magnitude and breadth of hepatitis C virus-specific CD8+ T cells depend on absolute CD4+ T-cell count in individuals coinfected with HIV-1. *Blood* **105**:1170–1178.

2191. Kim, C. H., B. Johnston, and E. C. Butcher. 2002. Trafficking machinery of NKT cells: shared and differential chemokine receptor expression among V alpha 24(+)V beta 11(+) NKT cell subsets with distinct cytokine-producing capacity. *Blood* **100**:11–16.

2192. Kim, C. H., H. W. Lim, J. R. Kim, L. Rott, P. Hillsamer, and E. C. Butcher. 2004. Unique gene expression program of human germinal center T helper cells. *Blood* **104**:1952–1960.

2193. Kim, E. Y., M. Busch, K. Abel, L. Fritts, P. Bustamante, J. Stanton, D. Lu, S. Wu, J. Glowczwskie, T. Rourke, D. Bogdan, M. Piatak, Jr., J. D. Lifson, R. C. Desrosiers, S. Wolinsky, and C. J. Miller. 2005. Retroviral recombination in vivo: viral replication patterns and genetic structure of simian immunodeficiency virus (SIV) populations in rhesus macaques after simultaneous or sequential intravaginal inoculation with SIVmac239Deltavpx/Deltavpr and SIVmac239Deltanef. *J. Virol.* **79**:4886–4895.

2194. Kim, J. H., J. D. Mosca, M. T. Vahey, R. J. McLinden, D. S. Burke, and R. R. Redfield. 1993. Consequences of human immunodeficiency virus type 1 superinfection of chronically infected cells. *AIDS Res. Hum. Retrovir.* **9**:875–882.

2195. Kim, J. J., and D. B. Weiner. 1999. Development of multicomponent DNA vaccination strategies against HIV. *Curr. Opin. Mol. Ther.* **1**:43–49.

2196. Kim, S., K. Ikeuchi, R. Byrn, J. Groopman, and D. Baltimore. 1989. Lack of a negative influence on viral growth by the *nef* gene of human immunodeficiency virus type 1. *Proc. Natl. Acad. Sci. USA* **86**:9544–9548.

2197. Kim, S., K. Ikeuchi, J. Groopman, and D. Baltimore. 1990. Factors affecting cellular tropism of human immunodeficiency virus. *J. Virol.* **64**:5600–5604.

2198. Kim, W. K., X. Alvarez, J. Fisher, B. Bronfin, S. Westmoreland, J. McLaurin, and K. Williams. 2006. CD163 identifies perivascular macrophages in normal and viral encephalitic brains and potential precursors to perivascular macrophages in blood. *Am. J. Pathol.* **168**:822–834.

2199. Kimmel, P. L., A. Ferreira-Centeno, T. Farkas-Szallasi, A. A. Abraham, and C. T. Garrett. 1993. Viral DNA in microdissected renal biopsy tissue from HIV infected patients with nephrotic syndrome. *Kidney Int.* **43**:1347–1352.

2200. Kimmel, P. L., T. M. Phillips, A. Ferreira-Centeno, T. Farkas-Szallasi, A. A. Abraham, and C. T. Garrett. 1992. Idiotypic IgA nephropathy in patients with human immunodeficiency virus infection. *N. Engl. J. Med.* **327**:702–706.

2201. Kimpton, J., and M. Emerman. 1992. Detection of replication-competent and pseudotyped human immunodeficiency virus with a sensitive cell line on the basis of activation of an integrated beta-galactosidase gene. *J. Virol.* **66**:2232–2239.

2202. King, M. D., D. A. Reznik, C. M. O'Daniels, N. M. Larsen, D. Osterholt, and H. M. Blumberg. 2002. Human papillomavirus-associated oral warts among human immunodeficiency virus-seropositive patients in the era of highly active antiretroviral therapy: an emerging infection. *Clin. Infect. Dis.* **34**:641–648.

2203. Kinlen, L. J. 1982. Immunosuppressive therapy and cancer. *Cancer Survey* **1**:567–583.

2203a. Kinloch-de Loes, S. 2006. Treatment of acute HIV-1 infection: is it coming of age? *J. Infect. Dis.* **194**:721–724.

2204. Kinloch-de Loes, S., B. Hoen, D. E. Smith, B. Autran, F. C. Lampe, A. N. Phillips, L. E. Goh, J. Andersson, C. Tsoukas, A. Sonnerborg, G. Tambussi, P. M. Girard, M. Bloch, M. Battegay, N. Carter, R. El Habib, G. Theofan, D. A. Cooper, and L. Perrin. 2005. Impact of therapeutic immunization on HIV-1 viremia after discontinuation of antiretroviral therapy initiated during acute infection. *J. Infect. Dis.* **192**:607–617.

2205. Kinter, A., A. Catanzaro, J. Monaco, M. Ruiz, J. Justement, S. Moir, J. Arthos, A. Oliva, L. Ehler, S. Mizell, R. Jackson, M. Ostrowski, J. Hoxie, R. Offord, and A. S. Fauci. 1998. CC-chemokines enhance the replication of T-tropic strains of HIV-1 in CD4(+) T cells: role of signal transduction. *Proc. Natl. Acad. Sci. USA* **95**:11880–11885.

2206. Kinter, A. L., S. M. Bende, E. C. Hardy, R. Jackson, and A. S. Fauci. 1995. Interleukin 2 induces CD8+ T cell-mediated suppression of human immunodeficiency virus replication in CD4+ T cells and this effect overrides its ability to stimulate virus expression. *Proc. Natl. Acad. Sci. USA* **92**:10985–10989.

2207. Kinter, A. L., M. Hennessey, A. Bell, S. Kern, Y. Lin, M. Daucher, M. Planta, M. McGlaughlin, R. Jackson, S. F. Ziegler, and A. S. Fauci. 2004. CD25(+)CD4(+) regulatory T cells from the peripheral blood of asymptomatic HIV-infected individuals regulate CD4(+) and CD8(+) HIV-specific T cell immune responses in vitro and are associated with favorable clinical markers of disease status. *J. Exp. Med.* **200**:331–343.

2208. Kinter, A. L., M. Ostrowski, D. Goletti, A. Oliva, D. Weissman, K. Gantt, E. Hardy, R. Jackson, L. Ehler, and A. S. Fauci. 1996. HIV replication in CD4+ T cells of HIV-infected individuals is regulated by a balance between the viral suppressive effects of endogenous β-chemokines and the viral inductive effects of other endogenous cytokines. *Proc. Natl. Acad. Sci. USA* **93**:14076–14081.

2209. Kinter, A. L., G. Poli, L. Fox, E. Hardy, and A. S. Fauci. 1995. HIV replication in IL-2-stimulated peripheral blood mononuclear cells is driven in an autocrine/paracrine manner by endogenous cytokines. *J. Immunol.* **154**:2448–2459.

2210. Kinter, A. L., G. Poli, W. Maury, T. M. Folks, and A. S. Fauci. 1990. Direct and cytokine-mediated activation of protein kinase C induces human immunodeficiency virus expression in chronically infected promonocytic cells. *J. Virol.* **64**:4306–4312.

2211. Kinter, A. L., C. A. Umscheid, J. Arthos, C. Cicala, Y. Lin, R. Jackson, E. Donoghue, L. Ehler, J. Adelsberger, R. L. Rabin, and A. S. Fauci. 2003. HIV envelope induces virus expression from resting CD4+ T cells isolated from HIV-infected individuals in the absence of markers of cellular activation or apoptosis. *J. Immunol.* **170**:2449–2455.

2212. Kiprov, D., W. Pfaeffl, G. Parry, R. Lippert, W. Lang, and R. Miller. 1988. Antibody-mediated peripheral neuropathies associated with ARC and AIDS: successful treatment with plasmapheresis. *J. Clin. Apheresis* **4**:3–7.

2213. Kiprov, D. D., B. J. Kwiatkowska, and R. G. Miller. 1990. Therapeutic apheresis in human immunodeficiency virus-related syndromes. *Curr. Stud. Hematol. Blood Transfus.* **57**:184–197.

2214. Kirchhoff, F., T. C. Greenough, D. B. Brettler, J. L. Sullivan, and R. C. Desrosiers. 1995. Brief report: absence of intact nef sequences in a long-term survivor with nonprogressive HIV-1 infection. *N. Engl. J. Med.* **332**:228–232.

2215. Kirchhoff, F., T. C. Greenough, M. Hamacher, J. L. Sullivan, and R. C. Desrosiers. 1997. Activity of human immunodeficiency virus type 1 promoter/TAR regions and *tat* 1 genes derived from individuals with different rates of disease progression. *Virology* **232**:319–331.

2216. Kishi, M., K. Tokunaga, Y.-H. Zheng, M. K. Bahmani, M. Kakinuma, M. Nonoyama, P. K. Lai, and K. Ikuta. 1995. Superinfection of a defective human immunodeficiency virus type 1 provirus-carrying T cell clone with *vif* or *vpu* mutants gives cytopathic virus particles by homologous recombination. *AIDS Res. Hum. Retrovir.* **11**:45–53.

2217. Kitchen, S. G., Y. D. Korin, M. D. Roth, A. Landay, and J. A. Zack. 1998. Costimulation of naive CD8⁺ lymphoyctes induces CD4 expression and allows human immunodeficiency virus type 1 infection. *J. Virol.* **72**:9054–9060.

2218. Kiviat, N. B., C. W. Critchlow, S. E. Hawes, J. Kuypers, C. Surawicz, G. Goldbaum, J. van Burik, T. Lampinen, and K. K. Holmes. 1998. Determinants of human immunodeficiency virus DNA and RNA shedding in the anal-rectal canal of homosexual men. *J. Infect. Dis.* **177**:571–578.

2219. Kiviat, N. B., C. W. Critchlow, K. K. Holmes, J. Kuypers, J. Sayer, C. Dunphy, C. Surawicz, P. Kirby, R. Wood, and J. R. Daling. 1992. Association of anal dysplasia and human papillomavirus with immunosuppression and HIV infection among homosexual men. *AIDS* **7**:43–49.

2220. Klaassen, R. J. L., R. Goldschmeding, K. M. Dolman, A. B. J. Vlekke, H. M. Weigel, J. K. M. Eeftinck Schattenkerk, J. W. Mulder, M. L. Westedt, and A. E. G. K. von dem Borne. 1992. Anti-neutrophil cytoplasmic autoantibodies in patients with symptomatic HIV infection. *Clin. Exp. Immunol.* **87**:24–30.

2221. Klaassen, R. J. L., J. W. Mulder, A. B. J. Vlekke, J. K. M. Eeftinck Schattenkerk, H. M. Weigel, J. M. A. Lange, and A. E. G. K. von dem Borne. 1990. Autoantibodies against peripheral blood cells appear early in HIV infection and their prevalence increases with disease progression. *Clin. Exp. Immunol.* **81**:11–17.

2222. Klasse, P. J., J. A. McKeating, M. Schutten, M. S. Reitz, Jr., and M. Robert-Guroff. 1993. An immune-selected point mutation in the transmembrane protein of human immunodeficiency virus type 1 (HXB2-Env:Ala 582 (AEThr) decreases viral neutralization by monoclonal antibodies to the CD4-binding site. *Virology* **196**:332–337.

2223. Klasse, P. J., and J. P. Moore. 2004. Is there enough gp120 in the body fluids of HIV-1-infected individuals to have biologically significant effects? *Virology* **323**:1–8.

2224. Klatzmann, D., F. Barre-Sinoussi, M. T. Nugeyre, C. Dauquet, E. Vilmer, C. Griscelli, F. Brun-Vezinet, C. Rouzioux, J. C. Gluckman, and J. C. Chermann. 1984. Selective tropism of lymphadenopathy-associated virus (LAV) for helper-inducer T-lymphocytes. *Science* **225**:59–62.

2225. Klatzmann, D., E. Champagne, S. Chamaret, J. Gurest, D. Guetard, T. Hercend, J. C. Gluckman, and L. Montagnier. 1984. T-lymphocyte T4 molecule behaves as receptor for human retrovirus LAV. *Nature* **312**:767–778.

2226. Klausner, R. D., A. S. Fauci, L. Corey, G. J. Nabel, H. Gayle, S. Berkley, B. F. Haynes, D. Baltimore, C. Collins, R. G. Douglas, J. Esparza, D. P. Francis, N. K. Ganguly, J. L. Gerberding, M. I. Johnston, M. D. Kazatchkine, A. J. McMichael, M. W. Makgoba, G. Pantaleo, P. Piot, Y. Shao, E. Tramont, H. Varmus, and J. N. Wasserheit. 2003. The need for a global HIV/AIDS vaccine enterprise. *Science* **300**:2036–2039.

2227. Kleburtz, K. D., D. W. Giang, R. B. Schiffer, and N. Vakil. 1991. Abnormal vitamin B12 metabolism in human immunodeficiency virus infection: association with neurological dysfunction. *Arch. Neurol.* **48**:312–314.

2228. Kleim, J.-P., A. Ackermann, H. H. Brackmann, M. Gahr, and K. E. Schneweis. 1991. Epidemiologically closely related viruses from hemophilia B patients display high homology in two hypervariable regions of the HIV-1 env gene. *AIDS Res. Hum. Retrovir.* **7**:417–421.

2229. Klein, G. 1981. The role of gene dosage and genetic transpositions in carcinogenesis. *Nature* **294**:313–318.

2230. Klein, M. B., P. Willemot, T. Murphy, and R. G. Lalonde. 2004. The impact of initial highly active antiretroviral therapy on future treatment sequences in HIV infection. *AIDS* **18**:1895–1904.

2231. Klein, M. R., C. A. van Baalen, A. M. Holwerda, S. R. Kerkhof Garde, R. J. Bende, I. P. M. Keet, J. K. Eeftinck-Schattenkerk, A. D. M. E. Osterhaus, H. Schuitemaker, and F. Miedema. 1995. Kinetics of Gag-specific cytotoxic T lymphocyte responses during the clinical course of HIV-1 infection: a longitudinal analysis of rapid progressors and long-term asymptomatics. *J. Exp. Med.* **181**:1365–1372.

2232. **Klein, M. R., S. H. van der Burg, O. Pontesilli, and F. Miedema.** 1998. Cytotoxic T lymphocytes in HIV-1 infection: a killing paradox? *Immunol. Today* **19**:317–324.

2233. **Klein, S. A., J. M. Dobmeyer, T. S. Dobmeyer, M. Pape, O. G. Ottmann, E. B. Helm, D. Hoelzer, and R. Rossol.** 1997. Demonstration of the Th1 to TH2 cytokine shift during the course of HIV-1 infection using cytoplasmic cytokine detection on single cell level by flow cytometry. *AIDS* **11**:1111–1118.

2234. **Klenerman, P., R. Phillips, and A. McMichael.** 1996. Cytotoxic T cell antagonism in HIV. *Semin. Virol.* **7**:31–39.

2235. **Klenerman, P., R. E. Phillips, C. R. Rinaldo, L. M. Wahl, G. Ogg, R. M. May, A. J. McMichael, and M. A. Nowak.** 1996. Cytotoxic T lymphocytes and viral turnover in HIV type 1 infection. *Proc. Natl. Acad. Sci. USA* **93**:15323–15328.

2236. **Klenerman, P., S. Rowland-Jones, S. McAdam, J. Edwards, S. Daenke, D. Lalloo, B. Koppe, W. Rosenberg, D. Boyd, A. Edwards, P. Giangrande, R. E. Phillips, and A. J. McMichael.** 1994. Cytotoxic T-cell activity antagonized by naturally ocurring HIV-1 Gag variants. *Nature* **369**:403–407.

2237. **Klenerman, P., and R. M. Zinkernagel.** 1998. Original antigenic sin impairs cytotoxic T lymphocyte responses to viruses bearing variant epitopes. *Nature* **394**:482–485.

2237a. **Klesney-Tait, J., I. R. Turnbull, and M. Colonna.** 2006. The TREM receptor family and signal integration. *Nat. Immunol.* **7**:1266–1273.

2238. **Kliks, S., C. H. Contag, G. Corliss, G. Learn, A. Rodrigo, D. Wara, J. I. Mullins, and J. A. Levy.** 2000. Genetic analysis of viral variants selected in transmission of human immunodeficiency viruses to newborns. *AIDS Res. Hum. Retrovir.* **196**:1223–1233.

2239. **Kliks, S. C., T. Shioda, N. L. Haigwood, and J. A. Levy.** 1993. V3 variability can influence the ability of an antibody to neutralize or enhance infection by diverse strains of human immunodeficiency virus type 1. *Proc. Natl. Acad. Sci. USA* **90**:11518–11522.

2240. **Kliks, S. C., D. W. Wara, D. V. Landers, and J. A. Levy.** 1994. Features of HIV-1 that could influence maternal-child transmission. *JAMA* **272**:467–474.

2241. **Klimas, N., R. Patarca, J. Walling, R. Garcia, V. Mayer, D. Moody, T. Okarma, and M. A. Fletcher.** 1994. Clinical and immunological changes in AIDS patients following adoptive therapy with activated autologous CD8 T cells and interleukin-2 infusion. *AIDS* **8**:1073–1081.

2242. **Klimas, N. G., J. B. Page, R. Patarca, D. Chitwood, R. Morgan, and M. A. Fletcher.** 1993. Effects of retroviral infections on immune function in African-American intravenous drug users. *AIDS* **7**:331–335.

2243. **Kloster, B. E., R. H. Tomar, and T. J. Spira.** 1984. Lymphocytotoxic antibodies in the acquired immune deficiency syndrome (AIDS). *Clin. Immunol. Immunopathol.* **30**:330–335.

2244. **Knight, S. C.** 1996. Bone-marrow-derived dendritic cells and the pathogenesis of AIDS. *AIDS* **10**:807–817.

2245. **Knight, S. C., W. Elsley, and H. Wang.** 1997. Mechanisms of loss of functional dendritic cells in HIV-1 infection. *J. Leukoc. Biol.* **62**:78–81.

2246. **Knight, S. C., S. E. Macatonia, and S. Patterson.** 1993. Infection of dendritic cells with HIV-1: virus load regulates stimulation and suppression of T-cell activity. *Res. Virol.* **144**:75–80.

2247. **Knight, S. C., and S. Patterson.** 1997. Bone marrowderived dendritic cells, infection with human immunodeficiency virus, and immunopathology. *Annu. Rev. Immunol.* **15**:593–615.

2248. **Knuchel, M. C., T. J. Spira, A. U. Neumann, L. Xiao, D. L. Rudolph, J. Phair, S. M. Wolinsky, R. A. Koup, O. J. Cohen, T. M. Folks, and R. B. Lal.** 1998. Analysis of a biallelic polymorphism in the tumor necrosis factor alpha promoter and HIV type 1 disease progression. *AIDS Res. Hum. Retrovir.* **14**:305–309.

2249. **Kobayashi, J., A. Takeda, S. Green, C. U. Tuazon, and F. A. Ennis.** 1993. Direct detection of infectious human immunodeficiency virus type 1 (HIV-1) immune complexes in the sera of HIV-1-infected persons. *J. Infect. Dis.* **168**:729–732.

2250. **Kobayashi, M., A. Takaori-Kondo, K. Shindo, A. Abudu, K. Fukunaga, and T. Uchiyama.** 2004. APOBEC3G targets specific virus species. *J. Virol.* **78**:8238–8244.

2251. **Kodama, T., K. Mori, T. Kawahara, D. J. Ringler, and R. C. Desrosiers.** 1993. Analysis of simian immunodeficiency virus sequence variation in tissues of rhesus macaques with simian AIDS. *J. Virol.* **67**:6522–6534.

2252. **Koenig, S., H. E. Gendelman, J. M. Orenstein, M. C. Dal Canto, G. H. Pezeshkpour, M. Yungbluth, F. Janotta, A. Aksamit, M. A. Martin, and A. S. Fauci.** 1986. Detection of AIDS virus in macrophages in brain tissue from AIDS patients with encephalopathy. *Science* **233**:1089–1093.

2253. **Koga, Y., M. Sasaki, H. Yoshida, M. Oh-Tsu, G. Kimura, and K. Nomoto.** 1991. Disturbance of nuclear transport of proteins in CD4$^+$ cells expressing gp160 of human immunodeficiency virus. *J. Virol.* **65**:5609–5612.

2254. **Kohler, H., J. Goudsmit, and P. Nara.** 1992. Clonal dominance: cause for a limited and failing immune response to HIV-1 infection and vaccination. *J. Acquir. Immune Defic. Syndr.* **5**:1158–1168.

2255. **Kohler, H., S. Muller, and P. L. Nara.** 1994. Deceptive imprinting in the immune response against HIV-1. *Immunol. Today* **15**:475–478.

2256. **Kohlstaedt, L. A., J. Wang, J. M. Friedman, P. A. Rice, and T. A. Steitz.** 1992. Crystal structure at 3.5 angstrom resolution of HIV-1 reverse transcriptase complexed with an inhibitor. *Science* **256**:1783–1790.

2257. **Koito, A., G. Harrowe, J. A. Levy, and C. Cheng-Mayer.** 1994. Functional role of the V1/V2 region of human immunodeficiency virus type 1 envelope glycoprotein gp120 in infection of primary macrophages and sCD4 neutralization. *J. Virol.* **68**:2253–2259.

2258. **Koito, A., L. Stamatatos, and C. Cheng-Mayer.** 1995. Small amino acid sequence changes within the V2 domain can affect the function of a T-cell line-tropic human immunodeficiency virus type 1 envelope gp120. *Virology* **206**:878–884.

2259. **Koka, P. S., J. K. Fraser, Y. Bryson, G. C. Bristol, G. M. Aldrovandi, E. S. Daar, and J. A. Zack.** 1998. Human immunodeficiency virus inhibits multilineage hematopoiesis in vivo. *J. Virol.* **72**:5121–5127.

2260. **Kolchinsky, P., E. Kiprilov, P. Bartley, R. Rubinstein, and J. Sodroski.** 2001. Loss of a single N-linked glycan allows CD4-independent human immunodeficiency virus type 1 infection by altering the position of the gp120 V1/V2 variable loops. *J. Virol.* **75**:3435–3443.

2261. **Kolesnitchenko, V., L. M. Wahl, H. Tian, I. Sunila, Y. Tani, D.-P. Hartmann, J. Cossman, M. Raffeld, J. Orenstein,**

L. E. Samelson, and D. I. Cohen. 1995. Human immunodeficiency virus 1 envelope-initiated G2-phase programmed cell death. *Proc. Natl. Acad. Sci. USA* 92:11889–11893.

2262. Koletar, S. L., A. E. Heald, D. Finkelstein, R. Hafner, J. S. Currier, J. A. McCutchan, M. Vallee, F. J. Torriani, W. G. Powderly, R. J. Fass, and R. L. Murphy. 2001. A prospective study of discontinuing primary and secondary *Pneumocystis carinii* pneumonia prophylaxis after CD4 cell count increase to > 200 x 106 /l. *AIDS* 15:1509–1515.

2263. Koller, H., H.-J. von Giesen, H. Schaal, and G. Arendt. 2001. Soluble cerebrospinal fluid factors induce Ca2+ dysregulation in rat cultured cortical astrocytes in HIV-1-associated dementia complex. *AIDS* 15:1789–1792.

2264. Kollmann, T. R., M. Pettoello-Mantovani, N. F. Katopodis, M. Hachamovitch, A. Rubinstein, A. Kim, and H. Goldstein. 1996. Inhibition of acute *in vivo* human immunodeficiency virus infection by human interleukin 10 treatment of SCID mice implanted with human fetal thymus and liver. *Proc. Natl. Acad. Sci. USA* 93:3126–3131.

2265. Kolson, D. L., J. Buchhalter, R. Collman, B. Hellmig, C. F. Farrell, C. Debouck, and F. Gonzalez-Scarano. 1993. HIV-1 Tat alters normal oganization of neurons and astrocytes in primary rodent brain cell cultures: RGD sequence dependence. *AIDS Res. Hum. Retrovir.* 9:677–685.

2266. Kolte, L., A. M. Dreves, A. K. Ersboll, C. Strandberg, D. L. Jeppesen, J. O. Nielsen, L. P. Ryder, and S. D. Nielsen. 2002. Association between larger thymic size and higher thymic output in human immunodeficiency virus-infected patients receiving highly active antiretroviral therapy. *J. Infect. Dis.* 185:1578–1585.

2267. Kolter, D. P. 2005. HIV infection and the gastrointestinal tract. *AIDS* 19:107–117.

2268. Komanduri, K. V., J. A. Luce, M. S. McGrath, B. G. Herndier, and V. L. Ng. 1996. The natural history and molecular heterogeneity of HIV-associated primary malignant lymphomatous effusions. *J. Acquir. Immune Defic. Syndr. Hum. Retrovirol.* 13:215–226.

2269. Komuro, I., Y. Yokota, S. Yasuda, A. Iwamoto, and K. S. Kagawa. 2003. CSF-induced and HIV-1-mediated distinct regulation of Hck and C/EBPb represent a heterogeneous susceptibility of monocyte-derived macrophages to M-tropic HIV-1 infection. *J. Exp. Med.* 198:443–453.

2270. Kong, F. K., C. L. Chen, A. Six, R. D. Hockett, and M. D. Cooper. 1999. T cell receptor gene deletion circles identify recent thymic emigrants in the peripheral T cell pool. *Proc. Natl. Acad. Sci. USA* 96:1536–1540.

2271. Kong, L. I., S.-W. Lee, J. C. Kappes, J. S. Parkin, D. Decker, J. A. Hoxie, B. H. Hahn, and G. M. Shaw. 1988. West African HIV-2-related human retrovirus with attenuated cytopathicity. *Science* 240:1525–1529.

2272. Koning, F. A., D. Kwa, B. Boese-Nunnick, J. Dekker, J. Vingerhoed, H. Hiemstra, and H. Schuitemaker. 2003. Decreasing sensitivity to RANTES (regulated on activation, normally T cell-expressed and -secreted) neutralization of CC chemokine receptor 5-using, non-syncytium-inducing virus variants in the course of human immunodeficiency virus type 1 infection. *J. Infect. Dis.* 188:864–872.

2273. Koning, F. A., S. A. Otto, M. D. Hazenberg, L. Dekker, M. Prins, F. Miedema, and H. Schuitemaker. 2005. Low-level CD4+ T cell activation is associated with low susceptibility to HIV-1 infection. *J. Immunol.* 175:6117–6122.

2274. Kontorinis, N., K. Agarwal, and D. T. Dieterich. 2005. Treatment of hepatitis C virus in HIV patients: a review. *AIDS* 19(Suppl. 3):S166–S173.

2275. Koon, H. B., G. J. Bubley, L. Pantanowitz, D. Masiello, B. Smith, K. Crosby, J. Proper, W. Weeden, T. E. Miller, P. Chatis, M. J. Egorin, S. R. Tahan, and B. J. Dezube. 2005. Imatinib-induced regression of AIDS-related Kaposi's sarcoma. *J. Clin. Oncol.* 23:982–989.

2276. Koopman, G., A. G. M. Haaksma, F. Ten Velden, C. E. Hack, and J. L. Heeney. 1999. The relative resistance of HIV type 1-infected chimpanzees to AIDS correlates with the maintenance of follicular architecture and the absence of infiltration by CD8+ cytotoxic T lymphocytes. *AIDS Res. Hum. Retrovir.* 15:365–373.

2277. Koopman, G., P. C. Wever, M. D. Ramkema, F. Bellot, P. Reiss, R. M. Keehnen, I. J. Ten Berge, and S. T. Pals. 1997. Expression of granzyme B by cytotoxic T lymphocytes in the lymph nodes of HIV-infected patients. *AIDS Res. Hum. Retrovir.* 13:227–233.

2278. Koot, M., I. P. M. Keet, A. H. V. Vos, R. E. Y. de Goede, J. T. L. Roos, R. A. Coutinho, F. Miedema, P. T. A. Schellekens, and M. Tersmette. 1993. Prognostic value of HIV-1 syncytium-inducing phenotype for rate of CD4+ cell depletion and progression to AIDS. *Ann. Intern. Med.* 118:681–688.

2279. Koot, M., A. H. V. Vos, R. P. M. Keet, R. E. Y. de Goede, M. W. Dercksen, F. G. Terpstra, R. A. Coutinho, F. Miedema, and M. Tersmette. 1992. HIV-1 biological phenotype in long-term infected individuals evaluated with an MT-2 cocultivation assay. *AIDS* 6:49–54.

2280. Kootstra, N. A., A. B. van't Wout, H. G. Huisman, F. Miedema, and H. Schuitemaker. 1994. Interference of interleukin-10 with human immunodeficiency virus type 1 replication in primary monocyte-derived macrophages. *J. Virol.* 68:6967–6975.

2281. Kopf, M., G. Le Gros, M. Bachmann, M. C. Lamers, H. Bluethmann, and G. Köhler. 1993. Disruption of murine IL-4 gene blocks Th2 cytokine responses. *Science* 362:245–247.

2282. Korber, B., M. Muldoon, J. Theiler, F. Gao, R. Gupta, A. Lapedes, B. H. Hahn, S. Wolinsky, and T. Bhattacharya. 2000. Timing the ancestor of the HIV-1 pandemic strains. *Science* 288:1789–1796.

2283. Korber, B. T. M., K. J. Kunstman, B. K. Patterson, M. Furtado, M. M. McEvilly, R. Levy, and S. M. Wolinsky. 1994. Genetic differences between blood- and brain-derived viral sequences from human immunodeficiency virus type 1-infected patients: evidence of conserved elements in the V3 region of the envelope protein of brain-derived sequences. *J. Virol.* 68:7467–7481.

2284. Korber, B. T. M., K. MacInnes, R. F. Smith, and G. Myers. 1994. Mutational trends in V3 loop protein sequences observed in different genetic lineages of human immunodeficiency virus type 1. *J. Virol.* 68:6730–6744.

2285. Korin, Y. D., and J. A. Zack. 1998. Progression to the G_1b phase of the cell cycle is required for completion of human immunodeficiency virus type 1 reverse transcription in T cells. *J. Virol.* 72:3161–3168.

2286. Kornfeld, C., M. J. Ploquin, I. Pandrea, A. Faye, R. Onanga, C. Apetrei, V. Poaty-Mavoungou, P. Rouquet, J. Estaquier, L. Mortara, J. F. Desoutter, C. Butor, R. Le Grand, P. Roques, F. Simon, F. Barre-Sinoussi, O. M. Diop, and M. C. Muller-Trutwin. 2005. Antiinflammatory profiles during primary SIV infection in African green monkeys are associated with protection against AIDS. *J. Clin. Investig.* 115:1082–1091.

2287. Kornfeld, H., W. W. Cruikshank, S. W. Pyle, J. S. Berman, and D. M. Center. 1988. Lymphocyte activation by HIV-1 envelope glycoprotein. *Nature* 335:445–448.

2288. Kos, F. J., and E. G. Engleman. 1995. Requirement for natural killer cells in the induction of cytotoxic T cells. *J. Immunol.* 155:578–584.

2289. Kosalaraksa, P., M. F. Kavlick, V. Maroun, R. Le, and H. Mitsuya. 1999. Comparative fitness of multidideoxynucleoside-resistant human immunodeficiency virus type 1 (HIV-1) in an in vitro competitive HIV-1 replication assay. *J. Virol.* 73:5356–5363.

2290. Kostense, S., K. Vandenberghe, J. Joling, D. Van Baarle, N. Nanlohy, E. Manting, and F. Miedema. 2002. Persistent numbers of tetramer+ CD8(+) T cells, but loss of interferon-gamma+ HIV-specific T cells during progression to AIDS. *Blood* 99:2505–2511.

2291. Kostrikis, L. G., E. Bagdades, Y. Cao, L. Zhang, D. Dimitriou, and D. D. Ho. 1995. Genetic analysis of human immunodeficiency virus type 1 strains from patients in Cyprus: identification of a new subtype designated subtype I. *J. Virol.* 69:6122–6130.

2292. Kostrikis, L. G., Y. Huang, J. P. Moore, S. M. Wolinsky, L. Zhang, Y. Guo, L. Deutsch, J. Phair, A. U. Neumann, and D. D. Ho. 1998. A chemokine receptor CCR2 allele delays HIV-1 disease progression and is associated with a CCR5 promoter mutation. *Nat. Med.* 4:350–353.

2293. Kostrikis, L. G., A. U. Neumann, B. Thomson, B. T. Korber, P. McHardy, R. Karanicolas, L. Deutsch, Y. Huang, J. F. Lew, K. McIntosh, H. Pollack, W. Borkowsky, H. M. Spiegel, P. Palumbo, J. Oleske, A. Bardeguez, K. Luzuriaga, J. Sullivan, S. M. Wolinsky, R. A. Koup, D. D. Ho, and J. P. Moore. 1999. A polymorphism in the regulatory region of the CC-chemokine receptor 5 gene influences perinatal transmission of human immunodeficiency virus type 1 to African-American infants. *J. Virol.* 73:10264–10271.

2294. Kotler, D. P. 2005. HIV infection and the gastrointestinal tract. *AIDS* 19:107–117.

2295. Kotler, D. P., H. P. Gaetz, M. Lange, E. B. Klein, and P. R. Holt. 1984. Enteropathy associated with the acquired immunodeficiency syndrome. *Ann. Intern. Med.* 101:421–428.

2296. Kotler, D. P., S. Reka, A. Borcich, and W. J. Cronin. 1991. Detection, localization, and quantitation of HIV-associated antigens in intestinal biopsies from patients with AIDS. *Am. J. Pathol.* 139:823–830.

2297. Kotler, D. P., T. Shimada, G. Snow, G. Winson, W. Chen, M. Zhao, Y. Inada, and F. Clayton. 1998. Effect of combination antiretroviral therapy upon rectal mucosal HIV RNA burden and mononuclear cell apoptosis. *AIDS* 12:597–604.

2298. Kotov, A., J. Zhou, P. Flicker, and C. Aiken. 1999. Association of Nef with the human immunodeficiency virus type 1 core. *J. Virol.* 73:8824–8830.

2299. Kottilil, S., T. S. Chun, S. Moir, S. Liu, M. McLaughlin, C. W. Hallahan, F. Maldarelli, L. Corey, and A. S. Fauci. 2003. Innate immunity in HIV infection: effect of HIV viremia on natural killer cell function. *J. Infect. Dis.* 187:1038–1045.

2300. Kottilil, S., K. Shin, M. Planta, M. McLaughlin, C. W. Hallahan, M. Ghany, T.-W. Chun, M. C. Sneller, and A. S. Fauci. 2004. Expression of chemokine and inhibitory receptors on natural killer cells: effect of immune activation and HIV viremia. *J. Infect. Dis.* 189:1193–1198.

2301. Koulinska, I. N., E. Villamor, B. Chaplin, G. Msamanga, W. Fawzi, B. Renjifo, and M. Essex. 2006. Transmission of cell-free and cell-associated HIV-1 through breast-feeding. *J. Acquir. Immune Defic. Syndr.* 41:93–99.

2302. Koup, R. A., J. T. Safrit, Y. Cao, C. A. Andrews, G. McLeod, W. Borkowsky, C. Farthing, and D. D. Ho. 1994. Temporal association of cellular immune responses with the initial control of viremia in primary human immunodeficiency virus type 1 syndrome. *J. Virol.* 68:4650–4655.

2303. Koup, R. A., J. L. Sullivan, P. H. Levine, D. Brettler, A. Mahr, G. Mazzara, S. McKenzie, and D. Panicali. 1989. Detection of major histocompatibility complex Class I-restricted, HIV-specific cytotoxic T lymphocytes in the blood of infected hemophiliacs. *Blood* 73:1909–1914.

2304. Kourtis, A. P., M. Buherys, S. R. Nesheim, and F. K. Lee. 2001. Understanding the timing of HIV transmission from mother to infant. *JAMA* 285:709–712.

2305. Kourtis, A. P., C. Ibegbu, A. J. Nahmias, F. K. Lee, W. S. Clark, M. K. Sawyer, and S. Nesheim. 1996. Early progression of disease in HIV-infected infants with thymus dysfunction. *N. Engl. J. Med.* 335:1431–1436.

2306. Koutsky, L. A., K. A. Ault, C. M. Wheeler, D. R. Brown, E. Barr, F. B. Alvarez, L. M. Chiacchierini, and K. U. Jansen. 2002. A controlled trial of a human papillomavirus type 16 vaccine. *N. Engl. J. Med.* 347:1645–1651.

2307. Kovacs, A., S. S. Wasserman, D. Burns, D. J. Wright, J. Cohn, A. Landay, K. Weber, M. Cohen, A. Levine, H. Minkoff, P. Miotti, J. Palefsky, M. Young, and P. Reichelderfer. 2001. Determinants of HIV-1 shedding in the genital tract of women. *Lancet* 358:1593–1601.

2308. Kovacs, J. A., M. Baseler, R. J. Dewar, S. Vogel, R. T. Davey, Jr., J. Falloon, M. A. Polis, R. E. Walker, R. Stevens, N. P. Salzman, J. A. Metcalf, H. Masur, and C. C. Lane. 1995. Increases in CD4 T lymphocytes with intermittent courses of interleukin-2 in patients with human immunodeficiency virus infection. *N. Engl. J. Med.* 332:567–575.

2309. Kovacs, J. A., R. A. Lempicki, I. A. Sidorov, J. W. Adelsberger, B. Herpin, J. A. Metcalf, I. Sereti, M. A. Polis, R. T. Davey, J. Tavel, J. Falloon, R. Stevens, L. Lambert, R. Dewar, D. J. Schwartzentruber, M. R. Anver, M. W. Baseler, H. Masur, D. S. Dimitrov, and H. C. Lane. 2001. Identification of dynamically distinct subpopulations of T lymphocytes that are differentially affected by HIV. *J. Exp. Med.* 194:1731–1741.

2310. Kovacs, J. A., R. A. Lempicki, I. A. Sidorov, J. W. Adelsberger, I. Sereti, W. Sachau, G. Kelly, J. A. Metcalf, R. T. Davey, J. Falloon, M. A. Polis, J. Tavel, R. Stevens, L. Lambert, D. A. Hosack, M. Bosche, H. J. Issaq, S. D. Fox, S. Leitman, M. W. Baseler, H. Masur, M. Di Mascio, D. S. Dimitrov, and H. C. Lane. 2005. Induction of prolonged survival of CD4 T lymphocytes by intermittent IL-2 therapy in HIV-infected patients. *J. Clin. Investig.* 115:2139–2148.

2311. Kovacs, J. A., M. B. Vasudevachari, M. Easter, R. T. Davey, J. Falloon, M. A. Polis, J. A. Metcalf, N. Salzman, M. Baseler, G. E. Smith, F. Volvovitz, H. Masur, and H. C. Lane. 1993. Induction of humoral and cell-mediated anti-human immunodeficiency virus (HIV) responses in HIV sero-negative volunteers by immunization with recombinant gp160. *J. Clin. Investig.* 92:919–928.

2312. Kovacs, J. A., S. Vogel, J. M. Albert, J. Falloon, R. T. Davey, Jr., R. E. Walker, M. A. Polis, K. Spooner, J. A. Metcalf, M. Baseler, G. Fyfe, and H. C. Lane. 1996. Controlled trial of interleukin-2 infusions in patients infected with the human immunodeficiency virus. *N. Engl. J. Med.* 335:1350–1356.

2313. Koval, V., C. Clark, M. Vaishnav, S. A. Spector, and D. H. Spector. 1991. Human cytomegalovirus inhibits human immunodeficiency virus replication in cells productively infected by both viruses. *J. Virol.* 65:6969–6978.

2314. Kowalski, M., L. Bergeron, T. Dorfman, W. Haseltine, and J. Sodroski. 1991. Attenuation of human immunodeficiency virus type 1 cytopathic effect by a mutation affecting the transmembrane envelope glycoprotein. *J. Virol.* 65:281–291.

2315. Kowalski, M., J. Potz, L. Basiripour, T. Dorfman, W. C. Goh, E. Terwilliger, A. Dayton, C. Rosen, W. Haseltine, and J. Sodroski. 1987. Functional regions of the envelope glycoprotein of human immunodeficiency virus type 1. *Science* 237:1351–1355.

2316. Koyanagi, Y., S. Miles, R. T. Mitsuyasu, J. E. Merrill, H. V. Vinters, and I. S. Y. Chen. 1987. Dual infection of the central nervous system by AIDS viruses with distinct cellular tropisms. *Science* 236:819–822.

2317. Koyanagi, Y., W. A. O'Brien, J. Q. Zhao, D. W. Golde, J. C. Gasson, and I. S. Y. Cheng. 1988. Cytokines alter production of HIV-1 from primary mononuclear phagocytes. *Science* 241:1673–1675.

2318. Kozak, C. A., and A. Chakraborti. 1996. Single amino acid changes in the murine leukemia virus capsid protein gene define the target of Fv1 resistance. *Virology* 225:300–305.

2319. Kozak, S. L., E. J. Platt, N. Madani, F. E. Ferro, K. Peden, and D. Kabat. 1997. CD4, CXCR-4, and CCR-5 dependencies for infections by primary patient and laboratory-adapted isolates of human immunodeficiency virus type 1. *J. Virol.* 71:873–882.

2320. Kozal, M. J., R. W. Shafer, M. A. Winters, D. A. Katzenstein, and T. C. Merigan. 1993. A mutation in human immunodeficiency virus reverse transcriptase and decline in CD4 lymphocyte numbers in long-term zidovudine recipients. *J. Infect. Dis.* 167:526–532.

2321. Kozlowski, P. A., K. P. Black, L. Shen, and S. Jackson. 1995. High prevalence of serum IgA HIV-1 infection-enhancing antibodies in HIV-infected persons. Masking by IgG. *J. Immunol.* 154:6163–6173.

2322. Kozlowski, P. A., D. Chen, J. H. Eldridge, and S. Jackson. 1994. Contrasting IgA and IgG neutralization capacities and responses to HIV type 1 gp120 V3 loop in HIV-infected individuals. *AIDS Res. Hum. Retrovir.* 10:813–822.

2323. Kozlowski, P. A., S. B. Williams, R. M. Lynch, T. P. Flanigan, R. R. Patterson, S. Cu-Uvin, and M. R. Neutra. 2002. Differential induction of mucosal and systemic antibody responses in women after nasal, rectal, or vaginal immunization: influence of the menstrual cycle. *J. Immunol.* 169:566–574.

2324. Kramer, B., A. Pelchen-Matthews, M. Deneka, E. Garcia, V. Piguet, and M. Marsh. 2005. HIV interaction with endosomes in macrophages and dendritic cells. *Blood Cells Mol. Dis.* 35:136–142.

2325. Kramer-Hammerle, S., I. Rothenaigner, H. Wolff, J. E. Bell, and R. Brack-Werner. 2005. Cells of the central nervous system as targets and reservoirs of the human immunodeficiency virus. *Virus Res.* 111:194–213.

2326. Kreiss, J. K., R. Coombs, F. Plummer, K. K. Holmes, B. Nikora, W. Cameron, E. Ngugu, J. O. N. Achola, and L. Corey. 1989. Isolation of human immunodeficiency virus from genital ulcers in Nairobi prostitutes. *J. Infect. Dis.* 160:380–384.

2327. Kremer, M., and B. S. Schnierle. 2005. HIV-1 Vif: HIV's weapon against the cellular defense factor APOBEC3G. *Curr. HIV Res.* 3:339–344.

2328. Krieg, A. M. 2002. CpG motifs in bacterial DNA and their immune defects. *Annu. Rev. Immunol.* 20:709–760.

2329. Krieger, J. N., R. W. Coombs, A. C. Collier, S. O. Ross, K. Chaloupka, D. K. Cummings, V. L. Murphy, and L. Corey. 1991. Recovery of human immunodeficiency virus type 1 from semen: minimal impact of stage of infection and current antiviral chemotherapy. *J. Infect. Dis.* 163:386–388.

2330. Krieger, J. N., R. W. Coombs, A. C. Collier, S. O. Ross, C. Speck, and L. Corey. 1995. Seminal shedding of human immunodeficiency virus type 1 and human cytomegalovirus: evidence for different immunologic controls. *J. Infect. Dis.* 171:1018–1022.

2331. Krishnan, A., A. Molina, J. Zaia, D. Smith, D. Vasquez, N. Kogut, P. M. Falk, J. Rosenthal, J. Alvarnas, and S. J. Forman. 2005. Durable remissions with autologous stem cell transplantation for high-risk HIV-associated lymphomas. *Blood* 105:874–878.

2332. Kroon, F. P., G. F. Rimmelzwaan, M. T. L. Roos, A. M. E. Osterhaus, D. Hamann, F. Miedema, and J. T. vanDissel. 1998. Restored humoral immune response to influenza vaccination in HIV-infected adults treated with highly active antiretroviral therapy. *AIDS* 12:F217–F223.

2333. Krown, S. E. 1988. AIDS-associated Kaposi's sarcoma: pathogenesis, clinical course and treatment. *AIDS* 2:71–80.

2334. Krzysiek, R., A. Rudent, L. Bouchet-Delbos, A. Foussat, C. Boutillion, A. Porter, D. Ingrand, D. Sereni, L. Galanaud-Keros, D. Emile, and the AR-NRS 086 PRIMOFERON A Study Group. 2001. Preferential and persistent depletion of CCR5+ T-helper lymphocytes with nonlymphoid homing potential despite early treatment of primary HIV infection. *Blood* 98:3169–3171.

2335. Kuchtey, J., P. J. Chefalo, R. C. Gray, L. Ramachandra, and C. V. Harding. 2005. Enhancement of dendritic cell antigen cross-presentation by CpG DNA involves type I IFN and stabilization of class I MHC mRNA. *J. Immunol.* 175:2244–2251.

2336. Kuhmann, S. E., E. J. Platt, S. L. Kozak, and D. Kabat. 2000. Cooperation of multiple CCR5 coreceptors is required for infections by human immunodeficiency virus type 1. *J. Virol.* 74:7005–7015.

2337. Kuhn, L., E. J. Abrams, P. B. Matheson, P. A. Thomas, G. Lambert, M. Bamji, B. Greenberg, R. W. Steketee, and D. M. Thea. 1997. Timing of maternal-infant HIV transmission: associations between intrapartum factors and early polymerase chain reaction results. *AIDS* 11:429–435.

2338. Kuhnel, H., H. von Briesen, U. Dietrich, M. Adamski, D. Mix, L. Biesert, R. Kreutz, A. Immelmann, K. Henco, C. Meichsner, R. Adreesen, H. Gelderblom, and H. Rubsamen-Waigmann. 1989. Molecular cloning of two West African human immunodeficiency virus type 2 isolates that replicate well in macrophages: a Gambian isolate, from a patient with neurologic acquired immunodeficiency syndrome, and a highly divergent Ghanian isolate. *Proc. Natl. Acad. Sci. USA* 86:2383–2387.

2339. Kuiken, C. A., J.-J. deJong, E. Baan, W. Keulen, M. Tersmette, and J. Goudsmit. 1992. Evolution of the V3 envelope domain in proviral sequences and isolates of human immunodeficiency virus type 1 during transition of the viral biological phenotype. *J. Virol.* 66:4622–4627.

2340. **Kuiken, C. I., B. Foley, E. Freed, B. Hahn, B. Korber, P. A. Marx, F. McCutchan, J. W. Mellors, and S. Wolinsky.** 2002. *Sequence Compendium LA-UR 03–3564.* Los Alamos National Laboratory, Los Alamos, N.M.

2341. **Kuiken, C. L., G. Zwart, E. Baan, R. A. Coutinho, A. R. van den Hoek, and J. Goudsmit.** 1993. Increasing antigenic and genetic diversity of the V3 variable domain of the human immunodeficiency virus envelope protein in the course of the AIDS epidemic. *Proc. Natl. Acad. Sci. USA* 90:9061–9065.

2342. **Kulkosky, J., and R. J. Pomerantz.** 2002. Approaching eradication of highly active antiretroviral therapy—persistent human immunodeficiency virus type 1 reservoirs with immune activation therapy. *Clin. Infect. Dis.* 35:1520–1526.

2343. **Kumar, A., S. Mukherjee, J. Shen, S. Buch, Z. Li, I. Adany, Z. Liu, W. Zhuge, M. Piatak, J. Lifson, H. McClure, and O. Narayan.** 2002. Immunization of macaques with live simian human immunodeficiency virus (SHIV) vaccines conferred protection against AIDS induced by homologous and heterologous SHIVs and simian immunodeficiency virus. *Virology* 301:189–205.

2344. **Kumar, M., L. Resnick, D. Loewenstein, J. Berger, and C. Eisdorfer.** 1989. Brain reactive antibodies and the AIDS dementia complex. *J. Acquir. Immune Defic. Syndr.* 2:469–471.

2345. **Kumar, P., H. X. Hui, J. C. Kappes, B. S. Haggarty, J. A. Hoxie, S. K. Arya, G. M. Shaw, and B. H. Hahn.** 1990. Molecular characterization of an attenuated human immunodeficiency virus type 2 isolate. *J. Virol.* 64:890–901.

2346. **Kumar, R., C. Torres, Y. Yamamura, I. Rodriguez, M. Martinez, S. Staprans, R. M. Donahoe, E. Kraiselburd, E. B. Stephens, and A. Kumar.** 2004. Modulation by morphine of viral set point in rhesus macaques infected with simian immunodeficiency virus and simian-human immunodeficiency virus. *J. Virol.* 78:11425–11428.

2347. **Kundu, S. K., D. Katzenstein, L. E. Moses, and T. C. Merigan.** 1992. Enhancement of human immunodeficiency virus HIV-specific CD4+ and CD8+ cytotoxic T-lymphocyte activities in HIV-infected asymptomatic patients given recombinant gp160 vaccine. *Proc. Natl. Acad. Sci. USA* 89:11204–11208.

2347a. **Kundu, S. K., and T. C. Merigan.** 1992. Equivalent recognition of HIV proteins, *env*, *gag* and *RT* by CD4+ and CD8+ cytotoxic T lymphocytes. *AIDS* 6:643–649.

2348. **Kunkel, E. J., J. Boisvert, K. Murphy, M. A. Vierra, M. C. Genovese, A. J. Wardlaw, H. B. Greenberg, M. R. Hodge, L. Wu, E. C. Butcher, and J. J. Campbell.** 2002. Expression of the chemokine receptors CCR4, CCR5, and CXCR3 by human tissue-infiltrating lymphocytes. *Am. J. Pathol.* 160:347–355.

2349. **Kuno, S., R. Ueno, and O. Hayaishi.** 1986. Prostaglandin E2 administered via anus causes immunosuppression in male but not female rats: a possible pathogenesis of acquired immune deficiency syndrome in homosexual males. *Proc. Natl. Acad. Sci. USA* 83:2682–2683.

2350. **Kuno, S., R. Ueno, O. Hayaishi, H. Nakashima, S. Harada, and N. Yamamoto.** 1986. Prostaglandin E2, a seminal constituent, facilitates the replication of acquired immune deficiency syndrome virus in vitro. *Proc. Natl. Acad. Sci. USA* 83:3487–3490.

2351. **Kunsch, C., H. T. Hartle, and B. Wigdahl.** 1989. Infection of human fetal dorsal root ganglion glial cells with human immunodeficiency virus type 1 involves an entry mechanism independent of the CD4 T4A epitope. *J. Virol.* 63:5054–5061.

2352. **Kunzi, M. S., H. Farzadegan, J. B. Margolick, D. Vlahov, and P. M. Pitha.** 1995. Identification of human immunodeficiency virus primary isolates resistant to interferon-α and correlation of prevalence to disease progression. *J. Infect. Dis.* 171:822–828.

2353. **Kunzi, M. S., and J. E. Groopman.** 1993. Identification of a novel human immunodeficiency virus strain cytopathic to megakaryocytic cells. *Blood* 81:3336–3342.

2353a. **Kurtz, J.** 2005. Specific memory within innate immune systems. *Trends Immunol.* 26:186–192.

2354. **Kusumi, K., B. Conway, S. Cunningham, A. Berson, C. Evans, A. K. N. Iversen, D. Colvin, M. V. Gallo, S. Coutre, E. G. Shpaer, D. V. Faulkner, A. DeRonde, S. Volkman, C. Williams, M. S. Hirsch, and J. I. Mullins.** 1992. Human immunodeficiency virus type 1 envelope gene structure and diversity in vivo and after cocultivation in vitro. *J. Virol.* 66:875–885.

2355. **Kutsch, O., J. Oh, A. Nath, and E. N. Benveniste.** 2000. Induction of the chemokines interleukin-8 and IP-10 by human immunodeficiency virus type 1 tat in astrocytes. *J. Virol.* 74:9214–9221.

2356. **Kutza, J., L. Crim, S. Feldman, M. P. Hayes, M. Gruber, J. Beeler, and K. A. Clouse.** 2000. Macrophage colony-stimulating factor antagonists inhibit replication of HIV-1 in human macrophages. *J. Immunol.* 164:4955–4960.

2357. **Kutza, J., M. P. Hayes, and K. A. Clouse.** 1998. Interleukin-2 inhibits HIV-1 replication in human macrophages by modulating expression of CD4 and CC-chemokine receptor-5. *AIDS* 12:F59–F64.

2358. **Kutzler, M. A., and D. B. Weiner.** 2004. Developing DNA vaccines that call to dendritic cells. *J. Clin. Investig.* 114:1241–1244.

2359. **Kuznetsov, Y. G., J. G. Victoria, W. E. Robinson, Jr., and A. McPherson.** 2003. Atomic force microscopy investigation of human immunodeficiency virus (HIV) and HIV-infected lymphocytes. *J. Virol.* 77:11896–11909.

2360. **Kwa, D., B. Boeser-Nunnink, and H. Schuitemaker.** 2003. Lack of evidence for an association between a polymorphism in CX3CR1 and the clinical course of HIV infection or virus phenotype evolution. *AIDS* 17:759–777.

2361. **Kwa, D., R. P. van Rij, B. Boeser-Nunnink, J. Vingerhoed, and H. Schuitemaker.** 2003. Association between an interleukin-4 promoter polymorphism and the acquisition of CXCR4 using HIV-1 variants. *AIDS* 17:981–985.

2362. **Kwa, D., J. Vingerhoed, B. Boeser, and H. Schuitemaker.** 2003. Increased in vitro cytopathicity of CC chemokine receptor 5-restricted human immunodeficiency virus type 1 primary isolates correlates with a progressive clinical course of infection. *J. Infect. Dis.* 187:1397–1403.

2363. **Kwa, D., J. Vingerhoed, B. Boeser-Nunnink, S. Broersen, and H. Schuitemaker.** 2001. Cytopathic effects of non-syncytium-inducing and syncytium-inducing human immunodeficiency virus type 1 variants on different CD4(+)-T-cell subsets are determined only by coreceptor expression. *J. Virol.* 75:10455–10459.

2364. **Kwak, L. W., M. Wilson, L. M. Weiss, S. J. Horning, R. A. Warnke, and R. F. Dorfman.** 1991. Clinical significance of morphologic subdivision in diffuse large cell lymphoma. *Cancer* 68:1988–1993.

2365. Kwok, S., D. H. Mack, K. B. Mullis, B. Poiesz, G. Ehrlich, D. Blair, A. Friedman-Kien, and J. J. Sninksy. 1987. Identification of human immunodeficiency virus sequences by using in vitro enzymatic amplification and oligomer cleavage detection. *J. Virol.* 61:1690–1694.

2366. Kwon, D. S., G. Gregorio, N. Bitton, W. A. Hendrickson, and D. R. Littman. 2002. DC-SIGN-mediated internalization of HIV is required for trans-enhancement of T cell infection. *Immunity* 16:135–144.

2367. Kwong, P. D., M. L. Doyle, D. J. Casper, C. Cicala, S. A. Leavitt, S. Majeed, T. D. Steenbeke, M. Venturi, I. Chaiken, M. Fung, H. Katinger, P. W. Parren, J. Robinson, D. Van Ryk, L. Wang, D. R. Burton, E. Freire, R. Wyatt, J. Sodroski, W. A. Hendrickson, and J. Arthos. 2002. HIV-1 evades antibody-mediated neutralization through conformational masking of receptor-binding sites. *Nature* 420:678–682.

2368. Kwong, P. D., R. Wyatt, J. Robinson, R. W. Sweet, J. Sodroski, and W. A. Hendrickson. 1998. Structure of an HIV gp120 envelope glycoprotein in complex with the CD4 receptor and a neutralizing human antibody. *Nature* 393:648–659.

2369. Kwong, P. D., R. Wyatt, Q. J. Sattentau, J. Sodroski, and W. A. Hendrickson. 2000. Oligomeric modeling and electrostatic analysis of the gp120 envelope glycoprotein of human immunodeficiency virus. *J. Virol.* 74:1961–1972.

2370. LaBonte, J. A., N. Madani, and J. Sodroski. 2003. Cytolysis by CCR5-using human immunodeficiency virus type 1 envelope glycoproteins is dependent on membrane fusion and can be inhibited by high levels of CD4 expression. *J. Virol.* 77:6645–6659.

2371. LaBranche, C. C., T. L. Hoffman, J. Romano, B. S. Haggarty, T. G. Edwards, T. J. Matthews, R. W. Doms, and J. A. Hoxie. 1999. Determinants of CD4 independence for a human immunodeficiency virus type 1 variant map outside regions required for coreceptor specificity. *J. Virol.* 73:10310–10319.

2372. Lacey, S. F., C. B. McDanal, R. Horuk, and M. L. Greenberg. 1997. The CXC chemokine stromal cell-derived factor 1 is not responsible for CD8+ T cell suppression of syncytia-inducing strains of HIV-1. *Proc. Natl. Acad. Sci. USA* 94:9842–9847.

2373. Lafeuillade, A., C. Poggi, G. Higginger, E. Counillon, and D. Emilie. 2003. Predictors of plasma human immunodeficiency virus type 1 RNA control after discontinuation of highly active antiretroviral therapy initiated at acute infection combined with structured treatment interruptions and immune based therapies. *J. Infect. Dis.* 188:1426–1492.

2374. Lafeuillade, A., C. Poggi, and C. Tamalet. 1996. GM-CSF increases HIV-1 load. *Lancet* 347:1123–1124.

2375. Lafeuillade, A., C. Tamalet, P. Pellegrino, C. Tourres, N. Yahi, C. Vignoli, R. Quilichini, and P. de Micco. 1993. High viral burden in lymph nodes during early stages of HIV-1 infection. *AIDS* 11:1527–1541.

2376. Lafeuillade, A., C. Tamalet, C. Poggi, P. Pellegrino, C. Tourres, and J. Izopet. 1997. Antiretroviral effect of zidovudine-didanosine combination on blood and lymph nodes. *AIDS* 11:67–72.

2377. Lafon, M.-E., A.-M. Steffan, C. Royer, D. Jaeck, A. Beretz, A. Kirn, and J.-L. Gendrault. 1994. HIV-1 infection induces functional alterations in human liver endothelial cells in primary culture. *AIDS* 8:747–752.

2378. Lafrenie, R. M., L. M. Wahl, J. S. Epstein, I. K. Hewlett, K. M. Yamada, and S. Dhawan. 1996. HIV-1-Tat modulates the function of monocytes and alters their interactions with microvessel endothelial cells. *J. Immunol.* 156:1638–1645.

2379. Laga, M., A. Manoka, M. Kivuvu, B. Malele, M. Tuliza, N. Nzila, J. Goeman, F. Behets, V. Batter, M. Alary, W. L. Heyward, R. W. Ryder, and P. Piot. 1993. Non-ulcerative sexually transmitted diseases as risk factors for HIV-1 transmission in women: results from a cohort study. *AIDS* 7:95–102.

2380. Lagaye, S., M. Derrien, E. Menu, C. Coito, E. Tresoldi, P. Mauclere, G. Scarlatti, G. Chaouat, F. Barre-Sinoussi, and M. Bomsel. 2001. Cell-to-cell contact results in a selective translocation of maternal human immunodeficiency virus type 1 quasispecies across a trophoblastic barrier by both transcytosis and infection. *J. Virol.* 75:4780–4791.

2381. Lahdevirta, J., C. P. J. Maury, A. M. Teppo, and H. Repo. 1988. Elevated levels of circulating cachectin/tumor necrosis factor in patients with acquired immunodeficiency syndrome. *Am. J. Med.* 85:289–291.

2382. Lai, H., S. Lai, G. Shor-Posner, F. Ma, E. Trapido, and M. K. Baum. 2001. Plasma zinc, copper, copper:zinc ratio, and survival in a cohort of HIV- 1-infected homosexual men. *J. Acquir. Immune Defic. Syndr.* 27:56–62.

2383. Lajoie, J., J. Hargrove, L. S. Zijenah, J. H. Humphrey, B. J. Ward, and M. Roger. 2006. Genetic variants in nonclassical major histocompatibility complex class I human leukocyte antigen (HLA)-E and HLA-G molecules are associated with susceptibility to heterosexual acquisition of HIV-1. *J. Infect. Dis.* 193:298–301.

2384. Lallemant, M., A. Baillou, S. Lallemant-Le Coeur, S. Nzingoula, M. Mampaka, P. M. Pele, F. Barin, and M. Essex. 1994. Maternal antibody response at delivery and perinatal transmission of human immunodeficiency virus type 1 in African women. *Lancet* 343:1001–1005.

2385. Lallemant, M., G. Jourdain, S. Le Coeur, S. Kim, S. Koetsawang, A. M. Comeau, W. Phoolcharoen, M. Essex, K. McIntosh, and V. Vithayasai. 2000. A trial of shortened zidovudine regimens to prevent mother-to-child transmission of human immunodeficiency virus type 1. *N. Engl. J. Med.* 343:982–991.

2386. Lamarre, D., A. Ashkenazi, S. Fleury, D. H. Smith, R.-P. Sekaly, and D. J. Capon. 1989. The MHC-binding and gp120-binding functions of CD4 are separable. *Science* 245:743–746.

2387. Lamb, R. A., and L. H. Pinto. 1997. Do Vpu and Vpr of human immunodeficiency virus type 1 and NB of influenza B virus have ion channel activities in the viral life cycles? *Virology* 229:1–11.

2388. Lambotte, O., M. Chaix, B. Gubler, N. Nasreddine, C. Wallon, C. Goujard, C. Rouzioux, Y. Taoufik, and J. Delfraissy. 2004. The lymphocyte HIV reservoir in patients on long-term HAART is a memory of virus evolution. *AIDS* 18:1147–1158.

2389. Lamers, S. L., J. W. Sleasman, J. X. She, K. A. Barrie, S. M. Pomeroy, D. J. Barrett, and M. M. Goodenow. 1993. Independent variation and positive selection in env V1 and V2 domains within maternal-infant strains of human immunodeficiency virus type 1 in vivo. *J. Virol.* 67:3951–3960.

2390. Lamhamedi-Cherradi, S., B. Culmann-Penciolelli, B. Guy, T. D. Ly, C. Goujard, J.-G. Guillet, and E. Gomard. 1995. Different patterns of HIV-1-specific cytotoxic T-lymphocyte activity after primary infection. *AIDS* 9:421–426.

2391. Lampinen, T. M., C. W. Critchlow, J. M. Kuypers, C. S. Hurt, P. J. Nelson, S. E. Hawes, R. W. Coombs, K. K. Holmes, and N. B. Kiviat. 2000. Association of antiretroviral therapy with detection of HIV-1 RNA and DNA in the anorectal mucosa of homosexual men. *AIDS* 14:F69–F75.

2392. Lampinen, T. M., S. Kulasingam, J. Min, M. Borok, L. Gwanzura, J. Lamb, K. Mahomed, G. B. Woelk, K. B. Strand, M. L. Bosch, D. C. Edelman, N. T. Constantine, D. Katzenstein, and M. A. Williams. 2000. Detection of Kaposi's sarcoma-associated herpesvirus in oral and genital secretions of Zimbabwean women. *J. Infect. Dis.* 181:1785–1790.

2393. Landau, N. R., K. A. Page, and D. R. Littman. 1991. Pseudotyping with human T-cell leukemia virus type I broadens the human immunodeficiency virus host range. *J. Virol.* 65:162–169.

2394. Landay, A., B. Ohlsson-Wilhelm, and J. V. Giorgi. 1990. Application of flow cytometry to the study of HIV infection. *AIDS* 4:479–497.

2395. Landay, A. L., M. Clerici, F. Hashemi, H. Kessler, J. A. Berzofsky, and G. M. Shearer. 1996. In vitro restoration of T cell immune function in human immunodeficiency virus-positive persons: effects of interleukin (IL)-12 and anti-IL-10. *J. Infect. Dis.* 173:1085–1091.

2396. Landay, A. L., C. Mackewicz, and J. A. Levy. 1993. An activated CD8+ T cell phenotype correlates with anti-HIV activity and asymptomatic clinical status. *Clin. Immunol. Immunopathol.* 69:106–116.

2397. Landesman, S. H., L. A. Kalish, D. N. Burns, H. Minkoff, H. E. Fox, C. Zorrilla, P. Garcia, M. G. Fowler, L. Mofenson, and R. Tuomala. 1996. Obstetrical factors and the transmission of human immunodeficiency virus type 1 from mother to child. *N. Engl. J. Med.* 334:1617–1623.

2398. Lane, H. C., J. M. Depper, W. C. Greene, G. Whalen, T. A. Walkmann, and A. S. Fauci. 1985. Qualitative analysis of immune function in patients with the acquired immunodeficiency syndrome. *N. Engl. J. Med.* 313:79–84

2399. Lane, H. C., H. Masur, L. C. Edgar, G. Whalen, A. H. Rook, and A. S. Fauci. 1983. Abnormalities of B-cell activation and immunoregulation in patients with the acquired immunodeficiency syndrome. *N. Engl. J. Med.* 309:453–458.

2400. Lane, T., A. Pettifor, S. Pascoe, A. Fiamma, and H. Rees. 2006. Heterosexual anal intercourse increases risk of HIV infection among young South African men. *AIDS* 20: 123–125.

2401. Lang, W., H. Perkins, R. E. Anderson, R. Royce, N. Jewell, and W. Winkelstein, Jr. 1989. Patterns of T lymphocyte changes with human immunodeficiency virus infection: from seroconversion to the development of AIDS. *J. Acquir. Immune Defic. Syndr.* 2:63–69.

2402. Lange, C. G., M. M. Lederman, K. Medvik, R. Asaad, M. Wild, R. Kalayjian, and H. Valdez. 2003. Nadir CD4+ T-cell count and numbers of CD28+ CD4+ T-cells predict functional responses to immunizations in chronic HIV-1 infection. *AIDS* 17:2015–2023.

2403. Lange, J. M. A., F. de Wolf, W. J. A. Krone, S. A. Danner, R. A. Coutinho, and J. Goudsmit. 1987. Decline of antibody reactivity to outer viral core protein p17 is an earlier serological marker of disease progression in human immunodeficiency virus infection than anti-p24 decline. *AIDS* 1:155–159.

2404. Lange, J. M. A., D. A. Paul, H. G. Huisman, F. de Wolf, H. van den Berg, R. A. Coutinho, S. A. Danner, J. van der Noordaa, and J. Goudsmit. 1986. Persistent HIV antigenaemia and decline of HIV core antibodies associated with transition to AIDS. *Br. Med. J.* 293:1459–1462.

2405. Langhoff, E., E. F. Terwilliger, H. J. Bos, K. H. Kalland, M. C. Poznansky, O. M. L. Bacon, and W. A. Haseltine. 1991. Replication of human immunodeficiency virus type 1 in primary dendritic cell cultures. *Proc. Natl. Acad. Sci. USA* 88: 7998–8002.

2406. Langlade-Demoyen, P., N. Ngo-Giang-Huong, F. Ferchal, and E. Oksenhendler. 1994. Human immunodeficiency virus (HIV) *nef*-specific cytotoxic T lymphocytes in noninfected heterosexual contact of HIV-infected patients. *J. Clin. Investig.* 93:1293–1297.

2407. Langlois, A. J., K. J. Weinhold, T. J. Matthews, M. L. Greenberg, and D. P. Bolognesi. 1992. The ability of certain SIV vaccines to provoke reactions against normal cells. *Science* 255:292–293.

2408. Lanier, L. L. 2005. NK cell recognition. *Annu. Rev. Immunol.* 23:225–274.

2409. Lanzavecchia, A., E. Roosnek, T. Gregory, P. Berman, and S. Abrignani. 1988. T cells can present antigens such as HIV gp120 targeted to their own surface molecules. *Nature* 334:530–532.

2410. Lapenta, C., M. Boirivant, M. Marini, S. M. Santini, M. Logozzi, M. Viora, F. Belardelli, and S. Fais. 1999. Human intestinal lamina propria lymphocytes are naturally permissive to HIV-1 infection. *Eur. J. Immunol.* 29:1202–1208.

2411. Reference deleted.

2412. Larder, B. A., P. Kellam, and S. D. Kemp. 1993. Convergent combination therapy can select viable multidrug-resistant HIV-1 in vitro. *Nature* 365:451–453.

2413. Larder, B. A., and S. D. Kemp. 1989. Multiple mutations in HIV-1 reverse transcriptase confer high-level resistance to zidovudine (AZT). *Science* 246:1155–1158.

2414. Larke, N., A. Murphy, C. Wirblich, D. Teoh, M. J. Estcourt, A. J. McMichael, P. Roy, and T. Hanke. 2005. Induction of human immunodeficiency virus type 1-specific T cells by a bluetongue virus tubule-vectored vaccine prime-recombinant modified virus Ankara boost regimen. *J. Virol.* 79:14822–14833.

2415. LaRosa, G. J., J. P. Davide, K. Weinhold, J. A. Waterbury, A. T. Profy, J. A. Lewis, A. J. Langlois, G. R. Dreesman, R. N. Boswell, P. Shadduck, L. H. Holley, M. Karplus, D. P. Bolognesi, T. J. Matthews, E. A. Emini, and S. D. Putney. 1990. Conserved sequence and structural elements in the HIV-1 principal neutralizing determinant. *Science* 249:932–935.

2416. Lascar, R. M., A. R. Lopes, R. J. Gilson, C. Dunn, R. Johnstone, A. Copas, S. Reignat, G. Webster, A. Bertoletti, and M. K. Maini. 2005. Effect of HIV infection and antiretroviral therapy on hepatitis B virus (HBV)-specific T cell responses in patients who have resolved HBV infection. *J. Infect. Dis.* 191:1169–1179.

2417. Lasky, L. A., G. Nakamura, D. H. Smith, C. Fennie, C. Shimasaki, E. Patzer, P. Berman, T. Gregory, and D. J. Capon. 1987. Delineation of a region of the human immunodeficiency virus type 1 gp120 glycoprotein critical for interaction with the CD4 receptor. *Cell* 50:975–985.

2418. Lassman, H., M. Schmied, K. Vass, and W. F. Hickey. 1993. Bone marrow derived elements and resident microglia in brain inflammation. *Glia* 7:19–24.

2419. Lassoued, K., J. P. Clauvel, S. Fegueux, S. Matheron, I. Gorin, and E. Oksenhandler. 1991. AIDS-associated Kaposi's sarcoma in female patients. *AIDS* 5:877–880.

2420. Lathey, J. L., R. D. Pratt, and S. A. Spector. 1997. Appearance of autologous neutralizing antibody correlates with reduction in virus load and phenotype switch during primary infection with human immunodeficiency virus type 1. *J. Infect. Dis.* 175:231–232.

2421. Latz, E., A. Schoenemeyer, A. Visintin, K. A. Fitzgerald, B. G. Monks, C. F. Knetter, E. Lien, N. J. Nilsen, T. Espevik, and D. T. Golenbock. 2004. TLR9 signals after translocating from the ER to CpG DNA in the lysosome. *Nat. Immunol.* 5:190–198.

2422. Lauener, R. P., S. Huttner, M. Buisoon, J. P. Hossle, M. Albisetti, J.-M. Seigneurin, R. A. Seger, and D. Nadal. 1995. T-cell death by apoptosis in vertically human immunodeficiency virus-infected children coincides with expansion of CD8+/interleukin-2 receptor-/HLA-DR+ T cells: sign of a possible role for herpes viruses as cofactors? *Blood* 86:1400–1407.

2423. Laughlin, M. A., S. Zeichner, D. Kolson, J. C. Alwine, T. Seshamma, R. J. Pomerantz, and F. Gonzalez-Scarano. 1993. Sodium butyrate treatment of cells latently infected with HIV-1 results in the expression of unspliced viral RNA. *Virology* 196:496–505.

2424. Laukkanen, T., J. Albert, K. Liitsola, S. D. Green, J. K. Carr, T. Leitner, F. E. McCutchan, and M. O. Salminen. 1999. Virtually full-length sequences of HIV type 1 subtype J reference strains. *AIDS Res. Hum. Retrovir.* 15:293–297.

2425. Launay, S., O. Hermine, M. Fontenay, G. Kroemer, E. Solary, and C. Garrido. 2005. Vital functions for lethal caspases. *Oncogene* 24:5137–5148.

2426. Laurence, J. 1990. Molecular interactions among herpesviruses and human immunodeficiency viruses. *J. Infect. Dis.* 162:338–346.

2427. Laurence, J., and S. M. Astrin. 1991. Human immunodeficiency virus induction of malignant transformation in human B lymphocytes. *Proc. Natl. Acad. Sci. USA* 88:7635–7639.

2428. Laurence, J., A. B. Gottlieb, and H. G. Kunkel. 1983. Soluble suppressor factors in patients with acquired immune deficiency syndrome and its prodrome. *J. Clin. Investig.* 72:2072–2081.

2429. Laurence, J., A. S. Hodtsev, and D. N. Posnett. 1992. Superantigen implicated in dependence of HIV-1 replication in T cells on TCR V beta expression. *Nature* 358:255–259.

2430. Laurence, J., A. Saunders, E. Early, and J. E. Salmon. 1990. Human immunodeficiency virus infection of monocytes: relationship to Fc-gamma receptors and antibody-dependent viral enhancement. *Immunology* 70:338–343.

2431. Laurence, J., M. B. Sellers, and S. Sikder. 1989. Effect of glucocorticoids on chronic human immunodeficiency virus (HIV) infection and HIV promoter-mediated transcription. *Blood* 74:291–297.

2432. Laurent-Crawford, A. G., B. Krust, S. Muller, Y. Riviere, M.-A. Rey-Cuille, J.-M. Bechet, L. Montagnier, and A. G. Hovanessian. 1991. The cytopathic effect of HIV is associated with apoptosis. *Virology* 185:829–839.

2433. Laurent-Crawford, A. G., B. Krust, Y. Riviere, C. Desgranges, S. Muller, M. P. Kieny, C. Dauguet, and A. G. Hovanessian. 1993. Membrane expression of HIV envelope glycoproteins triggers apoptosis in CD4 cells. *AIDS Res. Hum. Retrovir.* 9:761–773.

2434. Lauvau, G., K. Kakimi, G. Niedermann, M. Ostankovitch, P. Yotnda, H. Firat, F. V. Chisari, and P. M. van Endert. 1999. Human transporters associated with antigen processing (TAPs) select epitope precursor peptides for processing in the endoplasmic reticulum and presentation to T cells. *J. Exp. Med.* 190:1227–1240.

2435. Lavreys, L., M. L. Thompson, H. L. Martin, Jr, K. Mandaliya, J. O. Ndinya-Achola, J. J. Bwayo, and J. Kreiss. 2000. Primary human immunodeficiency virus type 1 infection: clinical manifestations among women in Mombasa, Kenya. *Clin. Infect. Dis.* 30:486–490.

2436. Lavrik, I., A. Golks, and P. H. Krammer. 2005. Death receptor signaling. *J. Cell Sci.* 118:265–267.

2436a. Lawrence, J., K. H. B. Hullsiek, L. M. Thackeray, D. I. Abrams, L. R. Crane, D. L. Mayers, M. C. Jones, J. M. Saldanha, B. S. Schmetter, and J. D. Baxter. 2006. Disadvantages of structured treatment interruption persist in patients with multidrug-resistant HIV-1: final results of the CPCRA 064 study. *J. Acquir. Immune Defic. Syndr.* 43:169–178.

2437. Lawrence, J., D. L. Mayers, K. H. Hullsiek, G. Collins, D. I. Abrams, R. B. Reisler, L. R. Crane, B. S. Schmetter, T. J. Dionne, J. M. Saldanha, M. C. Jones, and J. D. Baxter. 2003. Structured treatment interruption in patients with multi-drug-resistant human immunodeficiency virus. *N. Engl. J. Med.* 349:837–846.

2438. Layne, S. P., M. J. Merges, M. Dembo, J. L. Spouge, S. R. Conley, J. P. Moore, J. L. Raina, H. Renz, H. R. Gelderblom, and P. L. Nara. 1992. Factors underlying spontaneous inactivation and susceptibility to neutralization of human immunodeficiency virus. *Virology* 189:695–714.

2439. Layne, S. P., M. J. Merges, J. L. Spouge, M. Dembo, and P. L. Nara. 1991. Blocking of human immunodeficiency virus infection depends on cell density and viral stock age. *J. Virol.* 65:3293–3300.

2440. Layton, G. T., S. J. Harris, A. J. H. Gearing, M. Hill-Perkins, J. S. Cole, J. C. Griffiths, N. R. Burns, A. J. Kingsman, and S. E. Adams. 1993. Induction of HIV-specific cytotoxic T lymphocytes in vivo with hybrid HIV-1 V3: Ty-virus-like particles. *J. Immunol.* 151:1097–1107.

2441. Lazzarin, A., B. Clotet, D. Cooper, J. Reynes, K. Arastéh, M. Nelson, C. Katlama, H.-J. Stellbrink, J.-F. Delfraissy, J. Lange, L. Huson, R. DeMasi, C. Wat, J. Delehanty, C. Drobnes, and M. Salgo. 2003. Efficacy of enfuvirtide in patients infected with drug-resistant HIV-1 in Europe and Australia. *N. Engl. J. Med.* 35:2186–2195.

2442. Le Bon, A., and D. F. Tough. 2002. Links between innate and adaptive immunity via type I interferon. *Curr. Opin. Immunol.* 14:432–436.

2443. Le Borgne, S., M. Fevrier, C. Callebaut, S. P. Lee, and Y. Riviere. 2000. CD8+ cell antiviral factor activity is not restricted to human immunodeficiency virus (HIV)-specific T cells and can block HIV replication after initiation of reverse transcription. *J. Virol.* 74:4456–4464.

2444. Le Gall, S., M.-C. Prevost, J.-M. Heard, and O. Schwartz. 1997. Human immunodeficiency virus type 1 Nef independently affects virion incorporation of major histocompatibility complex class I molecules and virus infectivity. *Virology* 229:295–301.

2445. Le Rouzic, E., A. Mousnier, C. Rustum, F. Stutz, E. Hallberg, C. Dargemont, and S. Benichou. 2002. Docking of HIV-1 Vpr to the nuclear envelope is mediated by the interaction with the nucleoporin hCG1. *J. Biol. Chem.* 277:45091–45098.

2446. Leandersson, A., G. Gilljam, M. Fredriksson, J. Hinkula, A. Alaeus, K. Lidman, J. Albert, G. Bratt, E. Sandstrom, and B. Wahren. 2000. Cross-reactive T-helper responses in patients infected with different subtypes of human immunodeficiency virus type 1. *J. Virol.* 74:4888–4890.

2447. Learmont, J. C., A. F. Geczy, J. Mills, L. J. Ashton, C. H. Raynes-Greenow, R. J. Garsia, W. B. Dyer, L. McIntyre, R. B. Oelrichs, D. I. Rhodes, N. J. Deacon, and J. S. Sullivan. 1999. Immunologic and virologic status after 14 to 18 years of infection with an attenuated strain of HIV-1. A report from the Sydney Blood Bank Cohort. *N. Engl. J. Med.* 340:1715–1722.

2448. Learn, G. H., D. Muthui, S. J. Brodie, T. Zhu, K. Diem, J. I. Mullins, and L. Corey. 2002. Virus population homogenization following acute human immunodeficiency virus type 1 infection. *J. Virol.* 76:11953–11959.

2449. Lecatsas, G., S. Houff, A. Macher, E. Gelman, R. Steis, C. Reichert, H. Masur, and J. L. Sever. 1985. Retrovirus-like particles in salivary glands, prostate and testes of AIDS patients. *Proc. Soc. Exp. Biol. Med.* 178:653–655.

2450. Lech, W. J., G. Wang, Y. L. Yang, Y. Chee, K. Dorman, D. McCrae, L. C. Lazzeroni, J. W. Erickson, J. S. Sinsheimer, and A. H. Kaplan. 1996. In vivo sequence diversity of the protease of human immunodeficiency virus type 1: presence of protease inhibitor-resistant variants in untreated subjects. *J. Virol.* 70:2038–2043.

2451. Lecossier, D., F. Bouchonnet, F. Clavel, and A. J. Hance. 2003. Hypermutation of HIV-1 DNA in the absence of the Vif protein. *Science* 300:1112.

2452. Lederman, M. M., L. A. Kalish, D. Asmuth, E. Fiebig, M. Mileno, and M. P. Busch. 2000. 'Modeling' relationships among HIV-1 replication, immune activation and CD4+ T-cell losses using adjusted correlative analyses. *AIDS* 14:951–958.

2453. Lederman, M. M., S. F. Purvis, E. I. Walter, J. T. Carey, and M. E. Medof. 1989. Heightened complement sensitivity of acquired immunodeficiency syndrome lymphocytes related to diminished expression of decay-accelerating factor. *Proc. Natl. Acad. Sci. USA* 86:4205–4209.

2453a. Lederman, M. M., L. Smeaton, K. Y. Smith, B. Rodriguez, M. Pu, H. Wang, A. Sevin, P. Tebas, S. F. Sieg, K. Medvik, D. M. Margolis, R. Pollard, H. C. Ertl, and H. Valdez. 2006. Cyclosporin A provides no sustained immunologic benefit to persons with chronic HIV-1 infection starting suppressive antiretroviral therapy: results of a randomized, controlled trial of the AIDS Clinical Trials Group A5138. *J. Infect. Dis.* 194:1677–1685.

2454. Lederman, M. M., R. S. Veazey, R. Offord, D. E. Mosier, J. Dufour, M. Mefford, M. Piatak, Jr., J. D. Lifson, J. R. Salkowitz, B. Rodriguez, A. Baluvelt, and O. Hartley. 2004. Prevention of vaginal SHIV transmission in rhesus macaques through inhibition of CCR5. *Science* 306:485–487.

2455. Ledru, E., N. Christeff, O. Patey, P. de Truchis, J. C. Melchior, and M. L. Gougeon. 2000. Alteration of tumor necrosis factor-alpha T-cell homeostasis following potent antiretroviral therapy: contribution to the development of human immunodeficiency virus-associated lipodystrophy syndrome. *Blood* 95:3191–3198.

2456. Ledru, E., H. Lecoeur, S. Garcia, T. Debord, and M. L. Gougeon. 1998. Differential susceptibility to activation-induced apoptosis among peripheral Th1 subsets: correlation with Bcl-2 expression and consequences for AIDs pathogenesis. *J. Immunol.* 160:3194–3206.

2457. Lee, B., B. J. Doranz, S. Rana, Y. Yi, M. Mellado, J. M. R. Frade, C. Martinez-A, S. J. O'Brien, J. Dean, R. G. Collman, and R. W. Doms. 1998. Influence of the CCR2-V64I polymorphism on human immunodeficiency virus type 1 coreceptor activity and on chemokine receptor function of CCR2b, CCR3, CCR5, and CXCR4. *J. Virol.* 72:7450–7458.

2458. Lee, B., M. Sharron, L. J. Montaner, D. Weissman, and R. W. Doms. 1999. Quantification of CD4, CCR5, and CXCR4 levels on lymphocyte subsets, dendritic cells, and differentially conditioned monocyte-derived macrophages. *Proc. Natl. Acad. Sci. USA* 96:5215–5220.

2459. Lee, E. J., R. Kantor, L. Zijenah, W. Sheldon, L. Emel, P. Mateta, E. Johnston, J. Wells, A. K. Shetty, H. Coovadia, Y. Maldonado, S. A. Jones, L. M. Mofenson, C. Contag, M. Bassett, and D. A. Katzenstein. 2005. Breast-milk shedding of drug-resistant HIV-1 subtype C in women exposed to single-dose nevirapine. *J. Infect. Dis.* 192:126–1264.

2460. Lee, G. A., M. N. Rao, and C. Grunfeld. 2004. The effects of HIV protease inhibitors on carbohydrate and lipid metabolism. *Curr. Infect. Dis. Rep.* 6:471–482.

2461. Lee, G. A., T. Seneviratne, M. A. Noor, J. C. Lo, J. Schwatz, F. T. Aweeka, K. Mulligan, M. Schambelan, and C. Grunfeld. 2004. The metabolic effects of lopinavir/ritonavir in HIV-negative men. *AIDS* 18:641–649.

2462. Lee, H., R. Veazey, K. Williams, M. Li, J. Guo, F. Neipel, B. Fleckenstein, A. Lackner, R. C. Desrosiers, and J. U. Jung. 1998. Deregulation of cell growth by the K1 gene of Kaposi's sarcoma-associated herpesvirus. *Nat. Med.* 4:435–440.

2463. Lee, S., C. K. Lapham, H. Chen, L. King, J. Manischewitz, T. Romantseva, H. Mostowski, T. S. Stantchev, C. C. Broder, and H. Golding. 2000. Coreceptor competition for association with CD4 may change the susceptibility of human cells to infection with T-tropic and macrophagetropic isolates of human immunodeficiency virus type 1. *J. Virol.* 74:5016–5023.

2464. Lee, S., H. L. Tiffany, L. King, P. M. Murphy, H. Golding, and M. B. Zaitseva. 2000. CCR8 on human thymocytes functions as a human immunodeficiency virus type 1 coreceptor. *J. Virol.* 74:6946–6952.

2465. Lee, S. K., D. M. Dykxhoorn, P. Kumar, S. Ranjbar, E. Song, L. E. Maliszewski, V. Francois-Bongarcon, A. Goldfeld, N. M. Swamy, J. Lieberman, and P. Shankar. 2005. Lentiviral delivery of short hairpin RNAs protects CD4 T cells from multiple clades and primary isolates of HIV. *Blood* 106:818–826.

2466. Lee, S. K., Z. Xu, J. Lieberman, and P. Shankar. 2002. The functional CD8 T cell response to HIV becomes type-specific in progressive disease. *J. Clin. Investig.* 110:1339–1347.

2467. Lee, T. H., H. W. Sheppard, M. Reis, D. Dondero, D. Osmond, and M. P. Busch. 1994. Circulating HIV-1-infected cell burden from seroconversion to AIDS: importance of postseroconversion viral load on disease course. *J. Acquir. Immune Defic. Syndr.* 7:381–388.

2468. Lee, W.-R., W.-J. Syu, B. Du, M. Matsuda, S. Tan, A. Wolf, M. Essex, and T.-H. Lee. 1992. Nonrandom distribution of gp120 N-linked glycosylation sites important for infectivity of human immunodeficiency virus type 1. *Proc. Natl. Acad. Sci. USA* 89:2213–2217.

2469. Lee, W. T., G. Pasos, L. Cecchini, and J. N. Mittler. 2002. Continued antigen stimulation is not required during CD4(+) T cell clonal expansion. *J. Immunol.* 168:1682–1689.

2470. Lefevre, E. A., R. Krzysiek, E. P. Loret, P. Galanaud, and Y. Richard. 1999. Cutting edge: HIV-1 Tat protein differentially modulates the B cell response of naive, memory, and germinal center B cells. *J. Immunol.* 163:1119–1122.

2471. Lefrere, J. J., F. Roudot-Thoraval, M. Mariotti, M. Thauvin, J. Lerable, J. Salpetrier, and L. Morand-Joubert. 1998. The risk of disease progression is determined during the first year of human immunodeficiency virus type 1 infection. *J. Infect. Dis.* 177:1541–1548.

2472. Legac, E., B. Autran, H. Merle-Beral, C. Katlama, and P. Debre. 1992. CD4+CD7-CD57+ T cells: a new T-lymphocyte subset expanded during human immunodeficiency virus infection. *Blood* 79:1746–1753.

2473. Legrain, P., B. Goud, and G. Buttin. 1986. Increase of retroviral infection in vitro by the binding of antiretrovirus antibodies. *J. Virol.* 60:1141–1144.

2474. LeGuern, M., and J. A. Levy. 1992. HIV-1 can superinfect HIV-2-infected cells: pseudotype virions produced with expanded cellular host range. *Proc. Natl. Acad. Sci. USA* 89:363–367.

2475. LeGuern, M., T. Shioda, J. A. Levy, and C. Cheng-Mayer. 1993. Single amino acid change in Tat determines the different rates of replication of two sequential HIV-1 isolates. *Virology* 195:441–447.

2476. Lehmann-Che, J., and A. Saib. 2004. Early stages of HIV replication: how to hijack cellular functions for a successful infection. *AIDS Rev.* 6:199–207.

2477. Lehner, T., L. A. Bergmeier, C. Panagiotidi, L. Tao, R. Brookes, L. S. Klavinskis, P. Walker, J. Walker, R. G. Ward, L. Hussain, A. J. H. Gearing, and S. E. Adams. 1992. Induction of mucosal and systemic immunity to a recombinant simian immunodeficiency viral protein. *Science* 258:1365–1369.

2478. Lehner, T., R. Brookes, C. Panagiotodi, L. Tao, L. S. Klavinskis, J. Walker, P. Walker, R. Ward, L. Hussain, A. J. H. Gearing, S. E. Adams, and L. A. Bergmeier. 1993. T- and B-cell functions and epitope expression in nonhuman primates immunized with simian immunodeficiency virus antigen by the rectal route. *Proc. Natl. Acad. Sci. USA* 90:8638–8642.

2479. Lehner, T., G. M. Shearer, C. J. Hackett, A. Schultz, and O. K. Sharma. 2000. Alloimmunization as a strategy for vaccine design against HIV/AIDS. *AIDS Res. Hum. Retrovir.* 16:309–313.

2480. Lehner, T., Y. Wang, L. Ping, L. Bergmeier, E. Mitchell, M. Cranage, G. Hall, M. Dennis, N. Cook, C. Doyle, and I. Jones. 1999. The effect of route of immunization on mucosal immunity and protection. *J. Infect. Dis.* 179:S489–S492.

2481. Lehrman, G., I. B. Hogue, S. Palmer, C. Jennings, C. A. Spina, A. Wiegand, A. L. Landay, R. W. Coombs, D. D. Richman, J. W. Mellors, J. M. Coffin, R. J. Bosch, and D. M. Margolis. 2005. Depletion of latent HIV-1 infection in vivo: a proof-of-concept study. *Lancet* 366:549–555.

2482. Leigh Brown, A. J., S. D. W. Frost, W. C. Mathews, K. Dawson, N. S. Hellmann, E. S. Daar, D. D. Richman, and S. J. Little. 2003. Transmission fitness of drug-resistant human immunodeficiency virus and the prevalence of resistance in the antiretroviral-treated population. *J. Infect. Dis.* 187:683–686.

2483. Leigh Brown, A. J., and E. C. Holmes. 1994. Evolutionary biology of human immunodeficiency virus. *Annu. Rev. Ecol. Syst.* 25:127–165.

2484. Leis, J., D. Baltimore, J. M. Bishop, J. Coffin, E. Fleissner, S. P. Goff, S. Oroszlan, H. Robinson, A. M. Skalka, H. M. Temin, and V. Vogt. 1988. Standardized and simplified nomenclature for proteins common to all retroviruses. *J. Virol.* 62:1808–1809.

2485. Leith, J. G., K. F. T. Copeland, P. J. McKay, C. D. Richards, and K. L. Rosenthal. 1997. CD8+ T-cell-mediated suppression

of HIV-1 long terminal repeat-driven gene expression is not modulated by the CC chemokines RANTES, macrophage inflammatory protein (MIP)-1α and MIP-1β. *AIDS* 11:575–580.

2486. Lekutis, C., J. W. Shiver, M. A. Liu, and N. L. Letvin. 1997. HIV-1 env DNA vaccine administered to rhesus monkeys elicits MHC class II-restricted CD4+ T helper cells that secrete IFN-γ and TNF-α. *J. Immunol.* 158:4471–4477.

2487. Lemey, P., O. G. Pybus, B. Wang, N. K. Saksena, M. Salemi, and A.-M. Vandamme. 2003. Tracing the origin and history of the HIV-2 epidemic. *Proc. Natl. Acad. Sci. USA* 100:6588–6592.

2488. Lempicki, R. A., J. A. Kovacs, M. W. Baseler, J. W. Adelsberger, R. L. Dewar, V. Natarajan, M. C. Bosche, J. A. Metcalf, R. A. Stevens, L. A. Lambert, W. G. Alvord, M. A. Polis, R. T. Davey, D. S. Dimitrov, and H. C. Lane. 2000. Impact of HIV-1 infection and highly active antiretroviral therapy on the kinetics of CD4+ and CD8+ T cell turnover in HIV-infected patients. *Proc. Natl. Acad. Sci. USA* 97:13778–13783.

2489. Lenardo, M. J., S. B. Angleman, V. Bounkeua, J. Dimas, M. G. Duvall, M. B. Graubard, F. Hornung, M. C. Selkirk, C. K. Speirs, C. Trageser, J. O. Orenstein, and D. L. Bolton. 2002. Cytopathic killing of peripheral blood CD4(+) T lymphocytes by human immunodeficiency virus type 1 appears necrotic rather than apoptotic and does not require env. *J. Virol.* 76:5082–5093.

2490. Lenberg, M. E., and N. R. Landau. 1993. Vpu-induced degradation of CD4: requirement for specific amino acid residues in the cytoplasmic domain of CD4. *J. Virol.* 67:7238–7245.

2491. Leng, Q., Z. Bentwich, E. Magen, A. Kalinkovich, and G. Borkow. 2002. CTLA-4 upregulation during HIV infection: association with anergy and possible target for therapeutic intervention. *AIDS* 16:519–529.

2492. Leng, Q., G. Borkow, Z. Weisman, M. Stein, A. Kalinkovich, and Z. Bentwich. 2001. Immune activation correlates better than HIV plasma viral load with CD4 T-cell decline during HIV infection. *J. Acquir. Immune Defic. Syndr.* 27:389–397.

2493. Lenkei, R., G. Bratt, V. Holmberg, K. Muirhead, and E. Sandstrom. 1998. Indicators of T-cell activation: correlation between quantitative CD38 expression and soluble CD8 levels in asymptomatic HIV+ individuals and healthy controls. *Cytometry* 33:115–122.

2494. Lennert, K., E. Kaiserling, and H. K. Muller-Hermelink. 1975. T-associated plasma-cells. *Lancet* i:1031–1032.

2495. Lennette, E. T., D. J. Blackbourn, and J. A. Levy. 1996. Antibodies to human herpesvirus type 8 in the general population and in Kaposi's sarcoma patients. *Lancet* 348:858–861.

2496. Lennette, E. T., M. P. Busch, F. M. Hecht, and J. A. Levy. 2005. Potential herpesvirus interaction during HIV type 1 primary infection. *AIDS Res. Hum. Retrovir.* 21:869–875.

2497. Leonard, C. K., M. W. Spellman, L. Riddle, R. J. Harris, J. N. Thomas, and T. J. Gregory. 1990. Assignment of intrachain disulfide bonds and characterization of potential glycosylation sites of the type 1 recombinant human immunodeficiency virus envelope glycoprotein (gp120) expressed in Chinese hamster ovary cells. *J. Biol. Chem.* 265:10373–10382.

2498. Leonard, G., A. Chaput, V. Courgnaud, A. Sangare, F. Denis, and C. Brechot. 1993. Characterization of dual HIV-1 and HIV-2 serological profiles by polymerase chain reaction. *AIDS* 7:1185–1189.

2499. Leonard, J., C. Parrott, A. J. Buckler-White, W. Turner, E. K. Ross, M. A. Martin, and A. B. Rabson. 1989. The NF-kappa B binding sites in the human immunodeficiency virus type 1 long terminal repeat are not required for virus infectivity. *J. Virol.* **63**:4919–4924.

2500. Leslie, A. J., K. J. Pfafferott, P. Chetty, R. Draenert, M. M. Addo, M. Feeney, Y. Yang, E. C. Holmes, T. Allen, J. G. Prado, M. Altfeld, C. Brander, C. Dixon, D. Ramduth, P. Jeena, S. A. Thomas, A. St. John, T. A. Roach, B. Kupfer, G. Luzzi, A. Edwards, G. Taylor, H. Lyall, G. Tudor-Williams, V. Novelli, J. Martinez-Picado, P. Kiepiela, B. D. Walker, and P. J. R. Goulder. 2004. HIV evolution: CTL escape mutation and reversion after transmission. *Nat. Med.* **10**:282–289.

2501. Lesner, A., Y. Li, J. Nitkiewicz, G. Li, A. Kartvelishvili, M. Kartvelishvili, and M. Simm. 2005. A soluble factor secreted by an HIV-1-resistant cell line blocks transcription through inactivating the DNA-binding capacity of the NF-kappa B p65/p50 dimer. *J. Immunol.* **175**:2548–2554.

2502. Letvin, N. L., J. Li, M. Halloran, M. P. Cranage, E. W. Rud, and J. Sodroski. 1995. Prior infection with a nonpathogenic chimeric simian-human immunodeficiency virus does not efficiently protect macaques against challenge with simian immunodefiency virus. *J. Virol.* **69**:4569–4571.

2503. Letvin, N. L., D. C. Montefiori, Y. Yasutomi, H. C. Perry, M. E. Davies, C. Lekutis, M. Alroy, D. C. Freed, C. I. Lord, L. K. Handt, M. A. Liu, and J. W. Shiver. 1997. Potent, protective anti-HIV immune responses generated by bimodal HIV Envelope DNA plus protein vaccination. *Proc. Natl. Acad. Sci. USA* **94**:9378–9383.

2504. Leung, L., I. K. Srivastava, E. Kan, H. Legg, Y. Sun, C. Greer, D. C. Montefiori, J. zur Megede, and S. W. Barnett. 2004. Immunogenicity of HIV-1 Env and Gag in baboons using a DNA prime/protein boost regimen. *AIDS* **18**:991–1001.

2505. Levacher, M., F. Hulstaert, S. Tallet, S. Ullery, J. J. Pocidalo, and B. A. Bach. 1992. The significance of activation markers on CD8 lymphocytes in human immunodeficiency syndrome: staging and prognostic value. *Clin. Exp. Immunol.* **90**:376–382.

2506. Levi, G., M. Patrizio, A. Bernardo, T. C. Petrucci, and C. Agresti. 1993. Human immunodeficiency virus coat protein gp120 inhibits the beta-adrenergic regulation of astroglial and microglial functions. *Proc. Natl. Acad. Sci. USA* **90**:1541–1545.

2507. Levine, A. M. 1992. Acquired immunodeficiency syndrome-related lymphoma. *Blood* **80**:8–20.

2508. Levine, A. M., S. Groshen, J. Allen, K. M. Munson, D. J. Carlo, A. E. Daigle, F. Ferre, F. C. Jensen, S. P. Richieri, R. J. Trauger, J. W. Parker, P. L. Salk, and J. Salk. 1996. Initial studies on active immunization of HIV-infected subjects using a gp120-depleted HIV-1 immunogen: long-term follow-up. *J. Acquir. Immune Defic. Syndr. Hum. Retrovirol.* **11**:351–364.

2509. Levine, B. L., W. B. Bernstein, N. E. Aronson, K. Schlienger, J. Cotte, S. Perfetto, M. J. Humphries, S. Ratto-Kim, D. L. Birx, C. Steffens, A. Landay, R. G. Carroll, and C. H. June. 2002. Adoptive transfer of costimulated CD4+ T cells induces expansion of peripheral T cells and decreased CCR5 expression in HIV infection. *Nat. Med.* **8**:47–53.

2510. Levy, D. N., G. M. Aldrovandi, O. Kutsch, and G. M. Shaw. 2004. Dynamics of HIV-1 recombination in its natural target cells. *Proc. Natl. Acad. Sci. USA* **101**:4204–4209.

2511. Levy, D. N., Y. Refaeli, and D. B. Weiner. 1995. Extracellular Vpr protein increases cellular permissiveness to human immunodeficiency virus replication and reactivates virus from latency. *J. Virol.* **69**:1243–1252.

2512. Levy, J. A. 1977. Type C RNA viruses and autoimmune disease, p. 403–453. *In* N. Talal (ed.), *Autoimmunity: Genetic, Immunologic, Virology and Clinical Aspects.* Academic Press, New York, N.Y.

2513. Levy, J. A. 1978. Xenotropic type C viruses. *Curr. Top. Microbiol. Immunol.* **79**:111–213.

2514. Levy, J. A. 1986. The multifaceted retrovirus. *Cancer Res.* **46**:5457–5468.

2515. Levy, J. A. 1988. Can an AIDS vaccine be developed? *Transfus. Med. Rev.* **2**:265–271.

2516. Levy, J. A. 1988. The mysteries of HIV: challenges for therapy and prevention. *Nature* **333**:519–522.

2517. Levy, J. A. 1988. The transmission of AIDS: the case of the infected cell. *JAMA* **259**:3037–3038.

2518. Levy, J. A. 1989. Human immunodeficiency viruses and the pathogenesis of AIDS. *JAMA* **261**:2997–3006.

2519. Levy, J. A. 1990. Changing concepts in HIV infection: challenges for the 1990's. *AIDS* **4**:1051–1058.

2520. Levy, J. A. 1993. HIV pathogenesis and long-term survival. *AIDS* **7**:1401–1410.

2521. Levy, J. A. 1993. The transmission of HIV and factors influencing progression to disease. *Am. J. Med.* **95**:86–100.

2522. Levy, J. A. 1995. HIV research: a need to focus on the right target. *Lancet* **345**:1619–1621.

2523. Levy, J. A. 1995. A new human herpesvirus: KSHV or HHV8? *Lancet* **346**:786.

2524. Levy, J. A. 1996. Infection by human immunodeficiency virus—CD4 is not enough. *N. Engl. J. Med.* **335**:1528–1530.

2525. Levy, J. A. 1996. Surrogate markers in AIDS research. Is there truth in numbers? *JAMA* **276**:161–162.

2526. Levy, J. A. 1996. The value of primate models for studying human immunodeficiency virus pathogenesis. *J. Med. Primatol.* **25**:163–174.

2527. Levy, J. A. 1997. Three new human herpesviruses (HHV6, 7, and 8). *Lancet* **349**:558–563.

2528. Levy, J. A. 2001. The importance of the innate immune system in controlling HIV infection and disease. *Trends Immunol.* **22**:312–316.

2529. Levy, J. A. 2001. What can be achieved with an HIV vaccine? *Lancet* **357**:223–224.

2530. Levy, J. A. 2002. HIV-1: hitching a ride on erythrocytes. *Lancet* **359**:2212–2213.

2531. Levy, J. A. 2003. Is HIV superinfection worrisome? *Lancet* **361**:98–99.

2532. Levy, J. A. 2003. The search for the CD8+ cell anti-HIV factor (CAF). *Trends Immunol.* **24**:628–632.

2533. Levy, J. A. 2004. Prospects for an AIDS vaccine: encourage innate immunity. *AIDS* **18**:2085–2086.

2534. Levy, J. A., C. Cheng-Mayer, D. Dina, and P. A. Luciw. 1986. AIDS retrovirus (ARV-2) clone replicates in transfected human and animal fibroblasts. *Science* **232**:998–1001.

2535. Levy, J. A., L. Evans, C. Cheng-Mayer, L.-Z. Pan, A. Lane, C. Staben, D. Dina, C. Wiley, and J. Nelson. 1987. The biologic and molecular properties of the AIDS-associated retrovirus that affect antiviral therapy. *Ann. Inst. Pasteur* **138**:101–111.

2536. Levy, J. A., and D. Greenspan. 1988. HIV in saliva. *Lancet* ii:1248.

2537. Levy, J. A., A. D. Hoffman, S. M. Kramer, J. A. Landis, J. M. Shimabukuro, and L. S. Oshiro. 1984. Isolation of lymphocytopathic retroviruses from San Francisco patients with AIDS. *Science* 225:840–842.

2538. Levy, J. A., H. Hollander, J. Shimabukuro, J. Mills, and L. Kaminsky. 1985. Isolation of AIDS-associated retrovirus from cerebrospinal fluid and brain of patients with neurological symptoms. *Lancet* ii:586–588.

2539. Levy, J. A., H. Hollander, J. Shimabukuro, J. Mills, and L. Kaminsky. 1985. Isolation of AIDS-associated retroviruses from cerebrospinal fluid and brain of patients with neurological symptoms. *Lancet* ii:586–588.

2540. Levy, J. A., F. Hsueh, D. J. Blackbourn, D. Wara, and P. S. Weintrub. 1998. CD8 cell noncytotoxic antiviral activity in human immunodeficiency virus-infected and -uninfected children. *J. Infect. Dis.* 177:470–472.

2541. Levy, J. A., L. S. Kaminsky, W. J. W. Morrow, K. Steimer, P. Luciw, D. Dina, J. Hoxie, and L. Oshiro. 1985. Infection by the retrovirus associated with the acquired immunodeficiency syndrome. *Ann. Intern. Med.* 103:694–699.

2542. Levy, J. A., A. Landay, and E. T. Lennette. 1990. HHV-6 inhibits HIV-1 replication in cell culture. *J. Clin. Microbiol.* 28:2362–2364.

2543. Levy, J. A., C. E. Mackewicz, and E. Barker. 1996. Controlling HIV pathogenesis: the role of noncytotoxic anti-HIV activity of CD8+ cells. *Immunol. Today* 17:217–224.

2544. Levy, J. A., W. Margaretten, and J. Nelson. 1989. Detection of HIV in enterochromaffin cells in the rectal mucosa of an AIDS patient. *Am. J. Gastroenterol.* 84:787–789.

2545. Levy, J. A., G. Mitra, and M. M. Mozen. 1984. Recovery and inactivation of infectious retroviruses added to factor VIII concentrates. *Lancet* ii:722–723.

2546. Levy, J. A., G. A. Mitra, M. F. Wong, and M. M. Mozen. 1985. Inactivation by wet and dry heat procedures of AIDS-associated retrovirus (ARV) during factor VIII purification from plasma. *Lancet* i:1456–1457.

2547. Levy, J. A., L.-Z. Pan, B. Beth-Giraldo, L. Kaminsky, G. Henle, W. Henle, and G. Giraldo. 1986. Absence of antibodies to the human immunodeficiency virus in sera from Africa prior to 1975. *Proc. Natl. Acad. Sci. USA* 83:7935–7937.

2548. Levy, J. A., B. Ramachandran, E. Barker, J. Guthrie, and T. Elbeik. 1996. Plasma viral load, CD4+ cell counts, and HIV-1 production by cells. *Science* 271:670–671.

2549. Levy, J. A., I. Scott, and C. Mackewicz. 2003. Protection from HIV/AIDS: the importance of innate immunity. *Clin. Immunol.* 108:167–174.

2550. Levy, J. A., and J. Shimabukuro. 1985. Recovery of AIDS-associated retroviruses from patients with AIDS or AIDS-related conditions, and from clinically healthy individuals. *J. Infect. Dis.* 152:734–738.

2551. Levy, J. A., J. Shimabukuro, T. McHugh, C. Casavant, D. Stites, and L. Oshiro. 1985. AIDS-associated retroviruses (ARV) can productively infect other cells besides human T helper cells. *Virology* 147:441–448.

2552. Levy, J. A., and J. Ziegler. 1983. Acquired immune deficiency syndrome (AIDS) is an opportunistic infection and Kaposi's sarcoma results from secondary immune stimulation. *Lancet* ii:78–81.

2553. Levy, S. B., and B. Marshall. 2004. Antibacterial resistance worldwide: causes, challenges and responses. *Nat. Med.* 10:S122–S129.

2554. Levy, Y., and J. C. Brouet. 1994. Interleukin-10 prevents spontaneous death of germinal center B cells by induction of the bcl-1 protein. *J. Clin. Investig.* 93:424–428.

2555. Levy, Y., C. Durier, R. Krzysiek, C. Rabian, C. Capitant, A. S. Lascaux, C. Michon, E. Oksenhendler, L. Weiss, J. A. Gastaut, C. Goujard, C. Rouzioux, J. Maral, J. F. Delfraissy, D. Emilie, and J. P. Aboulker. 2003. Effects of interleukin-2 therapy combined with highly active antiretroviral therapy on immune restoration in HIV-1 infection: a randomized controlled trial. *AIDS* 17:343–351.

2555a. Lévy, Y., C. Durier, A. S. Lascaux, V. Meiffredy, H. Gahery-Segard, C. Goujard, C. Rouzioux, M. Resch, J. G. Guillet, M. Kazatchkine, J. F. Delfraissy, and J. P. Aboulker. 2006. Sustained control of viremia following therapeutic immunization in chronically HIV-1-infected individuals. *AIDS* 20:405–413.

2555b. Lévy, Y., H. Gahery-Segard, C. Durier, A.-S. Lascaux, C. Goujard, V. Meiffrédy, C. Rouzioux, R. El Habib, M. Beumont-Mauviel, J.-G. Guillet, J.-F. Delfraissy, and J.-P. Aboulker. 2005. Immunological and virological efficacy of a therapeutic immunization combined with interleukin-2 in chronically HIV-1 infected patients. *AIDS* 19:279–286.

2556. Lewin, S. R., P. Lambert, N. J. Deacon, J. Mills, and S. M. Crowe. 1997. Constitutive expression of p50 homodimer in freshly isolated human monocytes decreases with in vitro and in vivo differentiation: a possible mechanism influencing human immunodeficiency virus replication in monocytes and mature macrophages. *J. Virol.* 71:2114–2119.

2557. Lewinski, M. K., D. Bisgrove, P. Shinn, H. Chen, C. Hoffmann, S. Nannenhalli, E. Verdin, C. C. Berry, J. R. Ecker, and F. D. Bushman. 2005. Genome-wide analysis of chromosomal features repressing human immunodeficiency virus transcription. *J. Virol.* 79:6610–6619.

2558. Lewinski, M. K., and F. D. Bushman. 2005. Retroviral DNA integration—mechanism and consequences. *Adv. Genet.* 55:147–181.

2559. Lewis, D. E., D. S. N. Tang, A. Adu-Oppong, W. Schober, and J. R. Rodgers. 1994. Anergy and apoptosis in CD8+ T cells from HIV-infected persons. *J. Immunol.* 153:412–420.

2560. Lewis, M. G., J. Yalley-Ogunro, J. J. Greenhouse, T. P. Brennan, J. B. Jiang, T. C. VanCott, Y. Lu, G. A. Eddy, and D. L. Birx. 1999. Limited protection from a pathogenic chimeric simian-human immunodeficiency virus challenge following immunization with attenuated simian immunodeficiency virus. *J. Virol.* 73:1262–1270.

2561. Lewis, P., M. Hensel, and M. Emerman. 1992. Human immunodeficiency virus infection of cells arrested in the cell cycle. *EMBO J.* 11:3053–3058.

2562. Lewis, P. F., and M. Emerman. 1994. Passage through mitosis is required for oncoretroviruses but not for the human immunodeficiency virus. *J. Virol.* 68:510–516.

2563. Lewis, S. H., C. Reynolds-Kohler, H. E. Fox, and J. A. Nelson. 1990. HIV-1 in trophoblastic and villous Hofbauer cells, and haematological precursors in eight-week fetuses. *Lancet* 335:565–568.

2564. Li, B., M. D. Rossman, T. Imir, A. F. Oner-Eyuboglu, C. W. Lee, R. Biancaniello, and S. R. Carding. 1996. Disease-specific changes in gamma delta T cell repertoire and function in patients with pulmonary tuberculosis. *J. Immunol.* 157: 4222–4229.

2565. Li, C. J., D. J. Friedman, C. Wang, V. Metelev, and A. B. Pardee. 1995. Induction of apoptosis in uninfected lympho-cytes by HIV-1 Tat protein. *Science* 268:429–431.

2566. Li, C. J., L. J. Zhang, B. J. Dezube, C. S. Crumpacker, and A. B. Pardee. 1993. Three inhibitors of type 1 human im-munodeficiency virus long terminal repeat-directed gene ex-pression and virus replication. *Proc. Natl. Acad. Sci. USA* 90:1839–1842.

2567. Li, F., R. Goila-Gaur, K. Salzwedel, N. R. Kilgore, M. Reddick, C. Matallana, A. Castillo, D. Zoumplis, D. E. Martin, J. M. Orenstein, G. P. Allaway, E. O. Freed, and C. T. Wild. 2003. PA-457: a potent HIV inhibitor that disrupts core condensation by targeting a late step in Gag processing. *Proc. Natl. Acad. Sci. USA* 100:13555–13560.

2568. Li, G., M. Simm, M. J. Potash, and D. J. Volsky. 1993. Human immunodeficiency virus type 1 DNA synthesis, inte-gration, and efficient viral replication in growth-arrested T cells. *J. Virol.* 67:3969–3977.

2569. Li, J. J., A. E. Friedman-Kien, Y.-Q. Huang, M. Mirabile, and Y. Z. Cao. 1990. HIV-1 DNA proviral sequences in fresh urine pellets from HIV-1 seropositive persons. *Lancet* 335: 1590–1591.

2570. Li, J. J., Y. Q. Huang, C. J. Cockerell, and A. E. Friedman-Kien. 1996. Localization of human herpes-like virus type 8 in vascular endothelial cells and perivascular spindle-shaped cells of Kaposi's sarcoma lesions by *in situ* hybridization. *Am. J. Pathol.* 148:1741–1748.

2571. Li, J. Z., E. C. Mack, and J. A. Levy. 2003. Virucidal efficacy of soap and water against human immunodeficiency virus in genital secretions. *Antimicrob. Agents Chemother.* 47:3321–3322.

2572. Li, M., R. Song, S. Masciotra, V. Soriano, T. J. Spira, R. B. Lal, and C. Yang. 2005. Association of CCR5 human hap-logroup E with rapid HIV type 1 disease progression. *AIDS Res. Hum. Retrovir.* 21:111–114.

2573. Li, P., L. J. Kuiper, A. J. Stephenson, and C. J. Burrell. 1992. *De novo* reverse transcription is a crucial event in cell-to-cell transmission of human immunodeficiency virus. *J. Gen. Virol.* 73:955–959.

2574. Li, Q., L. Duan, J. D. Estes, Z.-M. Ma, T. Rourke, Y. Wang, C. Reilly, J. Carlis, C. J. Miller, and A. T. Haase. 2005. Peak SIV replication in resting memory CD4+ T cells depletes gut lamina propria CD4+ T cells. *Nature* 434:1148–1152.

2575. Li, S., C. P. Hill, W. I. Sundquist, and J. T. Finch. 2000. Image reconstructions of helical assemblies of the HIV-1 CA protein. *Nature* 407:409–413.

2576. Li, S., J. Juarez, M. Alali, D. Dwyer, R. Collman, A. Cun-ningham, and H. M. Naif. 1999. Persistent CCR5 utilization and enhanced macrophage tropism by primary blood human immunodeficiency virus type 1 isolates from advanced stages of disease and comparison to tissue-derived isolates. *J. Virol.* 73:9741–9755.

2577. Li, S., V. Polonis, H. Isobe, H. Zaghouani, R. Guinea, T. Moran, C. Bona, and P. Palese. 1993. Chimeric influenza virus induces neutralizing antibodies and cytotoxic T cells against human immunodeficiency virus type 1. *J. Virol.* 67:6659–6666.

2578. Li, W., D. Galey, M. P. Mattson, and A. Nath. 2005. Mol-ecular and cellular mechanisms of neuronal cell death in HIV dementia. *Neurotox. Res.* 8:119–134.

2579. Li, X. C., G. Demirci, S. Ferrari-Lacraz, C. Groves, A. Coyle, T. R. Malek, and T. B. Strom. 2001. IL-15 and IL-2: a matter of life and death for T cells in vivo. *Nat. Med.* 7:114–118.

2580. Li, X. D., B. Moore, and M. W. Cloyd. 1996. Gradual shutdown of virus production resulting in latency is the norm during the chronic phase of human immunodeficiency virus replication and differential rates and mechanisms of shutdown are determined by viral sequences. *Virology* 225:196–212.

2581. Li, Y., L. Li, R. Wadley, S. W. Reddel, J. C. Qi, C. Archis, A. Collins, E. Clark, M. Cooley, S. Kouts, H. M. Naif, M. Alali, A. Cunningham, G. W. Wong, R. L. Stevens, and S. A. Krilis. 2001. Mast cells/basophils in the peripheral blood of allergic individuals who are HIV-1 susceptible due to their surface ex-pression of CD4 and the chemokine receptors CCR3, CCR5, and CXCR4. *Blood* 97:3484–3490.

2582. Li, Y., X. Wang, S. Tian, C.-J. Guo, S. D. Douglas, and W.-Z. Ho. 2002. Methadone enhances human immunodefi-ciency virus infection of human immune cells. *J. Infect. Dis.* 185:118–122.

2583. Liang, J. S., O. Distler, D. A. Cooper, H. Jamil, R. J. Deck-elbaum, H. N. Ginsberg, and S. L. Sturley. 2001. HIV protease inhibitors protect apolipoprotein B from degradation by the proteasome: a potential mechanism for protease inhibitor-induced hyperlipidemia. *Nat. Med.* 7:1327–1331.

2584. Liang, X., D. R. Casimiro, W. A. Schleif, F. Wang, M. E. Davies, Z. Q. Zhang, T. M. Fu, A. C. Finnefrock, L. Handt, M. P. Citron, G. Heidecker, A. Tang, M. Chen, K. A. Wilson, L. Gabryelski, M. McElhaugh, A. Carella, C. Moyer, L. Huang, S. Vitelli, D. Patel, J. Lin, E. A. Emini, and J. W. Shiver. 2005. Vec-tored Gag and Env but not Tat show efficacy against simian-human immunodeficiency virus 89.6P challenge in Mamu-A*01-negative rhesus monkeys. *J. Virol.* 79:12321–12331.

2585. Lichtenstein, K. A. 2005. Redefining lipodystrophy syn-drome: risks and impact on clinical decision making. *J. Acquir. Immune Defic. Syndr.* 39:395–400.

2586. Lichtenstein, K. A., K. M. Delaney, C. Armon, D. J. Ward, A. C. Moorman, K. C. Wood, and S. D. Holmberg. 2002. Incidence of and risk factors for lipoatrophy (abnormal fat loss) in ambulatory HIV-1-infected patients. *J. Acquir. Immune Defic. Syndr.* 32:48–56.

2587. Lichterfeld, M., D. E. Kaufmann, X. G. Yu, S. K. Mui, M. M. Addo, M. N. Johnston, D. Cohen, G. K. Robbins, E. Pae, G. Alter, A. Wurcel, D. Stone, E. S. Rosenberg, B. D. Walker, and M. Altfeld. 2004. Loss of HIV-1-specific CD8+ T cell proliferation after acute HIV-1 infection and restoration by vaccine-induced HIV-1-specific CD4+ T cells. *J. Exp. Med.* 200:701–712.

2588. Lichterfeld, M., X. G. Uy, D. Cohen, M. M. Addo, J. Malenfant, B. Perkins, E. Pae, M. N. Johnston, D. Strick, T. M. Allen, E. S. Rosenberg, B. Korber, B. D. Walker, and M. Altfeld. 2004. HIV-1 Nef is preferentially recognized by CD8 T cells in primary HIV-1 infection despite a relatively high degree of ge-netic diversity. *AIDS* 18:1383–1392.

2589. Lichterfeld, M., X. G. Yu, S. Le Gall, and M. Altfeld. 2005. Immunodominance of HIV-1-specific CD8+ T-cell re-sponses in acute HIV-1 infection: at the crossroads of viral and host genetics. *Trends Immunol.* 26:166–171.

2590. Lichterfeld, M., X. G. Yu, M. T. Waring, S. K. Mui, M. N. Johnston, D. Cohen, M. M. Addo, J. Zaunders, G. Alter, E. Pae, D. Strick, T. M. Allen, E. S. Rosenberg, B. D. Walker, and M. Altfeld. 2004. HIV-1-specific cytotoxicity is preferentially mediated by a subset of CD8(+) T cells producing both interferon-gamma and tumor necrosis factor-alpha. *Blood* 104:487–494.

2590a. Lichtner, M., C. Maranon, P. Vidalain, O. Azocar, D. Hanau, P. Lebom, M. Burgard, C. Rouzioux, V. Vullo, H. Yagita, C. Rabourdin-Combe, C. Servet, and A. Hosmalin. 2004. HIV type 1-infected dendritic cells induce apoptotic death in infected and uninfected primary CD4+ T lymphocytes. *AIDS Res. Hum. Retroviruses* 20:175–182.

2591. Lieberman, A. P., P. M. Pitha, H. S. Shin, and M. L. Shin. 1989. Production of tumor necrosis factor and other cytokines by astrocytes stimulated with lipopolysaccharide of a neurotropic virus. *Proc. Natl. Acad. Sci. USA* 86:6348–6352.

2592. Lieberman, J. 2004. Tracking the killers: how should we measure CD8 T cells in HIV infection? *AIDS* 18:1489–1493.

2593. Lieberman, J., O. Shankar, N. Manjunath, and J. Andersson. 2001. Dressed to kill? A review of why antiviral CD8 T lymphocytes fail to prevent progressive immunodeficiency in HIV-1 infection. *Blood* 98:1667–1677.

2594. Lieberman, J., P. R. Skolnik, G. R. Parkerson, J. A. Fabry, B. Landry, J. Bethel, and J. Kagan. 1997. Safety of autologous, *ex vivo*-expanded human immunodeficiency virus (HIV)-specific cytotoxic T-lymphocyte infusion in HIV-infected patients. *Blood* 90:2196–2206.

2595. Lieberman, J., E. Song, S. K. Lee, and P. Shankar. 2003. Interfering with disease: opportunities and roadblocks to harnessing RNA interference. *Trends Mol. Med.* 9:397–403.

2596. Liegler, T. J., W. Yonemoto, T. Elbelk, E. Wittingoff, S. G. Buchbinder, and W. C. Greene. 1998. Diminished spontaneous apoptosis in lymphocytes from human immunodeficiency virus-infected long-term nonprogressors. *J. Infect. Dis.* 178:669–679.

2597. Lifson, A. R., S. P. Buchbinder, H. W. Sheppard, A. C. Mawle, J. C. Wilber, M. Stanley, C. E. Hart, N. A. Hessol, and S. D. Holmberg. 1991. Long-term human immunodeficiency virus infection in asymptomatic homosexual and bisexual men with normal CD4+ lymphocyte counts: immunologic and virologic characteristics. *J. Infect. Dis.* 163:959–965.

2598. Lifson, A. R., N. A. Hessol, S. P. Buchbinder, P. M. O'Malley, L. Barnhart, M. Segal, M. H. Katz, and S. D. Holmberg. 1992. Serum beta$_2$-microglobulin and prediction of progression to AIDS in HIV infection. *Lancet* 339:1436–1440.

2599. Lifson, J., S. Coutre, E. Huang, and E. Engleman. 1986. Role of envelope glycoprotein carbohydrate in human immunodeficiency virus (HIV) infectivity and virus-induced cell fusion. *J. Exp. Med.* 164:2101–2106.

2600. Lifson, J. D., M. B. Feinberg, G. R. Reyes, L. Rabin, B. Banapour, S. Chakrabarti, B. Moss, F. Wong-Staal, K. S. Steimer, and E. G. Engleman. 1986. Induction of CD4-dependent cell fusion by the HTLV-III/LAV envelope glycoprotein. *Nature* 323:725–728.

2601. Lifson, J. D., K. M. Hwang, P. L. Nara, B. Fraser, M. Padgett, N. M. Dunlop, and L. E. Eiden. 1988. Synthetic CD4 peptide derivatives that inhibit HIV infection and cytopathicity. *Science* 241:712–716.

2602. Lifson, J. D., M. Piatak, Jr., A. N. Cline, J. L. Rossio, J. Purcell, I. Pandrea, N. Bischofberger, J. Blanchard, and R. S. Veazey. 2003. Transient early post-inoculation anti-retroviral treatment facilitates controlled infection with sparing of CD4+ T cells in gut-associated lymphoid tissues in SIVmac239-infected rhesus macaques, but not resistance to rechallenge. *J. Med. Primatol.* 32:201–211.

2603. Lifson, J. D., D. M. Rausch, V. S. Kalyanaraman, K. M. Hwang, and L. E. Eiden. 1991. Synthetic peptides allow discrimination of structural features of CD4 (81–92) important for HIV-1 infection versus HIV-1-induced syncytium formation. *AIDS Res. Hum. Retrovir.* 7:449–455.

2604. Lifson, J. D., G. R. Reyes, M. S. McGrath, B. S. Stein, and E. G. Engleman. 1986. AIDS retrovirus induced cytopathology: giant cell formation and involvement of CD4 antigen. *Science* 232:1123–1127.

2605. Liles, W. C., and W. C. Van Voorhis. 1995. Review: nomenclature and biologic significance of cytokines involved in inflammation and the host immune response. *J. Infect. Dis.* 172:1573–1580.

2606. Lim, S. G., A. Condez, C. A. Lee, M. A. Johnson, C. Elia, and L. W. Poulter. 1993. Loss of mucosal CD4 lymphocytes is an early feature of HIV infection. *Clin. Exp. Immunol.* 92:448–454.

2607. Lim, S. G., A. Condez, and L. W. Poulter. 1993. Mucosal macrophage subsets of the gut in HIV: decrease in antigen-presenting cell phenotype. *Clin. Exp. Immunol.* 92:442–447.

2608. Lim, S. T., R. Karim, B. N. Nathwani, A. Tulpule, B. Espina, and A. M. Levine. 2005. AIDS-related Burkitt's lymphoma versus diffuse large-cell lymphoma in the pre-highly active antiretroviral therapy (HAART) and HAART eras: significant differences in survival with standard chemotherapy. *J. Clin. Oncol.* 23:4430–4438.

2609. Lin, J. C., S. C. Lin, E. C. Mar, P. E. Pellett, F. R. Stamey, J. A. Stewart, and T. J. Spira. 1995. Is Kaposi's sarcoma-associated herpesvirus detectable in semen of HIV-infected homosexual men? *Lancet* 346:1601–1602.

2610. Lin, X., D. Irwin, S. Kanazawa, L. Huang, J. Romeo, T. S. Yen, and B. M. Peterlin. 2003. Transcriptional profiles of latent human immunodeficiency virus in infected individuals: effects of Tat on the host and reservoir. *J. Virol.* 77:8227–8236.

2611. Lindboe, C. F., S. S. Froland, K. W. Wefring, P. J. Linnestad, T. Bohmer, A. Foerster, and A. C. Loken. 1986. Autopsy findings in three family members with a presumably acquired immunodeficiency syndrome of unknown etiology. *Acta Pathol. Microbiol. Immunol. Scand.* 94:117–123.

2612. Lindenmann, J. 1974. Viruses as immunological adjuvants in cancer. *Biochim. Biophys. Acta* 355:49–75.

2613. Linette, G. P., R. J. Hartzmann, J. A. Ledbetter, and C. H. June. 1988. HIV-1-infected T cells show a selective signaling defect after perturbation of CD3/antigen receptor. *Science* 241:573–576.

2614. Ling, B., C. Apetrei, I. Pandrea, R. S. Veazey, A. A. Lackner, B. Gormus, and P. A. Marx. 2004. Classic AIDS in a sooty mangabey after an 18-year natural infection. *J. Virol.* 78:8902–8908.

2615. Ling, E. A., and W.-C. Wong. 1993. The origin and nature of ramified and amoeboid microglia: a historical review and current concepts. *Glia* 7:9–18.

2616. Linhart, H., B. R. Gundlach, S. Sopper, U. Dittmer, K. Matz-Rensing, E.-M. Kuhn, J. Muller, G. Hunsmann, C. Stahl-Henning, and K. Uberla. 1997. Live attenuated SIV vaccines are not effective in a postexposure vaccination model. *AIDS Res. Hum. Retrovir.* 13:593–599.

2617. Linsley, P. S., J. L. Greene, P. Tan, J. Bradshaw, J. A. Ledbetter, C. Anasetti, and N. K. Damle. 1992. Coexpression and functional cooperation of CTLA-4 and CD28 on activated T lymphocytes. *J. Exp. Med.* 176:1595–1604.

2618. Linsley, P. S., and J. A. Ledbetter. 1993. The role of the CD28 receptor during T cell responses to antigen. *Annu. Rev. Immunol.* **11**:191–212.

2619. Liou, L. Y., C. H. Herrmann, and A. P. Rice. 2002. Transient induction of cyclin T1 during human macrophage differentiation regulates human immunodeficiency virus type 1 Tat transactivation function. *J. Virol.* **76**:10579–10587.

2620. Lipshultz, S. E., K. A. Easley, E. J. Orav, S. Kaplan, T. J. Strac, J. T. Bricker, W. W. Lai, D. S. Moodie, G. Sopko, M. D. Schlucher, and S. D. Colan. 2002. Cardiovascular status of infants and children of women infected with HIV-1 (P^2C^2 HIV): a cohort study. *Lancet* **360**:368–373.

2621. Lipshultz, S. E., C. H. Fox, A. R. Perez-Atayde, S. P. Sanders, S. D. Colan, K. McIntosh, and H. S. Winter. 1990. Identification of human immunodeficiency virus-1 RNA and DNA in the heart of a child with cardiovascular abnormalities and congenital acquired immune deficiency syndrome. *Am. J. Cardiol.* **66**:246–250.

2622. Lipton, S. A. 1991. Calcium channel antagonists and human immunodeficiency virus coat protein-mediated neuronal injury. *Ann. Neurol.* **30**:110–114.

2623. Lipton, S. A., N. J. Sucher, P. K. Kaiser, and E. B. Dreyer. 1991. Synergistic effects of HIV coat protein and NMDA receptor-mediated neurotoxicity. *Neuron* **7**:111–118.

2624. Lisignoli, G., M. C. Monaco, A. Degrassi, S. Toneguzzi, E. Ricchi, P. Costigliola, and A. Facchini. 1993. In vitro immunotoxicity of +/− 2'-deoxy-3'-thiacytidine, a new anti-HIV agent. *Clin. Exp. Immunol.* **92**:455–459.

2625. Little, S. J., S. Holte, J. P. Routy, E. S. Daar, M. Markowitz, A. C. Collier, R. A. Koup, J. W. Mellors, E. Connick, B. Conway, M. Kilby, L. Wang, J. M. Whitcomb, N. S. Hellmann, and D. D. Richman. 2002. Antiretroviral-drug resistance among patients recently infected with HIV. *N. Engl. J. Med.* **347**:385–394.

2625a. Little, S. J., A. R. McLean, C. A. Spina, D. D. Richman, and D. V. Havlir. 1999. Viral dynamics of acute HIV-1 infection. *J. Exp. Med.* **190**:841–850.

2626. Liu, B., X. Yu, K. Luo, Y. Yu, and X. Yu. 2004. Influence of primate lentiviral Vif and proteasome inhibitors on human immunodeficiency virus type 1 virion packaging of APOBEC3G. *J. Virol.* **78**:2072–2081.

2627. Liu, C., M. Carrington, R. A. Kaslow, X. Gao, C. R. Rinaldo, L. P. Jacobson, J. B. Margolick, J. Phair, S. J. O'Brien, and R. Detels. 2003. Association of polymorphisms in human leukocyte antigen class I and transporter associated with antigen processing genes with resistance to human immunodeficiency virus type 1 infection. *J. Infect. Dis.* **187**:1404–1410.

2628. Liu, H., M. Carrington, C. Wang, S. Holte, J. Lee, B. Greene, F. Hladik, D. M. Koelle, A. Wald, K. Kurosawa, C. R. Rinaldo, C. Celum, R. Detels, L. Corey, M. J. McElrath, and T. Zhu. 2006. Repeat-region polymorphisms in the gene for the dendritic cell-specific intercellular adhesion molecule-3-grabbing nonintegrin-related molecule: effects on HIV-1 susceptibility. *J. Infect. Dis.* **193**:698–702.

2629. Liu, H., D. Chao, E. E. Nakayama, H. Taguchi, M. Goto, X. Xin, J. K. Takamatsu, H. Saito, Y. Ishikawa, T. Akaza, T. Juji, Y. Takebe, T. Ohishi, K. Fukutake, Y. Maruyama, S. Yashiki, S. Sonoda, T. Nakamura, Y. Nagai, A. Iwamoto, and T. Shioda. 1999. Polymorphism in RANTES chemokine promoter affects HIV-1 disease progression. *Proc. Natl. Acad. Sci. USA* **96**:4581–4585.

2630. Liu, H., Y. Hwangbo, S. Holte, J. Lee, C. Wang, N. Kaupp, H. Zhu, C. Celum, L. Corey, M. J. McElrath, and T. Zhu. 2004. Analysis of genetic polymorphisms in CCR5, CCR2, stromal cell-derived factor-1, RANTES, and dendritic cell-specific intracellular adhesion molecule-3-grabbing nonintegrin in seronegative individuals repeatedly exposed to HIV-1. *J. Infect. Dis.* **190**:1055–1058.

2631. Liu, H., X. Wu, M. Newman, G. M. Shaw, B. H. Hahn, and J. C. Kappes. 1995. The Vif protein of human and simian immunodeficiency viruses is packaged into virions and associates with viral core structures. *J. Virol.* **69**:7630–7638.

2632. Liu, N. Q., A. S. Lossinsky, W. Popik, X. Li, G. Gujuluva, B. Kriederman, J. Roberts, T. Pushkarsky, M. Bukrinsky, M. Witte, M. Weinand, and M. Fiala. 2002. Human immunodeficiency virus type 1 enters brain microvascular endothelia by macropinocytosis dependent on lipid rafts and the mitogen-activated protein kinase signaling pathway. *J. Virol.* **76**:6689–6700.

2633. Liu, P. T., S. Stenger, H. Li, L. Wenzel, B. H. Tan, S. R. Krutzik, M. T. Ochoa, J. Schauber, K. Wu, C. Meinken, D. L. Kamen, M. Wagner, R. Bals, A. Steinmeyer, U. Zugel, R. L. Gallo, D. Eisenberg, M. Hewison, B. W. Hollis, J. S. Adams, B. R. Bloom, and R. L. Modlin. 2006. Toll-like receptor triggering of a vitamin D-mediated human antimicrobial response. *Science* **311**:1770–1773.

2634. Liu, Q. N., S. Reddy, J. W. Sayre, V. Pop, M. C. Graves, and M. Fiala. 2001. Essential role of HIV type 1-infected and cyclooxygenase 2-activated macrophages and T cells in HIV type 1 myocarditis. *AIDS Res. Hum. Retrovir.* **17**:1423–1433.

2635. Liu, R., W. A. Paxton, S. Choe, D. Ceradini, S. R. Martin, R. Horuk, M. E. MacDonald, H. Stuhlmann, R. A. Koup, and N. R. Landau. 1996. Homozygous defect in HIV-1 coreceptor accounts for resistance for some multiply-exposed individuals to HIV-1 infection. *Cell* **86**:367–377.

2636. Liu, X., J. Zha, H. Chen, J. Nishitani, P. Camargo, S. W. Cole, and J. A. Zack. 2003. Human immunodeficiency virus type 1 infection and replication in normal human oral keratinocytes. *J. Virol.* **77**:3470–3476.

2637. Liu, X., J. Zha, J. Nishitani, H. Chen, and J. A. Zack. 2003. HIV-1 infection in peripheral blood lymphocytes (PBLs) exposed to alcohol. *Virology* **307**:37–44.

2638. Liu, Y., M. Jones, C. M. Hingtgen, G. Bu, N. Laribee, R. E. Tanzi, R. D. Moir, A. Nath, and J. J. He. 2000. Uptake of HIV-1 Tat protein mediated by low-density lipoprotein receptor-related protein disrupts the neuronal metabolic balance of the receptor ligands. *Nat. Med.* **6**:1380–1387.

2639. Liu, Y., H. Liu, B. Kim, V. H. Gattone, J. Li, A. Nath, J. Blum, and J. J. He. 2004. CD4-independent infection of astrocytes by human immunodeficiency virus type 1: requirement for the human mannose receptor. *J. Virol.* **78**:4120–4133.

2640. Liu, Y. J. 2001. Dendritic cell subsets and lineages, and their functions in innate and adaptive immunity. *Cell* **106**:259–262.

2641. Liu, Y. J. 2005. IPC: professional type 1 interferon-producing cells and plasmacytoid dendritic cell precursors. *Annu. Rev. Immunol.* **23**:275–306.

2642. Liu, Z.-Q., C. Wood, J. A. Levy, and C. Cheng-Mayer. 1990. The viral envelope gene is involved in the macrophage tropism of an HIV-1 strain isolated from the brain. *J. Virol.* **64**:6143–6153.

2643. Liuzzi, G., P. Bagnarelli, A. Chirianni, M. Clementi, S. Nappa, P. T. Cataldo, A. Valenza, and M. Piazza. 1995. Quantitation of HIV-1 genome copy number in semen and saliva. *AIDS* 9:651–653.

2644. Livingstone, W. J., M. Moore, D. Innes, J. E. Bell, and P. Simmonds. 1996. Frequent infection of peripheral blood CD8-positive T-lymphocytes with HIV-1. *Lancet* 348:649–654.

2645. Ljunggren, K., G. Biberfeld, M. Jondal, and E.-M. Fenyo. 1989. Antibody-dependent cellular cytotoxicity detects type- and strain-specific antigens among human immunodeficiency virus types 1 and 2 and simian immunodeficiency virus SIV$_{mac}$ isolates. *J. Virol.* 63:3376–3381.

2646. Ljunggren, K., P. A. Broliden, Morfeldt, L. Manson, M. Jondal, and B. Wahren. 1988. IgG subclass response to HIV in relation to antibody-dependent cellular cytotoxicity at different clinical stages. *Clin. Exp. Immunol.* 73:343–347.

2647. Lloyd, T. E., L. Yang, D. N. Tang, T. Bennett, W. Schober, and D. E. Lewis. 1997. Regulation of CD28 costimulation in human CD8+ T cells. *J. Immunol.* 158:1551–1558.

2648. Locher, C. P., B. M. Ashlock, P. Polacino, S. H. Hu, S. Shiboski, A. M. Schmidt, M. B. Agy, D. M. Anderson, S. I. Staprans, J. zur Megede, and J. A. Levy. 2004. Human immunodeficiency virus type 2 DNA vaccine provides partial protection from acute baboon infection. *Vaccine* 22:2261–2272.

2649. Locher, C. P., D. J. Blackbourn, S. W. Barnett, K. K. Murthy, E. K. Cobb, S. Rouse, G. Greco, G. Reyes-Teran, K. M. Brasky, K. D. Carey, and J. A. Levy. 1997. Superinfection with HIV-2 can reactivate virus production in baboons but is contained by a CD8+ T-cell antiviral response. *J. Infect. Dis.* 176:948–959.

2650. Locher, C. P., S. A. Witt, R. Kassel, N. L. Dowell, S. Fujimura, and J. A. Levy. 2005. Differential effects of R5 and X4 human immunodeficiency virus type 1 infection on CD4+ cell proliferation and activation. *J. Gen. Virol.* 86:1171–1179.

2651. Locher, C. P., S. A. Witt, and J. A. Levy. 2001. The nuclear factor kappa B and Sp1 binding sites do not appear to be involved in virus suppression by CD8 T lymphocytes. *AIDS* 15:2455–2457.

2652. Loetscher, P., M. Uguccioni, L. Bordoli, M. Baggiolini, and B. Moser. 1998. CCR5 is characteristic of Th1 lymphocytes. *Nature* 391:344–345.

2653. Lohman, B. L., M. B. McChesney, C. J. Miller, E. McGowan, S. M. Joye, K. K. A. Van Rompay, E. Reay, L. Antipa, N. C. Pedersen, and M. L. Marthas. 1994. A partially attenuated simian immunodeficiency virus induces host immunity that correlates with resistance to pathogenic virus challenge. *J. Virol.* 68:7021–7029.

2654. Lohman, B. L., M. B. McChesney, C. J. Miller, M. Otsyula, C. J. Berardi, and M. L. Marthas. 1994. Mucosal immunization with a live, virulence-attenuated simian immunodeficiency virus (SIV) vaccine elicits antiviral cytotoxic T lymphocytes and antibodies in rhesus macaques. *J. Med. Primatol.* 23:95–101.

2655. Lohman, B. L., C. J. Miller, and M. B. McChesney. 1995. Antiviral cytotoxic T lymphocytes in vaginal mucosa of simian immunodeficiency virus-infected rhesus macaques. *J. Immunol.* 155:5855–5860.

2656. Lohman, B. L., J. Slyker, D. Mbori-Ngacha, R. Bosire, C. Farquhar, E. Obimbo, P. Otieno, R. Nduati, S. Rowland-Jones, and G. John-Stewart. 2003. Prevalence and magnitude of human immunodeficiency virus (HIV) type 1-specific lymphocyte responses in breast milk from HIV-1-seropositive women. *J. Infect. Dis.* 188:1666–1674.

2657. Lohse, A. W., F. Mor, N. Karin, and I. R. Cohen. 1989. Control of experimental autoimmune encephalomyelitis by T cells responding to activated T cells. *Science* 239:181–184.

2658. Lokensgard, J. R., G. Gekkar, L. C. Ehrlich, S. Hu, C. C. Chao, and P. K. Peterson. 1997. Proinflammatory cytokines inhibit HIV-1$_{SF162}$ expression in acutely infected human brain cell cultures. *J. Immunol.* 158:2449–2455.

2659. Long, E. M., H. L. Martin, Jr., J. K. Kreiss, S. M. J. Rainwater, L. Lavreys, D. J. Jackson, J. Rakwar, K. Mandaliya, and J. Overbaugh. 2000. Gender differences in HIV-1 diversity at time of infection. *Nat. Med.* 6:71–75.

2660. Long, E. O., and S. Rajagopalan. 2000. HLA class I recognition by killer cell Ig-like receptors. *Semin. Immunol.* 12:101–118.

2661. Lopalco, L. 2004. Humoral immunity in HIV-1 exposure: cause or effect of HIV resistance? *Curr. HIV Res.* 2:127–139.

2662. Lopalco, L., C. Barassi, C. Pastori, R. Longhi, S. E. Burastero, G. Tambussi, F. Mazzotta, A. Lazzarin, M. Clerici, and A. G. Siccardi. 2000. CCR5-reactive antibodies in seronegative partners of HIV-seropositive individuals down-modulate surface CCR5 in vivo and neutralize the infectivity of R5 strains of HIV-1 In vitro. *J. Immunol.* 164:3426–3433.

2663. Lopalco, L., C. De Sanito, R. Meneveri, R. Loughi, E. Gihelli, F. Grassi, A. Siccardi, and A. Beretta. 1993. Human immunodeficiency virus type 1 gp120 CS region mimics the HLA class 1 alpha 1 peptide-binding. *Eur. J. Immunol.* 23:2016–2021.

2664. Lopalco, L., C. Pastori, A. Cosma, S. E. Burastero, B. Capiluppi, E. Boeri, A. Beretta, A. Lazzarin, and A. G. Siccardi. 2000. Anti-cell antibodies in exposed seronegative individuals with HIV type 1-neutralizing activity. *AIDS Res. Hum. Retrovir.* 16:109–115.

2665. Lopes, A. R., A. Jaye, L. Dorrell, S. Sabally, A. Alabi, N. A. Jones, D. R. Flower, A. De Groot, P. Newton, R. M. Lascar, I. Williams, H. Whittle, A. Bertoletti, P. Borrow, and M. K. Maini. 2003. Greater CD8+ TCR heterogeneity and functional flexibility in HIV-2 compared to HIV-1 infection. *J. Immunol.* 171:307–316.

2666. Lopez, C., P. A. Fitzgerald, and F. P. Siegal. 1983. Severe acquired immune deficiency syndrome in male homosexuals: diminished capacity to make interferon-alpha in vitro associated with severe opportunistic infections. *J. Infect. Dis.* 148:962–966.

2667. Lopez-Vazquez, A., A. Mina-Blanco, J. Martinez-Borra, P. D. Njobvu, B. Suarez-Alvarez, M. A. Blanco-Gelaz, S. Gonzalez, L. Rodrigo, and C. Lopez-Larrea. 2005. Interaction between KIR3DL1 and HLA-B*57 supertype alleles influences the progression of HIV-1 infection in a Zambian population. *Hum. Immunol.* 66:285–289.

2667a. Lopez-Verges, S., G. Camus, G. Blot, R. Beauvoir, R. Benarous, and C. Berlioz-Torrent. 2006. Tail-interacting protein TIP47 is a connector between Gag and Env and is required for Env incorporation into HIV-1 virions. *Proc. Natl. Acad. Sci. USA* 103:14947–14952.

2668. Lori, F. 1999. Hydroxyurea and HIV: 5 years later—from antiviral to immune-modulating effects. *AIDS* 13:1433–1442.

2669. Lori, F., F. Veronese, A. L. de Vico, P. Lusso, M. S. Reitz, Jr., and R. C. Gallo. 1992. Viral DNA carried by human immunodeficiency virus type 1 virions. *J. Virol.* 66:5067–5074.

2670. Lortholary, O., A. Fontanet, N. Memain, A. Martin, K. Sitbon, and F. Dromer. 2005. Incidence and risk factors of immune reconstitution inflammatory syndrome complicating HIV-associated cryptococcosis in France. *AIDS* 19:1043–1049.

2671. Louder, M. K., A. Sambor, E. Chertova, T. Hunte, S. Barrett, F. Ojong, E. Sanders-Buell, S. Zolla-Pazner, F. E. McCutchan, J. D. Roser, D. Gabuzda, J. D. Lifson, and J. R. Mascola. 2005. HIV-1 envelope pseudotyped viral vectors and infectious molecular clones expressing the same envelope glycoprotein have a similar neutralization phenotype, but culture in peripheral blood mononuclear cells is associated with decreased neutralization sensitivity. *Virology* 339:226–238.

2672. Louwagie, J., W. Janssens, J. Mascola, L. Heyndrickx, P. Hegerich, G. van der Groen, F. E. McCutchan, and D. S. Burke. 1995. Genetic diversity of the envelope glycoprotein from human immunodeficiency virus type 1 isolates of African origin. *J. Virol.* 69:263–271.

2673. Louwagie, J., F. E. McCutchan, M. Peeters, T. P. Brennan, E. Sanders-Buell, G. A. Eddy, G. van der Groen, K. Fransen, G.-M. Gershy-Damet, R. Deleys, and D. S. Burke. 1993. Phylogenetic analysis of gag genes from 70 international HIV-1 isolates provides evidence for multiple genotypes. *AIDS* 7:769–780.

2674. Lowe, S. H., S. U. C. Sankatsing, S. Repping, F. van der Veen, P. Reiss, J. M. A. Lange, and J. M. Prins. 2004. Is the male genital tract really a sanctuary site for HIV? Arguments that it is not. *AIDS* 18:1353–1362.

2675. Lu, A. C., E. C. Jones, C. Chow, K. D. Miller, B. Herpin, D. Rock-Kress, J. A. Metcalf, H. C. Lane, and J. A. Kovacs. 2003. Increases in CD4+ T lymphocytes occur without increases in thymic size in HIV-infected subjects receiving interleukin-2 therapy. *J. Acquir. Immune Defic. Syndr.* 34:299–303.

2676. Lu, S., J. Arthos, D. C. Montefiori, Y. Yasutomi, K. Manson, F. Mustafa, E. Johnson, J. C. Santoro, J. Wissink, J. I. Mullins, J. R. Haynes, N. L. Letvin, M. Wyand, and H. L. Robinson. 1996. Simian immunodeficiency virus DNA vaccine trial in macaques. *J. Virol.* 70:3978–3991.

2677. Lu, W., L. C. Arraes, W. T. Ferreira, and J. M. Andrieu. 2004. Therapeutic dendritic-cell vaccine for chronic HIV-1 infection. *Nat. Med.* 10:1359–1365.

2678. Lu, W., J. W. Shih, J. M. Tourani, D. Eme, H. J. Alter, and J. M. Andrieu. 1993. Lack of isolate-specific neutralizing activity is correlated with an increased viral burden in rapidly progressing HIV-1-infected patients. *AIDS* 7:S91-S99.

2679. Lu, X., X. Wu, A. Plemenitas, H. Yu, E. T. Sawai, A. Abo, and B. M. Peterlin. 1996. DCD42 and Rac1 are implicated in the activation of the Nef-associated kinase and replication of HIV-1. *Curr. Biol.* 6:1677–1684.

2680. Lu, Y., P. Brosio, M. Lafaile, J. Li, R. G. Collman, J. Sodroski, and C. J. Miller. 1996. Vaginal transmission of chimeric simian/human immunodeficiency viruses in rhesus macaques. *J. Virol.* 70:3045–3050.

2681. Lu, Y., M. S. Salvato, C. D. Pauza, J. Li, J. Sodroski, K. Manson, M. Wyand, N. Letvin, S. Jenkins, N. Touzjian, C. Chutkowski, N. Kushner, M. LeFaile, L. G. Payne, and B. Roberts. 1996. Utility of SHIV for testing HIV-1 vaccine candidates in macaques. *J. Acquir. Immune Defic. Syndr. Hum. Retrovirol.* 12:99–106.

2682. Lu, Y. L., P. Spearman, and L. Ratner. 1993. Human immunodeficiency virus type 1 viral protein R localization in infected cells and virions. *J. Virol.* 67:6542–6550.

2683. Lu, Y. Y., Y. Koga, K. Tanaka, M. Sasaki, G. Kimura, and K. Nomoto. 1994. Apoptosis induced in CD4+ cells expressing gp160 of human immunodeficiency virus type 1. *J. Virol.* 68:390–399.

2684. Lu, Z., J. F. Berson, Y. H. Chen, J. D. Turner, T. Zhang, M. Sharron, M. H. Jenks, Z. Wang, J. Kim, J. Rucker, J. A. Hoxie, S. C. Peiper, and R. W. Doms. 1997. Evolution of HIV-1 coreceptor usage through interactions with distinct CCR5 and CXCR4 domains. *Proc. Natl. Acad. Sci. USA* 94:6426–6431.

2685. Luban, J. 1996. Absconding with the chaperone: essential cyclophilin-gag interaction in HIV-1 virions. *Cell* 87:1157–1159.

2686. Luban, J., K. L. Bossolt, E. K. Franke, G. V. Kalpana, and S. P. Goff. 1993. Human immunodeficiency virus type 1 Gag protein binds to cyclophilins A and B. *Cell* 73:1067–1078.

2687. Lubeck, M. D., R. Natuk, M. Myagkikh, N. Kalyan, K. Aldrich, F. Sinangil, S. Alipanah, S. C. Murthy, P. K. Chanda, S. M. Nigida, Jr., P. D. Markham, S. Zolla-Pazner, K. Steimer, M. Wade, M. S. Reitz, Jr., L. O. Arthur, S. Mizutani, A. Davis, P. P. Ung, R. C. Gallo, J. Eichberg, and M. Robert-Guroff. 1997. Long-term protection of chimpanzees against high-dose HIV-1 challenge induced by immunization. *Nat. Med.* 3:651–658.

2688. Lucey, D. R., M. Clerici, and G. M. Shearer. 1996. Type 1 and type 2 cytokine dysregulation in human infectious, neoplastic, and inflammatory diseases. *Clin. Microbiol. Rev.* 9:532–562.

2689. Luciw, P. A., C. Cheng-Mayer, and J. A. Levy. 1987. Mutational analysis of the human immunodeficiency virus (HIV): the orf-B region down-regulates virus replication. *Proc. Natl. Acad. Sci. USA* 84:1434–1438.

2690. Luciw, P. A., S. J. Potter, K. Steimer, D. Dina, and J. A. Levy. 1984. Molecular cloning of AIDS-associated retrovirus. *Nature* 312:760–763.

2691. Luciw, P. A., E. Pratt-Lowe, K. E. S. Shaw, J. A. Levy, and C. Cheng-Mayer. 1995. Persistent infection of rhesus macaques with T-cell-line-tropic and macrophage-tropic clones of simian/human immunodeficiency viruses (SHIV). *Proc. Natl. Acad. Sci. USA* 92:7490–7494.

2692. Ludvigsen, A., T. Werner, W. Gimbel, V. Erfle, and R. Brack-Werner. 1996. Down-modulation of HIV-1 LTR activity by an extra-LTR *nef* gene fragment. *Virology* 216:245–251.

2693. Luizzi, G. M., C. M. Mastroinni, V. Vullo, E. Jirillo, S. Delia, and P. Riccio. 1992. Cerebrospinal fluid myelin basic protein as predictive marker of demyelination in AIDS dementia complex. *J. Neuroimmunol.* 36:251–254.

2694. Lukashov, V. V., and J. Goudsmit. 1995. Increasing genotypic and phenotypic selection from the original genomic RNA populations of HIV-1 strains LAI and MN (NM) by peripheral blood mononuclear cell culture, B-cell-line propagation and T-cell-line adaptation. *AIDS* 9:1307–1311.

2695. Lukashov, V. V., C. L. Kuiken, and J. Goudsmit. 1995. Intrahost human immunodeficiency virus type 1 evolution is related to length of the immunocompetent period. *J. Virol.* 69:6911–6916.

2696. Luke, W., C. Coulibaly, U. Dittmer, G. Voss, R. Oesterle, B. Makoschey, U. Sauermann, E. Jurkiewicz, C. Stahl-Henning, H. Petry, and G. Hunsmann. 1996. Simian immunodeficiency virus (SIV) gp130 oligomers protect rhesus macaques (Macaca mulatta) against the infection with SIVmac32H grown on T-cells or derived *ex vivo*. *Virology* 216:444–450.

2697. Lum, J. J., O. J. Cohen, Z. Nie, J. G. Weaver, T. S. Gomez, X. Yao, D. Lynch, A. A. Pilon, N. Haley, J. E. Kim, Z. Chen, M. Montpetit, J. Sanchez-Dardon, E. A. Cohen, and A. D. Badley. 2003. Vpr R77Q is associated with long-term nonprogressive HIV infection and impaired induction of apoptosis. *J. Clin. Investig.* 111:1547–1554.

2697a. Lunardi-Iskandar, Y., J. L. Bryant, W. A. Blattner, C. L. Hung, L. Flamand, P. Gill, P. Hermans, S. Birken, and R. C. Gallo. 1998. Effects of a urinary factor from women in early pregnancy on HIV-1, SIV and associated disease. *Nat. Med.* 4:428–434.

2698. Lund, J., A. Sata, S. Akira, R. Medzhitov, and A. Iwasaki. 2003. Toll-like receptor 9-mediated recognition of Herpes simplex virus-2 by plasmacytoid dendritic cells. *J. Exp. Med.* 198:513–520.

2699. Lund, J. M., L. Alexopoulou, A. Sato, M. Karow, N. C. Adams, N. W. Gale, A. Iwasaki, and R. A. Flavell. 2004. Recognition of single-stranded RNA viruses by Toll-like receptor 7. *Proc. Natl. Acad. Sci. USA* 101:5598–5603.

2700. Lundquist, C. A., J. Zhou, and C. Aiken. 2004. Nef stimulates human immunodeficiency virus type 1 replication in primary T cells by enhancing virion-associated gp120 levels: coreceptor-dependent requirement for Nef in viral replication. *J. Virol.* 78:6287–6296.

2701. Luo, L., Y. Li, P. M. Cannon, S. Kim, and C. Yong Kang. 1992. Chimeric gag-V3 virus-like particles of human immunodeficiency virus induce virus-neutralizing antibodies. *Proc. Natl. Acad. Sci. USA* 89:10527–10531.

2702. Luo, T., J. L. Douglas, R. L. Livingston, and J. V. Garcia. 1998. Infectivity enhancement by HIV-1 Nef is dependent on the pathway of virus entry: implications for HIV-based gene transfer systems. *Virology* 241:224–233.

2703. Luria, S., I. Chambers, and P. Berg. 1991. Expression of the type 1 human immunodeficiency virus Nef protein in T cells prevents antigen receptor-mediated induction of interleukin 2 mRNA. *Proc. Natl. Acad. Sci. USA* 88:5326–5330.

2704. Lusso, P., A. DeMaria, M. Malnati, and F. Lori. 1991. Induction of CD4 and susceptibility to HIV-1 infection in human CD8+ T lymphocytes by human herpesvirus-6. *Nature* 349:533–535.

2705. Lusso, P., B. Ensoli, P. D. Markham, D. V. Ablashi, S. Z. Salahuddin, E. Tschachler, F. Wong-Staal, and R. C. Gallo. 1989. Productive dual infection of human CD4+ T lymphocytes by HIV-1 and HHV-6. *Nature* 337:370–373.

2706. Lusso, P., M. S. Malnati, A. Garzino-Demo, R. W. Crowley, E. O. Long, and R. C. Gallo. 1993. Infection of natural killer cells by human herpesvirus 6. *Nature* 362:458–462.

2707. Lusso, P., P. Secchiero, R. W. Crowley, A. Garzino-Demo, Z. N. Berneman, and R. C. Gallo. 1994. CD4 is a critical component of the receptor for human herpesvirus 7: interference with human immunodeficiency virus. *Proc. Natl. Acad. Sci. USA* 91:3872–3876.

2708. Lusso, P., F. di Marzo Veronese, B. Ensoli, G. Franchini, C. Jemma, S. E. de Rocco, V. S. Kalyanaraman, and R. C. Gallo. 1990. Expanded HIV-1 cellular tropism by phenotypic mixing with murine endogenous retroviruses. *Science* 247:848–852.

2709. Luzuriaga, K., M. McManus, M. Catalina, S. Mayack, M. Sharkey, M. Stevenson, and J. L. Sullivan. 2000. Early therapy of vertical human immunodeficiency virus type 1 (HIV-1) infection: control of viral replication and absence of persistent HIV-1-specific immune responses. *J. Virol.* 74:6984–6991.

2710. Ly, A., and L. Stamatatos. 2000. V2 loop glycosylation of the human immunodeficiency virus type 1 SF162 envelope facilitates interaction of this protein with CD4 and CCR5 receptors and protects the virus from neutralization by anti-V3 loop and anti-CD4 binding site antibodies. *J. Virol.* 74:6769–6776.

2711. Lyketsos, C. G., D. R. Hoover, M. Guccione, W. Senterfitt, M. A. Dew, J. Wesch, M. J. VanRaden, G. J. Treisman, and H. Morgenstern. 1993. Depressive symptoms as predictors of medical outcomes in HIV infection. *JAMA* 270:2563–2567.

2712. Lyles, R. H., A. Munoz, T. E. Yamashita, H. Bazmi, R. Detels, C. R. Rinaldo, J. B. Margolick, J. P. Phair, and J. W. Mellors. 2000. Natural history of human immunodeficiency virus type 1 viremia after seroconversion and proximal to AIDS in a large cohort of homosexual men. Multicenter AIDS Cohort Study. *J. Infect. Dis.* 181:872–880.

2713. Lynn, W. S., A. Tweedale, and M. W. Cloyd. 1988. Human immunodeficiency virus (HIV-1) cytotoxicity: perturbation of the cell membrane and depression of phospholipid synthesis. *Virology* 163:43–51.

2714. Lyter, D. W., J. Bryant, R. Thackeray, C. R. Rinaldo, and L. A. Kingsley. 1995. Incidence of human immunodeficiency virus-related and nonrelated malignancies in a large cohort of homosexual men. *J. Clin. Oncol.* 13:2540–2546.

2715. Reference deleted.

2716. Reference deleted.

2717. Ma, Z., F. X. Lu, M. Torten, and C. J. Miller. 2001. The number and distribution of immune cells in the cervicovaginal mucosa remain constant throughout the menstrual cycle of rhesus macaques. *Clin. Immunol.* 100:240–249.

2718. Macallan, D. C., D. Wallace, Y. Zhang, C. De Lara, A. T. Worth, H. Ghattas, G. E. Griffin, P. C. Beverley, and D. F. Tough. 2004. Rapid turnover of effector-memory CD4(+) T cells in healthy humans. *J. Exp. Med.* 200:255–260.

2719. Macatonia, S. E., M. Compels, A. J. Pinching, S. Patterson, and S. C. Knight. 1992. Antigen presentation by macrophages but not by dendritic cells in human immunodeficiency virus (HIV) infection. *Immunology* 75:576–581.

2720. Macatonia, S. E., R. Lau, S. Patterson, J. Pinching, and S. C. Knight. 1990. Dendritic cell infection, depletion and dysfunction in HIV-infected individuals. *Immunology* 71:38–45.

2721. Macatonia, S. E., S. Patterson, and S. C. Knight. 1989. Suppression of immune responses by dendritic cells infected with HIV. *Immunology* 67:285–289.

2722. Macatonia, S. E., P. M. Taylor, S. C. Knight, and B. A. Askonas. 1989. Primary stimulation by dendritic cells induces antiviral proliferative and cytotoxic T cell responses in vitro. *J. Exp. Med.* 169:1255–1264.

2723. Macchia, D., C. Simonelli, P. Parronchi, M. P. Piccinni, P. Biswas, A. Mazzetti, A. Ravina, E. Maggi, and S. Romagnani. 1991. In vitro infection with HIV of antigen-specific T cell clones derived from HIV-seronegative individuals. Effects on cytokine production and helper function. *Ric. Clin. Lab.* 21:85–90.

2724. MacDonald, K. P., D. J. Munster, G. J. Clark, A. Dzionek, J. Schmitz, and D. N. Hart. 2002. Characterization of human blood dendritic cell subsets. *Blood* 100:4512–4520.

2725. MacDonald, K. S., J. Embree, S. Njenga, N. J. D. Nagelkerke, I. Ngatia, Z. Mohammed, B. H. Barber, J. Ndinya-Achola, J. Bwayo, and F. A. Plummer. 1998. Mother-child class I HLA concordance increases perinatal human immunodeficiency virus type 1 transmission. *J. Infect. Dis.* 177:551–556.

2726. MacDonald, K. S., J. E. Embree, N. J. D. Nagelkerke, J. Castillo, S. Ramhadin, S. Njenga, J. Oyug, J. Ndinya-Achola, B. H. Barber, J. J. Bwayo, and F. A. Plummer. 2001. The HLA A2/6802 supertype is associated with reduced risk of perinatal human immunodeficiency virus type 1 transmission. *J. Infect. Dis.* **183**:503–506.

2727. MacDonald, K. S., K. R. Fowke, J. Kimani, V. A. Dunand, N. J. D. Nagelkerke, T. B. Ball, J. Oyugi, E. Njagi, L. K. Gaur, R. C. Brunham, J. Wade, M. A. Luscher, P. Krausa, S. Rowland-Jones, E. Ngugi, J. J. Bwayo, and F. A. Plummer. 2000. Influence of HLA supertypes on susceptibility and resistance to human immunodeficiency virus type 1 infection. *J. Infect. Dis.* **181**:1581–1589.

2728. MacDonald, K. S., I. Malonza, D. K. Chen, N. J. Nagelkerke, J. M. Nasio, J. Ndinya-Achola, J. J. Bwayo, D. S. Sitar, F. Y. Aoki, and F. A. Plummer. 2001. Vitamin A and risk of HIV-1 seroconversion among Kenyan men with genital ulcers. *AIDS* **15**:635–639.

2729. MacDonald, T. T., and J. Spencer. 1992. Cell-mediated immune injury in the intestine. *Gastroenterol. Clin. N. Am.* **21**:367–386.

2730. Machuca, A., L. Ding, R. Taffs, S. Lee, W. Wood, J. Hu, and I. Hewlett. 2004. HIV type 2 primary isolates induce a lower degree of apoptosis "in vitro" compared with HIV type 1 primary isolates. *AIDS Res. Hum. Retrovir.* **20**:507–512.

2731. Maciaszek, J. W., S. J. Coniglio, D. A. Talmage, and G. A. Viglianti. 1998. Retinoid-induced repression of human immunodeficiency virus type 1 core promoter activity inhibits virus replication. *J. Virol.* **72**:5862–5869.

2732. Maciejewski, J. P., F. F. Weichold, and N. S. Young. 1994. HIV-1 suppression of hematopoiesis in vitro mediated by envelope glycoprotein and TNF-alpha. *J. Immunol.* **153**:4303–4310.

2733. Mackall, C. L., T. A. Fleisher, M. R. Brown, M. P. Andrich, C. C. Chen, I. M. Feuerstein, M. E. Horowitz, I. T. Magrath, A. T. Shad, S. M. Steinberg, L. H. Wexler, and R. E. Gress. 1995. Age, thymopoiesis, and CD4+ T-lymphocyte regeneration after intensive chemotherapy. *N. Engl. J. Med.* **332**:143–149.

2734. Mackay, G. A., Z. Liu, D. K. Singh, M. S. Smith, S. Mukherjee, D. Sheffer, F. Jia, I. Adany, K. H. Sun, S. Dhillon, W. Zhuge, and O. Narayan. 2004. Protection against late-onset AIDS in macaques prophylactically immunized with a live simian HIV vaccine was dependent on persistence of the vaccine virus. *J. Immunol.* **173**:4100–4107.

2735. Mackewicz, C., and J. A. Levy. 1992. CD8+ cell anti-HIV activity: nonlytic suppression of virus replication. *AIDS Res. Hum. Retrovir.* **8**:1039–1050.

2736. Mackewicz, C. E., E. Barker, G. Greco, G. Reyes-Teran, and J. A. Levy. 1997. Do β-chemokines have clinical relevance in HIV infection? *J. Clin. Investig.* **100**:921–930.

2737. Mackewicz, C. E., E. Barker, and J. A. Levy. 1996. Role of β-chemokines in suppressing HIV replication. *Science* **274**:1393–1395.

2738. Mackewicz, C. E., D. J. Blackbourn, and J. A. Levy. 1995. CD8+ cells suppress human immunodeficiency virus replication by inhibiting viral transcription. *Proc. Natl. Acad. Sci. USA* **92**:2308–2312.

2739. Mackewicz, C. E., C. S. Craik, and J. A. Levy. 2003. The CD8+ cell noncytotoxic anti-HIV response can be blocked by protease inhibitors. *Proc. Natl. Acad. Sci. USA* **100**:3433–3438.

2740. Mackewicz, C. E., M. R. Garovoy, and J. A. Levy. 1998. HLA compatibility requirements for CD8+ T-cell-mediated suppression of human immunodeficiency virus replication. *J. Virol.* **72**:10165–10170.

2741. Mackewicz, C. E., A. Landay, H. Hollander, and J. A. Levy. 1994. Effect of zidovudine therapy on CD8+ T cell anti-HIV activity. *Clin. Immunol. Immunopathol.* **73**:80–87.

2742. Mackewicz, C. E., J. A. Levy, W. W. Cruikshank, H. Kornfeld, and D. M. Center. 1996. Role of IL-16 in HIV replication. *Nature* **383**:488–489.

2743. Mackewicz, C. E., J. Lieberman, C. Froelich, and J. A. Levy. 2000. HIV virions and HIV infection in vitro are unaffected by human granzymes A and B. *AIDS Res. Hum. Retrovir.* **16**:367–372.

2744. Mackewicz, C. E., H. Ortega, and J. A. Levy. 1994. Effect of cytokines on HIV replication in CD4+ lymphocytes: lack of identity with the CD8+ cell antiviral factor. *Cell. Immunol.* **153**:329–343.

2745. Mackewicz, C. E., H. W. Ortega, and J. A. Levy. 1991. CD8+ cell anti-HIV activity correlates with the clinical state of the infected individual. *J. Clin. Investig.* **87**:1462–1466.

2746. Mackewicz, C. E., B. K. Patterson, S. A. Lee, and J. A. Levy. 2000. CD8(+) cell noncytotoxic anti-human immunodeficiency virus response inhibits expression of viral RNA but not reverse transcription or provirus integration. *J. Gen. Virol.* **81**:1261–1264.

2747. Mackewicz, C. E., S. Ridha, and J. A. Levy. 2000. HIV virions and HIV replication are unaffected by granulysin. *AIDS* **14**:328–330.

2748. Mackewicz, C. E., B. Wang, S. Metkar, M. Richey, C. Froelich, and J. A. Levy. 2003. Lack of the CD8+ cell anti-HIV factor in CD8+ cell granules. *Blood* **102**:180–183.

2749. Mackewicz, C. E., L. C. Yang, J. D. Lifson, and J. A. Levy. 1994. Non-cytolytic CD8 T-cell anti-HIV responses in primary infection. *Lancet* **344**:1671–1673.

2750. Mackewicz, C. E., J. Yuan, P. Tran, L. Diaz, E. Mack, M. E. Selsted, and J. A. Levy. 2003. α-defensins can have anti-HIV activity but are not CD8+ cell anti-HIV factors. *AIDS* **17**:F23-F32.

2751. Maclean, C., P. J. Flegg, and D. C. Kilpatrick. 1990. Anticardiolipin antibodies and HIV infection. *Clin. Exp. Immunol.* **81**:263–266.

2752. MacMahon, E. M. E., J. D. Glass, S. D. Hayward, R. B. Mann, P. S. Becker, P. Charache, J. C. McArthur, and R. F. Ambinder. 1991. Epstein-Barr virus in AIDS-related primary central nervous system lymphoma. *Lancet* **338**:969–973.

2753. Maddon, P. J., A. G. Dalgleish, J. S. McDougal, P. R. Clapham, R. A. Weiss, and R. Axel. 1986. The T4 gene encodes the AIDS virus receptor and is expressed in the immune system and the brain. *Cell* **47**:333–348.

2754. Madec, Y., F. Boufassa, C. Rouzioux, J.-F. Delfraissy, and L. Meyer. 2005. Undetectable viremia without antiretroviral therapy in patients with HIV seroconversion: an uncommon phenomenon? *Clin. Infect. Dis.* **40**:1350–1354.

2755. Maecker, H. T. 2005. The role of immune monitoring in evaluating cancer immunotherapy, p. 59–72. *In* M. L. Disis (ed.), *Immunotherapy of Cancer.* Humana Press, Totowa, N.J.

2756. Maeda, Y., S. Matsushita, T. Hattori, T. Murakami, and K. Takatsuki. 1992. Changes in the reactivity and neutralizing activity of a type-specific neutralizing monoclonal antibody induced by interaction of soluble CD4 with gp120. *AIDS Res. Hum. Retrovir.* **8**:2049–2054.

2757. Maertens, G., P. Cherepanov, W. Pluymers, K. Busschots, E. De Clercq, Z. Debyser, and Y. Engelborghs. 2003. LEDGF/p75 is essential for nuclear and chromosomal targeting of HIV-1 integrase in human cells. *J. Biol. Chem.* 278:33528–33539.

2758. Maggi, E., M. G. Giudizi, R. Biagiotti, F. Annunziato, R. Manetti, M.-P. Piccinni, P. Parronchi, S. Sampognaro, L. Giannarini, G. Zuccati, and S. Romagnani. 1994. Th2-like CD8+ T cells showing B cell helper function and reduced cytolytic activity in human immunodeficiency virus type 1 infection. *J. Exp. Med.* 180:489–495.

2759. Maggi, E., D. Macchia, P. Parronchi, M. Mazzatti, A. Ravina, D. Milo, and S. Romagnani. 1987. Reduced production of interleukin 2 and interferon-gamma and enhanced helper activity for IgG synthesis by cloned CD4+ T cells from patients with AIDS. *Eur. J. Immunol.* 17:1685–1690.

2760. Maggiolo, F., D. Ripamonti, G. Gregis, G. Quinzan, A. Callegaro, and F. Suter. 2004. Effect of prolonged discontinuation of successful antiretroviral therapy on CD4 T cells: a controlled, prospective trial. *AIDS* 18:439–446.

2761. Magierowska, M., I. Theodorou, P. Debre, F. Sanson, B. Autran, Y. Riviere, D. Charron, French ALT and IMMUNOCO Study Groups, and D. Costagliola. 1999. Combined genotypes of CCR5, CCR2, SDF1, and HLA genes can predict the long-term nonprogressor status in human immunodeficiency virus-1-infected individuals. *Blood* 93:936–941.

2762. Magiorkinis, G., D. Paraskevis, E. Magiorkinis, A. M. Vandamme, and A. Hatzakis. 2002. Reanalysis of the HIV-1 circulating recombinant form A/E (CRF01_AE): evidence of A/E/G recombination. *J. Acquir. Immune Defic. Syndr.* 30:124–129.

2763. Magnuson, D. S. K., B. E. Knudsen, J. D. Geiger, R. M. Brownstone, and A. Nath. 1995. Human immunodeficiency virus type 1 Tat activates non-N-methyl-D-aspartate excitatory amino acid receptors and causes neurotoxicity. *Ann. Neurol.* 37:373–380.

2764. Magrath, I. 1990. The pathogenesis of Burkitt's lymphoma. *Adv. Cancer Res.* 55:133–270.

2765. Mahlknecht, U., C. Deng, M. C. Lu, T. C. Greenough, J. L. Sullivan, W. A. O'Brien, and G. Herbein. 2000. Resistance to apoptosis in HIV-infected CD4(+) T lymphocytes is mediated by macrophages: role for nef and immune activation in viral persistence. *J. Immunol.* 165:6437–6446.

2766. Maiman, M., R. G. Fruchter, M. Clark, C. D. Arrastia, R. Matthews, and E. J. Gates. 1997. Cervical cancer as an AIDS-defining illness. *Obstet. Gynecol.* 89:76–80.

2767. Maiman, M., R. G. Fruchter, L. Guy, S. Cuthill, P. Levine, and E. Serur. 1993. Human immunodeficiency virus infection and invasive cervical carcinoma. *Cancer* 71:402–406.

2768. Makedonas, G., J. Bruneau, M. Alary, C. M. Tsoukas, C. M. Lowndes, F. Lamothe, and N. F. Bernard. 2005. Comparison of HIV-specific CD8 T-cell responses among uninfected individuals exposed to HIV parenterally and mucosally. *AIDS* 19:251–259.

2769. Makedonas, G., J. Bruneau, H. Lin, R. P. Sekaly, F. Lamothe, and N. F. Bernard. 2002. HIV-specific CD8 T-cell activity in uninfected injection drug users is associated with maintenance of seronegativity. *AIDS* 16:1595–1602.

2770. Malamud, D., C. Davis, P. Berthold, E. Roth, and H. Friedman. 1993. Human submandibular saliva aggregates HIV. *AIDS Res. Hum. Retrovir.* 9:633–637.

2771. Malaspina, A., S. Moir, S. Kottilil, C. W. Hallahan, L. A. Ehler, S. Liu, M. A. Planta, T. Chun, and A. S. Fauci. 2003. Deleterious effect of HIV-1 plasma viremia on B cell costimulatory function. *J. Immunol.* 170:5965–5972.

2772. Malaspina, A., S. Moir, D. C. Nickle, E. T. Donoghue, K. M. Ogwaro, L. A. Ehler, S. Liu, J. M. Mican, M. Dybul, T. Chun, J. I. Mullins, and A. S. Fauci. 2002. Human immunodeficiency virus type 1 bound to B cells: relationship to virus replicating in CD4+ T cells and circulating in plasma. *J. Virol.* 76:8855–8863.

2773. Malaspina, A., S. Moir, S. M. Orsega, J. Vasquez, N. J. Miller, E. T. Donoghue, S. Kottilil, M. Gezmu, D. Follmann, G. M. Vodeiko, R. A. Levandowski, J. M. Mican, and A. S. Fauci. 2005. Compromised B cell responses to influenza vaccination in HIV-infected individuals. *J. Infect. Dis.* 191:1442–1450.

2774. Maldarelli, F., H. Sato, E. Berthold, J. Orenstein, and M. A. Martin. 1995. Rapid induction of apoptosis by cell-to-cell transmisssion of human immunodeficiency virus type 1. *J. Virol.* 69:6457–6465.

2775. Malenbaum, S. E., D. Yang, L. Cavacini, M. Posner, J. Robinson, and C. Cheng-Mayer. 2000. The N-terminal V3 loop glycan modulates the interaction of clade A and B human immunodeficiency virus type 1 envelopes with CD4 and chemokine receptors. *J. Virol.* 74:11008–11016.

2776. Malhotra, U., M. M. Berrey, Y. Huang, J. Markee, D. J. Brown, S. Ap, L. Musey, T. Schacker, L. Corey, and M. J. McElrath. 2000. Effect of combination antiretroviral therapy on T-cell immunity in acute human immunodeficiency virus type 1 infection. *J. Infect. Dis.* 181:121–131.

2777. Malhotra, U., S. Holte, S. Dutta, M. M., Berrey, E. Delpit, D. M. Koelle, A. Sette, L. Corey, and M. J. McElrath. 2001. Role for HLA class II molecules in HIV-1 suppression and cellular immunity following antiretroviral treatment. *J. Clin. Investig.* 107:505–517.

2778. Malhotra, U., S. Holte, T. Zhu, E. Delpit, C. Huntsberry, A. Sette, R. Shankarappa, J. Maenze, L. Corey, and M. J. McElrath. 2003. Early induction and maintenance of Env-specific T-helper cells following human immunodeficiency virus type 1 infection. *J. Virol.* 77:2663–2674.

2778a. Malkevitch, N. V., L. J. Patterson, M. K. Aldrich, Y. Wu, D. Venzon, R. H. Florese, V. S. Kalyanaraman, R. Pal, E. M. Lee, J. Zhao, A. Cristillo, and M. Robert-Guroff. 2006. Durable protection of rhesus macaques immunized with a replicating adenovirus-SIV multigene prime/protein boost vaccine regimen against a second SIVmac251 rectal challenge: role of SIV-specific CD8+ T cell responses. *Virology* 353:83–98.

2779. Malkovsky, M., M. Wallace, J.-J. Fournié, P. Fisch, F. Poccia, and M.-L. Gougeon. 2000. Alternative cytotoxic effector mechanisms in infections with immunodeficiency viruses: γδ T lymphocytes and natural killer cells. *AIDS* 14(Suppl. 3): S175–S186.

2780. Mallal, S., D. Nolan, C. Witt, G. Masel, A. M. Martin, C. Moore, D. Sayer, A. Castley, C. Mamotte, D. Maxwell, I. James, and F. T. Christiansen. 2002. Association between presence of HLA-B*5701, HLA-DR7, and HLA-DQ3 and hypersensitivity to HIV-1 reverse-transcriptase inhibitor abacavir. *Lancet* 359:727–732.

2781. Malley, S. D., J. M. Grange, F. Hamedi-Sangsari, and J. R. Vila. 1994. Synergistic anti-human immunodeficiency virus type 1 effect of hydroxamate compounds with 2′,3′-dideoxyinosine in infected resting human lymphocytes. *Proc. Natl. Acad. Sci. USA* 91:11017–11021.

2782. Managlia, E. Z., D. Carroll, A. Zloza, and L. Al-Harthi. 2004. Immune modulation of HIV replication: relevance to

HIV immuno- and neuro-pathogenesis. *Curr. HIV Res.* **2**: 395–401.

2783. Managlia, E. Z., A. Landay, and L. Al-Harthi. 2005. Interleukin-7 signalling is sufficient to phenotypically and functionally prime human CD4 naive T cells. *Immunology* **114**:322–335.

2784. Mandelbrot, L., M. Burgard, J. P. Teglas, J. L. Benifla, C. Khan, P. Blot, E. Vilmer, S. Matheron, G. Firtion, S. Blanche, M. J. Mayaux, and C. Rouzioux. 1999. Frequent detection of HIV-1 in the gastric aspirates of neonates born to HIV-infected mothers. *AIDS* **13**:2143–2149.

2785. Manes, S., G. del Real, R. A. Lacalle, P. Lucas, C. Gomez-Mouton, S. Sanchez-Palomino, R. Delgado, J. Alcami, E. Mira, and C. Martinez-A. 2000. Membrane raft microdomains mediate lateral assemblies required for HIV-1 infection. *EMBO Rep.* **1**:190–196.

2786. Manetti, R., P. Parronchi, M. G. Giudizi, M.-P. Piccinni, E. Maggi, G. Trinchieri, and S. Romagnani. 1993. Natural killer cell stimulatory factor (interleukin 12 [IL-12]) induces T helper type 1 (Th1)-specific immune responses and inhibits the development of IL-4-producing Th cells. *J. Exp. Med.* **177**:1199–1204.

2787. Mangan, D. F., B. Robertson, and S. M. Wahl. 1992. IL-4 enhances programmed cell death (apoptosis) in stimulated human monocytes. *J. Immunol.* **148**:1812–1816.

2788. Mangeat, B., P. Turelli, G. Caron, M. Friedli, L. Perrin, and D. Trono. 2003. Broad antiretroviral defence by human APOBEC3G through lethal editing of nascent reverse transcripts. *Nature* **424**:99–103.

2789. Mangkornkanok-Mark, M., A. S. Mark, and J. Dong. 1984. Immunoperoxidase evaluation of lymph nodes from acquired immune deficiency patients. *Clin. Exp. Immunol.* **55**: 581–586.

2790. Manigart, O., V. Courgnaud, O. Sanou, D. Valea, N. Bagot, N. Meda, E. Delaporte, M. Peeters, and P. Van de Perre. 2004. HIV-1 superinfections in a cohort of commercial sex workers in Burkina Faso as assessed by an autologous heteroduplex mobility procedure. *AIDS* **18**:1645–1651.

2791. Mankowski, J. L., J. P. Spelman, H. G. Ressetar, J. D. Strandberg, J. Laterra, D. L. Carter, J. E. Clements, and M. C. Zink. 1994. Neurovirulent simian immunodeficiency virus replicates productively in endothelial cells of the central nervous system in vivo and in vitro. *J. Virol.* **68**:8202–8208.

2792. Mann, D. L., F. Lasane, M. Popovic, L. O. Arthur, W. G. Robey, W. A. Blattner, and M. J. Newman. 1987. HTLV-III large envelope protein (gp120) suppresses PHA-induced lymphocyte blastogenesis. *J. Immunol.* **138**:2640–2644.

2793. Mann, D. L., C. Murray, R. Yarchoan, W. A. Blattner, and J. J. Goedert. 1988. HLA antigen frequencies in HIV-1 seropositive disease-free individuals and patients with AIDS. *J. Acquir. Immune Defic. Syndr.* **1**:13–17.

2794. Mann, J., and D. Tarantola. 1996. *AIDS in the World II.* Oxford University Press, New York, N. Y.

2795. Mann, J. M., H. Francis, F. Davachi, P. Baudoux, T. C. Quinn, N. Nzilambi, N. Bosenge, R. L. Colebunders, N. Kabote, P. Piot, et al. 1986. Human immunodeficiency virus seroprevalence in pediatric patients 2 to 14 years of age at Mama Yemo Hospital, Kinshasa, Zaire. *Pediatrics* **78**:673–677.

2796. Mannie, M. D., and M. S. Norris. 2001. MHC class-II-restricted antigen presentation by myelin basic protein-specific CD4+ T cells causes prolonged desensitization and outgrowth of CD4- responders. *Cell. Immunol.* **212**:51–62.

2797. Manninen, A., G. H. Renkema, and K. Saksela. 2000. Synergistic activation of NFAT by HIV-1 Nef and the Ras/MAPK pathway. *J. Biol. Chem.* **275**:16513–16517.

2798. Marandin, A., A. Katz, E. Oksenhendler, M. Tulliez, F. Picard, W. Vainchenker, and F. Louache. 1996. Loss of primitive hematopoietic progenitors in patients with human immunodeficiency virus infection. *Blood* **88**:4568–4578.

2799. Marasco, W. A., W. A. Haseltine, and S. Chen. 1993. Design, intracellular expression, and activity of a human anti-human immunodeficiency virus type 1 gp120 single-chain antibody. *Proc. Natl. Acad. Sci. USA* **90**:7889–7893.

2800. Marchant, D., S. J. Neil, K. Aubin, C. Schmitz, and A. McKnight. 2005. An envelope-determined, pH-independent endocytic route of viral entry determines the susceptibility of human immunodeficiency virus type 1 (HIV-1) and HIV-2 to Lv2 restriction. *J. Virol.* **79**:9410–9418.

2801. Marchetti, G., L. Meroni, S. Varchetta, V. Terzieva, A. Bandera, D. Manganaro, C. Molteni, D. Trabattoni, S. Fossati, M. Clerici, M. Galli, M. Moroni, F. Franzetti, and A. Gori. 2002. Low-dose prolonged intermittent interleukin-2 adjuvant therapy: results of a randomized trial among human immunodeficiency virus-positive patients with advanced immune impairment. *J. Infect. Dis.* **186**:606–616.

2802. Marchio, S., M. Alfano, L. Primo, D. Gramaglia, L. Butini, L. Gennero, E. De Vivo, W. Arap, M. Giacca, R. Pasqualini, and F. Bussolino. 2005. Cell surface-associated Tat modulates HIV-1 infection and spreading through a specific interaction with gp120 viral envelope protein. *Blood* **105**:2802–2811.

2803. Marcon, L., and J. Sodroski. 1994. gp120-independent fusion mediated by the human immunodeficiency virus type 1 gp41 envelope glycoprotein: a reassessment. *J. Virol.* **68**: 1977–1982.

2804. Marechal, V., F. Arenzana-Seisdedos, J.-M. Heard, and O. Schwartz. 1999. Opposite effects of SDF-1 on human immunodeficiency virus type 1 replication. *J. Virol.* **73**:3608–3615.

2805. Margalith, M., E. Levy, C. R. Rinaldo, R. Detels, J. Phair, R. Kaslow, A. J. Saah, and B. Sarov. 2001. HIV-1 IgA specific serum antibodies and disease progression during HIV-1 infection. *J. Hum. Virol.* **4**:269–277.

2806. Margolick, J. B., A. Munoz, A. D. Donnenberg, L. P. Park, N. Galai, J. V. Giorgi, M. R. G. O'Gorman, and J. Ferbas. 1995. Failure of T-cell homeostasis preceding AIDS in HIV-1 infection. *Nat. Med.* **1**:674–680.

2807. Margolick, J. B., D. J. Volkman, T. M. Folks, and A. S. Fauci. 1987. Amplification of HTLV-III/LAV infection by antigen-induced activation of T cells and direct suppression by virus of lymphocyte blastogenic responses. *J. Immunol.* **138**: 1719–1723.

2808. Margolis, D. M., S. Kewn, J. J. Coull, L. Ylisastigui, D. Turner, H. Wise, M. M. Hossain, E. R. Lanier, L. M. Shaw, and D. Back. 2002. The addition of mycophenolate mofetil to antiretroviral therapy including abacavir is associated with depletion of intracellular deoxyguanosine triphosphate and a decrease in plasma HIV-1 RNA. *J. Acquir. Immune Defic. Syndr.* **31**:45–49.

2809. Margolis, D. M., M. Somasundaran, and M. R. Green. 1994. Human transcription factor YY1 represses human immunodeficiency virus type 1 transcription and virion production. *J. Virol.* **68**:905–910.

2810. Mariani, R., G. Rutter, M. E. Harris, T. J. Hope, H. G. Krausslich, and N. R. Landau. 2000. A block to human immunodeficiency virus type 1 assembly in murine cells. *J. Virol.* 74:3859–3870.

2811. Mariani, R., and J. Skowronski. 1993. CD4 downregulation by nef alleles isolated from human immunodeficiency virus type 1-infected individuals. *Proc. Natl. Acad. Sci. USA* 90:5549–5553.

2812. Marin, M., K. M. Rose, S. L. Kozak, and D. Kabat. 2003. HIV-1 Vif protein binds the editing enzyme APOBEC3G and induces its degradation. *Nat. Med.* 9:1398–1403.

2813. Markel, G., H. Mussaffi, K. L. Ling, M. Salio, S. Gadola, G. Steuer, H. Blau, H. Achdout, M. de Miguel, T. Gonen-Gross, J. Hanna, T. I. Arnon, U. Qimron, I. Volovitz, L. Eisenbach, R. S. Blumberg, A. Porgador, V. Cerundolo, and O. Mandelboim. 2004. The mechanisms controlling NK cell autoreactivity in TAP2-deficient patients. *Blood* 103:1770–1778.

2814. Markert, M. L., D. D. Kostyu, F. E. Ward, T. M. McLaughlin, T. J. Watson, R. H. Buckley, S. E. Schiff, R. M. Ungerleider, J. W. Gaynor, K. T. Oldham, S. M. Mahaffey, M. Ballow, D. A. Driscoll, L. P. Hale, and B. F. Haynes. 1997. Successful formation of a chimeric human thymus allograft following transplantation of cultured postnatal human thymus. *J. Immunol.* 158:998–1005.

2815. Markham, R. B., J. Coberly, A. J. Ruff, D. Hoover, J. Gomez, E. Holt, J. Desormeaux, R. Boulos, T. C. Quinn, and N. A. Halsey. 1994. Maternal IgG1 and IgA antibody to V3 loop consensus sequence and maternal-infant HIV-1 transmission. *Lancet* 343:390–391.

2816. Markowitz, M., X. Jin, A. Hurley, V. Simon, B. Ramratnam, M. Louie, G. R. Deschenes, M. Ramanathan, Jr., S. Barsoum, J. Vanderhoeven, T. He, C. Chung, J. Murray, A. S. Perelson, L. Zhang, and D. D. Ho. 2002. Discontinuation of antiretroviral therapy commenced early during the course of human immunodeficiency virus type 1 infection, with or without adjunctive vaccination. *J. Infect. Dis.* 186:634–643.

2817. Markowitz, M., H. Mohri, S. Mehandru, A. Shet, L. Berry, R. Kalyanaraman, A. Kim, C. Chung, P. Jean-Pierre, A. Horowitz, M. LaMar, T. Wrin, N. Parkin, M. Poles, C. Petropoulos, M. Mullen, D. Boden, and D. D. Ho. 2005. Infection with multidrug resistant, dual-tropic HIV-1 and rapid progression to AIDS: a case report. *Lancet* 365:1031–1038.

2818. Markowitz, M., M. Vesanen, K. Tenner-Racz, Y. Cao, J. M. Binley, A. Talal, A. Hurley, X. Ji, M. R. Chaudhry, M. Yaman, S. Frankel, M. Heath-Chiozzi, J. M. Leonard, J. P. Moore, P. Racz, D. F. Nixon, and D. D. Ho. 1999. The effect of commencing combination antiretroviral therapy soon after human immunodeficiency virus type 1 infection on viral replication and antiviral immune responses. *J. Infect. Dis.* 179:525–537.

2819. Markwell, M. A. K., L. Svennerholm, and J. C. Paulson. 1981. Specific gangliosides function as host cell receptors for Sendai virus. *Proc. Natl. Acad. Sci. USA* 78:5406–5410.

2820. Marlink, R. 1996. Lessons from the second AIDS virus, HIV-2. *AIDS* 10:689–699.

2821. Marodon, G., D. Warren, M. C. Filomio, and D. N. Posnett. 1999. Productive infection of double-negative T cells with HIV in vivo. *Proc. Natl. Acad. Sci. USA* 96:11958–11963.

2822. Marozsan, A. J., D. M. Moore, M. A. Lobritz, E. Fraundorf, A. Abraha, J. D. Reeves, and E. J. Arts. 2005. Differences in the fitness of two diverse wild-type human immunodeficiency

virus type 1 isolates are related to the efficiency of cell binding and entry. *J. Virol.* 79:7121–7134.

2823. Marras, D., L. A. Bruggeman, F. Gao, N. Tanji, M. M. Mansukhani, A. Cara, M. D. Ross, G. L. Gusella, G. Benson, V. D. D'Agati, B. H. Hahn, M. E. Klotman, and P. E. Klotman. 2002. Replication and compartmentalization of HIV-1 in kidney epithelium of patients with HIV-associated nephropathy. *Nat. Med.* 8:522–526.

2824. Marriott, D. J. E., and M. McMurchie. 1996. Managing HIV. Part 2. Phases of disease. 2.4. HIV and advanced immune deficiency. *Med. J. Aust.* 164:111–112.

2825. Marschang, P., U. Kruger, C. Ochsenbauer, L. Gurtler, A. Hittmair, V. Bosch, J. R. Patsch, and M. P. Dierich. 1997. Complement activation by HIV-1-infected cells: the role of transmembrane glycoprotein gp41. *J. Acquir. Immune Defic. Syndr. Hum. Retrovirol.* 14:102–109.

2826. Marsh, J. W., B. Herndier, A. Tsuzuki, V. L. Ng, B. Shiramizu, N. Abbey, and M. S. McGrath. 1995. Cytokine expression in large cell lymphoma associated with acquired immunodeficiency syndrome. *J. Interferon Cytokine Res.* 15: 261–268.

2827. Marthas, M. L., S. Sutjipto, J. Higgins, B. Lohman, J. Torten, P. A. Luciw, P. A. Marx, and N. C. Pedersen. 1990. Immunization with a live, attenuated simian immunodeficiency virus (SIV) prevents early disease but not infection in rhesus macaques challenged with pathogenic SIV. *J. Virol.* 64:3694–3700.

2828. Martin, A. M., D. Nolan, I. James, P. Cameron, J. Keller, C. Moore, E. Phillips, F. T. Christiansen, and S. Mallal. 2005. Predisposition to nevirapine hypersensitivity associated with HLA-DRB1*0101 and abrogated by low CD4 T-cell counts. *AIDS* 19:97–99.

2829. Martin, M. P., and M. Carrington. 2005. Immunogenetics of viral infections. *Curr. Opin. Immunol.* 17:510–516.

2830. Martin, M. P., M. Dean, M. W. Smith, C. Winkler, B. Gerrard, N. L. Michael, B. Lee, R. W. Doms, J. Margolick, S. Buchbinder, J. J. Goedert, T. R. O'Brien, M. W. Hilgartner, D. Vlahov, S. J. O'Brien, and M. Carrington. 1998. Genetic acceleration of AIDS progression by a promoter variant of CCR5. *Science* 282:1907–1911.

2831. Martin, M. P., X. Gao, J. Lee, G. W. Nelson, R. Detels, J. J. Goedert, S. Buchbinder, K. Hoots, D. Vlahov, J. Trowsdale, M. Wilson, S. J. O'Brien, and M. Carrington. 2002. Epistatic interaction between KIR3DS1 and HLA-B delays the progression to AIDS. *Nat. Genet.* 31:429–434.

2832. Martin, M. P., M. M. Lederman, H. B. Hutcheson, J. J. Goedert, G. W. Nelson, Y. van Kooyk, R. Detels, S. Buchbinder, K. Hoots, D. Vlahov, S. O'Brien, and M. Carrington. 2004. Association of DC-SIGN promoter polymorphism with increased risk for parenteral, but not mucosal, acquisition of human immunodeficiency type 1 infection. *J. Infect. Dis.* 78:14053–14056.

2833. Martin, N. L., J. A. Levy, H. S. Legg, P. S. Weintrub, M. J. Cowan, and D. W. Wara. 1991. Detection of infection with human immunodeficiency virus (HIV) type 1 in infants by an anti-immunoglobulin A assay using recombinant proteins. *J. Pediatr.* 118:354–358.

2834. Martin, S. J., P. M. Matear, and A. Vyakarnam. 1994. HIV-1 infection of human CD4+ T cells in vitro. *J. Immunol.* 152:330–342.

2835. Martinez, E., A. Mocroft, A. A. Garcia-Viejo, J. B. Perez-Cuevas, J. L. Blanco, J. Mallolas, L. Bianchi, I. Conget, J. Blanch,

A. Phillips, and J. M. Gatell. 2005. Risk of lipodystrophy in HIV-1-infected patients treated with protease inhibitors: a prospective cohort study. *Lancet* 357:592–598.

2836. Martinez, M.-A., M. Cabana, A. Ibanez, C. Bonaventura, A. Arno, and L. Ruiz. 1999. Human immunodeficiency virus type 1 genetic evolution in patients with prolonged suppression of plasma viremia. *Virology* 256:180–187.

2837. Martinez, O. M., R. S. Gibbons, M. R. Garavoy, and F. R. Aronson. 1990. IL-4 inhibits IL-2 receptor expression and Il-2 dependent proliferation of human T-cells. *J. Immunol.* 144:2211–2215.

2838. Martinez, V., D. Costaglioloa, O. Bonduelle, N. N'Go, A. Schnuriger, I. Theodorou, J. Clauvel, D. Sicard, H. Agut, P. Debre, C. Rouzioux, and B. Autran. 2005. Combination of HIV-1-specific CD4 Th1 cell responses and IgG2 antibodies is the best predictor for persistence of long-term nonprogression. *J. Infect. Dis.* 191:2053–2063.

2839. Martinez-Marino, B., B. M. Ashlock, S. Shiboski, F. M. Hecht, and J. A. Levy. 2004. Effect of IL-2 therapy on CD8+ cell non-cytotoxic anti-HIV response during primary HIV-1 infection. *J. Clin. Immunol.* 24:135–144.

2840. Martinez-Marino, B., S. Shiboski, F. M. Hecht, J. O. Kahn, and J. A. Levy. 2004. Interleukin-2 therapy restores CD8 cell non-cytotoxic anti-HIV responses in primary infection subjects receiving HAART. *AIDS* 18:1991–1999.

2841. Martinez-Picado, J., K. Morales-Lopetegi, T. Wrin, J. G. Prado, S. D. Frost, C. J. Petropoulos, B. Clotet, and L. Ruiz. 2002. Selection of drug-resistant HIV-1 mutants in response to repeated structured treatment interruptions. *AIDS* 16:895–899.

2842. Martinez-Picado, J., A. V. Savara, L. Sutton, and R. T. D'Aquila. 1999. Replicative fitness of protease inhibitor-resistant mutants of human immunodeficiency virus type 1. *J. Virol.* 73:3744–3752.

2843. Martini, F., M. G. Paglia, C. Montesano, P. J. Enders, M. Gentile, C. D. Pauza, C. Gioia, V. Colizzi, P. Narciso, L. P. Pucillo, and F. Poccia. 2003. V gamma 9V delta 2 T-cell anergy and complementarity-determining region 3-specific depletion during paroxysm of nonendemic malaria infection. *Infect. Immun.* 71:2945–2949.

2844. Martini, F., F. Poccia, D. Goletti, S. Carrara, D. Vincenti, G. D'Offizi, C. Agrati, G. Ippolito, V. Colizzi, L. Pucillo, and C. Montesano. 2002. Acute human immunodeficiency virus replication causes a rapid and persistent impairment of Vγ9Vδ2 T cells in chronically infected patients undergoing structured treatment interruption. *J. Infect. Dis.* 186:847–850.

2845. Martini, F., R. Urso, C. Gioia, A. De Felici, P. Narciso, A. Amendola, M. G. Paglia, V. Colizzi, and F. Poccia. 2000. gammadelta T-cell anergy in human immunodeficiency virus-infected persons with opportunistic infections and recovery after highly active antiretroviral therapy. *Immunology* 100:481–486.

2846. Martins, L. P., N. Chenciner, B. Asjo, A. Meyerhans, and S. Wain-Hobson. 1991. Independent fluctuation of human immunodeficiency virus type 1 *rev* and gp41 quasispecies in vivo. *J. Virol.* 65:4502–4507.

2847. Martinson, J. J., N. H. Chapman, D. C. Rees, Y. T. Liu, and J. B. Clegg. 1997. Global distribution of the CCR5 gene 32-basepair deletion. *Nat. Genet.* 16:100–103.

2848. Marusic, C., P. Rizza, L. Lattanzi, C. Mancini, M. Spada, F. Belardelli, E. Benvenuto, and I. Capone. 2001. Chimeric plant virus particles as immunogens for inducing murine and human immune responses against human immunodeficiency virus type 1. *J. Virol.* 75:8434–8439.

2849. Marx, P. A. 2005. Unresolved questions over the origin of HIV and AIDS. *ASM News* 71:15–20.

2850. Marx, P. A., R. W. Compans, A. Gettie, J. K. Staas, R. M. Gilley, M. J. Mulligan, G. V. Yamshchikov, D. Chen, and J. H. Eldridge. 1993. Protection against vaginal SIV transmission with microencapsulated vaccine. *Science* 260:1323–1327.

2851. Marx, P. A., Y. Li, N. W. Lerche, S. Sutjipto, A. Gettie, J. A. Yee, B. H. Brotman, A. M. Prince, A. Hanson, R. G. Webster, and R. C. Desrosiers. 1991. Isolation of a simian immunodeficiency virus related to human immunodeficiency virus type 2 from a West African pet sooty mangabey. *J. Virol.* 65:4480–4485.

2852. Marx, P. A., A. I. Spira, A. Gettie, P. J. Dailey, R. S. Veazey, A. A. Lackner, C. J. Mahoney, C. J. Miller, L. E. Claypool, D. D. Ho, and N. J. Alexander. 1996. Progesterone implants enhance SIV vaginal transmission and early virus load. *Nat. Med.* 2:1084–1089.

2853. Mary-Krause, M., L. Cotte, A. Simon, M. Partisani, and D. Costagliola. 2003. Increased risk of myocardial infarction with duration of protease inhibitor therapy in HIV-infected men. *AIDS* 17:2479–2486.

2854. Marzolini, C., A. Telenti, L. A. Decosterd, G. Greub, J. Biollaz, and T. Buclin. 2001. Efavirenz plasma levels can predict treatment failure and central nervous system side effects in HIV-1-infected patients. *AIDS* 15:71–75.

2855. Masciotra, S., S. M. Owen, D. Rudolph, C. Yang, B. Wang, N. Saksena, T. Spira, S. Dhawan, and R. B. Lal. 2002. Temporal relationship between V1V2 variation, macrophage replication, and coreceptor adaptation during HIV-1 disease progression. *AIDS* 16:1887–1898.

2856. Mascola, J. R., P. D'Souza, P. Gilbert, B. H. Hahn, N. L. Haigwood, L. Morris, C. J. Petropoulos, V. R. Polonis, M. Sarzotti, and D. C. Montefiori. 2005. Recommendations for the design and use of standard virus panels to assess neutralizing antibody responses elicited by candidate human immunodeficiency virus type 1 vaccines. *J. Virol.* 79:10103–10107.

2857. Mascola, J. R., M. K. Louder, S. R. Surman, T. C. Vancott, X. F. Yu, J. Bradac, K. R. Porter, K. E. Nelson, M. Girard, J. G. McNeil, F. E. McCutchan, D. L. Birx, and D. S. Burke. 1996. Human immunodeficiency virus type 1 neutralizing antibody serotyping using serum pools and an infectivity reduction assay. *AIDS Res. Hum. Retrovir.* 12:1319–1328.

2858. Mascola, J. R., J. Louwagie, F. E. McCutchen, C. L. Fischer, P. A. Hegerich, K. F. Wagner, A. K. Fowler, J. G. McNeil, and D. S. Burke. 1994. Two antigenically distinct subtypes of human immunodeficiency virus type 1: viral genotype predicts neutralization serotype. *J. Infect. Dis.* 169:48–54.

2859. Mascola, J. R., B. J. Mathieson, P. M. Zack, M. C. Walker, S. B. Halstead, and D. S. Burke. 1993. Summary report: workshop on the potential risks of antibody-dependent enhancement in human HIV vaccine trials. *AIDS Res. Hum. Retrovir.* 9:1175–1184.

2860. Mascola, J. R., G. Stiegler, T. C. VanCott, H. Katinger, C. B. Carpenter, C. E. Hanson, H. Beary, D. Hayes, S. S. Frankel, D. L. Birx, and M. G. Lewis. 2000. Protection of macaques against vaginal transmission of a pathogenic HIV-1/SIV chimeric virus by passive infusion of neutralizing antibodies. *Nat. Med.* 6:207–210.

2861. Masliah, E., R. M. DeTeresa, M. E. Mallory, and L. A. Hansen. 2000. Changes in pathological findings at autopsy in AIDS cases for the last 15 years. *AIDS* 14:69–74.

2862. Masood, R., Y. Zhang, M. W. Bond, D. T. Scadden, T. Moudgil, R. E. Law, M. H. Kaplan, B. Jung, B. M. Espina, and Y. Lunardi-Iskandar. 1995. Interleukin-10 is an autocrine growth factor for acquired immunodeficiency syndrome-related B-cell lymphoma. *Blood* 85:3423–3430.

2863. Massad, L. S., K. A. Riester, K. M. Anastos, R. G. Fruchter, J. M. Palefsky, R. D. Burk, D. Burns, R. M. Greenblatt, L. I. Muderspach, P. Miotti, et al. 1999. Prevalence and predictors of squamous cell abnormalities in Papanicolaou smears from women infected with HIV-1. *J. Acquir. Immune Defic. Syndr.* 21:33–41.

2864. Massiah, M. A., M. R. Starich, C. Paschall, M. F. Summers, A. M. Christensen, and W. I. Sundquist. 1994. Three-dimensional structure of the human immunodeficiency virus type 1 matrix protein. *J. Mol. Biol.* 244:198–223.

2865. Master, S., J. Taylor, S. Kyalwazi, and J. L. Ziegler. 1970. Immunological studies in Kaposi's sarcoma in Uganda. *Br. Med. J.* 1:600–602.

2866. Mastroianni, C. M., G. d'Ettorre, G. Forcina, M. Lichtner, F. Mengoni, C. D'Agostino, A. Corpolongo, A. P. Massetti, and V. Vullo. 2000. Interleukin-15 enhances neutrophil functional activity in patients with human immunodeficiency virus infection. *Blood* 96:1979–1984.

2867. Masuda, M., P. M. Hoffman, and S. K. Ruscetti. 1993. Viral determinants that control the neuropathogenicity of PVC-211 murine leukemia virus in vivo determine brain capillary endothelial cell tropism of the virus in vitro. *J. Virol.* 67:4580–4587.

2868. Masur, H., M. A. Michelis, and J. B. Greene. 1981. An outbreak of community-acquired *Pneumocystis carinii* pneumonia. *N. Engl. J. Med.* 305:1431–1438.

2869. Matano, T., R. Shibata, C. Siemon, M. Connors, H. C. Lane, and M. A. Martin. 1998. Administration of an anti-CD8 monoclonal antibody interferes with the clearance of chimeric simian/human immunodeficiency virus during primary infections of rhesus macaques. *J. Virol.* 72:164–169.

2870. Mathijs, J. M., M. C. Hing, J. Grierson, D. E. Dwyer, C. Goldschmidt, D. A. Cooper, and A. L. Cunningham. 1988. HIV infection of rectal mucosa. *Lancet* i:1111.

2871. Matsuyama, T., N. Kobayashi, and N. Yamamoto. 1991. Cytokines and HIV infection: is AIDS a tumor necrosis factor disease? *AIDS* 5:1405–1417.

2872. Mattapallil, J. J., D. C. Douek, B. Hill, Y. Nishimura, M. Martin, and M. Roederer. 2005. Massive infection and loss of memory CD4+ T cells in multiple tissues during acute SIV infection. *Nature* 434:1093–1097.

2873. Matte, C., J. Lajoie, J. Lacaille, L. S. Zijenah, B. J. Ward, and M. Roger. 2004. Functionally active HLA-G polymorphisms are associated with the risk of heterosexual HIV-1 infection in African women. *AIDS* 18:427–431.

2874. Matte, C., L. S. Zijenah, J. Lacaille, B. Ward, and M. Roger. 2002. Mother-to-child leukocyte antigen G concordance: no impact on the risk of vertical transmission of HIV-1. *Lancet* 16:2491–2914.

2875. Matteucci, D., M. Pistello, P. Mazzetti, S. Giannecchini, D. Del Mauro, L. Zaccaro, P. Bandecchi, F. Tozzini, and M. Bendinelli. 1996. Vaccination protects against in vivo-grown feline immunodeficiency virus even in the absence of detectable neutralizing antibodies. *J. Virol.* 70:617–622.

2876. Matteucci, D., A. Poli, P. Mazzetti, S. Sozzi, F. Bonci, P. Isola, L. Zaccaro, S. Giannecchini, M. Calandrella, M. Pistello, S. Specter, and M. Bendinelli. 2000. Immunogenicity of an anti-clade B feline immunodeficiency fixed-cell virus vaccine in field cats. *J. Virol.* 74:10911–10919.

2877. Matthews, T. J., A. J. Langlois, W. G. Robey, N. T. Chang, R. C. Gallo, P. J. Fischinger, and D. P. Bolognesi. 1986. Restricted neutralization of divergent human T-lymphotropic virus type III isolates by antibodies to the major envelope glycoprotein. *Proc. Natl. Acad. Sci. USA* 83:9709–9713.

2878. Matthews, T. J., K. J. Weinhold, H. K. Lyerly, A. J. Langlois, H. Wigzell, and D. P. Bolognesi. 1987. Interaction between the human T-cell lymphotropic virus type IIIB envelope glycoprotein gp120 and the surface antigen CD4: role of carbohydrate in binding and cell fusion. *Proc. Natl. Acad. Sci. USA* 84:5424–5428.

2879. Maury, W., B. J. Potts, and A. B. Rabson. 1989. HIV-1 infection of first-trimester and term human placental tissue: a possible mode of maternal-fetal transmission. *J. Infect. Dis.* 160:583–588.

2880. Mauskopf, J., M. Kitahata, T. Kauf, A. Richter, and J. Tolson. 2005. HIV antiretroviral treatment: early versus later. *J. Acquir. Immune Defic. Syndr.* 39:562–569.

2881. Mavilio, D., J. Benjamin, M. Daucher, G. Lombardo, S. Kottilil, M. A. Planta, E. Marcenaro, C. Bottino, L. Moretta, A. Moretta, and A. S. Fauci. 2003. Natural killer cells in HIV-1 infection: dichotomous effects of viremia on inhibitory and activating receptors and their functional correlates. *Proc. Natl. Acad. Sci. USA* 100:15011–15016.

2881a. Mavilio, D., G. Lombardo, A. Kinter, M. Fogli, A. La Sala, S. Ortolano, A. Farschi, D. Follmann, R. Gregg, C. Kovacs, E. Marcenaro, D. Pende, A. Moretta, and A. S. Fauci. 2006. Characterization of the defective interaction between a subset of natural killer cells and dendritic cells in HIV-1 infection. *J. Exp. Med.* 203:2339–2350.

2882. Mayaux, M.-J., M. Burgard, J.-P. Teglas, J. Cottalorda, A. Krivine, F. Simon, J. Puel, C. Tamalet, D. Dormont, B. Masquelier, A. Doussin, C. Rouzioux, and S. Blanche. 1996. Neonatal characteristics in rapidly progressive perinatally acquired HIV-1 disease. *JAMA* 275:606–610.

2883. Mayer, K. H., and D. J. Anderson. 1995. Heterosexual HIV transmission. *Infect. Agents Dis.* 4:273–284.

2884. Mayer, K. H., S. Boswell, R. Goldstein, W. Lo, C. Xu, L. Tucker, M. P. DePasquale, R. D'Aquila, and D. J. Anderson. 1999. Persistence of human immunodeficiency virus in semen after adding indinavir to combination antiretroviral therapy. *Clin. Infect. Dis.* 28:1252–1259.

2885. Mazzoli, S., L. Lopalco, A. Salvi, D. Trabattoni, S. Lo Caputo, F. Semplici, M. Biasin, C. Bl, A. Cosma, C. Pastori, F. Meacci, F. Mazzotta, M. L. Villa, A. G. Siccardi, and M. Clerici. 1999. Human immunodeficiency virus (HIV)-specific IgA and HIV neutralizing activity in the serum of exposed seronegative partners of HIV-seropositive persons. *J. Infect. Dis.* 180:871–875.

2886. Mazzoli, S., D. Trabattoni, S. L. Caputo, S. Piconi, C. Cle, F. Meacci, S. Ruzzante, A. Salvi, F. Semplici, R. Longhi, M. L. Fusi, N. Tofani, M. Biasin, M. L. Villa, F. Mazzotta, and M. Clerici. 1997. HIV-specific mucosal and cellular immunity in HIV-seronegative partners of HIV-seropositive individuals. *Nat. Med.* 3:1250–1257.

2887. Mbulaiteye, S. M., R. M. Pfeiffer, D. Whitby, G. R. Brubaker, J. Shao, and R. J. Biggar. 2003. Human herpesvirus 8 infection within families in rural Tanzania. *J. Infect. Dis.* 187:1780–1785.

2888. McArthur, J. C., N. Haughey, S. Gartner, K. Conant, C. Pardo, A. Nath, and N. Sacktor. 2003. Human immunodeficiency virus-associated dementia: an evolving disease. *J. Neurovirol.* 9:205–221.

2889. McBreen, S., S. Imlach, T. Shirafuji, G. R. Scott, C. Leen, J. E. Bell, and P. Simmonds. 2001. Infection of the CD45RA⁺ (naive) subset of peripheral CD8⁺ lymphocytes by human immunodeficiency virus type 1 in vivo. *J. Virol.* 75:4091–4102.

2890. McClain, K. L., C. T. Leach, H. B. Jenson, V. V. Joshi, B. H. Pollock, R. T. Parmley, F. J. DiCarlo, E. G. Chadwick, and S. B. Murphy. 1995. Association of Epstein-Barr virus with leiomyosarcomas in young people with AIDS. *N. Engl. J. Med.* 332:12–18.

2891. McClelland, R. S., L. Lavreys, W. M. Hassan, K. Mandaliya, J. O. Ndinya-Achola, and J. M. Baeten. 2006. Vaginal washing and increased risk of HIV-1 acquisition among African women: a 10-year prospective study. *AIDS* 20:269–273.

2892. McCloskey, T. W., M. Ott, E. Tribble, S. A. Khan, S. Teichberg, M. O. Paul, S. Pahwa, E. Verdin, and N. Chirmule. 1997. Dual role of HIV Tat in regulation of apoptosis in T cells. *J. Immunol.* 158:1014–1019.

2893. McClure, C. P., P. J. Tighe, R. A. Robins, D. Bansal, C. A. Bowman, M. Kingston, and J. K. Ball. 2005. HIV coreceptor and chemokine ligand gene expression in the male urethra and female cervix. *AIDS* 19:1257–1265.

2894. McClure, M. O., J. P. Moore, D. F. Blanc, P. Scotting, G. M. W. Cook, R. J. Keynes, J. N. Weber, D. Davies, and R. A. Weiss. 1992. Investigations into the mechanism by which sulfated polysaccharides inhibit HIV infection *in vitro*. *AIDS Res. Hum. Retrovir.* 8:19–26.

2895. McCoig, C., G. Van Dyke, C. S. Chou, L. J. Picker, O. Ramilo, and E. S. Vitetta. 1999. An anti-CD45RO immunotoxin eliminates T cells latently infected with HIV-1 in vitro. *Proc. Natl. Acad. Sci. USA* 96:11482–11485.

2896. McComsey, G. A., and E. Leonard. 2004. Metabolic complications of HIV therapy in children. *AIDS* 18:1753–1768.

2897. McCormick, C., and D. Ganem. 2005. The kaposin B protein of KSHV activates the p38/MK2 pathway and stabilizes cytokine mRNAs. *Science* 307:739–741.

2898. McCoy, J. L., R. B. Herberman, E. B. Rosenberg, F. C. Donnelly, P. H. Levine, and C. Alford. 1973. 51 Chromium-release assay for cell-mediated cytotoxicity of human leukemia and lymphoid tissue-culture cells. *Natl. Cancer Inst. Monogr.* 37:59–67.

2899. McCune, J. M. 1995. Viral latency in HIV disease. *Cell* 82:183–188.

2900. McCune, J. M. 1997. Thymic function in HIV-1 disease. *Semin. Immunol.* 9:397–404.

2901. McCune, J. M. 2001. The dynamics of CD4+ T-cell depletion in HIV disease. *Nature* 410:974–979.

2902. McCune, J. M., M. B. Hanley, D. Cesar, R. Halvorsen, R. Hoh, D. Schmidt, E. Wieder, S. Deeks, S. Siler, R. Neese, and M. Hellerstein. 2000. Factors influencing T-cell turnover in HIV-1-seropositive patients. *J. Clin. Investig.* 105:R1–R8.

2903. McCune, J. M., R. Loftus, D. K. Schmidt, P. Carroll, D. Webster, L. B. Swor-Yim, I. R. Francis, B. H. Gross, and R. M. Grant. 1998. High prevalence of thymic tissue in adults with human immunodeficiency virus-1 infection. *J. Clin. Investig.* 101:2301–2308.

2904. McCune, J. M., L. B. Rabin, M. B. Feinberg, M. Lieberman, J. C. Kosek, G. R. Reyes, and I. L. Weissman. 1988. Endoproteolytic cleavage of gp160 is required for the activation of human immunodeficiency virus. *Cell* 53:55–67.

2905. McCusker, J., A. M. Stoddard, K. H. Mayer, D. N. Cowan, and J. E. Groopman. 1988. Behavioral risk factors for HIV infection among homosexual men at a Boston community health center. *Am. J. Public Health* 78:68–71.

2906. McCutchan, F. E. 2000. Understanding the genetic diversity of HIV-1. *AIDS* 14(Suppl. 3):S31–S44.

2907. McCutchan, F. E., P. A. Hegerich, T. P. Brennan, P. Phanuphak, P. Singharaj, A. Jugsudee, P. W. Berman, A. M. Gray, A. K. Fowler, and D. S. Burke. 1992. Genetic variants of HIV-1 in Thailand. *AIDS Res. Hum. Retrovir.* 8:1887–1895.

2908. McCutchan, F. E., M. Hoelscher, S. Tovanabutra, S. Piyasirisilp, E. Sanders-Buell, G. Ramos, L. Jagodzinski, V. Polonis, L. Maboko, D. Mmbando, O. Hoffmann, G. Riedner, F. von Sonnenburg, M. Robb, and D. L. Birx. 2005. In-depth analysis of a heterosexually acquired human immunodeficiency virus type 1 superinfection: evolution, temporal fluctuation, and intercompartment dynamics from the seronegative window period through 30 months postinfection. *J. Virol.* 79:11693–11704.

2909. McCutchan, F. E., E. Sanders-Buell, C. W. Oster, R. R. Redfield, S. K. Hira, P. L. Perine, B. L. P. Ungar, and D. S. Burke. 1991. Genetic comparison of human immunodeficiency virus (HIV-1) isolates by polymerase chain reaction. *J. Acquir. Immune Defic. Syndr.* 4:1241–1250.

2910. McDermott, A. B., D. H. O'Connor, S. Fuenger, S. Piaskowski, S. Martin, J. Loffredo, M. Reynolds, J. Reed, J. Furlott, T. Jacoby, C. Riek, E. Dodds, K. Krebs, M. E. Davies, W. A. Schleif, D. R. Casimiro, J. W. Shiver, and D. I. Watkins. 2005. Cytotoxic T-lymphocyte escape does not always explain the transient control of simian immunodeficiency virus SIVmac239 viremia in adenovirus-boosted and DNA-primed Mamu-A*01-positive rhesus macaques. *J. Virol.* 79:15556–15566.

2911. McDermott, D. H., M. J. Beecroft, C. A. Kleeberger, F. M. Al-Sharif, W. E. R. Ollier, P. A. Zimmerman, B. A. Boatin, S. F. Leitman, R. Detels, A. H. Hajeer, and P. M. Murphy. 2000. Chemokine RANTES promoter polymorphism affects risk of both HIV infection and disease progression in the Multicenter AIDS Cohort Study. *AIDS* 14:2671–2678.

2912. McDermott, D. H., P. A. Zimmerman, F. Guignard, C. A. Kleeberger, S. F. Leitman, and P. M. Murphy. 1998. CCR5 promoter polymorphism and HIV-1 disease progression. *Lancet* 352:866–870.

2913. McDonald, D., M. A. Vodicka, G. Lucero, T. M. Svitkina, G. G. Borisy, M. Emerman, and T. J. Hope. 2002. Visualization of the intracellular behavior of HIV in living cells. *J. Cell Biol.* 159:441–452.

2914. McDonald, D., L. Wu, S. M. Bohks, V. N. KewalRamani, D. Unutmaz, and T. J. Hope. 2003. Recruitment of HIV and its receptors to dendritic cell-T cell junctions. *Science* 300:1295–1296.

2915. McDonald, R. A., D. L. Mayers, R. C. Y. Chung, K. F. Wagner, S. Ratto-Kim, D. L. Birx, and N. L. Michael. 1997. Evolution of human immunodeficiency virus type 1 *env* sequence variation in patients with diverse rates of disease progression and T-cell function. *J. Virol.* 71:1871–1879.

2916. McDougal, J. S., M. S. Kennedy, J. K. A. Nicholson, T. J. Spira, H. W. Jaffe, J. E. Kaplan, D. B. Fishbein, P. O'Malley, C. H. Aloisio, C. M. Black, M. Hubbard, and C. B. Reimer. 1987. Antibody response to human immunodeficiency virus in homosexual men. *J. Clin. Investig.* 80:316–324.

2917. McDougal, J. S., M. S. Kennedy, S. L. Orloff, J. K. A. Nicholson, and T. J. Spira. 1996. Mechanisms of human immunodeficiency virus type 1 (HIV-1) neutralization: irreversible inactivation of infectivity by anti-HIV-1 antibody. *J. Virol.* 70:5236–5245.

2918. McDougal, J. S., M. S. Kennedy, J. M. Sligh, S. P. Cort, A. Mawle, and J. K. A. Nicholson. 1986. Binding of HTLV-III/LAV to T4+ T cells by a complex of the 110K viral protein and the T4 molecule. *Science* 231:382–385.

2919. McDougal, J. S., L. S. Martin, S. P. Cort, M. Mozen, C. M. Heldebrant, and B. L. Evatt. 1985. Thermal inactivation of the acquired immunodeficiency syndrome virus, human T lymphotropic virus-III, lymphadenopathy-associated virus, with special reference to antihemophilic factor. *J. Clin. Investig.* 76:875–877.

2920. McDougal, J. S., C. D. Pilcher, B. S. Parekh, G. Gershy-Damet, B. M. Branson, K. Marsh, and S. Z. Wiktor. 2005. Surveillance for HIV-1 incidence using tests for recent infection in resource-constrained countries. *AIDS* 19(Suppl. 2):S25–S30.

2921. McElrath, M. J., J. E. Pruett, and Z. A. Cohn. 1989. Mononuclear phagocytes of blood and bone marrow: comparative roles as viral reservoirs in human immunodeficiency virus type 1 infections. *Proc. Natl. Acad. Sci. USA* 86:675–679.

2922. McElroy, M. D., M. Elrefaei, N. Jones, F. Ssali, P. Mugyenyi, B. Barugahare, and H. Cao. 2005. Coinfection with Schistosoma mansoni is associated with decreased HIV-specific cytolysis and increased IL-10 production. *J. Immunol.* 174:5119–5123.

2923. McGeoch, D. J., and A. J. Davison. 1999. The descent of human herpesvirus 8. *Semin. Cancer Biol.* 9:201–209.

2924. McGeoch, D. J., F. J. Rixon, and A. J. Davison. 2006. Topics in herpesvirus genomics and evolution. *Virus Res.* 117:90–104.

2925. McGhee, J. R., J. Mestecky, M. T. Dertzbaugh, J. H. Eldridge, M. Hirasawa, and H. Kiyono. 1992. The mucosal immune system: from fundamental concepts to vaccine development. *Vaccine* 10:75–88.

2926. McGuire, T. C., D. S. Adams, G. C. Johnson, P. Klevjer-Anderson, D. D. Barbee, and J. R. Gorham. 1986. Acute arthritis after caprine arthritis-encephalitis virus challenge exposure of vaccinated or persistently infected goats. *Am. J. Vet. Res.* 47:537–540.

2927. McIlroy, D., B. Autran, R. Cheynier, S. Wain-Hobson, J.-P. Clauvel, E. Oksenhendler, P. Debre, and A. Hosmalin. 1995. Infection frequency of dendritic cells and CD4+ T lymphocytes in spleens of human immunodeficiency virus-positive patients. *J. Virol.* 69:4737–4745.

2928. McInerney, T. L., L. McLain, S. J. Armstrong, and N. J. Dimmock. 1997. A human IgG1 (b12) specific for the CD4 binding site of HIV-1 neutralizes by inhibiting the virus fusion entry process, but b12 Fab neutralizes by inhibiting a postfusion event. *Virology* 233:313–326.

2929. McKeating, J., A. McKnight, and J. P. Moore. 1991. Differential loss of envelope glycoprotein gp120 from virions of human immunodeficiency virus type 1 isolates: effects on infectivity and neutralization. *J. Virol.* 65:852–860.

2930. McKeating, J. A., J. Bennett, S. Zolla-Pazner, M. Schutten, S. Ashelford, A. Leigh Brown, and P. Balfe. 1993. Resistance of a human serum-selected human immunodeficiency virus type 1 escape mutant to neutralization by CD4 binding site monoclonal antibodies is conferred by a single amino acid change in gp120. *J. Virol.* 67:5216–5225.

2931. McKeating, J. A., J. Cordell, C. J. Dean, and P. Balfe. 1992. Synergistic interaction between ligands binding to the CD4 binding site and V3 domain of human immunodeficiency virus type 1 gp120. *Virology* 191:732–742.

2932. McKeating, J. A., J. Gow, J. Goudsmit, L. H. Pearl, C. Mulder, and R. A. Weiss. 1989. Characterization of HIV-1 neutralization escape mutants. *AIDS* 3:777–784.

2933. McKeating, J. A., P. D. Griffiths, and R. A. Weiss. 1990. HIV susceptibility conferred to human fibroblasts by cytomegalovirus-induced Fc receptor. *Nature* 343:659–661.

2934. McKeating, J. A., C. Shotton, J. Cordell, S. Graham, P. Balfe, N. Sullivan, M. Charles, M. Page, A. Bolmstedt, S. Olofsson, S. C. Kayman, Z. Wu, A. Pinter, C. Dean, J. Sodroski, and R. A. Weiss. 1993. Characterization of neutralizing monoclonal antibodies to linear and conformation-dependent epitopes within the first and second variable domains of human immunodeficiency virus type 1 gp120. *J. Virol.* 67:4932–4944.

2935. McKenna, K., A. S. Beignon, and N. Bhardwaj. 2005. Plasmacytoid dendritic cells: linking innate and adaptive immunity. *J. Virol.* 79:17–27.

2936. McKenna, P. M., R. J. Pomerantz, B. Dietzschold, J. P. McGettigan, and M. J. Schnell. 2003. Covalently linked human immunodeficiency virus type 1 gp120/gp41 is stably anchored in Rhabdovirus particles and exposes critical neutralizing epitopes. *J. Virol.* 77:12782–12794.

2937. McKenzie, S. W., G. Dallalio, M. North, P. Frame, and R. T. Means, Jr. 1996. Serum chemokine levels in patients with non-progressing HIV infection. *AIDS* 10:F29-F33.

2938. McKnight, A., M. T. Dittmar, J. Moniz-Periera, K. Ariyoshi, J. D. Reeves, S. Hibbitts, D. Whitby, E. Aarons, A. E. Proudfoot, H. Whittle, and P. R. Clapham. 1998. A broad range of chemokine receptors are used by primary isolates of human immunodeficiency virus type 2 as coreceptors with CD4. *J. Virol.* 72:4065–4071.

2939. McKnight, A., C. Shotton, J. Cordell, I. Jones, G. Simmons, and P. R. Clapham. 1996. Location, exposure, and conservation of neutralizing and nonneutralizing epitopes on human immunodeficiency virus type 2 SU glycoprotein. *J. Virol.* 70:4598–4606.

2940. McKnight, A., R. A. Weiss, C. Shotton, Y. Takeuchi, H. Hoshino, and P. R. Clapham. 1995. Change in tropism upon immune escape by human immunodeficiency virus. *J. Virol.* 69:3167–3170.

2941. McKnight, A., D. Wilkinson, G. Simmons, S. Talbot, L. Picard, M. Ahuja, M. Marsh, J. A. Hoxie, and P. R. Clapham. 1997. Inhibition of human immunodeficiency virus fusion by a monoclonal antibody to a coreceptor (CXCR4) is both cell type and virus strain dependent. *J. Virol.* 71:1692–1696.

2942. McMichael, A. J., and T. Hanke. 2003. HIV vaccines 1983–2003. *Nat. Med.* 9:874–880.

2943. McMichael, A. J., and S. L. Rowland-Jones. 2001. Cellular immune responses to HIV. *Nature* 410:980–987.

2944. McMillan, A., P. E. Bishop, D. Aw, and J. F. Peutherer. 1989. Immunohistology of the skin rash associated with acute HIV infection. *AIDS* 3:309–312.

2945. McNearney, T., Z. Hornickova, R. Markham, A. Birdwell, M. Arens, A. Saah, and L. Ratner. 1992. Relationship of human immunodeficiency virus type 1 sequence heterogeneity to stage of disease. *Proc. Natl. Acad. Sci. USA* 89:10247–10251.

2946. McNearney, T., P. Westervelt, B. J. Thielan, D. B. Trowbridge, J. Garcia, R. Whittier, and L. Ratner. 1990. Limited sequence heterogeneity among biologically distinct human immunodeficiency virus type 1 isolates from individuals involved in a clustered infectious outbreak. *Proc. Natl. Acad. Sci. USA* 87:1917–1921.

2947. McNearney, T. A., C. Odell, V. M. Holers, P. G. Spear, and J. P. Atkinson. 1987. Herpes simplex virus glycoproteins gC-1 and gC-2 bind to the third component of complement and provide protection against complement-mediated neutralization of viral infectivity. *J. Exp. Med.* 166:1525–1535.

2948. McNeely, T. B., M. Dealy, D. J. Dripps, J. M. Orenstein, S. P. Eisenberg, and S. M. Wahl. 1995. Secretory leukocyte protease inhibitor: a human saliva protein exhibiting anti-human immunodeficiency virus 1 activity *in vitro*. *J. Clin. Investig.* 96:456–464.

2949. McNeely, T. B., D. C. Shugars, M. Rosendahl, C. Tucker, S. P. Eisenberg, and S. M. Wahl. 1997. Inhibition of human immunodeficiency virus type 1 infectivity by secretory leukocyte protease inhibitor occurs prior to viral reverse transcriptase. *Blood* 90:1141–1149.

2950. McNeil, A. C., W. L. Shupert, C. A. Iyasere, C. W. Hallahan, J. A. Mican, R. T. Davey, Jr., and M. Connors. 2001. High-level HIV-1 viremia suppresses viral antigen-specific CD4+ T cell proliferation. *Proc. Natl. Acad. Sci. USA* 98:13878–13883.

2951. Medina, D. J., P. P. Tung, M. B. Lerner-Tung, C. J. Nelson, J. W. Mellors, and R. K. Strair. 1995. Sanctuary growth of human immunodeficiency virus in the presence of 3'-azido-3'deoxythymidine. *J. Virol.* 69:1606–1611.

2952. MedLine. 2006. *MedLine Search of the AIDS Subset.* [online.] http://med-libwww.bu.edu/library/biomedlit.html.

2953. Medzhitov, R., and C. Janeway, Jr. 2000. Innate immunity. *N. Engl. J. Med.* 343:338–344.

2954. Meeker, T. C., B. Shiramizu, L. Kaplan, B. Herndier, H. Sanchez, J. C. Grimaldi, J. Baumgartner, J. Rachlin, E. Feigal, M. Rosenblum, and M. S. McGrath. 1991. Evidence for molecular subtypes of HIV-associated lymphoma: division into peripheral monoclonal lymphoma, peripheral polyclonal lymphoma, and central nervous system lymphoma. *AIDS* 5:669–674.

2955. Meerloo, T., H. K. Parmentier, A. D. M. E. Osterhaus, J. Goudsmit, and H. J. Schuurman. 1992. Modulation of cell surface molecules during HIV-1 infection of H9 cells. An immunoelectron microscopic study. *AIDS* 6:1105–1116.

2956. Meerloo, T., M. A. Sheikh, A. C. Bloem, A. de Ronde, M. Schutten, C. A. C. van Els, P. J. M. Rohol, P. Joling, J. Goudsmit, and H.-J. Schuurman. 1993. Host cell membrane proteins on human immunodeficiency virus type 1 after in vitro infection of H9 cells and blood mononuclear cells. An immuno-electron microscopic study. *J. Gen. Virol.* 74:129–135.

2957. Mehandru, S., M. A. Poles, K. Tenner-Racz, A. Horowitz, A. Hurley, C. Hogan, D. Boden, P. Racz, and M. Markowitz. 2004. Primary HIV-1 infection is associated with preferential depletion of CD4+ T lymphocytes from effector sites in the gastrointestinal tract. *J. Exp. Med.* 200:761–770.

2958. Mehendale, S. M., M. E. Shepherd, R. S. Brookmeyer, R. D. Semba, A. D. Divekar, R. R. Gangakhedkar, S. Joshi, A. R. Risbud, R. S. Paranjape, D. A. Gadkari, and R. C. Bollinger. 2001. Low carotenoid concentration and the risk of HIV seroconversion in Pune, India. *J. Acquir. Immune Defic. Syndr.* 26:352–359.

2959. Mehta, S. H., J. Astemborski, T. R. Sterling, D. L. Thomas, and D. Vlahov. 2006. Serum albumin as a prognostic indicator for HIV disease progression. *AIDS Res. Hum. Retrovir.* 22:14–21.

2960. Meier, U.-C., P. Klenerman, P. Griffin, W. James, B. Koppe, B. Larder, A. McMichael, and R. Phillips. 1995. Cytotoxic T lymphocyte lysis inhibited by viable HIV mutants. *Science* 270:1360–1362.

2961. Meier, U. C., R. E. Owen, E. Taylor, A. Worth, N. Naoumov, C. Willberg, K. Tang, P. Newton, P. Pellegrino, I. Williams, P. Klenerman, and P. Borrow. 2005. Shared alterations in NK cell frequency, phenotype, and function in chronic human immunodeficiency virus and hepatitis C virus infections. *J. Virol.* 79:12365–12374.

2962. Mela, C. M., C. T. Burton, N. Imami, M. Nelson, A. Steel, B. G. Gazzard, F. M. Gotch, and M. R. Goodier. 2005. Switch from inhibitory to activating NKG2 receptor expression in HIV-1 infection: lack of reversion with highly active antiretroviral therapy. *AIDS* 19:1761–1769.

2963. Melendez-Guerrero, L. D., J. K. A. Nicholson, and J. S. McDougal. 1991. Infection of human monocytes with HIV-1$_{Ba-L}$. Effect on accessory cell function for T-cell proliferation *in vitro*. *AIDS Res. Hum. Retrovir.* 7:465–474.

2964. Melikyan, G. B., R. M. Markosyan, H. Hemmati, M. K. Delmedico, D. M. Lambert, and F. S. Cohen. 2000. Evidence that the transition of HIV-1 gp41 into a six-helix bundle, not the bundle configuration, induces membrane fusion. *J. Cell Biol.* 151:413–423.

2965. Mellert, W., A. Kleinschmidt, J. Schmidt, H. Festl, S. Elmer, W. K. Roth, and V. Erfle. 1990. Infection of human fibroblasts and osteoblast-like cells with HIV-1. *AIDS* 4:527–535.

2966. Mellor, A. L., D. Munn, P. Chandler, D. Keskin, T. Johnson, B. Marshall, K. Jhaver, and B. Baban. 2003. Tryptophan catabolism and T cell responses. *Adv. Exp. Med. Biol.* 527:27–35.

2967. Mellor, A. L., and D. H. Munn. 2004. IDO expression by dendritic cells: tolerance and tryptophan catabolism. *Nat. Rev. Immunol.* 4:762‑774.

2968. Mellors, J. W., L. A. Kingsley, C. R. Rinaldo, Jr., J. A. Todd, B. S. Hoo, R. P. Kokka, and P. Gupta. 1995. Quantitation of HIV-1 RNA in plasma predicts outcome after seroconversion. *Ann. Intern. Med.* 122:573–579.

2969. Mellors, J. W., C. R. Rinaldo, Jr., P. Gupta, R. M. White, J. A. Todd, and L. A. Kingsley. 1996. Prognosis in HIV-1 infection predicted by the quantity of virus in plasma. *Science* 272:1167–1170.

2970. Menez-Bautista, R., S. M. Fikrig, S. Pahwa, M. G. Sarngadharan, and R. L. Stoneburner. 1986. Monozygotic twins discordant for the acquired immunodeficiency syndrome. *Am. J. Dis. Child.* 140:678–679.

2971. Meng, G., M. T. Sellers, M. Mosteller-Barnum, T. S. Rogers, G. M. Shaw, and P. D. Smith. 2000. Lamina propria lymphocytes, not macrophages, express CCR5 and CXCR4 and are the likely target cell for human immunodeficiency virus type 1 in the intestinal mucosa. *J. Infect. Dis.* 182:785–791.

2972. Meng, G., X. Wei, X. Wu, M. T. Sellers, J. M. Decker, Z. Moldoveanu, J. M. Orenstein, M. F. Graham, J. C. Kappes, J. Mestecky, G. M. Shaw, and P. D. Smith. 2002. Primary intestinal epithelial cells selectively transfer R5 HIV-1 to CCR5+ cells. *Nat. Med.* 8:150–156.

2973. Menu, E., F. X. Mbopi-Keou, S. Lagaye, S. Pissard, P. Mauclere, G. Scarlatti, J. Martin, M. Goossens, G. Chaouat, F. Barre-Sinoussi, F. X. M'Bopi Keou, and the European Network for In Utero Transmission of HIV-1. 1999. Selection of maternal human immunodeficiency virus type 1 variants in human placenta. *J. Infect. Dis.* 179:44–51.

2974. Menzo, S., P. Bagnarelli, M. Giacca, A. Manzin, P. E. Varaldo, and M. Clementi. 1992. Absolute quantitation of viremia in human immunodeficiency virus infection by competitive reverse transcription and polymerase chain reaction. *J. Clin. Microbiol.* 30:1752–1757.

2975. Merigan, T. C., R. L. Hirsch, A. C. Fisher, L. A. Meyerson, G. Goldstein, and M. A. Winters. 1996. The prognostic significance of serum viral load, codon 215 reverse transcriptase mutation and CD4+ T cells on progression of HIV disease in a double-blind study of thymopentin. *AIDS* 10:159–165.

2976. Mermin, J. H., M. Holodniy, D. A. Katzenstein, and T. C. Merigan. 1991. Detection of human immunodeficiency virus DNA and RNA in semen by the polymerase chain reaction. *J. Infect. Dis.* 164:769–772.

2977. Merrill, J. E., Y. Koyanagi, and I. S. Y. Chen. 1989. Interleukin-1 and tumor necrosis factor alpha can be induced from mononuclear phagocytes by human immunodeficiency virus type 1 binding to the CD4 receptor. *J. Virol.* 63:4404–4408.

2978. Merrill, J. E., Y. Koyanagi, J. Zack, L. Thomas, F. Martin, and I. S. Y. Chen. 1992. Induction of interleukin-1 and tumor necrosis factor alpha in brain cultures by human immunodeficiency virus type 1. *J. Virol.* 66:2217–2225.

2979. Merry, C., M. G. Barry, F. Mulcahy, M. Ryan, J. Heavey, J. D. Tjia, S. E. Gibbons, A. M. Breckenridge, and D. J. Back. 1997. Saquinavir pharmacokinetics alone and in combination with ritonavir in HIV-infected patients. *AIDS* 11:F29-F33.

2980. Merson, M. H., E. A. Feldman, R. Bayer, and J. Stryker. 1996. Rapid self testing for HIV infection. *Lancet* 349:352–353.

2981. Mestecky, J., and S. Jackson. 1994. Reassessment of the impact of mucosal immunity in infection with the human immunodeficiency virus (HIV) and design of relevant vaccines. *J. Clin. Immunol.* 14:259–272.

2982. Mestecky, J., S. Jackson, Z. Moldoveanu, L. R. Nesbit, R. Kulhavy, S. J. Prince, S. Sabbaj, M. J. Mulligan, and P. A. Goepfert. 2004. Paucity of antigen-specific IgA responses in sera and external secretions of HIV-type 1-infected individuals. *AIDS Res. Hum. Retrovir.* 20:972–988.

2983. Metzner, K. J., P. Rauch, H. Walter, C. Boesecke, B. Zollner, H. Jessen, K. Schewe, S. Fenske, H. Gellermann, and H. J. Stellbrink. 2005. Detection of minor populations of drug-resistant HIV-1 in acute seroconverters. *AIDS* 19:1819–1825.

2984. Meyaard, L., S. A. Otto, R. R. Jonker, M. J. Mijnster, R. P. M. Keet, and F. Miedema. 1992. Programmed death of T cells in HIV-1 infection. *Science* 257:217–219.

2985. Meyaard, L., H. Schuitemaker, and F. Miedema. 1993. T-cell dysfunction in HIV infection: anergy due to defective antigen-presenting cell function? *Immunol. Today* 14:161–164.

2986. Meyenhofer, M. F., L. G. Epstein, E.-S. Cho, and L. R. Sharer. 1987. Ultrastructural morphology and intracellular production of human immunodeficiency virus (HIV) in brain. *J. Neuropathol. Exp. Neurol.* 46:474–484.

2987. Meyerhans, A., R. Cheynier, J. Albert, M. Seth, S. Kwok, J. Sninsky, L. Morfeldt-Manson, B. Asjo, and S. Wain-Hobson. 1989. Temporal fluctuations in HIV quasispecies *in vivo* are not reflected by sequential HIV isolations. *Cell* 58:901–910.

2988. Meyerhans, A., G. Dadaglio, J. P. Vartanian, P. Langlade-Demoyan, R. Frank, B. Asjo, F. Plata, and S. Wain-Hobson. 1991. *In vivo* persistence of an HIV-1-encoded HLA-B27-restricted cytotoxic T lymphocyte epitope despite specific *in vitro* reactivity. *Eur. J. Immunol.* 21:2637–2640.

2989. Meylan, P. R. A., J. C. Guatelli, J. R. Munis, D. D. Richman, and R. S. Kornbluth. 1993. Mechanisms for the inhibition of HIV replication by interferons-alpha, -beta, and -gamma in primary human macrophages. *Virology* 193:138–148.

2990. Meyohas, M. C., L. Morand-Joubert, P. Van de Wiel, M. Mariotti, and J. J. Lefrere. 1995. Time to HIV seroconversion after needlestick injury. *Lancet* 345:1634–1635.

2991. Miao, Y. M., P. J. Hayes, F. M. Gotch, M. C. Barrett, N. D. Francis, and B. G. Gazzard. 2002. Elevated mucosal addressin cell adhesion molecule-1 expression in acquired immunodeficiency syndrome is maintained during antiretroviral therapy by intestinal pathogens and coincides with increased duodenal CD4 T cell densities. *J. Infect. Dis.* 185:1043–1050.

2992. Michael, N. L., A. E. Brown, R. F. Voigt, S. S. Frankel, J. R. Mascola, K. S. Brothers, M. Louder, D. L. Birx, and S. A. Cassol. 1997. Rapid disease progression without seroconversion following primary human immunodeficiency virus type 1 infection—evidence for highly susceptible human hosts. *J. Infect. Dis.* 175:1352–1359.

2993. Michael, N. L., G. Chang, L. A. d'Arcy, C. J. Tseng, D. L. Birx, and H. W. Sheppard. 1995. Functional characterization of human immunodeficiency virus type 1 *nef* genes in patients with divergent rates of disease progression. *J. Virol.* 69:6758–6769.

2994. Michael, N. L., L. G. Louie, A. L. Rohrbaugh, K. A. Schultz, D. E. Dayhoff, C. E. Wang, and H. W. Sheppard. 1997. The role of CCR5 and CCR2 polymorphisms in HIV-1 transmission and disease progression. *Nat. Med.* 3:1160–1162.

2995. Michael, N. L., P. Morrow, J. Mosca, M. Vahey, D. S. Burke, and R. R. Redfield. 1991. Induction of human immunodeficiency virus type 1 expression in chronically infected cells is associated primarily with a shift in RNA splicing patterns. *J. Virol.* 65:1291–1303.

2996. Michaelis, B., and J. A. Levy. 1987. Recovery of human immunodeficiency virus from serum. *JAMA* 257:1327.

2997. Michaelis, B., and J. A. Levy. 1989. HIV replication can be blocked by recombinant human interferon beta. *AIDS* 3:27–31.

2998. Michaels, J., L. R. Sharer, and L. G. Epstein. 1988. Human immunodeficiency virus type 1 (HIV-1) infection of the nervous system: a review. *Immunodefic. Rev.* 1:71–104.

2999. Michel, M. L., M. Mancini, Y. Riviere, D. Dormont, and P. Tiollais. 1990. T- and B-lymphocyte responses to human immunodeficiency virus (HIV) type 1 in macaques immunized with hybrid HIV-hepatitis B surface antigen particles. *J. Virol.* 64:2452–2455.

3000. Michel, P., A. T. Balde, C. Roussilhon, G. Aribot, J. L. Sarthou, and M. L. Gougeon. 2000. Reduced immune activation and T cell apoptosis in human immunodeficiency virus type 2 compared with type 1: correlation of T cell apoptosis with beta2 microglobulin concentration and disease evolution. *J. Infect. Dis.* 181:64–75.

3001. Michie, C. A., A. McLean, C. Alcock, and P. C. L. Beverley. 1992. Lifespan of human lymphocyte subsets defined by CD45 isoforms. *Nature* 360:264–265.

3002. Micoli, K. J., O. Mamaeva, S. C. Piller, J. L. Barker, G. Pan, E. Hunter, and J. M. McDonald. 2006. Point mutations in the C-terminus of HIV-1 gp160 reduce apoptosis and calmodulin binding without affecting viral replication. *Virology* 344: 468–479.

3003. Miedema, F., L. Meyaard, M. Koot, M. R. Klein, M. T. Roos, M. Groenink, R. A. Fouchier, A. B. Van't Wout, M. Tersmette, and P. T. Schellekens. 1994. Changing virus-host interactions in the course of HIV-1 infection. *Immunol. Rev.* 140:35–72.

3004. Miedema, F., A. J. C. Petit, F. G. Terpstra, J. K. M. Eeftinck Schattenkerk, F. de Wolf, B. J. M. Al, M. Roos, J. M. A. Lange, S. A. Danner, J. Goudsmit, and P. T. A. Schellenkens. 1988. Immunological abnormalities in human immunodeficiency virus (HIV)-infected asymptomatic homosexual men. *J. Clin. Investig.* 82:1908–1914.

3005. Migueles, S. A., A. C. Laborico, W. L. Shupert, M. S. Sabbaghian, R. Rabin, C. W. Hallahan, S. Van Baarle, S. Kostense, F. Miedema, M. McLaughlin, L. Ehler, J. Metcalf, S. Liu, and M. Connors. 2002. HIV-specific CD8+ T cell proliferation is coupled to perforin expression and is maintained in nonprogressors. *Nat. Immunol.* 3:1061–1068.

3006. Migueles, S. A., M. S. Sabbaghian, W. L. Shupert, M. P. Bettinotti, F. M. Marincola, L. Martino, C. W. Hallahan, S. M. Selig, D. Schwartz, J. Sullivan, and M. Connors. 2000. HLA B*5701 is highly associated with restriction of virus replication in a subgroup of HIV-infected long term nonprogressors. *Proc. Natl. Acad. Sci. USA* 97:2709–2714.

3007. Mikovits, J. A., D. D. Taub, S. M. Turcovski-Corrales, and F. W. Ruscetti. 1998. Similar levels of human immunodeficiency virus type 1 replication in human TH1 and TH2 clones. *J. Virol.* 72:5231–5238.

3008. Mildvan, D., U. Mathur, and R. W. Enlow. 1982. Opportunistic infections and immune deficiency in homosexual men. *Ann. Intern. Med.* 96:700–704.

3009. Mildvan, D., J. Spritzler, S. E. Grossberg, J. L. Fahey, D. M. Johnston, B. R. Schrock, and K. Kagan. 2005. Serum neopterin, an immune activation marker, independently predicts disease progression in advanced HIV-1 infection. *Clin. Infect. Dis.* 40:853–858.

3010. Miles, S. A., A. R. Rezai, J. F. Salazar-Gonzalez, M. Vander Mayden, R. H. Stevens, D. M. Logan, R. T. Mitsuyasu, T. Taga, T. Hirano, and T. Kishimoto. 1990. AIDS Kaposi's sarcoma-derived cells produce and respond to interleukin 6. *Proc. Natl. Acad. Sci. USA* 87:4068–4072.

3011. Miller, C., and M. B. Gardner. 1991. AIDS and mucosal immunity: usefulness of the SIV macaque model of genital mucosal transmission. *J. Acquir. Immune Defic. Syndr.* 4:1169–1172.

3012. Miller, C. J., N. J. Alexander, S. Sutjipto, A. A. Lackner, A. Gettie, A. G. Hendrickx, L. J. Lowenstine, M. Jennings, and P. A. Marx. 1989. Genital mucosal transmission of simian immunodeficiency virus: animal model for heterosexual transmission of human immunodeficiency virus. *J. Virol.* 63:4277–4284.

3013. Miller, C. J., Q. Li, K. Abel, E. Y. Kim, Z. M. Ma, S. Wietgrefe, L. La Franco-Scheuch, L. Compton, L. Duan, M. D.

Shore, M. Zupancic, M. Busch, J. Carlis, S. Wolinsky, and A. T. Haase. 2005. Propagation and dissemination of infection after vaginal transmission of simian immunodeficiency virus. *J. Virol.* 79:9217–9227.

3014. Miller, D. G., and A. D. Miller. 1993. Inhibitors of retrovirus infection are secreted by several hamster cell lines and are also present in hamster sera. *J. Virol.* 67:5346–5352.

3015. Miller, G., M. O. Rigsby, L. Heston, E. Grogan, R. Sun, C. Metroka, J. A. Levy, S. J. Gao, Y. Chang, and P. Moore. 1996. Antibodies to butyrate-inducible antigens of Kaposi's sarcoma-associated herpesvirus in patients with HIV-1 infection. *N. Engl. J. Med.* 334:1292–1297.

3015a. Miller, J. D., D. Masopust, E. J. Wherry, S. Kaech, G. Silvestri, and R. Ahmed. 2005. Differentiation of CD8 T cells in response to acute and chronic viral infections: implications for HIV vaccine development. *Curr. Drug Targets Infect. Disord.* 5:121–129.

3016. Miller, M. A., M. W. Cloyd, J. Liebmann, C. R. Rinaldo, Jr., K. R. Islam, S. Z. S. Wang, T. A. Mietzner, and R. C. Montelaro. 1993. Alterations in cell membrane permeability by the lentivirus lytic peptide (LLP-1) of HIV-1 transmembrane protein. *Virology* 196:89–100.

3017. Miller, M. A., R. F. Garry, J. M. Jaynes, and R. C. Montelaro. 1991. A structural correlation between lentivirus transmembrane proteins and natural cytolytic peptides. *AIDS Res. Hum. Retrovir.* 7:511–519.

3018. Miller, M. D., C. M. Farnet, and F. D. Bushman. 1997. Human immunodeficiency virus type 1 preintegration complexes: studies of organization and composition. *J. Virol.* 71:5382–5390.

3019. Miller, M. D., M. T. Warmerdam, I. Gaston, W. C. Greene, and M. B. Feinberg. 1994. The human immunodeficiency virus-1 *nef* gene product: a positive factor for viral infection and replication in primary lymphocytes and macrophages. *J. Exp. Med.* 179:101–113.

3020. Miller, R. A. 1996. The aging immune system: primer and prospectus. *Science* 273:70–74.

3021. Milligan, S., M. Robinson, E. O'Donnell, and D. J. Blackbourn. 2004. Inflammatory cytokines inhibit Kaposi's sarcoma-associated herpesvirus lytic gene transcription in in vitro-infected endothelial cells. *J. Virol.* 78:2591–2596.

3022. Milone, M. C., and P. Fitzgerald-Bocarsly. 1998. The mannose receptor mediates induction of IFN-alpha in peripheral blood dendritic cells by enveloped RNA and DNA viruses. *J. Immunol.* 161:2391–2399.

3023. Mink, M., S. M. Mosier, S. Janumpalli, D. Davison, L. Jin, T. Melby, P. Sista, J. Erickson, D. Lambert, S. A. Stanfield-Oakley, M. Salgo, N. Cammack, T. Matthews, and M. L. Greenberg. 2005. Impact of human immunodeficiency virus type 1 gp41 amino acid substitutions selected during enfuvirtide treatment on gp41 binding and antiviral potency of enfuvirtide in vitro. *J. Virol.* 79:12447–12454.

3024. Minkoff, H., L. Ahdieh, L. S. Massad, K. Anastos, D. H. Watts, S. Melnick, L. Muderspach, R. Burk, and J. Palefsky. 2001. The effect of highly active antiretroviral therapy on cervical cytologic changes associated with oncogenic HPV among HIV-infected women. *AIDS* 15:2157–2164.

3025. Miro, O., S. Lopez, E. Martinez, E. Pedrol, A. Milinkovic, E. Deig, G. Garrabou, J. Casademont, J. M. Gatell, and F. Cardellach. 2004. Mitochondrial effects of HIV infection on the peripheral blood mononuclear cells of HIV-infected patients who were never treated with antiretrovirals. *Clin. Infect. Dis.* **39**:710–716.

3026. Mische, C. C., W. Yuan, B. Strack, S. Craig, M. Farzan, and J. Sodroski. 2005. An alternative conformation of the gp41 heptad repeat 1 region coiled coil exists in the human immunodeficiency virus (HIV-1) envelope glycoprotein precursor. *Virology* **338**:133–143.

3027. Miskovsky, E. P., A. Y. Liu, W. Pavlat, R. Viveen, P. E. Stanhope, D. Finzi, W. M. Fox III, R. H. Hruban, E. R. Podack, and R. F. Siliciano. 1994. Studies of the mechanism of cytolysis by HIV-1-specific CD4+ human CTL clones induced by candidate AIDS vaccines. *J. Immunol.* **153**:2787–2799.

3028. Misrahi, M., J. P. Teglas, N. N'Go, M. Burgard, M. J. Mayaux, C. Rouzioux, J. F. Delfraissy, and S. Blanche. 1998. CCR5 chemokine receptor variant in HIV-1 mother-to-child transmission and disease progression in children. *JAMA* **279**:277–280.

3029. Misumi, S., D. Nakayama, M. Kusaba, T. Iiboshi, R. Mukai, K. Tachibana, T. Nakasone, M. Umeda, H. Shibata, M. Endo, N. Takamune, and S. Shoji. 2006. Effects of immunization with CCR5-based cycloimmunogen on simian/HIVSF162P3 challenge. *J. Immunol.* **176**:463–471.

3030. Mitchell, R. S., B. F. Beitzel, A. R. W. Schroder, P. Shinn, H. Chen, C. C. Berry, J. R. Ecker, and F. D. Bushman. 2004. Retroviral DNA integration: ASLV, HIV, and MLV show distinct target site preferences. *PLoS Biol.* **2**:e234.

3031. Mitchell, W. M., J. Torres, P. R. Johnson, V. Hirsch, T. Yilma, M. B. Gardner, and W. E. Robinson, Jr. 1995. Antibodies to the putative SIV infection-enhancing domain diminish beneficial effects of an SIV gp160 vaccine in rhesus macaques. *AIDS* **9**:27–34.

3032. Mitsuya, H., K. J. Weinhold, P. A. Furman, M. H. St. Clair, S. N. Lehrman, R. C. Gallo, D. Bolognesi, D. W. Barry, and S. Broder. 1985. 3'-azido-3'-deoxythymidine (BW A509U): an antiviral agent that inhibits the infectivity and cytopathic effect of human T-lymphotropic virus type III/lymphadenopathy-associated virus *in vitro*. *Proc. Natl. Acad. Sci. USA* **82**:7096–7100.

3033. Mitsuyasu, R. 1999. Oncological complications of human immunodeficiency virus disease and hematologic consequences of their treatment. *Clin. Infect. Dis.* **29**:35–43.

3034. Miyauchi, K., J. Kumano, Y. Yokomake, W. Sugiura, N. Yamamoto, and Z. Matsuda. 2005. Role of the specific amino acid sequence of the membrane-spanning domain of human immunodeficiency virus type 1 in membrane fusion. *J. Virol.* **79**:4720–4729.

3035. Miyoshi, I., I. Kubonishi, S. Yoshimoto, T. Akagi, Y. Ohtsuki, Y. Shiraishi, K. Nagata, and Y. Hinuma. 1981. Type C virus particles in a cord T-cell line derived by co-cultivating normal human cord leukocytes and human leukaemic T cells. *Nature* **294**:770–771.

3036. Mizukami, T., T. R. Fuerst, E. A. Berger, and B. Moss. 1988. Binding region for human immunodeficiency virus (HIV) and epitopes for HIV-blocking monoclonal antibodies of the CD4 molecule defined by site-directed mutagenesis. *Proc. Natl. Acad. Sci. USA* **85**:9273–9277.

3037. Mocroft, A. 2000. Highly active antiretroviral therapy and incidence of cancer in HIV infected adults. *J. Natl. Cancer Inst.* **92**:1823–1830.

3038. Mocroft, A., M. Bofill, M. Lipman, E. Medina, N. Borthwick, A. Timms, L. Batista, M. Winter, C. A. Sabin, M. Johnson, C. A. Lee, A. Phillips, and G. Janossy. 1997. CD8+, CD38+ lymphocyte percent: a useful immunological marker for monitoring HIV-1-infected patients. *J. Acquir. Immune Defic. Syndr. Hum. Retrovirol.* **14**:158–162.

3039. Mocroft, A., C. Katlama, C. Pradier, F. Antunes, F. Mulcahy, A. Chiesi, A. N. Phillips, O. Kirk, and J. D. Lundgren. 2000. AIDS across Europe, 1994–98, the EuroSIDA study. *Lancet* **356**:291–296.

3040. Mocroft, A., L. Ruiz, P. Reiss, B. Ledergerber, C. Katlama, A. Lazzarin, F.-D. Goebel, A. N. Phillips, B. Clotet, and J. D. Lungren. 2003. Virological rebound after suppression on highly active antiretroviral therapy. *AIDS* **17**:1741–1751.

3041. Modi, W. S., J. J. Goedert, S. Strathdee, S. Buchbinder, R. Detels, S. Donfield, S. J. O'Brien, and C. Winkler. 2003. MCP-1-MCP-3-Eotaxin gene cluster influences HIV-1 transmission. *AIDS* **17**:2357–2365.

3042. Moebius, U., L. K. Clayton, S. Abraham, S. C. Harrison, and E. L. Reinherz. 1992. The human immunodeficiency virus gp120 binding site on CD4: delineation by quantitative equilibrium and kinetic binding studies of mutants in conjunction with a high-resolution CD4 atomic structure. *J. Exp. Med.* **176**:507–517.

3043. Mofenson, L., J. Lamber, R. Stiehm, J. Bethel, W. Meyer, J. Whitehouse, J. Moye, P. Reichelderfer, R. Harris, M. Fowler, B. Mathieson, and G. Nemo. 1999. Risk factors for perinatal transmission of human immunodeficiency virus type 1 in women treated with zidovudine. *N. Engl. J. Med.* **341**:385–393.

3044. Mofenson, L. M., D. R. Harris, J. Moye, J. Bethel, J. Korelitz, J. S. Read, R. Nugent, W. Meyer, and NICHD IVIG Clinical Trial Study Group. 2003. Alternatives to HIV-1 RNA concentration and CD4 count to predict mortality in HIV-1-infected children in resource-poor settings. *Lancet* **362**:1625–1627.

3045. Moffet-King, A. 2002. Natural killer cells and pregnancy. *Nat. Rev. Immunol.* **2**:656–663.

3046. Mohamed, O. A., R. Ashley, A. Goldstein, J. McElrath, J. Dalessio, and L. Corey. 1994. Detection of rectal antibodies to HIV-1 by a sensitive chemiluminescent Western blot immunodetection method. *J. Acquir. Immune Defic. Syndr.* **7**:375–380.

3047. Mohri, H., S. Bonhoeffer, S. Monard, A. S. Perelson, and D. D. Ho. 1998. Rapid turnover of T lymphocytes in SIV-infected rhesus macaques. *Science* **279**:1223–1227.

3048. Moir, S., A. Malaspina, Y. Li, T. W. Chun, T. Lowe, J. Adelsberger, M. Baseler, L. A. Ehler, S. Liu, R. T. Davey, Jr., J. A. Mican, and A. S. Fauci. 2000. B cells of HIV-1-infected patients bind virions through CD21-complement interactions and transmit infectious virus to activated T cells. *J. Exp. Med.* **192**:637–646.

3049. Moir, S., A. Malaspina, K. M. Ogwaro, E. T. Donoghue, C. W. Hallahan, L. A. Ehler, S. Liu, J. Adelsberger, R. Lapointe, P. Hwu, M. Baseler, J. M. Orenstein, T. W. Chun, J. A. Mican, and A. S. Fauci. 2001. HIV-1 induces phenotypic and functional perturbations of B cells in chronically infected individuals. *Proc. Natl. Acad. Sci. USA* **98**:10362–10367.

3050. Moir, S., A. Malaspina, O. K. Pickeral, E. T. Donoghue, J. Vasquez, N. J. Miller, S. R. Krishnan, M. A. Planta, J. F. Turney, J. S. Justement, S. Kottilil, M. Dybul, J. M. Mican, C. Kovacs, T. W. Chun, C. E. Birse, and A. S. Fauci. 2004. Decreased survival of B cells of HIV-viremic patients mediated by altered expression of receptors of the TNF superfamily. *J. Exp. Med.* **200**:587–599.

3051. Mole, L., S. Ripich, D. Margolis, and M. Holodniy. 1997. The impact of active herpes simplex virus infection on human immunodeficiency virus load. *J. Infect. Dis.* **176**:766–770.

3052. Molina, J.-M., D. T. Scadden, M. Sakaguchi, B. Fuller, A. Woon, and J. E. Groopman. 1990. Lack of evidence for infection of or effect on growth of hematopoietic progenitor cells after *in vivo* or *in vitro* exposure to human immunodeficiency virus. *Blood* 76:2476–2482.

3053. Molina, J.-M., R. Schindler, R. Ferriani, M. Sakaguchi, E. Vannier, C. A. Dinarello, and J. E. Groopman. 1990. Production of cytokines by peripheral blood monocytes/macrophages infected with human immunodeficiency virus type 1 (HIV-1). *J. Infect. Dis.* 161:888–893.

3054. Moll, M., J. Snyder-Cappione, G. Spotts, F. M. Hecht, J. K. Sandberg, and D. F. Nixon. 2006. Expansion of CD1d-restricted NKT cells in patients with primary HIV-1 infection treated with interleukin-2. *Blood* 107:3081–3083. (First published 20 December 2005.)

3055. Mologni, D., P. Citterio, B. Menzaghi, B. Z. Poma, C. Riva, V. Broggini, A. Sinicco, L. Milazzo, F. Adorni, S. Rusconi, M. Galli, and A. Riva. 2006. Vpr and HIV-1 disease progression: R77Q mutation is associated with long-term control of HIV-1 infection in different groups of patients. *AIDS* 20:567–574.

3056. Monie, D., R. P. Simmons, R. E. Nettles, T. L. Kieffer, Y. Zhou, H. Zhang, S. Karmon, R. Ingersoll, K. Chadwick, H. Zhang, J. B. Margolick, T. C. Quinn, S. C. Ray, M. Wind-Rotolo, M. Miller, D. Persaud, and R. F. Siliciano. 2005. A novel assay allows genotyping of the latent reservoir for human immunodeficiency virus type 1 in the resting CD4+ T cells of viremic patients. *J. Virol.* 79:5185–5205.

3057. Monini, P., L. de Lellis, M. Fabris, F. Rigolin, and E. Cassai. 1996. Kaposi's sarcoma-associated herpesvirus DNA sequences in prostate tissue and human semen. *N. Engl. J. Med.* 334:1168–1172.

3058. Monroe, J. E., A. Calender, and C. Mulder. 1988. Epstein-Barr virus-positive and -negative B-cell lines can be infected with human immunodeficiency virus types 1 and 2. *J. Virol.* 62:3497–3500.

3059. Montagnier, L., J. Chermann, F. Barre-Sinoussi, S. Chamaret, J. Gruest, M. T. Nugeyre, F. Rey, C. Dauguet, C. Axler-Blin, F. Vezinet-Brun, C. Rouzioux, A. G. Saimot, W. Rozenbaum, J. C. Gluckman, D. Klatzmann, E. Vilmer, C. Griselli, C. Gazengel, and J. B. Brunet. 1984. A new human T-lymphotropic retrovirus: characterization and possible role in lymphadenopathy and acquired immune deficiency syndromes, p. 363–379. *In* R. C. Gallo, M. E. Essex, and L. Gross (ed.), *Human T-cell Leukemia/Lymphoma Virus.* Cold Spring Harbor Laboratory, Cold Spring Harbor, N.Y.

3060. Montagnier, L., J. Gruest, S. Chamaret, C. Dauguet, C. Axler, D. Guetard, M. T. Nugeyre, F. Barre-Sinoussi, J. C. Chermann, and J. B. Brunet. 1984. Adaption of lymphadenopathy associated virus (LAV) to replication in EBV-transformed B lymphoblastoid cell lines. *Science* 225:63–66.

3061. Montaner, J. S. G., M. Harris, T. Mo, and P. R. Harrigan. 1998. Rebound of plasma HIV viral load following prolonged suppression with combination therapy. *AIDS* 12:1398–1399.

3062. Montaner, J. S. G., C. Zala, B. Conway, J. Raboud, P. Patenaude, S. Rae, M. V. O'Shaughnessy, and M. T. Schechter. 1997. A pilot study of hydroxyurea among patients with advanced human immunodeficiency virus (HIV) disease receiving chronic didanosine therapy: Canadian HIV trials network protocol 080. *J. Infect. Dis.* 175:801–806.

3063. Montaner, L. J., A. G. Doyle, M. Collin, G. Herbein, P. Illei, W. James, A. Minty, D. Caput, P. Ferrara, and S. Gordon. 1993. Interleukin 13 inhibits human immunodeficiency virus type 1 production in primary blood-derived human macrophages in vitro. *J. Exp. Med.* 178:743–747.

3064. Montano, M. A., C. P. Nixon, T. Ndung'u, H. Bussmann, V. A. Novitsky, D. Dickman, and M. Essex. 2000. Elevated tumor necrosis factor-alpha activation of human immunodeficiency virus type 1 subtype C in Southern Africa is associated with an NF-kappaB enhancer gain-of-function. *J. Infect. Dis.* 181:76–81.

3065. Montano, M. A., V. A. Novitsky, J. T. Blackard, N. L. Cho, D. A. Katzenstein, and M. Essex. 1997. Divergent transcriptional regulation among expanding human immunodeficiency virus type 1 subtypes. *J. Virol.* 71:8657–8665.

3066. Montefiori, D. C., M. Altfeld, P. K. Lee, M. Bilska, J. Zhou, M. N. Johnston, F. Gao, B. D. Walker, and E. S. Rosenberg. 2003. Viremia control despite escape from a rapid and potent autologous neutralizing antibody response after therapy cessation in an HIV-1-infected individual. *J. Immunol.* 170:3906–3914.

3067. Montefiori, D. C., B. S. Graham, S. Kliks, and P. F. Wright. 1992. Serum antibodies to HIV-1 in recombinant vaccinia virus recipients boosted with purified recombinant gp160. *J. Clin. Immunol.* 12:429–439.

3068. Montefiori, D. C., B. S. Graham, J. Zhou, J. Zhou, R. A. Bucco, D. H. Schwartz, L. A. Cavacini, and M. R. Posner. 1993. V3-specific neutralizing antibodies in sera from HIV-1 gp160-immunized volunteers block virus fusion and act synergistically with human monoclonal antibody to the conformation-dependent CD4 binding site of gp120. *J. Clin. Investig.* 92:840–847.

3069. Montefiori, D. C., L. B. Lefkowitz, Jr., R. E. Keller, V. Holmberg, E. Sandstrom, and J. P. Phair. 1991. Absence of a clinical correlation for complement-mediated, infection-enhancing antibodies in plasma or sera from HIV-1-infected individuals. *AIDS* 5:513–517.

3070. Montefiori, D. C., G. Pantaleo, L. M. Fink, J. T. Zhou, J. Y. Zhou, M. Bilska, G. D. Miralles, and A. S. Fauci. 1996. Neutralizing and infection-enhancing antibody responses to human immunodeficiency virus type 1 in long-term nonprogressors. *J. Infect. Dis.* 173:60–67.

3071. Montefiori, D. C., K. A. Reimann, N. L. Letvin, J. Zhou, and S.-L. Hu. 1995. Studies of complement-activating antibodies in the SIV/macaque model of acute primary infection and vaccine protection. *AIDS Res. Hum. Retrovir.* 11:963–970.

3072. Montefiori, D. C., W. E. Robinson, Jr., V. M. Hirsch, A. Modliszewski, W. M. Mitchell, and P. R. Johnson. 1990. Antibody dependent enhancement of simian immunodeficiency virus (SIV) infection in vitro by plasma from SIV-infected rhesus macaques. *J. Virol.* 64:113–119.

3073. Montefiori, D. C., W. E. Robinson, Jr., and W. M. Mitchell. 1988. Role of protein N-glycosylation in pathogenesis of human immunodeficiency virus type 1. *Proc. Natl. Acad. Sci. USA* 85:9248–9252.

3074. Montelaro, R. C., J. M. Ball, and K. E. Rushlow. 1993. Equine retroviruses, p. 257–360. *In* J. A. Levy (ed.), *The Retroviridae*, vol. 2. Plenum Press, New York, N.Y.

3075. Montelaro, R. C., and D. P. Bolognesi. 1995. Vaccines against retroviruses, p. 605–656. *In* J. A. Levy (ed.), *The Retroviridae*, vol. 4. Plenum, New York, N.Y.

3076. Moog, C., H. J. A. Fleury, I. Pellegrin, A. Kirn, and A. M. Aubertin. 1997. Autologous and heterologous neutralizing antibody responses following initial seroconversion in human immunodeficiency virus type 1-infected individuals. *J. Virol.* 71:3734–3741.

3077. Mooij, P., W. M. Bogers, H. Oostermeijer, W. Koornstra, P. J. Ten Haaft, B. E. Verstrepen, G. Van Der Auwera, and J. L. Heeney. 2000. Evidence for viral virulence as a predominant factor limiting human immunodeficiency virus vaccine efficacy. *J. Virol.* 74:4017–4027.

3078. Mooij, P., M. van der Kolk, W. M. Bogers, P. J. ten Haaft, P. Van Der Meide, N. Almond, J. Stott, M. Deschamps, D. Labbe, P. Momin, G. Voss, P. Von Hoegen, C. Bruck, and J. L. Heeney. 1998. A clinically relevant HIV-1 subunit vaccine protects rhesus macaques from in vivo passaged simian-human immunodeficiency virus infection. *AIDS* 12:F15–F22.

3079. Moonis, M., B. Lee, R. T. Bailer, Q. Luo, and L. J. Montaner. 2001. CCR5 and CXCR4 expression correlated with X4 and R5 HIV-1 infection yet not sustained replication in Th1 and Th2 cells. *AIDS* 15:1941–1949.

3080. Moore, C. B., M. John, I. R. James, F. T. Christiansen, C. S. Witt, and S. A. Mallal. 2002. Evidence of HIV-1 adaptation to HLA-restricted immune responses at a population level. *Science* 296:1439–1443.

3081. Moore, J. P. 1993. A monoclonal antibody to the CDR-3 region of CD4 inhibits soluble CD4 binding to virions of human immunodeficiency virus type 1. *J. Virol.* 67:3656–3659.

3082. Moore, J. P. 1993. The reactivities of HIV-1+ human sera with solid-phase V3 loop peptides can be poor predictors of their reactivities with V3 loops on native gp120 molecules. *AIDS Res. Hum. Retrovir.* 9:209–219.

3083. Moore, J. P. 1997. Coreceptors: implications for HIV pathogenesis and therapy. *Science* 276:51–52.

3084. Moore, J. P., Y. Cao, D. D. Ho, and R. A. Koup. 1994. Development of the anti-gp120 antibody response during seroconversion to human immunodeficiency virus type 1. *J. Virol.* 68:5142–5155.

3085. Moore, J. P., Y. Cao, J. Leu, L. Qin, B. Korber, and D. D. Ho. 1996. Inter- and intraclade neutralization of human immunodeficiency virus type 1: genetic clades do not correspond to neutralization serotypes but partially correspond to gp120 antigenic serotypes. *J. Virol.* 70:427–444.

3086. Moore, J. P., and D. D. Ho. 1993. Antibodies to discontinuous or conformationally sensitive epitopes on the gp120 glycoprotein of human immunodeficiency virus type 1 are highly prevalent in sera of infected humans. *J. Virol.* 67:863–875.

3087. Moore, J. P., and D. D. Ho. 1995. HIV-1 neutralization: the consequences of viral adaptation to growth on transformed T cells. *AIDS* 9:S117–S136.

3088. Moore, J. P., S. G. Kitchen, P. Pugach, and Z. A. Zack. 2004. The CCR5 and CXCR4 coreceptors—central to understanding the transmission and pathogenesis of human immunodeficiency virus type 1 infection. *AIDS Res. Hum. Retrovir.* 20:111–126.

3089. Moore, J. P., J. A. McKeating, Y. X. Huang, A. Ashkenazi, and D. D. Ho. 1992. Virions of primary human immunodeficiency virus type 1 isolates resistant to soluble CD4 (sCD4) neutralization differ in sCD4 binding and glycoprotein gp120 retention from sCD4-sensitive isolates. *J. Virol.* 66:235–243.

3090. Moore, J. P., J. A. McKeating, W. A. Norton, and Q. J. Sattentau. 1991. Direct measurement of soluble CD4 binding to

human immunodeficiency virus type 1 virions: gp120 dissociation and its implications for virus-cell binding and fusion reactions and their neutralization by soluble CD4. *J. Virol.* 65:1133–1140.

3091. Moore, J. P., J. A. McKeating, R. A. Weiss, and Q. J. Sattentau. 1990. Dissociation of gp120 from HIV-1 virions induced by soluble CD4. *Science* 250:1139–1142.

3092. Moore, J. P., Q. J. Sattentau, R. Wyatt, and J. Sodroski. 1994. Probing the structure of the human immunodeficiency virus surface glycoprotein gp120 with a panel of monoclonal antibodies. *J. Virol.* 68:469–484.

3093. Moore, J. P., and R. W. Sweet. 1993. The HIV gp120-CD4 interaction: a target for pharmacological or immunological intervention? *Perspect. Drug Discov. Des.* 1:235–250.

3094. Moore, J. P., R. L. Willey, G. K. Lewis, J. Robinson, and J. Sodroski. 1994. Immunological evidence for interactions between the first, second, and fifth conserved domains of the gp120 surface glycoprotein of human immunodeficiency virus type 1. *J. Virol.* 68:6836–6847.

3095. Moore, J. P., H. Yoshiyama, D. D. Ho, J. E. Robinson, and J. Sodroski. 1993. Antigenic variation in gp120s from molecular clones of HIV-1 LAI. *AIDS Res. Hum. Retrovir.* 9:1185–1193.

3096. Moore, J. S., F. Rahemtulla, L. W. Kent, S. T. Hall, M. R. Ikizler, P. F. Wright, H. H. Nguyen, and S. Jackson. 2003. Oral epithelial cells are susceptible to cell-free and cell-associated HIV-1 infection in vitro. *Virology* 313:343–353.

3097. Moore, P. L., E. T. Crooks, L. Porter, P. Zhu, C. S. Cayanan, H. Grise, P. Corcoran, M. B. Zwick, M. Franti, L. Morris, K. H. Roux, D. R. Burton, and J. M. Binley. 2006. Nature of nonfunctional envelope proteins on the surface of human immunodeficiency virus type 1. *J. Virol.* 80:2515–2528.

3098. Moore, P. S., C. Boshoff, R. A. Weiss, and Y. Chang. 1996. Molecular mimicry of human cytokine and cytokine response pathway genes by KSHV. *Science* 274:1739–1744.

3099. Moore, P. S., and Y. Chang. 2003. Kaposi's sarcoma-associated herpesvirus immunoevasion and tumorigenesis: two sides of the same coin? *Annu. Rev. Microbiol.* 57:609–639.

3100. Moore, P. S., L. A. Kingsley, S. D. Holmberg, T. Spira, P. Gupta, D. R. Hoover, J. P. Parry, L. J. Conley, H. W. Jaffe, and Y. Chang. 1996. Kaposi's sarcoma-associated herpesvirus infection prior to onset of Kaposi's sarcoma. *AIDS* 10:175–180.

3101. Morein, B., B. Sundquist, S. Hoglund, K. Dalsgaard, and A. Osterhaus. 1984. ISCOM, a novel structure for antigenic presentation of membrane proteins from enveloped viruses. *Nature* 308:457.

3102. Moreno, M. R., R. Pascual, and J. Villalain. 2004. Identification of membrane-active regions of the HIV-1 envelope glycoprotein gp41 using a 15-mer gp41-peptide scan. *Biochim. Biophys. Acta* 1661:97–105.

3103. Moreno, P., M. J. Rebollo, F. Pulido, R. Rubio, A. R. Noriega, and R. Delgado. 1996. Alveolar macrophages are not an important source of viral production in HIV-1 infected patients. *AIDS* 10:682–684.

3104. Morgan, J. R., J. M. LeDoux, R. G. Snow, R. G. Tompkins, and M. L. Yarmush. 1995. Retrovirus infection: effect of time and target cell number. *J. Virol.* 69:6994–7000.

3105. Mori, K., D. J. Ringler, and R. C. Desrosiers. 1993. Restricted replication of simian immunodeficiency virus strain 239 in macrophages is determined by *env* but is not due to restricted entry. *J. Virol.* 67:2807–2814.

3106. Morikawa, Y., J. P. Moore, A. J. Wilkinson, and I. M. Jones. 1991. Reduction in CD4 binding affinity associated with removal of a single glycosylation site in the external glycoprotein of HIV-2. *Virology* **180**:853–856.

3107. Moriuchi, H., and M. Moriuchi. 1999. Dichotomous effects of macrophage-derived chemokine on HIV infection. *AIDS* **13**:994–996.

3108. Moriuchi, H., M. Moriuchi, C. Combadiere, P. M. Murphy, and A. S. Fauci. 1996. CD8+ T-cell-derived soluble factor(s), but not beta-chemokines RANTES, MIP-1a, and MIP-1b, suppress HIV-1 replication in monocyte/macrophages. *Proc. Natl. Acad. Sci. USA* **93**:15341–15345.

3109. Moriuchi, M., and H. Moriuchi. 2001. A milk protein lactoferrin enhances human T cell leukemia virus type 1 and suppresses HIV-1 infection. *J. Immunol.* **166**:4231–4236.

3110. Moriuchi, M., H. Moriuchi, W. Turner, and A. S. Fauci. 1998. Exposure to bacterial products renders macrophages highly susceptible to T-tropic HIV-1. *J. Clin. Investig.* **102**: 1540–1550.

3111. Moriuchi, M., H. Yoshimine, K. Oishi, and H. Moriuchi. 2006. Norepinephrine inhibits human immunodeficiency virus type-1 infection through the NF-kappa B inactivation. *Virology* **345**:167–173.

3112. Morris, L., J. M. Binley, B. A. Clas, S. Bonhoeffer, T. P. Astill, R. Kost, A. Hurley, Y. Cao, M. Markowitz, D. D. Ho, and J. P. Moore. 1998. HIV-1 antigen-specific and -nonspecific B cell responses are sensitive to combination antiretroviral therapy. *J. Exp. Med.* **188**:233–245.

3113. Morris, L., D. J. Martin, H. Bredell, S. N. Nyoka, L. Sacks, S. Pendle, L. Page-Shipp, C. L. Karp, T. R. Sterling, T. C. Quinn, and R. E. Chaisson. 2003. Human immunodeficiency virus-1 RNA levels and CD4 lymphocyte counts, during treatment for active tuberculosis, in South African patients. *J. Infect. Dis.* **187**:1967–1971.

3114. Morrow, W. J. W., D. A. Isenberg, R. E. Sobol, R. B. Stricker, and T. Kieber-Emmons. 1991. AIDS virus infection and autoimmunity: a perspective of the clinical, immunological, and molecular origins of the autoallergic pathologies associated with HIV disease. *Clin. Immunol. Immunopathol.* **58**:163–180.

3115. Morrow, W. J. W., M. Wharton, R. B. Stricker, and J. A. Levy. 1986. Circulating immune complexes in patients with acquired immune deficiency syndrome contain the AIDS-associated retrovirus. *Clin. Immunol. Immunopathol.* **40**: 515–524.

3116. Morse, H. C. I., S. K. Chattopadhyay, M. Makino, T. N. Frederickson, A. W. Hügin, and J. W. Hartley. 1992. Retrovirus-induced immunodeficiency in the mouse: MAIDS as a model for AIDS. *AIDS* **6**:607–621.

3117. Mosca, J. D., D. P. Bednarik, N. B. K. Raj, C. A. Rosen, J. G. Sodroski, W. A. Haseltine, and P. M. Pitha. 1987. Herpes simplex virus type 1 can reactivate transcription of latent human immunodeficiency virus. *Nature* **325**:67–70.

3118. Moscicki, A.-B., Y. Ma, C. Holland, and S. H. Vermund. 2001. Cervical ectopy in adolescent girls with and without human immunodeficiency virus infection. *J. Infect. Dis.* **183**: 865–870.

3119. Moseman, E. A., X. Liang, A. J. Dawson, A. Panoskaltsis-Mortari, A. M. Krieg, Y. J. Liu, B. R. Blazar, and W. Chen. 2004. Human plasmacytoid dendritic cells activated by CpG oligodeoxynucleotides induce the generation of CD4+CD25+ regulatory T cells. *J. Immunol.* **173**:4433–4442.

3120. Moser, B., and M. Brandes. 2006. gammadelta T cells: an alternative type of professional APC. *Trends Immunol.* **27**: 112–118.

3121. Moser, B., P. Schaerli, and P. Loetscher. 2002. CXCR5(+) T cells: follicular homing takes center stage in T-helper-cell responses. *Trends Immunol.* **23**:250–254.

3122. Moses, A., J. Nelson, and G. C. Bagby. 1998. The influence of human immunodeficiency virus-1 on hematopoiesis. *Blood* **91**:1479–1495.

3123. Moses, A. V., F. E. Bloom, C. D. Pauza, and J. A. Nelson. 1993. Human immunodeficiency virus infection of human brain capillary endothelial cells occurs via a CD4/galactosyl ceramide-independent mechanism. *Proc. Natl. Acad. Sci. USA* **90**:10474–10478.

3124. Moses, A. V., K. N. Fish, R. Ruhl, P. P. Smith, J. G. Strussenberg, L. Zhu, B. Chandran, and J. A. Nelson. 1999. Long-term infection and transformation of dermal microvascular endothelial cells by human herpesvirus 8. *J. Virol.* **73**:6892–6902.

3125. Moses, A. V., M. A. Jarvis, C. Raggo, Y. C. Bell, R. Ruhl, B. G. M. Luukkonen, D. J. Griffith, C. L. Wait, B. J. Druker, M. C. Heinrich, and J. A. Nelson. 2002. Kaposi's sarcoma-associated herpesvirus-induced upregulation of the c-kit proto-oncogene, as identified by gene expression profiling, is essential for the transformation of endothelial cells. *J. Virol.* **76**:8383–8399.

3126. Moses, A. V., S. G. Stenglein, J. G. Strussenberg, K. Wehrly, B. Chesebro, and J. A. Nelson. 1996. Sequences regulating tropism of human immunodeficiency virus type 1 for brain capillary endothelial cells map to a unique region on the viral genome. *J. Virol.* **70**:3401–3406.

3127. Moses, A. V., S. Williams, M. L. Heneveld, J. Strussenberg, M. Rarick, M. Loveless, G. Bagby, and J. A. Nelson. 1996. Human immunodeficiency virus infection of bone marrow endothelium reduces induction of stromal hematopoietic growth factors. *Blood* **87**:919–925.

3128. Moses, A. V., S. E. Williams, J. G. Strussenberg, J. L. Heneveld, R. A. Ruhl, A. C. Bakke, G. C. Bagby, and J. A. Nelson. 1997. HIV-1 induction of CD40 on endothelial cells promotes the outgrowth of AIDS-associated B-cell lymphomas. *Nat. Med.* **3**:1242–1249.

3129. Moses, S., F. A. Plummer, E. N. Ngugi, N. J. Nagelkerke, A. O. Anzala, and J. O. Ndinya-Achola. 1991. Controlling HIV in Africa: effectiveness and cost of an intervention in a high frequency STD transmitter core group. *AIDS* **5**:407–411.

3130. Mosier, D. E., R. J. Gulizia, S. M. Baird, and D. B. Wilson. 1988. Transfer of a functional human immune system to mice with severe combined immunodeficiency. *Nature* **335**:256–259.

3131. Mosier, D. E., R. J. Gulizia, S. M. Baird, D. B. Wilson, D. H. Spector, and S. A. Spector. 1991. Human immunodeficiency virus infection of human-PBL-SCID mice. *Science* **251**:791–794.

3132. Mosier, D. E., R. J. Gulizia, P. D. MacIsaac, L. Corey, and P. D. Greenberg. 1993. Resistance to human immunodeficiency virus 1 infection of SCID mice reconstituted with peripheral blood leukocytes from donors vaccinated with vaccinia-gp160 and recombinant gp160. *Proc. Natl. Acad. Sci. USA* **90**:2443–2447.

3133. Mosier, D. E., R. J. Gulizia, P. D. MacIsaac, B. E. Torbett, and J. A. Levy. 1993. Rapid loss of CD4+ T cells in human-PBL-SCID mice by noncytopathic HIV isolates. *Science* **260**:689–692.

3134. Mosmann, T. R., H. Cherwinski, M. W. Bond, M. A. Giedlin, and R. L. Coffman. 1986. Two types of murine helper T cell clones. I. Definition according to profiles of lymphokine activities and secreted proteins. *J. Immunol.* **136:**2348–2357.

3135. Mosmann, T. R., and S. Sad. 1996. The expanding universe of T-cell subsets: Th1, Th2 and more. *Immunol. Today* **17:**138–146.

3136. Mosoian, A., A. Teixeira, E. Caron, J. Piqoz, and M. E. Klotman. 2000. CD8+ cell lines isolated from HIV-1-infected children have potent soluble HIV-1 inhibitory activity that differs from β-chemokines. *Viral Immunol.* **13:**481–495.

3136a. Mosoian, A., A. Teixeira, A. A. High, R. E. Christian, D. F. Hunt, J. Shabanowitz, X. Liu, and M. Klotman. 2006. Novel function of prothymosin alpha as a potent inhibitor of human immunodeficiency virus type 1 gene expression in primary macrophages. *J. Virol.* **80:**9200–9206.

3137. Moss, A. R., K. Vranizan, and R. Gorter. 1994. HIV seroconversion in intravenous drug users in San Francisco, 1985–1990. *AIDS* **8:**223–231.

3138. Moss, G. B., D. Clemetson, L. D'Costa, F. A. Plummer, J. O. Ndinya-Achola, M. Reilly, K. K. Holmes, P. Piot, G. M. Maitha, S. L. Hillier, N. C. Kiviat, C. W. Cameron, I. A. Wamola, and J. K. Kreiss. 1991. Association of cervical ectopy with heterosexual transmission of human immunodeficiency virus: results of a study of couples in Nairobi, Kenya. *J. Infect. Dis.* **164:**588–591.

3139. Moss, G. B., J. Overbaugh, M. Wlech, M. Reilly, J. Bwayo, F. A. Plummer, J. O. Ndinya-Achola, M. A. Malisa, and J. K. Kreiss. 1995. Human immunodeficiency virus DNA in urethral secretions in men: association with gonococcal urethritis and CD4 cell depletion. *J. Infect. Dis.* **172:**1469–1474.

3140. Moss, P. A. H. 1995. Persistent high frequency of human immunodeficiency virus-specific cytotoxic T cells in peripheral blood of infected donors. *Proc. Natl. Acad. Sci. USA* **92:**5773–5777.

3141. Moss, W. J., J. J. Ryon, M. Monze, F. Cutts, T. C. Quinn, and D. E. Griffin. 2002. Suppression of human immunodeficiency virus replication during acute measles. *J. Infect. Dis.* **185:**1035–1042.

3142. Mossman, S. P., F. Bex, P. Berglund, J. Arthos, S. P. O'Neil, D. Riley, D. H. Maul, C. Bruck, P. Momin, A. Burny, P. N. Fultz, J. I. Mullins, P. Liljestrom, and E. A. Hoover. 1996. Protection against lethal simian immunodeficiency virus SIVsmmPBj14 disease by a recombinant Semliki Forest virus gp160 vaccine and by a gp120 subunit vaccine. *J. Virol.* **70:**1953–1960.

3143. Mostad, S. B., and J. K. Kreiss. 1996. Shedding of HIV-1 in the genital tract. *AIDS* **10:**1305–1315.

3144. Motsinger, A., D. W. Haas, A. K. Stanic, L. Van Kaer, S. Joyce, and D. Unutmaz. 2002. CD1d-restricted human natural killer T cells are highly susceptible to human immunodeficiency virus 1 infection. *J. Exp. Med.* **195:**869.

3145. Motti, P. G., G. A. Dallabetta, R. W. Daniel, J. K. Canner, J. D. Chiphangwi, G. N. Liomba, L. P. Yang, and K. V. Shah. 1996. Cervical abnormalities, human papillomavirus, and human immunodeficiency virus infections in women in Malawi. *J. Infect. Dis.* **173:**714–717.

3146. Moulton, H. M., M. C. Hase, K. M. Smith, and P. L. Iversen. 2003. HIV Tat peptide enhances cellular delivery of antisense morpholino oligomers. *Antisense Nucleic Acid Drug Dev.* **13:**31–43.

3147. Moulton, H. M., M. H. Nelson, S. A. Hatlevig, M. T. Reddy, and P. L. Iversen. 2004. Cellular uptake of antisense morpholino oligomers conjugated to arginine-rich peptides. *Bioconjug. Chem.* **15:**290–299.

3148. Mount, A. M., V. Mwapasa, S. R. Elliott, J. G. Beeson, E. Tadesse, V. M. Lema, M. E. Molyneux, S. R. Meshnick, and S. J. Rogerson. 2004. Impairment of humoral immunity to Plasmodium falciparum malaria in pregnancy by HIV infection. *Lancet* **363:**1860–1867.

3149. Mourich, D. V., S. Lee, G. Reyes-Teran, C. E. Mackewicz, and J. A. Levy. 1999. Lack of differences in nef alleles among HIV-infected asymptomatic long-term survivors and those who progressed to disease. *AIDS Res. Hum. Retrovir.* **15:**1573–1575.

3150. Mowat, A. M., and J. L. Viney. 1997. The anatomical basis of intestinal immunity. *Immunol. Rev.* **156:**145–166.

3151. Mowen, K. A., and L. H. Glimcher. 2004. Signaling pathways in Th2 development. *Immunol. Rev.* **202:**203–222.

3152. Mowen, K. A., B. T. Schurter, J. W. Fathman, M. David, and L. H. Glimcher. 2004. Arginine methylation of NIP45 modulates cytokine gene expression in effector T lymphocytes. *Mol. Cell* **15:**559–571.

3153. Moyer, M. P., R. I. Juot, A. Ramirez, Jr., S. Joe, M. S. Meltzer, and H. E. Gendelman. 1990. Infection of human gastrointestinal cells by HIV-1. *AIDS Res. Hum. Retrovir.* **6:**1409–1415.

3153a. Moyle, G. J., C. A. Sabin, J. Cartledge, M. Johnson, E. Wilkins, D. Churchill, P. Hay, A. Fakoya, M. Murphy, G. Scullard, C. Leen, and G. Reilly. 2006. A randomized comparative trial of tenofovir DF or abacavir as replacement for a thymidine analogue in persons with lipoatrophy. *AIDS* **20:**2043–2050.

3154. Mrus, J. M., S. J. Goldie, M. C. Weinstein, and J. Tsevat. 2000. The cost-effectiveness of elective Cesarean delivery for HIV-infected women with detectable HIV RNA during pregnancy. *AIDS* **14:**2543–2552.

3155. Mueller, Y. M., C. Petrovas, P. M. Bojczuk, I. D. Dimitriou, B. Beer, P. Silvera, F. Villinger, J. S. Cairns, E. J. Gracely, M. G. Lewis, and P. D. Katsikis. 2005. Interleukin-15 increases effector memory CD8⁺ T cells and NK cells in simian immunodeficiency virus-infected macaques. *J. Virol.* **79:**4877–4885.

3156. Muesing, M. A., D. H. Smith, C. D. Cabradilla, C. V. Benton, L. A. Lasky, and D. J. Capon. 1985. Nucleic acid structure and expression of the human AIDS/lymphadenopathy retrovirus. *Nature* **313:**450–458.

3157. Mugnaini, E. N., A. M. Syversen, M. Sannes, A. Freng, and J. E. Brinchmann. 1999. Normal CD4 T-cell receptor repertoire in tonsillar tissue despite perturbed repertoire in peripheral blood in HIV-1 infected individuals. *AIDS* **13:**2507–2513.

3158. Mukhtar, M., S. Harley, P. Chen, M. BouHandan, C. Patel, E. Acheampong, and R. Pomerantz. 2002. Primary isolated human brain microvascular endothelial cells express diverse HIV/SIV-associated chemokine coreceptors and DC-SIGN and L-SIGN. *Virology* **297:**78–88.

3159. Mulherin, S. A., T. R. O'Brien, J. P. A. Ioannidis, J. J. Goedert, S. P. Buchbinder, R. A. Coutinho, B. D. Jamieson, L. Meyer, N. L. Michael, G. Pantaleo, G. P. Rizzardini, H. Schuitemaker, H. W. Sheppard, I. D. Theodorou, D. Vlahov, and P. S. Rosenberg. 2003. Effects of CCR-5Δ32 and CCR2-41 alleles on HIV-1 disease progression: the protection varies with duration of infection. *AIDS* **17:**377–387.

3160. Muller, B., U. Tessmer, U. Schubert, and H. G. Krausslich. 2000. Human immunodeficiency virus type 1 Vpr protein is incorporated into the virion in significantly smaller amounts than gag and is phosphorylated in infected cells. *J. Virol.* 74:9727–9731.

3161. Muller, C., S. Kukel, and R. Bauer. 1993. Relationship of antibodies against CD4+ T cells in HIV-infected patients to markers of activation and progression: autoantibodies are closely associated with CD4 cell depletion. *Immunology* 79:248–254.

3162. Muller, V., B. Ledergerber, L. Perrin, T. Klimkait, H. Furrer, A. Telenti, E. Bernasconi, P. Vernazza, H. F. Gunthard, and S. Bonhoeffer. 2006. Stable virulence levels in the HIV epidemic of Switzerland over two decades. *AIDS* 20:889–894.

3163. Mulroney, S. E., K. J. McDonnell, C. B. Pert, M. R. Ruff, Z. Resch, W. K. Samson, and M. D. Lumpkin. 1998. HIV gp120 inhibits the somatotropic axis: a possible GH-releasing hormone receptor mechanism for the pathogenesis of AIDS wasting. *Proc. Natl. Acad. Sci. USA* 95:1927–1932.

3164. Mummidi, S., S. S. Ahuja, E. Gonzalez, S. A. Anderson, E. N. Santiago, K. T. Stephan, F. E. Craig, P. O'Connell, V. Tryon, R. A. Clark, M. J. Dolan, and S. K. Ahuja. 1998. Genealogy of the CCR5 locus and chemokine system gene variants associated with altered rates of HIV-1 disease progression. *Nat. Med.* 4:786–793.

3165. Mundy, D. C., R. F. Schinazi, A. Ressell-Gerber, A. J. Nahmias, and H. W. Randal. 1987. Human immunodeficiency virus isolated from amniotic fluid. *Lancet* ii:459–460.

3166. Munier, S., A. Borjabad, M. Lemaire, V. Mariot, and U. Hazan. 2003. In vitro infection of human primary adipose cells with HIV-1: a reassessment. *AIDS* 17:2537–2541.

3167. Munis, J. R., R. S. Kornbluth, J. C. Guatelli, and D. D. Richman. 1992. Ordered appearance of human immunodeficiency virus type 1 nucleic acids following high multiplicity infection of macrophages. *J. Gen. Virol.* 73:1899–1906.

3168. Munk, C., S. M. Brandt, G. Lucero, and N. R. Landau. 2002. A dominant block to HIV-1 replication at reverse transcription in simian cells. *Proc. Natl. Acad. Sci. USA* 99:13843–13848.

3168a. Munn, D. H., M. D. Sharma, and A. L. Mellor. 2004. Ligation of B7–1/B7–2 by human CD4+ T cells triggers indoleamine 2,3-dioxygenase activity in dendritic cells. *J. Immunol.* 172:4100–4110.

3169. Munoz, A., A. J. Kirby, Y. D. He, J. B. Margolick, B. R. Visscher, C. R. Rinaldo, R. A. Kaslow, and J. P. Phair. 1995. Long-term survivors with HIV-1 infection: incubation period and longitudinal patterns of CD4+ lymphocytes. *J. Acquir. Immune Defic. Syndr. Hum. Retrovirol.* 8:496–505.

3170. Munoz, J. F., S. Salmen, L. R. Berueta, M. P. Carlos, J. A. Cova, J. H. Donis, M. R. Hernandez, and J. V. Torres. 1999. Effect of human immunodeficiency virus type 1 on intracellular activation and superoxide production by neutrophils. *J. Infect. Dis.* 180:206–210.

3171. Munteanu, A., J. M. Zingg, R. Ricciarelli, and A. Azzi. 2005. CD36 overexpression in ritonavir-treated THP-1 cells is reversed by alpha-tocopherol. *Free Radic. Biol. Med.* 38:1047–1056.

3172. Munz, C., R. M. Steinman, and S. Fujii. 2005. Dendritic cell maturation by innate lymphocytes: coordinated stimulation of innate and adaptive immunity. *J. Exp. Med.* 202:203–207.

3173. Murakami, T., and E. O. Freed. 2000. The long cytoplasmic tail of gp41 is required in a cell type-dependent manner for HIV-1 envelope glycoprotein incorporation into virions. *Proc. Natl. Acad. Sci. USA* 97:343–348.

3174. Murakami, T., T. Hattori, and K. Takatsuki. 1991. A principal neutralizing domain of human immunodeficiency virus type 1 interacts with proteinase-like molecule(s) at the surface of Molt-4 clone 8 cells. *Biochim. Biophys. Acta* 1079:279–284.

3175. Muralidhar, S., A. Pumfrey, M. Hassani, M. Sadaie, N. Azumi, M. Kishishita, J. Brady, J. Doniger, P. Medveczky, and L. Rosenthal. 1998. Identification of Kaposin (open reading frame K12) as a human herpesvirus 8 (Kaposi's sarcoma-associated herpesvirus) transforming gene. *J. Virol.* 72:4980–4988.

3176. Muro-Cacho, C. A., G. Pantaleo, and A. S. Fauci. 1995. Analysis of apoptosis in lymph nodes of HIV-infected persons. *J. Immunol.* 154:5555–5566.

3177. Murphey-Corb, M., L. N. Martin, B. Davison-Fairburn, R. C. Montelaro, M. Miller, M. West, S. Ohkawa, G. B. Baskin, J.-Y. Zhang, S. D. Putney, A. C. Allison, and D. A. Eppstein. 1989. A formalin-inactivated whole SIV vaccine confers protection in macaques. *Science* 246:1293–1297.

3178. Murphey-Corb, M., R. C. Montelaro, M. A. Miller, M. West, L. N. Martin, B. Davison-Fairburn, S. Ohkawa, G. B. Baskin, J.-Y. Zhang, G. B. Miller, S. D. Putney, A. C. Allison, and D. A. Eppstein. 1991. Efficacy of SIV/deltaB670 glycoprotein-enriched and glycoprotein-depleted subunit vaccines in protecting against infection and disease in rhesus monkeys. *AIDS* 5:655–662.

3179. Murri, R., A. C. Lepri, P. Cicconi, A. Poggio, M. Arlotti, G. Tositti, D. Santoro, M. L. Soranzo, G. Rizzardini, V. Colangeli, M. Montroni, and A. D. Monforte. 2006. Is moderate HIV viremia associated with a higher risk of clinical progression in HIV-infected people treated with highly active antiretroviral therapy: evidence from the Italian cohort of antiretroviral-naive patients study. *J. Acquir. Immune Defic. Syndr.* 41:23–30.

3180. Musey, L., Y. Hu, L. Eckert, M. Christensen, T. Karchmer, and M. J. McElrath. 1997. HIV-1 induces cytotoxic T lymphocytes in the cervix of infected women. *J. Exp. Med.* 185:293–303.

3181. Musey, L. K., J. N. Krieger, J. P. Hughes, T. W. Schacker, L. Corey, and M. J. McElrath. 1999. Early and persistent human immunodeficiency virus type 1 (HIV-1)- specific T helper dysfunction in blood and lymph nodes following acute HIV-1 infection. *J. Infect. Dis.* 180:278–284.

3182. Musicco, M., A. Lazzarin, A. Nicolosi, M. Gasparini, P. Costigliola, C. Arici, and A. Saracco. 1994. Antiretroviral treatment of men infected with human immunodeficiency virus type 1 reduces the incidence of heterosexual transmission. *Arch. Intern. Med.* 154:1971–1976.

3183. Muster, T., F. Steindl, M. Purtscher, A. Trkola, A. Klima, G. Himmler, F. Ruker, and H. Katinger. 1993. A conserved neutralizing epitope on gp41 of human immunodeficiency virus type 1. *J. Virol.* 67:6642–6647.

3184. Myagkikh, M., S. Alipanah, P. D. Markham, J. Tartaglia, E. Paoletti, R. C. Gallo, G. Franchini, and M. Robert-Guroff. 1996. Multiple immunizations with attenuated poxvirus HIV type 2 recombinants and subunit boosts required for protection of rhesus macaques. *AIDS Res. Hum. Retrovir.* 12:985–992.

3185. Myers, G. 1991. Analysis. Protein information summary, p. III–4. *In* G. Myers, J. A. Berzofsky, B. Korber, R. F. Smith, and G. Pavlakis (ed.), *Human Retroviruses and AIDS 1991. A Compilation and Analysis of Nucleic Acid and Amino Acid Sequences.* Theoretical Biology and Biophysics, Los Alamos National Laboratory, Los Alamos, N.M.

3186. **Myers, G.** 1994. Tenth anniversary perspectives on AIDS. HIV: between past and future. *AIDS Res. Hum. Retrovir.* **10:**1317–1324.

3187. **Myers, G., B. Korber, S. Wain-Hobson, R. F. Smith, and G. N. Pavlakis.** 1993. *Human Retroviruses and AIDS 1993, I–V. A Compilation and Analysis of Nucleic Acid and Amino Acid Sequences.* Los Alamos National Laboratory, Los Alamos, N.M.

3188. **Myers, G., K. MacInnes, and B. Korber.** 1992. The emergence of simian/human immunodeficiency viruses. *AIDS Res. Hum. Retrovir.* **8:**373–386.

3189. **Myers, G., and G. N. Pavlakis.** 1992. Evolutionary potential of complex retroviruses, p. 51–105. *In* J. A. Levy (ed.), *The Retroviridae,* vol. I. Plenum Press, New York, N.Y.

3190. **Mynarcik, D. C., M. A. McNurlan, R. T. Steigbigel, J. Fuhrer, and M. C. Gelato.** 2000. Association of severe insulin resistance with both loss of limb fat and elevated serum tumor necrosis factor receptor levels in HIV lipodystrophy. *J. Acquir. Immune Defic. Syndr.* **25:**312–321.

3191. **Myszka, D. G., R. W. Sweet, P. Hensley, M. Brigham-Burke, P. D. Kwong, W. A. Hendrickson, R. Wyatt, J. Sodroski, and M. L. Doyle.** 2000. Energetics of the HIV gp120-CD4 binding reaction. *Proc. Natl. Acad. Sci. USA* **97:**9026–9031.

3192. **Nabel, E. G., L. Shum, V. J. Pompili, Z. Y. Yang, H. San, H. B. Shu, S. Liptay, L. Gold, D. Gordon, R. Derynck, and G. J. Nabel.** 1993. Direct transfer of transforming growth factor beta-1 gene into arteries stimulates fibrocellular hyperplasia. *Proc. Natl. Acad. Sci. USA* **90:**10759–10763.

3193. **Nabel, G., and D. Baltimore.** 1987. An inducible transcription factor activates expression of human immunodeficiency virus in T cells. *Nature* **326:**711–713.

3194. **Nabel, G. J.** 2005. Immunology. Close to the edge: neutralizing the HIV-1 envelope. *Science* **308:**1878–1879.

3195. **Nabel, G. J., S. A. Rice, D. M. Knipe, and D. Baltimore.** 1988. Alternative mechanisms for activation of human immunodeficiency virus enhancer in T cells. *Science* **239:**1299–1302.

3196. **Nacher, M., S. Serrano, A. Gonzalez, A. Hernandez, M. L. Marinoso, A. Vilella, P. Hinarejos, A. Diez, and J. Aubia.** 2001. Osteoblasts in HIV-infected patients: HIV-1 infection and cell infection. *AIDS* **15:**2239–2243.

3197. **Nag, P., J. Kim, V. Sapiega, A. L. Landay, J. W. Bremer, J. Mestecky, P. Reichelderfer, A. Kovacs, J. Cohn, B. Weiser, and L. L. Baum.** 2004. Women with cervicovaginal antibody-dependent cell-mediated cytotoxicity have lower genital HIV-1 RNA loads. *J. Infect. Dis.* **190:**1970–1978.

3198. **Nagashunmugam, T., H. M. Friedman, C. Davis, S. Kennedy, L. T. Goldstein, and D. Malamud.** 1997. Human submandibular saliva specifically inhibits HIV type 1. *AIDS Res. Hum. Retrovir.* **13:**371–376.

3199. **Nahmias, A. J., J. Weiss, X. Yao, F. Lee, R. Kodsi, M. Schanfield, T. Matthews, D. Bolognesi, D. Durack, A. Motulsky, P. Kanki, and M. Essex.** 1986. Evidence for human infection with an HTLV III/LAV-like virus in Central Africa, 1959. *Lancet* **i:**1279–1280.

3200. **Naif, H. M., A. L. Cunnningham, M. Alali, S. Li, N. Nasr, M. M. Buhler, D. Schols, E. de Clerq, and G. Stewart.** 2002. A human immunodeficiency virus type 1 isolate from an infected person homozygous for CCR5Δ32 exhibits dual tropism by infecting macrophages and MT2 cells via CXCR4. *J. Virol.* **76:**3114–3124.

3201. **Najera, R., E. Delgado, L. Perez-Alvarez, and M. M. Thomson.** 2002. Genetic recombination and its role in the development of the HIV-1 pandemic. *AIDS* **16**(Suppl.) 4:S3–S16.

3202. **Nakajima, K., O. Martinez-Maza, T. Hirano, E. C. Breen, P. G. Nishanian, J. F. Salazar-Gonzalez, J. L. Fahey, and T. Kishimoto.** 1989. Induction of IL-6 (B cell stimulatory factor-2/IFN-beta-2) production by human immunodeficiency virus. *J. Immunol.* **142:**531–536.

3203. **Nakamura, G. R., R. Byrn, D. M. Wilkes, J. A. Fox, M. R. Hobbs, R. Hastings, H. C. Wessling, M. A. Norcross, B. M. Fendly, and P. W. Berman.** 1993. Strain specificity and binding affinity requirements of neutralizing monoclonal antibodies to the CD4 domain of gp120 from human immunodeficiency virus type 1. *J. Virol.* **67:**6179–6191.

3204. **Nakano, H., M. Yanagita, and M. D. Gunn.** 2001. CD11c(+)B220(+)Gr-1(+) cells in mouse lymph nodes and spleen display characteristics of plasmacytoid dendritic cells. *J. Exp. Med.* **194:**1171–1178.

3205. **Nakashima, H., N. Yamamoto, M. Masuda, and N. Fujii.** 1993. Defensins inhibit HIV replication in vitro. *AIDS* **7:**1129.

3206. **Nakayama, E. E., Y. Hoshino, X. Xin, H. Liu, M. Goto, N. Watanabe, H. Taguchi, A. Hitani, A. Kawana-Tachikawa, M. Fukushima, K. Yamada, W. Sugiura, S. I. Oka, A. Ajisawa, H. Sato, Y. Takebe, T. Nakamura, Y. Nagai, A. Iwamoto, and T. Shioda.** 2000. Polymorphism in the interleukin-4 promoter affects acquisition of human immunodeficiency virus type 1 syncytium-inducing phenotype. *J. Virol.* **74:**5452–5459.

3207. **Nakayama, E. E., L. Meyer, A. Iwamoto, A. Persoz, Y. Nagai, C. Rouzioux, J. F. Delfraissy, P. Debre, D. McIlroy, I. Theodorou, and T. Shioda.** 2002. Protective effect of interleukin-4 -589T polymorphism on human immunodeficiency virus type 1 disease progression: relationship with virus load. *J. Infect. Dis.* **185:**1183–1186.

3208. **Nakayama, E. E., H. Miyoshi, Y. Nagai, and T. Shioda.** 2005. A specific region of 37 amino acid residues in the SPRY (B30.2) domain of African green monkey TRIM5alpha determines species-specific restriction of simian immunodeficiency virus SIVmac infection. *J. Virol.* **79:**8870–8877.

3209. **Nakayama, E. E., Y. Tanaka, Y. Nagai, A. Iwamoto, and T. Shioda.** 2004. A CCR2-V64I polymorphism affects stability of CCR2A isoform. *AIDS* **18:**729–738.

3210. **Namikawa, R., H. Kaneshima, M. Lieberman, I. L. Weissman, and J. M. McCune.** 1988. Infection of the SCID-hu mouse by HIV-1. *Science* **242:**1684–1686.

3211. **Naora, H., and M. L. Gougeon.** 1999. Interleukin-15 is a potent survival factor in the prevention of spontaneous but not CD95-induced apoptosis in CD4 and CD8 T lymphocytes of HIV-infected individuals. Correlation with its ability to increase BCL-2 expression. *Cell Death Differ.* **6:**1002–1011.

3212. **Napolitano, L. A., R. M. Grant, S. G. Deeks, D. Schmidt, S. C. De Rosa, L. A. Herzenberg, B. G. Herndier, J. Andersson, and J. M. McCune.** 2001. Increased production of IL-7 accompanies HIV-1-mediated T-cell depletion: implications for T-cell homeostasis. *Nat. Med.* **7:**73–79.

3213. **Napolitano, L. A., J. C. Lo, M. B. Gotway, K. Mulligan, J. D. Barbour, D. Schmidt, R. M. Grant, R. A. Halvorsen, M. Schambelan, and J. M. McCune.** 2002. Increased thymic mass and circulating naive CD4 T cells in HIV-1-infected adults treated with growth hormone. *AIDS* **16:**1103–1111.

3214. Nappi, F., R. Schneider, A. Zolotukhin, S. Smulevitch, D. Michalowski, J. Bear, B. K. Felber, and G. N. Pavlakis. 2001. Identification of a novel posttranscriptional regulatory element by using a rev- and RRE-mutated human immunodeficiency virus type 1 DNA proviral clone as a molecular trap. *J. Virol.* 75:4558–4569.

3215. Nara, P. L., R. R. Garrity, and J. Goudsmit. 1991. Neutralization of HIV-1: a paradox of humoral proportions. *FASEB J.* 5:2437–2455.

3216. Nara, P. L., W. G. Robey, L. O. Arthur, D. M. Asher, A. V. Wolff, J. C. Gibbs, Jr., D. C. Gajdusek, and P. J. Fischinger. 1987. Persistent infection of chimpanzees with human immunodeficiency virus: serological responses and properties of reisolated viruses. *J. Virol.* 61:3173–3180.

3217. Nara, P. L., L. Smit, N. Dunlop, W. Hatch, M. Merges, D. Waters, J. Kelliher, R. C. Gallo, P. G. Fischinger, and J. Goudsmit. 1990. Emergence of viruses resistant to neutralization by V3-specific antibodies in experimental human immunodeficiency virus type 1 IIIB infection of chimpanzees. *J. Virol.* 64:3779–3791.

3218. Naranatt, P. P., H. H. Krishnan, S. R. Svojanovsky, C. Bloomer, S. Mathur, and B. Chandran. 2004. Host gene induction and transcriptional reprogramming in Kaposi's sarcoma-associated herpesvirus (KSHV/HHV-8)-infected endothelial, fibroblast, and B cells: insights into modulation events early during infection. *Cancer Res.* 64:72–84.

3219. Narimatsu, R., D. Wolday, and B. K. Patterson. 2005. IL-8 increases transmission of HIV type 1 in cervical explant tissue. *AIDS Res. Hum. Retrovir.* 21:228–233.

3220. Natarajan, V., R. A. Lempicki, I. Sereti, Y. Badralmaa, J. W. Adelsberger, J. A. Metcalf, D. A. Prieto, R. Stevens, M. W. Baseler, J. A. Kovacs, and H. C. Lane. 2002. Increased peripheral expansion of naive CD4+ T cells *in vivo* after IL-2 treatment of patients with HIV infection. *Proc. Natl. Acad. Sci. USA* 99:10712–10717.

3221. Natterman, J., H. Nischalke, B. Kupfer, J. Rockstroh, L. Hess, T. Sauerbruch, and U. Spengler. 2003. Regulation of CC chemokine receptor 5 in hepatitis G virus infection. *AIDS* 17:1457–1462.

3222. Navarro, F., B. Bollman, H. Chen, R. Konig, Q. Yu, K. Chiles, and N. R. Landau. 2005. Complementary function of the two catalytic domains of APOBEC3G. *Virology* 333:374–386.

3223. Navia, B. A., and R. W. Price. 1987. The acquired immunodeficiency syndrome dementia complex as the presenting or sole manifestation of human immunodeficiency virus infection. *Arch. Neurol.* 44:65–69.

3224. Navia, M. A., P. M. Fitzgerald, B. M. McKeever, C. T. Leu, J. C. Heimbach, W. K. Herber, I. S. Sigal, P. L. Darke, and J. P. Springer. 1989. Three-dimensional structure of aspartyl protease from human immunodeficiency virus HIV-1. *Nature* 337:615–620.

3225. Naylor, P. H., C. W. Naylor, M. Badamchian, S. Wada, A. L. Goldstein, S.-S. Wang, D. K. Sun, A. H. Thornton, and P. S. Sarin. 1987. Human immunodeficiency virus contains an epitope immunoreactive with thymosin alpha-1 and the 30-amino acid synthetic p17 group-specific antigen peptide HGP-30. *Proc. Natl. Acad. Sci. USA* 84:2951–2955.

3226. Nduati, R., G. John, D. Mbori-Ngacha, B. Richardson, J. Overbaugh, A. Mwatha, J. Ndinya-Achola, J. Bwayo, F. E. Onyango, J. Hughes, and J. Kreiss. 2000. Effect of breastfeeding and formula feeding on transmission of HIV-1: a randomized clinical trial. *JAMA* 283:1167–1174.

3227. Nduati, R. W., G. C. John, B. A. Richardson, J. Overbaugh, M. Welch, J. Ndinya-Achola, S. Moses, K. Holmes, F. Onyango, and J. K. Kreiss. 1995. Human immunodeficiency virus type 1-infected cells in breast milk: association with immunosuppression and vitamin A deficiency. *J. Infect. Dis.* 172:1461–1468.

3228. Neal, T. F., H. K. Holland, C. M. Baum, F. Villinger, A. A. Ansari, R. Saral, J. R. Wingard, and W. H. Fleming. 1995. CD34+ progenitor cells from asymptomatic patients are not a major reservoir for human immunodeficiency virus-1. *Blood* 86:1749–1756.

3229. Neil, S. J., M. M. Aasa-Chapman, P. R. Clapham, R. J. Nibbs, A. McKnight, and R. A. Weiss. 2005. The promiscuous CC chemokine receptor D6 is a functional coreceptor for primary isolates of human immunodeficiency virus type 1 (HIV-1) and HIV-2 on astrocytes. *J. Virol.* 79:9618–9624.

3230. Neildez, O., R. Le Grand, P. Caufour, B. Vaslin, A. Chéret, F. Matheux, F. Théodoro, P. Roques, and D. Dormont. 1998. Selective quasispecies transmission after systemic or mucosal exposure of macaques to simian immunodeficiency virus. *Virology* 243:12–20.

3231. Nelbock, P., P. J. Dillon, A. Perkins, and C. A. Rosen. 1990. A cDNA for a protein that interacts with the human immunodeficiency virus Tat transactivator. *Science* 248:1650–1653.

3232. Nelson, J. A., P. Ghazal, and C. A. Wiley. 1990. Role of opportunistic viral infections in AIDS. *AIDS* 4:1–10.

3233. Nelson, J. A., C. Reynolds-Kohler, M. B. A. Oldstone, and C. A. Wiley. 1988. HIV and HCMV coinfect brain cells in patients with AIDS. *Virology* 165:286–290.

3234. Nelson, J. A., C. A. Wiley, C. Reynolds-Kohler, C. E. Reese, W. Margaretten, and J. A. Levy. 1988. Human immunodeficiency virus detected in bowel epithelium from patients with gastrointestinal symptoms. *Lancet* i:259–262.

3235. Nerrienet, E., M. L. Santiago, Y. Foupouapouognigni, E. Bailes, N. I. Mundy, B. Njinku, A. Kfutwah, M. C. Muller-Trutwin, F. Barre-Sinoussi, G. M. Shaw, P. M. Sharp, B. H. Hahn, and A. Ayouba. 2005. Simian immunodeficiency virus infection in wild-caught chimpanzees from Cameroon. *J. Virol.* 79:1312–1319.

3236. Nettles, R. E., T. L. Kieffer, P. Kwon, D. Monie, Y. Han, T. Parsons, J. Cofrancesco, Jr., J. E. Gallant, T. C. Quinn, B. Jackson, C. Flexner, K. Carson, S. Ray, D. Persaud, and R. F. Siliciano. 2005. Intermittent HIV-1 viremia (Blips) and drug resistance in patients receiving HAART. *JAMA* 293:817–829.

3237. Neumann, A. U., R. Tubiana, V. Calvez, C. Robert, T. Li, H. Agut, R. Autran, C. Katlama, and C. S. Group. 1999. HIV-1 rebound during interruption of highly active antiviral therapy has no deleterious effect on reinitiated treatment. *AIDS* 13:677–683.

3238. Neumann, M., B. K. Felber, A. Kleinschmidt, B. Froese, V. Erfle, G. N. Pavlakis, and R. Brack-Werner. 1995. Restriction of human immunodeficiency virus type 1 production in a human astrocytoma cell line is associated with a cellular block in Rev function. *J. Virol.* 69:2159–2167.

3239. Neville, M., F. Stutz, L. Lee, L. I. Davis, and M. Rosbash. 1997. The importin-beta family member Crm1p bridges the interaction between Rev and the nuclear pore complex during nuclear export. *Curr. Biol.* 7:767–775.

3240. Newburg, D. S., R. P. Viscidi, A. Ruff, and R. H. Yolken. 1992. A human milk factor inhibits binding of human immunodeficiency virus to the CD4 receptor. *Pediatr. Res.* 31:22–28.

3241. Newell, M. L., D. Dunn, C. S. Peckham, A. E. Ades, G. Pardi, and A. E. Semprini. 1992. Risk factors for mother-to-child transmission of HIV-1. *Lancet* 339:1007–1012.

3242. Newman, E. N., R. K. Holmes, H. M. Craig, K. C. Klein, J. R. Lingappa, M. H. Malim, and A. M. Sheehy. 2005. Antiviral function of APOBEC3G can be dissociated from cytidine deaminase activity. *Curr. Biol.* 15:166–170.

3243. Newman, M. J., K. J. Munroe, C. A. Anderson, C. I. Murphy, D. L. Panicali, J. R. Seals, J.-Y. Wu, M. S. Wyand, and C. R. Kensil. 1994. Induction of antigen-specific killer T lymphocyte responses using subunit SIVmac251 gag and env vaccines containing QS-21 saponin adjuvant. *AIDS Res. Hum. Retrovir.* 10:853–861.

3244. Newstein, M., E. J. Stanbridge, G. Casey, and P. R. Shank. 1990. Human chromosome 12 encodes a species-specific factor which increases human immunodeficiency virus type 1 *tat*-mediated *trans* activation in rodent cells. *J. Virol.* 64:4565–4567.

3245. Newton, P. J., I. V. D. Weller, I. G. Williams, R. F. Miller, A. Copas, R. S. Tedder, D. R. Katz, and B. M. Chain. 2006. Monocyte derived dendritic cells from HIV-1 infected individuals partially reconstitute CD4 T-cell responses. *AIDS* 20:171–180.

3246. Ngo-Giang-Huong, N., D. Candotti, A. Goubar, B. Autran, M. Maynart, D. Sicard, J. P. Clauvel, H. Agut, D. Costagliola, and C. Rouzioux. 2001. HIV type 1-specific IgG2 antibodies: markers of helper T cell type 1 response and prognostic marker of long-term nonprogression. *AIDS Res. Hum. Retrovir.* 17:1435–1446.

3247. Ngugi, E. N., F. A. Plummer, J. N. Simonsen, D. W. Cameron, M. Bosire, P. Waiyaki, A. R. Ronald, and J. O. Ndinya-Achola. 1988. Prevention of transmission of human immunodeficiency virus in Africa: effectiveness of condom promotion and health education among prostitutes. *Lancet* ii:887–890.

3248. Nguyen, D. G., and J. E. Hildreth. 2003. Involvement of macrophage mannose receptor in the binding and transmission of HIV by macrophages. *Eur. J. Immunol.* 33:483–493.

3249. Nguyen, D. H., and J. E. Hildreth. 2000. Evidence for budding of human immunodeficiency virus type 1 selectively from glycolipid-enriched membrane lipid rafts. *J. Virol.* 74:3264–3272.

3250. Nguyen, D. H., N. Hurtado-Ziola, P. Gagneux, and A. Varki. 2006. Loss of Siglec expression on T lymphocytes during human evolution. *Proc. Natl. Acad. Sci. USA* 103:7765–7770.

3251. Nicholas, J. 2005. Human gammaherpesvirus cytokines and chemokine receptors. *J. Interferon Cytokine Res.* 25:373–383.

3252. Nick, S., J. Kalws, K. Friebel, C. Birr, G. Hunsmann, and H. Bayer. 1990. Virus neutralizing and enhancing epitopes characterized by synthetic oligopeptides derived from the feline leukemia virus glycoprotein sequence. *J. Gen. Virol.* 71:77–83.

3253. Nickoloff, B. J., and C. E. M. Griffiths. 1989. The spindle-shaped cells in cutaneous Kaposi's sarcoma. *Am. J. Pathol.* 135:793–800.

3254. Niederman, T. M. J., W. R. Hastings, S. Luria, J. C. Bandres, and L. Ratner. 1993. HIV-1 nef protein inhibits the recruitment of AP-1 DNA-binding activity in human T-cells. *Virology* 194:338–344.

3255. Niederman, T. M. J., W. Hu, and L. Ratner. 1991. Simian immunodeficiency virus negative factor suppresses the level of viral mRNA in COS cells. *J. Virol.* 65:3538–3546.

3256. Niederman, T. M. J., B. J. Thielan, and L. Ratner. 1989. Human immunodeficiency virus type 1 negative factor is a transcriptional silencer. *Proc. Natl. Acad. Sci. USA* 86:1128–1132.

3257. Nielsen, C., C. Pedersen, J. D. Lundgren, and J. Gerstoft. 1993. Biological properties of HIV isolates in primary HIV infection: consequences for the subsequent course of infection. *AIDS* 7:1035–1040.

3258. Nielsen, K., P. Boyer, M. Dillon, D. Wafer, L. S. Wei, E. Garratty, R. E. Dickover, and Y. J. Bryson. 1996. Presence of human immunodeficiency virus (HIV) type 1 and HIV-1-specific antibodies in cervicovaginal secretions of infected mothers and in the gastric aspirates of their infants. *J. Infect. Dis.* 173:1001–1004.

3259. Nielsen, S. D., A. K. Ersboll, L. Mathiesen, J. O. Nielsen, and J. E. S. Hansen. 1998. Highly active antiretroviral therapy normalizes the function of progenitor cells in human immunodeficiency virus-infected patients. *J. Infect. Dis.* 178:1299–1305.

3260. Nieman, R. B., J. Fleming, R. J. Coker, J. R. W. Harris, and D. M. Mitchell. 1993. The effect of cigarette smoking on the development of AIDS in HIV-1 seropositive individuals. *AIDS* 7:705–710.

3261. Nijhuis, M., R. Schuurman, D. de Jong, J. Erickson, E. Gustchina, J. Albert, P. Schipper, S. Gulnik, and C. A. Boucher. 1999. Increased fitness of drug resistant HIV-1 protease as a result of acquisition of compensatory mutations during suboptimal therapy. *AIDS* 13:2349–2359.

3261a. Nilsson, J., A. Boasso, P. A. Velilla, R. Zhang, M. Vaccari, G. Franchini, G. M. Shearer, J. Andersson, and C. Chougnet. 2006. HIV-1 driven regulatory T cell accumulation in lymphoid tissues is associated with disease progression in HIV/AIDS. *Blood* [Epub ahead of print].

3262. Nishioka, K., and I. Katayama. 1978. Angiogenic activity in culture supernatant of antigen-stimulated lymph node cells. *J. Pathol.* 126:63–69.

3263. Nisini, R., A. Aiuti, P. M. Matricardi, A. Fattorossi, C. Ferlini, R. Biselli, I. Mazzaroma, E. Pinter, and R. D'Amelio. 1994. Lack of evidence for a superantigen in lymphocytes from HIV-discordant monozygotic twins. *AIDS* 8:443–449.

3264. Nisole, S., C. Lynch, J. P. Stoye, and M. W. Yap. 2004. A Trim5-cyclophilin A fusion protein found in owl monkey kidney cells can restrict HIV-1. *Proc. Natl. Acad. Sci. USA* 101:13324–13328.

3265. Nisole, S., J. P. Stoye, and A. Saib. 2005. TRIM family proteins: retroviral restriction and antiviral defence. *Nat. Rev. Microbiol.* 3:799–808.

3266. Niu, M. T., D. S. Stein, and S. M. Schnittman. 1993. Primary human immunodeficiency virus type 1 infection: review of pathogenesis and early treatment intervention in humans and animal retrovirus infections. *J. Infect. Dis.* 168:1490–1501.

3267. Nixon, D. F., K. Broliden, G. Ogg, and P. A. Broliden. 1992. Cellular and humoral antigenic epitopes in HIV and SIV. *Immunology* 76:515–534.

3268. Nobile, C., C. Petit, A. Moris, K. Skrabal, J.-P. Abastado, F. Mammano, and O. Schwartz. 2005. Covert human immunodeficiency virus replication in dendritic cells and in DC-SIGN-expression cells promotes long-term transmission to lymphocytes. *J. Virol.* 79:5386–5399.

3269. Nolan, D., S. Gauddieri, M. John, and S. Mallal. 2004. Impact of host genetics on HIV disease progression and treatment: new conflicts on an ancient battleground. *AIDS* 18:1231–1240.

3270. Nolan, D., E. Hammond, A. Martin, L. Taylor, S. Herrmann, E. McKinnon, C. Metcalf, B. Latham, and S. Mallal. 2003. Mitochondrial DNA depletion and morphologic changes in adipocytes associated with nucleoside reverse transcriptase inhibitor therapy. *AIDS* 17:1329–1338.

3271. Nolan, D., P. Reiss, and S. Mallal. 2005. Adverse effects of antiretroviral therapy for HIV infection: a review of selected topics. *Expert Opin. Drug. Saf.* 4:201–218.

3272. Nolan, G. P., S. Ghosh, H. C. Liou, P. Tempst, and D. Baltimore. 1991. DNA binding and IkB inhibition of the cloned p65 subunit of NF-kB, rel-related polypeptide. *Cell* 65:961–969.

3273. Noor, M. A., J. C. Lo, K. Mulligan, J.-M. Schwarz, R. A. Halvorsen, M. Schambelan, and C. Grunfeld. 2001. Metabolic effects of indinavir in healthy HIV-seronegative men. *AIDS* 15:F11–F15.

3274. Noor, M. A., R. A. Parker, E. O'Mara, D. M. Grasela, A. Currie, S. L. Hodder, F. T. Fiedorek, and D. W. Haas. 2004. The effects of HIV protease inhibitors atazanavir and lopinavir/ritonavir on insulin sensitivity in HIV-seronegative healthy adults. *AIDS* 18:2137–2144.

3275. Noraz, N., J. Gozlan, J. Corbeil, T. Brunner, and S. A. Spector. 1997. HIV-induced apoptosis of activated primary CD4+ T lymphocytes is not mediated by Fas-Fas ligand. *AIDS* 11:1671–1680.

3276. Norley, S., B. Beer, D. Binninger-Schinzel, C. Cosma, and R. Kurth. 1996. Protection from pathogenic SIVmac challenge following short-term infection with a nef-deficient attenuated virus. *Virology* 219:195–205.

3277. Norley, S. G., U. Mikschy, A. Werner, S. Staszewski, E. B. Helm, and R. Kurth. 1990. Demonstration of cross-reactive antibodies able to elicit lysis of both HIV-1- and HIV-2-infected cells. *J. Immunol.* 145:1700–1705.

3278. Noronha, I. L., V. Daniel, K. Schimpf, and G. Opelz. 1992. Soluble IL-2 receptor and tumour necrosis factor-alpha in plasma of haemophilia patients infected with HIV. *Clin. Exp. Immunol.* 87:287–292.

3279. Norris, P. J., H. F. Moffett, O. O. Yang, D. E. Kaufmann, M. J. Clark, M. M. Addo, and E. S. Rosenberg. 2004. Beyond help: direct effector functions of human immunodeficiency virus type 1-specific CD4+ T cells. *J. Virol.* 78:8844–8851.

3280. Norris, P. J., and E. S. Rosenberg. 2002. CD4(+) T helper cells and the role they play in viral control. *J. Mol. Med.* 80:397–405.

3281. Norris, P. J., M. Sumaroka, C. Brander, H. F. Moffett, S. L. Boswell, T. Nguyen, Y. Sykulev, B. D. Walker, and E. S. Rosenberg. 2001. Multiple effector functions mediated by human immunodeficiency virus-specific CD4(+) T-cell clones. *J. Virol.* 75:9771–9779.

3282. Norton, S. D., L. Zuckerman, K. B. Urdahl, R. Shefner, J. Miller, and M. K. Jenkins. 1992. The CD28 ligand, B7, enhances IL2 production by providing a costimulatory signal to T cells. *J. Immunol.* 149:1556–1561.

3283. Notkins, A., S. Mergenhagen, and R. Howard. 1970. Effect of virus infections on the function of the immune system. *Annu. Rev. Microbiol.* 24:525–537.

3284. Nottet, H. S., Y. Persidsky, V. G. Sasseville, A. N. Nukana, P. Bock, Q. H. Zhai, L. R. Sharer, R. D. McComb, S. Swindells, and C. Soderland. 1996. Mechanisms for the transendothelial migration of HIV-1-infected monocytes into brain. *J. Immunol.* 156:1284–1295.

3285. Nottet, H. S. L. M., L. deGraaf, N. M. de Vos, L. J. Bakker, J. A. G. van Strijp, M. R. Visser, and J. Verhoef. 1993. Downregulation of human immunodeficiency virus type 1(HIV-1) production after stimulation of monocyte-derived macrophages infected with HIV-1. *J. Infect. Dis.* 167:810–817.

3286. Nottet, H. S. L. M., M. Jett, C. R. Flanagan, Q.-H. Zhai, Y. Persidsky, A. Rizzino, E. W. Bernton, P. Genis, T. Baldwin, J. Schwartz, C. J. LaBenz, and H. E. Gendelman. 1994. A regulatory role for astrocytes in HIV-1 encephalitis. *J. Immunol.* 154:3567–3581.

3287. Novina, C. D., M. F. Murray, D. M. Dykxhoorn, P. J. Beresford, J. Riess, S. Lee, R. G. Collman, J. Lieberman, P. Shankar, and P. A. Sharp. 2002. siRNA-directed inhibition of HIV-1 infection. *Nat. Med.* 8:681–686.

3288. Numazaki, K., X.-Q. Bai, H. Goldman, I. Wong, B. Spira, and M. A. Wainberg. 1989. Infection of cultured human thymic epithelial cells by human immunodeficiency virus. *Clin. Immunol. Immunopathol.* 51:185–195.

3289. Nunn, M. F., and J. W. Marsh. 1996. Human immunodeficiency virus type 1 Nef associates with a member of the p21-activated kinase family. *J. Virol.* 70:6157–6161.

3290. Nunnari, G., M. Oero, G. Dornadula, M. Vanella, H. Zhang, I. Frank, and R. J. Pomerantz. 2002. Residual HIV-1 disease in seminal cells of HIV-1-infected men on suppressive HAART: latency without on-going cellular infections. *AIDS* 16:39–45.

3291. Nunnari, G., J. Sullivan, Y. Xu, P. Nyirjesy, J. Kulkosky, W. Cavert, I. Frank, and R. J. Pomerantz. 2005. HIV type 1 cervicovaginal reservoirs in the era of HAART. *AIDS Res. Hum. Retrovir.* 21:714–718.

3292. Nuovo, G. J., J. Becker, M. W. Burk, M. Margiotta, J. Fuhrer, and R. T. Steigbigel. 1994. *In situ* detection of PCR-amplified HIV-1 nucleic acids in lymph nodes and peripheral blood in patients with asymptomatic HIV-1 infection and advanced stage AIDS. *J. Acquir. Immune Defic. Syndr.* 7:916–923.

3293. Nuovo, G. J., J. Becker, A. Simsir, M. Margiotta, G. Khalife, and M. Shevchuk. 1994. HIV-1 nucleic acids localize to the spermatogonia and their progeny: a study by PCR *in situ* hybridization. *Am. J. Pathol.* 145:1–7.

3294. Nuovo, G. J., A. Forde, P. MacConnell, and R. Fahrenwald. 1993. *In situ* detection of PCR-amplified HIV-1 nucleic acids and tumor necrosis factor cDNA in cervical tissues. *Am. J. Pathol.* 143:40–48.

3295. Nuovo, G. J., F. Gallery, P. MacConnell, and A. Braun. 1994. *In situ* detection of PCR-amplified HIV-1 nucleic acids and tumor necrosis factor alpha RNA in the central nervous system. *Am. J. Pathol.* 144:659–666.

3296. Nuvor, S. V., M. van der Sande, S. Rowland-Jones, H. Whittle, and A. Jaye. 2006. Natural killer cell function is well preserved in asymptomatic human immunodeficiency virus type 2 (HIV-2) infection but similar to that of HIV-1 infection when CD4 T-cell counts fall. *J. Virol.* 80:2529–2538.

3297. Nyambi, P. N., A. Nadas, H. A. Mbah, S. Burda, C. Williams, M. K. Gorny, and S. Zolla-Pazner. 2000. Immunoreactivity of intact virions of human immunodeficiency virus type 1 (HIV-1) reveals the existence of fewer HIV-1 immunotypes than genotypes. *J. Virol.* 74:10670–10680.

3298. Nyambi, P. N., J. Nkengasong, M. Peeters, F. Simon, J. Eberle, W. Janssens, K. Fransen, B. Willems, K. Vereecken, L. Heyndrickx, P. Piot, and G. van der Groen. 1995. Reduced capacity of antibodies from patients infected with human immunodeficiency virus type 1 (HIV-1) Group O to neutralize primary isolates of HIV-1 Group M viruses. *J. Infect. Dis.* 172:1228–1237.

3299. Nyambi, P. N., B. Willems, W. Janssens, K. Fransen, J. Nkengasong, M. Peeters, K. Vereecken, L. Heyndrickx, P. Piot, and G. Van der Groen. 1997. The neutralization relationship of HIV type 1, HIV type 2, and SIVcpz is reflected in the genetic diversity that distinguishes them. *AIDS Res. Hum. Retrovir.* 13:7–17.

3300. Nygren, A., T. Bergman, T. Matthews, H. Jornvall, and H. Wigzell. 1988. 95- and 25-kDa fragments of the human immunodeficiency virus envelope glycoprotein gp120 bind to the CD4 receptor. *Proc. Natl. Acad. Sci. USA* 85:6543–6546.

3301. Nyland, S. B., C. Cao, Y. Bai, T. P. Loughran, and K. E. Ugen. 2003. Modulation of infection and type 1 cytokine expression parameters by morphine during in vitro coinfection with human T-cell leukemia virus type 1 and HIV-1. *J. Acquir. Immune Defic. Syndr.* 32:406–416.

3302. Nzilambi, N., K. M. DeCock, D. N. Forthal, H. Francis, R. W. Ryder, I. Malebe, J. Getchell, M. Laga, P. Piot, and J. B. McCormick. 1988. The prevalence of infection with human immunodeficiency virus over a 10-year period in rural Zaire. *N. Engl. J. Med.* 318:276–279.

3303. O'Brien, S. J., and J. P. Moore. 2000. The effect of genetic variation in chemokines and their receptors on HIV transmission and progression to AIDS. *Immunol. Rev.* 177:99–111.

3304. O'Brien, T. R., J. R. George, and S. D. Holmberg. 1992. Human immunodeficiency virus type 2 infection in the United States. *JAMA* 267:2775–2779.

3305. O'Brien, T. R., C. Winkler, M. Dean, J. A. E. Nelson, M. Carrington, N. L. Michael, and G. C. White. 1997. HIV-1 infection in a man homozygous for CCR5Δ32. *Lancet* 340:1219–1220.

3306. O'Brien, W. A., I. S. Y. Chen, D. D. Ho, and E. S. Daar. 1992. Mapping genetic determinants for human immunodeficiency virus type 1 resistance to soluble CD4. *J. Virol.* 66:3125–3130.

3307. O'Brien, W. A., K. Grovit-Ferbas, A. Namazi, S. Ovcak-Derzic, H.-J. Wang, J. Park, C. Yeramian, S.-H. Mao, and J. Zack. 1995. Human immunodeficiency virus-type 1 replication can be increased in peripheral blood of seropositive patients after influenza vaccination. *Blood* 86:1082–1089.

3308. O'Brien, W. A., Y. Koyanagi, A. Namazie, J.-Q. Zhao, A. Diagne, K. Idler, J. A. Zack, and I. S. Y. Chen. 1990. HIV-1 tropism for mononuclear phagocytes can be determined by regions of gp120 outside the CD4-binding domain. *Nature* 348:69–73.

3309. O'Brien, W. A., S.-H. Mao, Y. Cao, and J. P. Moore. 1994. Macrophage-tropic and T-cell line-adapted chimeric strains of human immunodeficiency virus type 1 differ in their susceptibilities to neutralization by soluble CD4 at different temperatures. *J. Virol.* 68:5264–5269.

3310. O'Brien, W. A., A. Namazi, H. Kalhor, S. H. Mao, J. A. Zack, and I. S. Y. Chen. 1994. Kinetics of human immunodeficiency virus type 1 reverse trancription in blood mononuclear phagocytes are slowed by limitations of nucleotide precursors. *J. Virol.* 68:1258–1263.

3311. O'Connor, T. J., D. Kinchington, H. O. Gangro, and D. J. Jeffries. 1995. The activity of candidate virucidal agents, low pH and genital secretions against HIV-1 *in vitro*. *Int. J. STD AIDS* 6:267–272.

3312. O'Doherty, U., R. M. Steinman, M. Peng, P. U. Cameron, S. Gezelter, I. Kopeloff, W. J. Swiggard, M. Pope, and N. Bhardwaj. 1993. Dendritic cells freshly isolated from human blood express CD4 and mature into typical immunostimulatory dendritic cells after culture in monocyte-conditioned medium. *J. Exp. Med.* 178:1067–1078.

3313. O'Sullivan, C. E., W. L. Drew, D. J. McMullen, R. Miner, J. Y. Lee, R. A. Kaslow, J. G. Lazar, and M. S. Saag. 1999. Decrease of cytomegalovirus replication in human immunodeficiency virus infected-patients after treatment with highly active antiretroviral therapy. *J. Infect. Dis.* 180:847–849.

3314. O'Toole, C. M., S. Graham, M. W. Lowdell, D. Chargelegue, H. Marsden, and B. T. Colvin. 1992. Decline in CTL and antibody responses to HIV-1 p17 and p24 antigens in HIV-1-infected hemophiliacs irrespective of disease progression. A 5-year follow-up study. *AIDS Res. Hum. Retrovir.* 8:1361–1368.

3315. Oberlin, E., A. Amara, F. Bachelerie, C. Bessia, J. L. Virelizier, F. Arenzana-Seisdedos, O. Schwartz, J. M. Heard, I. Clark-Lewis, M. Loetscher, M. Baggiolini, and B. Moser. 1996. The CXC chemokine SDF-1 is the ligand for LESTR/fusin and prevents infection by T-cell-line adapted HIV-1. *Nature* 382:833–835.

3316. Ochsenbein, A. F., and R. M. Zinkernagel. 2000. Natural antibodies and complement link innate and acquired immunity. *Immunol. Today* 21:624–630.

3317. Ogg, G. S., X. Jin, S. Bonhoeffer, P. R. Dunbar, M. A. Nowak, S. Monard, J. P. Segal, Y. Cao, S. L. Rowland-Jones, V. Cerundolo, A. Hurley, M. Markowitz, D. D. Ho, D. F. Nixon, and A. J. McMichael. 1998. Quantitation of HIV-1-specific cytotoxic T lymphocytes and plasma load of viral RNA. *Science* 279:2103–2106.

3318. Ogg, G. S., X. Jin, S. Bonhoeffer, P. Moss, M. A. Nowak, S. Monard, J. P. Segal, Y. Cao, S. L. Rowland-Jones, A. Hurley, M. Markowitz, D. D. Ho, A. J. McMichael, and D. F. Nixon. 1999. Decay kinetics of human immunodeficiency virus-specific effector cytotoxic T lymphocytes after combination antiretroviral therapy. *J. Virol.* 73:797–800.

3319. Ogg, G. S., S. Kostense, M. R. Klein, S. Jurriaans, D. Hamann, A. J. McMichael, and F. Miedema. 1999. Longitudinal phenotypic analysis of human immunodeficiency virus type 1-specific cytotoxic T lymphocytes: correlation with disease progression. *J. Virol.* 73:9153–9160.

3320. Ohagen, A., S. Ghosh, J. L. He, K. Huang, Y. Z. Chen, M. L. Yuan, R. Osathanondh, S. Gartner, B. Shi, G. Shaw, and D. Gabuzda. 1999. Apoptosis induced by infection of primary brain cultures with diverse human immunodeficiency virus type 1 isolates: evidence for a role of the envelope. *J. Virol.* 73:897–906.

3321. Ohashi, T., M. Arai, H. Kato, M. Kubo, M. Fujii, N. Yamamoto, A. Iwamoto, and M. Kannagi. 1998. High SDF-1 expression in HIV-1 carriers does not correlate with CD8+ T-cell-mediated suppression of viral replication. *Virology* 244:467–472.

3322. Ohki, K., M. Kishi, K. Ohmura, Y. Morikawa, I. M. Jones, I. Azuma, and K. Ikuta. 1992. Human immunodeficiency virus type 1 (HIV-1) superinfection of a cell clone converting it from production of defective to infectious HIV-1 is mediated predominantly by CD4 regions other than the major binding site for HIV-1 glycoproteins. *J. Gen. Virol.* 73:1761–1772.

3323. Ohnimus, H., M. Heinkelein, and C. Jassoy. 1997. Apoptotic cell death upon contact of CD4+ T lymphocytes with HIV glycoprotein-expressing cells is mediated by caspases but bypasses CD95 (Fas/Apo-1) and TNF receptor 1. *J. Immunol.* 159:5246–5252.

3324. Okada, E., S. Sasaki, N. Ishii, I. Aoki, T. Yasuda, K. Nishioka, J. Fukushima, J. Miyazaki, B. Wahren, and K. Okuda. 1997. Intranasal immunization of a DNA vaccine with IL-12- and granulocyte-macrophage colony-stimulating factor (GM-CSF)-expressing plasmids in liposomes induces strong mucosal and cell-mediated immune responses against HIV-1 antigens. *J. Immunol.* 159:3638–3647.

3325. Okada, H., R. Takei, and M. Tashiro. 1997. HIV-1 Nef protein induced apoptotic cytolysis of a broad spectrum of uninfected human blood cells independently of CD95 (Fas). *FEBS Lett.* 414:603–606.

3326. Okamoto, Y., D. C. Douek, R. D. McFarland, and R. A. Koup. 2002. Effects of exogenous interleukin-7 on human thymus function. *Blood* 99:2851–2858.

3327. Olafsson, K., M. S. Smith, P. Marshburn, S. G. Carter, and S. Haskill. 1991. Variation of HIV infectibility of macrophages as a function of donor, stage of differentiation, and site of origin. *J. Acquir. Immune Defic. Syndr.* 4:154–164.

3328. Oldstone, M. B. A. 1987. Molecular mimicry and autoimmune disease. *Cell* 50:819–820.

3328a. O'Leary, J. G., M. Goodarzi, D. L. Drayton, and U. H. von Andrian. 2006. T cell- and B cell-independent adaptive immunity mediated by natural killer cells. *Nat. Immunol.* 7:507–516.

3329. Oleske, J., A. Minnefor, R. Cooper, Jr., K. Thomas, A. de la Cruz, H. Ahdieh, I. Guerrero, V. V. Joshi, and F. Desposito. 1983. Immune deficiency syndrome in children. *JAMA* 249:2345–2349.

3330. Olinger, G. G., M. Saifuddin, and G. T. Spear. 2000. CD4-Negative cells bind human immunodeficiency virus type 1 and efficiently transfer virus to T cells. *J. Virol.* 74:8550–8557.

3331. Oliver, R. E., J. R. Gorham, S. F. Parish, W. J. Hadlow, and O. Narayan. 1981. Studies on ovine progressive pneumonia. I. Pathologic and virology studies on the naturally occurring disease. *Am. J. Vet. Res.* 42:1554–1558.

3332. Olsen, G. P., and J. W. Shields. 1984. Seminal lymphocytes, plasma and AIDS. *Nature* 309:116.

3333. Olshevsky, U., E. Helseth, C. Furman, J. Li, W. Haseltine, and J. Sodroski. 1990. Identification of individual human immunodeficiency virus type 1 gp120 amino acids important for CD4 receptor binding. *J. Virol.* 64:5701–5707.

3334. Ometto, L., C. Zanotto, A. Maccabruni, D. Caselli, D. Truscia, C. Giaquinto, E. Ruga, L. Chieco-Bianchi, and A. De Rossi. 1995. Viral phenotype and host-cell susceptibility to HIV-1 infection as risk factors for mother-to-child HIV-1 transmission. *AIDS* 9:427–434.

3335. Ondoa, P., J. Vingerhoets, C. Vereecken, G. van der Groen, J. L. Heeney, and L. Kestens. 2002. In vitro replication of SIVcpz is suppressed by beta-chemokines and CD8+ T cells but not by natural killer cells of infected chimpanzees. *AIDS Res. Hum. Retrovir.* 18:373–382.

3336. Ong, C. L., J. C. Thorpe, P. R. Gorry, S. Bannwarth, A. Jaworowski, J. L. Howard, S. Chung, S. Campbell, H. S. Christensen, G. Clerzius, A. J. Mouland, A. Gatignol, and D. F. Purcell. 2005. Low TRBP levels support an innate human immunodeficiency virus type 1 resistance in astrocytes by enhancing the PKR antiviral response. *J. Virol.* 79:12763–12772.

3337. Ono, A., and E. O. Freed. 2001. Plasma membrane rafts play a critical role in HIV-1 assembly and release. *Proc. Natl. Acad. Sci. USA* 98:13925–13930.

3338. Operskalski, E. A., M. P. Busch, J. W. Mosley, and D. O. Stram. 1997. Comparative rates of disease progression among persons infected with the same or different HIV-1 strains. *J. Acquir. Immune Defic. Syndr. Hum. Retrovirol.* 15:145–150.

3339. Oppenheim, J. J., E. J. Kovacs, K. Matsushima, and S. K. Durum. 1986. There is more than one interleukin-1. *Immunol. Today* 7:45–56.

3340. Oppenheim, J. J., C. O. C. Zachariae, N. Mukaida, and K. Matsushima. 1991. Properties of the novel proinflammatory supergene "intercrine" cytokine family. *Annu. Rev. Immunol.* 9:617–648.

3341. Oravecz, T., M. Pall, and M. A. Norcross. 1996. Beta-chemokine inhibition of monocytotropic HIV-1 infection. Interference with a postbinding fusion step. *J. Immunol.* 157:1329–1332.

3342. Orenstein, J. M., S. Alkan, A. Blauvelt, K. T. Jeang, M. D. Weinstein, D. Ganem, and B. Herndier. 1997. Visualization of human herpesvirus type 8 in Kaposi's sarcoma by light and transmission electron microscopy. *AIDS* 11:F35–F45.

3343. Orentas, R. J., J. E. K. Hildreth, E. Obah, M. Polydefkis, G. E. Smith, M. L. Clements, and R. F. Siliciano. 1990. Induction of CD4+ human cytolytic T cells specific for HIV-infected cells by a gp160 subunit vaccine. *Science* 248:1234–1237.

3344. Oriss, T. B., S. A. McCarthy, B. F. Morel, M. A. K. Campana, and P. A. Morel. 1997. Crossregulation between T helper cell (Th)1 and Th2. *J. Immunol.* 158:3666–3672.

3345. Orloff, G. M., M. S. Kennedy, C. Dawson, and J. S. McDougal. 1991. HIV-1 binding to CD4 T cells does not induce a Ca^{2+} influx or lead to activation of protein kinases. *AIDS Res. Hum. Retrovir.* 7:587–593.

3346. Orloff, G. M., S. L. Orloff, M. S. Kennedy, P. J. Maddon, and J. S. McDougal. 1991. The CD4 receptor does not internalize with HIV, and CD4-related signal transduction events are not required for entry. *J. Immunol.* 146:2578–2587.

3347. Oroszlan, S., and R. B. Luftig. 1990. Retroviral proteinases. *Curr. Top. Microbiol. Immunol.* 157:153–185.

3348. Ortiz, G. M., J. Hu, J. A. Goldwitz, M. Larsson, N. Bhardwaj, S. Bonhieffer, B. Ramratnam, L. Zhang, M. S. Markowitz, and D. F. Nixon. 2002. Residual viral replication during antiretroviral therapy boosts human immunodeficiency virus type 1-specific CD8$^+$ T-cell responses in subjects treated early after infection. *J. Virol.* 76:411–415.

3349. Ortiz, G. M., D. F. Nixon, A. Trkola, J. Binley, X. Jin, S. Bonhoeffer, P. J. Kuebler, S. M. Donahoe, M. A. Demoitie, W. T. Kakimoto, T. Ketas, B. Clas, J. J. Heymann, L. Zhang, Y. Cao, A. Hurley, J. P. Moore, D. D. Ho, and M. Markowitz. 1999. HIV-1-specific immune responses in subjects who temporarily contain virus replication after discontinuation of highly active antiretroviral therapy. *J. Clin. Investig.* 104:R13–R18.

3350. Osborn, L., S. Kunkel, and G. J. Nabel. 1989. Tumor necrosis factor alpha and interleukin 1 stimulate the human immunodeficiency virus enhancer by activation of the nuclear factor kappa B. *Proc. Natl. Acad. Sci. USA* 86:2336–2340.

3351. Osmond, D., P. Bacchetti, R. E. Chaisson, T. Kelly, R. Stempel, J. Carlson, and A. R. Moss. 1988. Time of exposure and risk of HIV infection in homosexual partners of men with AIDS. *Am. J. Public Health* 78:944–948.

3352. Osmond, D. H., K. Page, J. Wiley, K. Garrett, H. W. Sheppard, A. R. Moss, L. Schrager, and W. Winkelstein. 1994. HIV infection in homosexual and bisexual men 18–29 years of age: The San Francisco Young Men's Health Study. *Am. J. Public Health* 84:1933–1937.

3353. Osmond, D. H., S. Shiboski, P. Bacchetti, E. E. Winger, and A. R. Moss. 1991. Immune activation markers and AIDS prognosis. *AIDS* 5:505–511.

3354. Ostrove, J. M., J. Leonard, K. E. Weck, A. B. Rabson, and H. E. Gendelman. 1987. Activation of the human immunodeficiency virus by herpes simplex virus type 1. *J. Virol.* 61:3726–3732.

3355. Ostrowski, M. A., T. W. Chun, S. J. Justement, I. Motola, M. A. Spinelli, J. Adelsberger, L. A. Ehler, S. B. Mizell, C. W. Hallahan, and A. S. Fauci. 1999. Both memory and CD45RA+/CD62L+ naive CD4(+) T cells are infected in human immunodeficiency virus type 1-infected individuals. *J. Virol.* 73:6430–6435.

3356. Ostrowski, M. A., S. J. Justement, A. Catanzaro, C. A. Hallahan, L. A. Ehler, S. B. Mizell, P. N. Kumar, J. Mican, T. Chun, and A. S. Fauci. 1998. Expression of chemokine receptors CXCR4 and CCR5 in HIV-1-infected and uninfected individuals. *J. Immunol.* 161:3195–3201.

3356a. Oswald-Richter, K., S. M. Grill, N. Shariat, M. Leelawong, M. S. Sundrud, D. W. Haas, and D. Unutmaz. 2004. HIV infection of naturally occurring and genetically reprogrammed human regulatory T-cells. *PLOS Biol.* 2:E198.

3357. Otsyula, M. G., C. J. Miller, A. F. Tarantal, M. L. Marthas, T. P. Greene, J. R. Collins, K. K. A. van Rompay, and M. B. McChesney. 1996. Fetal or neonatal infection with attenuated simian immunodeficiency virus results in protective immunity against oral challenge with pathogenic SIVmac251. *Virology* 222:275–278.

3358. Ott, D. E., L. V. Coren, B. P. Kane, L. K. Busch, D. G. Johnson, B. C. Sowder, E. N. Chertova, L. O. Arthur, and L. E. Henderson. 1996. Cytoskeletal proteins inside human immunodeficiency virus type 1 virions. *J. Virol.* 70:7734–7743.

3359. Otten, R. A., D. L. Ellenberger, D. R. Adams, C. A. Fridlund, E. Jackson, D. Pieniazek, and M. A. Rayfield. 1999. Identification of a window period for susceptibility to dual infection with two distinct human immunodeficiency virus type 2 isolates in a Macaca nemestrina (pig-tailed macaque) model. *J. Infect. Dis.* 180:673–684.

3360. Ou, C.-Y., C. A. Ciesielski, G. Myers, C. I. Bandea, C.-H. Luo, B. T. M. Korber, J. I. Mullins, G. Schochetman, R. L. Berkelman, A. N. Economou, J. J. Witte, L. J. Furman, G. A. Satten, K. A. MacInnes, J. W. Curran, and H. W. Jaffe. 1992. Molecular epidemiology of HIV transmission in a dental practice. *Science* 256:1165–1171.

3361. Ou, C.-Y., S. Kwok, S. W. Mitchell, D. H. Mack, J. J. Sninsky, J. W. Krebs, P. Feorino, D. Warfield, and G. Schochetman. 1988. DNA amplification for direct detection of HIV-1 in DNA of peripheral blood mononuclear cells. *Science* 239:295–297.

3362. Ou, S. H. I., and R. B. Gaynor. 1995. Intracellular factors involved in gene expression of human retroviruses, p. 97–187. *In* J. A. Levy (ed.), *The Retroviridae*, vol. 4. Plenum Press, New York, N.Y.

3363. Ouellet, M., S. Mercier, I. Pelletier, S. Bounou, J. Roy, J. Hirabayashi, S. Sato, and M. J. Tremblay. 2005. Galectin-1 acts as a soluble host factor that promotes HIV-1 infectivity through stabilization of virus attachment to host cells. *J. Immunol.* 174:4120–4126.

3364. Overbaugh, J., E. A. Hoover, J. I. Mullins, D. P. W. Burns, L. Rudensey, S. L. Quackenbush, V. Stallard, and P. R. Donohue. 1992. Structure and pathogenicity of individual variants within an immunodeficiency disease-inducing isolate of FeLV. *Virology* 188:558–569.

3365. Overholser, E. D., G. D. Coleman, J. L. Bennett, R. J. Casaday, M. C. Zink, S. A. Barber, and J. E. Clements. 2003. Expression of simian immunodeficiency virus (SIV) Nef in astrocytes during acute and terminal infection and requirement of Nef for optimal replication of neurovirulent SIV in vitro. *J. Virol.* 77:6855–6866.

3365a. Owens, B. J., G. M. Anantharamaiah, J. B. Kahlon, R. V. Srinivas, R. W. Compans, and J. P. Segrest. 1990. Aoplipoprotein A–I and its amphipathic helix peptide analogues inhibit human immunodeficiency virus-induced syncytium formation. *J. Clin. Investig.* 86:1142–1150.

3366. Owens, C. M., P. C. Yang, H. Gottlinger, and J. Sodroski. 2003. Human and simian immunodeficiency virus capsid proteins are major viral determinants of early, postentry replication blocks in simian cells. *J. Virol.* 77:726–731.

3367. Owens, R. J., J. W. Dubay, E. Hunter, and R. W. Compans. 1991. Human immunodeficiency virus envelope protein determines the site of virus release in polarized epithelial cells. *Proc. Natl. Acad. Sci. USA* 88:3987–3991.

3368. Oxenius, A., D. A. Price, P. J. Easterbrook, C. A. O'Callaghan, A. D. Kelleher, J. A. Whelan, G. Sontag, A. K. Sewell, and R. E. Phillips. 2000. Early highly active antiretroviral therapy for acute HIV-1 infection preserves immune function of CD8+ and CD4+ T lymphocytes. *Proc. Natl. Acad. Sci. USA* 97:3382–3387.

3369. Oxenius, A., D. A. Price, H. F. Gunthard, S. J. Dawson, C. Fagard, L. Perrin, M. Fischer, R. Weber, M. Plana, F. Garcia, B. Hirschel, A. McLean, and R. E. Phillips. 2002. Stimulation of HIV-specific cellular immunity by structured treatment interruption fails to enhance viral control in chronic HIV infection. *Proc. Natl. Acad. Sci. USA* 99:13747–13752.

3370. Oxenius, A., D. A. Price, M. Hersberger, E. Schlaepfer, R. Weber, M. Weber, T. M. Kundig, J. Boni, H. Joller, R. E. Philips, M. Flepp, M. Opravil, and R. F. Speck. 2004. HIV-specific cellular immune response is inversely correlated with disease progression as defined by decline of CD4+ T cells in relation to HIV RNA load. *J. Infect. Dis.* 189:1199–1208.

3371. Oxenius, A., S. Yerly, E. Ramirez, R. E. Phillips, D. A. Price, and L. Perrin. 2001. Distribution of functional HIV-specific CD8 T lymphocytes between blood and secondary lymphoid organs after 8–18 months of antiretroviral therapy in acutely infected patients. *AIDS* 15:1653–1656.

3372. Oyaizu, N., N. Chirmule, V. S. Kalyanaraman, W. W. Hall, R. Pahwa, M. Shuster, and S. Pahwa. 1990. Human immunodeficiency virus type 1 envelope glycoprotein gp120 produces immune defects in CD4+ T lymphocytes by inhibiting interleukin 2 mRNA. *Proc. Natl. Acad. Sci. USA* 87:2379–2383.

3373. Oyaizu, N., T. W. McCloskey, M. Coronesi, N. Chirmule, V. S. Kalyanaraman, and S. Pahwa. 1993. Accelerated apoptosis in peripheral blood mononuclear cells (PBMCs) from human immunodeficiency virus type-1 infected patients and in CD4 cross-linked PBMCs from normal individuals. *Blood* 82:3392–3400.

3374. Pacanowski, J., L. Develioglu, I. Kamga, M. Sinet, M. Desvarieux, P. M. Girard, and A. Hosmalin. 2004. Early plasmacytoid dendritic cell changes predict plasma HIV load rebound during primary infection. *J. Infect. Dis.* 190:1889–1892.

3375. Pacanowski, J., S. Kahi, M. Baillet, P. Lebon, C. Deveau, C. Goujard, L. Meyer, E. Oksenhendler, M. Sinet, and A. Hosmalin. 2001. Reduced blood CD123+ (lymphoid) and CD11c+ (myeloid) dendritic cell numbers in primary HIV-1 infection. *Blood* 98:3016–3021.

3376. Padian, N. S., S. Shiboski, and N. P. Jewell. 1991. Female-to-male transmission of human immunodeficiency virus. *JAMA* 266:1664–1667.

3377. Padian, N. S., S. C. Shiboski, S. O. Glass, and E. Vittinghoff. 1997. Heterosexual transmission of human immunodeficiency virus (HIV) in northern California: results from a ten-year study. *Am. J. Epidemiol.* 146:350–357.

3378. Padian, N. S., S. C. Shiboski, and N. P. Jewell. 1990. The effect of number of exposures on the risk of heterosexual HIV transmission. *J. Infect. Dis.* 161:883–887.

3379. Paganin, C., D. S. Monos, J. D. Marshall, I. Frank, and G. Trinchieri. 1997. Frequency and cytokine profile of HPRT mutant T cells in HIV-infected and healthy donors: implications for T cell proliferation in HIV disease. *J. Clin. Investig.* 99:663–668.

3380. Page, J. B., S. Lai, D. D. Chitwood, N. G. Klimas, P. C. Smith, and M. A. Fletcher. 1990. HTLV-I/II seropositivity and death from AIDS among HIV-1 seropositive intravenous drug users. *Lancet* 335:1439–1441.

3381. Page, K. A., S. M. Stearns, and D. R. Littman. 1992. Analysis of mutations in the V3 domain of gp160 that affect fusion and infectivity. *J. Virol.* 66:524–533.

3382. Pahwa, S., N. Chirmule, C. Leombruno, W. Lim, R. Harper, R. Bhalla, R. Rahwa, R. P. Nelson, and R. A. Good. 1989. *In vitro* synthesis of human immunodeficiency virus-specific antibodies in peripheral blood lymphocytes of infants. *Proc. Natl. Acad. Sci. USA* 86:7532–7536.

3383. Pahwa, S., R. Pahwa, C. Saxinger, R. C. Gallo, and R. A. Good. 1985. Influence of the human T-lymphotropic virus/lymphadenopathy-associated virus on functions of human lymphoctyes: evidence for immunosuppressive effects and polyclonal B-cell activation by banded viral preparations. *Proc. Natl. Acad. Sci. USA* 82:8198–8202.

3384. Paiardini, M., B. Cervasi, H. Albrecht, A. Muthukumar, R. Dunham, S. Gordon, H. Radziewicz, G. Piedimonte, M. Magnani, M. Montroni, S. M. Kaech, A. Weintrob, J. D. Altman, D. L. Sodora, M. B. Feinberg, and G. Silvestri. 2005. Loss of CD127 expression defines an expansion of effector CD8+ T cells in HIV-infected individuals. *J. Immunol.* 174:2900–2909.

3385. Pal, R., A. Garzino-Demo, P. D. Markham, J. Burns, M. Brown, R. C. Gallo, and A. L. DeVico. 1997. Inhibition of HIV-1 infection by the beta-chemokine MDC. *Science* 278:695–698.

3386. Pal, R., V. S. Kalyanaraman, B. C. Nair, S. Whitney, T. Keen, L. Hocker, L. Hudacik, N. Rose, I. Mboudjeka, S. Shen, T. H. Wu-Chou, D. Montefiori, J. Mascola, P. Markham, and S. Lu. 2006. Immunization of rhesus macaques with a polyvalent DNA prime/protein boost human immunodeficiency virus type 1 vaccine elicits protective antibody response against simian human immunodeficiency virus of R5 phenotype. *Virology* 348:341–353.

3387. Palasanthiran, P., J. B. Ziegler, G. J. Stewart, M. Stuckey, J. A. Armstrong, D. A. Cooper, R. Penny, and J. Gold. 1993. Breast-feeding during primary maternal human immunodeficiency virus infection and risk of transmission from mother to infant. *J. Infect. Dis.* 167:441–444.

3388. Palefsky, J. M. 1994. Anal human papillomavirus infection and anal cancer in HIV-positive individuals: an emerging problem. *AIDS* 8:283–295.

3389. Palefsky, J. M., E. A. Holly, J. T. Efirdc, M. Da Costa, N. Jay, J. M. Berry, and T. M. Darragh. 2005. Anal intraepithelial neoplasia in the highly active antiretroviral therapy era among HIV-positive men who have sex with men. *AIDS* 19:1407–1414.

3390. Palefsky, J. M., E. A. Holly, J. Gonzales, K. Lamborn, and H. Hollander. 1992. Natural history of anal cytologic abnormalities and papillomavirus infection among homosexual men with Group IV HIV disease. *J. Acquir. Immune Defic. Syndr.* 5:1258–1265.

3391. Palefsky, J. M., E. A. Holly, M. L. Ralston, M. Da Costa, and R. M. Greenblatt. 2001. Prevalence and risk factors for anal human papillomavirus infection in human immunodeficiency virus (HIV)-positive and high-risk HIV-negative women. *J. Infect. Dis.* 183:383–391.

3392. Paliard, X., A. Y. Lee, and C. M. Walker. 1996. RANTES, MIP-1α and MIP-1β are not involved in the inhibition of HIV-1_{SF33} replication mediated by CD8+ T-cell clones. *AIDS* 10:1317–1321.

3393. Palmer, B. E., N. Blyveis, A. P. Fontenot, and C. C. Wilson. 2005. Functional and phenotypic characterization of CD57+CD4+ T cells and their association with HIV-1-induced T cell dysfunction. *J. Immunol.* 175:8415–8423.

3394. Palmer, B. E., E. Boritz, and C. C. Wilson. 2004. Effects of sustained HIV-1 plasma viremia on HIV-1 gag-specific CD4+ T cell maturation and function. *J. Immunol.* 172:3337–3347.

3395. Palmer, S., A. P. Wiegand, F. Maldarelli, H. Bazmi, J. M. Mican, M. Polis, R. L. Dewar, A. Planta, S. Liu, J. A. Metcalf, J. W. Mellors, and J. M. Coffin. 2003. New real-time reverse transcriptase-initiated PCR assay with single-copy sensitivity for human immunodeficiency virus type 1 RNA in plasma. *J. Clin. Microbiol.* 41:4531–4536.

3396. Pan, L.-Z., A. Werner, and J. A. Levy. 1993. Detection of plasma viremia in HIV-infected individuals at all clinical stages. *J. Clin. Microbiol.* 31:283–288.

3397. Pande, V., and M. J. Ramos. 2003. Nuclear factor kappa B: a potential target for anti-HIV chemotherapy. *Curr. Med. Chem.* 10:1603–1615.

3398. Pandolfi, F., M. Pierdominici, A. Oliva, G. D'Offizi, I. Mezzarima, B. Mollicone, A. Giovannetti, L. Rainaldi, I. Quinti, and F. Aiuti. 1995. Apoptosis-related mortality in vitro of mononuclear cells from patients with HIV infection correlates with disease severity and progression. *J. Acquir. Immune Defic. Syndr. Hum. Retrovirol.* 9:450–458.

3399. Pandori, M. W., N. J. Fitch, H. M. Craig, D. D. Richman, C. A. Spina, and J. C. Guatelli. 1995. Nef stimulates human immunodeficiency virus type 1 proviral DNA synthesis. *J. Virol.* 70:4283–4290.

3400. Pandori, M. W., N. J. S. Fitch, H. M. Craig, D. D. Richman, C. A. Spina, and J. C. Guatelli. 1996. Producer-cell modification of human immunodeficiency virus type 1: Nef is a virion protein. *J. Virol.* 70:4283–4290.

3401. Pang, S., Y. Koyanagi, S. Miles, C. Wiley, H. V. Vinters, and I. S. Y. Chen. 1990. High levels of unintegrated HIV-1 DNA in brain tissue of AIDS dementia patients. *Nature* 343:85–89.

3402. Pang, S., H. V. Vinters, T. Akashi, W. A. O'Brien, and I. S. Y. Chen. 1991. HIV-1 *env* sequence variation in brain tissue of patients with AIDS-related neurologic disease. *J. Acquir. Immune Defic. Syndr.* 4:1082–1092.

3403. Pang, S., D. Yu, D. S. An, G. C. Baldwin, Y. Xie, B. Poon, Y. H. Chow, N. H. Park, and I. S. Y. Chen. 2000. Human immunodeficiency virus *env*-independent infection of human CD4(−) cells. *J. Virol.* 74:10994–11000.

3404. Pantaleo, G. 1997. How immune-based interventions can change HIV therapy. *Nat. Med.* 3:483–490.

3405. Pantaleo, G., L. Butini, C. Graziosi, G. Poli, S. M. Schnittman, J. J. Greenhouse, J. I. Gallin, and A. S. Fauci. 1991. Human immunodeficiency virus (HIV) infection in CD4+ T lymphocytes genetically deficient in LFA-1: LFA-1 is required for HIV-mediated cell fusion but not for viral transmission. *J. Exp. Med.* 173:511–514.

3406. Pantaleo, G., R. J. Cohen, D. J. Schwartzentruber, C. Graziosi, M. Vaccarezza, and A. S. Fauci. 1995. Pathogenic insights from studies of lymphoid tissue from HIV-infected individuals. *J. Acquir. Immune Defic. Syndr. Hum. Retrovirol.* 10(Suppl. 1):S6–S14.

3407. Pantaleo, G., A. De Maria, S. Koenig, L. Butini, B. Moss, M. Baseler, H. C. Lane, and A. S. Fauci. 1990. CD8+ T lymphocytes of patients with AIDS maintain normal broad cytolytic function despite the loss of human immunodeficiency virus-specific cytotoxicity. *Proc. Natl. Acad. Sci. USA* 87:4818–4822.

3408. Pantaleo, G., J. F. Demarest, T. Schacker, M. Vaccarezza, O. J. Cohen, M. Daucher, C. Graziosi, S. S. Schnittman, T. C. Quinn, G. M. Shaw, L. Perrin, G. Tambussi, A. Lazzarin, R. P. Sekaly, H. Soudeyns, L. Corey, and A. S. Fauci. 1997. The qualitative nature of the primary immune response to HIV infection is a prognosticator of disease progression independent of the initial level of plasma viremia. *Proc. Natl. Acad. Sci. USA* 94:254–258.

3409. Pantaleo, G., J. F. Demarest, H. Soudeyns, C. Graziosi, F. Denis, J. W. Adelsberger, P. Borrow, M. S. Saag, G. M. Shaw, R. P. Sekaly, and A. S. Fauci. 1994. Major expansion of CD8+ T cells with a predominant Vβ usage during the primary immune response to HIV. *Nature* 370:463–467.

3410. Pantaleo, G., C. Garziosi, and A. S. Fauci. 1993. The role of lymphoid organs in the immunopathogenesis of HIV infection. *AIDS* 7:S19–S23.

3411. Pantaleo, G., C. Graziosi, L. Butini, P. A. Pizzo, S. M. Schnittman, D. P. Kotler, and A. S. Fauci. 1991. Lymphoid organs function as major reservoirs for human immunodeficiency virus. *Proc. Natl. Acad. Sci. USA* 88:9838–9842.

3412. Pantaleo, G., C. Graziosi, J. F. Demarest, L. Butini, M. Montroni, C. H. Fox, J. M. Orenstein, D. P. Kotler, and A. S. Fauci. 1993. HIV infection is active and progressive in lymphoid tissue during the clinically latent stage of disease. *Nature* 362:355–358.

3413. Pantaleo, G., C. Graziosi, and A. S. Fauci. 1993. Mechanisms of disease: the immunopathogenesis of human immunodeficiency virus infection. *N. Engl. J. Med.* 328:327–336.

3414. Pantaleo, G., C. Graziosi, and A. S. Fauci. 1993. The role of lymphoid organs in the pathogenesis of HIV infection. *Semin. Immunol.* 5:157–163.

3415. Pantaleo, G., S. Koenig, M. Baseler, H. C. Lane, and A. S. Fauci. 1990. Defective clonogenic potential of CD8+ T-lymphocytes in patients with AIDS: expansion in vivo of a non-clonogenic CD3+CD8+CD25- T cell population. *J. Immunol.* 144:1696–1704.

3416. Pantaleo, G., S. Menzo, M. Vaccarazza, C. Graziosi, O. J. Cohen, J. F. Demarest, D. Montefiori, J. M. Orenstein, C. Fox, L. K. Schrager, J. B. Margolick, S. Buchbinder, J. V. Giorgi, and A. S. Fauci. 1995. Studies in subjects with long-term nonprogressive human immunodeficiency virus infection. *N. Engl. J. Med.* 332:209–216.

3417. Pantaleo, G., H. Soudeyns, J. F. Demarest, M. Vaccarezza, C. Graziosi, S. Paolucci, M. Daucher, O. J. Cohen, F. Denis, W. E. Biddison, R. P. Sekaly, and A. S. Fauci. 1997. Evidence for rapid disappearance of initially expanded HIV-specific CD8+ T cell clones during primary HIV infection. *Proc. Natl. Acad. Sci. USA* 94:9848–9853.

3418. Papagno, L., V. Appay, J. Sutton, T. Rostron, G. M. Gillespie, G. S. Ogg, A. King, A. T. Makadzanhge, A. Waters, C. Balotta, A. Vyakarnam, P. J. Easterbrook, and S. L. Rowland-Jones. 2002. Comparison between HIV- and CMV-specific T cell responses in long-term HIV infected donors. *Clin. Exp. Immunol.* 130:509–517.

3419. Papagno, L., C. A. Spina, A. Marchant, M. Salio, N. Rufer, S. Little, T. Dong, G. Chesney, A. Waters, P. Easterbrook, P. R. Dunbar, D. Shepherd, V. Cerundolo, V. Emery, P. Griffiths, C. Conlon, A. J. McMichael, D. D. Richman, S. L. Rowland-Jones, and V. Appay. 2004. Immune activation and CD8+ T-cell differentiation towards senescence in HIV-1 infection. *PLoS Biol.* 2:1–13.

3420. Papasavvas, E., J. Sun, Q. Luo, E. C. Moore, B. Thiel, R. R. MacGregor, A. Minty, K. Mounzer, J. R. Kostman, and L. J. Montaner. 2005. IL-13 acutely augments HIV-specific and recall responses from HIV-1-infected subjects in vitro by modulating monocytes. *J. Immunol.* 175:5532–5540.

3421. Parada, N. A., D. A. Center, H. Kornfeld, W. L. Rodriguez, J. Cook, M. Vallen, and W. W. Cruikshank. 1998. Synergistic activation of CD4+ T cells by IL-16 and IL-2. *J. Immunol.* 160:2115–2120.

3422. Paranjpe, S., J. Craigo, B. Patterson, M. Ding, P. Barroso, L. Harrison, R. Montelaro, and P. Gupta. 2002. Subcompartmentalization of HIV-1 quasispecies between seminal cells and seminal plasma indicates their origin in distinct genital tissues. *AIDS Res. Hum. Retrovir.* 18:1271–1280.

3423. Paraskevis, D., P. Lemey, M. Salemi, M. Suchard, Y. Van De Peer, and A. M. Vandamme. 2003. Analysis of the evolutionary relationships of HIV-1 and SIVcpz sequences using bayesian inference: implications for the origin of HIV-1. *Mol. Biol. Evol.* 20:1986–1996.

3424. Parato, K. G., A. Kuman, A. D. Badley, J. L. Sanchez-Dardon, K. A. Chambers, C. D. Young, W. T. Lim, S. Kravcik, D. W. Cameron, and J. B. Angel. 2002. Normalization of natural killer cell function and phenotype with effective anti-HIV therapy and the role of IL-10. *AIDS* 16:1251–1256.

3425. Pardoll, D. 1992. New strategies for active immunotherapy with genetically engineered tumor cells. *Curr. Opin. Immunol.* 4:619–623.

3426. Parekh, B. S., M. S. Kennedy, T. Dobbs, C.-P. Pau, R. Byers, T. Green, D. J. Hu, S. Vanichseni, N. L. Young, K. Choopanya, T. D. Mastro, and J. S. McDougal. 2002. Quantitative detection of increasing HIV type 1 antibodies after seroconversion: a simple assay for detecting recent HIV infection and estimating incidence. *AIDS Res. Hum. Retrovir.* **18**:295–307.

3427. Parekh, B. S., N. Shaffer, R. Coughlin, C. H. Hung, K. Krasinski, E. Abrams, M. Bamji, P. Thomas, D. Hutson, G. Schochetman, M. Rogers, and J. R. George. 1993. Dynamics of maternal IgG antibody decay and HIV-specific antibody synthesis in infants born to seropositive mothers. *AIDS Res. Hum. Retrovir.* **9**:907–912.

3428. Parish, C. R., and F. Y. Liew. 1972. Immune response to chemically modified flagellin. III. Enhanced cell-mediated immunity during high and low zone antibody tolerance to flagellin. *J. Exp. Med.* **135**:298–311.

3429. Parra, E., A. G. Wingren, G. Hedlund, T. Kalland, and M. Dohlsten. 1997. The role of B7-1 and LFA-3 in costimulation of CD8+ T cells. *J. Immunol.* **158**:637–642.

3430. Parravicini, C. L., D. Klatzmann, P. Jaffray, G. Costanzi, and J.-C. Gluckman. 1988. Monoclonal antibodies to the human immunodeficiency virus p18 protein cross-react with normal human tissues. *AIDS* **2**:171–177.

3431. Pascual, R., M. R. Moreno, and J. Villalain. 2005. A peptide pertaining to the loop segment of human immunodeficiency virus gp41 binds and interacts with model biomembranes: implications for the fusion mechanism. *J. Virol.* **79**:5142–5152.

3432. Pashenkov, M., Y. M. Huang, V. Kostulas, M. Haglund, M. Soderstrom, and H. Link. 2001. Two subsets of dendritic cells are present in human cerebrospinal fluid. *Brain* **124**:480–492.

3433. Pashine, A., N. M. Valiante, and J. B. Ulmer. 2005. Targeting the innate immune response with improved vaccine adjuvants. *Nat. Med.* **11**:S63–S68.

3434. Pastinen, T., K. Liitsola, P. Niini, M. Salminen, and A.-C. Syvanen. 1998. Contribution of the CCR5 and MBL genes to susceptibility to HIV type 1 infection in the Finnish population. *AIDS Res. Hum. Retrovir.* **14**:695–698.

3435. Pastore, C., R. Nedellec, A. Ramos, S. Pontow, L. Ratner, and D. E. Mosier. 2006. Human immunodeficiency virus type 1 coreceptor switching: V1/V2 gain-of-fitness mutations compensate for V3 loss-of-fitness mutations. *J. Virol.* **80**:750–758.

3435a. Pastori, C., B. Weiser, C. Barassi, C. Uberti-Foppa, S. Ghezzi, R. Longhi, G. Calori, H. Burger, K. Kemal, G. Poli, A. Lazzarin, and L. Lopalco. 2006. Long-lasting CCR5 internalization by antibodies in a subset of long-term nonprogressors: a possible protective effect against disease progression. *Blood* **107**:4825–4833.

3436. Patarroyo, M. E., R. Amador, P. Clavijo, A. Moreno, F. Guzman, P. Romero, R. Tascon, A. Franco, L. A. Murillo, G. Ponton, and G. Trujillo. 1988. A synthetic vaccine protects humans against challenge with asexual blood stages of *Plasmodium falciparum* malaria. *Nature* **332**:158–161.

3437. Patick, A. K., H. Mo, M. Markowitz, K. Appelt, B. Wu, L. Musick, V. Kalish, S. Kaldor, S. Reich, D. Ho, and S. Webber. 1996. Antiviral and resistance studies of AG1343, an orally bioavailable inhibitor of human immunodeficiency virus protease. *Antimicrob. Agents and Chemother.* **40**:292–297.

3438. Patki, A. H., D. L. Georges, and M. M. Lederman. 1997. CD4+ T-cell counts, spontaneous apoptosis, and Fas expression in peripheral blood mononuclear cells obtained from human immunodeficiency virus type 1-infected subjects. *Clin. Diagn. Lab. Immunol.* **4**:736–741.

3439. Patki, A. H., M. E. Quinones-Mateu, D. Dorazio, B. Yen-Lieberman, W. H. Boom, E. K. Thomas, and M. M. Lederman.

1996. Activation of antigen-induced lymphocyte proliferation by interleukin-15 without the mitogenic effect of interleukin-2 that may induce human immunodeficiency virus-1 expression. *J. Clin. Investig.* **98**:616–621.

3440. Patterson, B. K., H. Behbahani, W. J. Kabat, Y. Sullivan, M. R. O'Gorman, A. Landay, Z. Flener, N. Khan, R. Yogev, and J. Andersson. 2001. Leukemia inhibitory factor inhibits HIV-1 replication and is upregulated in placentae from nontransmitting women. *J. Clin. Investig.* **107**:287–294.

3441. Patterson, B. K., M. Czerniewski, J. Andersson, Y. Sullivan, F. Su, D. Jiyamapa, Z. Burki, and A. Landay. 1999. Regulation of CCR5 and CXCR4 expression by type 1 and type 2 cytokines: CCR5 expression is downregulated by IL-10 in CD4-positive lymphocytes. *Clin. Immunol.* **91**:254–262.

3442. Patterson, B. K., M. Till, P. Otto, C. Goolsby, M. R. Furtado, L. J. McBride, and S. M. Wolinsky. 1993. Detection of HIV-1 DNA and messenger RNA in individual cells by PCR-driven in situ hybridization and flow cytometry. *Science* **260**:976–979.

3442a. Patterson, L. J., N. Malkevitch, D. Venzon, J. Pinczewski, V. R. Gomez-Roman, L. Wang, V. S. Kalyanaraman, P. D. Markham, F. A. Robey, and M. Robert-Guroff. 2004. Protection against mucosal simian immunodeficiency virus SIV(mac251) challenge by using replicating adenovirus-SIV multigene vaccine priming and subunit boosting. *J. Virol.* **78**:2212–2221.

3443. Patterson, S., and S. C. Knight. 1987. Susceptibility of human peripheral blood dendritic cells to infection by human immunodeficiency virus. *J. Gen. Virol.* **68**:1177–1181.

3444. Patton, H. K., Z. H. Zhou, J. K. Bubien, E. N. Benveniste, and D. J. Benos. 2000. gp120-induced alterations of human astrocyte function: Na(+)/H(+) exchange, K(+) conductance, and glutamate flux. *Am. J. Physiol. Cell Physiol.* **279**:C700–C708.

3445. Paul, M. O., S. Tetali, M. L. Lesser, E. J. Abrams, X. P. Wang, R. Kowalski, M. Bamji, B. Napolitano, L. Gulick, S. Bakshi, and S. Pahwa. 1996. Laboratory diagnosis of infection status in infants perinatally exposed to human immunodeficiency virus type 1. *J. Infect. Dis.* **173**:68–76.

3446. Paul, N. L., M. Marsh, J. A. McKeating, T. F. Schulz, P. Liljestrom, H. Garoff, and R. A. Weiss. 1993. Expression of HIV-1 envelope glycoproteins by Semliki Forest virus vectors. *AIDS Res. Hum. Retrovir.* **9**:963–970.

3447. Pauza, C. D., J. E. Galindo, and D. D. Richman. 1990. Reinfection results in accumulation of unintegrated viral DNA in cytopathic and persistent human immunodeficiency virus type 1 infection of CEM cells. *J. Exp. Med.* **172**:1035–1042.

3448. Pauza, C. D., and T. M. Price. 1988. Human immunodeficiency virus infection of T cells and monocytes proceeds via receptor-mediated endocytosis. *J. Cell Biol.* **107**:959–968.

3449. Pauza, C. D., P. Trivedi, M. Wallace, T. J. Ruckwardt, H. Le Buanec, W. Lu, B. Bizzini, A. Burny, D. Zagury, and R. C. Gallo. 2000. Vaccination with tat toxoid attenuates disease in simian/HIV-challenged macaques. *Proc. Natl. Acad. Sci. USA* **97**:3515–3519.

3450. Paxton, W., R. I. Connor, and N. R. Landau. 1993. Incorporation of Vpr into human immunodeficiency virus type 1 virions: requirement for the p6 region of gag and mutational analysis. *J. Virol.* **67**:7229–7237.

3451. Pazmany, L., O. Mandelboim, M. Valés-Gomez, D. M. Davis, H. T. Reyfurn, and J. L. Stromenger. 1996. Protection from natural killer cell-mediated lysis by HLA-G expression on target cells. *Science* **274**:792–795.

3452. **Pearce-Pratt, R., and D. M. Phillips.** 1993. Studies of adhesion of lymphocytic cells: implications for sexual transmission of HIV. *Biol. Reprod.* 48:431–435.

3453. **Peden, K., M. Emerman, and L. Montagnier.** 1991. Changes in growth properties on passage in tissue culture of viruses derived from infectious molecular clones of HIV-1$_{LAI}$, HIV-1$_{MAL}$, and HIV-1$_{ELI}$. *Virology* 185:661–672.

3454. **Pedersen, N. C., and J. F. Boyle.** 1980. Immunologic phenomena in the effusive form of feline infectious peritonitis. *Am. J. Vet. Res.* 44:868–876.

3455. **Peeters, M., K. Fransen, F. Delaporte, M. Van den Haesevelde, G. M. Gershy-Damet, L. Kestens, G. van der Groen, and P. Piot.** 1992. Isolation and characterization of a new chimpanzee lentivirus (simian immunodeficiency virus isolate cpzant) from a wild-captured chimpanzee. *AIDS* 6:447–452.

3456. **Peeters, M., C.-Y. Gershy-Damet, K. Fransen, K. Koffi, M. Coulibaly, E. Delaporte, P. Piot, and G. van der Groen.** 1992. Virological and polymerase chain reaction studies of HIV-1/HIV-2 dual infection in Cote d'Ivoire. *Lancet* 340:339–340.

3457. **Peeters, M., A. Gueye, S. Mboup, F. Bibollet-Ruche, E. Ekaza, C. Mulanga, R. Ouedrago, R. Gandji, P. Mpele, G. Dibanga, B. Koumare, M. Saidou, E. Esu-Williams, J.-P. Lombart, W. Badombena, N. Luo, M. Vanden Haesevelde, and E. Delaporte.** 1997. Geographical distribution of HIV-1 group O viruses in Africa. *AIDS* 11:493–498.

3458. **Peeters, M., W. Janssens, M. Vanden Haesevelde, K. Fransen, B. Willems, L. Heyndrickx, L. Kestens, P. Piot, G. van der Groen, and J. Heeney.** 1995. Virologic and serologic characteristics of a natural chimpanzee lentivirus infection. *Virology* 211:312–315.

3459. **Peeters, M., P. Piot, and G. van der Groen.** 1991. Variability among HIV and SIV strains of African origin. *AIDS* 5:S29–S36.

3460. **Peeters, M., C. Toure-Kane, and J. N. Nkengasong.** 2003. Genetic diversity of HIV in Africa: impact on diagnosis, treatment, vaccine development and trials. *AIDS* 17:2547–2560.

3461. **Peiris, J. S. M., and J. S. Porterfield.** 1979. Antibody-mediated enhancement of flavivirus replication in macrophage-like cell lines. *Nature* 282:509–511.

3462. **Pelchen-Matthews, A., B. Kramer, and M. Marsh.** 2003. Infectious HIV-1 assembles in late endosomes in primary macrophages. *J. Cell Biol.* 162:443–455.

3463. **Pelliccia, P., L. Galli, M. de Martino, F. Chiarelli, A. Verrotti, G. Sabatino, B. Fornarini, S. Iacobelli, and C. Natoli.** 2000. Lack of mother-to-child HIV-1 transmission is associated with elevated serum levels of 90 K immune modulatory protein. *AIDS* 14:F41–F45.

3464. **Pellici, P.-G., D. M. Knowles, I. Magrath, and R. Dalla-Favera.** 1986. Chromosomal breakpoints and structural alterations of the c-myc locus differ in endemic and sporadic forms of Burkitt's lymphoma. *Proc. Natl. Acad. Sci. USA* 83:2984–2988.

3465. **Peng, H., D. E. Callison, P. Li, and C. J. Burrell.** 1997. Enhancement or inhibition of HIV-1 replication by intracellular expression of sense or antisense RNA targeted at different intermediates of reverse transcription. *AIDS* 11:587–595.

3466. **Penn, I.** 1979. Kaposi's sarcoma in organ transplant recipients: report of 20 cases. *Transplantation* 27:8–11.

3467. **Penn, I.** 1981. Depressed immunity and the development of cancer. *Clin. Exp. Immunol.* 46:459–474.

3468. **Penn, I.** 1986. Cancers of the anogenital region in renal transplant recipients. Analysis of 65 cases. *Am. J. Obstet. Gynecol.* 58:611–616.

3469. **Pennington, D. J., D. Vermijlen, E. L. Wise, S. L. Clarke, R. E. Tigelaar, and A. C. Hayday.** 2005. The integration of conventional and unconventional T cells that characterizes cell-mediated responses. *Adv. Immunol.* 87:27–59.

3469a. **Pereira, L. A., K. Bentley, A. Peeters, M. J. Churchill, and N. J. Deacon.** 2000. A compilation of cellular transcription factor interactions with the HIV-1 LTR promoter. *Nucleic Acids Res.* 28:663–668.

3470. **Perelson, A. S., P. Essunger, Y. Cao, M. Vesanen, A. Hurley, K. Saksela, M. Markowitz, and D. D. Ho.** 1997. Decay characteristics of HIV-1-infected compartments during combination therapy. *Nature* 387:188–191.

3471. **Perelson, A. S., A. U. Neumann, M. Markowitz, J. M. Leonard, and D. D. Ho.** 1996. HIV-1 dynamics *in vivo*: virion clearance rate, infected cell life-span, and viral generation time. *Science* 271:1582–1586.

3472. **Peretz, Y., G. Alter, M.-P. Boisvert, G. Hatzakis, C. M. Tsoukas, and N. F. Bernard.** 2005. Human immunodeficiency virus (HIV)-specific gamma interferon secretion directed against all expressed HIV genes: relationship to rate of CD4 decline. *J. Virol.* 79:4908–4917.

3473. **Perez, L. G., M. A. O'Donnell, and E. B. Stephens.** 1992. The transmembrane glycoprotein of human immunodeficiency virus type 1 induces syncytium formation in the absence of the receptor binding glycoprotein. *J. Virol.* 66:4134–4143.

3474. **Perkins, H. A., S. Samsen, J. Garner, D. Echenberg, J. R. Allen, M. Cowan, and J. A. Levy.** 1987. Risk of acquired immunodeficiency syndrome (AIDS) for recipients of blood components from donors who subsequently developed AIDS. *Blood* 70:1604–1610.

3475. **Perl, A.** 1999. Mechanisms of viral pathogenesis in rheumatic disease. *Ann. Rheum. Dis.* 58:454–461.

3476. **Perno, C.-F., M. W. Baseler, S. Broder, and R. Yarchoan.** 1990. Infection of monocytes by human immunodeficiency virus type 1 blocked by inhibitors of CD4-gp120 binding, even in the presence of enhancing antibodies. *J. Exp. Med.* 171:1043–1056.

3477. **Perotti, M. E., X. Tan, and D. M. Phillips.** 1996. Directional budding of human immunodeficiency virus from monocytes. *J. Virol.* 70:5916–5921.

3478. **Perry, V. H., and S. Gordon.** 1988. Macrophages and microglia in the nervous system. *Trends Neurosci.* 11:273–277.

3479. **Persaud, D., Y. Zhou, J. M. Siliciano, and R. F. Siliciano.** 2003. Latency in human immunodeficiency virus type 1 infection: no easy answers. *J. Virol.* 77:1659–1665.

3480. **Persidsky, Y., M. Stins, D. Way, M. H. Witte, M. Weinand, K. S. Kim, P. Bock, H. E. Gendelman, and M. Fiala.** 1997. A model for monocyte migration through the blood-brain barrier during HIV-1 encephalitis. *J. Immunol.* 158:3499–3510.

3481. **Peruzzi, M., C. Azzari, M. E. Rossi, M. De Martino, and A. Vierucci.** 2000. Inhibition of natural killer cell cytotoxicity and interferon γ production by the envelope protein of HIV and prevention by vasoactive intestinal peptide. *AIDS* 16:1067–1073.

3482. **Pestka, S., J. A. Lander, K. C. Zoon, and C. E. Samuel.** 1987. Interferons and their actions. *Annu. Rev. Biochem.* 56:727–777.

3483. **Peterlin, B. M.** 1995. Molecular biology of HIV, p. 185–238. *In* J. A. Levy (ed.), *The Retroviridae*, vol. 4. Plenum Press, New York, N.Y.

3484. Peterman, T. A., H. W. Jaffe, and V. Beral. 1993. Epidemiologic clues to the etiology of Kaposi's sarcoma. *AIDS* 7:605–611.

3485. Peters, B., T. Whittall, K. Babbahmady, K. Gray, R. Vaughan, and T. Lehner. 2004. Effect of heterosexual intercourse on mucosal alloimmunisation and resistance to HIV-1 infection. *Lancet* 363:518–524.

3486. Peters, B. S., E. J. Beck, D. G. Coleman, M. J. H. Wadsworth, O. McGuinness, J. R. W. Harris, and A. J. Pinching. 1991. Changing disease patterns in patients with AIDS in a referral center in the United Kingdom: the changing face of AIDS. *BMJ* 302:203–207.

3487. Peters, P. J., W. M. Sullivan, M. J. Duenas-Decamp, J. Bhattacharya, C. Ankghuambom, R. Brown, K. Luzuriaga, J. Bell, P. Simmonds, J. Ball, and P. R. Clapham. 2006. Non-macrophage-tropic human immunodeficiency virus type 1 r5 envelopes predominate in blood, lymph nodes, and semen: implications for transmission and pathogenesis. *J Virol.* 80:6324–6332.

3488. Peterson, P. K., G. Gekker, C. C. Chao, S. Hu, C. Edelman, H. H. Balfour, Jr., and J. Verhoef. 1992. Human cytomegalovirus-stimulated peripheral blood mononuclear cells induce HIV-1 replication via a tumor necrosis factor-alpha-mediated mechanism. *J. Clin. Investig.* 89:574–580.

3489. Peterson, P. K., G. Gekker, C. C. Chao, R. Schut, J. Verhoef, C. K. Edelman, A. Erice, and H. H. Balfour. 1992. Cocaine amplifies HIV-1 replication in cytomegalovirus-stimulated peripheral blood mononuclear cell coculture. *J. Immunol.* 149:676–680.

3490. Petito, C. K., B. A. Navia, E.-S. Cho, B. D. Jordan, D. C. George, and R. W. Price. 1985. Vacuolar myelopathy pathologically resembling subacute combined degeneration in patients with the acquired immunodeficiency syndrome. *N. Engl. J. Med.* 312:874–879.

3490a. Petrovas, C., J. P. Casazza, J. M. Brenchley, D. A. Price, E. Gostick, W. C. Adams, M. L. Precopio, T. Schacker, M. Roederer, D. C. Douek, and R. A. Koup. 2006. PD-1 is a regulator of virus-specific CD8+ T cell survival in HIV infection. *J. Exp. Med.* 203:2281–2292.

3491. Petrovas, C., Y. M. Mueller, I. D. Dimitriou, P. M. Bojczuk, K. C. Mounzer, J. Witek, J. D. Altman, and P. D. Katsikis. 2004. HIV-specific CD8+ T cells exhibit markedly reduced levels of Bcl-2 and Bcl-xL. *J. Immunol.* 172:4444–4453.

3492. Petry, H., U. Dittmer, C. Stahl-Hennig, C. Coulibaly, B. Makoschey, D. Fuchs, H. Wachter, T. Tolle, C. Morys-Wortmann, F.-J. Kaup, E. Jurkiewicz, W. Luke, and G. Hunsmann. 1995. Reactivation of human immunodeficiency virus type 2 in macaques after simian immunodeficiency virus SIV-mac superinfection. *J. Virol.* 69:1564–1574.

3493. Peudenier, S., C. Hery, L. Montagnier, and M. Tardieu. 1991. Human microglial cells: characterization in cerebral tissue and in primary culture, and study of their susceptibility to HIV-1 infection. *Ann. Neurol.* 29:152–161.

3494. Phillips, A. N. 1996. Reduction of HIV concentration during acute infection: independence from a specific immune response. *Science* 271:497–499.

3495. Phillips, A. N., P. Pezzotti, A. C. Lepri, and G. Rezza. 1994. CD4 lymphocyte count as a determinant of the time from HIV seroconversion to AIDS and death from AIDS: evidence from the Italian Seroconversion Study. *AIDS* 8:1299–1305.

3496. Phillips, A. N., C. A. Sabin, J. Elford, M. Bofill, C. A. Lee, and G. Janossy. 1993. CD8 lymphocyte counts and serum immunoglobulin A levels early in HIV infection as predictors of CD4 lymphocyte depletion during 8 years of follow-up. *AIDS* 7:975–980.

3496a. Phillips, A. N., D. Dunn, C. Sabin, A. Pozniak, R. Matthias, A. M. Geretti, J. Clarke, D. Churchill, I. Williams, T. Hill, H. Green, K. Porter, G. Scullard, M. Johnson, P. Easterbrook, R. Gilson, M. Fischer, C. Loveday, B. Gazzard, and D. Pillay. 2005. Long term probability of detection of HIV-1 drug resistance after starting antiretroviral therapy in routine clinical practice. *AIDS* 19:487–494.

3497. Phillips, D. M., and A. S. Bourinbaiar. 1992. Mechanism of HIV spread from lymphocytes to epithelia. *Virology* 186:261–273.

3498. Phillips, K. D., and M. Groer. 2002. Differentiation and treatment of anemia in HIV disease. *J. Assoc. Nurses AIDS Care* 13:47–72.

3499. Phillips, R. E., S. Rowland-Jones, D. F. Nixon, F. M. Gotch, J. P. Edwards, A. O. Ogunlesi, J. G. Elvin, J. A. Rothbard, C. R. M. Bangham, C. R. Rizza, and A. J. McMichael. 1991. Human immunodeficiency virus genetic variation that can escape cytotoxic T cell recognition. *Nature* 354:453–459.

3500. Philpott, S., H. Burger, C. Tsoukas, B. Foley, K. Anastos, C. Kitchen, and B. Weiser. 2005. Human immunodeficiency virus type 1 genomic RNA sequences in the female genital tract and blood: compartmentalization and intrapatient recombination. *J. Virol.* 79:353–363.

3501. Philpott, S., B. Weiser, K. Anastos, C. M. Ramirez Kitchen, E. Robison, W. A. Meyer, H. S. Sacks, U. Mathur-Wagh, C. Brunner, and H. Burger. 2001. Preferential suppression of CXCR4-specific strains of HIV-1 by antiviral therapy. *J. Clin. Investig.* 107:431–438.

3502. Piatak, M., Jr., S. Saag, L. C. Yang, J. C. Kappes, K.-C. Luk, B. H. Hahn, G. M. Shaw, and J. D. Lifson. 1993. High levels of HIV-1 in plasma during all stages of infection determined by competitive PCR. *Science* 259:1749–1754.

3503. Piazza, C., M. S. Gilardini Montani, S. Moretti, E. Cundari, and E. Piccolella. 1997. CD4+ T cells kill CD8+ T cells via Fas/Fas ligand-mediated apoptosis. *J. Immunol.* 158:1503–1506.

3504. Picard, L., D. A. Wilkinson, A. McKnight, P. W. Gray, J. A. Hoxie, P. R. Clapham, and R. A. Weiss. 1997. Role of the amino-terminal extracellular domain of CXCR-4 in human immunodeficiency virus type 1 entry. *Virology* 231:105–111.

3505. Picker, L. J., S. I. Hagen, R. Lum, E. F. Reed-Inderbitzin, L. M. Daly, A. W. Sylwester, J. M. Walker, D. C. Siess, M. Piatak, Jr., C. Wang, D. B. Allison, V. C. Maino, J. D. Lifson, T. Kodama, and M. K. Axthelm. 2004. Insufficient production and tissue delivery of CD4+ memory T cells in rapidly progressive simian immunodeficiency virus infection. *J. Exp. Med.* 200:1299–1314.

3506. Picker, L. J., and V. C. Maino. 2000. The CD4(+) T cell response to HIV-1. *Curr. Opin. Immunol.* 12:381–386.

3507. Picker, L. J., and D. I. Watkins. 2005. HIV pathogenesis: the first cut is the deepest. *Nat. Immunol.* 6:430–432.

3508. Pierson, T., T. L. Hoffman, J. Blankson, D. Finzi, K. Chadwick, J. B. Margolick, C. Buck, J. D. Siliciano, R. W. Doms, and R. F. Siliciano. 2000. Characterization of chemokine receptor utilization of viruses in the latent reservoir for human immunodeficiency virus type 1. *J. Virol.* 74:7824–7833.

3509. Pierson, T. C., Y. Zhou, T. L. Kieffer, C. T. Ruff, C. Buck, and R. F. Siliciano. 2002. Molecular characterization of preintegration latency in human immunodeficiency virus type 1 infection. *J. Virol.* 76:8518–8531.

3510. Piketty, C., T. M. Drragh, M. Da Costa, P. Bruneval, I. Heard, M. D. Kazathckine, and J. M. Palefsky. 2003. High prevalence of anal human papillomavirus infection and anal cancer precursors among HIV-infected persons in the absence of anal intercourse. *Ann. Intern. Med.* 183:453–459.

3511. Pilcher, C. D., H. C. Tien, J. J. Eron, Jr., P. L. Vernazza, S. Y. Leu, P. W. Stewart, L. E. Goh, and M. S. Cohen. 2004. Brief but efficient: acute HIV infection and the sexual transmission of HIV. *J. Infect. Dis.* 189:1785–1792.

3512. Pillai, S. K., B. Good, S. K. Pond, J. K. Wong, M. C. Strain, D. D. Richman, and D. M. Smith. 2005. Semen-specific genetic characteristics of human immunodeficiency virus type 1 *env. J. Virol.* 79:1734–1742.

3513. Pillay, D., A. S. Walker, D. M. Gibb, A. de Rossi, S. Kaye, M. Ait-Khaled, M. Munoz-Fernandez, and A. Babiker. 2002. Impact of human immunodeficiency virus type 1 subtypes on virologic response and emergence of drug resistance among children in the Paediatric European Network for Treatment of AIDS (PENTA) 5 trial. *J. Infect. Dis.* 186:617–625.

3514. Pillay, K., A. Coutsoudis, A. K. Agadzi-Naqvi, L. Kuhn, H. M. Coovadia, and E. N. Janoff. 2001. Secretory leukocyte protease inhibitor in vaginal fluids and perinatal human immunodeficiency virus type 1 transmission. *J. Infect. Dis.* 183:653–656.

3515. Ping, L. H., M. S. Cohen, I. Hoffman, P. Vernazza, F. Seillier-Moiseiwitsch, H. Chakraborty, P. Kazembe, D. Zimba, M. Maida, S. A. Fiscus, J. J. Eron, R. Swanstrom, and J. A. Nelson. 2000. Effects of genital tract inflammation on human immunodeficiency virus type 1 V3 populations in blood and semen. *J. Virol.* 74:8946–8952.

3516. Pinkerton, S. D., J. N. Martin, M. E. Roland, M. H. Katz, T. J. Coates, and J. O. Kahn. 2004. Cost-effectiveness of HIV postexposure prophylaxis following sexual or injection drug exposure in 96 metropolitan areas in the United States. *AIDS* 18:2065–2073.

3517. Pinter, A., W. J. Honnen, P. D'Agostino, M. K. Gorny, S. Zolla-Pazner, and S. C. Kayman. 2005. The C108g epitope in the V2 domain of gp120 functions as a potent neutralization target when introduced into envelope proteins derived from human immunodeficiency virus type 1 primary isolates. *J. Virol.* 79:6909–6917.

3518. Pinter, A., W. J. Honnen, M. E. Racho, and S. A. Tilley. 1993. A potent, neutralizing human monoclonal antibody against a unique epitope overlapping the CD4-binding site of HIV-1 gp120 that is broadly conserved across North American and African virus isolates. *AIDS Res. Hum. Retrovir.* 9:985–996.

3519. Pinter, A., W. J. Honnen, and S. A. Tilley. 1993. Conformational changes affecting the V3 and CD4-binding domains of human immunodeficiency virus type 1 gp120 associated with env processing and with binding of ligands to these sites. *J. Virol.* 67:5692–5697.

3520. Pinto, L. A., V. Blazevic, B. K. Patterson, C. M. Trubey, M. J. Dolan, and G. M. Shearer. 2000. Inhibition of human immunodeficiency virus type 1 replication prior to reverse transcriptase by influenza virus stimulation. *J. Virol.* 74:4505–4511.

3521. Pinto, L. A., V. Blazevic, G. M. Shearer, B. K. Patterson, and M. J. Dolan. 2000. Alloantigen-induced anti-HIV activity occurs prior to reverse transcription and can be generated by leukocytes from HIV-infected individuals. *Blood* 95:1875–1876. (Letter.)

3522. Pinto, L. A., S. Sharpe, D. I. Cohen, and G. M. Shearer. 1998. Alloantigen-stimulated anti-HIV activity. *Blood* 92:3346–3354.

3523. Pinto, L. A., J. Sullivan, J. A. Berzofsky, M. Clerici, H. A. Kessler, A. L. Landay, and G. M. Shearer. 1995. ENV-specific cytotoxic T lymphocyte responses in HIV seronegative health care workers occupationally exposed to HIV-contaminated body fluids. *J. Clin. Investig.* 96:867–876.

3523a. Pion, M., A. Granelli-Piperno, B. Mangeat, R. Stalder, R. Correa, R. M. Steinman, and V. Piguet. 2006. APOBEC3G/3F mediates intrinsic resistance of monocyte-derived dendritic cells to HIV-1 infection. *J. Exp. Med.* 203:2887–2893.

3524. Piroth, L., M. Duong, C. Quantin, M. Abrahamowicz, R. Michardiere, L.-S. Aho, M. Grappin, M. Buisson, A. Waldner, H. Portier, and P. Chavanet. 1998. Does hepatitis C virus coinfection accelerate clinical and immunological evolution of HIV-infected patients? *AIDS* 12:381–388.

3525. Piscitelli, S. C., A. H. Burstein, N. Welden, K. D. Gallicano, and J. Falloon. 2002. The effect of garlic supplements on the pharmacokinetics of saquinavir. *Clin. Infect. Dis.* 34:234–238.

3526. Piscitelli, S. C., and K. D. Gallicano. 2001. Interactions among drugs for HIV and opportunistic infections. *N. Engl. J. Med.* 344:984–996.

3527. Pitcher, C. J., C. Quittner, D. M. Peterson, M. Connors, R. A. Koup, V. C. Maino, and L. J. Picker. 1999. HIV-1-specific CD4+ T cells are detectable in most individuals with active HIV-1 infection, but decline with prolonged viral suppression. *Nat. Med.* 5:518–525.

3528. Pitrak, E. L., P. M. Bak, P. DeMarais, R. M. Novak, and B. R. Andersen. 1993. Depressed neutrophil superoxide production in human immunodeficiency virus infection. *J. Infect. Dis.* 167:1406–1410.

3529. Pizzato, N., M. Derrien, and F. Lenfant. 2004. The short cytoplasmic tail of HLA-G determines its resistance to HIV-1 Nef-mediated cell surface downregulation. *Hum. Immunol.* 65:1389–1396.

3530. Plaeger, S., S. Bermudez, Y. Mikyas, N. Harawa, R. Dickover, D. Mark, M. Dillon, Y. J. Bryson, P. J. Boyer, and J. S. Sinsheimer. 1999. Decreased CD8 cell-mediated viral suppression and other immunologic characteristics of women who transmit human immunodeficiency virus to their infants. *J. Infect. Dis.* 179:1388–1394.

3531. Plaeger-Marshall, S., M. A. Hausner, V. Isacescu, and J. V. Giorgi. 1992. CD8 T-cell-mediated inhibition of HIV replication in HIV infected adults and children. *AIDS Res. Hum. Retrovir.* 8:1375–1376.

3532. Planelles, V., J. B. Jowett, Q. X. Li, Y. Xie, B. Hahn, and I. S. Chen. 1996. Vpr-induced cell cycle arrest is conserved among primate lentiviruses. *J. Virol.* 70:2516–2524.

3533. Planz, O., P. Seiler, H. Hengartner, and R. M. Zinkernagel. 1996. Specific cytotoxic T cells eliminate B cells producing virus-neutralizing antibodies. *Nature* 382:726–729.

3534. Plata, F. 1989. HIV-specific cytotoxic T lymphocytes. *Res. Immunol.* 140:89–91.

3535. Plata, F., F. Garcia-Pons, A. Ryter, F. Lebargy, M. M. Goodenow, M. H. Q. Dat, B. Autran, and C. Mayaud. 1990. HIV-1 infection of lung alveolar fibroblasts and macrophages in humans. *AIDS Res. Hum. Retrovir.* 6:979–986.

3536. Platt, E. J., J. P. Durnin, and D. Kabat. 2005. Kinetic factors control efficiencies of cell entry, efficacies of entry inhibitors, and mechanisms of adaptation of human immunodeficiency virus. *J. Virol.* 79:4347–4356.

3537. Pleskoff, O., C. Treboute, A. Brelot, N. Heveker, M. Seman, and M. Alizon. 1997. Identification of a chemokine receptor encoded by human cytomegalovirus as a cofactor for HIV-1 entry. *Science* 276:1874–1878.

3538. Plummer, F. A., J. N. Simonsen, D. W. Cameron, J. O. Ndinya-Achola, J. K. Kreiss, M. N. Gakinya, P. Waiyaki, M. Cheang, P. Piot, A. R. Ronald, and E. N. Ngugi. 1991. Cofactors in male-female sexual transmission of human immunodeficiency virus type 1. *J. Infect. Dis.* 163:233–239.

3539. Plymale, D. R., D. S. Tang, A. M. Comardelle, C. D. Fermin, D. E. Lewis, and R. F. Garry. 1999. Both necrosis and apoptosis contribute to HIV-1-induced killing of CD4 cells. *AIDS* 13:1827–1839.

3540. Poccia, F., L. Battistini, B. Cipriani, G. Mancino, F. Martini, M. L. Gougeon, and V. Colizzi. 1999. Phosphoantigen-reactive Vgamma9Vdelta2 T lymphocytes suppress in vitro human immunodeficiency virus type 1 replication by cell-released antiviral factors including CC chemokines. *J. Infect. Dis.* 180:858–861.

3541. Poccia, F., S. Boullier, H. Lecoeur, M. Cochet, Y. Poquet, V. Colizzi, J. J. Fournie, and M. L. Gougeon. 1996. Peripheral V gamma 9/V delta 2 T cell deletion and anergy to nonpeptidic mycobacterial antigens in asymptomatic HIV-1-infected persons. *J. Immunol.* 157:449–461.

3542. Poccia, F., M. L. Gougeon, C. Agrati, C. Montesano, F. Martini, C. D. Pauza, P. Fisch, M. Wallace, and M. Malkovsky. 2002. Innate T-cell immunity in HIV infection: the role of Vgamma9Vdelta2 T lymphocytes. *Curr. Mol. Med.* 2:769–781.

3543. Podda, A., and G. Del Giudice. 2003. MF59-adjuvanted vaccines: increased immunogenicity with an optimal safety profile. *Expert Rev. Vaccines* 2:197–203.

3544. Poggi, A., R. Carosio, D. Fenoglio, S. Brenci, G. Murdaca, M. Setti, F. Indiveri, S. Scabini, E. Ferrero, and M. R. Zocchi. 2004. Migration of V delta 1 and V delta 2 T cells in response to CXCR3 and CXCR4 ligands in healthy donors and HIV-1-infected patients: competition by HIV-1 Tat. *Blood* 103:2205–2213.

3545. Pohlmann, S., G. J. Leslie, T. G. Edwards, T. MacFarlan, J. D. Reeves, K. Hiebenthal-Millow, F. Kirchhoff, F. Baribaud, and R. W. Doms. 2001. DC-SIGN interactions with human immunodeficiency virus: virus binding and transfer are dissociable functions. *J. Virol.* 75:10523–10526.

3546. Pohlmann, S., E. J. Soilleux, F. Baribaud, G. J. Leslie, L. S. Morris, J. Trowsdale, B. Lee, N. Coleman, and R. W. Doms. 2001. DC-SIGNR, a DC-SIGN homologue expressed in endothelial cells, binds to human and simian immunodeficiency viruses and activates infection in trans. *Proc. Natl. Acad. Sci. USA* 98:2670–2675.

3547. Poiesz, B. J., F. W. Ruscetti, A. F. Gazdar, P. A. Bunn, J. D. Minna, and R. C. Gallo. 1980. Detection and isolation of type C retrovirus particles from fresh and cultured lymphocytes of a patient with cutaneous T cell lymphoma. *Proc. Natl. Acad. Sci. USA* 77:7415–7418.

3548. Poignard, P., T. Fouts, D. Naniche, J. P. Moore, and Q. J. Sattentau. 1996. Neutralizing antibodies to human immunodeficiency virus type-1 gp120 induce envelope glycoprotein subunit dissociation. *J. Exp. Med.* 183:473–484.

3549. Poinar, H., M. Kuch, and S. Paabo. 2001. Molecular analyses of oral polio vaccine samples. *Science* 292:743–744.

3550. Polacino, P., V. Stallard, J. E. Klanecki, D. C. Montefiori, A. J. Langlois, B. A. Richardson, J. Overbaugh, W. R. Morton, R. E. Benveniste, and S. L. Hu. 1999. Limited breadth of the protective immunity elicited by simian immunodeficiency virus SIVmne gp160 vaccines in a combination immunization regimen. *J. Virol.* 73:618–630.

3551. Polacino, P., V. Stallard, D. C. Montefiori, C. R. Brown, B. A. Richardson, W. R. Morton, R. E. Benveniste, and S. L. Hu. 1999. Protection of macaques against intrarectal infection by a combination immunization regimen with recombinant simian immunodeficiency virus SIVmne gp160 vaccines. *J. Virol.* 73:3134–3146.

3552. Polacino, P. S., V. Stallard, J. E. Klanecki, S. Pennathur, D. C. Montefiori, A. J. Langlois, B. A. Richardson, W. R. Morton, R. E. Benveniste, and S. L. Hu. 1999. Role of immune responses against the envelope and the core antigens of simian immunodeficiency virus SIVmne in protection against homologous cloned and uncloned virus challenge in Macaques. *J. Virol.* 73:8201–8215.

3553. Polak, J. M., A. G. E. Pearse, and C. M. Heath. 1975. Complete identification of endocrine cells in the gastrointestinal tract using semithin-thin sections to identify motilin cells in human and animal intestine. *Gut* 16:225–229.

3554. Poland, S. D., G. P. A. Rice, and G. A. Dekaban. 1995. HIV-1 infection of human brain-derived microvascular endothelial cells in vitro. *J. Acquir. Immune Defic. Syndr. Hum. Retrovirol.* 8:437–445.

3555. Poles, M. A., S. Barsoum, W. Yu, J. Yu, P. Sun, J. Daly, T. He, S. Mehandru, A. Talal, M. Markowitz, A. Hurley, D. Ho, and L. Zhang. 2003. Human immunodeficiency virus type 1 induces persistent changes in mucosal and blood gammadelta T cells despite suppressive therapy. *J. Virol.* 77:10456–10467.

3556. Poli, G., B. Bottazzi, R. Acero, L. Bersani, V. Rossi, M. Introna, A. Lazzarini, M. Galli, and A. Mantovani. 1985. Monocyte function in intravenous drug abusers with acquired immunodeficiency syndrome: selective impairment of chemotaxis. *Clin. Exp. Immunol.* 62:136–142.

3557. Poli, G., and A. S. Fauci. 1992. The effect of cytokines and pharmacologic agents on chronic HIV infection. *AIDS Res. Hum. Retrovir.* 8:191–197.

3558. Poli, G., and A. S. Fauci. 1993. Cytokine modulation of HIV expression. *Semin. Immunol.* 5:165–173.

3559. Poli, G., A. Kinter, J. S. Justement, J. H. Kehrl, P. Bressler, S. Stanley, and A. S. Fauci. 1990. Tumor necrosis factor alpha functions in an autocrine manner in the induction of human immunodeficiency virus expression. *Proc. Natl. Acad. Sci. USA* 87:782–785.

3560. Poli, G., J. M. Orenstein, A. Kinter, T. M. Folks, and A. S. Fauci. 1989. Interferon-alpha but not AZT suppresses HIV expression in chronically infected cell lines. *Science* 244:575–577.

3561. Polis, M. A., I. A. Sidorov, C. Yoder, S. Jankelevich, J. Metcalf, B. U. Mueller, M. A. Dimitrov, P. Pizzo, R. Yarchoan, and D. S. Dimitrov. 2001. Correlation between reduction in plasma HIV-1 RNA concentration 1 week after start of antiretroviral treatment and longer-term efficacy. *Lancet* 358:1760–1765.

3562. Pollack, H., M. X. Zhan, J. T. Safrit, S. H. Chen, G. Rochford, P. Z. Tao, R. Koup, K. Krasinski, and W. Borkowsky. 1997. CD8+ T-cell-mediated suppression of HIV replication in the first year of life: association with lower viral load and favorable early survival. *AIDS* 11:F9-F13.

3563. Polo, S., F. Veglia, M. S. Malnati, C. Gobbi, P. Farci, R. Raiteri, A. Sinicco, and P. Lusso. 1999. Longitudinal analysis of serum chemokine levels in the course of HIV-1 infection. *AIDS* 13:447–454.

3564. Polyak, S., H. Chen, D. Hirsch, I. George, R. Hershberg, and K. Sperber. 1997. Impaired class II expression and antigen uptake in monocytic cells after HIV-1 infection. *J. Immunol.* **159:**2177–2188.

3565. Polycarpou, A., C. Ntais, B. T. Korber, H. A. Elrich, R. Winchester, P. Krogstad, S. Wolinsky, T. Rostron, S. L. Rowland-Jones, A. J. Ammann, and J. P. Ioannidis. 2002. Association between maternal and infant class I and II HLA alleles and of their concordance with the risk of perinatal HIV type 1 transmission. *AIDS Res. Hum. Retrovir.* **18:**741–746.

3566. Pomerantz, R. J. 2001. Residual HIV-1 infection during antiretroviral therapy: the challenge of viral persistence. *AIDS* **15:**1201–1211.

3567. Pomerantz, R. J., S. M. de la Monte, S. P. Donegan, T. R. Rota, M. W. Vogt, D. E. Craven, and M. S. Hirsch. 1988. Human immunodeficiency virus (HIV) infection of the uterine cervix. *Ann. Intern. Med.* **108:**321–327.

3568. Pomerantz, R. J., D. R. Kuritzkes, S. M. de la Monte, T. R. Rota, A. S. Baker, D. Albert, D. H. Bor, E. L. Feldman, R. T. Schooley, and M. S. Hirsch. 1987. Infection of the retina by human immunodeficiency virus type 1. *N. Engl. J. Med.* **317:**1643–1647.

3569. Pomerantz, R. J., D. Trono, M. B. Feinberg, and D. Baltimore. 1990. Cells nonproductively infected with HIV-1 exhibit an aberrant pattern of viral RNA expression: a molecular model for latency. *Cell* **61:**1271–1276.

3570. Pontesilli, O., P. Carotenuto, S. R. Kerkhof-Gared, M. T. M. Roos, I. P. M. Keet, R. A. Coutinho, J. Goudsmit, and F. Miedema. 1999. Lymphoproliferative response to HIV type 1 p24 in long-term survivors of HIV type 1 infection is predictive of persistent AIDS-free infection. *AIDS Res. Hum. Retrovir.* **15:**973–981.

3571. Poon, B., and I. S. Y. Chen. 2003. Human immunodeficiency virus type 1 (HIV-1) Vpr enhances expression from unintegrated HIV-1 DNA. *J. Virol.* **77:**3962–3972.

3572. Poon, B., J. T. Safrit, H. McClure, C. Kitchen, J. F. Hsu, V. Gudeman, C. Petropoulos, T. Wrin, I. S. Y. Chen, and K. Grovit-Ferbas. 2005. Induction of humoral immune responses following vaccination with envelope-containing, formaldehyde-treated, thermally inactivated human immunodeficiency virus type 1. *J. Virol.* **79:**4927–4935.

3573. Poonia, B., S. Nelson, G. J. Bagby, P. Zhang, L. Quniton, and R. S. Veazey. 2005. Chronic alcohol consumption results in higher simian immunodeficiency virus replication in mucosally inoculated rhesus macaques. *AIDS Res. Hum. Retrovir.* **21:**863–868.

3574. Pope, M., S. Gezelter, N. Gallo, L. Hoffman, and R. M. Steinman. 1995. Low levels of HIV-1 infection in cutaneous dendritic cells promote extensive viral replication upon binding to memory CD4+ T cells. *J. Exp. Med.* **182:**2045–2056.

3575. Pope, M., and A. T. Haase. 2003. Transmission, acute HIV-1 infection and the quest for strategies to prevent infection. *Nat. Med.* **9:**847–852.

3576. Popik, W., J. E. Hesselgesser, and P. M. Pitha. 1998. Binding of a human immunodeficiency virus type 1 to CD4 and CXCR4 receptors differentially regulates expression of inflammatory genes and activates the MEK/ERK signaling pathway. *J. Virol.* **72:**6406–6413.

3577. Popik, W., and P. M. Pitha. 2000. Exploitation of cellular signaling by HIV-1: unwelcome guests with master keys that signal their entry. *Virology* **276:**1–6.

3578. Popik, W., and P. M. Pitha. 2000. Inhibition of CD3/CD28-mediated activation of the MEK/ERK signaling pathway represses replication of X4 but not R5 human immunodeficiency virus type 1 in peripheral blood CD4(+) T lymphocytes. *J. Virol.* **74:**2558–2566.

3579. Popov, S., M. Rexach, L. Ratner, G. Blobel, and M. Bukrinsky. 1998. Viral protein R regulates docking of the HIV-1 reintegration complex to the nuclear pore complex. *J. Biol. Chem.* **273:**13347–13352.

3580. Popovic, M., M. G. Sarngadharan, E. Read, and R. C. Gallo. 1984. Detection, isolation, and continuous production of cytopathic retroviruses (HTLV-III) from patients with AIDS and pre-AIDS. *Science* **224:**497–500.

3581. Popper, S. J., A. D. Sarr, A. Guèye-Ndiaye, S. Mboup, M. E. Essex, and P. J. Kanki. 2000. Low plasma human immunodeficiency virus type 2 viral load is independent of proviral load: low virus production in vivo. *J. Virol.* **74:**1554–1557.

3582. Porco, T. C., J. N. Martin, K. A. Page-Shafer, A. Cheng, E. Charlebois, R. M. Grant, and D. H. Osmond. 2004. Decline in HIV infectivity following the introduction of highly active antiretroviral therapy. *AIDS* **18:**81–88.

3583. Portales, P., J. Reynes, V. Pinet, R. Rouzier-Panis, V. Baillat, J. Clot, and P. Corbeau. 2003. Interferon-α restores HIV-induced alteration of natural killer cell perforin expression *in vivo*. *AIDS* **17:**495–504.

3584. Portegies, P. 1994. AIDS dementia complex: a review. *J. Acquir. Immune Defic. Syndr.* **7:**S38-S48.

3585. Portegies, P., J. de Gans, J. M. A. Lange, M. M. A. Derix, H. Speelman, M. Bakker, S. A. Danner, and J. Goudsmit. 1989. Declining incidence of AIDS dementia complex after introduction of zidovudine treatment. *BMJ* **299:**819–821.

3586. Porter, D. C., D. C. Ansardi, W. S. Choi, and C. D. Morrow. 1993. Encapsidation of genetically engineered poliovirus minireplicons which express human immunodeficiency virus type 1 Gag and Pol proteins upon infection. *J. Virol.* **67:**3712–3719.

3587. Posnett, D. N., S. Kabak, A. S. Hodtsev, E. A. Goldberg, and A. Asch. 1993. T-cell antigen receptor V-beta subsets are not preferentially deleted in AIDS. *AIDS* **7:**625–631.

3588. Poss, M., H. L. Matrin, J. K. Kreiss, L. Granville, B. Chohan, P. Nyange, K. Mandaliya, and J. Overbaugh. 1995. Diversity in virus populations from genital secretions and peripheral blood from women recently infected with human immunodeficiency virus type 1. *J. Virol.* **69:**8118–8122.

3589. Potash, M. J., M. Zeira, Z.-B. Huang, T. E. Pearce, E. Eden, H. E. Gendelman, and D. J. Volsky. 1992. Virus-cell membrane fusion does not predict efficient infection of alveolar macrophages by human immunodeficiency virus type 1 (HIV-1). *Virology* **188:**864–868.

3590. Potempa, S., L. Picard, J. D. Reeves, D. Wilkinson, R. A. Weiss, and S. J. Talbot. 1997. CD4-independent infection by human immunodeficiency virus type 2 strain ROD/B: the role of the N-terminal domain of CXCR-4 in fusion and entry. *J. Virol.* **71:**4419–4424.

3591. Potts, K. E., M. L. Kalish, T. Lott, G. Orloff, C. C. Luo, M. A. Bernard, C. B. Alves, R. Badaro, J. Suleiman, O. Ferreira, G. Schochetman, W. D. Johnson, Jr., C. Y. Ou, and J. L. Ho. 1993. Genetic heterogeneity of the principal neutralizing determinant of the human immunodeficiency virus type 1 (HIV-1) in Brazil. *AIDS* **7:**1191–1197.

3592. Potula, R., L. Poluektova, B. Knipe, J. Chrastil, D. Heilman, H. Dou, O. Takikawa, D. H. Munn, H. E. Gendelman, and Y. Persidsky. 2005. Inhibition of indoleamine 2,3-dioxygenase

(IDO) enhances elimination of virus-infected macrophages in an animal model of HIV-1 encephalitis. *Blood* 106:2382–2390.

3593. Poulin, L., L. A. Evans, S. Tang, A. Barboza, H. Legg, D. R. Littman, and J. A. Levy. 1991. Several CD4 domains can play a role in human immunodeficiency virus infection of cells. *J. Virol.* 65:4893–4901.

3594. Poulin, L., and J. A. Levy. 1992. The HIV-1 nef gene product is associated with phosphorylation of a 46 kD cellular protein. *AIDS* 6:787–791.

3595. Poulsen, A. G., B. Kvinesdal, P. Aaby, K. Molbak, K. Frederiksen, F. Dias, and E. Lauritzen. 1989. Prevalence of and mortality from human immunodeficiency virus type 2 in Bissau, West Africa. *Lancet* ii:827–830.

3596. Powell, D. J., D. P. Bednarik, T. M. Folks, T. Jehuda-Cohen, F. Villinger, K. W. Sell, and A. A. Ansari. 1993. Inhibition of cellular activity of retroviral replication by CD8 T cells derived from non-human primates. *Clin. Exp. Immunol.* 91:473–481.

3597. Powell, J. D., T. Yehuda-Cohen, F. Villinger, H. M. McClure, K. W. Sell, and A. Ahmed-Ansari. 1990. Inhibition of SIV-SMM replication *in vitro* by CD8+ cells from SIV/SMM infected seropositive clinically asymptomatic sooty mangabeys. *J. Med. Primatol.* 19:239–249.

3598. Power, C., J. C. McArthur, R. T. Johnson, D. E. Griffin, J. D. Glass, S. Perryman, and B. Chesebro. 1994. Demented and nondemented patients with AIDS differ in brain-derived human immunodeficiency virus type 1 envelope sequences. *J. Virol.* 68:4643–4649.

3599. Power, C., J. C. McArthur, A. Nath, K. Wehrly, M. Mayne, J. Nishio, T. Langelier, R. T. Johnson, and B. Chesebro. 1998. Neuronal death induced by brain-derived human immunodeficiency virus type 1 envelope genes differs between demented and nondemented AIDS patients. *J. Virol.* 72:9045–9053.

3600. Prabhakar, B. S., and N. Nathanson. 1981. Acute rabies death mediated by antibody. *Nature* 290:590–591.

3601. Pratt, R. D., J. F. Shapiro, N. McKinney, S. Kwok, and S. A. Spector. 1995. Virologic characterization of primary human immunodeficiency virus type 1 infection in a health care worker following needlestick injury. *J. Infect. Dis.* 172:851–854.

3602. Preston, B. D., B. J. Poiesz, and L. A. Loeb. 1988. Fidelity of HIV-1 reverse transcriptase. *Science* 242:1168–1171.

3603. Price, D. A., P. J. R. Goulder, P. Klenerman, A. K. Sewell, P. J. Easterbrook, M. Troop, C. R. M. Bangham, and R. E. Phillips. 1997. Positive selection of HIV-1 cytotoxic T lymphocyte escape variants during primary infection. *Proc. Natl. Acad. Sci. USA* 94:1890–1895.

3604. Price, P., G. Morahan, D. Huang, E. Stone, K. Y. Cheong, A. Castley, M. Rodgers, M. Q. McIntyre, L. J. Abraham, and M. A. French. 2002. Polymorphisms in cytokine genes define subpopulations of HIV-1 patients who experienced immune restoration diseases. *AIDS* 16:2043–2047.

3605. Price, R. W. 1996. Neurological complications of HIV infection. *Lancet* 348:445–452.

3606. Price, R. W., B. Brew, J. Sidtis, M. Rosenblum, A. G. Scheck, and P. Clearly. 1988. The brain in AIDS: central nervous system HIV-1 infection and AIDS dementia complex. *Science* 239:586–592.

3607. Prince, A. M., B. Horowitz, L. Baker, R. W. Shulman, H. Ralph, J. Valinsky, A. Cundell, B. Brotman, W. Boehle, F. Rey, M. Piet, H. Reesink, N. Lelie, M. Tersmette, F. Miedema, L. Barbosa,

G. Nemo, C. L. Nastala, J. S. Allan, D. R. Lee, and J. W. Eichberg. 1988. Failure of a human immunodeficiency virus (HIV) immune globulin to protect chimpanzees against experimental challenge with HIV. *Proc. Natl. Acad. Sci. USA* 85:6944–6948.

3608. Prince, A. M., H. Reesink, D. Pascual, B. Horowitz, I. Hewlett, K. K. Murthy, K. E. Cobb, and J. W. Eichberg. 1991. Prevention of HIV infection by passive immunization with HIV immunoglobulin. *AIDS Res. Hum. Retrovir.* 7:971–973.

3609. Prince, H. E., and E. R. Jensen. 1991. HIV-related alterations in CD8 cell subsets defined by in vitro survival characteristics. *Cell. Immunol.* 134:276–286.

3610. Prins, M., L. Meyer, and N. A. Hessol. 2005. Sex and the course of HIV infection in the pre- and highly active antiretroviral therapy eras. *AIDS* 19:357–370.

3611. Psallidopoulos, M. C., S. M. Schnittman, L. M. Thompson III, M. Baseler, A. S. Fauci, H. C. Lane, and N. P. Salzman. 1989. Integrated proviral human immunodeficiency virus type 1 is present in CD4+ peripheral blood lymphocytes in healthy seropositive individuals. *J. Virol.* 63:4626–4631.

3612. Pu, R., S. Okada, E. R. Little, B. Xu, W. V. Stoffs, and J. K. Yamamoto. 1995. Protection of neonatal kittens against feline immunodeficiency virus infection with passive maternal antiviral antibodies. *AIDS* 9:235–242.

3613. Pudney, J., M. Oneta, K. Mayer, G. Seage III, and D. Anderson. 1992. Pre-ejaculatory fluid as potential vector for sexual transmission of HIV-1. *Lancet* 340:1470.

3614. Puerta-Fernandez, E., A. B. Jesus, C. Romero-Lopez, N. Tapia, M. A. Martinez, and A. Berzal-Herranz. 2005. Inhibition of HIV-1 replication by RNA targeted against the LTR region. *AIDS* 19:863–870.

3615. Pulakhandam, U., and H. P. Dincsoy. 1990. Cytomegaloviral adrenalitis and adrenal insufficiency in AIDS. *Am. J. Clin. Pathol.* 93:651–656.

3615a. Pulendran, B., and R. Ahmed. 2006. Translating innate immunity into immunological memory: implications for vaccine development. *Cell* 124:849–863.

3616. Pulendran, B., J. Bancherau, S. Burkeholder, E. Kraus, E. Guinet, C. Chalouni, D. Caron, C. Maliszewski, J. Davoust, J. Fay, and K. Palucka. 2000. Flt3-ligand and granulocyte colony-stimulating factor mobilize distinct human dendritic cell subsets in vivo. *J. Immunol.* 165:566–572.

3617. Pulendran, B., K. Palucka, and J. Bancherau. 2001. Sensing pathogens and tuning immune responses. *Science* 293:253–256.

3618. Pulliam, L., R. Gascon, M. Stubblebine, D. McGuire, and M. S. McGrath. 1997. Unique monocyte subset in patients with AIDS dementia. *Lancet* 349:692–695.

3619. Pulliam, L., B. G. Herndier, N. M. Tang, and M. S. McGrath. 1991. Human immunodeficiency virus-infected macrophages produce soluble factors that cause histological and neurochemical alterations in cultured human brains. *J. Clin. Investig.* 87:503–512.

3620. Pulliam, L., B. Sun, and H. Rempel. 2004. Invasive chronic inflammatory monocyte phenotype in subjects with high HIV-1 viral load. *J. Neuroimmunol.* 157:93–98.

3621. Pulliam, L., D. West, N. Haigwood, and R. A. Swanson. 1993. HIV-1 envelope gp120 alters astrocytes in human brain cultures. *AIDS Res. Hum. Retrovir.* 9:439–444.

3622. Pumarola-Sune, T., B. A. Navia, C. Cordon-Cardo, E. S. Cho, and R. W. Price. 1987. HIV antigen in the brains of patients with the AIDS dementia complex. *Ann. Neurol.* **21**: 490–496.

3623. Puoti, M., F. Gargiulo, E. Q. Roldan, A. Chiodera, L. Palvarini, A. Spinetti, S. Zaltron, V. Putzolu, B. Zanini, F. Favilli, A. Turano, and G. Carosi. 2000. Liver damage and kinetics of hepatitis C virus and human immunodeficiency virus replication during the early phases of combination antiretroviral treatment. *J. Infect. Dis.* **181**:2033–2036.

3624. Puri, A., J. L. Riley, D. Kim, D. W. Ritchey, P. Hug, K. Jernigan, P. Rose, R. Blumenthal, and R. G. Carroll. 2000. Influenza virus upregulates CXCR4 expression in CD4+ cells. *AIDS Res. Hum. Retrovir.* **16**:19–25.

3625. Purtscher, M., A. Trkola, G. Gruber, A. Buchacher, R. Predl, F. Steindl, C. Tauer, R. Berger, N. Barrett, A. Jungbauder, and H. Katinger. 1994. A broadly neutralizing human monoclonal antibody against gp41 of human immunodeficiency virus type 1. *AIDS Res. Hum. Retrovir.* **10**:1651–1658.

3626. Putkonen, P., R. Thorstensson, L. Ghavamzadeh, J. Albert, K. Hild, G. Biberfeld, and E. Norrby. 1991. Prevention of HIV-2 and SIVsm infection by passive immunization in cynomolgus monkeys. *Nature* **352**:436–438.

3627. Putkonen, P., R. Thorstensson, L. Walther, J. Albert, L. Akerblom, O. Granquist, G. Wadell, E. Norrby, and G. Biberfeld. 1991. Vaccine protection against HIV-2 infection in cynomolgus monkeys. *AIDS Res. Hum. Retrovir.* **7**:271–277.

3628. Qi, J. C., R. L. Stevens, R. Wadley, A. Collins, M. Cooley, H. M. Naif, N. Nasr, A. Cunningham, G. Katsoulotos, Y. Wanigasek, B. Roufogalis, and S. A. Krilis. 2002. IL-16 regulation of human mast cells/basophils and their susceptibility to HIV-1. *J. Immunol.* **168**:4127–4134.

3629. Qian, J., V. Bours, J. Manischewitz, R. Blackburn, U. Siebenlist, and H. Golding. 1994. Chemically selected subclones of the CEM cell line demonstrate resistance to HIV-1 infection resulting from a selective loss of NF-kB DNA binding proteins. *J. Immunol.* **152**:4183–4191.

3630. Qiao, X., B. He, A. Chiu, D. M. Knowles, A. Chadburn, and A. Cerutti. 2006. Human immunodeficiency virus 1 Nef suppresses CD40-dependent immunoglobulin class switching in bystander B cells. *Nat. Immunol.* **7**:302–310.

3631. Qing, M., T. Li, Y. Han, Z. Qiu, and Y. Jiao. 2006. Accelerating effect of human leukocyte antigen-Bw6 homozygosity on disease progression in Chinese HIV-1-infected patients. *J. Acquir. Immune Defic. Syndr.* **41**:137–139.

3632. Qiu, J. T., R. Song, M. Dettenhofer, C. Tian, T. August, B. K. Felber, G. N. Pavlakis, and X. F. Yu. 1999. Evaluation of novel human immunodeficiency virus type 1 Gag DNA vaccines for protein expression in mammalian cells and induction of immune responses. *J. Virol.* **73**:9145–9152.

3633. Quesada-Rolander, M., B. Makitalo, R. Thorstensson, Y. J. Zhang, E. Castanos-Velez, G. Biberfeld, and P. Pukonen. 1996. Protection against mucosal SIV$_{sm}$ challenge in macaques infected with a chimeric SIV that expresses HIV type 1 envelope. *AIDS Res. Hum. Retrovir.* **12**:993–999.

3634. Quillent, C., E. Oberlin, J. Braun, D. Rousset, G. GonzalezCanali, P. Metais, L. Montagnier, J. L. Virelizier, F. ArenzanaSeisdedos, and A. Beretta. 1998. HIV-1-resistance phenotype conferred by combination of two separate inherited mutations of CCR5 gene. *Lancet* **351**:14–18.

3635. Quinn, T. C. 1996. Global burden of the HIV pandemic. *Lancet* **348**:99–106.

3636. Quinn, T. C., M. J. Wawer, N. Sewankambo, D. Serwadda, C. Li, F. Wabwire-Mangen, M. O. Meehan, T. Lutalo, R. H. Gray, et al. 2000. Viral load and heterosexual transmission of human immunodeficiency virus type 1. *N. Engl. J. Med.* **342**:921–929.

3637. Quinones-Mateu, M. E., S. C. Ball, A. J. Marozsan, V. S. Torre, J. L. Albright, G. Vanham, G. van Der Groen, R. L. Colebunders, and E. J. Arts. 2000. A dual infection/competition assay shows a correlation between ex vivo human immunodeficiency virus type 1 fitness and disease progression. *J. Virol.* **74**:9222–9233.

3638. Quiñones-Mateu, M. E., M. M. Lederman, Z. Feng, B. Chakraborty, J. Weber, H. R. Rangel, M. L. Marotta, M. Mirza, B. Jiang, P. Kiser, K. Medvik, S. F. Sieg, and A. Weinberg. 2003. Human epithelial β-defensins 2 and 3 inhibit HIV-1 replication. *AIDS* **17**:F39-F48.

3639. Qureshi, M. N., C. E. Barr, T. Seshamma, J. Reidy, R. J. Pomerantz, and O. Bagasra. 1995. Infection of oral mucosal cells by human immunodeficiency virus type 1 in seropositive persons. *J. Infect. Dis.* **171**:190–193.

3640. Qureshi, N. M., D. H. Coy, R. F. Garry, and L. A. Henderson. 1990. Characterization of a putative cellular receptor for HIV-1 transmembrane glycoprotein using synthetic peptides. *AIDS* **4**:553–558.

3641. Qurishi, N., C. Kreuzberg, G. Luchters, W. Effenberger, B. Kupfer, T. Sauerbruch, J. K. Rockstroh, and U. Spengler. 2003. Effect of antiretroviral therapy on liver-related mortality in patients with HIV and hepatitis C virus coinfection. *Lancet* **362**:1708–1713.

3642. Rabeneck, L., M. Popovic, S. Gartner, D. M. McLean, W. A. McLeod, E. Read, K. K. Wong, and W. J. Boyko. 1990. Acute HIV infection presenting with painful swallowing and esophageal ulcers. *JAMA* **263**:2318–2322.

3643. Rabkin, C. S., J. J. Goedert, R. J. Biggar, F. Yellin, and W. A. Blattner. 1990. Kaposi's sarcoma in three HIV-1 infected cohorts. J. Acquir. Immune Defic. Syndr. **3** (Suppl. 1):S38–S43.

3644. Rabkin, C. S., S. Janz, A. Lash, A. E. Coleman, E. Musaba, L. Liotta, R. J. Biggar, and Z. Zhuang. 1997. Monoclonal origin of multicentric Kaposi's sarcoma lesions. *N. Engl. J. Med.* **336**:988–993.

3645. Rabkin, C. S., Q. Yang, J. J. Goedert, G. Nguyen, H. Mitsuya, and S. Sei. 1999. Chemokine and chemokine receptor gene variants and risk of non-Hodgkin's lymphoma in human immunodeficiency virus-1-infected individuals. *Blood* **93**:1838–1842.

3646. Rabkin, C. S., and F. Yellin. 1994. Cancer incidence in a population with a high prevalence of infection with human immunodeficiency virus type 1. *J. Natl. Cancer Inst.* **86**:1711–1716.

3647. Rabkin, J. G., J. B. W. Williams, R. H. Remien, R. Goetz, R. Kertzner, and J. M. Gorman. 1991. Depression, distress, lymphocyte subsets, and human immunodeficiency virus symptoms on two occasions in HIV-positive homosexual men. *Arch. Gen. Psychiatry* **48**:111–119.

3648. Raboud, J. M., J. S. G. Montaner, B. Conway, L. Haley, C. Sherlock, M. V. O'Shaughnessy, and M. T. Schecter. 1996. Variation in plasma RNA levels, CD4 cell counts, and p24 antigen levels in clinically stable men with human immunodeficiency virus infection. *J. Infect. Dis.* **174**:191–194.

3649. Rabson, A., and M. Martin. 1985. Molecular organization of the AIDS retrovirus. *Cell* **40**:477–480.

3650. Racz, P., K. Tenner-Racz, C. Kahl, A. C. Feller, P. Kern, and M. Dietrich. 1986. Spectrum of morphologic changes of lymph nodes from patients with AIDS or AIDS-related complexes. *Prog. Allergy* 37:81–181.

3651. Radja, F., D. G. Kay, S. Albrecht, and P. Jolicoeur. 2003. Oligodendrocyte-specific expression of human immunodeficiency virus Type 1 Nef in transgenic mice leads to vacuolar myelopathy and alters oligodendrocyte phenotype in vitro. *J. Virol.* 77:11745–11753.

3652. Radkov, S. A., P. Kellam, and C. Boshoff. 2000. The latent nuclear antigen of Kaposi sarcoma-associated herpesvirus targets the retinoblastoma-E2F pathway and with the oncogene Hras transforms primary rat cells. *Nat. Med.* 6:1121–1127.

3653. Raffanti, S. P., J. S. Fusco, B. H. Sherrill, N. I. Hansen, A. C. Justice, R. D'Aquila, E. J. Mangialardi, and G. P. Fusco. 2004. Effect of persistent moderate viremia on disease progression during HIV therapy. *J. Acquir. Immune Defic. Syndr.* 37:1147–1154.

3654. Rahman, A. A., M. Teschner, K. K. Sethi, and H. Brandis. 1976. Appearance of IgG (Fc) receptor(s) on cultured human fibroblasts infected with human cytomegalovirus. *J. Immunol.* 117:253–258.

3655. Rambaut, A., D. L. Robertson, O. G. Pybus, M. Peeters, and E. C. Holmes. 2001. Human immunodeficiency virus. Phylogeny and the origin of HIV-1. *Nature* 410:1047–1048.

3656. Rameshwar, P., T. N. Denny, and P. Gascon. 1996. Enhanced HIV-1 activity in bone marrow can lead to myelopoietic suppression partially contributed by gag p24. *J. Immunol.* 157:4244–4250.

3657. Ramilo, O., K. D. Bell, J. W. Uhr, and E. S. Vitetta. 1993. Role of CD25+ and CD25− T cells in acute HIV infection in vitro. *J. Immunol.* 150:5202–5208.

3658. Rammensee, H. G., K. Falk, and O. Rotzschke. 1993. Peptides naturally presented by MHC class I molecules. *Annu. Rev. Immunol.* 11:213–244.

3659. Ramos, A., D. J. Hu, L. Nguyen, K. O. Phan, S. Vanichseni, N. Promadej, K. Choopanya, M. Callahan, N. L. Young, J. McNicholl, T. D. Mastro, T. M. Folks, and S. Subbarao. 2002. Intersubtype human immunodeficiency virus type 1 superinfection following seroconversion to primary infection in two injection drug users. *J. Virol.* 76:7444–7452.

3660. Ramratnam, B., S. Bonhoeffer, J. Binley, A. Hurley, L. Zhang, J. E. Mittler, M. Markowitz, J. P. Moore, A. S. Perelson, and D. D. Ho. 1999. Rapid production and clearance of HIV-1 and hepatitis C virus assessed by large volume plasma apheresis. *Lancet* 354:1782–1785.

3661. Rana, S., G. Besson, D. G. Cook, J. Rucker, R. J. Smyth, Y. Yi, J. D. Turner, H. H. Guo, J. G. Du, S. C. Peiper, E. Lavi, M. Samson, F. Libert, C. Liesnard, G. Vassart, R. W. Doms, M. Parmentier, and R. G. Collman. 1997. Role of CCR5 in infection of primary macrophages and lymphocytes by macrophage-tropic strains of human immunodeficiency virus: resistance to patient-derived and prototype isolates resulting from the Δccr5 mutation. *J. Virol.* 71:3219–3227.

3662. Rando, R. F., A. Srinivasan, J. Feingold, E. Gonczol, and S. Plotkin. 1990. Characterization of multiple molecular interactions between human cytomegalovirus (HCMV) and human immunodeficiency virus type 1 (HIV-1). *Virology* 176:87–97.

3663. Ranki, A., S. Mattinen, R. Yarchoan, S. Broder, J. Ghrayeb, J. Lahdevirta, and K. Krohn. 1989. T-cell response towards HIV in infected individuals with and without zidovudine therapy, and in HIV-exposed sexual partners. *AIDS* 3:63–69.

3664. Ranki, A., M. Nyberg, V. Ovod, M. Haltia, I. Elovaara, R. Raininko, H. Haapasalo, and K. Krohn. 1995. Abundant expression of HIV Nef and Rev proteins in brain astrocytes in vivo is associated with dementia. *AIDS* 9:1001–1008.

3664a. Rao, P. E., A. L. Petrone, and P. D. Ponath. 2005. Differentiation and expansion of T cells with regulatory function from human peripheral lymphocytes by stimulation in the presence of TGF-{beta}. *J. Immunol.* 174:1446–1455.

3665. Rao, T. K. S., E. J. Filippone, A. D. Nicastri, S. H. Landesman, E. Frank, C. K. Chen, and E. A. Friedman. 1984. Associated focal and segmental glomerulosclerosis in the acquired immunodeficiency syndrome. *N. Engl. J. Med.* 310:669–673.

3666. Rappaport, J., J. B. Kopp, and P. E. Klotman. 1994. Host virus interactions and the molecular regulation of HIV-1: role in the pathogenesis of HIV-associated nephropathy. *Kidney Int.* 46:16–27.

3667. Rappersberger, K., S. Gartner, P. Schenk, G. Stingl, V. Groh, E. Tschachler, D. L. Mann, K. Wolff, K. Konrad, and M. Popovic. 1988. Langerhans's cells are an actual site of HIV-1 replication. *Intervirology* 29:185–194.

3668. Rappocciolo, G., F. J. Jenkins, H. R. Hensler, P. Piazza, M. Jais, L. Borowski, S. C. Watkins, and C. R. Rinaldo, Jr. 2006. DC-SIGN Is a receptor for human herpesvirus 8 on dendritic cells and macrophages. *J. Immunol.* 176:1741–1749.

3669. Rappocciolo, G., P. Piazza, C. L. Fuller, T. A. Reinhart, S. C. Watkins, D. T. Rowe, M. Jais, P. Gupta, and C. R. Rinaldo, Jr. 2006. DC-SIGN on B lymphocytes is required for transmission of HIV-1 to T lymphocytes. *PLoS Pathogens* 2:e70.

3670. Rasheed, S., A. A. Gottlieb, and R. F. Garry. 1986. Cell killing by ultraviolet-inactivated human immunodeficiency virus. *Virology* 154:395–400.

3671. Rasheed, S., Z. Li, D. Xu, and A. Kovacs. 1996. Presence of cell-free human immunodeficiency virus in cervicovaginal secretions is independent of viral load in the blood of human immunodeficiency virus-infected women. *Am. J. Obstet. Gynecol.* 175:122–129.

3672. Ratner, L. 1992. Glucosidase inhibitors for treatment of HIV-1 infection. *AIDS Res. Hum. Retrovir.* 8:165–173.

3673. Ratner, L., W. Haseltine, R. Patarca, K. J. Livak, B. Starcich, S. F. Josephs, E. R. Doran, A. Rafalski, E. A. Whitehorn, K. Baumeister, L. Ivanoff, S. R. Petteway, Jr., M. L. Pearson, J. A. Lautenberger, T. S. Papas, J. Ghrayeb, N. T. Chang, R. C. Gallo, and F. Wong-Staal. 1985. Complete nucleotide sequence of the AIDS virus, HTLV-III. *Nature* 313:277–284.

3674. Rautonen, J., N. Rautonen, N. L. Martin, and D. W. Wara. 1994. HIV type 1 tat protein induces immunoglobulin and interleukin 6 synthesis by uninfected peripheral blood mononuclear cells. *AIDS Res. Hum. Retrovir.* 10:781–785.

3675. Rautonen, N., J. Rautonen, N. L. Martin, and D. W. Wara. 1994. HIV-1 Tat induces cytokine synthesis by uninfected mononuclear cells. *AIDS* 8:1504–1506.

3675a. Rawal, B.D., A. Degula, L. Lebedeva, R. S. Janssen, F. M. Hecht, H. W. Sheppard, and M. P. Busch. 2003. Development of a new less-sensitive enzyme immunoassay for detection of early HIV-1 infection. *J. Acquir. Immune Defic. Syndr.* 33:349–355.

3676. Ray, P. E., X. H. Liu, D. Henry, L. D. Dye, L. Xu, J. M. Orenstein, and T. E. Schuztbank. 1998. Infection of human primary renal epithelial cells with HIV-1 from children with HIV-associated nephropathy. *Kidney Int.* 53:1217–1229.

3677. Rayfield, M., K. De Cock, W. Heyward, L. Goldstein, J. Krebs, S. Kwok, S. Lee, J. McCormick, J. M. Moreau, K. Odehouri, G. Schochetman, J. Sninsky, and C.-Y. Ou. 1988. Mixed human immunodeficiency virus (HIV) infection in an individual: demonstration of both HIV type 1 and type 2 proviral sequences by using polymerase chain reaction. *J. Infect. Dis.* **158:**1170–1176.

3678. Razvi, E. S., and R. M. Welsh. 1993. Programmed cell death of T lymphocytes during acute viral infection: a mechanism for virus-induced immune deficiency. *J. Virol.* **67:**5754–5765.

3679. Re, F., D. Braaten, E. K. Franke, and J. Luban. 1995. Human immunodeficiency virus type 1 Vpr arrests the cell cycle in G_2 by inhibiting the activation of $p34^{cdc2}$-cyclin B. *J. Virol.* **69:**6859–6864.

3680. Re, M. C., G. Zauli, D. Gibellini, G. Furlini, E. Ramazzotti, P. Monari, S. Ranieri, S. Capitani, and M. La Placa. 1993. Uninfected haematopoietic progenitor (CD34+) cells purified from the bone marrow of AIDS patients are committed to apoptotic cell death in culture. *AIDS* **7:**1049–1055.

3681. Real, F. X., and S. E. Krown. 1985. Spontaneous regression of Kaposi's sarcoma in patients with AIDS. *N. Engl. J. Med.* **313:**1659.

3682. Reddy, M. M., and M. H. Grieco. 1989. Neopterin and alpha and beta interleukin-1 levels in sera of patients with human immunodeficiency virus infection. *J. Clin. Microbiol.* **27:**1919–1923.

3683. Redfield, R. R., D. L. Birx, N. Ketter, E. Tramont, V. Polonis, C. Davis, J. F. Brundage, G. Smith, S. Johnson, A. Fowler, T. Wierzba, A. Shafferman, F. Volvoyitz, C. Oster, and D. S. Burke. 1991. A phase I evaluation of the safety and immunogenicity of vaccination with recombinant gp160 in patients with early human immunodeficiency virus infection. *N. Engl. J. Med.* **324:**1677–1684.

3684. Reeves, J. D., and R. W. Doms. 2002. Human immunodeficiency virus type 2. *J. Gen. Virol.* **83:**1253–1265.

3685. Reeves, J. D., S. A. Gallo, N. Ahmad, J. L. Miamidian, P. E. Harvey, M. Sharron, S. Pohlmann, J. N. Sfakianos, C. A. Derdeyn, R. Blumenthal, E. Hunter, and R. W. Doms. 2002. Sensitivity of HIV-1 to entry inhibitors correlates with envelope/coreceptor affinity, receptor density, and fusion kinetics. *Proc. Natl. Acad. Sci. USA* **99:**16249–16254.

3686. Reeves, J. D., S. Hibbitts, G. Simmons, A. Mcknight, J. M. Azevedo-Pereira, J. Moniz-Pereira, and P. R. Clapham. 1999. Primary human immunodeficiency virus type 2 (HIV-2) isolates infect CD4-negative cells via CCR5 and CXCR4: comparison with HIV-1 and simian immunodeficiency virus and relevance to cell tropism in vivo. *J. Virol.* **73:**7795–7804.

3687. Reeves, J. D., F.-H. Lee, J. L. Miamidian, C. B. Jabara, M. M. Juntilla, and R. W. Doms. 2005. Enfuvirtide resistance mutations: impact on human immunodeficiency virus envelope function, entry inhibitor sensitivity, and virus neutralization. *J. Virol.* **79:**4991–4999.

3688. Reeves, J. D., and T. F. Schulz. 1997. The CD4-independent tropism of human immunodeficiency virus type 2 involves several regions of the envelope protein and correlates with a reduced activation threshold for envelope-mediated fusion. *J. Virol.* **71:**1453–1465.

3689. Reichelderfer, P. S., R. W. Coombs, D. J. Wright, J. Cohn, D. N. Burns, S. Cu-Uvin, P. A. Baron, M. H. Coheng, A. L. Landay, S. K. Beckner, S. R. Lewis, A. A. Kovacs, and the WHS 001 Study Team. 2000. Effect of menstrual cycle on HIV-1 levels in the peripheral blood and genital tract. *AIDS* **14:**2101–2107.

3690. Reiher, W. E. I., J. E. Blalock, and T. K. Brunck. 1986. Sequence homology between acquired immunodeficiency syndrome virus envelope protein and interleukin 2. *Proc. Natl. Acad. Sci. USA* **83:**9188–9192.

3691. Reil, H., A. A. Bukovsky, H. R. Gelderblom, and H. G. Gottlinger. 1998. Efficient HIV-1 replication can occur in the absence of the viral matrix protein. *EMBO J.* **17:**2699–2708.

3691a. Reilly, C., S. Wietgrefe, G. Sedgewick, and A. Haase. 2007. Determination of simian immunodeficiency virus production by infected activated and resting cells. *AIDS* **21:**163–168.

3692. Reimann, K. A., J. T. Li, R. Veazey, M. Halloran, I.-W. Park, G. B. Karlsson, J. Sodroski, and N. L. Letvin. 1996. A chimeric simian/human immunodeficiency virus expressing a primary patient human immunodeficiency virus type 1 isolate env causes an AIDS-like disease after in vivo passage in rhesus monkeys. *J. Virol.* **70:**6922–6928.

3693. Reimann, K. A., K. Tenner-Racz, P. Racz, D. C. Montefiori, Y. Yasutomi, W. Lin, B. J. Ransil, and N. L. Letvin. 1994. Immunopathogenic events in acute infection of rhesus monkeys with simian immunodeficiency virus of macaques. *J. Virol.* **68:**2362–2370.

3694. Reimer, L., S. Mottice, C. Schable, P. Sullivan, A. Nakashima, M. Rayfield, R. Den, and C. Brokopp. 1997. Absence of detectable antibody in a patient infected with human immunodeficiency virus. *Clin. Infect. Dis.* **25:**98–100.

3695. Reinhardt, P. P., B. Reinhardt, J. L. Lathey, and S. A. Spector. 1995. Human cord blood mononuclear cells are preferentially infected by non-syncytium-inducing macrophage-tropic human immunodeficiency virus type 1 isolates. *J. Clin. Microbiol.* **33:**292–297.

3696. Reinhart, T. A., M. J. Rogan, G. A. Viglianti, D. M. Rausch, L. E. Eiden, and A. T. Haase. 1997. A new approach to investigating the relationship between productive infection and cytopathicity *in vivo*. *Nat. Med.* **3:**218–221.

3697. Reinherz, E. L., P. C. Kung, G. Goldstein, R. H. Levey, and S. F. Schlossman. 1980. Discrete stages of human intrathymic differentiation: analysis of normal thymocytes and leukemic lymphoblasts of T-cell lineage. *Proc. Natl. Acad. Sci. USA* **77:**1588–1592.

3698. Reiser, H., and M. J. Stadecker. 1996. Costimulatory B7 molecules in the pathogenesis of infectious and autoimmune diseases. *N. Engl. J. Med.* **335:**1369–1377.

3699. Reiser, J., G. Harmison, S. Kluepfel-Stahl, R. O. Brady, S. Karlsson, and M. Schubert. 1996. Transduction of nondividing cells using pseudotyped defective high-titer HIV type 1 particles. *Proc. Natl. Acad. Sci. USA* **93:**15266–15271.

3700. Reisinger, E. C., W. Vogetseder, D. Berzow, D. Kofler, G. Bitterlich, H. A. Lehr, H. Wachter, and M. P. Dierich. 1990. Complement-mediated enhancement of HIV-1 infection of the monoblastoid cell line U937. *AIDS* **4:**961–965.

3701. Reitz, M. S., Sr., C. Wilson, C. Naugle, R. C. Gallo, and M. Robert-Guroff. 1988. Generation of a neutralization-resistant variant of HIV-1 is due to selection for a point mutation in the envelope gene. *Cell* **54:**57–63.

3702. Rempel, H. C., and L. Pulliam. 2005. HIV-1 Tat inhibits neprilysin and elevates amyloid β. *AIDS* **19:**127–135.

3703. Renjifo, B., P. Gilbert, B. Chaplin, G. Msamanga, D. Mwakagile, W. Fawzi, and M. Essex. 2004. Preferential in-utero transmission of HIV-1 subtype C as compared to HIV-1 subtype A or D. *AIDS* **18:**1629–1636.

3704. Renne, R., W. Zhong, B. Herndier, M. McGrath, N. Abbey, D. Kedes, and D. Ganem. 1996. Lytic growth of Kaposi's sarcoma-associated herpesvirus (human herpesvirus 8) in culture. *Nat. Med.* **2**:342–346.

3705. Renzi, C., J. M. Douglas, Jr., M. Foster, C. W. Critchlow, R. Ashley-Morrow, S. P. Buchbinder, B. A. Koblin, D. J. McKirnan, K. H. Mayer, and C. L. Celum. 2003. Herpes simplex virus type 2 infection as a risk factor for human immunodeficiency virus acquisition in men who have sex with men. *J. Infect. Dis.* **187**:19–25.

3706. Rerks-Ngarm, S., A. E. Brown, C. Khamboonruang, P. Thongcharoen, and P. Kunasol. 2006. HIV/AIDS prevention vaccine "prime-boost" Phase III Trial: foundations and initial lessons learned from Thailand. *AIDS* **20**:1471–1479.

3707. Resch, W., N. Hoffman, and R. Swanstrom. 2001. Improved success of phenotype prediction of the human immunodeficiency virus type 1 from envelope variable loop 3 sequence using neural networks. *Virology* **288**:51–62.

3708. Resch, W., R. Ziermann, N. Parkin, A. Gamarnik, and R. Swanstrom. 2002. Nelfinavir-resistant, amprenavir-hypersusceptible strains of human immunodeficiency virus type 1 carrying an N88S mutation in protease have reduced infectivity, reduced replication capacity, and reduced fitness and process the Gag-polyprotein precursor aberrantly. *J. Virol.* **76**:8659–8666.

3709. Resnick, D. A., A. D. Smith, S. C. Gesiler, A. Zhang, E. Arnold, and G. F. Arnold. 1995. Chimeras from a human rhinovirus 14-human immunodeficiency virus type 1 (HIV-1) V3 loop seroprevalence library induce neutralizing responses against HIV-1. *J. Virol.* **69**:2406–2411.

3710. Rethi, B., C. Fluur, A. Atlas, M. Krzyzowska, F. Mowafi, S. Grutzmeier, A. De Milito, R. Bellocco, K. I. Falk, E. Rajnavolgyi, and F. Chiodi. 2005. Loss of IL-7Ralpha is associated with CD4 T-cell depletion, high interleukin-7 levels and CD28 down-regulation in HIV infected patients. *AIDS* **19**:2077–2086.

3711. Rey, F., G. Donker, I. Hirsch, and J.-C. Chermann. 1991. Productive infection of CD4+ cells by selected HIV strains is not inhibited by anti-CD4 monoclonal antibodies. *Virology* **181**:165–171.

3712. Reyes-Teran, G., J. G. Sierra-Madero, V. Martinez del Cerro, H. Arroyo-Figueroa, A. Pasquetti, J. J. Calva, and G. M. Ruiz-Palacios. 1996. Effects of thalidomide on HIV-associated wasting syndrome: a randomized, double-blind, placebo-controlled clinical trial. *AIDS* **10**:1501–1507.

3713. Reynes, J., P. Portales, M. Segondy, V. Baillat, P. Ande, B. Reant, O. Avinens, G. Couderc, M. Benkirane, J. Clot, J. Eliaou, and P. Corbeau. 2000. CD4+ T cell surface CCR5 density as a determining factor of virus load in persons infected with human immunodeficiency virus type 1. *J. Infect. Dis.* **181**:927–932.

3714. Reynolds, M. R., E. Rakasz, P. J. Skinner, C. White, K. Abel, Z. M. Ma, L. Compton, G. Napoe, N. Wilson, C. J. Miller, A. Haase, and D. I. Watkins. 2005. CD8+ T-lymphocyte response to major immunodominant epitopes after vaginal exposure to simian immunodeficiency virus: too late and too little. *J. Virol.* **79**:9228–9235.

3715. Reynolds, S. J., M. E. Shepherd, A. R. Risbud, R. R. Gangakhedker, R. S. Brookmeyer, A. Divekar, S. M. Mehendale, and R. C. Bollinger. 2004. Male circumcision and risk of HIV-1 and other sexually transmitted infections in India. *Lancet* **363**:1039–1040.

3716. Rezaee, S. A., C. Cunningham, A. J. Davison, and D. J. Blackbourn. 2006. Kaposi's sarcoma-associated herpesvirus immune modulation: an overview. *J. Gen. Virol.* **87**:1781–1804.

3717. Rezza, G., V. Fiorelli, M. Dorrucci, M. Ciccozzi, A. Tripiciano, A. Scoglio, B. Collacchi, M. Ruiz-Alvarez, C. Giannetto, A. Caputo, L. Tomasoni, F. Castelli, M. Sciandra, A. Sinicco, F. Ensoli, S. Butto, and B. Ensoli. 2005. The presence of anti-Tat antibodies is predictive of long-term nonprogression to AIDS or severe immunodeficiency: findings in a cohort of HIV-1 seroconverters. *J. Infect. Dis.* **191**:1321–1324.

3718. Ribaudo, H. J., D. W. Haas, C. Tierney, R. B. Kim, G. R. Wilkinson, R. M. Gulick, D. B. Clifford, C. Marzolini, C. V. Fletcher, K. T. Tashima, D. R. Kuritzkes, and E. P. Acosta. 2006. Pharmacogenetics of plasma efavirenz exposure after treatment discontinuation: an Adult AIDS Clinical Trials Group Study. *Clin. Infect. Dis.* **42**:401–407.

3719. Ribeiro, A., A. Maia e Silva, M. Santa-Marta, A. Pombo, J. Moniz-Pereira, J. Goncalves, and I. Barahona. 2005. Functional analysis of Vif protein shows less restriction of human immunodeficiency virus type 2 by APOBEC3G. *J. Virol.* **79**:823–833.

3720. Rice, W. G., and J. P. Bader. 1995. Discovery and in vitro development of AIDS antiviral drugs as biopharmaceuticals. *Adv. Pharmacol.* **33**:389–438.

3721. Rice, W. G., J. G. Supko, L. Malspeis, R. W. Buckheit, Jr., D. Clanton, M. Bu, L. Graham, C. A. Schaeffer, J. A. Turpin, J. Domagala, R. Gogliotti, J. P. Bader, S. M. Halliday, L. Coren, R. C. Sowder II, L. O. Arthur, and L. E. Henderson. 1995. Inhibitors of HIV nucleocapsid protein zinc fingers as candidates for the treatment of AIDS. *Science* **270**:1194–1197.

3722. Rich, E. A., I. S. Y. Chen, J. A. Zack, M. L. Leonard, and W. A. O'Brien. 1992. Increased susceptibility of differentiated mononuclear phagocytes to productive infection with human immunodeficiency virus-1 (HIV-1). *J. Clin. Investig.* **89**:176–183.

3723. Richards, R. L., M. D. Hayre, W. T. Hockmeyer, and C. R. Alving. 1988. Liposomes, lipid A, and aluminum hydroxide enhance the immune response to a synthetic malaria sporozoite antigen. *Infect. Immun.* **56**:682–686.

3724. Richardson, B. A., G. C. John-Stewart, J. P. Hughes, R. Nduati, D. Mbori-Ngacha, J. Overbaugh, and J. K. Kreiss. 2003. Breast-milk infectivity in human immunodeficiency virus type 1-infected mothers. *J. Infect. Dis.* **187**:736–740.

3725. Richardson, B. A., D. Mbori-Ngacha, L. Lavreys, G. C. John-Stewart, R. Nduati, D. D. Panteleeff, S. Emery, J. K. Kreiss, and J. Overbaugh. 2003. Comparison of human immunodeficiency virus type 1 viral loads in Kenyan women, men, and infants during primary and early infection. *J. Virol.* **77**:7120–7123.

3726. Richardson, J., A. Moraillon, S. Baud, A.-M. Cuisinier, P. Sonigo, and G. Pancino. 1997. Enhancement of feline immunodeficiency virus (FIV) infection after DNA vaccination with the FIV envelope. *J. Virol.* **71**:9640–9649.

3727. Richman, D. D., and S. A. Bozzette. 1994. The impact of the syncytium-inducing phenotype of human immunodeficiency virus on disease progression. *J. Infect. Dis.* **169**:968–974.

3728. Richman, D. D., R. S. Kornbluth, and D. A. Carson. 1987. Failure of dideoxynucleosides to inhibit human immunodeficiency virus replication in cultured human macrophages. *J. Exp. Med.* **166**:1144–1149.

3729. Richman, D. D., T. Wrin, S. J. Little, and C. J. Petropoulos. 2003. Rapid evolution of the neutralizing antibody response to HIV type 1 infection. *Proc. Natl. Acad. Sci. USA* **100**:4144–4149.

3730. Rickman, L. S., D. M. Gordon, R. Wistar, Jr., U. Krzych, M. Gross, M. R. Hollingale, J. E. Egan, J. D. Chulay, and S. L. Hoffman. 1991. Use of adjuvant containing mycobacterial cell-wall skeleton, monophosphoryl lipid A and squalene in malaria circumsporozoite protein vaccine. *Lancet* **337**:998–1001.

3730a. **Rietmeijer, C. A., and M. W. Thrun.** 2006. Mainstreaming HIV testing. *AIDS* **20**:1667–1668.

3731. **Rinaldo, C., L. Kingsley, J. Neumann, D. Reed, P. Gupta, and D. Lyter.** 1989. Association of human immunodeficiency virus (HIV) p24 antigenemia with decrease in CD4$^+$ lymphocytes and onset of acquired immunodeficiency syndrome during the early phase of HIV infection. *J. Clin. Microbiol.* **27**:880–884.

3732. **Rinaldo, C. R., Jr.** 1994. Modulation of major histocompatibility complex antigen expression by viral infection. *Am. J. Pathol.* **144**:637–650.

3733. **Rinaldo, C. R., Jr., L. A. Beltz, X. L. Huang, P. Gupta, Z. Fan, and D. J. Torpey III.** 1995. Anti-HIV type 1 cytotoxic T lymphocyte effector activity and disease progression in the first 8 years of HIV type 1 infection of homosexual men. *AIDS Res. Hum. Retrovir.* **11**:481–489.

3734. **Rissoan, M. C., V. Soumelis, N. Kadowaki, G. Grouard, F. Briere, R. de Waal Malefyt, and Y. J. Liu.** 1999. Reciprocal control of T helper cell and dendritic cell differentiation. *Science* **283**:1183–1186.

3735. **Ritola, K., C. D. Pilcher, S. A. Fiscus, N. G. Hoffman, J. A. E. Nelson, K. M. Kitrinos, C. B. Hicks, J. J. Eron, Jr, and R. Swanstrom.** 2004. Multiple V1/V2 *env* variants are frequently present during primary infection with human immunodeficiency virus type 1. *J. Virol.* **78**:11208–11218.

3736. **Rivera, H., N. G. Nikitakis, J. Castillo, H. Siavash, J. C. Papadimitriou, and J. J. Sauk.** 2003. Histopathological analysis and demonstration of EBV and HIV p-24 antigen but not CMV expression in labial minor salivary glands of HIV patients affected by diffuse infiltrative lymphocytosis syndrome. *J. Oral Pathol. Med.* **32**:431–437.

3737. **Riviere, Y., M. B. McChesney, F. Porrot, F. Tanneau-Salvadori, P. Sansonetti, O. Lopez, G. Pialoux, V. Feuillie, M. Mollereau, S. Chamaret, E. Tekaia, and L. Montagnier.** 1995. Gag-specific cytotoxic responses to HIV type 1 are associated with a decreased risk of progression to AIDS-related complex or AIDS. *AIDS Res. Hum. Retrovir.* **11**:903–907.

3738. **Riviere, Y., F. Tanneau-Salvadori, A. Regnault, O. Lopez, P. Sansonetti, B. Guy, M.-P. Kieny, J.-J. Fournel, and L. Montagnier.** 1989. Human immunodeficiency virus-specific cytotoxic responses of seropositive individuals: distinct types of effector cells mediate killing of targets expressing *gag* and *env* proteins. *J. Virol.* **63**:2270–2277.

3739. **Rizzardi, G. P., W. Barcellini, G. Tambussi, F. Lillo, M. Malnati, L. Perrin, and A. Lazzarin.** 1996. Plasma levels of soluble CD30, tumour necrosis factor (TNF)-α and TNF receptors during primary HIV-1 infection: correlation with HIV-1 RNA and the clinical outcome. *AIDS* **10**:F45-F50.

3740. **Rizzardi, G. P., A. Harari, B. Capiluppi, G. Tambussi, K. Ellefsen, D. Ciuffreda, P. Champagne, P.-A. Bart, J.-P. Chave, A. Lazzarin, and G. Pantaleo.** 2002. Treatment of primary HIV-1 infection with cyclosporin A coupled with highly active antiretroviral therapy. *J. Clin. Investig.* **109**:681–688.

3741. **Rizzardini, G., S. Piconi, S. Ruzzante, M. L. Fusi, M. Lukwiya, S. Declich, M. Tamburini, M. L. Villa, M. Fabiani, F. Milazzo, and M. Clerici.** 1996. Immunological activation markers in the serum of African and European HIV-seropositive and seronegative individuals. *AIDS* **10**:1535–1542.

3742. **Rizzuto, C. D., and J. G. Sodroski.** 1997. Contribution of virion ICAM-1 to human immunodeficiency virus infectivity and sensitivity to neutralization. *J. Virol.* **71**:4847–4851.

3743. **Rizzuto, C. D., R. Wyatt, N. Hernandez-Ramos, Y. Sun, P. D. Kwong, W. A. Hendrickson, and J. Sodroski.** 1998. A conserved HIV gp120 glycoprotein structure involved in chemokine receptor binding. *Science* **280**:1949–1953.

3744. **Robain, M., F. Boufassa, J. Hubert, A. Persoz, M. Burgard, and L. Meyer.** 2001. Cytomegalovirus seroconversion as a cofactor for progression to AIDS. *AIDS* **15**:251–256.

3745. **Robbins, D. S., Y. Shirazi, B. E. Drysdale, A. Lieberman, H. S. Shin, and M. L. Shin.** 1987. Production of cytotoxic factor for oligodendrocytes by stimulated astrocytes. *J. Immunol.* **139**:2593–2597.

3746. **Robbins, G. K., M. M. Addo, H. Troung, A. Rathod, K. Habeeb, B. Davis, H. Heller, N. Basgoz, B. D. Walker, and E. S. Rosenberg.** 2003. Augmentation of HIV-1-specific T helper cell responses in chronic HIV-1 infection by therapeutic immunization. *AIDS* **17**:1121–1126.

3747. **Robbins, K. E., P. Lemey, O. G. Pybus, H. W. Jaffe, A. S. Youngpairoj, T. M. Brown, M. Salemi, A. Vandamme, and M. L. Kalish.** 2003. U.S. human immunodeficiency virus type 1 epidemic: date of origin, population history, and characterization of early strains. *J. Virol.* **77**:6359–6366.

3748. **Robert-Guroff, M., K. Aldrich, R. Muldoon, T. L. Stern, G. P. Bansal, T. J. Matthews, P. D. Markham, R. C. Gallo, and G. Franchini.** 1992. Cross-neutralization of human immunodeficiency virus type 1 and 2 and simian immunodeficiency virus isolates. *J. Virol.* **66**:3602–3608.

3749. **Robert-Guroff, M., M. Brown, and R. Gallo.** 1985. HTLV-III neutralizing antibodies in patients with AIDS and AIDS-related complex. *Nature* **316**:72–74.

3750. **Robert-Guroff, M., M. Popovic, S. Gartner, P. Markham, R. C. Gallo, and M. S. Reitz.** 1990. Structure and expression of Tat-, Rev-, and Nef-specific transcripts of human immunodeficiency virus type 1 in infected lymphocytes and macrophages. *J. Virol.* **64**:3391–3398.

3751. **Robert-Guroff, M., M. S. Reitz, Jr., W. G. Robey, and R. C. Gallo.** 1986. *In vitro* generation of an HTLV-III variant by neutralizing antibody. *J. Immunol.* **137**:3306–3309.

3752. **Roberts, E. S., E. Masliah, and H. S. Fox.** 2004. CD163 identifies a unique population of ramified microglia in HIV encephalitis (HIVE). *J. Neuropathol. Exp. Neurol.* **63**:1255–1264.

3753. **Roberts, J. D., K. Bebenek, and T. A. Kunkel.** 1988. The accuracy of reverse transcriptase from HIV-1. *Science* **242**:1171–1173.

3754. **Roberts, N. A., J. A. Martin, D. Kinchington, A. V. Broadhurst, J. C. Craig, I. B. Duncan, S. A. Galpin, B. J. Handa, J. Kay, A. Krohn, R. W. Lambert, J. H. Merrett, J. S. Mills, K. E. B. Parkes, S. Redshaw, A. J. Ritchie, D. L. Taylor, G. J. Thomas, and P. J. Machin.** 1990. Rational design of peptide-based HIV proteinase inhibitors. *Science* **248**:358–361.

3755. **Robertson, D. L., J. P. Anderson, J. A. Bradac, J. K. Carr, B. Foley, R. K. Funkhouser, F. Gao, B. H. Hahn, M. L. Kalish, C. Kuiken, G. H. Learn, T. Leitner, F. McCutchan, S. Osmanov, M. Peeters, D. Pieniazek, M. Salminen, P. M. Sharp, S. Wolinsky, and B. Korber.** 2000. HIV-1 nomenclature proposal. *Science* **288**:55–56.

3756. **Robertson, D. L., P. M. Sharp, F. E. McCutchan, and B. H. Hahn.** 1995. Recombination in HIV-1. *Nature* **374**:124–126.

3757. **Robinson, E. K., and B. G. Evans.** 1999. Oral sex and HIV transmission. *AIDS* **13**:737–738.

3758. **Robinson, F. P., H. L. Mathews, and L. Witek-Janusek.** 2000. Stress reduction and HIV disease: a review of intervention studies using a psychoneuroimmunology framework. *J. Assoc. Nurses AIDS Care* 11:87–96.

3759. **Robinson, H. L.** 1997. DNA vaccines for immunodeficiency viruses. *AIDS* 11:S109-S119.

3760. **Robinson, H. L.** 2002. New hope for an AIDS vaccine. *Nat. Rev. Immunol.* 2:239–250.

3761. **Robinson, H. L., and R. R. Amara.** 2005. T cell vaccines for microbial infections. *Nat. Med.* 11:S25-S32.

3761a. **Robinson, H. L., and K. J. Weinhold.** 2006. Phase 1 clinical trials of the National Institutes of Health Vaccine Research Center HIV/AIDS candidate vaccines. *J. Infect. Dis.* 194:1625–1627.

3762. **Robinson, H. L., and D. M. Zinkus.** 1990. Accumulation of human immunodeficiency virus type 1 DNA in T cells: results of multiple infection events. *J. Virol.* 64:4836–4841.

3762a. **Robinson, M. J., D. Sancho, E. C. Slack, S. Leibundgut-Landmann, and C. R. Sousa.** 2006. Myeloid C-type lectins in innate immunity. *Nat. Immunol.* 7:1258–1265.

3763. **Robinson, W. E., Jr., M. K. Gorny, J.-Y. Xu, W. M. Mitchell, and S. Zolla-Pazner.** 1991. Two immunodominant domains of gp41 bind antibodies which enhance human immunodeficiency virus type 1 infection in vitro. *J. Virol.* 65:4169–4176.

3764. **Robinson, W. E., Jr., T. Kawamura, M. K. Gorny, D. Lake, J.-Y. Xu, Y. Matsumoto, T. Sugano, Y. Masuho, W. M. Mitchell, E. Hersh, and S. Zolla-Pazner.** 1990. Human monoclonal antibodies to the human immunodeficiency virus type 1 (HIV-1) transmembrane glycoprotein gp41 enhance HIV-1 infection *in vitro. Proc. Natl. Acad. Sci. USA* 87:3185–3189.

3765. **Robinson, W. E., Jr., and W. M. Mitchell.** 1990. Neutralization and enhancement of *in vitro* and *in vivo* HIV and simian immunodeficiency virus infections. *AIDS* 4:S151-S162.

3766. **Robinson, W. E., Jr., D. C. Montefiori, and W. M. Mitchell.** 1988. Antibody-dependent enhancement of human immunodeficiency virus type 1 infection. *Lancet* i:790–794.

3767. **Robinson, W. E., Jr., D. C. Montefiori, and W. M. Mitchell.** 1990. Complement-mediated antibody-dependent enhancement of HIV-1 infection requires CD4 and complement receptors. *Virology* 175:600–604.

3768. **Rocha, B., N. Dautigny, and P. Pereira.** 1989. Peripheral T lymphocytes: expansion potential and homeostatic regulation of pool sizes and CD4/CD8 ratios *in vivo. Eur. J. Immunol.* 19:905–911.

3769. **Rodman, T. C., J. D. Lutton, S. Jiang, H. B. Al-Kouatly, and R. Winston.** 2001. Circulating natural IgM antibodies and their corresponding human cord blood cell-derived Mabs specifically combat the Tat protein of HIV. *Exp. Hematol.* 29:1004–1009.

3770. **Rodman, T. C., F. H. Pruslin, S. E. To, and R. Winston.** 1992. Human immunodeficiency virus (HIV) Tat-reactive antibodies present in normal HIV-negative sera and depleted in HIV-positive sera. Identification of the epitope. *J. Exp. Med.* 175:1247–1253.

3771. **Rodman, T. C., J. J. Sullivan, X. Bai, and R. Winston.** 1999. The human uniqueness of HIV: innate immunity and the viral Tat protein. *Hum. Immunol.* 60:631–639.

3772. **Rodman, T. C., S. E. To, H. Hashish, and K. Manchester.** 1993. Epitopes for natural antibodies of human immunodeficiency virus (HIV)-negative (normal) and HIV-positive sera are coincident with two key functional sequences of HIV Tat protein. *Proc. Natl. Acad. Sci. USA* 90:7719–7723.

3772a. **Rodriguez, B., M. M. Lederman, W. Jiang, D. A. Bazdar, K. Garate, C. V. Harding, and S. F. Sieg.** 2006. Interferon-alpha differentially rescues CD4 and CD8 T cells from apoptosis in HIV infection. *AIDS* 20:1379–1389.

3772b. **Rodriguez, B., A. K. Sethi, V. K. Cheruvu, W. Mackay, R. J. Bosch, M. Kitahata, S. L. Boswell, W. C. Mathews, D. R. Bangsberg, J. Martin, C. C. Whalen, S. Sieg, S. Yadavalli, S. G. Deeks, and M. M. Lederman.** 2006. Predictive value of plasma HIV RNA level on rate of CD4 T-cell decline in untreated HIV infection. *JAMA* 296:1498–1506.

3773. **Rodriguez, E. M., L. M. Mofenson, B.-H. Chang, K. C. Rich, M. G. Fowler, V. Smeriglio, S. Landesman, H. E. Fox, C. Diaz, K. Green, and I. C. Hanson.** 1996. Association of maternal drug use during pregnancy with maternal HIV culture positivity and perinatal HIV transmission. *AIDS* 10:273–282.

3774. **Rodriguez, E. R., S. Nasim, J. Hsia, R. L. Sandin, A. Ferreira, B. A. Hilliard, A. M. Ross, and C. T. Garrett.** 1991. Cardiac myocytes and dendritic cells harbor human immunodeficiency virus in infected patients with and without cardiac dysfunction: detection by multiplex, nested, polymerase chain reaction in individually microdissected cells from right ventricular endomyocardial biopsy tissue. *Am. J. Cardiol.* 68:1511–1520.

3775. **Rodriguez, M., K. D. Pavelko, M. K. Njenga, W. C. Logan, and P. J. Wettstein.** 1996. The balance between persistent virus infection and immune cells determines demyelination. *J. Immunol.* 157:5699–5709.

3775a. **Rodriguez, S. K., A. D. Sarr, O. Olorunnipa, S. J. Popper, A. Gueye-Ndiaye, I. Traore, M. C. Dia, S. Mboup, and P. J. Kanki.** 2006. The absence of anti-Tat antibodies is associated with risk of disease progression in HIV-2 infection. *J. Infect. Dis.* 194:760–763.

3776. **Rodriguez-Novoa, S., P. Barreiro, A. Rendon, I. Jimenez-Nacher, J. Gonzalez-Lahoz, and V. Soriano.** 2005. Influence of 516G>T polymorphisms at the gene encoding the CYP450–2B6 isoenzyme on efavirenz plasma concentrations in HIV-infected subjects. *Clin. Infect. Dis.* 40:1358–1361.

3777. **Roederer, M., J. G. Dubs, M. T. Anderson, P. A. Raju, L. A. Herzenberg, and L. A. Herzenberg.** 1995. CD8 naive T cell counts decrease progressively in HIV-infected adults. *J. Clin. Investig.* 95:2061–2066.

3778. **Roederer, M., P. A. Raju, D. K. Mitra, L. A. Herzenberg, and L. A. Herzenberg.** 1997. HIV does not replicate in naive CD4 T cells stimulated with CD3/CD28. *J. Clin. Investig.* 99:1555–1564.

3779. **Roeth, J. F., M. Williams, M. R. Kasper, T. M. Filzen, and K. L. Collins.** 2004. HIV-1 Nef disrupts MHC-I trafficking by recruiting AP-1 to the MHC-I cytoplasmic tail. *J. Cell Biol.* 167:903–913.

3780. **Rogers, M. F., C. R. White, R. Sanders, C. Schable, T. E. Ksell, R. L. Wasserman, J. A. Bellanti, S. M. Peters, and B. B. Wray.** 1990. Lack of transmission of human immunodeficiency virus from infected children to their household contacts. *Pediatrics* 85:210–214.

3781. **Rogge, L., L. Barberis-Maino, M. Biffi, N. Passini, D. H. Presky, U. Gubler, and F. Sinigaglia.** 1997. Selective expression of an interleukin-12 receptor component by human T helper 1 cells. *J. Exp. Med.* 185:825–831.

3782. **Rogge, L., D. D'Ambrosio, M. Biffi, G. Penna, L. J. Minetti, D. H. Presky, L. Adorini, and F. Sinigaglia.** 1998. The role of Stat4 in species-specific regulation of Th cell development by type I IFNs. *J. Immunol.* 161:6567–6574.

3783. **Roglic, M., R. D. MacPhee, S. R. Duncan, F. R. Sattler, and A. N. Theofilopoulos.** 1997. T cell receptor (TCR) BV gene repertoires and clonal expansions of CD4 cells in patients with HIV infections. *Clin. Exp. Immunol.* **107:**21–30.

3784. **Roland, M. E., and D. V. Havlir.** 2003. Responding to organ failure in HIV-infected patients. *N. Engl. J. Med.* **348:**2279–2281.

3785. **Roland, M. E., J. N. Martin, R. M. Grant, N. S. Hellmann, J. D. Bamberger, M. H. Katz, M. Chesney, K. Franses, T. J. Coates, and J. O. Kahn.** 2001. Postexposure prophylaxis for human immunodeficiency virus infection after sexual or injection drug use exposure: identification and characterization of the source of exposure. *J. Infect. Dis.* **184:**1608–1612.

3786. **Romagnani, S.** 1992. Human TH1 and TH2 subsets: regulation of differentiation and role in protection and immunopathology. *Int. Arch. Allergy Immunol.* **98:**279–285.

3787. **Romagnani, S.** 1992. Induction of TH1 and TH2 responses: a key role for the 'natural' immune response? *Immunol. Today* **13:**379–381.

3788. **Roman, M., J. W. Rodriguez, N. O. Pagan, E. Rios-Olivares, A. Amill, and R. Hunter.** 2002. Distribution of naive (CD45RA+) and memory (CD45RO+) T-cells in HIV-infected Puerto Rican population. *P. R. Health Sci. J.* **21:**195–201.

3789. **Romeria, F., M. N. Gabriel, and D. M. Margolis.** 1997. Repression of human immunodeficiency virus type 1 through the novel cooperation of human factors YY1 and LSF. *J. Virol.* **71:**9375–9382.

3790. **Rook, A. H., J. J. Hooks, G. V. Quinnan, H. C. Lane, J. F. Manischewitz, A. M. Macher, H. Masur, A. S. Fauci, and J. Y. Djeu.** 1985. Interleukin-2 enhances the natural killer cell activity of acquired immune deficiency syndrome patients through a gamma-interferon-independent mechanism. *J. Immunol.* **134:**1503–1507.

3791. **Rook, A. H., H. C. Lane, T. Folks, S. McCoy, H. Alter, and A. S. Fauci.** 1987. Sera from HTLV-III/LAV antibody-positive individuals mediate antibody-dependent cellular cytotoxicity against HTLV-III/LAV-infected T cells. *J. Immunol.* **138:**1064–1067.

3792. **Roos, M. T. L., J. M. A. Lange, R. E. Y. de Goede, R. A. Coutinho, P. T. A. Schellenkens, F. Miedema, and M. Termsette.** 1992. Viral phenotype and immune response in primary human immunodeficiency virus type 1 infection. *J. Infect. Dis.* **165:**427–432.

3793. **Roos, M. T. L., F. Miedema, M. Koot, M. Tersmette, W. P. Schaasberg, R. A. Coutinho, and P. T. A. Schellekens.** 1995. T cell function *in vitro* is an independent progression marker for AIDS in human immunodeficiency virus-infected asymptomatic subjects. *J. Infect. Dis.* **171:**531–536.

3794. **Roos, M. T. L., F. Miedema, A. A. P. Meinesz, N. A. S. M. De Leeuw, N. G. Pakker, J. M. A. Lange, R. A. Coutinho, and P. T. A. Schellekens.** 1996. Low T cell reactivity to combined CD3 plus CD28 stimulation is predictive for progression to AIDS: correlation with decreased CD28 expression. *Clin. Exp. Immunol.* **105:**409–415.

3795. **Roques, P., E. Menu, R. Narwa, G. Scarlatti, E. Tresoldi, F. Damond, P. Mauclere, D. Dormont, G. Chaouat, F. Simon, and F. Barre-Sinoussi.** 1999. An unusual HIV type 1 env sequence embedded in a mosaic virus from Cameroon: identification of a new env clade. European Network on the study of in utero transmission of HIV-1. *AIDS Res. Hum. Retrovir.* **15:**1585–1589.

3796. **Roques, P., D. L. Robertson, S. Souquiere, C. Apetrei, E. Nerrienet, F. Barre-Sinoussi, M. Muller-Trutwin, and F. Simon.** 2004. Phylogenetic characteristics of three new HIV-1 N strains and implications for the origin of group N. *AIDS* **18:**1371–1381.

3797. **Roques, P., D. L. Robertson, S. Souquiere, F. Damond, A. Ayouba, I. Farfara, C. Depienne, E. Nerrienet, D. Dormont, F. Brun-Vezinet, F. Simon, and P. Mauclere.** 2002. Phylogenetic analysis of 49 newly derived HIV-1 group O strains: high viral diversity but no group M-like subtype structure. *Virology* **302:**259–273.

3798. **Rosas-Taraco, A. G., A. Y. Arce-Mendoza, G. Caballero-Olin, and M. C. Salinas-Carmona.** 2006. *Mycobacterium tuberculosis* upregulates coreceptors CCR5 and CXCR4 while HIV modulates CD14 favoring concurrent infection. *AIDS Res. Hum. Retrovir.* **22:**45–51.

3799. **Rose, R. E., Y. F. Gong, J. A. Greytok, C. M. Bechtold, B. J. Terry, B. S. Robinson, M. Alam, R. J. Colonno, and P. F. Lin.** 1996. Human immunodeficiency virus type 1 viral background plays a major role in development of resistance to protease inhibitors. *Proc. Natl. Acad. Sci. USA* **93:**1648–1653.

3800. **Rose, T. M., K. B. Strand, E. R. Schultz, G. Schaefer, G. W. Randkin, Jr., M. E. Thouless, C. C. Tsai, and M. L. Bosch.** 1997. Identification of two homologs of the Kaposi's sarcoma-associated herpesvirus (human herpesvirus 8) in retroperitoneal fibromatosis of different macaque species. *J. Virol.* **71:**4138–4144.

3801. **Rosenberg, E. S., M. Altfeld, S. H. Poon, M. N. Phillips, B. M. Wilkes, R. L. Eldridge, G. K. Robbins, R. T. D'Aquila, P. J. Goulder, and B. D. Walker.** 2000. Immune control of HIV-1 after early treatment of acute infection. *Nature* **407:**523–526.

3802. **Rosenberg, E. S., J. M. Billingsley, A. M. Caliendo, S. L. Boswell, P. E. Sax, S. A. Kalams, and B. D. Walker.** 1997. Vigorous HIV-1-specific CD4+ T cell responses associated with control of viremia. *Science* **278:**1447–1450.

3803. **Rosenberg, Y. J., A. O. Anderson, and R. Pabst.** 1998. HIV-induced decline in blood CD4/CD8 ratios: viral killing or altered lymphocyte trafficking? *Immunol. Today* **19:**10–17.

3804. **Rosenberg, Y. J., P. M. Zack, E. C. Leon, B. D. White, S. F. Papermaster, E. Hall, J. J. Greenhouse, G. A. Eddy, and M. G. Lewis.** 1994. Immunological and virological changes associated with decline in CD4/CD8 ratios in lymphoid organs of SIV-infected macaques. *AIDS Res. Hum. Retrovir.* **10:**863–872.

3805. **Rosenwirth, B., P. ten Haaft, W. M. Bogers, I. G. Nieuwenhuis, H. Niphuis, E. M. Kuhn, N. Bischofberger, J. L. Heeney, and K. Uberla.** 2000. Antiretroviral therapy during primary immunodeficiency virus infection can induce persistent suppression of virus load and protection from heterologous challenge in rhesus macaques. *J. Virol.* **74:**1704–1711.

3806. **Rosler, C., J. Kock, M. H. Malim, H. E. Blum, and F. von Weizsacker.** 2004. Comment on "Inhibition of hepatitis B virus replication by APOBEC3G". *Science* **305:**1403.

3807. **Rosok, B., J. E. Brinchmann, P. Voltersvik, J. Olofsson, L. Bostad, and B. Asjo.** 1997. Correlates of latent and productive HIV type-1 infection in tonsillar CD4+ T cells. *Proc. Natl. Acad. Sci. USA* **94:**9332–9336.

3808. **Rosok, B., P. Voltersvik, B.-M. Larsson, J. Albert, J. E. Brinchmann, and B. Asjo.** 1997. CD8+ T cells from HIV type 1-seronegative individuals suppress virus replication in acutely infected cells. *AIDS Res. Hum. Retrovir.* **13:**79–85.

3809. **Rosok, B. I., L. Bostad, P. Voltersvik, R. Bjerknes, J. Olofsson, B. Asjo, and J. E. Brinchmann.** 1996. Reduced CD4 cell counts in blood do not reflect CD4 cell depletion in tonsillar tissue in asymptomatic HIV-1 infection. *AIDS* **10:**F35-F38.

3810. Ross, A., L. Van der Paal, R. Lubega, B. N. Mayanja, L. Shafer, and J. Whitworth. 2004. HIV-1 disease progression and fertility: the incidence of recognized pregnancy and pregnancy outcome in Uganda. *AIDS* 18:799–804.

3811. Ross, M. J., and P. E. Klotman. 2004. HIV-associated nephropathy. *AIDS* 18:1089–1099.

3812. Ross, M. J., P. E. Klotman, and J. A. Winston. 2000. HIV-associated nephropathy: case study and review of the literature. *AIDS Patient Care STDS* 14:637–645.

3813. Rossi, J. J., D. Elkins, J. A. Zaia, and S. Sullivan. 1992. Ribozymes as anti-HIV-1 therapeutic agents: principles, applications, and problems. *AIDS Res. Hum. Retrovir.* 8:183–189.

3814. Rossi, P., V. Moschese, P. A. Broliden, C. Fundaro, I. Quinti, A. Plebani, C. Giaquinto, P. A. Tovo, K. Ljunggren, J. Rosen, H. Wigzell, M. Jondal, and B. Wahren. 1989. Presence of maternal antibodies to human immunodeficiency virus 1 envelope glycoprotein gp120 epitopes correlates with the uninfected status of children born to seropositive mothers. *Proc. Natl. Acad. Sci. USA* 86:8055–8058.

3815. Rossio, J. L., M. T. Esser, K. Suryanarayana, D. K. Schneider, J. W. Bess, Jr., G. M. Vasquez, T. A. Wiltrout, E. Chertova, M. K. Grimes, Q. Sattentau, L. O. Arthur, L. E. Henderson, and J. D. Lifson. 1998. Inactivation of human immunodeficiency virus type 1 infectivity with preservation of conformational and functional integrity of virion surface proteins. *J. Virol.* 72:7992–8001.

3816. Roth, W. K. 1991. HIV-associated Kaposi's sarcoma: new developments in epidemiology and molecular pathology. *J. Cancer Res. Clin. Oncol.* 117:186–191.

3817. Roth, W. K., H. Brandstetter, and M. Sturzl. 1992. Cellular and molecular features of HIV-associated Kaposi's sarcoma. *AIDS* 6:895–913.

3818. Rothenberg, R. B., M. Scarlett, C. delRio, D. Reznik, and C. Odaniels. 1998. Oral transmission of HIV. *AIDS* 12:2095–2105.

3819. Rouse, B. T., and D. W. Horohov. 1986. Immunosuppression in viral infections. *Rev. Infect. Dis.* 8:850–873.

3820. Rousseau, C., R. W. Nduati, B. A. Richardson, G. C. John-Stewart, D. A. Mbori-Ngacha, J. K. Kreiss, and J. Overbaugh. 2004. Association of levels of HIV-1-infected breast milk cells and risk of mother-to-child transmission. *J. Infect. Dis.* 190:1880–1888.

3821. Rousseau, C. M., R. W. Nduati, B. A. Richardson, M. S. Steele, G. C. John-Stewart, D. A. Mbori-Ngacha, J. K. Kreiss, and J. Overbaugh. 2003. Longitudinal analysis of human immunodeficiency virus type 1 RNA in breast milk and of its relationship to infant infection and maternal disease. *J. Infect. Dis.* 187:741–747.

3822. Rousseau, F. S., C. Wakeford, H. Mommeja-Marin, I. Sanne, C. Moxham, J. Harris, L. Hulett, L. H. Wang, J. B. Quinn, and D. W. Barry. 2003. Prospective randomized trial of emtricitabine versus lamivudine short-term monotherapy in human immunodeficiency virus-infected patients. *J. Infect. Dis.* 188:1652–1658.

3823. Routy, J. P., P. Vanhems, D. Rouleau, C. Tsoukas, E. Lefebvre, P. Cote, R. LeBlanc, B. Conway, M. Alary, J. Bruneau, and R. P. Sekaly. 2000. Comparison of clinical features of acute HIV-1 infection in patients infected sexually or through injection drug use. *J. Acquir. Immune Defic. Syndr.* 24:425–432.

3824. Rovinski, B., L. Rodrigues, S. X. Cao, F. L. Yao, U. McGuinness, C. Sia, G. Cates, S. Zolla-Pazner, S. Karwowska, T. J. Matthews, C. B. McDanal, J. Mascola, and M. H. Klein. 1995. Induction of HIV type 1 neutralizing and *env*-CD4 blocking

antibodies by immunization with genetically engineered HIV type 1-like particles containing unprocessed gp160 glycoproteins. *AIDS Res. Hum. Retrovir.* 11:1187–1195.

3825. Rowland-Jones, S., and A. McMichael. 1993. Cytotoxic T lymphocytes in HIV infection. *Semin. Virol.* 4:83–94.

3826. Rowland-Jones, S., J. Sutton, K. Ariyoshi, T. Dong, F. Gotch, S. McAdam, D. Whitby, S. Sabally, A. Gallimore, T. Corrah, et al. 1995. HIV-specific cytotoxic T-cells in HIV-exposed but uninfected Gambian women. *Nat. Med.* 1:59–64.

3827. Rowland-Jones, S., R. Tan, and A. McMichael. 1997. Role of cellular immunity in protection against HIV infection. *Adv. Immunol.* 65:277.

3828. Rowland-Jones, S. L., and A. McMichael. 1995. Immune responses in HIV-exposed seronegatives: have they repelled the virus? *Curr. Opin. Immunol.* 7:448–455.

3829. Roy, A. M., B. Schweighardt, L. A. Eckstein, M. A. Goldsmith, and J. M. McCune. 2005. Enhanced replication of R5 HIV-1 over X4 HIV-1 in CD4(+)CCR5(+)CXCR4(+) T cells. *J. Acquir. Immune Defic. Syndr.* 40:267–275.

3830. Roy, S., L. Fitz-Gibbon, L. Poulin, and M. A. Wainberg. 1988. Infection of human monocytes/macrophages by HIV-1: effect on secretion of IL-1 activity. *Immunology* 64:233–239.

3831. Royce, R. A., A. Sena, W. Cates, Jr., and M. S. Cohen. 1997. Sexual transmission of HIV. *N. Engl. J. Med.* 336:1072–1078.

3832. Rubbert, A., C. Combadiere, M. Ostrowski, J. Arthos, M. Dybul, E. Machado, M. A. Cohn, J. A. Hoxie, P. M. Murphy, A. S. Fauci, and D. Weissman. 1998. Dendritic cells express multiple chemokine receptors used as coreceptors for HIV entry. *J. Immunol.* 160:3933–3941.

3833. Rubbert, A., D. Weissman, C. Combadiere, K. A. Pettrone, J. A. Daucher, P. M. Murphy, and A. S. Fauci. 1997. Multifactorial nature of noncytolytic CD8+ T cell-mediated suppression of HIV replication: β-chemokine-dependent and -independent effects. *AIDS Res. Hum. Retrovir.* 13:63–69.

3834. Rucker, J., A. L. Edinger, M. Sharron, M. Samson, B. Lee, J. F. Berson, Y. Yi, B. Margulies, R. G. Collman, B. J. Doranz, M. Parmentier, and R. W. Doms. 1997. Utilization of chemokine receptors, orphan receptors, and herpesvirus-encoded receptors by diverse human and simian immunodeficiency viruses. *J. Virol.* 71:8999–9007.

3835. Rucker, J., M. Samson, B. J. Doranz, F. Libert, J. F. Berson, Y. Yi, R. J. Smyth, R. G. Collman, C. C. Broder, G. Vassart, R. W. Doms, and M. Parmentier. 1996. Regions in beta-chemokine receptors CCR5 and CCR2b that determine HIV-1 cofactor specificity. *Cell* 87:437–446.

3836. Rudbach, J. A., J. L. Cantrell, and J. T. Ulrich. 1988. Molecularly engineered microbial immunostimulators, p. 443–454. *In* L. Lasky (ed.), *Technological Advances in Vaccine Development.* Alan R. Liss, Inc., New York, N.Y.

3837. Rudin, A., E. L. Johansson, C. Bergquist, and J. Holmgren. 1998. Differential kinetics and distribution of antibodies in serum and nasal and vaginal secretions after nasal and oral vaccination of humans. *Infect. Immun.* 66:3390–3396.

3838. Ruegg, C. L., C. R. Monell, and M. Strand. 1989. Inhibition of lymphoproliferation by a synthetic peptide with sequence identity to gp41 of human immunodeficiency virus type 1. *J. Virol.* 63:3257–3260.

3839. Ruegg, C. L., and M. Strand. 1991. A synthetic peptide with sequence identity to the transmembrane protein gp41 of HIV-1 inhibits distinct lymphocyte activation pathways dependent on protein kinase C and intracellular calcium influx. *Cell. Immunol.* 137:1–13.

3840. Ruff, A. J., J. Coberly, N. A. Halsey, R. Boulos, J. Desormeaux, A. Burnley, D. J. Joseph, M. McBrien, T. Quinn, P. Losikoff, K. L. O'Brien, M. A. Louis, and H. Farzadegan. 1994. Prevalence of HIV-1 DNA and p24 antigen in breast milk and correlation with maternal factors. *J. Acquir. Immune Defic. Syndr.* 7:68–73.

3841. Rugeles, M. R., C. M. Trubey, V. I. Bedoya, L. A. Pinto, J. J. Oppenheim, S. M. Rybak, and G. M. Shearer. 2003. Ribonuclease is partly responsible for the HIV-1 inhibitory effect activated by HLA alloantigen recognition. *AIDS* 17:481–486.

3842. Ruiz, L., J. Martinez-Picado, J. Romeu, R. Paredes, M. K. Zayat, S. Marfil, E. Negredo, G. Sirera, C. Tural, and B. Clotet. 2000. Structured treatment interruption in chronically HIV-1 infected patients after long-term viral suppression. *AIDS* 14:397–403.

3843. Ruppach, H., P. Nara, I. Raudonat, Z. Elanjikal, H. Rubsamen-Waigmann, and U. Dietrich. 2000. Human immunodeficiency virus (HIV)-positive sera obtained shortly after seroconversion neutralize autologous HIV type 1 isolates on primary macrophages but not on lymphocytes. *J. Virol.* 74:5403–5411.

3844. Ruprecht, R. M. 1999. Live attenuated AIDS viruses as vaccines: promise or peril? *Immunol. Rev.* 170:135–149.

3845. Ruprecht, R. M., T. W. Baba, R. Rasmussen, Y. Hu, and P. L. Sharma. 1996. Murine and simian retrovirus models: the threshold hypothesis. *AIDS* 10 (Suppl. A):S33–S40.

3846. Russell, M. W., S. R. Hedges, H. Y. Wu, E. W. Hook III, and J. Mestecky. 1999. Mucosal immunity in the genital tract: prospects for vaccines against sexually transmitted diseases—a review. *Am. J. Reprod. Immunol.* 42:58–63.

3847. Russell-Jones, R., and E. Wilson-Jones. 1988. The histogenesis of Kaposi's sarcoma. *Am. J. Dermatopathol.* 8:369–370.

3848. Russo, J. J., R. A. Bohenzky, M. C. Chien, J. Chen, M. Yan, D. Maddalena, J. P. Parry, D. Peruzzi, I. S. Edelman, Y. Chang, and P. S. Moore. 1996. Nucleotide sequence of Kaposi sarcoma-associated herpesvirus (HHV8). *Proc. Natl. Acad. Sci. USA* 93:14862–14867.

3849. Rutherford, G. W., A. R. Lifson, and N. A. Hessol. 1990. Course of HIV-1 infection in a cohort of homosexual and bisexual men: an 11 year follow up study. *BMJ* 301:1183–1188.

3850. Rutka, J. T., J. R. Giblin, M. E. Berens, E. Bar-Shiva, K. Tokuda, J. R. McCulloch, M. L. Rosenblum, T. E. Eessalu, B. B. Aggarwal, and W. J. Bodell. 1988. The effects of human recombinant tumor necrosis factor on glioma-derived cell lines: cellular proliferation, cytotoxicity, morphological and radioreceptor studies. *Int. J. Cancer* 41:573–582.

3851. Ryan-Graham, M. A., and K. W. C. Peden. 1995. Both virus and host components are important for the manifestation of Nef- phenotype in HIV-1 and HIV-2. *Virology* 213:158–168.

3852. Ryu, S. E., P. D. Kwong, A. Truneh, T. G. Porter, J. Arthos, M. Rosenberg, X. Dai, N. Xuong, R. Axel, R. W. Sweet, and W. A. Hendrickson. 1990. Crystal structure of an HIV-binding recombinant fragment of human CD4. *Nature* 348:419–426.

3853. Saada, M., J. Le Chenadec, A. Berrebi, A. Bongain, J.-F. Delfraissy, M.-J. Mayaux, and L. Meyer. 2000. Pregnancy and progression to AIDS: results of the French prospective cohorts. *AIDS* 14:2355–2360.

3854. Saag, M. S., B. H. Hahn, J. Gibbons, Y. Li, E. S. Parks, W. P. Parks, and G. M. Shaw. 1988. Extensive variation of human immunodeficiency virus type-1 *in vivo. Nature* 334:440–444.

3855. Saarloos, M.-N., B. L. Sullivan, M. A. Czerniewski, K. D. Parameswar, and G. T. Spear. 1997. Detection of HLA-DR associated with monocytotropic, primary, and plasma isolate of human immunodeficiency virus type 1. *J. Virol.* 71:1640–1643.

3856. Sabatier, J.-M., E. Vives, K. Mabrouk, A. Benjouad, H. Rochat, A. Duval, B. Hue, and E. Bahraoui. 1991. Evidence for neurotoxic activity of *tat* from human immunodeficiency virus type 1. *J. Virol.* 65:961–967.

3857. Sabbaj, S., B. H. Edwards, M. K. Ghosh, K. Semrau, S. Cheelo, D. M. Thea, L. Kuhn, G. D. Ritter, M. J. Mulligan, P. A. Goepfert, and G. M. Aldrovandi. 2002. Human immunodeficiency virus-specific CD8(+) T cells in human breast milk. *J. Virol.* 76:7365–7373.

3858. Sabin, A. B. 1992. Improbability of effective vaccination against human immunodeficiency virus because of its intracellular transmission and rectal portal of entry. *Proc. Natl. Acad. Sci. USA* 89:8852–8855.

3859. Sabin, E. A., M. I. Araujo, E. M. Carvalho, and E. J. Pearce. 1996. Impairment of tetanus toxoid-specific Th1-like immune responses in humans infected with *Schistosoma mansoni. J. Infect. Dis.* 173:269–272.

3860. Sabino, E., L. Z. Pan, C. Cheng-Mayer, and A. Mayer. 1994. Comparison of in vivo plasma and peripheral blood mononuclear cell HIV-1 quasispecies to short-term tissue culture isolates: an analysis of Tat and C2-V3 Env regions. *AIDS* 8:901–909.

3861. Sabri, F., F. Chiodi, and E. M. Fenyo. 1996. Lack of correlation between V3 amino acid sequence and syncytium-inducing capacity of some HIV type 1 isolates. *AIDS Res. Hum. Retrovir.* 12:855–858.

3862. Sabri, F., E. Tresoldi, M. Di Stefano, S. Polo, M. C. Monaco, A. Verani, J. R. Fiore, P. Lusso, E. Major, F. Chiodi, and G. Scarlatti. 1999. Nonproductive human immunodeficiency virus type 1 infection of human fetal astrocytes: independence from CD4 and major chemokine receptors. *Virology* 264:370–384.

3863. Sacktor, N. C. 1999. Advances in the treatment of HIV dementia. *AIDS Read.* 9:57–60, 62.

3864. Sad, S., and T. R. Mosmann. 1995. Interleukin (IL) 4, in the absence of antigen stimulation, induces an anergy-like state in differentiated CD8+ TC1 cells: loss of IL-2 synthesis and autonomous proliferation but retention of cytotoxicity and synthesis of other cytokines. *J. Exp. Med.* 182:1505–1515.

3865. Sadat-Sowti, B., P. Debre, T. Idziorek, J.-M. Guillon, F. Hadida, E. Okzenhendler, C. Katlama, C. Mayaud, and B. Autran. 1991. A lectin-binding soluble factor released by CD8+ CD57+ lymphocytes from AIDS inhibits T cell cytotoxicity. *Eur. J. Immunol.* 21:737–741.

3866. Sadat-Sowti, B., P. Debre, L. Mollet, L. Quint, F. Hadida, V. Leblond, G. Bismuth, and B. Autran. 1994. An inhibitor of cytotoxic functions produced by CD8+CD57+ T lymphocytes from patients suffering from AIDS and immunosuppressed bone marrow recipients. *Eur. J. Immunol.* 24:2882–2888.

3867. Saeland, S., V. Duvert, D. Pandrau, C. Caux, I. Durand, N. Wrighton, J. Wideman, F. Lee, and J. Banchereau. 1991. Interleukin-7 induces the proliferation of normal B cell precursors. *Blood* 78:2229–2238.

3868. Safai, B., and R. A. Good. 1981. Kaposi's sarcoma: a review and recent developments. *CA Cancer J. Clin.* **335:**2–12.

3869. Safrin, S., and C. Grunfeld. 1999. Fat distribution and metabolic changes in patients with HIV infection. *AIDS* **13:**2493–2505.

3870. Sagar, M., L. Lavreys, J. M. Baeten, B. A. Richardson, K. Mandaliya, B. H. Chohan, J. K. Kreiss, and J. Overbaugh. 2003. Infection with multiple human immunodeficiency virus type 1 variants is associated with faster disease progression. *J. Virol.* **77:**12921–12926.

3871. Saha, K., D. J. Volsky, and E. Matczak. 1999. Resistance against syncytium-inducing human immunodeficiency virus type 1 (HIV-1) in selected CD4+ T cells from an HIV-1-infected nonprogressor: evidence of a novel pathway of resistance mediated by a soluble factor(s) that acts after virus entry. *J. Virol.* **73:**7891–7898.

3872. Saha, K., J. Zhang, A. Gupta, R. Dave, M. Yimen, and R. Zerhouni. 2001. Isolation of primary HIV-1 that target CD8+ T lymphocytes using CD8 as a receptor. *Nat. Med.* **7:**65–72.

3873. Saha, K., J. Zhang, and B. Zerhouni. 2001. Evidence of productively infected CD8+ T cells in patients with AIDS: implications for HIV-1 pathogenesis. *J. Acquir. Immune Defic. Syndr.* **26:**199–207.

3874. Sahu, G. K., J. J. Chen, J. C. Huang, K. M. Ramsey, and M. W. Cloyd. 2001. Transient or occult HIV-1 infection in high-risk adults. *AIDS* **15:**1175–1177.

3875. Saito, Y., B. M. Blumberg, L. R. Sharer, J. Michaels, M. Minz, M. Louder, K. Golding, T. Cvetkovich, and L. Epstein. 1994. Overexpression of Nef is a marker for restricted HIV-1 infection of astrocytes in postmortem pediatric central nervous system tissue. *Neurology* **44:**474–481.

3876. Sakaguchi, M., T. Sato, and J. E. Groopman. 1991. Human immunodeficiency virus infection of megakaryocytic cells. *Blood* **77:**481–485.

3877. Sakaguchi, S., N. Sakaguchi, M. Asano, M. Itoh, and M. Toda. 1995. Immunologic self-tolerance maintained by activated T cells expressing IL-2 receptor alpha-chains (CD25). Breakdown of a single mechanism of self-tolerance causes various autoimmune diseases. *J. Immunol.* **155:**1151–1164.

3878. Sakaguchi, S., N. Sakaguchi, J. Shimizu, S. Yamazaki, T. Sakihama, M. Itoh, Y. Kuniyasu, T. Nomura, M. Toda, and T. Takahashi. 2001. Immunologic tolerance maintained by CD25+ CD4+ regulatory T cells: their common role in controlling autoimmunity, tumor immunity, and transplantation tolerance. *Immunol. Rev.* **182:**18–32.

3879. Sakai, H., M. Kawamura, J.-I. Sakuragi, S. Sakuragi, R. Shibata, A. Ishimoto, N. Ono, S. Ueda, and A. Adachi. 1993. Integration is essential for efficient gene expression of human immunodeficiency virus type 1. *J. Virol.* **67:**1169–1174.

3880. Sakai, K., S. Dewhurst, X. Ma, and D. J. Volsky. 1988. Differences in cytopathogenicity and host cell range among infectious molecular clones of human immunodeficiency virus type 1 simultaneously isolated from an individual. *J. Virol.* **62:**4078–4085.

3881. Sakai, K., J. Dimas, and M. J. Lenardo. 2006. The Vif and Vpr accessory proteins independently cause HIV-1-induced T cell cytopathicity and cell cycle arrest. *Proc. Natl. Acad. Sci. USA* **103:**3369–3374.

3882. Sakai, K., X. Ma, I. Gordienko, and D. J. Volsky. 1991. Recombinational analysis of a natural noncytopathic human immunodeficiency virus type 1 (HIV-1) isolate: role of the *vif* gene in HIV-1 infection kinetics and cytopathicity. *J. Virol.* **65:**5765–5773.

3883. Sakaida, H., T. Hori, A. Yonezawa, A. Sato, Y. Isaka, O. Yoshie, T. Hattori, and T. Uchiyama. 1998. T-tropic human immunodeficiency virus type 1 (HIV-1) derived V3 loop peptides directly bind to CXCR-4 and inhibit T-tropic HIV-1 infection. *J. Virol.* **72:**9763–9770.

3884. Saksela, K., G. Cheng, and D. Baltimore. 1995. Proline-rich (PxxP) motifs in HIV-1 Nef bind to SH3 domains of a subset of Src kinases and are required for the enhanced growth of Nef+ viruses but not for down-regulation of CD4. *EMBO J.* **14:**484–491.

3885. Saksela, K., E. Muchmore, M. Girard, P. Fultz, and D. Baltimore. 1993. High viral load in lymph nodes and latent human immunodeficiency virus (HIV) in peripheral blood cells of HIV-1-infected chimpanzees. *J. Virol.* **67:**7423–7427.

3886. Saksela, K., C. Stevens, P. Rubinstein, and D. Baltimore. 1994. Human immunodeficiency virus type 1 mRNA expression in peripheral blood cells predicts disease progression independently of the numbers of CD4+ lymphocytes. *Proc. Natl. Acad. Sci. USA* **91:**1104–1108.

3887. Sala, M., G. Zambruno, J.-P. Vartanian, A. Marconi, U. Bertazzoni, and S. Wain-Hobson. 1994. Spatial discontinuities in human immunodeficiency virus type 1 quasispecies derived from epidermal Langerhans cells of a patient with AIDS and evidence for double infection. *J. Virol.* **68:**5280–5283.

3888. Salahuddin, S. Z., P. D. Markham, M. Popovic, M. G. Sarngadharan, S. Orndorff, A. Fladagar, A. Patel, J. Gold, and R. C. Gallo. 1985. Isolation of infectious human T-cell leukemia/lymphotropic virus type III (HTLV-III) from patients with acquired immunodeficiency syndrome (AIDS) or AIDS-related complex (ARC) and from healthy carriers: a study of risk groups and tissue sources. *Proc. Natl. Acad. Sci. USA* **82:**5530–5534.

3889. Salahuddin, S. Z., A. G. Palestine, E. Heck, D. Ablashi, M. Luckenbach, J. P. McCulley, and R. B. Nussenblatt. 1986. Isolation of the human T-cell leukemia/lymphotropic virus type III from the cornea. *Am. J. Ophthalmol.* **101:**149–152.

3890. Salemi, M., K. Strimmer, W. W. Hall, M. Duffy, E. Delaporte, S. Mboup, M. Peeters, and A. Vandamme. 2001. Dating the common ancestor of SIVcpz and HIV-1 group M and the origin of HIV-1 subtypes using a new method to uncover clock-like molecular evolution. *FASEB J.* **15:**276–278.

3891. Salim, Y. S., V. Faber, A. Wiik, P. L. Andersen, H. Hoier-Madsen, and S. Mouritsen. 1988. Anti-corticosteroid antibodies in AIDS patients. *APMIS* **96:**889–894.

3892. Salinovich, O., S. L. Payne, R. C. Montelaro, K. A. Hussain, C. J. Issel, and K. L. Schnoor. 1986. Rapid emergence of novel antigenic and genetic variants of equine infectious anemia virus during persistent infection. *J. Virol.* **57:**71–80.

3893. Salk, J. 1987. Prospects for the control of AIDS by immunizing seropositive individuals. *Nature* **327:**473–476.

3894. Salk, J., P. A. Bretscher, P. L. Salk, M. Clerici, and G. M. Shearer. 1993. A strategy for prophylactic vaccination against HIV. *Science* **260:**1270–1272.

3895. Salkowitz, J. R., S. Purvis, H. Meyerson, P. Zimmerman, T. R. O'Brien, L. Aledort, M. E. Eyster, M. Hilgartner, C. Kessler, B. A. Konkle, G. C. White III, J. J. Goedert, and M. M. Lederman. 2001. Characterization of high-risk HIV-1 seronegative hemophiliacs. *Clin. Immunol.* **98:**200–211.

3896. Sallusto, F., J. Geginat, and A. Lanzavecchia. 2004. Central memory and effector memory T cell subsets: function, generation, and maintenance. *Annu. Rev. Immunol.* 22:745–763.

3897. Sallusto, F., D. Lenig, R. Forster, M. Lipp, and A. Lanzavecchia. 1999. Two subsets of memory T lymphocytes with distinct homing potentials and effector functions. *Nature* 401: 708–712.

3898. Sallusto, F., D. Lenig, C. R. Mackay, and A. Lanzavecchia. 1998. Flexible programs of chemokine receptor expression on human polarized T helper 1 and 2 lymphocytes. *J. Exp. Med.* 187:875–883.

3899. Salmon, P., R. Olivier, Y. Riviere, E. Brisson, J.-C. Gluckman, M.-P. Kieny, L. Montagnier, and D. Klatzmann. 1988. Loss of CD4 membrane expression and CD4 mRNA during acute human immunodeficiency virus replication. *J. Exp. Med.* 168:1953–1969.

3900. Salzwedel, K., E. D. Smith, B. Dey, and E. A. Berger. 2000. Sequential CD4–coreceptor interactions in human immunodeficiency virus type 1 Env function: soluble CD4 activates Env for coreceptor-dependent fusion and reveals blocking activities of antibodies against cryptic conserved epitopes on gp120. *J. Virol.* 74:326–333.

3901. Sampaio, E. P., E. N. Sarno, R. Galilly, Z. A. Cohn, and G. Kaplan. 1991. Thalidomide selectively inhibits tumor necrosis factor-alpha production by stimulated human monocytes. *J. Exp. Med.* 173:699–703.

3902. Samson, M., F. Libert, B. J. Doranz, J. Rucker, C. Liesnard, C. M. Farber, S. Saragosti, C. Lapoumeroulie, J. Cognaux, C. Forceille, G. Muyldermans, C. Verhofstede, G. Burtonboy, M. Georges, T. Imai, S. Rana, Y. Yi, R. J. Smyth, R. G. Collman, R. W. Doms, G. Vassart, and M. Parmentier. 1996. Resistance to HIV-1 infection in caucasian individuals bearing mutant alleles of the CCR-5 chemokine receptor gene. *Nature* 382:722–725.

3903. Samuel, C. E. 2001. Antiviral actions of interferons. *Clin. Microbiol. Rev.* 14:778–809.

3904. Samuel, K. P., A. Seth, A. Konopka, J. A. Lautenberger, and T. S. Papas. 1987. The 3'-orf protein of human immunodeficiency virus shows structural homology with the phosphorylation domain of human interleukin-2 receptor and the ATP-binding site of the protein kinase family. *FEBS Lett.* 218:81–86.

3905. Samuelsson, A., C. Brostrom, N. Van Dijk, A. Sonnerborg, and F. Chiodi. 1997. Apoptosis of CD4+ and CD19+ cells during human immunodeficiency virus type 1 infection: correlation with clinical progression. *Virology* 238:180–188.

3906. Sanchez, G., X. Xu, J. C. Chermann, and I. Hirsch. 1997. Accumulation of defective viral genomes in peripheral blood mononuclear cells of human immunodeficiency virus type 1-infected individuals. *J. Virol.* 71:2233–2240.

3907. Sanchez-Palomino, S., J. M. Rohas, M. A. Martinez, E. M. Fenyo, R. Najera, E. Domingo, and C. Lopez-Galindez. 1993. Dilute passage promotes expression of genetic and phenotypic variants of human immunodeficiency virus type 1 in cell culture. *J. Virol.* 67:2938–2943.

3908. Sanchez-Pescador, R., M. D. Power, P. J. Barr, K. S. Steimer, M. M. Stempien, S. L. Brown-Shimer, W. W. Gee, A. Renard, A. Randolph, J. A. Levy, D. Dina, and P. A. Luciw. 1985. Nucleotide sequence and expression of an AIDS-associated retrovirus (ARV-2). *Science* 227:484–492.

3909. Sandberg, J. K., N. M. Fast, E. H. Palacios, G. Fennelly, J. Dobroszycki, P. Palumbo, A. Wiznia, R. M. Grant, N. Bhardwaj, M. G. Rosenberg, and D. F. Nixon. 2002. Selective loss of innate CD4(+) V alpha 24 natural killer T cells in human immunodeficiency virus infection. *J. Virol.* 76:7528–7534.

3910. Sanders, R. W., M. Venturi, L. Schiffner, R. Kalyanaraman, H. Katinger, K. O. Lloyd, P. D. Kwong, and J. P. Moore. 2002. The mannose-dependent epitope for neutralizing antibody 2G12 on human immunodeficiency virus type 1 glycoprotein gp120. *J. Virol.* 76:7293–7305.

3911. Sandrin, V., and F. L. Cosset. 2006. Intracellular versus cell surface assembly of retroviral pseudotypes is determined by the cellular localization of the viral glycoprotein, its capacity to interact with Gag, and the expression of the Nef protein. *J. Biol. Chem.* 281:528–542.

3912. Sandstrom, P. A., D. Pardi, C. S. Goldsmith, D. Chengying, A. M. Diamond, and T. M. Folks. 1996. bcl-2 expression facilitates human immunodeficiency virus type 1-mediated cytopathic effects during acute spreading infections. *J. Virol.* 70:4617–4622.

3913. Sankale, J. L., R. S. De La Tour, R. G. Marlink, R. Scheib, S. Mboup, M. E. Essex, and P. J. Kanki. 1996. Distinct quasispecies in the blood and the brain of an HIV-2-infected individual. *Virology* 226:418–423.

3914. Sankale, J. L., R. S. de la Tour, B. Renjifo, T. Siby, S. Mboup, R. G. Marlink, M. E. Essex, and P. J. Kanki. 1995. Intrapatient variability of the human immunodeficiency virus type 2 envelope V3 loop. *AIDS Res. Hum. Retrovir.* 11:617–623.

3915. Sankaran, S., M. Guadalupe, E. Reay, M. D. George, J. Flamm, T. Prindiville, and S. Dandekar. 2005. Gut mucosal T cell responses and gene expression correlate with protection against disease in long-term HIV-1-infected nonprogressors. *Proc. Natl. Acad. Sci. USA* 102:9860–9865.

3916. Santiago, M. L., F. Bibollet-Ruche, E. Bailes, S. Kamenya, M. N. Muller, M. Lukasik, A. E. Pusey, D. A. Collins, R. W. Wrangham, J. Goodall, G. M. Shaw, P. M. Sharp, and B. H. Hahn. 2003. Amplification of a complete simian immunodeficiency virus genome from fecal RNA of a wild chimpanzee. *J. Virol.* 77:2233–2242.

3917. Santiago, M. L., F. Range, B. F. Keele, Y. Li, E. Bailes, F. Bibollet-Ruche, C. Fruteau, R. Noe, M. Peeters, J. F. Brookfield, G. M. Shaw, P. M. Sharp, and B. H. Hahn. 2005. Simian immunodeficiency virus infection in free-ranging sooty mangabeys (Cercocebus atys atys) from the Tai Forest, Cote d'Ivoire: implications for the origin of epidemic human immunodeficiency virus type 2. *J. Virol.* 79:12515–12527.

3918. Saphire, A. C. S., M. D. Bobardt, Z. Zhang, G. David, and P. A. Gallay. 2001. Syndecans serve as attachment receptors for human immunodeficiency virus type 1 on macrophages. *J. Virol.* 75:9187–9200.

3919. Saphire, E. O., P. W. Parren, R. Pantophlet, M. B. Zwick, G. M. Morris, P. M. Rudd, R. A. Dwek, R. L. Stanfield, D. R. Burton, and I. A. Wilson. 2001. Crystal structure of a neutralizing human IGG against HIV-1: a template for vaccine design. *Science* 293:1155–1159.

3920. Saracco, A., M. Musicco, A. Nicolosi, G. Angarano, C. Arici, G. Gavazzeni, P. Costigliola, S. Gafa, C. Gervasoni, R. Luzzati, F. Piccinino, F. Puppo, B. Salassa, A. Sinicco, R. Stellini, U. Tirelli, G. Turbessi, G. M. Vigevani, G. Visco, R. Zerboni, and A. Lazzarin. 1993. Man-to-woman sexual transmission of HIV: longitudinal study of 343 steady partners of infected men. *J. Acquir. Immune Defic. Syndr.* 6:497–502.

3921. Saravolatz, L. D., D. Winslow, G. Collins, J. S. Hodges, C. Pettinelli, D. S. Stein, N. Markowitz, R. Reves, M. O. Loveless, L. Crane, M. Thompson, and D. Abrams. 1996. Zidovudine alone or in combination with didanosine or zalcitabine in HIV-infected patients with the acquired immunodeficiency syndrome or fewer than 200 CD4 cells per cubic millimeter. *N. Engl. J. Med.* 335:1099–1106.

3921a. Sarkis, P. T., S. Ying, R. Xu, and X. F. Yu. 2006. STAT1-independent cell type-specific regulation of antiviral APOBEC3G by IFN-α. *J. Immunol.* 177:4530–4540.

3922. Sarngadharan, M. G., M. Popovic, L. Bruch, J. Schupbach, and R. C. Gallo. 1984. Antibodies reactive with human T-lymphotropic retroviruses (HTLV-III) in the serum of patients with AIDS. *Science* 224:506–508.

3923. Sarr, A. D., G. Eisen, A. Gueye-Ndiaye, C. Mullins, I. Traore, M. C. Dia, J. L. Sankale, D. Faye, S. Mboup, and P. Kanki. 2005. Viral dynamics of primary HIV-1 infection in Senegal, West Africa. *J. Infect. Dis.* 191:1460–1467.

3924. Sasada, A., A. Takaori-Kondo, K. Shirakawa, M. Kobayashi, A. Abudu, M. Hishizawa, K. Imada, Y. Tanaka, and T. Uchiyama. 2005. APOBEC3G targets human T-cell leukemia virus type 1. *Retrovirology* 2:32.

3925. Sato, A. I., F. B. Balamuth, K. E. Ugen, W. V. Williams, and D. B. Weiner. 1994. Identification of CD7 glycoprotein as an accessory molecule in HIV-1-mediated syncytium formation and cell-free infection. *J. Immunol.* 152:5142–5152.

3926. Sato, H., J. Orenstein, D. Dimitrov, and M. Martin. 1992. Cell-to-cell spread of HIV-1 occurs within minutes and may not involve the participation of virus particles. *Virology* 186:712–724.

3927. Sato, K., H. Kawasaki, H. Nagayama, M. Enomoto, C. Morimoto, K. Tadokoro, T. Juji, and T. A. Takahashi. 2000. TGF-beta 1 reciprocally controls chemotaxis of human peripheral blood monocyte-derived dendritic cells via chemokine receptors. *J. Immunol.* 164:2285–2295.

3928. Satomi, M., M. Shimizu, E. Shinya, E. Watari, A. Owaki, C. Hidaka, M. Ichikawa, T. Takeshita, and H. Takahashi. 2005. Transmission of macrophage-tropic HIV-1 by breast-milk macrophages via DC-SIGN. *J. Infect. Dis.* 191:174–181.

3929. Satow, Y.-I., M. Hashido, K.-I. Ishikawa, H. Honda, M. Mizuno, T. Kawana, and M. Hayami. 1991. Detection of HTLV-I antigen in peripheral and cord blood lymphocytes from carrier mothers. *Lancet* 338:915–916.

3930. Sattentau, Q. J., A. G. Dalgleish, R. A. Weiss, and P. C. L. Beverley. 1986. Epitopes of the CD4 antigen and HIV infection. *Science* 234:1120–1123.

3931. Sattentau, Q. J., and J. P. Moore. 1991. Conformational changes induced in the human immunodeficiency virus envelope glycoprotein by soluble CD4 binding. *J. Exp. Med.* 174:407–415.

3932. Sattentau, Q. J., and J. P. Moore. 1995. Human immunodeficiency virus type 1 neutralization is determined by epitope exposure on the gp120 oligomer. *J. Exp. Med.* 182:185–196.

3933. Sattentau, Q. J., J. P. Moore, F. Vignaux, F. Traincard, and P. Poignard. 1993. Conformational changes induced in the envelope glycoproteins of the human and simian immunodeficiency viruses by soluble receptor binding. *J. Virol.* 67:7383–7393.

3934. Saulsbury, F. T. 1997. The clinical course of human immunodeficiency virus infection in genetically identical children. *Clin. Infect. Dis.* 24:971–974.

3935. Saunders, C. J., R. A. McCaffrey, I. Zharkikh, Z. Kraft, S. E. Malenbaum, B. Burke, C. Cheng-Mayer, and L. Stamatatos. 2005. The V1, V2, and V3 regions of the human immunodeficiency virus type 1 envelope differentially affect the viral phenotype in an isolate-dependent manner. *J. Virol.* 79:9069–9080.

3936. Savarino, A., F. Bottarel, F. Malavasi, and U. Dianzani. 2000. Role of CD38 in HIV-1 infection: an epiphenomenon of T-cell activation or an active player in virus/host interactions? *AIDS* 14:1079–1089.

3937. Sawai, E. T., A. Baur, H. Struble, B. M. Peterlin, J. A. Levy, and C. Cheng-Mayer. 1994. Human immunodeficiency virus type 1 Nef associates with a cellular serine kinase in T lymphocytes. *Proc. Natl. Acad. Sci. USA* 91:1539–1543.

3938. Sawai, E. T., I. H. Khan, P. M. Montbriand, B. M. Peterlin, C. Cheng-Mayer, and P. A. Luciw. 1996. Activation of PAK by HIV and SIV Nef: importance for AIDS in rhesus macaques. *Curr. Biol.* 6:1519–1527.

3939. Sawyer, L. A., D. A. Katzenstein, R. M. Hendry, E. J. Boone, L. K. Vujcic, C. C. Williams, S. L. Zeger, A. J. Saah, C. R. Rinaldo, Jr., J. P. Phair, J. V. Giorgi, and G. V. Quinnan, Jr. 1990. Possible beneficial effects of neutralizing antibodies and antibody-dependent cell mediated cytotoxicity in human immunodeficiency virus infection. *AIDS Res. Hum. Retrovir.* 6:341–356.

3940. Sawyer, L. S. W., M. T. Wrin, L. Crawford-Miksza, B. Potts, Y. Wu, P. A. Weber, R. D. Alfonso, and C. V. Hanson. 1994. Neutralization sensitivity of human immunodeficiency virus type 1 is determined in part by the cells in which the virus is propagated. *J. Virol.* 68:1342–1349.

3941. Sayers, M. H., P. G. Beatty, and J. A. Hansen. 1986. HLA antibodies as a cause of false-positive reactions in screening enzyme immunoassays for antibodies to human T-lymphotropic virus type III. *Transfusion* (Paris) 26:113–115.

3942. Scadden, D. T., O. Pickus, S. M. Hammer, B. Stretcher, J. Bresnahan, J. Gere, J. McGrath, and J. M. Agosti. 1996. Lack of *in vivo* effect of granuloycte-macrophage colony-stimulating factor on human immunodeficiency virus type 1. *AIDS Res. Hum. Retrovir.* 12:1151–1159.

3943. Scadden, D. T., M. Zeira, A. Woon, Z. Wang, L. Schieve, K. Ikeuchi, B. Lim, and J. E. Groopman. 1990. Human immunodeficiency virus infection of human bone marrow stromal fibroblasts. *Blood* 76:317–322.

3943a. Scarborough, M., S. B. Gordon, N. French, C. Phiri, J. Musaya, and E. E. Zijlstra. 2006. Grey nails predict low CD4 cell count among untreated patients with HIV infection in Malawi. *AIDS* 20:1415–1417.

3944. Scarlatti, G., J. Albert, P. Rossi, V. Hodara, P. Biraghi, L. Muggiasca, and E. M. Fenyo. 1993. Mother-to-child transmission of human immunodeficiency virus type 1: correlation with neutralizing antibodies against primary isolates. *J. Infect. Dis.* 168:207–210.

3945. Scarlatti, G., V. Hodara, P. Rossi, L. Muggiasca, A. Bucceri, J. Albert, and E. M. Fenyo. 1993. Transmission of human immunodeficiency virus type 1 (HIV-1) from mother to child correlates with viral phenotype. *Virology* 197:624–629.

3946. Scarlatti, G., T. Leitner, E. Halapi, J. Wahlberg, P. Marchisio, M. A. Clerici-Schoeller, H. Wigzell, E. M. Fenyo, J. Albert, M. Uhlen, et al. 1993. Comparison of variable region 3 sequences of human immunodeficiency virus type 1 from infected children with the RNA and DNA sequences of the virus populations of their mothers. *Proc. Natl. Acad. Sci. USA* 90:1721–1725.

3947. Scarlatti, G., V. Lombardi, A. Plebani, N. Principi, C. Vegni, G. Ferraris, A. Bucceri, E. M. Fenyo, H. Wigzell, P. Rossi, and J. Albert. 1991. Polymerase chain reaction, virus isolation and antigen assay in HIV-1-antibody-positive mothers and their children. *AIDS* 5:1173–1178.

3948. Schacker, T., S. Little, E. Connick, K. Gebhard, Z.-Q. Zhang, J. Krieger, J. Pryor, D. Havlir, J. K. Wong, R. T. Schooley, D. Richman, L. Corey, and A. T. Haase. 2001. Productive infection of T cells in lymphoid tissues during primary and early human immunodeficiency virus infection. *J. Infect. Dis.* 183:555–562.

3949. Schacker, T., S. Little, E. Connick, K. Gebhard-Mitchell, Z. Q. Zhang, J. Krieger, J. Pryor, D. Havlir, J. K. Wong, D. Richman, L. Corey, and A. T. Haase. 2000. Rapid accumulation of human immunodeficiency virus (HIV) in lymphatic tissue reservoirs during acute and early HIV infection: implications for timing of antiretroviral therapy. *J. Infect. Dis.* 181:354–357.

3950. Schacker, T., A. J. Ryncarz, J. Goddard, K. Diem, M. Shaughnessy, and L. Corey. 1998. Frequent recovery of HIV-1 from genital herpes simplex virus lesions in HIV-1-infected men. *JAMA* 280:61–66.

3951. Schacker, T., J. Zeh, H. Hu, M. Shaughnessy, and L. Corey. 2002. Changes in plasma human immunodeficiency virus type 1 RNA associated with herpes simplex virus reactivation and suppression. *J. Infect. Dis.* 186:1718–1725.

3952. Schacker, T. W., J. P. Hughes, T. Shea, R. W. Coombs, and L. Corey. 1998. Biological and virologic characteristics of primary HIV infection. *Ann. Intern. Med.* 128:613–620.

3953. Schacker, T. W., P. L. Nguyen, G. J. Beilman, S. Wolinsky, M. Larson, C. Reilly, and A. T. Haase. 2002. Collagen deposition in HIV-1 infected lymphatic tissues and T cell homeostasis. *J. Clin. Investig.* 110:1133–1139.

3954. Schacker, T. W., C. Reilly, G. J. Beilman, J. Taylor, D. Skarda, D. Krason, M. Larson, and A. T. Haase. 2005. Amount of lymphatic tissue fibrosis in HIV infection predicts magnitude of HAART-associated change in peripheral CD4 cell count. *AIDS* 19:2169–2171.

3955. Schaeffer, E., R. Geleziunas, and W. C. Greene. 2001. Human immunodeficiency virus type 1 Nef functions at the level of virus entry by enhancing cytoplasmic delivery of virions. *J. Virol.* 75:2993–3000.

3956. Schambelan, M., C. A. Benson, A. Carr, J. S. Currier, M. P. Dube, J. G. Gerber, S. K. Grinspoon, C. Grunfeld, D. P. Kotler, K. Mulligan, W. G. Powderly, and M. S. Saag. 2002. Management of metabolic complications associated with antiretroviral therapy for HIV-1 infection: recommendations of an International AIDS Society-USA Panel. *J. Acquir. Immune Defic. Syndr.* 31:257–275.

3957. Schechter, M., L. H. Harrison, N. A. Halsey, G. Trade, M. Santino, L. H. Moulton, and T. C. Quinn. 1994. Coinfection with human T-cell lymphotropic virus type 1 and HIV in Brazil. *JAMA* 271:353–357.

3958. Schechter, M. T., K. J. P. Craib, T. N. Le, J. S. G. Montaner, B. Douglas, P. Sestak, B. Willoughby, and M. V. O'Shaughnessy. 1990. Susceptibility to AIDS progression appears early in HIV infection. *AIDS* 4:185–190.

3959. Scheffner, M., K. Munger, J. M. Huibregtse, and P. M. Howley. 1992. Targeted degradation of the retinoblastoma protein by human papillomavirus E7-E6 fusion proteins. *EMBO J.* 11:2425–2431.

3960. Scheffner, M., B. A. Werness, J. M. Huibregtse, A. J. Levine, and P. M. Howley. 1990. The E6 oncoprotein encoded by human papillomavirus types 16 and 18 promotes the degradation of p53. *Cell* 63:1129–1136.

3961. Schellekens, P. T., M. Tersmette, M. T. Roos, R. O. Keet, F. De Wolf, R. A. Coutinho, and F. Miedema. 1992. Biphasic rate of CD4+ cell count decline during progression to AIDS correlates with HIV-1 phenotype. *AIDS* 6:665–670.

3962. Scheppler, J. A., J. K. A. Nicholson, D. C. Swan, A. Ahmed-Ansari, and J. S. McDougal. 1989. Down-modulation of MHC-I in a CD4+ T cell line, CEM-E5, after HIV-1 infection. *J. Immunol.* 143:2858–2866.

3963. Schinazi, R. F. 1992. Progress in the development of natural products for human immunodeficiency viruses infections, p. 1–29. *In* C. K. Chu and H. G. Cutler (ed.), *Natural Products as Antiviral Agents.* Plenum Press, New York, N.Y.

3964. Schindler, M., J. Munch, O. Kutsch, H. Li, M. L. Santiago, F. Bibollet-Ruche, M. C. Muller-Trutwin, F. J. Novembre, M. Peeters, V. Courgnaud, E. Bailes, P. Roques, D. L. Sodora, G. Silvestri, P. M. Sharp, B. H. Hahn, and F. Kirchhoff. 2006. Nef-mediated suppression of T cell activation was lost in a lentiviral lineage that gave rise to HIV-1. *Cell* 125:1055–1067.

3965. Schito, A. M., E. Vittinghoff, F. M. Hecht, M. K. Elkins, J. O. Kahn, J. A. Levy, and J. R. Oksenberg. 2001. Longitudinal analysis of T-cell receptor gene use by CD8(+) T cells in early human immunodeficiency virus infection in patients receiving highly active antiretroviral therapy. *Blood* 97:214–220.

3966. Schlaak, J. F., C. Schramm, K. Radecke, K. H. zum Buschenfelde, and G. Gerken. 2002. Sustained suppression of HCV replication and inflammatory activity after interleukin-2 therapy in patients with HIV/hepatitis C virus coinfection. *J. Acquir. Immune Defic. Syndr.* 29:145–148.

3967. Schläpfer, E., M. Fischer, P. Ott, and R. F. Speck. 2003. Anti-HIV-1 activity of leflunomide: a comparison with mycophenolic acid and hydroxyurea. *AIDS* 17:1613–1620.

3968. Schlienger, K., M. Mancini, Y. Riviere, D. Dormont, P. Tiollais, and M. L. Michel. 1992. Human immunodeficiency virus type 1 major neutralizing determinant exposed on hepatitis B surface antigen particles is highly immunogenic in primates. *J. Virol.* 66:2570–2576.

3969. Schlienger, K., D. C. Montefiori, M. Mancini, Y. Riviere, P. Tiollais, and M. L. Michel. 1994. Vaccine-induced neutralizing antibodies directed in part to the simian immunodeficiency virus (SIV) V2 domain were unable to protect rhesus monkeys from SIV experimental challenge. *J. Virol.* 68:6578–6588.

3970. Schluns, K. S., W. C. Kieper, S. C. Jameson, and L. Lefrancois. 2001. Interleukin-7 mediates the homeostasis of naive and memory CD8 % cell *in vivo. Nat. Immunol.* 1:426–432.

3971. Schmidt, B., B. M. Ashlock, H. Foster, S. Fujimura, and J. A. Levy. 2005. HIV-infected cells are major inducers of plasmacytoid dendritic cells (PDC) interferon production, maturation and migration. *Virology* 343:256–266.

3972. Schmidt, B., S. H. Fujimura, J. M. Martin, and J. A. Levy. 2006. Variations in plasmacytoid dendritic cell (PDC) and myeloid dendritic cell (MDC) levels in HIV-infected subjects on and off antiretroviral therapy. *J. Clin. Immunol.* 26:55–64.

3973. Schmidt, B., I. Scott, R. G. Whitmore, H. Foster, S. Fujimura, J. Schmitz, and J. A. Levy. 2004. Low-level HIV infection of plasmacytoid dendritic cells: onset of cytopathic effects and cell death after PDC maturation. *Virology* 329:280–288.

3974. Schmidtmayerova, H., M. Alfano, G. Nuovo, and M. Bukrinsky. 1998. Human immunodeficiency virus type 1

T-lymphotropic strains enter macrophages via a CD4– and CXCR4-mediated pathway: replication is restricted at a postentry level. *J. Virol.* 72:4633–4642.

3975. **Schmidtmayerova, H., C. Bolmont, S. Baghdiguian, I. Hirsch, and J. C. Chermann.** 1992. Distinctive pattern of infection and replication of HIV-1 strains in blood-derived macrophages. *Virology* 190:124–133.

3976. **Schmidtmayerova, H., H. S. L. Nottet, G. Nuovo, T. Raabe, C. R. Flanagan, L. Dubrovsky, H. E. Gendelman, A. Cerami, M. Bukrinsky, and B. Sherry.** 1996. Human immunodeficiency virus type 1 infection alters chemokine beta peptide expression in human monocytes: implications for recruitment of leukocytes into brain and lymph nodes. *Proc. Natl. Acad. Sci. USA* 93:700–704.

3977. **Schmidtmayerova, H., B. Sherry, and M. Bukrinsky.** 1996. Chemokines and HIV replication. *Nature* 382:767.

3978. **Schmit, J.-C., J. Cogniaux, P. Hermans, C. Van Vaeck, S. Sprecher, B. Van Remoortel, M. Witvrouw, J. Balzarini, J. Desmyter, E. De Clercq, and A.-M. Vandamme.** 1996. Multiple drug resistance to nucleoside analogues and nonnucleoside reverse transcriptase inhibitors in an efficiently replicating human immunodeficiency virus type 1 patient strain. *J. Infect. Dis.* 174:962–968.

3979. **Schmitt, M. P., J. L. Gendrault, C. Schweitzer, A. M. Steffan, C. Beyer, C. Royer, D. Jaeck, J. L. Pasquali, A. Kirn, and A. M. Aubertin.** 1990. Permissivity of primary cultures of human Kupffer cells for HIV-1. *AIDS Res. Hum. Retrovir.* 6:987–991.

3980. **Schmitz, C., D. Marchant, S. J. D. Neil, K. Aubin, S. Reuter, M. T. Dittmar, and A. McKnight.** 2004. Lv2, a novel postentry restriction, is mediated by both capsid and envelope. *J. Virol.* 78:2006–2016.

3981. **Schmitz, J., J. van Lunzen, K. Tenner-Racz, G. Großschupff, P. Racz, H. Schmitz, M. Dietrich, and F. T. Hufert.** 1994. Follicular dendritic cells retain HIV-1 particles on their plasma membrane, but are not productively infected in asymptomatic patients with follicular hyperplasia. *J. Immunol.* 153:1352–1359.

3982. **Schmitz, J., J. P. Zimmer, B. Kluxen, S. Aries, M. Bogel, I. Gigli, and H. Schmitz.** 1995. Antibody-dependent complement-mediated cytotoxicity in sera from patients with HIV-1 infection is controlled by CD55 and CD59. *J. Clin. Investig.* 96:1520–1526.

3983. **Schmitz, J. E., M. J. Kuroda, S. Santra, V. G. Sasseville, M. A. Simon, M. A. Lifton, P. Racz, K. Tenner-Racz, M. Dalesandro, B. J. Scallon, J. Ghrayeb, M. A. Forman, D. C. Montefiori, E. P. Rieber, N. L. Letvin, and K. A. Reimann.** 1999. Control of viremia in simian immunodeficiency virus infection by CD8+ lymphocytes. *Science* 283:857–860.

3984. **Schmitz, T., R. Underwood, R. Khiroya, W. W. Bachovchin, and B. T. Huber.** 1996. Potentiation of the immune response in HIV-1+ individuals. *J. Clin. Investig.* 97:1545–1549.

3985. **Schneider, J., O. Kaaden, T. D. Copeland, S. Oroszlan, and G. Hunsmann.** 1986. Shedding and interspecies type seroreactivity of the envelope glycopolypeptide gp120 of the human immunodeficiency virus. *J. Gen. Virol.* 67:2533–2538.

3986. **Schneider, M. M., J. C. Borleffs, R. P. Stolk, C. A. Jaspers, and A. I. Hoepelman.** 1999. Discontinuation of prophylaxis for Pneumocystis carinii pneumonia in HIV-1-infected patients treated with highly active antiretroviral therapy. *Lancet* 353:201–203.

3987. **Schneider, R., M. Campbell, G. Nasioulas, B. K. Felber, and G. N. Pavlakis.** 1997. Inactivation of the human immunodeficiency virus type 1 inhibitory elements allows Rev-independent expression of Gag/protease and particle formation. *J. Virol.* 71:4892–4903.

3988. **Schneider, T., A. Beck, C. Ropke, R. Ullrich, H.-P. Harthis, M. Broker, and G. Pauli.** 1993. The HIV-1 Nef protein shares an antigenic determinant with a T-cell surface protein. *AIDS* 7:647–654.

3989. **Schneider-Schaulies, J., S. Schneider-Schaulies, R. Brinkman, P. Tas, M. Halbrugge, U. Walter, H. C. Holmes, and V. Ter Meulen.** 1992. HIV-1 gp120 receptor on CD4−negative brain cells activates a tyrosine kinase. *Virology* 191:765–772.

3990. **Schnittman, S. M., J. J. Greenhouse, M. C. Psallidopoulos, M. Baseler, N. P. Salzman, A. S. Fauci, and H. C. Lane.** 1990. Increasing viral burden in CD4+ T cells from patients with human immunodeficiency virus (HIV) infection reflects rapidly progressive immunosuppression and clinical disease. *Ann. Intern. Med.* 113:438–443.

3991. **Schnittman, S. M., H. C. Lane, J. Greenhouse, J. S. Justement, M. Baseler, and A. S. Fauci.** 1990. Preferential infection of CD4+ memory T cells by human immunodeficiency virus type 1: evidence for a role in the selective T-cell functional defects observed in infected individuals. *Proc. Natl. Acad. Sci. USA* 87:6058–6062.

3992. **Schnittman, S. M., H. C. Lane, S. E. Higgins, T. Folks, and A. S. Fauci.** 1986. Direct polyclonal activation of human B lymphocytes by the acquired immune deficiency syndrome virus. *Science* 233:1084–1086.

3993. **Schnittman, S. M., M. C. Psallidopoulos, H. C. Lane, L. Thompson, M. Baseler, F. Massari, C. H. Fox, N. P. Salzman, and A. S. Fauci.** 1989. The reservoir for HIV-1 in human peripheral blood is a T cell that maintains expression of CD4. *Science* 245:305–308.

3994. **Schols, D., and E. De Clercq.** 1996. Human immunodeficiency virus type 1 gp120 induces anergy in human peripheral blood lymphocytes by inducing interleukin-10 production. *J. Virol.* 70:4953–4960.

3995. **Schols, D., R. Pauwels, J. Desmyter, and E. De Clercq.** 1992. Presence of class II histocompatibility DR proteins on the envelope of human immunodeficiency virus demonstrated by FACS analysis. *Virology* 189:374–376.

3996. **Schrager, L. K., J. M. Young, M. G. Fowler, B. J. Mathieson, and S. H. Vermund.** 1994. Long-term survivors of HIV-1 infection: definitions and research challenges. *AIDS* 8(Suppl.):S95–S108.

3997. **Schreiber, G. B., M. P. Busch, S. H. Kleinman, and J. J. Korelitz.** 1996. The risk of transfusion-transmitted viral infections. *N. Engl. J. Med.* 334:1685–1690.

3998. **Schrier, R. D., J. A. McCutchan, J. C. Venable, J. A. Nelson, and C. A. Wiley.** 1990. T-cell-induced expression of human immunodeficiency virus in macrophages. *J. Virol.* 64:3280–3288.

3999. **Schrier, R. D., J. A. McCutchan, and C. A. Wiley.** 1993. Mechanisms of immune activation of human immunodeficiency virus in monocytes/macrophages. *J. Virol.* 67:5713–5720.

4000. **Schroder, A. R. W., P. Shinn, H. Chen, C. Berry, J. R. Ecker, and F. Bushman.** 2002. HIV-1 integration in the human genome favors active genes and local hotspots. *Cell* 110:521–529.

4001. Schrofelbauer, B., D. Chen, and N. R. Landau. 2004. A single amino acid of APOBEC3G controls its species-specific interaction with virion infectivity factor (Vif). *Proc. Natl. Acad. Sci. USA* **101**:3927–3932.

4002. Schubert, U., S. Bour, R. L. Willey, and K. Strebel. 1999. Regulation of virus release by the macrophage-tropic human immunodeficiency virus type 1 AD8 isolate is redundant and can be controlled by either Vpu or Env. *J. Virol.* **73**:887–896.

4003. Schuitemaker, H., M. Groenink, L. Meyaard, N. A. Kootstra, R. A. M. Fouchier, R. A. Gruters, H. G. Huisman, M. Tersmette, and F. Miedema. 1993. Early replication steps but not cell type-specific signalling of the viral long terminal repeat determine HIV-1 monocytotropism. *AIDS Res. Hum. Retrovir.* **9**:669–675.

4004. Schuitemaker, H., M. Koot, N. A. Kootstra, M. W. Dercksen, R. E. Y. de Goede, R. P. van Steenwijk, J. M. A. Lange, J. K. M. Schattenkerk, F. Miedema, and M. Tersmette. 1992. Biological phenotype of human immunodeficiency virus type 1 clones at different stages of infection: progression of disease is associated with a shift from monocytotropic to T-cell-tropic virus populations. *J. Virol.* **66**:1354–1360.

4005. Schuitemaker, H., N. A. Kootstra, M. H. G. M. Koppelman, S. M. Bruisten, H. G. Huisman, M. Tersmette, and F. Miedema. 1992. Proliferation-dependent HIV-1 infection of monocytes occurs during differentiation into macrophages. *J. Clin. Investig.* **89**:1154–1160.

4006. Schuitemaker, H., L. Meyaard, J. A. Kootstra, R. Dubbes, S. A. Otto, M. Tersmette, J. L. Heeney, and F. Miedema. 1993. Lack of T cell dysfunction and programmed cell death in human immunodeficiency virus type 1-infected chimpanzees correlates with absence of monocytotropic variants. *J. Infect. Dis.* **168**:1140–1147.

4007. Schultz, E. R., G. W. Rankin, Jr., M. P. Blanc, B. W. Raden, C. C. Tsai, and T. M. Rose. 2000. Characterization of two divergent lineages of macaque rhadinoviruses related to Kaposi's sarcoma-associated herpesvirus. *J. Virol.* **74**:4919–4928.

4008. Schulz, T. F., B. A. Jameson, L. Lopalco, A. G. Siccardi, R. A. Weiss, and J. P. Moore. 1992. Conserved structural features in the interaction between retroviral surface and transmembrane glycoproteins. *AIDS Res. Hum. Retrovir.* **8**:1571–1580.

4009. Schupbach, J., M. Popovic, R. V. Gilden, M. A. Gonda, M. G. Sangadharan, and R. C. Gallo. 1984. Serological analysis of a subgroup of human T-lymphotropic retroviruses (HTLV-III) associated with AIDS. *Science* **224**:503–505.

4010. Schutten, M., C. A. van Baalen, C. Guillon, R. C. Huisman, P. H. M. Boers, K. Sintnicolaas, R. A. Gruters, and A. D. M. E. Osterhaus. 2001. Macrophage tropism of human immunodeficiency virus type 1 facilitates in vivo escape from cytotoxic T-lymphocyte pressure. *J. Virol.* **75**:2706–2709.

4011. Schwartz, D. H., R. C. Castillo, S. Arango-Jaramillo, U. K. Sharma, H. F. Song, and G. Sridharan. 1997. Chemokine-independent in vitro resistance to human immunodeficiency virus (HIV-1) correlating with low viremia in long-term and recently infected HIV-1-positive persons. *J. Infect. Dis.* **176**:1168–1174.

4012. Schwartz, D. H., G. Gorse, M. L. Clements, R. Belshe, A. Izu, A.-M. Duliege, P. Berman, T. Twaddell, D. Stablein, R. Sposto, R. Siliciano, and T. Matthews. 1993. Induction of HIV-1-neutralising and syncytium-inhibiting antibodies in uninfected recipients of HIV-1IIIB rgp120 subunit vaccine. *Lancet* **342**:69–73.

4013. Schwartz, O., V. Marechal, O. Danos, and J.-M. Heard. 1995. Human immunodeficiency virus type 1 Nef increases the efficiency of reverse transcription in the infected cell. *J. Virol.* **69**:4053–4059.

4014. Schwartz, O., V. Marechal, S. Le Gall, F. Lemonnier, and J. M. Heard. 1996. Endocytosis of major histocompatibility complex class I molecules is induced by the HIV-1 Nef protein. *Nat. Med.* **2**:338–342.

4015. Schwartz, S., B. K. Felber, E.-M. Fenyo, and G. N. Pavlakis. 1989. Rapidly and slowly replicating human immunodeficiency virus type 1 isolates can be distinguished according to target-cell tropism in T-cell and monocyte cell lines. *Proc. Natl. Acad. Sci. USA* **86**:7200–7203.

4016. Schwartz, S., B. K. Felber, E. M. Fenyo, and G. N. Pavlakis. 1990. Env and Vpu proteins of human immunodeficiency virus type 1 are produced from multiple bicistronic mRNAs. *J. Virol.* **64**:5448–5456.

4017. Schwarz, A., G. Offermann, F. Keller, I. Bennhold, J. L'Age-Stehr, P. H. Krause, and M. J. Mihatsch. 1993. The effect of cyclosporine on the progression of human immunodeficiency virus type 1 infection transmitted by transplantation—data on four cases and review of the literature. *Transplantation* **55**:95–103.

4018. Schweighardt, B., A.-M. Roy, D. A. Meiklejohn, E. J. Grace, W. J. Moretto, J. J. Heymann, and D. F. Nixon. 2004. R5 human immunodeficiency virus type 1 (HIV-1) replicates more efficiently in primary CD4+ T-cell cultures than X4 HIV-1. *J. Virol.* **78**:9164–9173.

4019. Scoazec, J.-Y., and G. Feldmann. 1990. Both macrophages and endothelial cells of the human hepatic sinusoid express the CD4 molecule, a receptor for the human immunodeficiency virus. *Hepatology* **12**:505–510.

4020. Scoggins, R. M., J. R. Taylor, Jr., J. Patrie, A. B. van't Wout, H. Schuitemaker, and D. Camerini. 2000. Pathogenesis of primary R5 human immunodeficiency virus type 1 clones in SCID-hu mice. *J. Virol.* **74**:3205–3216.

4021. Scorza Smeraldi, R., G. Fabio, A. Lazzarin, N. B. Eisera, M. Moroni, and C. Zanussi. 1986. HLA-associated susceptibility to acquired immunodeficiency syndrome in Italian patients with human-immunodeficiency-virus infection. *Lancet* **2**:1187–1189.

4022. Scorziello, A., T. Florio, A. Bajetto, S. Thellung, and G. Schettini. 1997. TGF-beta1 prevents gp120-induced impairment of Ca2+ homeostasis and rescues cortical neurons from apoptotic death. *J. Neurosci. Res.* **49**:600–607.

4023. Scott, P. 1993. IL-12: initiation cytokine for cell-mediated immunity. *Science* **260**:496–497.

4024. Scott, W. A., D. Brambilla, E. Siwak, C. Beatty, J. Bremer, R. W. Coombs, H. Farzadegen, S. A. Fiscus, S. M. Hammer, F. B. Hollinger, N. Khan, S. Rasheed, and P. S. Reichelderfer. 1996. Evaluation of an infectivity standard for real-time quality control of human immunodeficiency virus type 1 quantitative micrococulture assays. *J. Clin. Microbiol.* **34**:2312–2315.

4025. Scott-Algara, D., L. X. Truong, P. Versmisse, A. David, T. T. Luong, N. V. Nguyen, I. Theodorou, F. Barre-Sinoussi, and G. Pancino. 2003. Increased NK cell activity in HIV-1 exposed but uninfected Vietnamese intravascular drug users. *J. Immunol.* **171**:5663–5667.

4026. Scott-Algara, D., F. Vuillier, A. Cayota, V. Rame, D. Guetard, M. L. J. Moncany, M. Marasescu, C. Dauguet, and G. Dighiero. 1993. In vitro non-productive infection of purified natural killer cells by the BRU isolate of the human immunodeficiency virus type 1. *J.Gen. Virol.* 74:725–731.

4027. Searles, R. P., E. P. Bergquam, M. K. Axthelm, and S. W. Wong. 1999. Sequence and genomic analysis of a Rhesus macaque rhadinovirus with similarity to Kaposi's sarcoma-associated herpesvirus/human herpesvirus 8. *J. Virol.* 73:3040–3053.

4028. Secchiero, P., D. Zella, O. Barabitskaja, M. S. Reitz, S. Capitani, R. Gallo, and G. Zauli. 1998. Progressive and persistent downregulation of surface CXCR4 in CD4+ T cells infected with human herpesvirus 7. *Blood* 92:4521–4528.

4029. Secchiero, P., D. Zella, S. Capitani, R. C. Gallo, and G. Zauli. 1999. Extracellular HIV-1 Tat protein up-regulates the expression of surface CXC-chemokine receptor 4 in resting CD4(+) T cells. *J. Immunol.* 162:2427–2431.

4030. Seddon, B., P. Tomlinson, and R. Zamoyska. 2003. Interleukin 7 and T cell receptor signals regulate homeostasis of CD4 memory cells. *Nat. Immunol.* 4:680–686.

4031. Seder, R. A., R. Gazzinelli, A. Sher, and W. E. Paul. 1993. Interleukin 12 acts directly on CD4+ T cells to enhance priming for interferon gamma production and diminishes interleukin 4 inhibition of such priming. *Proc. Natl. Acad. Sci. USA* 90:10188–10192.

4032. Sedgwick, J. D., D. S. Riminton, J. G. Cyster, and I. Korner. 2000. Tumor necrosis factor: a master-regulator of leukocyte movement. *Immunol. Today* 21:110–113.

4033. Sei, Y., P. H. Tsang, F. N. Chu, I. Wallace, J. P. Roboz, P. S. Sarin, and J. G. Bekesi. 1989. Inverse relationship between HIV-1 p24 antigenemia, anti-p24 antibody and neutralizing antibody response in all stages of HIV-1 infection. *Immunol. Lett.* 20:223–230.

4034. Sei, Y., P. H. Tsang, J. P. Roboz, P. S. Sarin, J. I. Wallace, and J. G. Bekesi. 1988. Neutralizing antibodies as a prognostic indicator in the progression of acquired immune deficiency syndrome (AIDS)-related disorders: a double-blind study. *J. Clin. Immunol.* 8:464–472.

4035. Seidman, R., N. S. Peress, and G. J. Nuovo. 1994. In situ detection of polymerase chain reaction-amplified HIV-1 nucleic acids in skeletal muscle in patients with myopathy. *Mod. Pathol.* 7:369–375.

4036. Sekigawa, I., H. Kaneko, L. P. Neoh, N. Takeda-Hirokawa, H. Akimoto, T. Hishikawa, H. Hashimoto, S. Hirose, N. Yamamoto, and Y. Kaneko. 1998. Differences of HIV envelope protein between HIV-1 and HIV-2: possible relation to the lower virulence of HIV-2. *Viral Immunol.* 11:1–8.

4037. Seligmann, M., D. A. Warrell, J. P. Aboulker, C. Carbon, J. H. Darbyshire, J. Dormont, E. Eschwege, D. J. Girling, D. R. James, J. P. Levy, T. E. A. Peto, D. Schwarz, A. B. Stone, I. V. D. Weller, and R. Withnall. 1994. Concorde: MRT/ANRS randomized double-blind controlled trial of immediate and deferred zidovudine in symptom-free HIV infection. *Lancet* 343:871–881.

4038. Selmaj, K., C. S. Raine, M. Farooq, W. T. Norton, and C. F. Brosnan. 1991. Cytokine cytotoxicity against oligodendrocytes. *J. Immunol.* 147:1522–1529.

4039. Selmaj, K. W., M. Farooq, W. T. Norton, C. S. Raine, and C. F. Brosnan. 1990. Proliferation of astrocytes in vitro in response to cytokines. *J. Immunol.* 144:129–135.

4040. Selmaj, K. W., and C. S. Raine. 1988. Tumor necrosis factor mediates myelin and oligodendrocyte damage *in vitro. Ann. Neurol.* 23:339–346.

4041. Selwyn, P. A., P. Alcabes, D. Hartel, D. Buono, E. E. Schoenbaum, R. S. Klein, K. Davenny, and G. H. Friedland. 1992. Clinical manifestations and predictors of disease progression in drug users with human immunodeficiency virus infection. *N. Engl. J. Med.* 327:1697–1703.

4042. Semba, R. D., N. Kumwenda, D. R. Hoover, T. E. Taha, T. C. Quinn, L. Mtimavalye, R. J. Biggar, R. Broadhead, P. G. Miotti, L. J. Sokoll, L. van der Hoeven, and J. D. Chiphangwi. 1999. Human immunodeficiency virus load in breast milk, mastitis, and mother-to-child transmission of human immunodeficiency virus type 1. *J. Infect. Dis.* 180:93–98.

4043. Semba, R. D., P. G. Miotti, J. D. Chiphangwi, A. J. Saah, J. K. Canner, G. A. Dallabetta, and D. R. Hoover. 1994. Maternal vitamin A deficiency and mother-to-child transmission of HIV-1. *Lancet* 343:1593–1597.

4044. Semenzato, G., C. Agostini, L. Ometto, R. Zambello, L. Trentin, L. Chieco-Bianchi, and A. De Rossi. 1995. CD8+ T lymphocytes in the lung of acquired immunodeficiency syndrome patients harbor human immunodeficiency virus type 1. *Blood* 85:2308–2314.

4045. Semple, M. G., C. Loveday, E. Preston, and R. S. Tedder. 1991. Detection of HIV-1 RNA in factor VIII concentrate. *AIDS* 5:597–598.

4046. Semprini, A., P. Levy-Setti, M. Bozzo, M. Ravizza, A. Taglioretti, P. Sulpizio, E. Albani, M. Oneta, and G. Pardi. 1992. Insemination of HIV-negative women with processed semen of HIV-positive partners. *Lancet* 340:1317–1319.

4047. Semprini, A. E., C. Castagna, M. Ravizza, S. Fiore, V. Savasi, M. L. Muggiasca, E. Grossi, B. Guerra, C. Tibaldi, G. Scaravelli, et al. 1995. The incidence of complications after caesarean section in 156 HIV-positive women. *AIDS* 9:913–917.

4048. Sereti, I., B. Herpin, J. A. Metcalf, R. Stevens, M. W. Baseler, C. W. Hallahan, J. A. Kovacs, R. T. Davey, and H. C. Lane. 2001. CD4 T cell expansions are associated with increased apoptosis rates of T lymphocytes during IL-2 cycles in HIV infected patients. *AIDS* 15:1765–1775.

4049. Sereti, I., H. Imamichi, V. Natarajan, T. Imamichi, M. S. Ramchandani, Y. Badralmaa, S. C. Berg, J. A. Metcalf, B. K. Hahn, J. M. Shen, A. Powers, R. T. Davey, J. A. Kovacs, E. M. Shevach, and H. C. Lane. 2005. In vivo expansion of CD4CD45RO-CD25 T cells expressing foxP3 in IL-2-treated HIV-infected patients. *J. Clin. Investig.* 115:1839–1847.

4050. Sereti, I., and H. C. Lane. 2001. Immunopathogenesis of human immunodeficiency virus: implications for immune-based therapies. *Clin. Infect. Dis.* 32:1738–1755.

4051. Sereti, I., H. Martinez-Wilson, J. A. Metcalf, M. W. Baselar, C. W. Hallahan, B. Hahn, R. L. Hengel, R. T. Davey, J. A. Kovacs, and H. C. Lane. 2002. Long-term effects of intermittent interleukin 2 therapy in patients with HIV infection: characterization of a novel subset of CD4(+)/CD25(+) T cells. *Blood* 100:2159–2167.

4051a. Serra, P., A. Amrani, J. Yamanouchi, B. Han, S. Thiessen, T. Utsugi, J. Verdaguer, and P. Santamaria. 2003. CD40 ligation releases immature dendritic cells from the control of regulatory CD4+CD25+ T cells. *Immunity* 19:877–889.

4052. Serraino, D. 1999. The spectrum of AIDS-associated cancers in Africa. *AIDS* 13:2589–2590.

4053. Serwadda, D., R. D. Mugerwa, N. K. Sewankambo, A. Lwegaba, J. W. Carswell, G. B. Kirya, A. C. Bayley, R. G. Downing, R. S. Tedder, S. A. Clayden, R. A. Weiss, and A. G.

Dalgleish. 1985. Slim disease: a new disease in Uganda and its association with HTLV-III infection. *Lancet* ii:849–852.

4054. **Serwold, T., S. Gaw, and N. Shastri.** 2001. ER aminopeptidases generate a unique pool of peptides for MHC class I molecules. *Nat. Immunol.* 2:644–651.

4055. **Seshamma, T., O. Bagasra, D. Trono, D. Baltimore, and R. J. Pomerantz.** 1992. Blocked early-stage latency in the peripheral blood cells of certain individuals infected with human immunodeficiency virus type 1. *Proc. Natl. Acad. Sci. USA* 89:10663–10667.

4056. **Shacklett, B. L., T. J. Beadle, P. A. Pacheco, J. H. Grendell, P. A. Haslett, A. S. King, G. S. Ogg, P. M. Basuk, and D. F. Nixon.** 2000. Characterization of HIV-1-specific cytotoxic T lymphocytes expressing the mucosal lymphocyte integrin CD103 in rectal and duodenal lymphoid tissue of HIV-1-infected subjects. *Virology* 270:317–327.

4057. **Shacklett, B. L., C. A. Cox, M. F. Quigley, C. Kreis, N. H. Stollman, M. A. Jacobson, J. Andersson, J. K. Sandberg, and D. F. Nixon.** 2004. Abundant expression of granzyme A, but not perforin, in granules of CD8+ T cells in GALT: implications for immune control of HIV-1 infection. *J. Immunol.* 173:641–648.

4058. **Shadduck, P. P., J. B. Weinberg, A. F. Haney, J. A. Bartlett, A. J. Langlois, D. P. Bolognesi, and T. J. Matthews.** 1991. Lack of enhancing effect of human anti-human immunodeficiency virus type 1 (HIV-1) antibody on HIV-1 infection of human blood monocytes and peritoneal macrophages. *J. Virol.* 65:4309–4316.

4059. **Shaffer, N., R. Chuachoowong, P. A. Mock, C. Bhadrakom, W. Siriwasin, N. L. Young, T. Chotpitayasunondh, S. Chearskul, A. Roongpisuthipong, P. Chinayon, J. Karon, T. D. Mastro, and R. J. Simonds.** 1999. Short-course zidovudine for perinatal HIV-1 transmission in Bangkok, Thailand: a randomised controlled trial. *Lancet* 353:773–780.

4060. **Shafferman, A., P. B. Jahrling, R. E. Benveniste, M. G. Lewis, T. J. Phipps, F. Eden-McCutchan, J. Sadoff, G. A. Eddy, and D. S. Burke.** 1991. Protection of macaques with a simian immunodeficiency virus envelope peptide vaccine based on conserved human immunodeficiency virus type 1 sequences. *Proc. Natl. Acad. Sci. USA* 88:7126–7130.

4061. **Shahabuddin, M., B. Volsky, M. C. Hsu, and D. J. Volsky.** 1992. Restoration of cell surface CD4 expression in human immunodeficiency virus type 1-infected cells by treatment with a Tat antagonist. *J. Virol.* 66:6802–6805.

4061a. **Shankar, P., M. Russo, B. Harnisch, M. Patterson, P. Skolnik, and J. Lieberman.** 2000. Impaired function of circulating HIV-specific CD8(+) T cells in chronic human immunodeficiency virus infection. *Blood* 96:3094–3101.

4062. **Shannon, K., M. J. Cowan, E. Ball, D. Abrams, P. Volberding, and A. J. Ammann.** 1985. Impaired mononuclear-cell proliferation in patients with the acquired immune deficiency syndrome results from abnormalities of both T lymphocytes and adherent mononuclear cells. *J. Clin. Immunol.* 5:239–245.

4063. **Shapiro, L., G. B. Pott, and A. H. Ralston.** 2001. Alpha-1-antitrypsin inhibits human immunodeficiency virus type 1. *FASEB J.* 15:115–122.

4064. **Shapiro, R. L., T. Ndung'u, S. Lockman, L. M. Smeaton, I. Thior, C. Wester, L. Stevens, G. Sebetso, S. Gaseitsiwe, T. Peter, and M. Essex.** 2005. Highly active antiretroviral therapy started during pregnancy or postpartum suppresses HIV-1 RNA, but not DNA, in breast milk. *J. Infect. Dis.* 192:713–719.

4065. **Shapshak, P., D. M. Segal, K. A. Crandall, R. K. Fujimura, B.-T. Zhang, K.-Q. Xin, K. Okuda, C. K. Pettito, C. Eisdorfer, and K. Goodkin.** 1999. Independent evolution of HIV type 1 in different brain regions. *AIDS Res. Hum. Retrovir.* 15:811–820.

4066. **Sharer, L. R.** 1992. Pathology of HIV-1 infection of the central nervous system. A review. *J. Neuropathol. Exp. Neurol.* 51:3–11.

4067. **Sharer, L. R., C. Eun-Sook, and L. G. Epstein.** 1985. Multinucleated giant cells and HTLV-III in AIDS encephalopathy. *Hum. Pathol.* 16:760.

4068. **Sharkey, M. E., I. Teo, T. Greenough, N. Sharova, K. Luzuriaga, J. L. Sullivan, R. P. Bucy, L. G. Kostrikis, A. Haase, C. Veryard, R. E. Davaro, S. H. Cheeseman, J. S. Daly, C. Bova, R. T. Ellison III, B. Mady, K. K. Lai, G. Moyle, M. Nelson, B. Gazzard, S. Shaunak, and M. Stevenson.** 2000. Persistence of episomal HIV-1 infection intermediates in patients on highly active anti-retroviral therapy. *Nat. Med.* 6:76–81.

4069. **Sharma, D. P., M. Anderson, M. C. Zink, R. J. Adams, A. D. Donnenberg, J. E. Clements, and O. Narayan.** 1992. Pathogenesis of acute infection in rhesus macaques with a lymphocyte-tropic strain of simian immunodeficiency virus. *J. Infect. Dis.* 166:738–746.

4070. **Sharma, D. P., M. C. Zink, M. Anderson, R. Adams, J. E. Clements, S. V. Joag, and O. Narayan.** 1992. Derivation of neurotropic simian immunodeficiency virus from exclusively lymphocytotropic parental virus: pathogenesis of infection in macaques. *J. Virol.* 66:3550–3556.

4071. **Sharma, U. K., J. Trujillo, H. F. Song, F. P. Saitta, O. B. Laeyendecker, R. Castillo, S. Arango-Jaramillo, G. Sridharan, M. Dettenhofer, K. Blakemore, X. F. Yu, and D. H. Schwartz.** 1998. A novel factor produced by placental cells with activity against HIV-1. *J. Immunol.* 161:6406–6412.

4072. **Sharon, M., N. Kessler, R. Levy, S. Zolla-Pazner, and J. Anglister.** 2003. Alternative conformations of HIV-1 V3 loops mimic beta hairpins in chemokines, suggesting a mechanism for coreceptor selectivity. *Structure* 11:225–236.

4073. **Sharp, P. M., E. Bailes, R. R. Chaudhuri, C. M. Rodenburg, M. O. Santiago, and B. H. Hahn.** 2001. The origins of acquired immune deficiency syndrome viruses: where and when? *Philos. Trans. R. Soc. Lond. B. Biol. Sci.* 356:867–876.

4074. **Sharp, P. M., G. M. Shaw, and B. H. Hahn.** 2005. Simian immunodeficiency virus infection of chimpanzees. *J. Virol.* 79:3891–3902.

4075. **Sharpless, N. E., W. A. O'Brien, E. Verdin, C. V. Kufta, I. S. Y. Chen, and M. Dubois-Dalcq.** 1992. Human immunodeficiency virus type 1 tropism for brain microglial cells is determined by a region of the *env* glycoprotein that also controls macrophage tropism. *J. Virol.* 66:2588–2593.

4076. **Shaw, G. M., B. H. Hahn, S. K. Arya, J. E. Groopman, R. C. Gallo, and F. Wong-Staal.** 1984. Molecular characterization of human T-cell leukemia (lymphotropic) virus type III in the acquired immune deficiency syndrome. *Science* 226:1165–1171.

4077. **Shaw, G. M., M. E. Harper, B. H. Hahn, L. G. Epstein, D. C. Gajdusek, R. W. Price, B. A. Navia, C. K. Petito, C. J. O'Hara, J. E. Groopman, E.-S. Cho, J. Oleske, M., F. Wong-Staal, and R. C. Gallo.** 1985. HTLV-III infection in brains of children and adults with AIDS encephalopathy. *Science* 227:177–182.

4078. **Shea, A., A. Dieng Sarr, N. Jones, L. Penning, G. Eisen, A. Gueye-Ndiaye, S. Mboup, P. Kanki, and H. Cao.** 2004. CCR5 receptor expression is down-regulated in HIV type 2 infection: implication for viral control and protection. *AIDS Res. Hum. Retrovir.* 20:630–635.

4079. Shearer, G. M., and M. Clerici. 1991. Early T-helper cell defects in HIV infection. *AIDS* **5**:245–253.

4080. Shearer, G. M., and M. Clerici. 1993. Abnormalities of immune regulation in human immunodeficiency virus infection. *Pediatr. Res.* **33**:S71–S74.

4081. Shearer, G. M., and M. Clerici. 1996. Protective immunity against HIV infection: has nature done the experiment for us? *Immunol. Today* **17**:21–24.

4082. Shearer, M. H., R. D. Dark, J. Chodosh, and R. C. Kennedy. 1999. Comparison and characterization of immunoglobulin G subclasses among primate species. *Clin. Diagn. Lab. Immunol.* **6**:953–958.

4083. Sheehy, A. M., N. C. Gaddis, J. D. Chol, and M. H. Malim. 2002. Isolation of a human gene that inhibits HIV-1 infection and is suppressed by the viral Vif protein. *Nature* **418**:646–650.

4084. Sheehy, A. M., N. C. Gaddis, and M. H. Malim. 2003. The antiretroviral enzyme APOBEC3G is degraded by the proteasome in response to HIV-1 Vif. *Nat. Med.* **9**:1404–1407.

4085. Shelburne, S. A., F. Visnegarwala, J. Darcourt, E. A. Graviss, T. P. Giordano, J. White, A.C., and R. J. Hamill. 2005. Incidence and risk factors from immune reconstitution inflammatory syndrome during highly active antiretroviral therapy. *AIDS* **19**:399–406.

4086. Shen, H. M., T. Cheng, F. I. Preffer, D. Dombkowski, M. H. Tomasson, D. E. Golan, O. Yang, W. Hofmann, J. G. Sodroski, A. D. Luster, and D. T. Scadden. 1999. Intrinsic human immunodeficiency virus type 1 resistance of hematopoietic stem cells despite coreceptor expression. *J. Virol.* **73**:728–737.

4087. Shen, L., G. P. Mazzara, S. O. DiSciullo, D. L. Panicali, and N. L. Letvin. 1993. Immunization with lentivirus-like particles elicits a potent SIV-specific recall cytotoxic T-lymphocyte response in rhesus monkeys. *AIDS Res. Hum. Retrovir.* **9**:129–132.

4088. Shepp, D. H., and A. Ashraf. 1993. Effect of didanosine on human immunodeficiency virus viremia and antigenemia in patients with advanced disease: correlation with clinical response. *J. Infect. Dis.* **167**:30–35.

4089. Sheppard, H. W., M. S. Ascher, and J. F. Krowka. 1993. Viral burden and HIV disease. *Nature* **364**:291–292.

4090. Sheppard, H. W., W. Lang, M. S. Ascher, E. Vittinghoff, and W. Winkelstein. 1993. The characterization of non-progressors: long-term HIV-1 infection with stable CD4+ T-cell levels. *AIDS* **7**:1159–1166.

4091. Sher, A., R. T. Gazzinelli, I. P. Oswald, M. Clerici, M. Kullberg, E. J. Pearce, J. A. Berzofsky, T. R. Mosmann, S. L. James, H. C. Morse III, and G. M. Shearer. 1992. Role of T cell derived cytokines in the downregulation of immune responses in parasitic and retroviral infection. *Immunol. Rev.* **127**:183–204.

4092. Sheridan, P. L., T. P. Mayall, E. Verdin, and K. A. Jones. 2005. Histone acetyltransferases regulate HIV-1 enhancer activity in vitro. *Genes Dev.* **11**:3327–3340.

4093. Sherman, M. P., C. M. C. de Noronnha, M. I. Heusch, S. Greene, and W. C. Greene. 2001. Nucleocytoplasmic shuttling by human immunodeficiency virus type 1 Vpr. *J. Virol.* **75**:1522–1532.

4094. Sheth, P. M., A. Danesh, K. Shahabi, A. Rebbapragada, C. Kovacs, R. Dimayuga, R. Halpenny, K. S. Macdonald, T. Mazzulli, D. Kelvin, M. Ostrowski, and R. Kaul. 2005. HIV-specific CD8+ lymphocytes in semen are not associated with reduced HIV shedding. *J. Immunol.* **175**:4789–4796.

4095. Sheth, P. M., A. Danesh, A. Sheung, A. Rebbapragada, K. Shahabi, C. Kovacs, R. Halpenny, D. Tilley, T. Mazzulli, K. MacDonald, D. Kelvin, and R. Kaul. 2006. Disproportionately high semen shedding of HIV is associated with compartmentalized cytomegalovirus reactivation. *J. Infect. Dis.* **193**:45–48.

4096. Shevach, E. M. 2000. Regulatory T cells in autoimmmunity*. *Annu. Rev. Immunol.* **18**:423–449.

4096a. Shevach, E. M. 2006. From vanilla to 28 flavors: multiple varieties of T regulatory cells. *Immunity* **25**:195–201.

4097. Shi, B., U. De Girolami, J. He, S. Wang, A. Lorenzo, J. Busciglio, and D. Gabuzda. 1996. Apoptosis induced by HIV-1 infection of the central nervous system. *J. Clin. Investig.* **98**:1979–1990.

4098. Shi, Y., E. Brandin, E. Vincic, M. Jansson, A. Blaxhult, K. Gyllensten, L. Moberg, C. Brostrom, E. M. Fenyo, and J. Albert. 2005. Evolution of human immunodeficiency virus type 2 coreceptor usage, autologous neutralization, envelope sequence and glycosylation. *J. Gen. Virol.* **86**:3385–3396.

4099. Shibata, D., L. M. Weiss, A. M. Hernandez, B. N. Nathwani, L. Bernstein, and A. M. Levine. 1993. Epstein-Barr virus-associated non-Hodgkin's lymphoma in patients infected with the human immunodeficiency virus. *Blood* **8**:2102–2109.

4100. Shibata, R., M. D. Hoggan, C. Broscius, G. Englund, T. S. Theodore, A. Buckler-White, L. O. Arthur, Z. Israel, A. Schultz, H. C. Lane, and M. A. Martin. 1995. Isolation and characterization of a syncytium-inducing, macrophage/T-cell line-tropic human immunodeficiency virus type 1 isolate that readily infects chimpanzee cells in vitro and in vivo. *J. Virol.* **69**:4453–4462.

4101. Shibata, R., H. Sakai, T. Kiyomasu, A. Ishimoto, M. Hayami, and A. Adachi. 1990. Generation and characterization of infectious chimeric clones between human immunodeficiency virus type 1 and simian immunodeficiency virus from an African Green monkey. *J. Virol.* **64**:5861–5868.

4102. Shibata, R., C. Siemon, M. W. Cho, L. O. Arthur, S. M. Nigida, Jr., T. Matthews, L. A. Sawyer, A. Schultz, K. K. Murthy, Z. Israel, A. Javadian, P. Frost, R. C. Kennedy, H. C. Lane, and M. A. Martin. 1996. Resistance of previously infected chimpanzees to successive challenges with a heterologous intraclade B strain of human immunodeficiency virus type 1. *J. Virol.* **70**:4361–4369.

4103. Shibata, R., C. Siemon, S. C. Czajak, R. C. Desrosiers, and M. A. Martin. 1997. Live, attenuated simian immunodeficiency virus vaccines elicit potential resistance against a challenge with a human immunodeficiency virus type 1 chimeric virus. *J. Virol.* **71**:8141–8148.

4104. Shibuya, H., K. Irie, J. Ninomiya-Tsuji, M. Goebl, T. Taniguchi, and K. Matsumoto. 1992. New human gene encoding a positive modulator of HIV Tat-mediated transactivation. *Nature* **357**:700–702.

4105. Shieh, J. T., J. Martin, G. Baltuch, M. H. Malim, and F. Gonzalez-Scarano. 2000. Determinants of syncytium formation in microglia by human immunodeficiency virus type 1: role of the V1/V2 domains. *J. Virol.* **74**:693–701.

4106. Shikuma, C. M., N. Hu, C. Milne, F. Yost, C. Waslien, S. Shimizu, and B. Shiramizu. 2001. Mitochondrial DNA decrease in subcutaneous adipose tissue of HIV-infected individuals with peripheral lipoatrophy. *AIDS* **15**:1801–1809.

4107. Shimizu, N., Y. Haraguchi, Y. Takeuchi, Y. Soda, K. Kanbe, and H. Hoshino. 1999. Changes in and discrepancies between cell tropisms and coreceptor uses of human immunodeficiency virus type 1 induced by single point mutations at the V3 tip of the env protein. *Virology* **259**:324–333.

4108. Shimizu, N., Y. Soda, K. Kanbe, H. Liu, R. Mukai, T. Kitamura, and H. Hoshino. 2000. A putative G protein-coupled receptor, RDC1, is a novel coreceptor for human and simian immunodeficiency viruses. *J. Virol.* **74:**619–626.

4109. Shimizu, N. S., N. G. Shimizu, Y. Takeuchi, and H. Hoshino. 1994. Isolation and characterization of human immunodeficiency virus type 1 variants infectious to brain-derived cells: detection of common point mutations in the V3 region of the *env* gene of the variants. *J. Virol.* **68:**6130–6135.

4110. Shin, H. D., C. Winkler, J. C. Stephens, J. Bream, H. Young, J. J. Goedert, T. R. O'Brien, D. Vlahov, S. Buchbinder, J. Giorgi, C. Rinaldo, S. Donfield, A. Willoughby, S. J. O'Brien, and M. W. Smith. 2000. Genetic restriction of HIV-1 pathogenesis to AIDS by promoter alleles of IL10. *Proc. Natl. Acad. Sci. USA* **97:**14467–14472.

4111. Shioda, T., J. A. Levy, and C. Cheng-Mayer. 1991. Macrophage and T-cell line tropisms of HIV-1 are determined by specific regions of the envelope gp120 gene. *Nature* **349:**167–169.

4112. Shioda, T., J. A. Levy, and C. Cheng-Mayer. 1992. Small amino acid changes in the V3 hypervariable region of gp120 can affect the T cell line and macrophage tropisms of human immunodeficiency virus type 1. *Proc. Natl. Acad. Sci. USA* **89:**9434–9438.

4113. Shioda, T., S. Oka, S. Ida, K. Nokihara, H. Toriyoshi, S. Mori, Y. Takebe, S. Kimura, K. Shimada, and Y. Nagai. 1994. A naturally occurring single basic amino acid substitution in the V3 region of the human immunodeficiency virus type 1 env protein alters the cellular host range and antigenic structure of the virus. *J. Virol.* **68:**7689–7696.

4114. Shioda, T., S. Oka, X. Xin, H. Liu, R. Harukuni, A. Kurotani, M. Fukushima, M. K. Hasan, T. Shiino, Y. Takebe, A. Iwamoto, and Y. Nagai. 1997. In vivo sequence variability of human immunodeficiency virus type 1 envelope gp120: association of V2 extension with slow disease progression. *J. Virol.* **71:**4871–4881.

4115. Shioda, T., and H. Shibuta. 1990. Production of human immunodeficiency virus (HIV)-like particles from cells infected with recombinant vaccinia viruses carrying the *gag* gene of HIV. *Virology* **175:**139–148.

4116. Shirai, A., M. Cosentino, S. F. Leitman-Klinman, and D. M. Klinman. 1992. Human immunodeficiency virus infection induces both polyclonal and virus-specific B cell activation. *J. Clin. Investig.* **89:**561–566.

4117. Shiramizu, B., B. Herndier, T. Meeker, L. D. Kaplan, and M. McGrath. 1992. Molecular and immunophenotypic characterization of AIDS-associated EBV-negative polyclonal lymphoma. *J. Clin. Oncol.* **10:**383–389.

4118. Shirasaka, T., S. Chokekijchai, A. Yamada, G. Gosselin, J. L. Imback, and H. Mitsuya. 1995. Comparative analysis of anti-human immunodeficiency virus type 1 activities of dideoxynucleoside analogs in resting and activated peripheral blood mononuclear cells. *Antimicrob. Agents Chemother.* **39:**2555–2559.

4119. Shiver, J. W., T. M. Fu, L. Chen, D. R. Casimiro, M. E. Davies, R. K. Evans, Z. Q. Zhang, A. J. Simon, W. L. Trigona, S. A. Dubey, L. Huang, V. A. Harris, R. S. Long, X. Liang, L. Handt, W. A. Schleif, L. Zhu, D. C. Freed, N. V. Persaud, L. Guan, K. S. Punt, A. Tang, M. Chen, K. A. Wilson, K. B. Collins, G. J. Heidecker, V. R. Fernandez, H. C. Perry, J. G. Joyce, K. M. Grimm, J. C. Cook, P. M. Keller, D. S. Kresock, H. Mach, R. D. Troutman, L. A. Isopi, D. M. Williams, Z. Xu, K. E. Bohannon, D. B. Volkin, D. C. Montefiori, A. Miura, G. R. Krivulka, M. A. Lifton, M. J. Kuroda, J. E. Schmitz, N. L. Letvin, M. J. Caulfield, A. J. Bett, R. Youil, D. C. Kaslow, and E. A. Emini. 2002. Replication-incompetent adenoviral vaccine vector elicits effective anti-immunodeficiency-virus immunity. *Nature* **415:**331–335.

4119a. Shiver, J. W., and E. A. Emini. 2004. Recent advances in the development of HIV-1 vaccines using replication-incompetent adenovirus vectors. *Annu. Rev. Med.* **55:**355–372.

4120. Shore, S. L., T. L. Cromeons, and T. J. Romano. 1976. Immune destruction of virus-infected cells early in the infection cycle. *Nature* **262:**695–696.

4121. Shotton, C., C. Arnold, Q. Sattentau, J. Sodroski, and J. A. McKeating. 1995. Identification and characterization of monoclonal antibodies specific for polymorphic antigenic determinants within the V2 region of the human immunodeficiency virus type 1 envelope glycoprotein. *J. Virol.* **69:**222–230.

4122. Shrestha, S., S. A. Strathdee, N. Galai, T. Oleksyk, M. D. Fallin, S. Mehta, D. Schaid, D. Vlahov, S. J. O'Brien, and M. W. Smith. 2006. Behavioral risk exposure and host genetics of susceptibility to HIV-1 infection. *J. Infect. Dis.* **193:**16–26.

4123. Shrikant, P., D. J. Benos, L. P. Tang, and E. N. Benveniste. 1996. HIV glycoprotein 120 enhances intercellular adhesion molecule-1 gene expression in glial cells. *J. Immunol.* **156:**1307–1314.

4124. Shrikant, P., and E. N. Benveniste. 1996. The central nervous system as an immunocompetent organ: role of glial cells in antigen presentation. *J. Immunol.* **157:**1819–1882.

4125. Si, Z., N. Madani, J. M. Cox, J. J. Chruma, J. C. Klein, A. Schon, N. Phan, L. Wang, A. C. Biorn, S. Cocklin, I. Chaiken, E. Freire, A. B. I. Smith, and J. G. Sodroski. 2004. Small-molecule inhibitors of HIV-1 entry block receptor-induced conformational changes in the viral envelope glycoproteins. *Proc. Natl. Acad. Sci. USA* **101:**5036–5041.

4126. Si-Mohamed, A., M. D. Kazatchkine, I. Heard, C. Goujon, T. Prazuck, G. Aymard, G. Cessot, Y. H. Kuo, M. C. Bernard, B. Diquet, J. E. Malkin, L. Gutmann, and L. Belec. 2000. Selection of drug-resistant variants in the female genital tract of human immunodeficiency virus type 1-infected women receiving antiretroviral therapy. *J. Infect. Dis.* **182:**112–122.

4127. Sica, A., A. Saccani, A. Borsatti, C. A. Power, T. N. Wells, W. Luini, N. Polentarutti, S. Sozzani, and A. Mantovani. 1997. Bacterial lipopolysaccharide rapidly inhibits expression of C-C chemokine receptors in human monocytes. *J. Exp. Med.* **185:**969–974.

4128. Siddiqi, M. A., M. Tachibana, S. Ohta, Y. Ikegami, S. Tahara-Hanaoka, Y. Y. Huang, and N. Shinohara. 1997. Comparative analysis of the gp120-binding area of murine and human CD4 molecules. *J. Acquir. Immune Defic. Syndr. Hum. Retrovirol.* **14:**7–12.

4129. Siddiqui, A., R. Gaynor, A. Srinivasan, J. Mapoles, and R. W. Farr. 1989. Trans-activation of viral enhancers including long terminal repeat of the human immunodeficiency virus by the hepatitis B virus X protein. *Virology* **169:**479–484.

4130. Sidenius, N., C. F. Sier, H. Ullum, B. K. Pedersen, A. C. Lepri, F. Blasi, and J. Eugen-Olsen. 2000. Serum level of soluble urokinase-type plasminogen activator receptor is a strong and independent predictor of survival in human immunodeficiency virus infection. *Blood* **96:**4091–4095.

4131. Siebelink, K. H. J., E. Tijhaar, R. C. Huisman, W. Huisman, A. de Ronde, I. H. Darby, M. J. Francis, G. F. Rimmelzwaan, and A. D. M. E. Osterhaus. 1995. Enhancement of feline immunodeficiency virus infection after immunization with envelope glycoprotein subunit vaccines. *J. Virol.* **69:**3704–3711.

4132. Sieg, S. F., C. V. Harding, and M. M. Lederman. 2001. HIV-1 infection impairs cell cycle progression of CD4+ T cells without affecting early activation responses. *J. Clin. Investig.* 108:757–764.

4133. Siegal, F. P., N. Kadowaki, M. Shodell, P. A. Fitzgerald-Bocarsly, K. Shah, S. Ho, S. Antonenko, and Y. J. Liu. 1999. The nature of the principal type 1 interferon-producing cells in human blood. *Science* 284:1835–1837.

4134. Siegal, F. P., C. Lopez, P. A. Fitzgerald, K. Shah, P. Baron, I. Z. Leiderman, D. Imperato, and S. Landesman. 1986. Opportunistic infections in acquired immune deficiency syndrome result from synergistic defects of both the natural and adaptive components of cellular immunity. *J. Clin. Investig.* 78:115–123.

4135. Siegal, F. P., C. Lopez, and G. S. Hammer. 1981. Severe acquired immunodeficiency in male homosexuals, manifested by chronic perianal ulcerative *herpes simplex* lesions. *N. Engl. J. Med.* 305:1439–1444.

4136. Siegal, F. P., and G. T. Spear. 2001. Innate immunity and HIV. *AIDS* 15:S127–S137.

4137. Siegel, F., R. Kurth, and S. Norley. 1995. Neither whole inactivated virus immunogen nor passive immunoglobulin transfer protects against SIVagm infection in the African Green monkey natural host. *J. Acquir. Immune Defic. Syndr. Hum. Retrovirol.* 8:217–226.

4138. Siegel, J. P., J. Y. Djeu, N. I. Stocks, H. Mazur, E. P. Gelman, and G. V. Quinnan. 1985. Sera from patients with the acquired immune deficiency syndrome inhibit production of interleukin-2 by normal lymphocytes. *J. Clin. Investig.* 75:1957–1964.

4139. Sieling, P. A., J. S. Abrams, M. Yamamura, P. Salgame, B. R. Bloom, T. H. Rea, and R. L. Modlin. 1993. Immunosuppressive roles for IL-10 and IL-4 in human infection: *in vitro* modulation of T-cell response in leprosy. *J. Immunol.* 150:5501–5510.

4140. Siliciano, J. D., J. Kajdas, D. Finzi, T. C. Quinn, K. Chadwick, J. B. Margolick, C. Kovacs, S. J. Gange, and R. F. Siliciano. 2003. Long-term follow-up studies confirm the stability of the latent reservoir for HIV-1 in resting CD4+ T cells. *Nat. Med.* 9:727–728.

4141. Siliciano, J. D., and R. F. Siliciano. 2000. Latency and viral persistence in HIV-1 infection. *J. Clin. Investig.* 106:823–825.

4142. Siliciano, R. F., T. Lawton, C. Knall, R. W. Karr, P. Berman, T. Gregory, and E. L. Reinherz. 1988. Analysis of host-virus interactions in AIDS with anti-gp120 T cell clones: effect of HIV sequence variation and a mechanism for CD4+ cell depletion. *Cell* 54:561–575.

4143. Silvestri, G., A. Fedanov, S. Germon, N. Kozyr, W. J. Kaiser, D. A. Garber, H. McClure, M. B. Feinberg, and S. I. Staprans. 2005. Divergent host responses during primary simian immunodeficiency virus SIVsm infection of natural sooty mangabey and nonnatural rhesus macaque hosts. *J. Virol.* 79:4043–4054.

4144. Silvestri, G., and M. B. Feinberg. 2003. Turnover of lymphocytes and conceptual paradigms in HIV infection. *J. Clin. Investig.* 112:821–824.

4145. Silvestri, G., D. L. Sodora, R. A. Koup, M. Paiardini, S. P. O'Neil, H. M. McClure, S. I. Staprans, and M. B. Feinberg. 2003. Nonpathogenic SIV infection of sooty mangabeys is characterized by limited bystander immunopathology despite chronic high-level viremia. *Immunity* 18:441–452.

4146. Silvestris, F., P. Cafforio, M. A. Frassanito, M. Tucci, A. Romito, S. Nagata, and F. Dammacco. 1996. Overexpression of Fas antigen on T cells in advanced HIV-1 infection: differential ligation constantly induces apoptosis. *AIDS* 10:131–141.

4147. Simm, M., L. S. Miller, H. G. Durkin, M. Allen, W. Chao, A. Lesner, M. J. Potash, and D. J. Volsky. 2002. Induction of secreted human immunodeficiency virus type 1 (HIV-1) resistance factors in CD4–positive T lymphocytes by attenuated HIV-1 infection. *Virology* 294:1–12.

4148. Simmonds, P., P. Balfe, J. F. Peutherer, C. A. Ludlam, J. O. Biship, and A. J. L. Brown. 1990. Human immunodeficiency virus-infected individuals contain provirus in small numbers of peripheral mononuclear cells and at low copy numbers. *J. Virol.* 64:864–872.

4149. Simmonds, P., L. Q. Zhang, F. McOmish, P. Balfe, C. A. Ludlam, and A. J. L. Brown. 1991. Discontinuous sequence change of human immunodeficiency virus (HIV) type 1 *env* sequences in plasma viral and lymphocyte-associated proviral populations in vivo: implications for models of HIV pathogenesis. *J. Virol.* 65:6266–6276.

4150. Simmons, G., P. R. Clapham, L. Picard, R. E. Offord, M. M. Rosenkilde, T. W. Schwartz, R. Buser, T. N. C. Wells, and A. E. I. Proudfoot. 1997. Potent inhibition of HIV-1 infectivity in macrophages and lymphocytes by a novel CCR5 antagonist. *Science* 276:276–279.

4151. Simmons, G., J. D. Reeves, A. McKnight, N. Dejucq, S. Hibbitts, C. A. Power, E. Aarons, D. Scholds, E. De Clercq, A. E. I. Proudfoot, and P. R. Clapham. 1998. CXCR4 as a functional coreceptor for human immunodeficiency virus type 1 infection of primary macrophages. *J. Virol.* 72:8453–8457.

4152. Simon, F., S. Matheron, C. Tamalet, I. Loussert-Ajaka, S. Bartczak, J. M. Pepin, C. Dhiver, E. Gamba, C. Elbim, J. A. Gastaut, A. G. Saimot, and F. Brun-Vezinet. 1993. Cellular and plasma viral load in patients infected with HIV-2. *AIDS* 7:1411–1417.

4153. Simon, F., P. Mauclere, P. Roques, I. Loussert-Ajaka, M. C. Muller-Trutwin, S. Saragosti, M. C. Georges-Courbot, F. Barre-Sinoussi, and F. Brun-Vezinet. 1998. Identification of a new human immunodeficiency virus type 1 distinct from group M and group O. *Nat. Med.* 4:1032–1037.

4154. Simon, J. H. M., D. L. Miller, R. A. M. Fouchier, and M. H. Malim. 1998. Virion incorporation of human immunodeficiency virus type-1 Vif is determined by intracellular expression level and may not be necessary for function. *Virology* 248:182–187.

4155. Sinangil, F., A. Loyter, and D. J. Volsky. 1988. Quantitative measurement of fusion between human immunodeficiency virus and cultured cells using membrane fluorescence dequenching. *FEBS Lett.* 239:88–92.

4156. Sindhu, S., R. Ahmad, R. Morisset, A. Ahmad, and J. Menezes. 2003. Peripheral blood cytotoxic gamma delta T lymphocytes from patients with human immunodeficiency virus type 1 infection and AIDS lyse uninfected CD4+ T cells, and their cytocidal potential correlates with viral load. *J. Virol.* 77:1848–1855.

4156a. Singh, I. P., A. K. Chopra, D. H. Coppenhaver, G. M. Ananatharamaiah, and S. Baron. 1999. Lipoproteins account for part of the broad non-specific antiviral activity of human serum. *Antiviral Res.* 42:211–218.

4157. Singh, K. K., M. D. Hughes, J. Chen, and S. A. Spector. 2005. Genetic polymorphisms in CX_3CR1 predict HIV-1 disease progression in children independently of CD4+ lymphocyte count and HIV-1 RNA load. *J. Infect. Dis.* 191:1971–1980.

4158. Singh, M. K., and C. D. Pauza. 1992. Extrachromosomal human immunodeficiency virus type 1 sequences are methylated in latently infected U937 cells. *Virology* **188**:451–458.

4159. Sinicco, A., R. Fora, M. Sciandra, A. Lucchini, P. Caramello, and P. Gioannini. 1993. Risk of developing AIDS after primary acute HIV-1 infection. *J. Acquir. Immune Defic. Syndr.* **6**:575–581.

4160. Sipsas, N. V., S. A. Kalams, A. Trocha, S. He, W. A. Blattner, B. D. Walker, and R. P. Johnson. 1997. Identification of type-specific cytotoxic T lymphocyte responses to homologous viral proteins in laboratory workers accidentally infected with HIV-1. *J. Clin. Investig.* **99**:752–762.

4161. Sipsas, N. V., S. I. Kokori, J. P. Ioannidis, D. Kyriaki, A. G. Tzioufas, and T. Kordossis. 1999. Circulating autoantibodies to erythropoietin are associated with human immunodeficiency virus type 1-related anemia. *J. Infect. Dis.* **180**:2044–2047.

4162. Sirianni, M. C., S. Uccini, A. Angeloni, A. Faggioni, F. Cottoni, and B. Ensoli. 1997. Circulating spindle cells: correlation with human herpesvirus-8 (HHV-8) infection and Kaposi's sarcoma. *Lancet* **349**:255.

4163. Skiest, D. J., and C. Crosby. 2003. Survival is prolonged by highly active antiretroviral therapy in AIDS patients with primary central nervous system lymphoma. *AIDS* **17**:1787–1793.

4164. Skiest, D. J., P. Morrow, B. Allen, J. McKinsey, C. Crosby, B. Foster, and R. D. Hardy. 2004. It is safe to stop antiretroviral therapy in patients with preantiretroviral CD4 cell counts >250 cells/microL. *J. Acquir. Immune. Defic. Syndr.* **37**:1351–1357.

4165. Skinner, M. A., A. J. Langlois, C. B. McDanal, J. S. McDougal, D. P. Bolognesi, and T. J. Matthews. 1988. Neutralizing antibodies to an immunodominant envelope sequence do not prevent gp120 binding to CD4. *J. Virol.* **62**:4195–4200.

4166. Sklar, P., and H. Masur. 2003. HIV infection and cardiovascular disease—is there really a link? *N. Engl. J. Med.* **349**:2065–2067.

4167. Skolnik, P. R., B. R. Kosloff, L. J. Bechtel, K. R. Huskins, T. Flynn, N. Karthas, K. McIntosh, and M. S. Hirsch. 1989. Absence of infectious HIV-1 in the urine of seropositive viremic subjects. *J. Infect. Dis.* **160**:1056–1060.

4168. Skolnik, P. R., B. R. Kosloff, and M. S. Hirsch. 1988. Bidirectional interactions between human immunodeficiency virus type 1 and cytomegalovirus. *J. Infect. Dis.* **157**:508–514.

4169. Skowronski, J., D. Parks, and R. Mariani. 1993. Altered T cell activation and development in transgenic mice expressing the HIV-1 nef gene. *EMBO J.* **12**:703–713.

4170. Skrabal, K., S. Saragosti, J. L. Labernardiere, F. Barin, F. Clavel, and F. Mammano. 2005. Human immunodeficiency virus type 1 variants isolated from single plasma samples display a wide spectrum of neutralization sensitivity. *J. Virol.* **79**:11848–11857.

4171. Skrabal, K., V. Trouplin, B. Labrosse, V. Obry, F. Damong, A. J. Hance, F. Clavel, and F. Mammano. 2003. Impact of antiretroviral treatment on the tropism of HIV-1 plasma virus populations. *AIDS* **17**:809–814.

4172. Slepushkin, V. A., G. V. Kornilaeva, S. M. Andreev, M. V. Sidorova, A. O. Petrukhina, G. R. Matsevich, S. V. Raduk, V. B. Grigoriev, T. V. Makarova, V. V. Lukashov, and E. V. Karamov. 1993. Inhibition of human immunodeficiency virus type 1 (HIV-1) penetration into target cells by synthetic peptides mimicking the N-terminus of the HIV-1 transmembrane glycoprotein. *Virology* **194**:294–301.

4173. Sloan, E. K., R. P. Tarara, J. P. Capitanio, and S. W. Cole. 2006. Enhanced replication of simian immunodeficiency virus adjacent to catecholaminergic varicosities in primate lymph nodes. *J. Virol.* **80**:4326–4335.

4174. Smed-Sorensen, A., K. Lore, J. Vasudevan, M. K. Louder, J. Andersson, J. R. Mascola, A. L. Spetz, and R. A. Koup. 2005. Differential susceptibility to human immunodeficiency virus type 1 infection of myeloid and plasmacytoid dendritic cells. *J. Virol.* **79**:8861–8869.

4175. Smith, A. J., N. Srinivasakumar, M.-L. Hammarskjold, and D. Rekosh. 1993. Requirements for incorporation of Pr160gag-pol from human immunodeficiency virus type 1 into virus-like particles. *J. Virol.* **67**:2266–2275.

4176. Smith, B. A., S. Gartner, Y. Liu, A. S. Perelson, N. I. Stilianakis, B. F. Keele, T. M. Kerkering, A. Ferreira-Gonzalez, A. K. Szakal, J. G. Tew, and G. F. Burton. 2001. Persistence of infectious HIV on follicular dendritic cells. *J. Immunol.* **166**:690–696.

4177. Smith, B. A., J. L. Neidig, J. T. Nickel, G. L. Mitchell, M. F. Para, and R. J. Fass. 2001. Aerobic exercise: effects on parameters related to fatigue, dyspnea, weight and body composition in HIV-infected adults. *AIDS* **15**:693–701.

4178. Smith, D. E., B. D. Walker, D. A. Cooper, E. S. Rosenberg, and J. M. Kaldor. 2004. Is antiretroviral treatment of primary HIV infection clinically justified on the basis of current evidence? *AIDS* **18**:709–718.

4179. Smith, D. M., D. D. Richman, and S. J. Little. 2005. HIV superinfection. *J. Infect. Dis.* **192**:438–444.

4180. Smith, D. M., J. K. Wong, G. K. Hightower, C. C. Ignacio, K. K. Koelsch, E. S. Daar, D. D. Richman, and S. J. Little. 2004. Incidence of HIV superinfection following primary infection. *JAMA* **292**:1177–1178.

4181. Smith, D. M., J. K. Wong, G. K. Hightower, C. C. Ignacio, K. K. Koelsch, C. J. Petropoulos, D. D. Richman, and S. J. Little. 2005. HIV drug resistance acquired through superinfection. *AIDS* **19**:1251–1256.

4182. Smith, K. Y., H. Valdez, A. Landay, J. Spritzler, H. A. Kessler, E. Connick, D. Kuritzkes, B. Gross, I. Francis, J. M. McCune, and M. M. Lederman. 2000. Thymic size and lymphocyte restoration in patients with human immunodeficiency virus infection after 48 weeks of zidovudine, lamivudine, and ritonavir therapy. *J. Infect. Dis.* **181**:141–147.

4183. Smith, M. W., M. Dean, M. Carrington, C. Winkler, G. A. Huttley, D. A. Lomb, J. J. Goedert, T. R. O'Brien, L. P. Jacobson, R. Kaslow, S. Buchbinder, E. Vittinghoff, D. Vlahov, K. Hoots, M. W. Hilgartner, and S. J. O'Brien. 1997. Contrasting genetic influence of CCR2 and CCR5 variants on HIV-1 infection and disease progression. *Science* **277**:959–965.

4184. Smith, M. W., M. Dean, M. Carrington, C. Winkler, G. A. Huttley, D. A. Lomb, J. J. Goedert, T. R. O'Brien, L. P. Jacobson, R. Kaslow, S. Buchbinder, E. Vittinghoff, D. Vlahov, K. Hoots, M. W. Hilgartner, and S. J. O'Brien. 1997. Contrasting genetic influence of CCR2 and CCR5 variants on HIV-1 infection and disease progression. Hemophilia Growth and Development Study (HGDS), Multicenter AIDS Cohort Study (MACS), Multicenter Hemophilia Cohort Study (MHCS), San Francisco City Cohort (SFCC), ALIVE Study. *Science* **277**:959–965.

4185. Smith, P. D., G. Meng, J. F. Salazar-Gonzalez, and G. M. Shaw. 2003. Macrophage HIV-1 infection and the gastrointestinal tract reservoir. *J. Leukoc. Biol.* **74**:642–649.

4186. Smith, P. D., G. Meng, M. T. Sellers, T. S. Rogers, and G. M. Shaw. 2000. Biological parameters of HIV-1 infection in primary intestinal lymphocytes and macrophages. *J. Leukoc. Biol.* 68:360–365.

4187. Smith, P. D., K. Ohura, H. Masur, H. C. Lane, A. S. Fauci, and S. M. Wahl. 1984. Monocyte function in the acquired immune deficiency syndrome: defective chemotaxis. *J. Clin. Investig.* 74:2121–2128.

4188. Smith, S. M., M. Khoroshev, P. A. Marx, J. Orenstein, and K. T. Jeang. 2001. Constitutively dead, conditionally live HIV-1 genomes. Ex vivo implications for a live virus vaccine. *J. Biol. Chem.* 276:32184–32190.

4189. Smith, S. M., M. Mefford, D. Sodora, Z. Klase, M. Singh, N. Alexander, D. Hess, and P. A. Marx. 2004. Topical estrogen protects against SIV vaginal transmission without evidence of systemic effect. *AIDS* 18:1637–1643.

4190. Smyth, M. J., K. Y. Thia, S. E. Street, E. Cretney, J. A. Trapani, M. Taniguchi, T. Kawano, S. B. Pelikan, N. Y. Crowe, and D. I. Godfrey. 2000. Differential tumor surveillance by natural killer (NK) and NKT cells. *J. Exp. Med.* 191:661–668.

4191. Snider, W. D., D. M. Simpson, K. E. Aronyk, and S. L. Nielsen. 1983. Primary lymphoma of the nervous system associated with acquired immune-deficiency syndrome. *N. Engl. J. Med.* 308:45.

4192. Snijders, F., P. C. Wever, S. A. Danner, C. E. Hack, F. J. W. ten Kate, and I. J. M. ten Berge. 1996. Increased numbers of granzyme-B-expressing cytotoxic T-lymphocytes in the small intestine of HIV-infected patients. *J. Acquir. Immune Defic. Syndr. Hum. Retrovirol.* 12:276–281.

4193. Snyder, G. A., J. Ford, P. Torabi-Parizi, J. A. Arthos, P. Schuck, M. Colonna, and P. D. Sun. 2005. Characterization of DC-SIGN/R interaction with human immunodeficiency virus type 1 gp120 and ICAM molecules favors the receptor's role as an antigen-capturing rather than an adhesion receptor. *J. Virol.* 79:4589–4598.

4194. So, Y. T., J. H. Beckstead, and R. L. Davis. 1986. Primary central nervous system lymphoma in acquired immune deficiency syndrome: a clinical and pathological study. *Ann. Neurol.* 20:566–572.

4195. Sodora, D. L., A. Gettie, C. J. Miller, and P. A. Marx. 1998. Vaginal transmission of SIV: assessing infectivity and hormonal influences in macaques inoculated with cell-free and cell-associated viral stocks. *AIDS Res. Hum. Retrovir.* 14(Suppl. 1):S119–S123.

4196. Sodroski, J., W. C. Goh, C. Rosen, K. Campbell, and W. A. Haseltine. 1986. Role of the HTLV-III/LAV envelope in syncytium formation and cytopathicity. *Nature* 322:470–474.

4197. Sodroski, J. G., W. C. Goh, C. Rosen, A. Dayton, E. Terwilliger, and W. A. Haseltine. 1986. A second posttranscriptional transactivator gene required for HTLV-III replication. *Nature* 321:412–417.

4198. Soeiro, R., A. Rubinstein, W. K. Rashbaum, and W. D. Lyman. 1992. Maternofetal transmission of AIDS: frequency of human immunodeficiency virus type 1 nucleic acid sequences in human fetal DNA. *J. Infect. Dis.* 166:699–703.

4199. Soilleux, E. J., R. Barten, and J. Trowsdale. 2000. DC-SIGN; a related gene, DC-SIGNR; and CD23 form a cluster on 19p13. *J. Immunol.* 165:2937–2942.

4200. Soilleux, E. J., L. S. Morris, G. Leslie, J. Chehimi, Q. Luo, E. Levroney, J. Trowsdale, L. J. Montaner, R. W. Doms, D. Weissman, N. Coleman, and B. Lee. 2002. Constitutive and induced expression of DC-SIGN on dendritic cell and macrophage subpopulations in situ and in vitro. *J. Leukoc. Biol.* 71:445–457.

4201. Solder, B. M., T. F. Schulz, P. Hengster, J. Lower, C. Larcher, G. Bitterlich, R. Kurth, H. Wachter, and M. P. Dierich. 1989. HIV and HIV-infected cells differentially activate the human complement system independent of antibody. *Immunol. Lett.* 22:135–145.

4202. Solomon, A., N. Lane, F. Wightman, P. R. Gorry, and S. R. Lewin. 2005. Enhanced replicative capacity and pathogenicity of HIV-1 isolated from individuals infected with drug-resistant virus and declining CD4+ T-cell counts. *J. Acquir. Immune. Defic. Syndr.* 40:140–148.

4203. Somasundaran, M., and H. L. Robinson. 1987. A major mechanism of human immunodeficiency virus-induced cell killing does not involve cell fusion. *J. Virol.* 61:3114–3119.

4204. Song, H., E. E. Nakayama, and T. Shioda. 2006. Effects of human interleukin 7 on HIV-1 replication in monocyte-derived human macrophages. *AIDS* 20:937–939.

4205. Song, S. K., H. Li, and M. W. Cloyd. 1996. Rates of shutdown of HIV-1 into latency: roles of the LTR and *tat/rev/vpu* gene region. *Virology* 225:377–386.

4206. Sonnerborg, A., B. Johansson, and O. Strannegard. 1991. Detection of HIV-1 DNA and infectious virus in cerebrospinal fluid. *AIDS Res. Hum. Retrovir.* 7:369–373.

4207. Sonnerborg, A. B., A. C. Ehrnst, S. K. M. Bergdahl, P. O. Pehrson, B. R. Skoldenberg, and O. O. Strannegard. 1988. HIV isolation from cerebrospinal fluid in relation to immunological deficiency and neurological symptoms. *AIDS Res. Hum. Retrovir.* 2:89–93.

4208. Sonza, S., A. Maerz, N. Deacon, J. Meanger, J. Mills, and S. Crowe. 1996. Human immunodeficiency virus type 1 replication is blocked prior to reverse transcription and integration in freshly isolated peripheral blood monocytes. *J. Virol.* 70:3863–3869.

4209. Soriano, V., C. Dona, R. Rodriguez-Rosado, P. Barreiro, and J. Gonzalez-Lahoz. 2000. Discontinuation of secondary prophylaxis for opportunistic infections in HIV-infected patients receiving highly active antiretroviral therapy. *AIDS* 14:383–386.

4210. Soriano, V., M. Puoti, M. Bonacini, G. Brook, A. Cargnel, J. Rockstroh, C. Thio, and Y. Benhamou. 2005. Care of patients with chronic hepatitis B and HIV co-infection: recommendations from an HIV-HBV International Panel. *AIDS* 19:221–240.

4211. Soros, V. B., H. V. Carvajal, S. Richard, and A. W. Cochrane. 2001. Inhibition of human immunodeficiency virus type 1 Rev function by a dominant-negative mutant of Sam68 through sequestration of unspliced RNA at perinuclear bundles. *J. Virol.* 75:8203–8215.

4212. Soto-Ramirez, L. E., B. Renjifo, M. F. McLane, R. Marlink, C. O'Hara, R. Sutthent, C. Wasi, P. Vithayasai, V. Vithayasai, C. Apichartpiyakul, P. Auewarakul, V. Pena Cruz, D. S. Chui, R. Osanthanondh, K. Mayer, T. H. Lee, and M. Essex. 1996. HIV-1 Langerhans' cell tropism associated with heterosexual transmission of HIV. *Science* 271:1291–1293.

4213. Soudeyns, H., S. Paolucci, C. Chappey, M. Daucher, C. Grazioso, M. Vaccarezza, O. J. Cohen, A. S. Fauci, and G. Pantaleo. 1999. Selective pressure exerted by immunodominant HIV-1-specific cytotoxic T lymphocyte responses during primary infection drives genetic variation restricted to the cognate epitope. *Eur. J. Immunol.* 29:2629–3635.

4214. Soulier, J., L. Grollet, E. Oksenhendler, P. Cacoub, D. Cazals-Hatem, P. Babinet, M. F. d'Agay, J. P. Clauvel, M. Raphael, L. Degos, and F. Sigaux. 1995. Kaposi's sarcoma-associated herpesvirus-like DNA sequences in multicentric Castleman's disease. *Blood* 86:1276–1280.

4215. Soumelis, V., I. Scott, F. Gheyas, D. Bouhour, G. Cozon, L. Cotte, L. Huang, J. Levy, and Y. J. Liu. 2001. Depletion of circulating natural type 1 interferon-producing cells in HIV-infected AIDS patients. *Blood* 98:906–912.

4216. Sousa, A. E., J. Carneiro, M. Meier-Schellersheim, Z. Grossman, and R. M. M. Victorino. 2002. CD4 T cell depletion is linked directly to immune activation in the pathogenesis of HIV-1 and HIV-2 but only indirectly to the viral load. *J. Immunol.* 169:3400–3406.

4217. Sozzani, S., S. Ghezzi, G. Iannolo, W. Luini, A. Borsatti, N. Polentarutti, A. Sica, M. Locati, C. Mackay, T. N. Wells, P. Biswas, E. Vicenzi, G. Poli, and A. Mantovani. 1998. Interleukin 10 increases CCR5 expression and HIV infection in human monocytes. *J. Exp. Med.* 187:439–444.

4218. Spear, G. T. 1993. Interaction of non-antibody factors with HIV in plasma. *AIDS* 7:1149–1157.

4219. Spear, G. T., J. R. Carlson, M. B. Jennings, D. M. Takefman, and A. L. Landay. 1992. Complement-mediated neutralizing activity of antibody from HIV-infected persons and HIV-vaccinated macaques. *AIDS* 6:1047. (Letter.)

4220. Spear, G. T., G. G. Olinger, M. Saifuddin, and H. M. Gebel. 2001. Human antibodies to major histocompatibility complex alloantigens mediate lysis and neutralization of HIV-1 primary isolate virions in the presence of complement. *J. Acquir. Immune Defic. Syndr.* 26:103–110.

4221. Spear, G. T., B. L. Sullivan, A. L. Landay, and T. F. Lint. 1990. Neutralization of human immunodeficiency virus type 1 by complement occurs by viral lysis. *J. Virol.* 64:5869–5873.

4222. Spear, G. T., D. M. Takefman, B. L. Sullivan, A. L. Landay, and S. Zolla-Pazner. 1993. Complement activation by human monoclonal antibodies to human immunodeficiency virus. *J. Virol.* 67:53–59.

4223. Spearman, P., J. J. Wang, N. Vander Heyden, and L. Ratner. 1994. Identification of human immunodeficiency virus type 1 Gag protein domains essential to membrane binding and particle assembly. *J. Virol.* 68:3232–3242.

4224. Speck, R. F., K. Wehrly, E. J. Platt, R. E. Atchison, I. F. Charo, D. Kabat, B. Chesebro, and M. A. Goldsmith. 1997. Selective employment of chemokine receptors as human immunodeficiency virus type 1 coreceptors determined by individual amino acids within the envelope V3 loop. *J. Virol.* 71:7136–7139.

4225. Spehar, T., and M. Strand. 1994. Cross-reactivity of anti-human immunodeficiency virus type 1 gp41 antibodies with human astrocytes and astrocytoma cell lines. *J. Virol.* 68:6262–6269.

4226. Speiser, D. E., D. Liénard, N. Rufer, V. Rubio-Godoy, D. Rimoldi, F. Lejeune, A. M. Krjieg, J.-C. Cerottini, and P. Romero. 2005. Rapid and strong human CD8+ T cell responses to vaccination with peptide, IFA, and CpG oligodeoxynucleotide 7909. *J. Clin. Investig.* 115:739–746.

4227. Spencer, L. T., M. T. Ogino, W. M. Dankner, and S. A. Spector. 1994. Clinical significance of human immunodeficiency virus type 1 phenotypes in infected children. *J. Infect. Dis.* 169:491–495.

4228. Sperduto, A. R., Y. J. Bryson, and I. S. Y. Chen. 1993. Increased susceptibility of neonatal monocyte/macrophages to HIV-1 infection. *AIDS Res. Hum. Retrovir.* 9:1277–1285.

4229. Speth, C., K. Williams, M. Hagleitner, S. Westmoreland, G. Rambach, I. Mohsenipour, J. Schmitz, R. Wurzner, C. Lass-Florl, H. Stoiber, M. P. Dierich, and H. Maier. 2004. Complement synthesis and activation in the brain of SIV-infected monkeys. *J. Neuroimmunol.* 151:45–54.

4230. Spiegel, H., H. Berbst, G. Niedobitek, H. D. Foss, and H. Stein. 1992. Follicular dendritic cells are a major reservoir for human immunodeficiency virus type 1 in lymphoid tissues facilitating infection of CD4+ T-helper cells. *Am. J. Pathol.* 140:15–22.

4231. Spiegel, H. M., E. DeFalcon, G. S. Ogg, M. Larsson, T. J. Beadle, P. Tao, A. J. McMichael, N. Bhardwaj, C. O'Callaghan, W. I. Cox, K. Krasinski, H. Pollack, W. Borkowsky, and D. F. Nixon. 1999. Changes in frequency of HIV-1-specific cytotoxic T cell precursors and circulating effectors after combination antiretroviral therapy in children. *J. Infect. Dis.* 180:359–368.

4232. Spiegel, H. M., G. S. Ogg, E. DeFalcon, M. E. Sheehy, S. Monard, P. A. Haslett, G. Gillespie, S. M. Donahoe, H. Pollack, W. Borkowsky, A. J. McMichael, and D. F. Nixon. 2000. Human immunodeficiency virus type 1- and cytomegalovirus-specific cytotoxic T lymphocytes can persist at high frequency for prolonged periods in the absence of circulating peripheral CD4(+) T cells. *J. Virol.* 74:1018–1022.

4233. Spijkerman, I. J. B., M. Koot, M. Prins, I. P. M. Keet, A. J. A. R. van den Hoek, F. Miedema, and R. A. Coutinho. 1995. Lower prevalence and incidence of HIV-1 syncytium-inducing phenotype among injecting drug users compared with homosexual men. *AIDS* 9:1085–1092.

4234. Spina, C. A., T. J. Kwoh, M. Y. Chowers, J. C. Guatelli, and D. D. Richman. 1994. The importance of Nef in the induction of human immunodeficiency virus type 1 replication from primary quiescent CD4 lymphocytes. *J. Exp. Med.* 179:115–123.

4235. Spina, C. A., H. E. Prince, and D. D. Richman. 1997. Preferential replication of HIV-1 in the CD45RO memory cell subset of primary CD4 lymphcytes *in vitro*. *J. Clin. Investig.* 99:1774–1785.

4236. Spina, M., U. Jaeger, J. A. Sparano, R. Talamini, C. Simonelli, M. Michieli, G. Rossi, E. Nigra, M. Berretta, C. Cattaneo, A. C. Rieger, E. Vaccher, and U. Tirelli. 2005. Rituximab plus infusional cyclophosphamide, doxorubicin, and etoposide in HIV-associated non-Hodgkin lymphoma: pooled results from 3 phase 2 trials. *Blood* 105:1891–1897.

4237. Spira, A. I., P. A. Marx, B. K. Patterson, J. Mahoney, R. A. Koup, S. M. Wolinsky, and D. D. Ho. 1996. Cellular targets of infection and route of viral dissemination after an intravaginal inoculation of simian immunodeficiency virus into rhesus macaques. *J. Exp. Med.* 183:215–225.

4238. Spits, H., F. Couwenberg, A. Q. Bakker, K. Weijer, and C. H. Uittenbogaart. 2000. Id2 and Id3 inhibit development of CD34(+) stem cells into predendritic cell (pre-DC)2 but not into pre-DC1. Evidence for a lymphoid origin of pre-DC2. *J. Exp. Med.* 192:1775–1784.

4239. Sprent, J., and D. F. Tough. 1994. Lymphocyte life-span and memory. *Science* 265:1395–1400.

4240. Spring, M., C. Stahl-Hennig, N. Nisslein, C. Locher, D. Fuchs, W. Bodemer, G. Hunsmann, and U. Dittmer. 1998. Suppression of viral replication in a long-term nonprogressing rhesus macaque experimentally infected with pathogenic simian immunodeficiency virus (SIV). *Clin. Immunol. Immunopathol.* 87:101–105.

4241. Spruth, M., H. Stoiber, L. Kacani, D. Schonitzer, and M. P. Dierich. 1999. Neutralization of HIV type 1 by alloimmune sera derived from polytransfused patients. *AIDS Res. Hum. Retrovir.* **15**:533–543.

4242. Srivastava, I. K., L. Stamatatos, E. Kan, M. Vajdy, Y. Lain, S. Hilt, L. Martin, C. Vita, P. Zhu, K. H. Roux, L. C. Vojtech, D. Montefiori, J. Donnelly, J. B. Ulmer, and S. W. Barnett. 2003. Purification, characterization, and immunogenicity of a soluble trimeric envelope protein containing a partial deletion of the V2 loop derived from SF162, an R5-tropic human immunodeficiency virus type 1 isolate. *J. Virol.* **77**:11244–11259.

4243. Srivastava, I. K., J. B. Ulmer, and S. W. Barnett. 2004. Neutralizing antibody responses to HIV: role in protective immunity and challenges for vaccine design. *Expert Rev. Vaccines* **3**:S33–52.

4244. St. Louis, M. E., M. Kamenga, C. Brown, A. M. Nelson, T. Manzila, V. Batter, F. Behets, U. Kabagabo, R. W. Ryder, M. Oxtoby, T. C. Quinn, and W. L. Heyward. 1993. Risk for perinatal HIV-1 transmission according to maternal immunologic, virologic, and placental factors. *JAMA* **269**:2853–2859.

4245. Staak, K., S. Prosch, J. Stein, C. Priemer, R. Ewert, W. D. Docke, D. H. Kruger, H. D. Volk, and P. Reinke. 1997. Pentoxifylline promotes replication of human cytomegalovirus *in vivo* and *in vitro*. *Blood* **89**:3682–3690.

4246. Stahl, R. E., A. Friedman-Kien, R. Dubin, M. Marmor, and S. Zolla-Pazner. 1982. Immunologic abnormalities in homosexual men. *Am. J. Med.* **73**:171–178.

4247. Stahl-Hennig, C., U. Dittmer, T. Nisslein, H. Petry, E. Jurkiewicz, D. Fuchs, H. Wachter, K. Matz-Rensing, E.-M. Kuhn, F.-J. Kaup, E. W. Rud, and G. Hunsmann. 1996. Rapid development of vaccine protection in macaques by live-attenuated simian immunodeficiency virus. *J. Gen. Virol.* **77**:2969–2981.

4248. Stahl-Hennig, C., G. Voss, S. Nick, H. Petry, D. Fuchs, H. Wachter, C. Coulibaly, W. Luke, and G. Hunsmann. 1992. Immunization with tween-ether-treated SIV adsorbed onto aluminum hydroxide protects monkeys against experimental SIV infection. *Virology* **186**:588–596.

4249. Stahmer, I., J. P. Zimmer, M. Ernst, T. Fenner, R. Finnern, H. Schmitz, H.-D. Flad, and J. Gerdes. 1991. Isolation of normal human follicular dendritic cells and CD4–independent *in vitro* infection by human immunodeficiency virus (HIV-1). *Eur. J. Immunol.* **21**:1873–1878.

4250. Stalmeijer, E. H. B., R. P. van Rij, B. Boeser-Nunnink, J. A. Visser, M. A. Naarding, D. Schols, and H. Schuitemaker. 2004. In vivo evolution of X4 human immunodeficiency virus type 1 variants in the natural course of infection coincides with decreasing sensitivity to CXCR4 antagonists. *J. Virol.* **78**:2722–2728.

4251. Stamatatos, L., and C. Cheng-Mayer. 1993. Evidence that the structural conformation of envelope gp120 affects human immunodeficiency virus type 1 infectivity, host range, and syncytium-forming ability. *J. Virol.* **67**:5635–5639.

4252. Stamatatos, L., and C. Cheng-Mayer. 1995. Structural modulations of the envelope gp120 glycoprotein of human immunodeficiency virus type 1 upon oligomerization and differential V3 loop epitope exposure of isolates displaying distinct tropism upon virion-soluble receptor binding. *J. Virol.* **69**:6191–6198.

4253. Stamatatos, L., and C. Cheng-Mayer. 1998. An envelope modification that renders a primary, neutralization-resistant clade B human immunodeficiency virus type 1 isolate highly susceptible to neutralization by sera from other clades. *J. Virol.* **72**:7840–7845.

4254. Stamatatos, L., and N. Duzgunes. 1993. Simian immunodeficiency virus (SIVmac251) membrane lipid mixing with human CD4+ and CD4– cell lines in vitro does not necessarily result in internalization of the viral core proteins and productive infection. *J. Gen. Virol.* **74**:1043–1054.

4255. Stamatatos, L., A. Werner, and C. Cheng-Mayer. 1994. Differential regulation of cellular tropism and sensitivity to sCD4 neutralization by the envelope gp120 of human immunodeficiency virus type 1. *J. Virol.* **68**:4973–4979.

4256. Stamatatos, L., S. Zolla-Pazner, M. K. Gorny, and C. Cheng-Mayer. 1997. Binding of antibodies to virion-associated gp120 molecules of primary-like human immunodeficiency virus type 1 (HIV-1) isolates: effect on HIV-1 infection of macrophages and peripheral blood mononuclear cells. *Virology* **229**:360–369.

4257. Stanley, S. K., T. M. Folks, and A. S. Fauci. 1989. Induction of expression of human immunodeficiency virus in a chronically infected promonocytic cell line by ultraviolet irradiation. *AIDS Res. Hum. Retrovir.* **5**:375–384.

4258. Stanley, S. K., S. W. Kessler, J. S. Justement, S. M. Schnittman, J. J. Greenhouse, C. C. Brown, L. Musongela, K. Musey, B. Kapita, and A. S. Fauci. 1992. CD34+ bone marrow cells are infected with HIV in a subset of seropositive individuals. *J. Immunol.* **149**:689–697.

4259. Stanley, S. K., J. M. McCune, H. Kaneshima, J. S. Justement, M. Sullivan, M. Baseler, J. Adelsberger, M. Bonyhadi, J. Orenstein, C. H. Fox, and A. S. Fauci. 1993. Human immunodeficiency virus infection of the human thymus and disruption of the thymic microenvironment in the SCID-hu mouse. *J. Exp. Med.* **178**:1151–1163.

4260. Stanley, S. K., M. A. Ostrowski, J. S. Justement, K. Gantt, S. Hedayati, M. Mannix, K. Roche, D. J. Schwartzentruber, C. H. Fox, and A. S. Fauci. 1996. Effect of immunization with a common recall antigen on viral expression in patients infected with human immunodeficiency virus type 1. *N. Engl. J. Med.* **334**:1222–1230.

4261. Staprans, S. I., A. P. Barry, G. Silvestri, J. T. Safrit, N. Kozyr, B. Sumpter, H. Nguyen, H. McClure, D. Montefiori, J. I. Cohen, and M. B. Feinberg. 2004. Enhanced SIV replication and accelerated progression to AIDS in macaques primed to mount a CD4 T cell response to the SIV envelope protein. *Proc. Natl. Acad. Sci. USA* **101**:13026–13031.

4262. Staprans, S. I., B. L. Hamilton, S. E. Follansbee, T. Elbeik, P. Barbosa, R. M. Grant, and M. B. Feinberg. 1995. Activation of virus replication after vaccination of HIV-1-infected individuals. *J. Exp. Med.* **182**:1727–1737.

4263. Starcich, B. R., B. H. Hahn, G. M. Shaw, R. D. McNeely, S. Morrow, H. Wolf, E. S. Parks, W. P. Parks, S. F. Josephs, and R. C. Gallo. 1986. Identification and characterization of conserved and variable regions in the envelope gene of HTLV-III/LAV, the retrovirus of AIDS. *Cell* **45**:637–648.

4264. Stark, L. A., and R. T. Hay. 1998. Human immunodeficiency virus type 1 (HIV-1) viral protein R (Vpr) interacts with Lys-tRNA synthetase: implications for priming of HIV-1 reverse transcription. *J. Virol.* **72**:3037–3044.

4265. Staszewski, S., J. Morales-Ramirez, K. T. Tashima, A. Rachlis, D. Skiest, J. Stanford, R. Stryker, P. Johnson, D. F. Labriola, D. Farina, D. J. Manion, N. M. Ruiz, et al. 1999. Efavirenz plus zidovudine and lamivudine, efavirenz plus indinavir, and indinavir plus zidovudine and lamivudine in the treatment of HIV-1 infection in adults. *N. Engl. J. Med.* **341:**1865–1873.

4266. Stebbings, R., N. Berry, H. Waldmann, P. Bird, G. Hale, J. Stott, D. North, R. Hull, J. Hall, J. Lines, S. Brown, N. D'Arcy, L. Davis, W. Elsley, C. Edwards, D. Ferguson, J. Allen, and N. Almond. 2005. CD8+ lymphocytes do not mediate protection against acute superinfection 20 days after vaccination with a live attenuated simian immunodeficiency virus. *J. Virol.* **79:**12264–12272.

4267. Steck, F. T., and H. Rubin. 1966. The mechanism of interference between an avian leukosis virus and Rous sarcoma virus. I. Establishment of interference. *Virology* **29:**628–641.

4268. Steckbeck, J. D., I. Orlov, A. Chow, H. Grieser, K. Miller, J. Bruno, J. E. Robinson, R. C. Montelaro, and K. S. Cole. 2005. Kinetic rates of antibody binding correlate with neutralization sensitivity of variant simian immunodeficiency virus strains. *J. Virol.* **79:**12311–12320.

4269. Steel, C. M., D. Beatson, R. J. G. Cuthbert, H. Morrison, C. A. Ludlam, J. F. Peutherer, P. Simmonds, and M. Jones. 1988. HLA haplotype A1 B8 DR3 as a risk factor for HIV-related disease. *Lancet* **i:**1185–1188.

4270. Steffan, A. M., M. E. Lafon, J. L. Gendrault, C. Schweitzer, C. Royer, D. Jaeck, J. P. Arnaud, M. P. Schmitt, A. M. Aubertin, and A. Kirn. 1992. Primary cultures of endothelial cells from the human liver sinusoid are permissive for human immunodeficiency virus type 1. *Proc. Natl. Acad. Sci. USA* **89:**1582–1586.

4271. Steffen, M., H. C. Reinecker, H. C. Petersen, C. Doehn, I. Pfluger, A. Voss, and A. Raedler. 1993. Differences in cytokine secretion by intestinal mononuclear cells, peripheral blood monocytes and alveolar macrophages from HIV-infected patients. *Clin. Exp. Immunol.* **91:**30–36.

4272. Steffens, C. M., E. Z. Managlia, A. Landay, and L. Al-Harthi. 2002. Interleukin-7-treated naive T cells can be productively infected by T-cell-adapted and primary isolates of human immunodeficiency virus 1. *Blood* **99:**3310–3318.

4273. Steffens, C. M., K. Y. Smith, A. Landay, S. Shott, A. Truckenbrod, M. Russert, and L. Al-Harthi. 2001. T cell receptor excision circle (TREC) content following maximum HIV suppression is equivalent in HIV-infected and HIV-uninfected individuals. *AIDS* **15:**1757–1764.

4274. Steffy, K. R., G. Kraus, D. J. Looney, and F. Wong-Staal. 1992. Role of the fusogenic peptide sequence in syncytium induction and infectivity of human immunodeficiency virus type 2. *J. Virol.* **66:**4532–4535.

4275. Steimer, K. S., P. J. Klasse, and J. A. McKeating. 1991. HIV-1 neutralization directed to epitopes other than linear V3 determinants. *AIDS* **5**(Suppl. 2):S135–S143.

4276. Steimer, K. S., C. J. Scandella, P. V. Skiles, and N. L. Haigwood. 1991. Neutralization of divergent HIV-1 isolates by conformation-dependent human antibodies to gp120. *Science* **254:**105–108.

4277. Stein, B., M. Kramer, H. J. Rahmsdorf, H. Ponta, and P. Herrlich. 1989. UV-induced transcription from the human immunodeficiency virus type 1 (HIV-1) long terminal repeat and UV-induced secretion of an extracellular factor that induces HIV-1 transcription in nonirradiated cells. *J. Virol.* **63:**4540–4544.

4278. Stein, B. S., S. F. Gowda, J. D. Lifson, R. C. Penhallow, K. G. Bensch, and E. G. Engleman. 1987. pH-independent HIV entry into CD4–positive T cells via virus envelope fusion to the plasma membrane. *Cell* **49:**659–668.

4279. Stein, D. S., J. A. Korvick, and S. H. Vermund. 1992. CD4+ lymphocyte cell enumeration for prediction of clinical course of human immunodeficiency virus disease: a review. *J. Infect. Dis.* **165:**352–363.

4280. Steinberg, H. N., J. Anderson, C. S. Crumpacker, and P. A. Chatis. 1993. HIV infection of the BS-1 human stroma cell line: effect on murine hematopoiesis. *Virology* **193:**524–527.

4281. Steinman, L. 1993. Connections between the immune system and the nervous system. *Proc. Natl. Acad. Sci. USA* **90:**7912–7914.

4282. Steinman, R. M., and Z. A. Cohn. 1973. Identification of a novel cell type in peripheral lymphoid organs of mice. I. Morphology, quantitation, tissue distribution. *J. Exp. Med.* **137:**1142–1162.

4283. Steketee, R. W., E. J. Abrams, D. M. Thea, T. M. Brown, G. Lambert, S. Orloff, J. Weedon, M. Bamji, E. E. Schoenbaum, J. Rapier, and M. L. Kalish. 1997. Early detection of perinatal human immunodeficiency virus (HIV) type 1 infection using HIV RNA amplification and detection. *J. Infect. Dis.* **175:**707–711.

4284. Stephens, E. B., H. M. McClure, and O. Narayan. 1995. The proteins of lymphocyte- and macrophage-tropic strains of simian immunodeficiency virus are processed differently in macrophages. *Virology* **206:**535–544.

4285. Stephens, E. B., C. Q. Tian, Z. Li, O. Narayan, and V. H. Gattone. 1998. Rhesus macaques infected with macrophage-tropic simian immunodeficiency virus (SIVmacR71/17E) exhibit extensive focal segmental and global glomerulosclerosis. *J. Virol.* **72:**8820–8832.

4286. Stephens, H. A. F. 2005. HIV-1 diversity versus HLA class 1 polymorphism. *Trends Immunol.* **26:**41–47.

4287. Sterling, T. R., D. Vlahov, J. Astemborski, D. R. Hoover, J. B. Margolick, and T. C. Quinn. 2001. Initial plasma HIV-1 RNA levels and progression to AIDS in women and men. *N. Engl. J. Med.* **344:**720–725.

4288. Steuler, H., B. Storch-Hagenlocher, and B. Wildemann. 1992. Distinct populations of human immunodeficiency virus type 1 in blood and cerebrospinal fluid. *AIDS Res. Hum. Retrovir.* **8:**53–59.

4289. Stevceva, L., X. Alvarez, A. A. Lackner, E. Tryniszewska, B. Kelsall, J. Nacsa, J. Tartaglia, W. Strober, and G. Franchini. 2002. Both mucosal and systemic routes of immunization with the live, attenuated NYVAC/simian immunodeficiency virus SIV(gpe) recombinant vaccine result in gag-specific CD8(+) T-cell responses in mucosal tissues of macaques. *J. Virol.* **76:**11659–11676.

4290. Stevenson, M. 1997. Molecular mechanisms for the regulation of HIV replication, persistence and latency. *AIDS* **11:**S25–S33.

4291. Stevenson, M., S. Haggerty, C. Lamonica, A. M. Mann, C. Meier, and A. Wasiak. 1990. Cloning and characterization of human immunodeficiency virus type 1 variants diminished in the ability to induce syncytium-independent cytolysis. *J. Virol.* **64:**3792–3803.

4292. Stevenson, M., C. Meier, A. M. Mann, N. Chapman, and A. Wasiak. 1988. Envelope glycoprotein of HIV induces interference and cytolysis resistance in CD4+ cells: mechanism for persistence in AIDS. *Cell* **53:**483–496.

4293. Stevenson, M., T. L. Stanwick, M. P. Dempsey, and C. A. Lamonica. 1990. HIV-1 replication is controlled at the level of T cell activation and proviral integration. *EMBO J.* **9:** 1551–1560.

4294. Stevenson, M., X. H. Zhang, and D. J. Volsky. 1987. Downregulation of cell surface molecules during noncytopathic infection of T cells with human immunodeficiency virus. *J. Virol.* **61:**3741–3748.

4295. Stewart, G. J., J. P. P. Tyler, A. L. Cunningham, J. A. Barr, G. L. Driscoll, J. Gold, and B. J. Lamont. 1985. Transmission of human T-cell lymphotropic virus type III (HTLV-III) by artificial insemination by donor. *Lancet* **ii:**581–585.

4296. Stewart, S. A., B. Poon, J. B. M. Jowett, and I. S. Y. Chen. 1997. Human immunodeficiency virus type 1 Vpr induces apoptosis following cell cycle arrest. *J. Virol.* **71:**5579–5592.

4297. Stoddart, C. A., T. J. Liegler, F. Mammano, V. D. Linquist-Stepps, M. S. Hayden, S. G. Deeks, R. M. Grant, F. Clavel, and J. M. McCune. 2001. Impaired replication of protease inhibitor-resistant HIV-1 in human thymus. *Nat. Med.* **7:**712–718.

4298. Stoiber, H., C. Pinter, A. G. Siccardi, A. Clivio, and M. P. Dierich. 1996. Efficient destruction of human immunodeficiency virus in human serum by inhibiting the protective action of complement factor H and decay accelerating factor (DAF, CD55). *J. Exp. Med.* **183:**307–310.

4299. Stone, S. F., P. Price, J. Brochier, and M. A. French. 2001. Plasma bioavailable interleukin-6 is elevated in human immunodeficiency virus-infected patients who experience herpesvirus-associated immune restoration disease after start of highly active antiretroviral therapy. *J. Infect. Dis.* **184:**1073–1077.

4300. Stone, T. W., G. M. Mackay, C. M. Forrest, C. J. Clark, and L. G. Darlington. 2003. Tryptophan metabolites and brain disorders. *Clin. Chem. Lab. Med.* **41:**852–859.

4301. Storey, D. F., M. J. Dolan, S. A. Anderson, P. A. Meier, and E. A. Walter. 1999. Seminal plasma RANTES levels positively correlate with seminal plasma HIV-1 RNA levels. *AIDS* **13:**2169–2171.

4302. Stott, E. J. 1991. Anti-cell antibody in macaques. *Nature* **353:**393.

4303. Stove, V., I. Van de Walle, E. Naessens, E. Coene, C. Stove, J. Plum, and B. Verhasselt. 2005. Human immunodeficiency virus Nef induces rapid internalization of the T-cell coreceptor CD8alphabeta. *J. Virol.* **79:**11422–11433.

4304. Stoye, J. P. 2002. An intracellular block to primate lentivirus replication. *Proc. Natl. Acad. Sci. USA* **99:**11549–11551.

4305. Strain, M. C., S. Letendre, S. K. Pillai, T. Russell, C. C. Ignacio, H. F. Gunthard, B. Good, D. M. Smith, S. M. Wolinsky, M. Furtado, J. Marquie-Beck, J. Durelle, I. Grant, D. D. Richman, T. Marcotte, J. A. McCutchan, R. J. Ellis, and J. K. Wong. 2005. Genetic composition of human immunodeficiency virus type 1 in cerebrospinal fluid and blood without treatment and during failing antiretroviral therapy. *J. Virol.* **79:**1772–1788.

4306. Strain, M. C., S. J. Little, E. S. Daar, D. V. Havlir, H. F. Gunthard, R. Y. Lam, O. A. Daly, J. Nguyen, C. C. Ignacio, C. A. Spina, D. D. Richman, and J. K. Wong. 2005. Effect of treatment, during primary infection, on establishment and clearance of cellular reservoirs of HIV-1. *J. Infect. Dis.* **191:**1394–1396.

4307. Stramer, S. L., S. A. Glynn, S. H. Kleinman, M. Strong, S. Caglioti, D. J. Wright, R. Y. Dodd, and M. P. Busch. 2004. Detection of HIV-1 and HCV infections among antibody-negative blood donors by nucleic acid-amplification testing. *N. Engl. J. Med.* **351:**760–768.

4308. Stranford, S., J. Skurnick, D. Louria, D. Osmond, S. Chang, J. Sninsky, G. Ferrari, K. Weinhold, C. Lindquist, and J. Levy. 1999. Lack of infection in HIV-exposed individuals is associated with a strong CD8+ cell noncytotoxic anti-HIV response. *Proc. Natl. Acad. Sci. USA* **96:**1030–1035.

4309. Stranford, S. A., J. C. Ong, B. Martinez-Marino, M. Busch, F. M. Hecht, J. Kahn, and J. A. Levy. 2001. Reduction in CD8+ cell noncytotoxic anti-HIV activity in individuals receiving highly active antiretroviral therapy during primary infection. *Proc. Natl. Acad. Sci. USA* **98:**597–602.

4310. Straus, D. J., J. Huang, M. A. Testa, A. M. Levine, L. D. Kaplan, and the National Institute of Allergy and Infectious Diseases. 1998. Prognostic factors in the treatment of human immunodeficiency virus-associated non-Hodgkin's lymphoma: analysis of AIDS Clinical Trials Group protocol 142–low-dose versus standard-dose m-BACOD plus granulocyte-macrophage colony-stimulating factor. *J. Clin. Oncol.* **16:**3601–3606.

4311. Strauss, W. M., T. Quertermous, and J. G. Seidman. 1987. Measuring the human T cell receptor gamma-chain locus. *Science* **237:**1217–1219.

4312. Strawford, A., T. Barbieri, M. Van Loan, E. Parks, D. Catlin, N. Barton, R. Neese, M. Christiansen, J. King, and M. K. Hellerstein. 1999. Resistance exercise and supraphysiologic androgen therapy in eugonadal men with HIV-related weight loss: a randomized controlled trial. *JAMA* **281:**1282–1290.

4313. Street, N. E., J. H. Schumacher, A. T. Fong, H. Bass, D. F. Fiorentino, J. A. Leverah, and T. R. Mosmann. 1990. Heterogeneity of mouse helper T cells. Evidence from bulk cultures and limiting dilution cloning for precursors of Th1 and Th2 cells. *J. Immunol.* **144:**1629–1639.

4314. Stremlau, M., C. M. Owens, M. J. Perron, M. Kiessling, P. Autissier, and J. Sodroski. 2004. The cytoplasmic body component TRIM5α restricts HIV-1 infection in Old World monkeys. *Nature* **427:**848–853.

4315. Stremlau, M., M. Perron, S. Welikala, and J. Sodroski. 2005. Species-specific variation in the B30.2(SPRY) domain of TRIM5a determines the potency of human immunodeficiency virus restriction. *J. Virol.* **79:**3139–3145.

4316. Strieter, R. M., T. J. Standiford, G. B. Huffnagle, L. M. Colletti, N. W. Lukacs, and S. L. Kunkel. 1996. "The good, the bad, and the ugly". The role of chemokines in models of human disease. *J. Immunol.* **156:**3583–3586.

4317. Strizki, J. M., A. V. Albright, H. Sheng, M. O'Connor, L. Perrin, and F. Gonzalez-Scarano. 1996. Infection of primary human microglia and monocyte-derived macrophages with human immunodeficiency virus type 1 isolates: evidence of differential tropism. *J. Virol.* **70:**7654–7662.

4318. Struble, K., J. Murray, B. Cheng, T. Gegeny, V. Miller, and R. Gulick. 2005. Antiretroviral therapies for treatment-experienced patients: current status and research challenges. *AIDS* **19:**747–756.

4319. Stryker, J., and T. J. Coates. 1997. Home access HIV testing. What took so long? *Arch. Intern. Med.* **157:**261–262.

4320. Stumptner-Cuvelette, P., S. Morchoisne, M. Dugast, S. Le Gall, G. Raposo, O. Schwartz, and P. Benaroch. 2001. HIV-1 Nef impairs MHC class II antigen presentation and surface expression. *Proc. Natl. Acad. Sci. USA* **98:**12144–12149.

4321. Su, H., and R. J. Boackle. 1991. Interaction of the envelope glycoprotein of human immunodeficiency virus with C1q and fibronectin under conditions present in human saliva. *Mol. Immunol.* **28:**811–817.

4322. Su, L., M. Graf, Y. Zhang, H. von Briesen, H. Xing, J. Kostler, H. Melzl, H. Wolf, Y. Shao, and R. Wagner. 2000. Characterization of a virtually full-length human immunodeficiency virus type 1 genome of a prevalent intersubtype (C/B') recombinant strain in China. *J. Virol.* 74:11367–11376.

4323. Subar, M., A. Neri, G. Inghirami, D. M. Knowles, and R. Dalla-Favera. 1988. Frequent c-myc oncogene activation and infrequent presence of Epstein-Barr viurs genome in AIDS-associated lymphoma. *Blood* 72:667–672.

4324. Subbramanian, R. A., J. Xu, E. Toma, R. Morisset, E. A. Cohen, J. Menezes, and A. Ahmad. 2002. Comparison of human immunodeficiency virus (HIV)-specific infection-enhancing and -inhibiting antibodies in AIDS patients. *J. Clin. Microbiol.* 40:2141–2146.

4325. Subramaniam, K. S., R. Segal, R. H. Lyles, M. C. Rodriguez-Barradas, and L. A. Pirofski. 2003. Qualitative change in antibody responses of human immunodeficiency virus-infected individuals to pneumococcal capsular polysaccharide vaccination associated with highly active antiretroviral therapy. *J. Infect. Dis.* 187:758–768.

4326. Subramanyam, M., W. G. Gutheil, W. W. Bachovchin, and B. T. Huber. 1993. Mechanism of HIV-1 tat induced inhibition of antigen-specific T cell responsiveness. *J. Immunol.* 150:2544–2553.

4327. Sugamura, K., and Y. Hinuma. 1993. Human retroviruses: HTLV-I and HTLV-II, p. 399–436. *In* J. A. Levy (ed.), *The Retroviridae*, vol. 2. Plenum Press, New York, N.Y.

4328. Suh, H.-S., M.-L. Zhao, M. Rivieccio, E. Connolly, Y. Zhao, O. Takikawa, C. F. Brosnan, and S. C. Lee. Astrocyte indoleamine 2, 3 dioxygenase (IDO) is induced by the TLR3 ligand poly IC: mechanism of induction and role in anti-viral response. Submitted for publication.

4329. Sulkowski, M. S., R. E. Chaisson, C. L. Karp, R. D. Moore, J. B. Margolick, and T. C. Quinn. 1998. The effect of acute infectious illnesses on plasma human immunodeficiency virus (HIV) type 1 load and the expression of serologic markers of immune activation among HIV-infected adults. *J. Infect. Dis.* 178:1642–1648.

4330. Sulkowski, M. S., E. E. Mast, L. B. Seeff, and D. L. Thomas. 2000. Hepatitis C virus infection as an opportunistic disease in persons infected with human immunodeficiency virus. *Clin. Infect. Dis.* 30(Suppl. 1):S77–S84.

4331. Sulkowski, M. S., R. D. Moore, S. H. Mehta, R. E. Chaisson, and D. L. Thomas. 2002. Hepatitis C and progression of HIV disease. *JAMA* 288:199–206.

4332. Sullivan, B. L., E. J. Knopoff, M. Saifuddin, D. M. Takefman, M. N. Saarloos, B. E. Sha, and G. T. Spear. 1996. Susceptibility of HIV-1 plasma virus to complement-mediated lysis. *J. Immunol.* 157:1791–1798.

4333. Sullivan, N., Y. Sun, J. Li, W. Hofmann, and J. Sodroski. 1995. Replicative function and neutralization sensitivity of envelope glycoproteins from primary and T-cell line-passaged human immunodeficiency virus type 1 isolates. *J. Virol.* 69:4413–4422.

4334. Sullivan, N., M. Thali, C. Furman, D. D. Ho, and J. Sodroski. 1993. Effect of amino acid changes in the V1/V2 region of the human immunodeficiency virus type 1 gp120 glycoprotein on subunit association, syncytium formation, and recognition by a neutralizing antibody. *J. Virol.* 67:3674–3679.

4335. Sumida, S. M., P. F. McKay, D. M. Truitt, M. G. Kishko, J. C. Arthur, M. S. Seaman, S. S. Jackson, D. A. Gorgone, M. A.

Lifton, N. L. Letvin, and D. H. Barouch. 2004. Recruitment and expansion of dendritic cells in vivo potentiate the immunogenicity of plasmid DNA vaccines. *J. Clin. Investig.* 114:1334–1342.

4336. Sumida, S. M., D. M. Truitt, M. G. Kishko, J. C. Arthur, S. S. Jackson, D. A. Gorgone, M. A. Lifton, W. Koudstaal, M. G. Pau, S. Kostense, M. J. Havenga, J. Goudsmit, N. L. Letvin, and D. H. Barouch. 2004. Neutralizing antibodies and CD8+ T lymphocytes both contribute to immunity and adenovirus serotype 5 vaccine vectors. *J. Virol.* 78:2666–2673.

4337. Summerfield, J. A., S. Ryder, M. Sumiya, M. Thursz, A. Gorchein, M. A. Monteil, and M. W. Turner. 1995. Mannose binding protein gene mutations associated with unusual and severe infections in adults. *Lancet* 345:886–889.

4338. Sun, J. C., and M. J. Bevan. 2003. Defective CD8 T cell memory following acute infection without CD4 T cell help. *Science* 300:339–342.

4339. Sun, N.-C., D. D. Ho, C. R. Y. Sun, R.-S. Liou, W. Gordon, M. S. C. Fung, X.-L. Li, R. C. Ting, T.-H. Lee, N. T. Chang, and T.-W. Chang. 1989. Generation and characterization of monoclonal antibodies to the putative CD4–binding domain of human immunodeficiency virus type 1 gp120. *J. Virol.* 63:3579–3585.

4340. Sun, S., L. M. Pinchuk, M. B. Agy, and E. A. Clark. 1997. Nuclear import of HIV-1 DNA in resting CD4+ T cells requires a cyclosporin A-sensitive pathway. *J. Immunol.* 158:512–517.

4341. Sun, Y., J. E. Schmitz, P. M. Acierno, S. Santra, R. A. Subbramanian, D. H. Barouch, D. A. Gorgone, M. A. Lifton, K. R. Beaudry, K. Manson, V. Philippon, L. Xu, H. T. Maecker, J. R. Mascola, D. Panicali, G. J. Nabel, and N. L. Letvin. 2005. Dysfunction of simian immunodeficiency virus/simian human immunodeficiency virus-induced IL-2 expression by central memory CD4+ T lymphocytes. *J. Immunol.* 174:4753–4760.

4341a. Sundaravaradan, V., S. K. Saxena, R. Ramakrishnan, V. R. Yedavalli, D. T. Harris, and N. Ahmad. 2006. Differential HIV-1 replication in neonatal and adult blood mononuclear cells is influenced at the level of HIV-1 gene expression. *Proc. Natl. Acad. Sci. USA* 103:11701–11706.

4342. Susal, C., M. Kirschfink, M. Kropelin, V. Daniel, and G. Opelz. 1994. Complement activation by recombinant HIV-1 glycoprotein gp120. *J. Immunol.* 152:6028–6034.

4343. Sutjipto, S., N. C. Pedersen, C. J. Miller, M. B. Gardner, C. V. Hanson, A. Gettie, M. Jennings, J. Higgins, and P. Marx. 1990. Inactivated simian immunodeficiency virus vaccine failed to protect rhesus macaques from intravenous or genital mucosal infection but delayed disease in intravenously exposed animals. *J. Virol.* 64:2290–2297.

4343a. Sutmuller, R. P., M. E. Morgan, M. G. Netea, O. Grauer, and G. J. Adema. 2006. Toll-like receptors on regulatory T cells: expanding immune regulation. *Trends Immunol.* 27:387–393.

4344. Swaggerty, C. L., H. Huang, W. S. Lim, F. Schroeder, and J. M. Ball. 2004. Comparison of SIVmac239$_{(352–382)}$ and SIVsmmPBj41$_{(360–390)}$ enterotoxic synthetic peptides. *Virology* 320:243–257.

4345. Swann, S. A., M. Williams, C. M. Story, K. R. Bobbitt, R. Fleis, and K. L. Collins. 2001. HIV-1 Nef blocks transport of MHC class I molecules to the cell surface via a PI 3-kinase-dependent pathway. *Virology* 282:267–277.

4346. Swart, P. J., M. E. Kuipers, C. Smit, R. Pauwels, M. P. de-Bethune, E. de Clercq, D. K. F. Meijer, and J. G. Huisman. 1996. Antiviral effects of milk proteins: acylation results in polyanionic compounds with potent activity against human immunodeficiency virus types 1 and 2 *in vitro. AIDS Res. Hum. Retrovir.* **12**:769–775.

4347. Sweet, R. W., A. Truneh, and W. A. Hendrickson. 1991. CD4: its structure, role in immune function and AIDS pathogenesis, and potential as a pharmacological target. *Curr. Opin. Biotechnol.* **2**:622–633.

4348. Swigut, T., N. Shohdy, and J. Skowronski. 2001. Mechanism for down-regulation of CD28 by Nef. *EMBO J.* **20**:1593–1604.

4349. Swingler, S., B. Brichacek, J.-M. Jacque, C. Ulich, J. Zhou, and M. Stevenson. 2003. HIV-1 Nef intersects the macrophage CD40L signalling pathway to promote resting-cell infection. *Nature* **424**:213–219.

4350. Swingler, S., A. Easton, and A. Morris. 1992. Cytokine augmentation of HIV-1 LTR-driven gene expression in neural cells. *AIDS Res. Hum. Retrovir.* **8**:487–493.

4351. Swingler, S., A. Mann, J. Jacque, B. Brichacek, V. G. Sasseville, K. Williams, A. A. Lackner, E. N. Janoff, R. Wang, D. Fisher, and M. Stevenson. 1999. HIV-1 Nef mediates lymphocyte chemotaxis and activation by infected macrophages. *Nat. Med.* **5**:997–103.

4352. Switzer, W. M., B. Parekh, V. Shanmugam, V. Bhullar, S. Phillips, J. J. Ely, and W. Heneine. 2005. The epidemiology of simian immunodeficiency virus infection in a large number of wild- and captive-born chimpanzees: evidence for a recent introduction following chimpanzee divergence. *AIDS Res Hum Retrovir.* **21**:335–342.

4353. Szabo, J., Z. Prohaszka, F. D. Toth, A. Gyuris, J. Segesdi, D. Banhegyi, E. Ujhelyi, J. Minarovits, and G. Fust. 1999. Strong correlation between the complement-mediated antibody-dependent enhancement of HIV-1 infection and plasma viral load. *AIDS* **13**:1841–1849.

4354. Szabo, S. J., A. S. Dighe, U. Gubler, and K. M. Murphy. 1997. Regulation of the interleukin (IL)-12R β2 subunit expression in developing T helper 1 (Th1) and Th2 cells. *J. Exp. Med.* **185**:817–824.

4355. Szawlowski, P. W. S., T. Hanke, and R. E. Randall. 1993. Sequence homology between HIV-1 gp120 and the apoptosis mediating protein Fas. *AIDS* **7**:1018.

4356. Szelc, C. M., C. Mitcheltree, R. L. Roberts, and E. R. Stiehm. 1992. Deficient polymorphonuclear cell and mononuclear cell antibody-dependent cellular cytotoxicity in pediatric and adult human immunodeficiency virus infection. *J. Infect. Dis.* **166**:486–493.

4357. Tachet, A., E. Dulioust, D. Salmon, M. De Almeida, S. Rivalland, L. Finkielsztejn, I. Heard, P. Jouannet, D. Sicard, and C. Rouzioux. 1999. Detection and quantification of HIV-1 in semen: identification of a subpopulation of men at high potential risk of viral sexual transmission. *AIDS* **13**:823–831.

4358. Taddeo, B., M. Federico, F. Titti, G. B. Rossi, and P. Verani. 1993. Homologous superinfection of both producer and nonproducer HIV-infected cells is blocked at a late retrotranscription step. *Virology* **194**:441–452.

4359. Takahashi, H., Y. Nakagawa, C. D. Pendleton, R. A. Houghten, K. Yokomuro, R. N. Germain, and J. A. Berzofsky. 1992. Induction of broadly cross-reactive cytotoxic T cells recognizing an HIV-1 envelope determinant. *Science* **255**:333–336.

4360. Takahashi, H., Y. Nakagawa, K. Yokomuro, and J. A. Berzofsky. 1993. Induction of CD8+ CTL by immunization

with syngeneic irradiated HIV-1 envelope derived peptide-pulsed dendritic cells. *Int. Immunol.* **5**:849–857.

4361. Takahashi, H., T. Takeshita, B. Morein, S. Putney, R. N. Germain, and J. A. Berzofsky. 1990. Induction of CD8+ cytotoxic T cells by immunization with purified HIV-1 envelope protein in ISCOMs. *Nature* **344**:873–875.

4362. Takamizawa, M., A. Rivas, F. Fagnoni, C. Benike, J. Kosek, H. Hyakawa, and E. G. Engleman. 1997. Dendritic cells that process and present nominal antigens to naive T lymphocytes are derived from CD2+ precursors. *J. Immunol.* **158**:2134–2142.

4363. Takeda, A., and F. A. Ennis. 1990. FcR-mediated enhancement of HIV-1 infection by antibody. *AIDS Res. Hum. Retrovir.* **6**:999–1004.

4364. Takeda, A., J. E. Robinson, D. D. Ho, C. Debouck, N. L. Haigwood, and F. A. Ennis. 1992. Distinction of human immunodeficiency virus type 1 neutralization and infection enhancement by human monoclonal antibodies to glycoprotein 120. *J. Clin. Investig.* **89**:1952–1957.

4365. Takeda, A., R. W. Sweet, and F. A. Ennis. 1990. Two receptors are required for antibody-dependent enhancement of human immunodeficiency virus type 1 infection: CD4 and Fc-gammaR. *J. Virol.* **64**:5605–5610.

4366. Takeda, A., C. V. Tuazon, and F. A. Ennis. 1988. Antibody-enhanced infection by HIV-1 via Fc receptor-mediated entry. *Science* **242**:580–583.

4367. Takehisa, J., L. Zekeng, E. Ido, I. Mboudjeka, H. Moriyama, T. Miura, M. Yamashita, L. G. Gürtler, M. Hayami, and L. Kaptué. 1998. Various types of HIV mixed infections in Cameroon. *Virology* **245**:1–10.

4368. Takehisa, J., L. Zekeng, E. Ido, Y. Yamaguchi-Kabata, I. Mboudjeka, Y. Harada, T. Miura, L. Kaptu, and M. Hayami. 1999. Human immunodeficiency virus type 1 intergroup (M/O) recombination in Cameroon. *J. Virol.* **73**:6810–6820.

4369. Takehisa, J., L. Zekeng, T. Miura, E. Ido, M. Yamashita, I. Mboudjeka, L. G. Gurtler, M. Hayami, and L. Kaptue. 1997. Triple HIV-1 infection with group O and group M of different clades in a single Cameroonian AIDS patient. *J. Acquir. Immune Defic. Syndr. Hum. Retrovirol.* **14**:81–82.

4370. Takeuchi, Y., M. Akutsu, K. Murayama, N. Shimizu, and H. Hoshino. 1991. Host range mutant of human immunodeficiency virus type 1: modification of cell tropism by a single point mutation at the neutralization epitope in the *env* gene. *J. Virol.* **65**:1710–1718.

4371. Takeuchi, Y., T. Nagumo, and H. Hoshino. 1988. Low fidelity of cell-free DNA synthesis by reverse transcriptase of human immunodeficiency virus. *J. Virol.* **62**:3900–3902.

4372. Takihara, Y., J. Reimann, E. Michalopoulos, E. Ciccone, L. Moretta, and T. W. Mak. 1989. Diversity and structure of human T cell receptor delta chain genes in peripheral blood gamma/delta-bearing T lymphocytes. *J. Exp. Med.* **169**:393–405.

4373. Tamalet, C., A. Lafeuillade, C. Tourres, N. Yahi, C. Vignoli, and P. De Micco. 1994. Inefficacy of neutralizing antibodies against lymph-node HIV-1 isolates in patients with early-stage HIV infection. *AIDS* **8**:388–389.

4374. Tambussi, G., S. Ghezzi, S. Nozza, G. Vallanti, L. Magenta, M. Guffanti, A. Brambilla, E. Vicenzi, P. Carrera, S. Racca, L. Soldini, N. Gianotti, M. Murone, F. Veglia, G. Poli, and A. Lazzarin. 2001. Efficacy of low-dose intermittent subcutaneous interleukin (IL)-2 in antiviral drug-experienced human immunodeficiency virus-infected persons with detectable virus load: a controlled study of 3 IL-2 regimens with antiviral drug therapy. *J. Infect. Dis.* **183**:1476–1784.

4375. Tan, X., R. Pearce-Pratt, and D. M. Phillips. 1993. Productive infection of a cervical epithelial cell line with human immunodeficiency virus: implications for sexual transmission. *J. Virol.* **67**:6447–6452.

4376. Tanaka, T., J. Hu-Li, R. A. Seder, B. F. De St.Groth, and W. E. Paul. 1993. Interleukin 4 suppresses interleukin 2 and interferon gamma production by naive T cells stimulated by accessory cell-dependent receptor engagement. *Proc. Natl. Acad. Sci. USA* **90**:5914–5918.

4377. Tanaka, Y., Y. Koyanagi, R. Tanaka, Y. Kumazawa, T. Nishimura, and N. Yamamoto. 1997. Productive and lytic infection of human CD4+ type 1 helper T cells with macrophage-tropic human immunodeficiency virus type 1. *J. Virol.* **71**:465–470.

4378. Tang, A. M., J. Lanzillotti, K. Hendricks, J. Gerrior, M. Ghosh, M. Woods, and C. Wanke. 2005. Micronutrients: current issues of HIV care providers. *AIDS* **19**:847–861.

4379. Tang, J., C. Costello, I. P. Keet, C. Rivers, S. Leblanc, E. Karita, S. Allen, and R. A. Kaslow. 1999. HLA class I homozygosity accelerates disease progression in human immunodeficiency virus type 1 infection. *AIDS Res. Hum. Retrovir.* **15**:317–324.

4380. Tang, J., A. Penman-Aguilar, E. Lobashevsky, A. Allen, and R. A. Kaslow. 2004. HLA-DRB1 and -DQB1 alleles and haplotypes in Zambian couples and their associations with heterosexual transmission of HIV type 1. *J. Infect. Dis.* **189**:1696–1704.

4381. Tang, J., S. Tang, E. Lobashevsky, A. D. Myracle, U. Fideli, G. Aldrovandi, S. Allen, R. Musonda, and R. A. Kaslow. 2002. Favorable and unfavorable HLA class I alleles and haplotypes in Zambians predominantly infected with clade C human immunodeficiency virus type 1. *J. Virol.* **76**:8276–8284.

4382. Tang, S., and J. A. Levy. 1990. Parameters involved in the cell fusion induced by HIV. *AIDS* **4**:409–414.

4383. Tang, S., B. Patterson, and J. A. Levy. 1995. Highly purified quiescent human peripheral blood CD4+ T cells are infectible by human immunodeficiency virus but do not release virus after activation. *J. Virol.* **69**:5659–5665.

4384. Tang, S., L. Poulin, and J. A. Levy. 1992. Lack of human immunodeficiency virus type-1 (HIV-1) replication and accumulation of viral DNA in HIV-1-infected T cells blocked in cell replication. *J. Gen. Virol.* **73**:933–939.

4385. Tang, Y. W., J. T. Huong, R. M. Lloyd, Jr., P. Spearman, and D. W. Haas. 2000. Comparison of human immunodeficiency virus type 1 RNA sequence heterogeneity in cerebrospinal fluid and plasma. *J. Clin. Microbiol.* **38**:4637–4639.

4386. Tarazona, R., J. G. Casado, O. Delarosa, J. Torre-Cisneros, J. L. Villanueva, B. Sanchez, M. D. Galiani, R. Gonzalez, R. Solana, and J. Pena. 2002. Selective depletion of CD56(dim) NK cell subsets and maintenance of CD56(bright) NK cells in treatment-naive HIV-1-seropositive individuals. *J. Clin. Immunol.* **22**:176–183.

4387. Tardieu, M., C. Hery, S. Peudenier, O. Boespflug, and L. Montagnier. 1992. Human immunodeficiency virus type 1-infected monocytic cells can destroy human neural cells after cell-to-cell adhesion. *Ann. Neurol.* **32**:11–17.

4388. Tardif, M. R., and M. J. Tremblay. 2005. LFA-1 is a key determinant for preferential infection of memory CD4+ T cells by human immunodeficiency virus type 1. *J. Virol.* **79**:13714–13724.

4389. Tartakovsky, B., M. Burke, N. Vardinon, F. Rosenberg, D. Hatiashvili, D. Turner, and I. Yust. 1998. Increased intracellular macrophage inflammatory protein-1 beta correlates with advanced HIV disease. *J. Acquir. Immune Defic. Syndr. Hum. Retrovirol.* **19**:1–5.

4390. Tas, M., H. A. Drexhage, and J. Goudsmit. 1988. A monocyte chemotaxis inhibiting factor in serum of HIV-infected men shares epitopes with HIV transmembrane protein gp41. *Clin. Exp. Immunol.* **71**:13–18.

4391. Tasca, S., G. Tambussi, S. Nozza, B. Capiluppi, M. R. Zocchi, L. Soldini, F. Veglia, G. Poli, A. Lazzarin, and C. Fortis. 2003. Escape of monocyte-derived dendritic cells of HIV-1 infected individuals from natural killer cell-mediated lysis. *AIDS* **17**:2291–2298.

4392. Tascini, C., F. Baldelli, C. Monari, C. Retini, D. Pietrella, D. Francisci, F. Bistoni, and A. Vecchiarelli. 1996. Inhibition of fungicidal activity of polymorphonuclear leukocytes from HIV-infected patients by interleukin (IL)-4 and IL-10. *AIDS* **10**:477–483.

4393. Tateno, M., F. Gonzalez-Scarano, and J. A. Levy. 1989. The human immunodeficiency virus can infect CD4-negative human fibroblastoid cells. *Proc. Natl. Acad. Sci. USA* **86**:4287–4290.

4394. Tateno, M., and J. A. Levy. 1988. MT-4 plaque formation can distinguish cytopathic subtypes of the human immunodeficiency virus (HIV). *Virology* **167**:299–301.

4395. Taylor, S., H. Reynolds, C. A. Sabin, S. M. Drake, D. J. White, D. J. Back, and D. Pillay. 2001. Penetration of efavirenz into the male genital tract: drug concentrations and antiviral activity in semen and blood of HIV-infected men. *AIDS* **15**:2051–2053.

4396. Tedla, N., P. Palladinetti, M. Kelly, R. K. Kumar, N. Di-Girolamo, U. Chattophadhay, B. Cooke, P. Truskett, J. Dwyer, D. Wakefield, and A. Lloyd. 1996. Chemokines and T lymphocyte recruitment to lymph nodes in HIV infection. *Am. J. Pathol.* **148**:1367–1373.

4397. Teixeira, L., H. Valdez, J. M. McCune, R. A. Koup, A. D. Badley, M. K. Hellerstein, L. A. Napolitano, D. C. Douek, S. Mbisa, S. Deeks, J. M. Harris, J. D. Barbour, B. H. Gross, I. R. Francis, R. Halvorsen, R. Asaad, and M. M. Lederman. 2001. Poor CD4 T cell restoration after suppression of HIV-1 replication may reflect lower thymic function. *AIDS* **15**:1749–1756.

4398. Tellier, M. C., G. Greco, M. Klotman, A. Mosoian, A. Cara, W. Arap, E. Ruoslahti, R. Pasqualini, and L. M. Schnapp. 2000. Superfibronectin, a multimeric form of fibronectin, increases HIV infection of primary CD4+ T lymphocytes. *J. Immunol.* **164**:3236–3245.

4399. Tenner-Racz, K., P. Racz, M. Dietrich, and P. Kern. 1985. Altered follicular dendritic cells and virus-like particles in AIDS and AIDS-related lymphadenopathy. *Lancet* **i**:105–106.

4400. Teppler, H., G. Kaplan, K. Smith, P. Cameron, A. Montana, P. Meyn, and Z. Cohn. 1993. Efficacy of low doses of polyethylene glycol derivative of interleukin-2 in modulating the immune response of patients with human immunodeficiency virus type 1 infection. *J. Infect. Dis.* **167**:291–298.

4401. Terai, C., R. S. Kornbluth, C. D. Pauza, D. D. Richman, and D. A. Carson. 1991. Apoptosis as a mechanism of cell death in cultured T lymphoblasts acutely infected with HIV-1. *J. Clin. Investig.* **87**:1710–1715.

4402. Tereskerz, P. M., M. Bentley, and J. Jagger. 1996. Risk of HIV-1 infection after human bites. *Lancet* **348**:1512.

4403. Tersmette, M., R. E. Y. de Goede, J. M. Bert, I. N. Al, R. A. Winkel, H. T. C. Gruters, H. G. Huisman, and F. Miedema. 1988. Differential syncytium-inducing capacity of human immunodeficiency virus isolates: frequent detection of syncytium-inducing isolates in patients with acquired immunodeficiency syndrome (AIDS) and AIDS-related complex. *J. Virol.* **62**:2026–2032.

4404. Tersmette, M., R. A. Gruters, F. de Wolf, R. E. Y. de Goede, J. M. A. Lange, P. T. A. Schellekens, J. Goudsmit, H. G. Huisman, and F. Miedema. 1989. Evidence for a role of virulent human immunodeficiency virus (HIV) variants in the pathogenesis of acquired immunodeficiency syndrome. *J. Virol.* **63**:2118–2125.

4405. Tersmette, M., J. M. A. Lange, R. E. Y. deGoede, F. de-Wolf, J. K. M. Eeftink-Schattenkerk, P. T. A. Schellekens, R. A. Coutinho, H. G. Huisman, J. Goudsmit, and F. Miedema. 1989. Association between biological properties of human immunodeficiency virus variants and risk for AIDS and AIDS mortality. *Lancet* **i**:983–985.

4406. Tersmette, M., J. J. M. Van Dongen, P. R. Clapham, R. E. Y. De Goede, I. L. M. Wolvers-Tettero, A. G. Van Kessel, J. G. Huisman, R. A. Weiss, and F. Miedema. 1989. Human immunodeficiency virus infection studied in CD4-expressing human-murine T-cell hybrids. *Virology* **168**:267–273.

4407. Terwilliger, E., J. G. Sodroski, C. A. Rosen, and W. A. Haseltine. 1986. Effects of mutations within the 3' orf open reading frame region of human T-cell lymphotropic virus type III on replication and cytopathogenicity. *J. Virol.* **60**:754–760.

4408. Terwilliger, E. F., E. Langhoff, D. Gabuzda, E. Zazopoulos, and W. A. Haseltine. 1991. Allelic variation in the effects of the *nef* gene on replication of human immunodeficiency virus type 1. *Proc. Natl. Acad. Sci. USA* **88**:10971–10975.

4409. Thakar, M. R., L. S. Bhonge, S. K. Lakhashe, U. Shankarkumar, S. S. Sane, S. S. Kulkarni, B. A. Mahajan, and R. S. Paranjape. 2005. Cytolytic T lymphocytes (CTLs) from HIV-1 subtype C-infected Indian patients recognize CTL epitopes from a conserved immunodominant region of HIV-1 Gag and Nef. *J. Infect. Dis.* **192**:749–759.

4410. Thali, M., A. Bukovsky, E. Kondo, B. Rosenwirth, C. T. Walsh, J. Sodroski, and H. G. Gottlinger. 1994. Functional association of cyclophilin A with HIV-1 virions. *Nature* **372**:363–365.

4411. Thali, M., M. Charles, C. Furman, L. Cavacini, M. Posner, J. Robinson, and J. Sodroski. 1994. Resistance to neutralization by broadly reactive antibodies to the human immunodeficiency virus type 1 gp120 glycoprotein conferred by a gp41 amino acid change. *J. Virol.* **68**:674–680.

4412. Thali, M., C. Furman, D. D. Ho, J. Robinson, S. Tilley, A. Pinter, and J. Sodroski. 1992. Discontinuous, conserved neutralization epitopes overlapping the CD4-binding region of human immunodeficiency virus type 1 gp120 envelope glycoprotein. *J. Virol.* **66**:5635–5641.

4413. Thali, M., J. P. Moore, C. Furman, M. Charles, D. D. Ho, J. Robinson, and J. Sodroski. 1993. Characterization of conserved human immunodeficiency virus type 1 gp120 neutralization epitopes exposed upon gp120-CD4 binding. *J. Virol.* **67**:3978–3988.

4414. Reference deleted.

4415. Reference deleted.

4416. Theodorou, I., L. Meyer, M. Magierowska, C. Katlama, and C. Rouzioux. 1997. HIV-1 infection in an individual homozygous for CCR5Δ32. *Lancet* **349**:1219–1220.

4417. Thieblemont, N., N. Haeffner-Cavaillon, A. Ledur, J. L'Age-Stehr, H. W. Ziegler-Heitbrock, and M. D. Kazatchkine. 1993. CR1 (CD35) and CR3 (CD11b/CD18) mediate infection of human monocytes and monocytic cell lines with complement-opsonized HIV independently of CD4. *Clin. Exp. Immunol.* **92**:106–113.

4418. Thielens, N. M., I. M. Bally, C. F. Ebenbichler, M. P. Dierich, and G. J. Arlaud. 1993. Further characterization of the interaction between the C1q subcomponent of human C1 and the transmembrane envelope glycoprotein gp41 of HIV-1. *J. Immunol.* **151**:6583–6592.

4419. Thiriart, C., J. Goudsmit, P. Schellekens, F. Barin, D. Zagury, M. De Wilde, and C. Bruck. 1988. Antibodies to soluble CD4 in HIV-1 infected individuals. *AIDS* **2**:345–351.

4420. Thomas, D. L., D. Vlahov, H. J. Alter, R. Marshall, J. Astemborski, and K. E. Nelson. 1998. Association of antibody to GB virus C (hepatitis G virus) with viral clearance and protection from re-infection. *J. Infect. Dis.* **177**:539–542.

4421. Thomas, E. R., C. Shotton, R. A. Weiss, P. R. Clapham, and A. McKnight. 2003. CD4–dependent and CD4–independent HIV-2: consequences for neutralization. *AIDS* **17**:291–300.

4421a. Thomas, S. M., D. B. Tse, D. S. Ketner, G. Rochford, D. A. Meyer, D. D. Zade, P. N. Halkitis, A. Nadas, W. Borkowsky, and M. Marmor. 2006. CCR5 expression and duration of high risk sexual activity among HIV-seronegative men who have sex with men. *AIDS* **20**:1879–1883.

4422. Thompson, K. A., M. J. Churchill, P. R. Gorry, J. Sterjovski, R. B. Oelrichs, S. L. Wesselingh, and C. A. McLean. 2004. Astrocyte specific viral strains in HIV dementia. *Ann. Neurol.* **56**:873–877.

4423. Thompson, P. M., R. A. Dutton, K. M. Hayashi, A. W. Toga, O. L. Lopez, H. J. Aizenstein, and J. T. Becker. 2005. Thinning of the cerebral cortex visualized in HIV/AIDS reflects CD4+ T lymphocyte decline. *Proc. Natl. Acad. Sci. USA* **102**:15647–15652.

4424. Thomson, M. M., E. Delgado, I. Herrero, M. Villahermosa, E. Vazquez-de Parga, L. Cuevas, and R. Najera. 2002. Diversity of mosaic structures and common ancestry of human immunodeficiency virus type 1 BF intersubtype recombinant viruses from Argentina revealed by analysis of near full-length genome sequences. *J. Gen. Virol.* **83**:107–119.

4425. Thornton, A. M., R. M. L. Buller, A. L. DeVico, I. Wang, and K. Ozato. 1996. Inhibition of human immunodeficiency virus type 1 and vaccinia virus infection by a dominant negative factor of the interferon regulatory factor family expressed in monocytic cells. *Proc. Natl. Acad. Sci. USA* **93**:383–387.

4426. Thornton, A. M., and E. M. Shevach. 1998. CD4+CD25+ immunoregulatory T cells suppress polyclonal T cell activation in vitro by inhibiting interleukin 2 production. *J. Exp. Med.* **188**:287–296.

4427. Tian, H., E. T. Donoghue, E. Fang, J. W. Newport, and D. I. Cohen. 1994. Cells expressing mutated CDC2 kinase undergo programmed cell death with striking similarities to HIV-directed cytopathicity. *J. Cell. Biochem. Suppl.* **18B**:143.

4428. Tien, P. C., and C. Grunfeld. 2004. What is HIV-associated lipodystrophy? Defining fat distribution changes in HIV infection. *Curr. Opin. Infect. Dis.* **17**:27–32.

4429. Tilley, S., W. Honnen, M. Racho, T.-C. Chou, and A. Pinter. 1992. Synergistic neutralization of HIV-1 by human monoclonal antibodies against the V3 loop and the CD4–binding site of gp120. *AIDS Res. Hum. Retrovir.* **8**:461–467.

4430. Tillmann, H. L., H. Heiken, A. Knapik-Botor, S. Her-inglake, J. Ockenga, J. C. Wilber, B. Goergen, N. Detmer, M. McMorrow, M. Stoll, R. E. Schmidt, and M. P. Manns. 2001. Infection with GB virus C and reduced mortality among HIV-infected patients. *N. Engl. J. Med.* **345:**715–724.

4431. Tilney, L. G., and D. A. Portnoy. 1989. Actin filaments and the growth, movement, and spread of the intracellular bacterial parasite, Listeria monocytogenes. *J. Cell Biol.* **109:**1597–1608.

4432. Tindall, B., S. Barker, B. Donovan, T. Barnes, J. Roberts, C. Kronenberg, J. Gold, R. Penny, and D. Cooper. 1988. Characterization of the acute clinical illness associated with human immunodeficiency virus infection. *Arch. Intern. Med.* **148:**945–949.

4433. Tindall, B., A. Carr, D. Goldstein, R. Penny, and D. A. Cooper. 1993. Administration of zidovudine during primary HIV-1 infection may be associated with a less vigorous immune response. *AIDS* **7:**127–128.

4434. Tindall, B., and D. A. Cooper. 1991. Primary HIV infection: host responses and intervention strategies. *AIDS* **5:**1–14.

4435. Tindall, B., L. Evans, P. Cunningham, P. McQueen, L. Hurren, E. Vasak, J. Mooney, and D. A. Cooper. 1992. Identification of HIV-1 in seminal fluid following primary HIV-1 infection. *AIDS* **6:**949–952.

4436. Tindall, B., H. Gaines, I. Imrie, M. A. E. von Sydow, L. A. Evans, O. Strannegard, M. L. Tsang, S. Lindback, and D. A. Cooper. 1991. Zidovudine in the management of primary HIV infection. *AIDS* **5:**477–484.

4437. Tirelli, U., M. Spina, G. Gaidano, E. Vaccher, S. Franceschi, and A. Carbone. 2000. Epidemiological, biological and clinical features of HIV-related lymphomas in the era of highly active antiretroviral therapy. *AIDS* **14:**1675–1688.

4438. Tissot, C., and N. Mechti. 1995. Molecular cloning of a new interferon-induced factor that represses human immunodeficiency virus type 1 long terminal repeat expression. *J. Biol. Chem.* **270:**14891–14898.

4439. Tissot, O., J.-P. Viard, C. Rabian, N. Ngo, M. Burgard, C. Rouzioux, and C. Penit. 1998. No evidence for proliferation in the blood CD4+ T-cell pool during HIV-1 infection and triple combination therapy. *AIDS* **12:**879–884.

4439a. Titanji, K., A. De Milito, A. Cagigi, R. Thorstensson, S. Grutzmeier, A. Atlas, B. Hejdeman, F. P. Kroon, L. Lopalco, A. Nilsson, and F. Chiodi. 2006. Loss of memory B cells impairs maintenance of long-term serologic memory during HIV-1 infection. *Blood* **108:**1580–1587.

4440. Tobiume, M., J. E. Lineberger, C. A. Lundquist, M. D. Miller, and C. Aiken. 2003. Nef does not affect the efficiency of human immunodeficiency virus type 1 fusion with target cells. *J. Virol.* **77:**10645–10650.

4441. Todd, B. J., P. Kedar, and J. H. Pope. 1995. Syncytium induction in primary CD4+ T-cell lines from normal donors by human immunodeficiency virus type 1 isolates with non-syncytium-inducing genotype and phenotype in MT-2 cells. *J. Virol.* **69:**7099–7105.

4442. Toggas, S. M., E. Masliah, E. M. Rockenstein, G. F. Rall, C. R. Abraham, and L. Mucke. 1994. Central nervous system damage produced by expression of the HIV-1 coat protein gp120 in transgenic mice. *Nature* **367:**188–193.

4443. Tokars, J. I., R. Marcus, D. H. Culver, C. A. Schable, P. S. McKibben, C. I. Bandea, and D. M. Bell. 1993. Surveillance of HIV infection and zidovudine use among health care workers after occupational exposure to HIV-infected blood. *Ann. Intern. Med.* **118:**913–919.

4444. Tomaras, G. D., S. F. Lacey, C. B. McDanal, G. Ferrari, K. J. Weinhold, and M. L. Greenberg. 2000. CD8+ T cell-mediated suppressive activity inhibits HIV-1 after virus entry with kinetics indicating effects on virus gene expression. *Proc. Natl. Acad. Sci. USA* **97:**3503–3508.

4445. Tong-Starksen, S. E., P. A. Luciw, and B. M. Peterlin. 1989. Signaling through T lymphocyte surface proteins, TCR/CD3 and CD28, activates the HIV-1 long terminal repeat. *J. Immunol.* **142:**702–707.

4446. Tong-Starksen, S. E., T. M. Welsh, and B. M. Peterlin. 1990. Differences in transcriptional enhancers of HIV-1 and HIV-2. Response to T cell activation signals. *J. Immunol.* **145:**4348–4354.

4447. Toniolo, A., C. Serra, P. G. Conaldi, F. Basolo, V. Falcone, and A. Dolei. 1995. Productive HIV-1 infection of normal human mammary epithelial cells. *AIDS* **9:**859–866.

4448. Toohey, K., K. Wehrly, J. Nishio, S. Perryman, and B. Chesebro. 1995. Human immunodeficiency virus envelope V1 and V2 regions influence replication efficiency in macrophages by affecting virus spread. *Virology* **213:**70–79.

4449. Tornatore, C., R. Chandra, J. R. Berger, and E. O. Major. 1994. HIV-1 infection of subcortical astrocytes in the pediatric central nervous system. *Neurology* **44:**481–487.

4450. Tornatore, C., K. Meyers, W. Atwood, K. Conant, and E. Major. 1994. Temporal patterns of human immunodeficiency virus type 1 transcripts in human fetal astrocytes. *J. Virol.* **68:**93–102.

4451. Tornatore, C., A. Nath, K. Amemiya, and E. O. Major. 1991. Persistent human immunodeficiency virus type 1 infection in human fetal glial cells reactivated by T cell factor(s) or by the cytokines tumor necrosis factor alpha and interleukin-1 beta. *J. Virol.* **65:**6094–6100.

4452. Torre, D., A. Pugliese, and G. Orofino. 2002. Effect of highly active antiretroviral therapy on ischemic cardiovascular disease in patients with HIV-1 infection. *Clin. Infect. Dis.* **35:**631–632.

4453. Toso, J. F., C. H. Chen, J. R. Mohr, L. Piglia, C. Oei, G. Ferrari, M. L. Greenberg, and K. J. Weinhold. 1995. Oligoclonal CD8 lymphocytes from persons with asymptomatic human immunodeficiency virus (HIV) type 1 infection inhibit HIV-1 replication. *J. Infect. Dis.* **172:**964–973.

4454. Toth, F. D., P. Mosborg-Petersen, J. Kiss, G. Aboagye-Mathiesen, M. Zdravkovic, H. Hager, J. Aranyosi, L. Lampe, and P. Ebbesen. 1994. Antibody-dependent enhancement of HIV-1 infection in human term syncytiotrophoblast cells cultured *in vitro*. *Clin. Exp. Immunol.* **96:**389–394.

4455. Tovo, P.-A., M. de Martino, C. Gabiano, L. Galli, C. Tibaldi, A. Vierucci, and F. Veglia. 1994. AIDS appearance in children is associated with the velocity of disease progression in their mothers. *J. Infect. Dis.* **170:**1000–1002.

4456. Tovo, P. A., M. deMartino, C. Gabiano, N. Cappello, R. D'Elia, A. Loy, A. Plebani, G. V. Zuccotti, P. Dallacasa, G. Ferraris, D. Caselli, C. Fundaro', P. D'Argenio, L. Galli, N. Principi, M. Stegagno, E. Ruga, and E. Palomba. 1992. Prognostic factors and survival in children with perinatal HIV-1 infection. *Lancet* **339:**1249–1253.

4457. Towers, G., M. Bock, S. Martin, Y. Takeuchi, J. P. Stoye, and O. Danos. 2000. A conserved mechanism of retrovirus restriction in mammals. *Proc. Natl. Acad. Sci. USA* 97:12295–12299.

4458. Towers, G. J., T. Hatziioannou, S. Cowan, S. P. Godd, J. Luban, and P. D. Bieniasz. 2003. Cyclophilin A modulates the sensitivity of HIV-1 to host restriction factors. *Nat. Med.* 9:1138–1143.

4458a. Townsend, C. L., P. A. Tookey, M. Cortina-Borja, and C. S. Peckham. 2006. Antiretroviral therapy and congenital abnormalities in infants born to HIV-1-infected women in the United Kingdom and Ireland, 1990 to 2003. *J. Acquir. Immune Defic. Syndr.* 42:91–94.

4459. Tozzi, V., P. Balestra, S. Galgani, P. Narciso, F. Ferri, G. Sebastiani, C. D'Amato, C. Affricano, F. Pigorini, F. M. Pau, A. De Felici, and A. Benedetto. 1999. Positive and sustained effects of highly active antiretroviral therapy on HIV-1-associated neurocognitive impairment. *AIDS* 13:1889–1897.

4459a. Trabattoni, D., M. Saresella, M. Biasin, A. Boasso, L. Piacentini, P. Ferrante, H. Dong, R. Maserati, G. M. Shearer, L. Chen, and M. Clerici. 2003. B7-H1 is upregulated in HIV infection and is a novel surrogate marker of disease progression. *Blood* 101:2514–2520.

4460. Trachtenberg, E., B. Korber, C. Sollars, T. B. Kepler, P. T. Hraber, E. Hayes, R. Funkhouser, M. Fugate, J. Theiler, Y. S. Hsu, K. Kunstman, S. Wu, J. Phair, H. Erlich, and S. Wolinsky. 2003. Advantage of rare HLA supertype in HIV disease progression. *Nat. Med.* 9:928–935.

4461. Trauger, R. J., F. Ferre, A. E. Diagle, F. C. Jensen, R. B. Moss, S. H. Mueller, S. P. Richieri, H. B. Slade, and D. J. Carlo. 1994. Effect of immunization with inactivated gp120-depleted human immunodeficiency virus type 1 (HIV-1) immunogen on HIV-1 immunity, viral DNA, and percentage of CD4 cells. *J. Infect. Dis.* 169:1256–1264.

4461a. Trautmann, L., L. Janbazian, N. Chomont, E. A. Said, S. Gimmig, B. Bessette, M. R. Boulassel, E. Delwart, H. Sepulveda, R. S. Balderas, J. P. Routy, E. K. Haddad, and R. P. Sekaly. 2006. Upregulation of PD-1 expression on HIV-specific CD8+ T cells leads to reversible immune dysfunction. *Nat. Med.* 12:1198–1202.

4462. Travers, K., S. Mboup, R. Marlink, A. Gueye-Ndiaye, T. Siby, I. Thior, I. Traore, A. Dieng-Sarr, J.-L. Sankale, C. Mullins, I. Ndoye, C.-C. Hsieh, M. Essex, and P. Kanki. 1995. Natural protection against HIV-1 infection provided by HIV-2. *Science* 268:1612–1615.

4463. Travers, S. A., J. P. Clewley, J. R. Glynn, P. E. M. Fine, A. C. Crampin, F. Sibande, D. Mulawa, J. O. McInerney, and G. P. McCormack. 2004. Timing and reconstruction of the most recent common ancestor of the subtype C clade of human immunodeficiency virus type 1. *J. Virol.* 78:10501–10506.

4464. Tremblay, M., S. Meloche, R.-P. Sekaly, and M. A. Wainberg. 1990. Complement receptor 2 mediates enhancement of human immunodeficiency virus 1 infection in Epstein-Barr virus-carrying B cells. *J. Exp. Med.* 171:1791–1796.

4465. Tremblay, M., K. Numazaki, X. G. Li, M. Gornitsky, J. Hiscott, and M. A. Wainberg. 1990. Resistance to infection by HIV-1 of peripheral blood mononuclear cells from HIV-1-infected patients is probably mediated by neutralizing antibodies. *J. Immunol.* 145:2896–2901.

4466. Tremblay, M., and M. A. Wainberg. 1990. Neutralization of multiple HIV-1 isolates from a single subject by autologous sequential sera. *J. Infect. Dis.* 162:735–737.

4467. Tresoldi, E., M. L. Romiti, M. Boniotto, S. Crovella, F. Salvatori, E. Palomba, A. Pastore, C. Cancrini, M. de Martino, A. Plebani, G. Castelli, P. Rossi, P. A. Tovo, A. Amoroso, and G. Scarlatti. 2002. Prognostic value of the stromal cell-derived factor 1 3'A mutation in pediatric human immunodeficiency virus type 1 infection. *J. Infect. Dis.* 185:696–700.

4468. Trial, J., H. H. Birdsall, J. A. Hallum, M. L. Crane, M. C. Rodriguez-Barradas, A. L. de Jong, B. Krishnan, C. E. Lacke, C. G. Figdor, and R. D. Rossen. 1995. Phenotypic and functional changes in peripheral blood monocytes during progression of human immunodeficiency virus infection. *J. Clin. Investig.* 95:1690–1701.

4469. Trinchieri, G. 1994. Interleukin-12: a cytokine produced by antigen-presenting cells with immunoregulatory functions in the generation of T-helper cells type 1 and cytotoxic lymphocytes. *Blood* 84:4008–4027.

4470. Trinchieri, G., and P. Scott. 1994. The role of interleukin 12 in the immune response, disease and therapy. *Immunol. Today* 15:460–463.

4471. Triozzi, P., W. Aldrich, H. Bresler, M. Para, and L. Flancbaum. 1999. Cellular immunotherapy of advanced human immunodeficiency virus type 1 infection using autologous lymph node lymphocytes: effects on chemokine production. *J. Infect. Dis.* 179:245–248.

4472. Triques, K., A. Bourgeois, N. Vidal, E. Mpudi-Ngole, C. Mulanga-Kaeya, N. Nzilambi, N. Torimiro, E. Saman, E. Delaporte, and M. Peeters. 2000. Near-full-length genome sequencing of divergent African HIV type 1 subtype F viruses leads to identification of a new HIV-1 subtype designated K. *AIDS Res. Hum. Retrovir.* 16:139–151.

4473. Triques, K., and M. Stevenson. 2004. Characterization of restrictions to human immunodeficiency virus type 1 infection of monocytes. *J. Virol.* 78:5523–5527.

4474. Trischmann, H., D. Davis, and P. J. Lachmann. 1995. Lymphocytotropic strains of HIV type 1 when complexed with enhancing antibodies can infect macrophages via FcγRIII, independently of CD4. *AIDS Res. Hum. Retrovir.* 11:343–352.

4475. Tristem, M., C. Marshall, A. Karpas, and F. Hill. 1992. Evolution of the primate lentiviruses: evidence from vpx and vpr. *EMBO J.* 11:3405–3412.

4476. Tristem, M., C. Marshall, A. Karpas, J. Petrik, and F. Hill. 1990. Origin of *vpx* in lentiviruses. *Nature* 347:341–342.

4477. Trkola, A., T. Dragic, J. Arthos, J. M. Binley, W. C. Olson, G. P. Allaway, C. Cheng-Mayer, J. Robinson, P. J. Maddon, and J. P. Moore. 1996. CD4-dependent, antibody-sensitive interactions between HIV-1 and its co-receptor CCR-5. *Nature* 384:184–187.

4478. Trkola, A., C. Gordon, J. Matthews, E. Maxwell, T. Ketas, L. Czaplewski, A. E. Proudfoot, and J. P. Moore. 1999. The CC-chemokine RANTES increases the attachment of human immunodeficiency virus type 1 to target cells via glycosaminoglycans and also activates a signal transduction pathway that enhances viral infectivity. *J. Virol.* 73:6370–6379.

4479. Trkola, A., S. E. Kuhmann, J. M. Strizki, E. Maxwell, T. Ketas, T. Morgan, P. Pugach, S. Xu, L. Wojcik, J. Tagat, A. Palani, S. Shapiro, J. W. Clader, S. McCombie, G. R. Reyes, B. M. Baroudy, and J. P. Moore. 2002. HIV-1 escape from a small molecule, CCR5-specific entry inhibitor does not involve CXCR4 use. *Proc. Natl. Acad. Sci. USA* 99:395–400.

4479a. Trkola, A., H. Kuster, C. Leemann, A. Oxenius, C. Fagard, H. Furrer, M. Battegay, P. Vernazza, E. Bernasconi, R.

Weber, B. Hirschel, S. Bonhoeffer, and H. F. Gunthard. 2004. Humoral immunity to HIV-1: kinetics of antibody responses in chronic infection reflects capacity of immune system to improve viral set point. *Blood* 104:1784–1792.

4480. Trkola, A., H. Kuster, C. Leemann, C. Ruprecht, B. Joos, A. Telenti, B. Hirschel, R. Weber, S. Bonhoeffer, H. F. Gunthard, and Swiss HIV Cohort Study. 2003. Human immunodeficiency virus type 1 fitness is a determining factor in viral rebound and set point in chronic infection. *J. Virol.* 77: 13146–13155.

4481. Trkola, A., H. Kuster, P. Rusert, B. Joos, M. Fischer, C. Leemann, A. Manrique, M. Huber, M. Rehr, A. Oxenius, R. Weber, G. Stiegler, B. Vcelar, H. Katinger, L. Aceto, and H. F. Gunthard. 2005. Delay of HIV-1 rebound after cessation of antiretroviral therapy through passive transfer of human neutralizing antibodies. *Nat. Med.* 11:615–622.

4482. Trkola, A., A. B. Pomales, H. Yuan, B. Korber, P. J. Maddon, G. P. Allaway, H. Katinger, C. F. Barbas III, D. R. Burton, D. D. Ho, and J. P. Moore. 1995. Cross-clade neutralization of primary isolates of human immunodeficiency virus type 1 by human monoclonal antibodies and tetrameric CD4-IgG. *J. Virol.* 69:6609–6617.

4483. Trkola, A., M. Purtscher, T. Muster, C. Ballaun, A. Buchacher, N. Sullivan, K. Srinivasan, J. Sodroski, J. P. Moore, and H. Katinger. 1996. Human monoclonal antibody 2G12 defines a distinctive neutralization epitope on the gp120 glycoprotein of human immunodeficiency virus type 1. *J. Virol.* 70:1100–1108.

4484. Trono, D. 1992. Partial reverse transcripts in virions from human immunodeficiency and murine leukemia viruses. *J. Virol.* 66:4893–4900.

4485. Trono, D., and C. Aiken. 1994. Nef induces CD4 endocytosis: requirement for a critical motif in the membrane-proximal CD4 cytoplasmic domain. *J. Cell. Biochem. Suppl.* 18B:143.

4486. Trono, D., and D. Baltimore. 1990. A human cell factor is essential for HIV-1 *rev* action. *EMBO J.* 9:4155–4160.

4487. Trubey, C. M., E. Chertova, L. V. Coren, J. M. Hilburn, C. V. Hixson, K. Nagashima, J. D. Lifson, and D. E. Ott. 2003. Quantitation of HLA class II protein incorporated into human immunodeficiency type 1 virions purified by anti-CD45 immunoaffinity depletion of microvesicles. *J. Virol.* 77: 12699–12709.

4488. Trujillo, J. R., M. F. McLane, T. H. Lee, and M. Essex. 1993. Molecular mimicry between the human immunodeficiency virus type 1 gp120 V3 loop and human brain proteins. *J. Virol.* 67:7711–7715.

4489. Truneh, A., D. Buck, D. R. Cassatt, R. Juszczak, S. Kassis, S. E. Ryu, D. Healey, R. Sweet, and Q. Sattentau. 1991. A region in domain 1 of CD4 distinct from the primary gp120 binding site is involved in HIV infection and virus-mediated fusion. *J. Biol. Chem.* 266:5942–5948.

4490. Truong, L. X., T. T. Luong, D. Scott-Algara, P. Versmisse, A. David, D. Perez-Bercoff, N. V. Nguyen, H. K. Tran, C. T. Cao, A. Fontanet, J.-Y. Follezou, I. Theodorou, F. Barre-Sinoussi, and G. Pancino. 2003. CD4 cell and CD8 cell-mediated resistance to HIV-1 infection in exposed uninfected intravascular drug users in Vietnam. *AIDS* 17:1423–1434.

4491. Truong, M. J., E. C. Darcissac, E. Hermann, J. Dewulf, A. Capron, and G. M. Bahr. 1999. Interleukin-16 inhibits human immunodeficiency virus type 1 entry and replication in macrophages and in dendritic cells. *J. Virol.* 73:7008–7013.

4492. Tsai, C. C., K. E. Follis, A. Sabo, T. W. Beck, R. F. Grant, N. Bischofberger, R. E. Benveniste, and R. Black. 1995. Prevention of SIV infection in macaques by (R)-9-(2-phosphonylmethoxypropyl) adenine. *Science* 270:1197–1199.

4493. Tsang, M. L., L. A. Evans, P. McQueen, L. Hurren, C. Byrne, R. Penny, B. Tindall, and D. A. Cooper. 1994. Neutralizing antibodies against sequential autologous human immunodeficiency virus type 1 isolates after seroconversion. *J. Infect. Dis.* 170:1141–1147.

4494. Tschlachler, E., V. Groh, M. Popovic, D. L. Mann, K. Konrad, B. Safai, L. Eron, F. d. M. Veronese, K. Wolff, and G. Stingl. 1987. Epidermal Langerhans cells—a target for HTLV-III/LAV infection. *J. Investig. Dermatol.* 88:233–237.

4495. Tsubota, H., D. J. Ringler, M. Kannagi, N. W. King, K. R. Solomon, J. J. MacKey, D. G. Walsh, and N. L. Letvin. 1989. CD8+CD4- lymphocyte lines can harbor the AIDS virus *in vitro. J. Immunol.* 143:858–863.

4496. Tsui, R., B. L. Herring, J. D. Barbour, R. M. Grant, P. Bacchetti, A. Kral, B. R. Edlin, and E. L. Delwart. 2004. Human immunodeficiency virus type 1 superinfection was not detected following 215 years of injection drug user exposure. *J. Virol.* 78:94–103.

4497. Tsuji, T., K. Hamajima, J. Fukushima, K. Q. Zin, N. Ishii, I. Aoki, Y. Ishigatsubo, K. Tani, S. Kawamoto, Y. Nitta, J. Miyazaki, W. C. Koff, T. Okubo, and K. Okuda. 1997. Enhancement of cell-mediated immunity against HIV-1 induced by coinoculation of plasmid-encoded HIV-1 antigen with plasmid expressing IL-12. *J. Immunol.* 158:4008–4013.

4498. Tsuji, T., K. Hamajima, N. Ishii, I. Aoki, J. Fukushima, K. Q. Xin, S. Kawamoto, S. Sasaki, K. Matsunaga, Y. Ishigatsubo, K. Tani, T. Okubo, and K. Okuda. 1997. Immunomodulatory effects of a plasmid expressing B7-2 on human immunodeficiency virus-1-specific cell-mediated immunity induced by a plasmid encoding the viral antigen. *Eur. J. Immunol.* 27:782–787.

4499. Tsunemi, S., T. Iwasaki, T. Imado, S. Higasa, F. Kakishita, T. Shirasaka, and H. Sano. 2005. Relationship of CD4+CD25+ regulatory T cells to immune status in HIV-infected patients. *AIDS* 19:879–886.

4500. Tsunetsugu-Yokota, Y., K. Akagawa, H. Kimoto, K. Suzuki, M. Iwasaki, S. Yasuda, G. Hausser, C. Hultgren, A. Meyerhans, and T. Takemori. 1995. Monocyte-derived cultured dendritic cells are susceptible to human immunodeficiency virus infection and transmit virus to resting T cells in the process of nominal antigen presentation. *J. Virol.* 69:4544–4547.

4501. Tsunetsugu-Yokota, Y., S. Matsuda, M. Maekawa, T. Saito, T. Takemori, and Y. Takebe. 1992. Constitutive expression of the *nef* gene suppresses human immunodeficiency virus type 1 (HIV-1) replication in monocytic cell lines. *Virology* 191:960–963.

4502. Tsunoda, R., K. Hashimoto, M. Baba, S. Shigeta, and N. Sugai. 1996. Follicular dendritic cells *in vitro* are not susceptible to infection by HIV-1. *AIDS* 10:595–602.

4503. Tummino, P. J., J. D. Scholten, P. J. Harvey, T. P. Holler, L. Maloney, R. Gogliotti, J. Domagala, and D. Hupe. 1996. The *in vitro* ejection of zinc from human immunodeficiency virus (HIV) type 1 nucleocapsid protein by disulfide benzamides with cellular anti-HIV activity. *Proc. Natl. Acad. Sci. USA* 93:969–973.

4504. Turci, M., E. Pilotti, P. Ronzi, G. Magnani, A. Boschini, S. G. Parisi, D. Zipeto, A. Lisa, C. Casoli, and U. Bertazzoni. 2006. Coinfection with HIV-1 and human T-cell lymphotropic virus type II in intravenous drug users is associated with delayed progression to AIDS. *J. Acquir. Immune Defic. Syndr.* 41:100–106.

4505. Turelli, P., B. Mangeat, S. Jost, S. Vianin, and D. Trono. 2004. Inhibition of hepatitis B virus replication by APOBEC3G. *Science* 303:1829.

4506. Turelli, P., and D. Trono. 2005. Editing at the crossroad of innate and adaptive immunity. *Science* 307:1061–1065.

4507. Turnbull, E. L., A. R. Lopes, N. A. Jones, D. Cornforth, P. Newton, D. Aldam, P. Pellegrino, J. Turner, I. Williams, C. M. Wilson, P. A. Goepfert, M. K. Maini, and P. Borrow. 2006. HIV-1 epitope-specific CD8+ T cell responses strongly associated with delayed disease progression cross-recognize epitope variants efficiently. *J. Immunol.* 176:6130–6146.

4508. Turner, D., B. Brenna, J.-P. Routy, D. Moisi, Z. Rosberger, M. Rober, and M. A. Wainberg. 2004. Diminished representation of HIV-1 variants containing select drug resistance-conferring mutations in primary HIV-1 infection. *J. Acquir. Immune Defic. Syndr.* 37:1627 1631.

4509. Turpin, J. A., M. Vaugo, and E. S. Meltzer. 1992. Enhanced HIV-1 replication in retinoid-treated monocytes. *J. Immunol.* 148:2539–2546.

4510. Turville, S. G., J. Arthos, K. M. Donald, G. Lynch, H. Naif, G. Clark, D. Hart, and A. L. Cunningham. 2001. HIV gp120 receptors on human dendritic cells. *Blood* 98:2482–2488.

4511. Turville, S. G., P. U. Cameron, A. Handley, G. Lin, S. Pohlmann, R. W. Doms, and A. L. Cunningham. 2002. Diversity of receptors binding HIV on dendritic cell subsets. *Nat. Immunol.* 3:975–983.

4512. Turville, S. G., J. J. Santos, I. Frank, P. U. Cameron, J. Wilkinson, M. Miranda-Saksena, J. Dable, H. Stossel, N. Romani, M. Piatak, Jr., J. D. Lifson, M. Pope, and A. L. Cunningham. 2004. Immunodeficiency virus uptake, turnover, and 2-phase transfer in human dendritic cells. *Blood* 103:2170–2179.

4513. Tuttle, D. L., C. B. Anders, M. J. Aquino-De Jesus, P. P. Poole, S. L. Lamers, D. R. Briggs, S. M. Pomeroy, L. Alexander, K. W. Peden, W. A. Andiman, J. W. Sleasman, and M. M. Goodenow. 2002. Increased replication of non-syncytium-inducing HIV type 1 isolates in monocyte-derived macrophages is linked to advanced disease in infected children. *AIDS Res. Hum. Retrovir.* 18:353–362.

4514. Twigg, H. L., III, D. M. Soliman, and B. A. Spain. 1994. Impaired alveolar macrophage accessory cell function and reduced incidence of lymphocytic alveolitis in HIV-infected patients who smoke. *AIDS* 8:611–618.

4515. Twu, C., N. Q. Liu, W. Popik, M. Bukrinsky, J. Sayre, J. Roberts, S. Rania, V. Bramhandam, K. P. Roos, W. R. MacLellan, and M. Fiala. 2002. Cardiomyocytes undergo apoptosis in human immunodeficiency virus cardiomyopathy through mitochondrion- and death receptor-controlled pathways. *Proc. Natl. Acad. Sci. USA* 99:14386–14391.

4516. Tyler, D. S., S. D. Stanley, C. A. Nastala, A. A. Austin, J. A. Bartlett, K. C. Stine, H. K. Lyerly, D. P. Bolognesi, and K. J. Weinhold. 1990. Alterations in antibody-dependent cellular cytotoxicity during the course of HIV-1 infection. *J. Immunol.* 144:3375–3384.

4517. Tyndall, M. W., A. R. Ronald, E. Agoki, W. Malisa, J. J. Bwayo, J. O. Ndinya-Achola, S. Moses, and F. A. Plummer. 1996. Increased risk of infection with human immunodeficiency virus type 1 among uncircumcised men presenting with genital ulcer disease in Kenya. *Clin. Infect. Dis.* 23:449–453.

4518. Tyor, W. R., J. D. Glass, J. W. Griffin, P. S. Becker, J. C. McArthur, L. Bezman, and D. E. Griffin. 1991. Cytokine expression in the brain during the acquired immunodeficiency syndrome. *Ann. Neurol.* 31:349–360.

4519. Ueda, H., O. M. Z. Howard, M. C. Grimm, S. B. Su, W. H. Gong, G. Evans, F. W. Ruscetti, J. J. Oppenheim, and J. M. Wang. 1998. HIV-1 envelope gp41 is a potent inhibitor of chemoattractant receptor expression and function in monocytes. *J. Clin. Investig.* 102:804–812.

4520. Uehara, T., T. Miyawaki, K. Ohta, Y. Tamaru, T. Yokio, S. Nakamura, and N. Taniguchi. 1992. Apoptotic cell death of primed CD45RO+ T lymphocytes in Epstein-Barr virus-induced infectious mononucleosis. *Blood* 80:452–458.

4521. Ugen, K. E., V. Srikantan, J. J. Goedert, R. P. Nelson, Jr., W. V. Williams, and D. B. Weiner. 1997. Vertical transmission of human immunodeficiency virus type 1: seroreactivity by maternal antibodies to the carboxy region of the gp41 envelope glycoprotein. *J. Infect. Dis.* 175:63–69.

4522. Ugolini, S., I. Mondor, and Q. J. Sattentau. 1999. HIV-1 attachment: another look. *Trends Microbiol.* 7:144–149.

4523. Uittenbogaart, C. H., D. J. Anisman, B. D. Jamieson, S. Kitchen, I. Schmid, J. A. Zack, and E. F. Hays. 1996. Differential tropism of HIV-1 isolates for distinct thymocyte subsets *in vitro. AIDS* 10:F9–F16.

4524. Ullum, H., P. C. Gotzsche, J. Victor, E. Dickmeiss, P. Skinhoj, and B. K. Pedersen. 1995. Defective natural immunity: an early manifestation of human immunodeficiency virus infection. *J. Exp. Med.* 182:789–799.

4525. Ullum, H., A. C. Lepri, J. Victor, H. Aladdin, A. N. Phillips, J. Gerstoft, P. Skinhoj, and B. K. Pedersen. 1998. Production of β-chemokines in human immunodeficiency virus (HIV) infection: evidence that high levels of macrophage inflammatory protein-1β are associated with a decreased risk of HIV disease progression. *J. Infect. Dis.* 177:331–336.

4526. Ullum, H., J. Palmo, J. Halkjaer-Kristensen, M. Diamant, M. Klokker, A. Kruuse, A. LaPerriere, and B. K. Pedersen. 1994. The effect of acute exercise on lymphocyte subsets, natural killer cells, proliferative responses, and cytokines in HIV-seropositive persons. *J. Acquir. Immune Defic. Syndr.* 7:1122–1133.

4527. UNAIDS. 2004, posting date. *XV International AIDS Conference Bangkok.* [online.] http://www.unaids.org/bangkok2004/factsheets.html. UNAIDS.

4527a. Unutmaz, D., V. N. Kewal Ramani, S. Marmon, and D. R. Littman. 1999. Cytokine signals are sufficient for HIV-1 infection of resting human T lymphocytes. *J. Exp. Med.* 189:1735–1746.

4528. Urdea, M. S. 1993. Synthesis and characterization of branched DNA (bDNA) for the direct and quantitative detection of CMV, HBV, HCV, and HIV. *Clin. Chem.* 39:725–726.

4529. Urschel, S., J. Ramos, M. Mellado, C. Giaquinto, G. Verweel, T. Schuster, T. Niehues, B. Belohradsky, and U. Wintergerst. 2005. Withdrawal of Pneumocystis jirovecii prophylaxis in HIV-infected children under highly active antiretroviral therapy. *AIDS* 19:2103–2108.

4530. Vaccher, E., M. Spina, R. Talamini, M. Zanetti, G. di Gennaro, G. Nasti, M. Tavio, D. Bernardi, C. Simonelli, and U. Tirelli. 2003. Improvement of systemic human immunodeficiency virus-related non-Hodgkin lymphoma outcome in the era of highly active antiretroviral therapy. *HIV/AIDS* 37:1556–1564.

4531. Valcour, V., C. Shikuma, B. Shiramizu, M. Watters, P. Poff, O. A. Selnes, J. Grove, Y. Liu, K. B. Abdul-Majid, S. Gartner, and N. Sacktor. 2004. Age, apolipoprotein E4, and the risk of HIV dementia: the Hawaii Aging with HIV Cohort. *J. Neuroimmunol.* 157:197–202.

4532. Valdez, H., R. Mitsuyasu, A. Landay, A. D. Sevin, E. S. Chan, J. Sprtizler, S. A. Kalams, R. B. Pollard, J. Fahey, L. Fox, A. Namking, S. Estep, R. Moss, D. Sahner, and M. M. Lederman. 2003. Interleukin-2 increases CD4+ lymphocyte numbers but does not enhance responses to immunization: results of A5046s. *J. Infect. Dis.* 187:320–325.

4533. Valdez, H., S. F. Purvis, M. M. Lederman, M. Fillingame, and P. A. Zimmerman. 1999. Association of the CCR5delta32 mutation with improved response to antiretroviral therapy. *JAMA* 282:734.

4533a. Valente, S. T., and S. P. Goff. 2006. Inhibition of HIV-1 gene expression by a fragment of hnRNP U. *Mol. Cell* 23:597–605.

4534. Valentin, A., J. Albert, E. M. Fenyo, and B. Asjo. 1994. Dual tropism for macrophages and lymphocytes is a common feature of primary human immunodeficiency virus type 1 and 2 isolates. *J. Virol.* 68:6684–6689.

4535. Valentin, A., K. Lundin, M. Patarroyo, and B. Asjo. 1990. The leukocyte adhesion glycoprotein CD18 participates in HIV-1-induced syncytia formation in monocytoid and T cells. *J. Immunol.* 144:934–937.

4536. Valentin, A., M. Rosati, D. J. Patenaude, A. Hatzakis, L. G. Kostrikis, M. Lazanas, K. M. Wyvill, R. Yarchoan, and G. N. Pavlakis. 2002. Persistent HIV-1 infection of natural killer cells in patients receiving highly active antiretroviral therapy. *Proc. Natl. Acad. Sci. USA* 99:7015–7020.

4537. Valentin, A., A. von Gegerfelt, S. Matsuda, K. Nilsson, and B. Asjo. 1991. *In vitro* maturation of mononuclear phagocytes and susceptibility to HIV-1 infection. *J. Acquir. Immune Defic. Syndr.* 4:751–759.

4538. Valentin, H., M. T. Nugeyre, F. Vuillier, L. Boumsell, and M. Schmid. 1994. Two subpopulations of human triple-negative thymic cells are susceptible to infection by human immunodeficiency virus type 1 in vitro. *J. Virol.* 68:3041–3050.

4539. Valeriano-Marcet, J., L. Ravichandran, and L. D. Kerr. 1990. HIV associated systemic necrotizing vasculitis. *J. Rheumatol.* 17:1091–1093.

4540. Valerie, K., A. Delers, C. Bruck, C. Thiriart, H. Rosenberg, C. Debouck, and C. M. Rosenberg. 1988. Activation of human immunodeficiency virus type 1 by DNA damage in human cells. *Nature* 333:78–81.

4541. Vallee, H., and H. Carre. 1904. Sur l'anemie infectieuse du cheval. *C. R. Acad. Sci.* 139:1239–1241.

4542. Van Damme, L., G. Ramjee, M. Alary, B. Vuylsteke, V. Chandeying, H. Rees, P. Sirivongrangson, L. Mukenge-Tshibaka, V. Ettiegne-Traore, C. Uaheowitchai, S. S. Karim, B. Masse, J. Perriens, and M. Laga. 2002. Effectiveness of COL-1492, a nonoxynol-9 vaginal gel, on HIV-1 transmission in female sex workers: a randomised controlled trial. *Lancet* 360:971–977.

4543. Van de Perre, P., A. Simonon, D. G. Hitimana, F. Dabis, P. Msellati, B. Mukamabano, J.-B. Butera, C. Van goethem, E. Karita, and P. Lepage. 1993. Infective and anti-infective properties of breastmilk from HIV-1-infected women. *Lancet* 341:914–918.

4544. Van de Perre, P., A. Simonon, P. Msellati, D.-G. Hitimana, D. Vaira, A. Bazubagira, C. Van Goethem, A.-M. Stevens, E. Karita, D. Sondag-Thull, F. Dabis, and P. Lepage. 1991. Postnatal transmission of human immunodeficiency virus type 1 from mother to infant. *N. Engl. J. Med.* 325:593–598.

4545. van der Burg, S. H., M. R. Klein, O. Pontesilli, A. M. Holwerda, J. W. Drijfhout, W. M. Kast, F. Miedema, and C. J. Melief. 1997. HIV-1 reverse transcriptase-specific CTL against conserved epitopes do not protect against progression to AIDS. *J. Immunol.* 159:3648–3654.

4546. van der Ende, M. E., M. Schutten, B. Raschdorff, G. Großschupff, P. Racz, A. D. M. E. Osterhaus, and K. Tenner-Racs. 1999. CD4 cells remain the major source of HIV-1 during end stage disease. *AIDS* 13:1015–1019.

4547. van der Hoek, L., R. Boom, J. Goudsmit, F. Snijders, and C. J. A. Sol. 1995. Isolation of human immunodeficiency virus type 1 (HIV-1) RNA from feces by a simple method and difference between HIV-1 subpopulations in feces and serum. *J. Clin. Microbiol.* 33:581–588.

4548. van der Loeff, M. F., P. Aaby, K. Aryioshi, T. Vincent, A. A. Awasana, C. Da Costa, L. Pembrey, F. Dias, E. Harding, H. A. Weiss, and H. C. Whittle. 2001. HIV-2 does not protect against HIV-1 infection in a rural community in Guinea-Bissau. *AIDS* 15:2303–2310.

4549. van der Straten, A., M. S. Kang, S. F. Posner, M. Kamba, T. Chipato, and N. S. Padian. 2005. Predictors of diaphragm use as a potential sexually transmitted disease/HIV prevention method in Zimbabwe. *Sex. Transm. Dis.* 32:64–71.

4550. van der Vliet, H. J., B. M. von Blomberg, M. D. Hazenberg, N. Nishi, S. A. Otto, B. H. van Benthem, M. Prins, F. A. Claessen, A. J. van den Eertwegh, G. Giaccone, F. Miedema, R. J. Scheper, and H. M. Pinedo. 2002. Selective decrease in circulating V alpha 24+V beta 11+ NKT cells during HIV type 1 infection. *J. Immunol.* 168:1490–1495.

4550a. Van Heuverswyn, F., Li, Y., Neel, C., Bailes, E., Keele, B. F., Liu, W., Loul, S., Butel, C., Liegeois, F., Bienvenue, Y., Ngolle, E. M., Sharp, P. M., Shaw, G. M., Delaporte, E., Halm, B. H., and Peeters, M. 2006. Human immunodeficiency viruses: SIV infection in wild gorillas. *Nature* 444:164.

4551. van Kerckhoven, I., K. Fransen, M. Peeters, H. De Beenhouwer, P. Piot, and G. van der Groen. 1994. Quantification of human immunodeficiency virus in plasma by RNA PCR, viral culture, and p24 antigen detection. *J. Clin. Microbiol.* 32:1669–1673.

4552. van Leth, F., S. Andrews, B. Grinsztejn, E. Wilkins, M. K. Lazanas, J. M. A. Lange, and J. Montaner. 2005. The effect of baseline CD4 cell count and HIV-1 viral load on the efficacy and safety of nevirapine or efavirenz-based first-line HAART. *AIDS* 19:463–471.

4553. Van Lint, C., S. Emiliani, M. Ott, and E. Verdin. 1996. Transcriptional activation and chromatin remodeling of the HIV-1 promoter in response to histone acetylation. *EMBO J.* 15:1112–1120.

4554. Van Nest, G. A., K. S. Steimer, N. L. Haigwood, R. L. Burke, and G. Ott. 1992. Advanced adjuvant formulations for use with recombinant subunit vaccines, p. 57–62. *In* R. M. Chanock, R. A. Lerner, F. Brown, and H. Ginsburg (ed.), *Vaccines 92: Modern Approaches to New Vaccines*. Cold Spring Harbor Laboratories, Cold Spring Harbor, N.Y.

4555. van Noesel, C. J. M., R. A. Gruters, F. G. Terpstra, P. T. A. Schellekens, R. A. W. van Lier, and F. Miedema. 1990. Functional and phenotypic evidence for a selective loss of memory

T cells in asymptomatic human immunodeficiency virus-infected men. *J. Clin. Investig.* 86:293–299.

4556. van Rij, R. P., H. Blaak, J. A. Visser, M. Brouwer, R. Rientsma, S. Broersen, A.-R. D. Husman, and H. Schuitemaker. 2000. Differential coreceptor expression allows for independent evolution of non-syncytium-inducing and syncytium-inducing HIV-1. *J. Clin. Investig.* 106:1039–1052.

4557. van Rij, R. P., S. Broersen, J. Goudsmit, R. A. Coutinho, and H. Schuitemaker. 1998. The role of a stromal cell-derived factor-1 chemokine gene variant in the clinical course of HIV-1 infection. *AIDS* 12:F85–F90.

4558. van Rij, R. P., A. de Roda Husman, M. Brouwer, J. Goudsmit, R. A. Coutinho, and H. Schuitemaker. 1998. Role of CCR2 genotype in the clinical course of syncytium-inducing (SI) or non-SI human immunodeficiency virus type 1 infection and in the time to conversion to SI virus variants. *J. Infect. Dis.* 178:1806–1811.

4559. van Rij, R. P., M. D. Hazenberg, B. H. van Benthem, S. A. Otto, M. Prins, F. Miedema, and H. Schuitemaker. 2003. Early viral load and CD4+ T cell count, but not percentage of CCR5+ or CXCR4+ CD4+ T cells, are associated with R5-to-X4 HIV type 1 virus evolution. *AIDS Res. Hum. Retrovir.* 19:389–398.

4560. Van Rompay, K. K., C. J. Berardi, S. Dillard-Telm, R. P. Tarara, D. R. Canfield, C. R. Valverde, D. C. Montefiori, K. S. Cole, R. C. Montelaro, C. J. Miller, and M. L. Marthas. 1998. Passive immunization of newborn rhesus macaques prevents oral simian immunodeficiency virus infection. *J. Infect. Dis.* 177:1247–1259.

4561. Van Rompay, K. K. A., J. M. Cherrington, M. L. Marthas, C. J. Berardi, A. S. Mulato, A. Spinner, R. P. Tarara, D. R. Canfield, S. Telm, N. Bischofberger, and N. C. Pedersen. 1996. 9-[2-(Phosphonomethoxy)propyl]adenine therapy of established simian immunodeficiency virus infection in infant rhesus macaques. *Antimicrob. Agents Chemother.* 40:2586–2591.

4562. Van Rompay, K. K. A., M. G. Otsylua, M. L. Marthas, C. J. Miller, M. B. McChesney, and N. C. Pedersen. 1995. Immediate zidovudine treatment protects simian immunodeficiency virus-infected newborn macaques against rapid onset of AIDS. *Antimicrob. Agents Chemother.* 39:125–131.

4563. Van Rompay, K. K. A., M. G. Otsyula, R. P. Tarara, D. R. Canfield, C. J. Berardi, M. B. McChesney, and M. L. Marthas. 1996. Vaccination of pregnant macaques protects newborns against mucosal simian immunodeficiency virus infection. *J. Infect. Dis.* 173:1327–1335.

4564. Van Voorhis, B. J., A. Martinez, K. Mayer, and D. J. Anderson. 1991. Detection of human immunodeficiency virus type 1 in semen from seropositive men using culture and polymerase chain reaction deoxyribonucleic acid amplification techniques. *Fertil. Steril.* 55:588–594.

4565. van't Wout, A. B., H. Blaak, L. J. Ran, M. Brouwer, C. Kuiken, and H. Schuitemaker. 1998. Evolution of syncytium-inducing and non-syncytium-inducing biological virus clones in relation to replication kinetics during the course of human immunodeficiency virus type 1 infection. *J. Virol.* 72:5099–5107.

4566. van't Wout, A. B., L. J. Ran, M. D. de Jong, M. Bakker, R. van Leeuwen, D. W. Notermans, A. E. Loeliger, F. de Wolf, S. A. Danner, P. Reiss, C. A. B. Boucher, J. M. A. Lange, and H. Schuitemaker. 1997. Selective inhibition of syncytium-inducing and nonsyncytium-inducing HIV-1 variants in individuals receiving didanosine or zidovudine, respectively. *J. Clin. Investig.* 100:2325–2332.

4567. VanCott, T. C., F. R. Bethke, V. R. Polonis, M. K. Gorny, S. Zolla-Pazner, R. R. Redfield, and D. L. Birx. 1994. Dissociation rate of antibody-gp120 binding interactions is predictive of V3-mediated neutralization of HIV-1. *J. Immunol.* 153:449–459.

4568. Vanden Haesevelde, M. M., M. Peeters, G. Jannes, W. Janssens, G. van der Groen, P. M. Sharp, and E. Saman. 1996. Sequence analysis of a highly divergent HIV-1-related lentivirus isolated from a wild captured chimpanzee. *Virology* 221:346–350.

4569. Vanham, G., L. Kestens, I. De Meester, J. Vingerhoets, G. Penne, G. Vanhoof, S. Scharpe, H. Heyligen, E. Bosmans, J. L. Ceuppens, and P. Gigase. 1993. Decreased expression of the memory marker CD26 on both CD4+ and CD8+ lymphocytes of HIV-infected subjects. *J. Acquir. Immune Defic. Syndr.* 6:749–757.

4570. Vanhems, P., B. Hirschel, A. N. Phillips, D. A. Cooper, J. Vizzard, J. Brassard, and L. Perrin. 2000. Incubation time of acute human immunodeficiency virus (HIV) infection and duration of acute HIV infection are independent prognostic factors of progression to AIDS. *J. Infect. Dis.* 182:334–337.

4571. Varthakavi, V., R. M. Smith, S. P. Bour, K. Strebel, and P. Spearman. 2003. Viral protein U counteracts a human host cell restriction that inhibits HIV-1 particle production. *Proc. Natl. Acad. Sci. USA* 100:15154–15159.

4572. Vasan, A., B. Renjifo, E. Hertzmark, B. Chaplin, G. Msamanga, M. Essex, W. Fawzi, and D. Hunter. 2006. Different rates of disease progression of HIV type 1 infection in Tanzania based on infecting subtype. *Clin. Infect. Dis.* 42:843–852.

4573. Vasu, S. K., and D. J. Forges. 2001. Nuclear pores and nuclear assembly. *Curr. Opin. Cell Biol.* 13:363–375.

4574. Veazey, R., P. J. Klasse, T. J. Ketas, J. D. Reeves, M. Piatak, K. Kunstman, S. E. Kuhmann, P. A. Marx, J. D. Lifson, J. Dufour, M. Mefford, I. Pandrea, S. M. Wolinsky, R. W. Doms, J. A. DeMartino, S. J. Siciliano, K. Lyons, M. S. Springer, and J. P. Moore. 2003. Use of a small molecule CCR5 inhibitor in macaques to treat simian immunodeficiency virus infection or prevent simian-human immunodeficiency virus infection. *J. Exp. Med.* 198:1551–1562.

4575. Veazey, R. S., M. A. DeMaria, L. V. Chalifoux, D. E. Shvetz, D. R. Pauley, H. L. Knight, M. Rosenzweig, R. P. Johnson, R. C. Desrosiers, and A. A. Lackner. 1998. Gastrointestinal tract as a major site of CD4+ T cell depletion and viral replication in SIV infection. *Science* 280:427–431.

4576. Veenstra, J., I. G. Williams, R. Colebunders, L. Dorrell, S. E. Tchamouroff, G. Patou, J. M. A. Lange, I. V. D. Weller, J. Goeman, S. Uthayakumar, I. R. Gow, J. N. Weber, and R. A. Coutinho. 1996. Immunization with recombinant p17/p24: Ty virus-like particles in human immunodeficiency virus-infected persons. *J. Infect. Dis.* 174:862–866.

4577. Vega, M. A., R. Guigdo, and T. F. Smith. 1990. Autoimmune response in AIDS. *Nature* 345:26.

4578. Velazquez-Campoy, A., M. J. Todd, S. Vega, and E. Freire. 2001. Catalytic efficiency and vitality of HIV-1 proteases from African viral subtypes. *Proc. Natl. Acad. Sci. USA* 98:6062–6067.

4579. Vella, S., M. Giuliano, M. Floridia, A. Chiesi, C. Tomino, A. Seeber, S. Barcherini, R. Bucciardini, and S. Mariotti. 1995. Effect of sex, age and transmission category on the progression to AIDS and survival of zidovudine-treated symptomatic patients. *AIDS* 9:51–56.

4580. Vella, S., and L. Palmisano. 2005. The global status of resistance to antiretroviral drugs. *Clin. Infect. Dis.* **41** (Suppl. 4):S239–S246.

4581. Venkataraman, N., A. L. Cole, P. Svoboda, J. Pohl, and A. M. Cole. 2005. Cationic polypeptides are required for anti-HIV-1 activity of human vaginal fluid. *J. Immunol.* 175:7560–7567.

4582. Vento, S., T. Garofano, C. Renzini, F. Casali, T. Ferraro, and E. Concia. 1997. Enhancement of hepatitis C virus replication and liver damage in HIV coinfected patients on antiretroviral combination therapy. *AIDS* 12:116–117.

4583. Verani, A., E. Pesenti, S. Polo, E. Tresoldi, G. Scarlatti, P. Lusso, A. G. Siccardi, and D. Vercelli. 1998. CXCR4 is a functional coreceptor for infection of human macrophages by CXCR4-dependent primary HIV-1 isolates. *J. Immunol.* 161:2084–2088.

4584. Verani, A., G. Scarlatti, M. Comar, E. Tresoldi, S. Polo, M. Giacca, P. Lusso, A. G. Siccardi, and D. Vercelli. 1997. C-C chemokines released by lipopolysaccharide (LPS)-stimulated human macrophages suppress HIV-1 infection in both macrophages and T cells. *J. Exp. Med.* 185:805–816.

4585. Verhofstede, C., S. Reniers, F. Van Wanzeele, and J. Plum. 1994. Evaluation of proviral copy number and plasma RNA level as early indicators of progression in HIV-1 infection: correlation with virological and immunological markers of disease. *AIDS* 8:1421–1427.

4586. Vernazza, P. L., J. R. Dyer, S. A. Fiscus, J. J. Eron, and M. S. Cohen. 1997. HIV-1 viral load in blood, semen and saliva. *AIDS* 11:1058–1059.

4587. Vernazza, P. L., J. J. Eron, M. S. Cohen, C. M. van der Horst, L. Troiani, and S. A. Fiscus. 1994. Detection and biologic characterization of infectious HIV-1 in semen of seropositive men. *AIDS* 8:1325–1329.

4588. Vernazza, P. L., J. J. Eron, and S. A. Fiscus. 1996. Sensitive method for the detection of infectious HIV in semen of seropositive individuals. *J. Virol. Methods* 56:33–40.

4589. Vernazza, P. L., J. J. Eron, S. A. Fiscus, and M. S. Cohen. 1999. Sexual transmission of HIV: infectiousness and prevention. *AIDS* 13:155–166.

4590. Vernazza, P. L., and J. J. Eron, Jr. 1997. Probability of heterosexual transmission of HIV. *J. Acquir. Immune Defic. Syndr. Hum. Retrovirol.* 14:85–86.

4591. Vernazza, P. L., L. Troiani, M. J. Flepp, R. W. Cone, J. Schock, F. Roth, K. Boggian, M. S. Cohen, S. A. Fiscus, J. J. Eron, and The Swiss HIV Cohort Study. 2000. Potent antiretroviral treatment of HIV-infection results in suppression of the seminal shedding of HIV. *AIDS* 14:117–121.

4592. Vernochet, C., S. Azoulay, D. Duval, G. Roger, G. Ailhaud, and C. Dani. 2003. Differential effect of HIV protease inhibitors on adipogenesis: intracellular Ritonavir is not sufficient to inhibit differentiation. *AIDS* 17:2177–2180.

4592a. VerPlank, L., F. Bouamr, T. J. LaGrassa, B. Agresta, A. Kikonyogo, J. Leis, and C. A. Carter. 2001. Tsg101, a homologue of ubiquitin-conjugating (E2) enzymes, binds the L domain in HIV type 1 Pr55(Gag). *Proc. Natl. Acad. Sci. USA* 98:7724–7729.

4593. Verthlyi, D., V. W. Wang, J. D. Lifson, and D. M. Klinman. 2004. CpG oligodeoxynucleotides improve the response to hepatitis B immunization in healthy and SIV-infected rhesus macaques. *AIDS* 18:1003–1008.

4594. Veugelers, P. J., J. M. Kaldor, S. A. Strathdee, K. A. Page-Shafer, M. T. Schechter, R. A. Coutinho, I. P. M. Keet, and G. J. P. van Griensven. 1997. Incidence and prognostic significance of symptomatic primary human immunodeficiency virus type 1 infection in homosexual men. *J. Infect. Dis.* 176:112–117.

4595. Veugelers, P. J., S. A. Strathdee, B. Tindall, K. A. Page, A. R. Moss, M. T. Schechter, J. S. G. Montaner, and G. J. P. van Griensven. 1994. Increasing age is associated with faster progression to neoplasms but not opportunistic infections in HIV-infected homosexual men. *AIDS* 8:1471–1475.

4596. Viard, J., M. Burgard, J. Hubert, L. Aaron, C. Rabian, N. Pertuiset, M. Lourenco, C. Rothschild, and C. Rouzioux. 2004. Impact of 5 years of maximally successful highly active antiretroviral therapy on CD4 cell count and HIV-1 DNA level. *AIDS* 18:45–49.

4597. Vicenzi, E., P. Bagnarelli, E. Santagostino, S. Ghezzi, M. Alfano, M. S. Sinnons, G. Fabio, L. Turchetto, G. Moretti, A. Lazzarin, A. Mantovani, P. M. Mannucci, M. Clementi, A. Gringeri, and G. Poli. 1997. Hemophilia and nonprogressing human immunodeficiency virus type 1 infection. *Blood* 89:191–200.

4598. Vicenzi, E., P. P. Bordignon, P. Biswas, A. Brambilla, C. Bovolenta, M. Cota, F. Sinigaglia, and G. Poli. 1999. Envelope-dependent restriction of human immunodeficiency virus type 1 spreading in CD4+ T lymphocytes: R5 but not X4 viruses replicate in the absence of T-cell receptor restimulation. *J. Virol.* 73:7515–7523.

4599. Vidal, F., J. Peraire, P. Domingo, M. Broch, H. Knobel, E. Pedrol, D. Dalmau, C. Vilades, M. A. Sambeat, C. Gutierrez, and C. Richart. 2005. Lack of association of SDF-1 3'A variant allele with long-term nonprogressive HIV-1 infection is extended beyond 16 years. *J. Acquir. Immune Defic. Syndr.* 40:276–279.

4600. Vidal, F., C. Vilades, P. Domingo, M. Broch, E. Pedrol, D. Dalmau, H. Knobel, J. Peraire, C. Gutierrez, M. A. Sambeat, A. Fontanet, E. Deig, M. Cairo, M. Montero, C. Richart, and S. Mallal. 2005. Spanish HIV-1-infected long-term nonprogressors of more than 15 years have an increased frequency of the CX3CR1 249I variant allele. *J. Acquir. Immune Defic. Syndr.* 40:527–531.

4601. Vidal, N., C. Mulanga-Kabeya, N. Nzilambi, E. Delaporte, and M. Peeters. 2000. Identification of a complex env subtype E HIV type 1 virus from the Democratic Republic of Congo, recombinant with A, G, H, J, K, and unknown subtypes. *AIDS Res. Hum. Retrovir.* 16:2059–2064.

4602. Vidal, N., M. Peeters, C. Mulanga-Kabeya, N. Nzilambi, D. Robertson, W. Ilunga, H. Sema, K. Tshimanga, B. Bongo, and E. Delaporte. 2000. Unprecedented degree of human immunodeficiency virus type 1 (HIV-1) group M genetic diversity in the Democratic Republic of Congo suggests that the HIV-1 pandemic originated in central Africa. *J. Virol.* 74:10498–10507.

4603. Vidmar, L., M. Poljak, J. Tomazic, K. Seme, and I. Klavs. 1996. Transmission of HIV-1 by human bite. *Lancet* 347:1762–1763.

4604. Vieillard, V., J. L. Strominger, and P. Debre. 2005. NK cytotoxicity against CD4+ T cells during HIV-1 infection: a gp41 peptide induces the expression of an NKp44 ligand. *Proc. Natl. Acad. Sci. USA* 102:10981–10986.

4605. Vieira, J., M. L. Huang, D. M. Koelle, and L. Corey. 1997. Transmissible Kaposi's sarcoma-associated herpesvirus (human herpesvirus 8) in saliva of men with a history of Kaposi's sarcoma. *J. Virol.* 71:7083–7087.

4606. Vigano, A., D. Trabattoni, L. Schneider, F. Ottaviani, A. Aliffi, E. Longhi, S. Rusconi, and M. Clerici. 2006. Failure to eradicate HIV despite fully successful HAART initiated in the first days of life. *J. Pediatr.* 148:389–391.

4607. **Vigano, A., S. Vella, M. Saresella, A. Vanzulli, D. Bricalli, S. Di Fabio, P. Ferrante, M. Andreotti, M. Pirillo, L. G. Dally, M. Clerici, and N. Principi.** 2000. Early immune reconstitution after potent antiretroviral therapy in HIV-infected children correlates with the increase in thymus volume. *AIDS* 14:251–261.

4608. **Vignoli, M., B. Stecca, G. Furlini, M. C. Re, V. Mantovani, G. Zauli, G. Visani, V. Colangeli, and M. La Placa.** 1998. Impaired telomerase activity in uninfected haematopoietic progenitors in HIV-1-infected patients. *AIDS* 12:999–1005.

4609. **Vignuzzi, M., J. K. Stone, J. J. Arnold, C. E. Cameron, and R. Andino.** 2006. Quasispecies diversity determines pathogenesis through cooperative interactions in a viral population. *Nature* 439:344–348.

4610. **Vigouroux, C., M. Maachi, N. T., C. Coussieu, S. Gharakhanian, T. Funahashi, Y. Matsuzawa, I. Shimomura, W. Rozenbaum, J. Capeau, and J. Bastard.** 2003. Serum adipocytokines are related to lipodystrophy and metabolic disorders in HIV-infected men under antiretroviral therapy. *AIDS* 17:1503–1511.

4611. **Villar-Arias, A., J. Pinilla-Moraza, P. Labarga-Echeverria, and F. Anton-Botella.** 1999. Changes in viral load during acute respiratory infections in HIV-infected patients. *AIDS* 13:1601–1602.

4612. **Villinger, F., G. T. Brice, A. E. Mayne, P. Bostik, K. Mori, C. H. June, and A. A. Ansari.** 2002. Adoptive transfer of simian immunodeficiency virus (SIV) naive autologous CD4+ cells to macaques chronically infected with SIV is sufficient to induce long-term nonprogressor status. *Blood* 99:590–599.

4613. **Viscidi, R. P., K. Mayur, H. M. Lederman, and A. D. Frankel.** 1989. Inhibition of antigen-induced lymphocyte proliferation by *tat* protein from HIV-1. *Science* 246:1606–1608.

4614. **Visconti, A., L. Visconti, R. Bellocco, N. Binkin, G. Colucci, L. Vernocchi, M. Amendola, and D. Ciaci.** 1993. HTLV-II/HIV-1 coinfection and risk for progression to AIDS among intravenous drug users. *J. Acquir. Immune Defic. Syndr.* 6:1228–1237.

4615. **Vittecoq, D., B. Mattlinger, F. Barre-Sinoussi, A. M. Courouce, C. Rouzioux, C. Doinel, M. Bary, J. P. Viard, J. F. Bach, P. Rouger, and J. J. Lefrere.** 1992. Passive immunotherapy in AIDS: a randomized trial of serial human immunodeficiency virus-positive transfusions of plasma rich in p24 antibodies versus transfusions of seronegative plasma. *J. Infect. Dis.* 165:364–368.

4616. **Vlahakis, S. R., A. Algeciras-Schimnich, G. Bou, C. J. Heppelmann, A. Villasis-Keever, R. G. Collman, and C. V. Paya.** 2001. Chemokine-receptor activation by *env* determines the mechanism of death in HIV-infected and uninfected T lymphocytes. *J. Clin. Investig.* 107:207–215.

4617. **Vogel, M., K. Cichutek, S. Norley, and R. Kurth.** 1993. Self-limiting infection by int/nef-double mutants of simian immunodeficiency virus. *Virology* 193:115–123.

4618. **Vogel, T. U., M. R. Reynolds, D. H. Fuller, K. Vielhuber, T. Shipley, J. T. Fuller, K. J. Kunstman, G. Sutter, M. L. Marthas, V. Erfle, S. M. Wolinsky, C. Wang, D. B. Allison, E. W. Rud, N. Wilson, D. Montefiori, J. D. Altman, and D. I. Watkins.** 2003. Multispecific vaccine-induced mucosal cytotoxic T lymphocytes reduce acute-phase viral replication but fail in long-term control of simian immunodeficiency virus SIVmac239. *J. Virol.* 77:13348–13360.

4619. **Vogt, M. W., D. J. Witt, D. E. Craven, R. Byington, D. F. Crawford, M. S. Hutchinson, R. T. Schooley, and M. S. Hirsch.** 1987. Isolation patterns of the human immunodeficiency virus from cervical secretions during the menstrual cycle of women at risk for the acquired immunodeficiency syndrome. *Ann. Intern. Med.* 106:380–382.

4620. **Vogt, M. W., D. J. Witt, D. E. Craven, R. Byington, D. F. Crawford, R. T. Schooley, and M. S. Hirsch.** 1986. Isolation of HTLV-III/LAV from cervical secretions of women at risk for AIDS. *Lancet* i:525–527.

4621. **Vogt, P. K., and R. Ishizaki.** 1966. Patterns of viral interference in the avian leukosis and sarcoma complex. *Virology* 30:368–374.

4622. **Volberding, P. A., S. W. Lagakos, M. A. Koch, C. Pettinelli, M. W. Myers, D. K. Booth, H. H. Balfour, R. C. Reichman, J. A. Bartlett, M. S. Hirsch, R. L. Murphy, W. D. Hardy, R. Soeiro, M. A. Fischl, J. G. Bartlett, T. C. Merigan, N. E. Hyslop, D. D. Richman, F. T. Valentine, and L. Corey.** 1990. Zidovudine in asymptomatic human immunodeficiency virus infection: a controlled trial in persons with fewer than 500 CD4-positive cells per cubic millimeter. *N. Engl. J. Med.* 322:941–949.

4623. **Volsky, D. J., M. Simm, M. Shahabuddin, G. Li, W. Chao, and M. J. Potash.** 1996. Interference to human immunodeficiency virus type 1 infection in the absence of downmodulation of the principal virus receptor, CD4. *J. Virol.* 70:3823–3833.

4624. **von Andrian, U. H., and C. R. Mackay.** 2000. T-cell function and migration. Two sides of the same coin. *N. Engl. J. Med.* 343:1020–1034.

4624a. **von Boehmer, H.** 2005. Mechanisms of suppression by suppressor T cells. *Nat. Immunol.* 6:338–344.

4625. **von Briesen, H., R. Andreesen, and H. Rubsamen-Waigmann.** 1990. Systematic classification of HIV biological subtypes on lymphocytes and monocytes/macrophages. *Virology* 178:597–602.

4626. **von Briesen, H., M. Grezl, H. Ruppach, I. Raudant, R. E. Unger, K. Becker, B. Panhans, U. Dietrich, and H. Rubsamen-Waigmann.** 1999. Selection of HIV-1 genotypes by cultivation in different primary cells. *AIDS* 13:307–315.

4627. **von Gegerfelt, A., J. Albert, L. Morfeldt-Manson, K. Broliden, and E. M. Fenyo.** 1991. Isolate-specific neutralizing antibodies in patients with progressive HIV-1-related disease. *Virology* 185:162–168.

4628. **von Gegerfelt, A., F. Chiodi, B. Keys, G. Norkrans, L. Hagberg, E.-M. Fenyo, and K. Broliden.** 1992. Lack of autologous neutralizing antibodies in the cerebrospinal fluid of HIV-1 infected individuals. *AIDS Res. Hum. Retrovir.* 8:1133–1138.

4629. **von Gegerfelt, A., C. Diaz-Pohl, E. M. Fenyo, and K. Broliden.** 1993. Specificity of antibody-dependent cellular cytotoxicity in sera from human immunodeficiency virus type 1-infected individuals. *AIDS Res. Hum. Retrovir.* 9:883–889.

4630. **von Laer, D., F. T. Hufert, T. E. Fenner, S. Schwander, M. Dietrich, H. Schmitz, and P. Kern.** 1990. CD34+ hematopoietic progenitor cells are not a major reservoir of the human immunodeficiency virus. *Blood* 76:1281–1286.

4631. **von Lindern, J. J., D. Rojo, K. Grovit-Ferbas, C. Yeramian, C. Deng, G. Herbein, M. R. Ferguson, T. C. Pappas, J. M. Decker, A. Singh, R. G. Collman, and W. A. O'Brien.** 2003. Potential role for CD63 in CCR5-mediated human immunodeficiency virus type 1 infection of macrophages. *J. Virol.* 77:3624–3633.

4632. von Schwedler, U., J. Song, C. Aiken, and D. Trono. 1993. Vif is crucial for human immunodeficiency virus type 1 proviral DNA synthesis in infected cells. *J. Virol.* **67:**4945–4955.

4633. von Schwedler, U. K., M. Stuchell, B. Muller, D. M. Ward, H. Y. Chung, E. Morita, H. E. Wang, T. Davis, G. P. He, D. M. Cimbora, A. Scott, H. G. Krausslich, J. Kaplan, S. G. Morham, and W. I. Sundquist. 2003. The protein network of HIV budding. *Cell* **114:**701–713.

4634. von Sydow, M., H. Gaines, A. Sonnerborg, M. Forsgren, P. O. Pehrson, and O. Strannegard. 1988. Antigen detection in primary HIV infection. *Br. Med. J.* **296:**238–240.

4635. von Sydow, M., A. Sonnerborg, H. Gaines, and O. Strannegard. 1991. Interferon-α and tumor necrosis factor-α in serum of patients in various stages of HIV-1 infection. *AIDS Res. Hum. Retrovir.* **7:**375–380.

4636. Voss, T. G., C. D. Fermin, J. A. Levy, S. Vigh, B. Choi, and R. F. Garry. 1996. Alteration of intracellular potassium and sodium concentrations correlates with induction of cytopathic effects by human immunodeficiency virus. *J. Virol.* **70:**5447–5454.

4637. Voulgaropoulou, F., S. E. Pontow, and L. Ratner. 2000. Productive infection of CD34+-cell-derived megakaryocytes by X4 and R5 HIV-1 isolates. *Virology* **269:**78–85.

4638. Reference deleted.

4639. Voulgaropoulou, F., B. Tan, M. Soares, B. Hahn, and L. Ratner. 1999. Distinct human immunodeficiency virus strains in the bone marrow are associated with the development of thrombocytopenia. *J. Virol.* **73:**3497–3504.

4640. Vyakarnam, A., J. Eyeson, I. Teo, M. Zuckerman, K. Babaahmady, H. Schuitemaker, S. Shaunak, T. Rostron, S. Rowland-Jones, G. Simmons, and P. Clapham. 2001. Evidence for a post-entry barrier to R5 HIV-1 infection of CD4 memory T cells. *AIDS* **15:**1613–1626.

4641. Vyakarnam, A., P. M. Matear, S. J. Martin, and M. Wagstaff. 1995. Th1 cells specific for HIV-1 gag p24 are less efficient than Th0 cells in supporting HIV replication, and inhibit virus replication in Th0 cells. *Immunology* **86:**85–96.

4641a. Wada, M., N. A. Wada, H. Shirono, K. Taniguchi, H. Tsuchie, and J. Koga. 2001. Amino-terminal fragment of urokinase-type plasminogen activator inhibits HIV-1 replication. *Biochem. Biophys. Res. Commun.* **284:**346–351.

4642. Wagner, L., O. O. Yang, E. A. Garcia-Zepeda, Y. Ge, S. A. Kalams, B. D. Walker, M. S. Pasternack, and A. D. Luster. 1998. β-chemokines are released from HIV-1-specific cytolytic T-cell granules complexed to proteoglycans. *Nature* **391:**908–911.

4643. Wagner, R., H. Fliessbach, G. Wanner, M. Motz, M. Niedrig, G. Deby, A. von Brunn, and H. Wolf. 1992. Studies on processing, particle formation, and immunogenicity of the HIV-1 gag gene product: a possible component of a HIV vaccine. *Arch. Virol.* **127:**117–137.

4644. Wagner, R., B. Leschonsky, E. Harrer, C. Paulus, C. Weber, B. D. Walker, S. Buchbinder, H. Wolf, J. R. Kalden, and T. Harrer. 1999. Molecular and functional analysis of a conserved CTL epitope in HIV-1 p24 recognized from a long-term nonprogressor: constraints on immune escape associated with targeting a sequence essential for viral replication. *J. Immunol.* **162:**3727–3734.

4645. Wahl, L. M., M. L. Corcoran, S. W. Pyle, L. O. Arthur, A. Harel-Bellan, and W. L. Farrar. 1989. Human immunodeficiency virus glycoprotein (gp120) induction of monocyte arachidonic acid metabolites and interleukin 1. *Proc. Natl. Acad. Sci. USA* **86:**621–625.

4646. Wahl, S. M., J. B. Allen, S. Gartner, J. M. Ornstein, M. Popovic, D. E. Chenoweth, L. O. Arthur, W. L. Farrar, and L. M. Wahl. 1989. HIV-1 and its envelope glycoprotein down-regulate chemotactic ligand receptors and chemotactic function of peripheral blood monocytes. *J. Immunol.* **142:**3553–3559.

4647. Wahl, S. M., J. B. Allen, N. McCartney-Francis, M. C. Morganti-Kossmann, T. Kossmann, L. Ellingsworth, U. E. H. Mai, S. E. Mergenhagen, and J. M. Orenstein. 1991. Macrophage- and astrocyte-derived transforming growth factor beta as a mediator of central nervous system dysfunction in acquired immune deficiency syndrome. *J. Exp. Med.* **173:**981–991.

4648. Wahl, S. M., T. Greenwell-Wild, G. Peng, P. Hale-Donze, T. M. Doherty, D. Mizel, and J. M. Orenstein. 1998. Mycobacterium avium complex augments macrophage HIV-1 production and increases CCR5 expression. *Proc. Natl. Acad. Sci. USA* **95:**12574–12579.

4649. Wahman, A., S. L. Melnick, F. S. Rhame, and J. D. Potter. 1991. The epidemiology of classic, African and immunosuppressed Kaposi's sarcoma. *Epidemiol. Rev.* **13:**178–199.

4650. Wahren, B., L. Morfeldt-Mansson, G. Biberfeld, L. Moberg, A. Sonnerborg, P. Ljungman, A. Werner, R. Kurth, R. Gallo, and D. Bolognesi. 1987. Characteristics of the specific cell-mediated immune response in human immunodeficiency virus infection. *J. Virol.* **61:**2017–2023.

4651. Wain-Hobson, S., P. Sonigo, O. Danos, S. Cole, and M. Alizon. 1985. Nucleotide sequence of the AIDS, LAV. *Cell* **40:**9–17.

4652. Wain-Hobson, S., J.-P. Vartanian, M. Henry, N. Chenciner, R. Cheynier, S. Delassus, L. P. Martins, M. Sala, M.-T. Nugeyre, D. Guitard, D. Kaltzmann, J.-C. Gluckman, W. Rozenbaum, F. Barre-Sinoussi, and L. Montagnier. 1991. LAV revisited: origins of the early HIV-1 isolates from Institut Pasteur. *Science* **252:**961–965.

4653. Wainberg, M., R. Beaulieu, C. Tsoukas, and R. Thomas. 1993. Detection of zidovudine-resistant variants of HIV-1 in genital fluids. *AIDS* **7:**433–444.

4654. Wainberg, M. A., W. C. Drosopoulos, H. Salomon, M. Hsu, G. Borkow, M. A. Parniak, Z. Gu, Q. Song, J. Manne, S. Islam, G. Castriota, and V. R. Prasad. 1996. Enhanced fidelity of 3TC-selected mutant HIV-1 reverse transcriptase. *Science* **271:**1282–1285.

4655. Wakrim, L., R. Le Grand, B. Vaslin, A. Cheret, F. Matheux, F. Theodoro, P. Roques, I. Nicol-Jourdain, and D. Dormont. 1996. Superinfection of HIV-2-preinfected macaques after rectal exposure to a primary isolate of SIV-mac251. *Virology* **221:**260–270.

4656. Waldmann, T. A., and Y. Tagaya. 1999. The multifaceted regulation of interleukin-15 expression and the role of this cytokine in NK cell differentiation and host response to intracellular pathogens. *Annu. Rev. Immunol.* **17:**19–49.

4656a. Walker, B. D., C. Flexner, T. J. Paradis, T. C. Fuller, M. S. Hirsch, R. T. Schooley, and B. Moss. 1988. HIV-1 reverse transcriptase is a target for cytotoxic T lymphocytes in infected individuals. *Science* **240:**64–66.

4657. Walker, B. D., and F. Plata. 1990. Cytotoxic T lymphocytes against HIV. *AIDS* **4:**177–184.

4658. Walker, C. M., A. L. Erikson, F. C. Hsueh, and J. A. Levy. 1991. Inhibition of human immunodeficiency virus replication in acutely infected CD4⁺ cells by CD8⁺ cells involves a noncytotoxic mechanism. *J. Virol.* **65**:5921–5927.

4659. Walker, C. M., and J. A. Levy. 1989. A diffusible lymphokine produced by CD8+ T lymphocytes suppresses HIV replication. *Immunology* **66**:628–630.

4660. Walker, C. M., D. J. Moody, D. P. Stites, and J. A. Levy. 1986. CD8+ lymphocytes can control HIV infection *in vitro* by suppressing virus replication. *Science* **234**:1563–1566.

4661. Walker, C. M., D. J. Moody, D. P. Stites, and J. A. Levy. 1989. CD8+ T lymphocyte control of HIV replication in cultured CD4+ cells varies among infected individuals. *Cell. Immunol.* **119**:470–475.

4662. Walker, C. M., G. A. Thomson-Honnebier, F. C. Hsueh, A. L. Erickson, L.-Z. Pan, and J. A. Levy. 1991. CD8+ T cells from HIV-1-infected individuals inhibit acute infection by human and primate immunodeficiency viruses. *Cell. Immunol.* **137**:420–428.

4663. Walker, L., D. Wilks, J. O'Brien, J. Habeshaw, and A. Dalgleish. 1992. Localized conformational changes in the N-terminal domain of CD4 identified in competitive binding assay of monoclonal antibodies and HIV-1 envelope glycoprotein. *AIDS Res. Hum. Retrovir.* **8**:1083–1090.

4663a. Walker, M. R., D. J. Kasprowicz, V. H. Gersuk, A. Benard, M. Van Landeghen, J. H. Buckner, and S. F. Ziegler. 2003. Induction of FoxP3 and acquisition of T regulatory activity by stimulated human CD4+CD25− T cells. *J. Clin. Investig.* **112**:1437–1443.

4664. Walker, R. E., C. S. Carter, L. Muul, V. Natarajan, B. R. Herpin, S. F. Leitman, H. G. Klein, C. A. Mullen, J. A. Metcalf, M. Baseler, J. Falloon, R. T. Davey, J. A. Kovacs, M. A. Polis, H. Masur, R. M. Blaese, and H. C. Lane. 1998. Peripheral expansion of pre-existing mature T cells is an important means of CD4(+) T-cell regeneration in HIV-infected adults. *Nat. Med.* **4**:852–856.

4665. Wallace, M., A. M. Scharko, C. D. Pauza, P. Fisch, K. Imaoka, S. Kawabata, K. Fujihashi, K. Kiyono, Y. Tanaka, B. R. Bloom, and M. Malkovsky. 1997. Functional gamma delta T-lymphocyte defect associated with human immunodeficiency virus infections. *Mol. Med.* **3**:60–71.

4666. Wallis, R. S., M. Vjecha, M. Amir-Tahmasseb, A. Okwera, F. Byekwaso, S. Nyole, S. Kabengera, R. D. Mugerwa, and J. J. Ellner. 1993. Influence of tuberculosis on human immunodeficiency virus (HIV-1): enhanced cytokine expression and elevated β2-microglobulin in HIV-1-associated tuberculosis. *J. Infect. Dis.* **167**:43–48.

4667. Walter, B. L., K. Wehrly, R. Swanstrom, E. Platt, D. Kabat, and B. Chesebro. 2005. Role of low CD4 levels in the influence of human immunodeficiency virus type 1 envelope V1 and V2 regions on entry and spread in macrophages. *J. Virol.* **79**:4828–4837.

4668. Wang, B., J. Boyer, V. Srikantan, K. Ugen, L. Gilbert, C. Phan, K. Dang, M. Merva, M. G. Agadjanyan, M. Newman, R. Carrano, D. McCallus, L. Coney, W. V. Williams, and D. B. Weiner. 1995. Induction of humoral and cellular immune responses to the human immunodeficiency type 1 virus in nonhuman primates by in vivo DNA inoculation. *Virology* **211**:102–112.

4669. Wang, C. C., R. S. McClelland, J. Overbaugh, M. Reilly, D. D. Panteleeff, K. Mandaliya, B. Chohan, L. Lavreys, J. Ndinya-Achola, and J. K. Kreiss. 2004. The effect of hormonal contraception on genital tract shedding of HIV-1. *AIDS* **18**:205–209.

4670. Wang, H., N. J. English, C. D. Reid, J. E. Merson, and S. C. Knight. 1999. Role of beta-chemokines in HIV-1 infection of dendritic cells maturing from CD34+ stem cells. *J. Acquir. Immune Defic. Syndr.* **21**:179–188.

4671. Wang, H. W., M. W. Trotter, D. Lagos, D. Bourboulia, S. Henderson, T. Makinen, S. Elliman, A. M. Flanagan, K. Alitalo, and C. Boshoff. 2004. Kaposi sarcoma herpesvirus-induced cellular reprogramming contributes to the lymphatic endothelial gene expression in Kaposi sarcoma. *Nat. Genet.* **36**:687–693.

4672. Wang, J., G. Roderiquez, T. Oravecz, and M. Norcross. 1998. Cytokine regulation of human immunodeficiency virus type 1 entry and replication in human monocytes/macrophages through modulation of CCR5 expression. *J. Virol.* **72**:7642–7647.

4673. Wang, J., Y. Yan, T. P. J. Garrett, J. Liu, D. W. Rodgers, R. L. Garlick, G. E. Tarr, Y. Husain, E. L. Reinherz, and S. C. Harrison. 1990. Atomic structure of a fragment of human CD4 containing two immunoglobulin-like domains. *Nature* **348**:411–418.

4674. Wang, R., S. I. Abrams, D. Y. Loh, C. S. Shieh, K. M. Murphy, and J. H. Russell. 1993. Separation of CD4+ functional responses by peptide dose in Th1 and Th2 subsets expressing the same transgenic antigen receptor. *Cell. Immunol.* **148**:357–370.

4674a. Wang, S., R. Pal, J. R. Mascola, T. H. Chou, I. Mboudjeka, S. Shen, Q. Liu, S. Whitney, T. Keen, B. C. Nair, V. S. Kalyanaraman, P. Markham, and S. Lu. 2006. Polyvalent HIV-1 Env vaccine formulations delivered by the DNA priming plus protein boosting approach are effective in generating neutralizing antibodies against primary human immunodeficiency virus type 1 isolates from subtypes A, B, C, D and E. *Virology* **350**:34–47.

4675. Wang, S. Z. S., K. E. Rushlow, C. J. Issel, R. F. Cook, S. J. Cook, M. L. Raabe, Y. H. Chong, L. Costa, and R. C. Montelaro. 1994. Enhancement of EIAV replication and disease by immunization with a baculovirus-expressed recombinant envelope surface glycoprotein. *Virology* **199**:247–251.

4676. Wang, W., S. M. Owen, D. L. Rudolph, A. M. Cole, T. Hong, A. J. Waring, R. B. Lal, and R. I. Lehrer. 2004. Activity of alpha- and theta-defensins against primary isolates of HIV-1. *J. Immunol.* **173**:515–520.

4677. Wang, Y., K. Abel, K. Lantz, A. M. Krieg, M. B. McChesney, and C. J. Miller. 2005. The Toll-like receptor 7 (TLR7) agonist, Imiquod, and the TLR9 agonst, CpG ODN, induce antiviral cytokines and chemokines but do not prevent vaginal transmission of simian immunodeficiency virus when applied intravaginally to rhesus macaques. *J. Virol.* **79**:14355–14370.

4678. Wang, Y., S. S. Kim, D. Lu, X. J. You, S. Joye, H. Fan, and C. J. Miller. 2004. Use of a replication-defective vector to track cells initially infected by SIV *in vivo*: infected mononuclear cells rapidly appear in the draining lymph node after intradermal inoculation of rhesus monkeys. *AIDS Res. Hum. Retrovir.* **20**:1298–1305.

4679. Wang, Y., L. Tao, E. Mitchell, C. Bravery, P. Berlingieri, P. Armstrong, R. Vaughan, J. Underwood, and T. Lehner. 1999. Allo-immunization elicits CD8+ T cell-derived chemokines, HIV suppressor factors and resistance to HIV infection in women. *Nat. Med.* **5**:1004–1009.

4680. Wang, Z., M. A. Golberg, and D. T. Scadden. 1993. HIV-1 suppresses erythropoietin production in vitro. *Exp. Hematol.* **21**:683–688.

4681. Wanke, C. A. 1999. Epidemiological and clinical aspects of the metabolic complications of HIV infection. The fat redistribution syndrome. *AIDS* **13**:1287–1293.

4682. Ward, J. P., M. I. Bonaparte, and E. Barker. 2004. HLA-C and HLA-E reduce antibody-dependent natural killer cell-mediated cytotoxicity of HIV-infected primary T cell blasts. *AIDS* 18:1769–1779.

4683. Ward, J. W., T. J. Bush, H. A. Perkins, L. E. Lieb, J. R. Allen, D. Goldfinger, S. M. Samson, S. H. Pepkowitz, L. P. Fernando, P. V. Holland, S. H. Kleinman, A. J. Grindon, J. L. Garner, G. W. Rutherford, and S. D. Holmberg. 1989. The natural history of transfusion-associated infection with human immunodeficiency virus: factors influencing the rate of progression to disease. *N. Engl. J. Med.* 321:947–952.

4684. Ward, J. W., S. D. Holmberg, J. R. Allen, D. L. Cohn, S. E. Critchley, S. H. Kleinman, B. A. Lenes, O. Ravenholt, J. R. Davis, M. G. Quinn, and H. W. Jaffe. 1988. Transmission of human immunodeficiency virus (HIV) by blood transfusions screened as negative for HIV antibody. *N. Engl. J. Med.* 318:473–478.

4685. Warren, M. K., W. L. Rose, J. L. Cone, W. G. Rice, and J. A. Turpin. 1997. Differential infection of CD34+ cell-derived dendritic cells and monocytes with lymphocyte-tropic and monocyte-tropic HIV-1 strains. *J. Immunol.* 158:5035–5042.

4686. Warren, R. Q., S. A. Anderson, W. M. Nkya, J. F. Shao, C. W. Hendrix, G. P. Melcher, R. R. Redfield, and R. C. Kennedy. 1992. Examination of sera from human immunodeficiency virus type 1 (HIV-1)-infected individuals for antibodies reactive with peptides corresponding to the principal neutralizing determinant of HIV-1 gp120 and for in vitro neutralizing activity. *J. Virol.* 66:5210–5215.

4687. Wasik, T. J., P. P. Jagodzinski, E. M. Hyjek, J. Wustner, G. Trinchieri, H. W. Lischner, and D. Kozbor. 1997. Diminished HIV-specific CTL activity is associated with lower type 1 and enhanced type 2 responses to HIV-specific peptides during perinatal HIV infection. *J. Immunol.* 158:6029–6036.

4688. Watkins, B. A., H. H. Dorn, W. B. Kelly, R. C. Armstrong, B. J. Potts, F. Michaels, C. V. Kufta, and M. Dubois-Dalcq. 1990. Specific tropism of HIV-1 for microglial cells in primary human brain cultures. *Science* 249:549–553.

4689. Watkins, B. A., M. S. Reitz, Jr., C. A. Wilson, K. Aldrich, A. E. Davis, and M. Robert-Guroff. 1993. Immune escape by human immunodeficiency virus type 1 from neutralizing antibodies: evidence for multiple pathways. *J. Virol.* 67:7493–7500.

4690. Watret, K. C., J. A. Whitelaw, K. S. Froebel, and A. G. Bird. 1993. Phenotypic characterization of CD8+ T cell populations in HIV disease and in anti-HIV immunity. *Clin. Exp. Immunol.* 92:93–99.

4691. Watson, A., J. McClure, J. Ranchalis, M. Scheibel, A. Schmidt, B. Kennedy, W. R. Morton, N. L. Haigwood, and S. L. Hu. 1997. Early post-infection antiviral treatment reduces viral load and prevents CD4+ cell decline in HIV-2 infected macaques. *AIDS Res. Hum. Retrovir.* 13:1375–1381.

4692. Watt, G., P. Kantipong, M. de Souza, P. Chanbancherd, K. Jongsakul, R. Ruangweerayud, L. D. Loomis-Price, V. Polonis, K. S. Myint, D. L. Birx, A. E. Brown, and S. Krishna. 2000. HIV-1 suppression during acute scrub-typhus infection. *Lancet* 356:475–479.

4693. Wawer, M. J., R. H. Gray, N. K. Sewankambo, D. Serwadda, X. Li, O. Laeyendecker, N. Kiwanuka, G. Kigozi, M. Kiddugavu, T. Lutalo, F. Nalugoda, F. Wabwire-Mangen, M. P. Meehan, and T. C. Quinn. 2005. Rates of HIV-1 transmission per coital act, by stage of HIV-1 infection, in Rakai, Uganda. *J. Infect. Dis.* 191:1403–1409.

4694. Weber, J., P. Clapham, J. McKeating, M. Stratton, E. Robey, and R. Weiss. 1989. Infection of brain cells by diverse human immunodeficiency virus isolates: role of CD4 as receptor. *J. Gen. Virol.* 70:2653–2660.

4695. Weber, J., E. M. Fenyo, S. Beddows, P. Kaleebu, and A. Bjorndal. 1996. Neutralization serotypes of human immunodeficiency virus type 1 field isolates are not predicted by genetic subtype. *J. Virol.* 70:7827–7832.

4696. Weber, K., D. Meyer, V. Grosse, M. Stoll, R. E. Schmidt, and H. Heiken. 2000. Reconstitution of NK cell activity in HIV-1 infected individuals receiving antiretroviral therapy. *Immunobiology* 202:172–178.

4697. Webster, A., C. A. Lee, D. G. Cook, J. E. Grundy, V. C. Emery, P. B. A. Kernoff, and P. D. Griffiths. 1989. Cytomegalovirus infection and progression towards AIDS in haemophiliacs with human immunodeficiency virus infection. *Lancet* ii:63–66.

4698. Weeratna, R. D., S. R. Makinen, M. J. McCluskie, and H. L. Davis. 2005. TLR agonists as vaccine adjuvants: comparison of CpG ODN and Resiquimod (R-848). *Vaccine* 23:5263–5270.

4698a. Wei, S., I. Kryczek, L. Zou, B. Daniel, P. Cheng, P. Mottram, T. Curiel, A. Lange, and W. Zou. 2005. Plasmacytoid dendritic cells induce CD8+ regulatory T cells in human ovarian carcinoma. *Cancer Res.* 65:5020–5026.

4699. Wei, X., J. M. Decker, S. Wang, H. Hui, J. C. Kappes, X. Wu, J. F. Salazar-Gonzalez, M. G. Salazar, J. M. Kilby, M. S. Saag, N. L. Komarova, M. A. Nowak, B. H. Hahn, P. D. Kwong, and G. M. Shaw. 2003. Antibody neutralization and escape by HIV-1. *Nature* 422:307–312.

4700. Wei, X., S. K. Ghosh, M. E. Taylor, V. A. Johnson, E. A. Emini, P. Deutsch, J. D. Lifson, S. Bonhoeffer, M. A. Nowak, B. H. Hahn, M. S. Saag, and G. M. Shaw. 1995. Viral dynamics in human immunodeficiency virus type 1 infection. *Nature* 373:117–122.

4701. Wei, X., C. Liang, M. Gotte, and M. A. Wainberg. 2002. The M184V mutation in HIV-1 reverse transcriptase reduces the restoration of wild-type replication by attenuated viruses. *AIDS* 16:2391–2398.

4702. Weiblen, B. J., F. K. Lee, E. R. Cooper, S. H. Landesman, K. McIntosh, J. A. Harris, S. Nieshman, H. Mendez, S. I. Pelton, and A. J. Nahmias. 1990. Early diagnosis of HIV infection in infants by detection of IgA HIV antibodies. *Lancet* 335:988–990.

4703. Weiden, M., N. Tanaka, Y. Qiao, B. Y. Zhao, Y. Honda, K. Nakata, A. Canova, D. E. Levy, W. M. Rom, and R. Pine. 2000. Differentiation of monocytes to macrophages switches the *Mycobacterium tuberculosis* effect on HIV-1 replication from stimulation to inhibition: modulation of interferon response and CCAAT/enhancer binding protein beta expresson. *J. Immunol.* 165:2028–2039.

4704. Weidle, P. J., T. D. Mastro, A. D. Grant, J. Nkengasong, and D. Macharia. 2002. HIV/AIDS treatment and HIV vaccines for Africa. *Lancet* 359:2261–2267.

4705. Weimer, R., V. Daniel, R. Zimmermann, K. Schimpf, and G. Opelz. 1991. Autoantibodies against CD4 cells are associated with CD4 helper defects in human immunodeficiency virus-infected patients. *Blood* 77:133–140.

4706. Weinberg, J. B., T. J. Matthews, B. R. Cullen, and M. H. Malim. 1991. Productive human immunodeficiency virus type 1 (HIV-1) infection of nonproliferating human monocytes. *J. Exp. Med.* 174:1477–1482.

4707. Weinhold, K. J., H. K. Lyerly, T. J. Matthews, D. S. Tyler, P. M. Ahearne, K. C. Stine, A. J. Langlois, D. T. Durack, and

D. P. Bolognesi. 1988. Cellular anti-gp120 cytolytic reactivities in HIV-1 seropositive individuals. *Lancet* i:902–905.

4708. Weinhold, K. J., H. K. Lyerly, S. D. Stanley, A. A. Austin, T. J. Matthews, and D. P. Bolognesi. 1989. HIV-1 gp120-mediated immune suppression and lymphocyte destruction in the absence of viral infection. *J. Immunol.* 142:3091–3097.

4709. Weiss, C. D., S. W. Barnett, N. Cacalano, N. Killeen, D. R. Littman, and J. M. White. 1996. Studies of HIV-1 envelope glycoprotein-mediated fusion using a simple fluorescence assay. *AIDS* 10:241–246.

4710. Weiss, C. D., J. A. Levy, and J. M. White. 1990. Oligomeric organization of gp120 on infectious human immunodeficiency virus type 1 particles. *J. Virol.* 64:5674–5677.

4711. Weiss, L., V. Donkova-Petrini, L. Caccavelli, M. Balbo, C. Carbonneil, and Y. Levy. 2004. Human immunodeficiency virus-driven expansion of CD4+CD25+ regulatory T cells, which suppress HIV-specific CD4 T-cell responses in HIV-infected patients. *Blood* 104:3249–3256.

4712. Weiss, L., N. Okada, N. Haeffner-Cavaillon, T. Hattori, C. Faucher, M. D. Kazatchkine, and H. Okada. 1992. Decreased expression of the membrane inhibitor of complement-mediated cytolysis CD59 on T-lymphocytes of HIV-infected patients. *AIDS* 6:379–385.

4713. Weiss, L., A. Si-Mohamed, P. Giral, P. Castiel, A. Ledur, C. Blondin, M. D. Kazatchkine, and N. Haeffner-Cavaillon. 1997. Plasma levels of monocyte chemoattractant protein-1 but not those of macrophage inhibitory protein-1α and RANTES correlate with virus load in human immunodeficiency virus infection. *J. Infect. Dis.* 176:1621–1624.

4714. Weiss, R. A. 1988. Receptor molecule blocks HIV. *Nature* 331:15.

4715. Weiss, R. A., P. R. Clapham, J. N. Weber, A. G. Dalgleish, L. A. Lasky, and P. W. Berman. 1986. Variable and conserved neutralization antigens of human immunodeficiency virus. *Nature* 324:572–575.

4716. Weiss, R. A., P. R. Clapham, J. N. Weber, D. Whitby, R. S. Tedder, T. O'Connor, S. Chamaret, and L. Montagnier. 1988. HIV-2 antisera cross-neutralize HIV-1. *AIDS* 2:95–100.

4717. Weiss, S. H., J. Lombardo, J. Michaels, L. R. Sharer, M. Rayyarah, J. Leonard, A. Mangia, P. Kloser, S. Sathe, R. Kapila, N. M. Williams, R. Altman, J. French, and W. E. Parkin. 1988. AIDS due to HIV-2 infection—New Jersey. *Morb. Mortal. Wkly. Rep.* 259:969–972.

4718. Weissenhorn, W., A. Dessen, S. C. Harrison, J. J. Skehel, and D. C. Wiley. 1997. Atomic structure of the ectodomain from HIV-1 gp41. *Nature* 387:426–430.

4719. Weissman, D., Y. Li, J. Ananworanich, L. J. Zhou, J. Adelsberger, T. F. Tedder, M. Baseler, and A. S. Fauci. 1995. Three populations of cells with dendritic morphology exist in peripheral blood only, one of which is infectable with human immunodeficiency virus type 1. *Proc. Natl. Acad. Sci. USA* 92:826–830.

4720. Weissman, D., Y. Li, J. M. Orenstein, and A. S. Fauci. 1995. Both a precursor and a mature population of dendritic cells can bind HIV. *J. Immunol.* 155:4111–4117.

4721. Weissman, D., G. Poli, and A. S. Fauci. 1994. Interleukin 10 blocks HIV replication in macrophages by inhibiting the autocrine loop of tumor necrosis factor α and interleukin 6 induction of virus. *AIDS Res. Hum. Retrovir.* 10:1199–1206.

4722. Weissman, D., G. Poli, and A. S. Fauci. 1995. IL-10 synergizes with multiple cytokines in enhancing HIV production in cells of monocytic lineage. *J. Acquir. Immune Defic. Syndr. Hum. Retrovirol.* 9:442–449.

4723. Weissman, D., R. L. Rabin, J. Arthos, A. Rubbert, M. Dybul, R. Swofford, S. Venkatesan, J. M. Farber, and A. S. Fauci. 1997. Macrophage-tropic HIV and SIV envelope proteins induce a signal through the CCR5 chemokine receptor. *Nature* 389:981–985.

4724. Wekerle, H., C. Unington, H. Lassmann, and R. Meyermann. 1986. Cellular immune reactivity within the CNS. *Trends Neurosci.* 9:271–277.

4725. Welker, R., H. Kottler, H. R. Kalbitzer, and H.-G. Krausslich. 1996. Human immunodeficiency virus type 1 Nef protein is incorporated into virus particles and specifically cleaved by the viral proteinase. *Virology* 219:228–236.

4725a. Welzel, T. M., X. Gao, R. M. Pfeiffer, M. P. Martin, J. O'Brien S, J. J. Goedert, M. Carrington, and R. O'Brien T. 2007. HLA-B Bw4 alleles and HIV-1 transmission in heterosexual couples. *AIDS* 21:225–229.

4726. Weniger, B. G., Y. Takebe, C.-Y. Ou, and S. Yamazaki. 1994. The molecular epidemiology of HIV in Asia. *AIDS* 8:S13-S28.

4727. Wenner, C. A., M. L. Guler, S. E. Macatonia, A. O'Garra, and K. M. Murphy. 1996. Roles of IFN-γ and IFN-α in IL-12 induced T helper cell-1 development. *J. Immunol.* 1156:1442–1447.

4728. Werner, A., and J. A. Levy. 1993. Human immunodeficiency virus type 1 envelope gp120 is cleaved after incubation with recombinant soluble CD4. *J. Virol.* 67:2566–2574.

4729. Werner, A., G. Winskowsky, and R. Kurth. 1990. Soluble CD4 enhances simian immunodeficiency virus SIV_{agm} infection. *J. Virol.* 64:6252–6256.

4730. Werner, E. R., D. Fuchs, A. Hausen, H. Jaeger, G. Reibnegger, G. Werner-Felmayer, M. P. Dierich, and H. Wachter. 1988. Tryptophan degradation in patients infected by human immunodeficiency virus. *Biol. Chem. Hoppe. Seyler* 369:337–340.

4731. Werner, T., S. Ferroni, T. Saermark, R. Brack-Werner, R. B. Banati, R. Mager, L. Steinaa, G. W. Kreutzberg, and V. Erfle. 1991. HIV-1 *nef* protein exhibits structural and functional similarity to scorpion peptides interacting with K+ channels. *AIDS* 5:1301–1308.

4732. Werness, B. A., A. J. Levine, and P. M. Howley. 1990. Association of human papillomavirus types 16 and 18 E6 proteins with p53. *Science* 248:76–79.

4733. Wesselborg, S., O. Janssen, and D. Kabelitz. 1993. Induction of activation-driven death (apoptosis) in activated but not resting peripheral blood T cells. *J. Immunol.* 150:4338–4345.

4734. Wesselingh, S. L., C. Power, J. D. Glass, W. R. Tyor, J. C. McArthur, J. M. Farber, J. W. Griffin, and D. E. Griffin. 1993. Intracerebral cytokine messenger RNA expression in acquired immunodeficiency syndrome dementia. *Ann. Neurol.* 33:576–582.

4735. Westby, M., F. Manca, and A. G. Dalgleish. 1996. The role of host immune responses in determining the outcome of HIV infection. *Immunol. Today* 17:120–126.

4736. Westendorp, M. O., R. Frank, C. Ochsenbauer, K. Stricker, J. Dhein, H. Walczak, K. M. Debatin, and P. H. Krammer. 1995. Sensitization of T cells to CD95-mediated apoptosis by HIV-1 Tat and gp120. *Nature* 375:497–500.

4737. Westermann, J., and R. Pabst. 1990. Lymphocyte subsets in the blood: a diagnostic window on the lymphoid system? *Immunol. Today* 11:406–410.

4738. Westervelt, P., T. Henkel, D. B. Trowbridge, J. Orenstein, J. Heuser, H. E. Gendelman, and L. Ratner. 1992. Dual regulation of silent and productive infection in monocytes by distinct human immunodeficiency virus type 1 determinants. *J. Virol.* 66:3925–3931.

4739. Westmoreland, S. V., D. Kolson, and F. Gonzalez-Scarano. 1996. Toxicity of TNF-α and platelet activating factor for human NT2N neurons: a tissue culture model for human immunodeficiency virus dementia. *J. Neurovirol.* 2:118–126.

4740. Wetzel, M. A., A. D. Steele, E. E. Henderson, and T. J. Rogers. 2002. The effect of X4 and R5 HIV-1 on C, C-C, and C-X-C chemokines during the early stages of infection in human PBMCs. *Virology* 292:6–15.

4741. Wherry, E. J., V. Teichgraber, T. C. Becker, D. Masopust, S. M. Kaech, R. Antia, U. H. von Andrian, and R. Ahmed. 2003. Lineage relationship and protective immunity of memory CD8 T cell subsets. *Nat. Immunol.* 4:225–234.

4742. Whitby, D., M. R. Howard, M. Tenant-Flowers, N. S. Brink, A. Copas, C. Boshoff, T. Hatzioannou, F. E. A. Suggett, D. M. Aldam, A. S. Denton, R. F. Miller, I. V. D. Weller, R. A. Weiss, R. S. Tedder, and T. F. Schulz. 1995. Detection of Kaposi's sarcoma associated herpesvirus (KSHV) in peripheral blood of HIV-infected individuals predicts progression to Kaposi's sarcoma. *Lancet* 346:799–802.

4743. Whitby, D., A. Stossel, C. Gamache, J. Papin, M. Bosch, A. Smith, D. H. Kedes, G. White, R. Kennedy, and D. P. Dittmer. 2003. Novel Kaposi's sarcoma-associated herpesvirus homolog in baboons. *J. Virol.* 77:8159–8165.

4744. Whitcomb, J. M., W. Huang, K. Limoli, E. Paxinos, T. Wrin, G. Skowron, S. G. Deeks, M. Bates, N. S. Hellmann, and C. J. Petropoulos. 2002. Hypersusceptibility to non-nucleoside reverse transcriptase inhibitors in HIV-1: clinical, phenotypic and genotypic correlates. *AIDS* 16:F41–F47.

4745. White, J. M. 1990. Viral and cellular membrane fusion proteins. *Annu. Rev. Physiol.* 52:675–697.

4746. Whitney, J. B., and R. M. Ruprecht. 2004. Live attenuated HIV vaccines: pitfalls and prospects. *Curr. Opin. Infect. Dis.* 17:17–26.

4747. Whittle, H., J. Morris, J. Todd, T. Corrah, S. Sabally, J. Bangali, P. T. Ngom, M. Rolfe, and A. Wilkins. 1994. HIV-2-infected patients survive longer than HIV-1-infected patients. *AIDS* 8:1617–1620.

4748. Whittle, H. C., K. Ariyoshi, and S. Rowland-Jones. 1998. HIV-2 and T cell recognition. *Curr. Opin. Immunol.* 10:382–387.

4749. WHO-IUIS Nomenclature Sub-Committee on TCR Designation. 1995. Nomenclature for T-cell receptor (TCR) gene segments of the immune system. *Immunogenetics* 42:451–453.

4750. Wichukchinda, N., E. E. Nakayama, A. Rojanawiwat, P. Pathipvanich, W. Auwanit, S. Vongsheree, K. Ariyoshi, P. Sawanpanyalert, and T. Shioda. 2006. Protective effects of IL4-589T and RANTES-28G on HIV-1 disease progression in infected Thai females. *AIDS* 20:189–196.

4751. Wick, W. D., O. O. Yang, L. Corey, and S. G. Self. 2005. How many human immunodeficiency virus type 1-infected target cells can a cytotoxic T-lymphocyte kill? *J. Virol.* 79:13579–13586.

4752. Widera, G., M. Austin, D. Rabussay, C. Goldbeck, S. W. Barnett, M. Chen, L. Leung, G. R. Otten, K. Thudium, M. J. Selby, and J. B. Ulmer. 2000. Increased DNA vaccine delivery and immunogenicity by electroporation in vivo. *J. Immunol.* 164:4635–4640.

4753. Wigdahl, B., R. Guyton, and P. S. Sarin. 1987. Human immunodeficiency virus infection of the developing human nervous system. *Virology* 159:440–445.

4754. Wiktor, S. Z., E. Ekpini, J. M. Karon, J. Nkengasong, C. Maurice, S. T. Severin, T. H. Roels, M. K. Kouassi, E. M. Lackritz, I. M. Coulibaly, and A. E. Greenberg. 1999. Short-course oral zidovudine for prevention of mother-to-child transmission of HIV-1 in Abidjan, Cote d'Ivoire: a randomised trial. *Lancet* 353:781–785.

4755. Wiktor, S. Z., J. N. Nkengasong, E. R. Ekpini, G. T. Adjorlolo-Johnson, P. D. Ghys, K. Brattegaard, O. Tossou, T. J. Dondero, K. M. De Cock, and A. E. Greenberg. 1999. Lack of protection against HIV-1 infection among women with HIV-2 infection. *AIDS* 13:695–699.

4756. Wild, C., T. Oas, C. McDanal, D. Bolognesi, and T. Matthews. 1992. A synthetic peptide inhibitor of human immunodeficiency virus replication: correlation between solution structure and viral inhibition. *Proc. Natl. Acad. Sci. USA* 89:10537–10541.

4757. Wiley, C. A., C. L. Achim, R. D. Schrier, M. P. Heyes, J. A. McCutchan, and I. Grant. 1992. Relationship of cerebrospinal fluid immune activation associated factors to HIV encephalitis. *AIDS* 6:1299–1307.

4758. Wiley, C. A., and J. A. Nelson. 1988. Role of human immunodeficiency virus and cytomegalovirus in AIDS encephalitis. *Am. J. Pathol.* 133:73–81.

4759. Wiley, C. A., R. D. Schrier, J. A. Nelson, P. W. Lambert, and M. B. A. Oldstone. 1986. Cellular localization of human immunodeficiency virus infection within the brains of acquired immune deficiency syndrome patients. *Proc. Natl. Acad. Sci. USA* 83:7089–7093.

4760. Wiley, C. A., R. D. Schrier, F. J. Denaro, J. A. Nelson, P. W. Lampert, and M. B. A. Oldstone. 1986. Localization of cytomegalovirus proteins and genome during fulminant central nervous system infection in an AIDS patient. *J. Neuropathol. Exp. Neurol.* 45:127–139.

4761. Wiley, J. A., S. J. Herschkorn, and N. S. Padian. 1989. Heterogeneity in the probability of HIV transmission per sexual contact: the case of male-to-female transmission in penile-vaginal intercourse. *Stat. Med.* 8:93–102.

4762. Wilfert, C. M., C. Wilson, K. Luzuriaga, and L. Epstein. 1994. Pathogenesis of pediatric human immunodeficiency virus type 1 infection. *J. Infect. Dis.* 170:286–292.

4763. Wilkinson, J., J. J. Zaunders, A. Carr, and D. A. Cooper. 1999. CD8+ anti-human immunodeficiency virus suppressor activity (CASA) in response to antiretroviral therapy: loss of CASA is associated with loss of viremia. *J. Infect. Dis.* 180:68–75.

4764. Wille-Reece, U., B. J. Flynn, K. Lore, R. A. Koup, R. M. Kedl, J. J. Mattapallil, W. R. Weiss, M. Roederer, and R. A. Seder. 2005. HIV Gag protein conjugated to a Toll-like receptor 7/8 agonist improves the magnitude and quality of Th1 and CD8+ T cell responses in nonhuman primates. *Proc. Natl. Acad. Sci. USA* 102:15190–15194.

4765. Willems, F., A. Marchant, J. P. Delville, C. Gerard, A. Delvaux, T. Velu, M. de Boer, and M. Goldman. 1994. Interleukin-10 inhibits B7 and intercellular adhesion molecule-1 expression on human monocytes. *Eur. J. Immunol.* 24:1007–1009.

4766. Willey, R. I., E. K. Ross, A. J. Buckler-White, T. S. Theodore, and M. A. Martin. 1989. Functional interaction of constant and variable domains of HIV-1 gp120. *J. Virol.* **63:**3595–3600.

4767. Willey, R. L., F. Maldarelli, M. A. Martin, and K. Strebel. 1992. Human immunodeficiency virus type 1 *vpu* protein regulates the formation of intracellular gp160-CD4 complexes. *J. Virol.* **66:**226–234.

4768. Willey, R. L., and M. A. Martin. 1993. Association of human immunodeficiency virus type 1 envelope glycoprotein with particles depends on interactions between the third variable and conserved regions of gp120. *J. Virol.* **67:**3639–3643.

4769. Willey, R. L., R. A. Rutledge, S. Dias, T. Folks, T. Theodore, C. E. Buckler, and M. A. Martin. 1986. Identification of conserved and divergent domains within the envelope gene of the acquired immunodeficiency syndrome retrovirus. *Proc. Natl. Acad. Sci. USA* **83:**5038–5042.

4770. Willey, R. L., R. Shibata, E. O. Freed, M. W. Cho, and M. A. Martin. 1996. Differential glycosylation, virion incorporation, and sensitivity to neutralizing antibodies of human immunodeficiency virus type 1 envelope produced from infected primary T-lymphocyte and macrophage cultures. *J. Virol.* **70:**6431–6436.

4771. Willey, R. L., D. H. Smith, L. A. Lasky, T. S. Theodore, P. L. Earl, B. Moss, D. J. Capon, and M. A. Martin. 1988. In vitro mutagenesis identifies a region within the envelope gene of the human immunodeficiency virus that is critical for infectivity. *J. Virol.* **62:**139–147.

4772. Willey, R. L., T. S. Theodore, and M. A. Martin. 1994. Amino acid substitutions in the human immunodeficiency virus type 1 gp120 V3 loop that change viral tropism also alter physical and functional properties of the virion envelope. *J. Virol.* **68:**4409–4419.

4773. Willey, S., V. Roulet, J. D. Reeves, M.-L. Kergadallan, E. Thomas, A. McKnight, B. Jegou, and N. Dejucq-Rainsford. 2003. Human Leydig cells are productively infected by some HIV-2 and SIV strains but not HIV-1. *AIDS* **17:**183–188.

4774. Williams, C. F., D. Klinzman, T. E. Yamashita, J. Xiang, P. M. Polgreen, C. Rinaldo, C. Liu, J. Phair, J. B. Margolick, D. Zdunek, G. Hess, and J. T. Stapleton. 2004. Persistent GB virus C infection and survival in HIV-infected men. *N. Engl. J. Med.* **350:**981–990.

4775. Williams, F. M., P. R. Cohen, J. Jumshyd, and J. D. Reveille. 1998. Prevalence of the diffuse infiltrative lymphocytosis syndrome among human immunodeficiency virus type 1-positive outpatients. *Arthritis Rheum.* **41:**863–868.

4776. Williams, M., J. F. Roeth, M. R. Kasper, T. M. Filzen, and K. L. Collins. 2005. Human immunodeficiency virus type 1 Nef domains required for disruption of major histocompatibility complex class I trafficking are also necessary for coprecipitation of Nef with HLA-A2. *J. Virol.* **79:**632–636.

4777. Williams, N. S., and V. H. Engelhard. 1997. Perforin-dependent cytotoxic activity and lymphokine secretion by CD4+ T cells are regulated by CD8+ T cells. *J. Immunol.* **159:**2091–2099.

4778. Williams, S. B., T. P. Flanigan, A. W. Artenstein, T. C. VanCott, D. Smith, K. Mayer, and R. A. Koup. 1999. CCR5 genotype and human immunodeficiency virus (HIV)-specific mucosal antibody in seronegative women at high risk for HIV infection. *J. Infect. Dis.* **179:**1310–1312.

4779. Williamson, C., S. A. Loubser, B. Brice, G. Joubert, T. Smit, R. Thomas, M. Visagie, M. Cooper, and E. van der Ryst. 2000. Allelic frequencies of host genetic variants influencing susceptibility to HIV-1 infection and disease in South African populations. *AIDS* **14:**449–451.

4780. Willumsen, J. F., M.-L. Newell, S. M. Filteau, A. Coutsoudis, S. Dwarika, D. York, A. M. Tomkins, and H. M. Coovadia. 2001. Variation in breastmilk HIV-1 viral load in left and right breasts during the first 3 months of lactation. *AIDS* **15:**1896–1898.

4781. Wilson, C., M. S. Reitz, K. Aldrich, P. J. Klasse, J. Blomberg, R. C. Gallo, and M. Robert-Guroff. 1990. The site of an immune-selected point mutation in the transmembrane protein of human immunodeficiency virus type 1 does not constitute the neutralization epitope. *J. Virol.* **64:**3240–3248.

4782. Wilson, C. C., R. C. Brown, B. T. Korber, B. M. Wilkes, D. J. Ruhl, D. Sakamoto, K. Kunstman, K. Luzuriaga, I. C. Hanson, S. M. Widmayer, A. Wiznia, S. Clapp, A. J. Ammann, R. A. Koup, S. M. Wolinsky, and B. D. Walker. 1999. Frequent detection of escape from cytotoxic T-lymphocyte recognition in perinatal human immunodeficiency virus (HIV) type 1 transmission: the ariel project for the prevention of transmission of HIV from mother to infant. *J. Virol.* **73:**3975–3985.

4783. Wilson, C. C., S. A. Kalams, B. M. Wilkes, D. J. Ruhl, F. Gao, B. H. Hahn, I. C. Hanson, K. Luzuriaga, S. Wolinsky, R. Koup, S. P. Buchbinder, R. P. Johnson, and B. D. Walker. 1997. Overlapping epitopes in human immunodeficiency virus type 1 gp120 presented by HLA A, B, and C molecules: effects of viral variation on cytotoxic T-lymphocyte recognition. *J. Virol.* **71:**1256–1264.

4784. Wilson, J. D., G. S. Ogg, R. L. Allen, C. Davis, S. Shaunak, J. Downie, W. Dyer, C. Workman, S. Sullivan, A. J. McMichael, and S. L. Rowland-Jones. 2000. Direct visualization of HIV-1-specific cytotoxic T lymphocytes during primary infection. *AIDS* **14:**225–233.

4785. Wilson, J. D. K., N. Imami, A. Watkins, J. Gill, P. Hay, B. Gazzard, M. Westby, and F. M. Gotch. 2000. Loss of CD4+ T cell proliferative ability but not loss of human immunodeficiency virus type 1 specificity equates with progression to disease. *J. Infect. Dis.* **182:**792–798.

4786. Wilson, K. M., E. I. M. Johnson, H. A. Croom, K. M. Richards, L. Doughty, P. H. Cunningham, B. E. Kemp, B. M. Branson, and E. M. Dax. 2004. Incidence immunoassay for distinguishing recent from established HIV-1 infection in therapy-naive populations. *AIDS* **18:**2253–2259.

4787. Wilson, S. B., and T. L. Delovitch. 2003. Janus-like role of regulatory iNKT cells in autoimmune disease and tumour immunity. *Nat. Rev. Immunol.* **3:**211–222.

4788. Winchester, R., J. Pitt, M. Charurat, L. S. Magder, H. H. H. Goring, A. Landay, J. S. Read, W. Shearer, E. Handelsman, K. Luzuriaga, G. V. Hillyer, and W. Blattner. 2004. Mother-to-child transmission of HIV-1: strong association with certain maternal HLA-B independent of viral load implicates innate immune mechanisms. *J. Acquir. Immune Defic. Syndr.* **36:**659–670.

4789. Winkelstein, W., Jr., D. M. Lyman, N. Padian, R. Grant, M. Samuel, J. A. Wiley, R. E. Anderson, W. Lang, J. Riggs, and J. A. Levy. 1987. Sexual practices and risk of infection by the human immunodeficiency virus: The San Francisco Men's Health Study. *JAMA* **257:**321–325.

4790. Winkler, C., W. Modi, M. W. Smith, G. W. Nelson, X. Wu, M. Carrington, M. Dean, T. Honjo, K. Tashiro, D. Yabe, S. Buchbinder, E. Vittinghoff, J. J. Goedert, T. R. O'Brien, L. P. Jacobson, R. Detels, S. Donfield, A. Willoughby, E. Gomperts, D. Vlahov, J. Phair, and S. J. O'Brien. 1998. Genetic restriction of AIDS pathogenesis by an SDF-1 chemokine gene variant. *Science* 279:389–393.

4791. Winslow, B. J., R. J. Pomerantz, O. Bagasra, and D. Trono. 1993. HIV-1 latency due to the site of proviral integration. *Virology* 196:849–854.

4792. Winslow, B. J., and D. Trono. 1993. The blocks to human immunodeficiency virus type 1 Tat and Rev functions in mouse cell lines are independent. *J. Virol.* 67:2349–2354.

4793. Winston, J. A., L. A. Bruggeman, M. D. Ross, J. Jacobson, L. Ross, V. D. D'Agati, P. E. Klotman, and M. E. Klotman. 2001. Nephropathy and establishment of a renal reservoir of HIV type 1 during primary infection. *N. Engl. J. Med.* 344:1979–1984.

4794. Wiskerchen, M., and M. A. Muesing. 1995. Human immunodeficiency virus type 1 integrase: effects of mutations on viral ability to integrate, direct viral gene expression from unintegrated viral DNA templates, and sustain viral propagation in primary cells. *J. Virol.* 69:376–386.

4795. Wistuba, I. I., C. Behrens, S. Milchgrub, A. K. Virmani, J. Jagirdar, B. Thomas, H. L. Ioachim, L. A. Litzky, E. M. Brambilla, J. D. Minna, and A. F. Gazdar. 1998. Comparison of molecular changes in lung cancers in HIV-positive and HIV-indeterminate subjects. *JAMA* 279:1554–1559.

4796. Wit, F. W., D. H. Blanckenberg, K. Brinkman, J. M. Prins, M. E. van der Ende, M. M. E. Schneider, J.-W. Mulder, F. de Wolf, and J. M. Lange. 2005. Safety of long-term interruption of successful antiretroviral therapy: The ATHENA cohort study. *AIDS* 19:345–347.

4797. Withrington, R. H., P. Cornes, J. R. W. Harris, M. H. Seifert, E. Berrie, D. Taylor-Robinson, and D. J. Jeffries. 1987. Isolation of human immunodeficiency virus from synovial fluid of a patient with reactive arthritis. *Br. Med. J.* 294:484.

4798. Wiviott, L. D., C. M. Walker, and J. A. Levy. 1990. CD8+ lymphocytes suppress HIV production by autologous CD4+ cells without eliminating the infected cells from culture. *Cell. Immunol.* 128:628–634.

4799. Wlodawer, A., M. Miller, M. Jaskolski, B. K. Sathyanarayana, E. Baldwin, I. T. Weber, L. M. Selk, L. Clawson, J. Schneider, and S. B. H. Kent. 1989. Conserved folding in retroviral proteases: crystal structure of a synthetic HIV-1 protease. *Science* 245:616–621.

4800. Wofsy, C. B., J. B. Cohen, L. B. Hauer, N. S. Padian, B. A. Michaelis, L. A. Evans, and J. A. Levy. 1986. Isolation of the AIDS-associated retrovirus from genital secretions from women with antibodies to the virus. *Lancet* i:527–529.

4801. Wolber, V., H. Rensland, B. Brandmeier, M. Sagemann, R. Hoffmann, H. R. Kalbitzer, and A. Wittinghofer. 1992. Expression, purification and biochemical characterization of the human immunodeficiency virus 1 *nef* gene product. *Eur. J. Biochem.* 205:1115–1121.

4802. Wolfe, N. D., W. M. Switzer, J. K. Carr, V. B. Bhullar, V. Shanmugam, U. Tamoufe, A. Prosser, J. N. Torimiro, A. Wright, E. Mpoudi-Ngole, F. E. McCutchan, D. L. Birx, T. M. Folks, D. S. Burke, and W. Heneine. 2004. Naturally acquired simian retrovirus infections in central African hunters. *Lancet* 363:932–937.

4803. Wolff, H., and D. J. Anderson. 1988. Immunohistologic characterization and quantitation of leukocyte subpopulations in human semen. *Fertil. Steril.* 49:497–504.

4804. Wolff, H., and D. J. Anderson. 1988. Potential human immunodeficiency virus-host cells in human semen. *AIDS Res. Hum. Retrovir.* 4:1–2.

4805. Wolff, J. A., R. W. Malone, P. Williams, W. Chong, G. Acsadi, A. Jani, and P. L. Felgner. 1990. Direct gene transfer into mouse muscle in vivo. *Science* 247:1465–1468.

4806. Wolfs, T. F. W., G. Zwart, M. Bakker, and J. Goudsmit. 1992. HIV-1 genomic RNA diversification following sexual and parenteral virus transmission. *Virology* 189:103–110.

4807. Wolfs, T. F. W., G. Zwart, M. Bakker, M. Valk, C. L. Kuiken, and J. Goudsmit. 1991. Naturally occurring mutations within HIV-1 V3 genomic RNA lead to antigenic variation dependent on a single amino acid substitution. *Virology* 185:195–205.

4808. Wolinsky, S. M., C. M. Wike, B. T. M. Korber, C. Hutto, W. P. Parks, L. L. Rosenblum, K. J. Kunstman, M. R. Furtado, and J. L. Munoz. 1992. Selective transmission of human immunodeficiency virus type 1 variants from mothers to infants. *Science* 255:1134–1137.

4809. Wolthers, K. C., G. Bea, A. Wisman, S. A. Otto, A. M. de Roda Husman, N. Schaft, F. de Wolf, J. Goudsmit, R. A. Coutinho, A. G. J. van der Zee, L. Meyaard, and F. Miedema. 1996. T cell telomere length in HIV-1 infection: no evidence for increased CD4+ T cell turnover. *Science* 274:1543–1547.

4810. Wong, J. K., H. F. Gunthard, D. V. Vavlir, Z. Q. Zhang, A. T. Haase, C. C. Ignacio, S. Kowk, E. Emini, and D. D. Richman. 1997. Reduction of HIV-1 in blood and lymph nodes following potent antiretroviral therapy and the virologic correlates of treatment failure. *Proc. Natl. Acad. Sci. USA* 94:12574–12579.

4811. Wong, J. K., M. Hezareh, H. F. Gunthard, D. V. Havlir, C. C. Ignacio, C. A. Spina, and D. D. Richman. 1997. Recovery of replication-competent HIV despite prolonged suppression of plasma viremia. *Science* 278:1291–1295.

4812. Wong, J. K., C. C. Ignacio, F. Torriani, D. Havlir, N. J. S. Fitch, and D. D. Richman. 1997. In vivo compartmentalization of human immunodeficiency virus: evidence from the examination of *pol* sequences from autopsy tissues. *J. Virol.* 71:2059–2071.

4813. Wong, S. W., E. P. Bergquam, R. M. Swanson, F. W. Lee, S. M. Shiigi, N. A. Avery, J. W. Fanton, and M. K. Axthelm. 1999. Induction of B cell hyperplasia in simian immunodeficiency virus-infected rhesus macaques with the simian homologue of Kaposi's sarcoma-associated herpesvirus. *J. Exp. Med.* 190:827–840.

4814. Wood, G. S., C. F. Garcia, R. F. Dorfman, and R. A. Warnke. 1985. The immunohistology of follicle lysis in lymph node biopsies from homosexual men. *Blood* 66:1092–1097.

4815. Woods, T. C., B. D. Roberts, S. T. Butera, and T. M. Folks. 1997. Loss of inducible virus in CD45RA naive cells after human immunodeficiency virus-1 entry accounts for preferential viral replication in CD45RO memory cells. *Blood* 89:1635–1641.

4816. Woodward, T. E. 1962. Chemosuppression of specific infections with antibiotics. *J. Chronic Dis.* 15:611–622.

4817. Wooley, D. P., R. A. Smith, S. Czajak, and R. C. Desrosiers. 1997. Direct demonstration of retroviral recombination in a rhesus monkey. *J. Virol.* 71:9650–9653.

4818. Worku, S., A. Bjorkman, M. Troye-Blomberg, L. Jemaneh, A. Farnert, and B. Christensson. 1997. Lymphocyte activation and subset redistribution in the peripheral blood in acute malaria illness: distinct gamma delta+ T cell patterns in Plasmodium falciparum and P. vivax infections. *Clin. Exp. Immunol.* **108**:34–41.

4819. **Wormser, G. P., S. Bittker, G. Forester, I. K. Hewlett, I. Argani, B. Joshi, J. S. Epstrin, and D. Bucher.** 1992. Absence of infectious human immunodeficiency virus type 1 in "natural" eccrine sweat. *J. Infect. Dis.* **165**:155–158.

4820. **Wright, S. C., A. Jewett, R. Mitsuyasu, and B. Bonavida.** 1988. Spontaneous cytotoxicity and tumor necrosis factor production by peripheral blood monocytes from AIDS patients. *J. Immunol.* **141**:99–104.

4821. **Wrin, T., L. Crawford, L. Sawyer, P. Weber, H. W. Sheppard, and C. V. Hanson.** 1994. Neutralizing antibody responses to autologous and heterologous isolates of human immunodeficiency virus. *J. Acquir. Immune Defic. Syndr.* **7**:211–219.

4822. **Wu, F., J. Garcia, D. Sigman, and R. Gaynor.** 1991. *Tat* regulates binding of the human immunodeficiency virus transactivating region RNA loop-binding protein TRP-185. *Genes Dev.* **5**:2128–2140.

4823. **Wu, J.-Y., B. H. Gardner, C. I. Murphy, J. R. Seals, C. R. Kensil, J. Recchia, G. A. Beltz, G. W. Newman, and M. J. Newman.** 1992. Saponin adjuvant enhancement of antigen-specific immune responses to an experimental HIV-1 vaccine. *J. Immunol.* **148**:1519–1525.

4824. **Wu, L., A. A. Bashirova, T. D. Martin, L. Villamide, E. Mehlhop, A. O. Chertov, D. Unutmaz, M. Pope, M. Carrington, and V. N. Kewal-Ramani.** 2002. Rhesus macaque dendritic cells efficiently transmit primate lentiviruses independently of DC-SIGN. *Proc. Natl. Acad. Sci. USA* **99**:1568–1573.

4825. **Wu, L., N. P. Gerard, R. Wyatt, H. Choe, C. Parolin, N. Ruffing, A. Borsetti, A. A. Cardoso, E. Desjardin, W. Newman, C. Gerard, and J. Sodroski.** 1996. CD4-induced interaction of primary HIV-1 gp120 glycoproteins with the chemokine receptor CCR-5. *Nature* **384**:179–183.

4826. **Wu, X., A. B. Parast, B. A. Richardson, R. Nduati, G. John-Stewart, D. Mbori-Ngacha, S. M. Rainwater, and J. Overbaugh.** 2006. Neutralization escape variants of human immunodeficiency virus type 1 are transmitted from mother to infant. *J. Virol.* **80**:835–844.

4827. **Wu, Y., and J. W. Marsh.** 2003. Early transcription from nonintegrated DNA in human immunodeficiency virus infection. *J. Virol.* **77**:10376–10382.

4828. **Wyand, M. S., K. H. Manson, M. Garcia-Moll, D. Montefiori, and R. C. Desrosiers.** 1996. Vaccine protection by a triple deletion mutant of simian immunodeficiency virus. *J. Virol.* **70**:3724–3733.

4829. **Wyatt, R., P. D. Kwong, E. Desjardins, R. W. Sweet, J. Robinson, W. A. Hendrickson, and J. G. Sodroski.** 1998. The antigenic structure of the HIV gp120 envelope glycoprotein. *Nature* **393**:705–711.

4830. **Wyatt, R., and J. Sodroski.** 1998. The HIV-1 envelope glycoproteins: fusogens, antigens, and immunogens. *Science* **280**:1884–1888.

4831. **Wyma, D. J., A. Kotov, and C. Aiken.** 2000. Evidence for a stable interaction of gp41 with Pr55(Gag) in immature human immunodeficiency virus type 1 particles. *J. Virol.* **74**:9381–9387.

4832. **Wynn, T. A., A. W. Cheever, D. Jankovic, R. W. Poindexter, P. Caspar, F. A. Lewis, and A. Sher.** 1995. An IL-12-based vaccination method for preventing fibrosis induced by schistosome infection. *Nature* **376**:594–596.

4833. **Wyss, S., A. S. Dimitrov, F. Baribaud, T. G. Edwards, R. Blumenthal, and J. A. Hoxie.** 2005. Regulation of human immunodeficiency virus type 1 envelope glycoprotein fusion by a membrane-interactive domain in the gp41 cytoplasmic tail. *J. Virol.* **79**:12231–12241.

4834. **Xiang, J., S. L. George, S. Wunschmann, Q. Chang, D. Klinzman, and J. T. Stapleton.** 2004. Inhibition of HIV-1 replication by GB virus C infection through increases in RANTES, MIP-1α, MIP-1β, and SDF-1. *Lancet* **363**:2040–2046.

4835. **Xiang, J., S. Wünschmann, D. J. Kiekema, K. D. Patrick, S. L. George, and J. T. Stapleton.** 2001. Effect of coinfection with GB virus C and reduced mortality among HIV-infected patients. *N. Engl. J. Med.* **345**:707–714.

4836. **Xiao, H., C. Neuveut, H. L. Tiffany, M. Benkirane, E. A. Rich, P. M. Murphy, and K. T. Jeang.** 2000. Selective CXCR4 antagonism by tat: implications for in vivo expansion of coreceptor use by HIV-1. *Proc. Natl. Acad. Sci. USA* **97**:11466–11471.

4837. **Xiao, L., S. M. Owen, D. L. Rudolph, R. B. Lal, and A. A. Lal.** 1998. *Plasmodium falciparum* antigen-induced human immunodeficiency virus type 1 replication is mediated through induction of tumor necrosis factor-alpha. *J. Infect. Dis.* **177**:437–445.

4838. **Xu, J., L. Whitman, F. Lori, and J. Lisziewicz.** 2002. Methods of using interleukin 2 to enhance HIV-specific immune responses. *AIDS Res. Hum. Retrovir.* **18**:289–293.

4839. **Xu, Y., J. Kulkosky, E. Acheampong, G. Nunnari, J. Sullivan, and R. J. Pomerantz.** 2004. HIV-1-mediated apoptosis of neuronal cells: proximal molecular mechanisms of HIV-1-induced encephalopathy. *Proc. Natl. Acad. Sci. USA* **101**:7070–7075.

4840. **Yagita, H., M. Nakata, A. Kawasaki, Y. Shinkai, and K. Okumura.** 1992. Role of perforin in lymphocyte-mediated cytolysis. *Adv. Immunol.* **51**:215–242.

4841. **Yahi, N., S. Baghdiguian, H. Moreau, and J. Fantini.** 1992. Galactosyl ceramide (or a closely related molecule) is the receptor for human immunodeficiency virus type 1 on human colon epithelial HT29 cells. *J. Virol.* **66**:4848–4854.

4842. **Yahi, N., J.-M. Sabatier, S. Baghdiguian, F. Gonzalez-Scarano, and J. Fantini.** 1995. Synthetic multimeric peptides derived from the principal neutralization domain (V3 loop) of human immunodeficiency virus type 1 (HIV-1) gp120 bind to galactosylceramide and block HIV-1 infection in a human CD4-negative mucosal epithelial cell line. *J. Virol.* **69**:320–325.

4843. **Yahi, N., S. L. Spitalnik, K. A. Stefano, P. De Micco, F. Gonzalez-Scarano, and J. Fantini.** 1994. Interferon-gamma decreases cell surface expression of galactosyl ceramide, the receptor for HIV-1 gp120 on human colonic epithelial cells. *Virology* **204**:550–557.

4844. **Yamada, M., A. Zurbriggen, M. B. A. Oldstone, and R. S. Fujinami.** 1991. Common immunologic determinant between human immunodeficiency virus type 1 gp41 and astrocytes. *J. Virol.* **65**:1370–1376.

4845. **Yamada, T., N. Watanabe, T. Nakamura, and A. Iwamoto.** 2004. Antibody-dependent cellular cytotoxicity via humoral immune epitope of Nef protein expressed on cell surface. *J. Immunol.* **172**:2401–2406.

4846. **Yamaguchi, J., P. Bodelle, l. Kaptue, L. Zekeng, L. G. Gurtler, S. G. Devare, and C. A. Brennan.** 2003. Near full-length genomes of 15 HIV Type 1 group O isolates. *AIDS Res. Hum. Retrovir.* **19**:979–988.

4847. Yamaguchi, J., R. Coffey, A. Vallari, C. Ngansop, D. Mbanya, N. Ndembi, L. Kaptue, L. G. Gurtler, P. Bodelle, G. Schochetman, S. G. Devare, and C. A. Brennan. 2006. Identification of HIV type 1 group N infections in a husband and wife in Cameroon: viral genome sequences provide evidence for horizontal transmission. *AIDS Res. Hum. Retrovir.* 22:83–92.

4848. Yamaguchi, J., A. S. Vallari, P. Swanson, P. Bodelle, L. Kaptue, C. Ngansop, L. Zekeng, L. G. Gurtler, S. G. Devare, and C. A. Brennan. 2002. Evaluation of HIV type 1 group O isolates: identification of five phylogenetic clusters. *AIDS Res. Hum. Retrovir.* 18:269–282.

4849. Yamamoto, J. K., F. Barre-Sinoussi, V. Bolton, N. C. Pedersen, and M. B. Gardner. 1986. Human alpha- and beta-interferon but not gamma- suppress the in vitro replication of LAV, HTLV-III, and ARV-2. *J. Interferon Res.* 6:143–152.

4850. Yamamoto, J. K., T. Hohdatsu, R. A. Olmsted, R. Pu, H. Louie, H. A. Zochlinski, V. Acevedo, H. M. Johnson, G. A. Soulds, and M. B. Gardner. 1993. Experimental vaccine protection against homologous and heterologous strains of feline immunodeficiency virus. *J. Virol.* 67:601–605.

4851. Yang, C., M. Li, R. D. Newman, Y.-P. Shi, J. Ayisi, A. M. van Eijk, J. Otieno, A. O. Misore, R. W. Steketee, B. L. Nahlen, and R. B. Lal. 2003. Genetic diversity of HIV-1 in western Kenya: subtype-specific differences in mother-to-child transmission. *AIDS* 17:1667–1674.

4852. Yang, J., H. P. Bogerd, P. J. Wang, D. C. Page, and B. R. Cullen. 2001. Two closely related human nuclear export factors utilize entirely distinct export pathways. *Mol. Cell* 8:397–406.

4853. Yang, L. P., J. L. Riley, R. G. Carroll, C. H. June, J. Hoxie, B. K. Patterson, Y. Ohshima, R. J. Hodes, and G. Delespesse. 1998. Productive infection of neonatal CD8(+) T lymphocytes by HIV-1. *J. Exp. Med.* 187:1139–1144.

4854. Yang, O. O., S. A. Kalams, M. Rosenzweig, A. Trocha, N. Jones, M. Koziel, B. D. Walker, and R. P. Johnson. 1996. Efficient lysis of human immunodeficiency virus type 1-infected cells by cytotoxic T lymphocytes. *J. Virol.* 70:5799–5806.

4855. Yang, O. O., S. A. Kalams, A. Trocha, H. Cao, A. Luster, R. P. Johnson, and B. D. Walker. 1997. Suppression of human immunodeficiency virus type 1 replication by CD8+ cells: evidence for HLA class I-restricted triggering of cytolytic and noncytolytic mechanisms. *J. Virol.* 71:3120–3128.

4856. Yang, O. O., H. Lin, M. Dagarag, H. L. Ng, R. B. Effros, and C. H. Uittenbogaart. 2005. Decreased perforin and granzyme B expression in senescent HIV-1-specific cytotoxic T lymphocytes. *Virology* 332:16–19.

4857. Yang, R., X. Xia, S. Kusagawa, C. Zhang, K. Ben, and Y. Takebe. 2002. On-going generation of multiple forms of HIV-1 intersubtype recombinants in the Yunnan province of China. *AIDS* 16:1401–1407.

4858. Yang, T. Y., S. C. Chen, M. W. Leach, D. Manfra, B. Homey, M. Wiekowski, L. Sullivan, C. H. Jenh, S. K. Narula, S. W. Chensue, and S. A. Lira. 2000. Transgenic expression of the chemokine receptor encoded by human herpesvirus 8 induces an angioproliferative disease resembling Kaposi's sarcoma. *J. Exp. Med.* 191:445–454.

4859. Yang, X., M. O. Gold, D. N. Tang, D. E. Lewis, E. Aguilar-Cordova, A. P. Rice, and C. H. Herrmann. 1997. TAK, an HIV Tat-associated kinase, is a member of the cyclin-dependent family of protein kinases and is induced by activation of peripheral blood lymphocytes and differentiation of promonocytic cell lines. *Proc. Natl. Acad. Sci. USA* 94:12331–12336.

4860. Yang, X., S. Kurteva, X. Ren, S. Lee, and J. Sodroski. 2005. Stoichiometry of envelope glycoprotein trimers in the entry of human immunodeficiency virus type 1. *J. Virol.* 79: 12132–12147.

4861. Yap, M. W., S. Nisole, C. Lynch, and J. P. Stoye. 2004. Trim5α protein restricts both HIV-1 and murine leukemia virus. *Proc. Natl. Acad. Sci. USA* 101:10786–10791.

4862. Yap, M. W., S. Nisole, and J. P. Stoye. 2005. A single amino acid change in the SPRY domain of human Trim5α leads to HIV-1 restriction. *Curr. Biol.* 15:73–78.

4863. Yarchoan, R., C. F. Perno, R. V. Thomas, R. W. Klecker, J.-P. Allain, R. J. Wills, N. McAtee, M. A. Fischl, R. Dubinsky, M. C. McNeely, H. Mitsuya, J. M. Pluda, T. J. Lawley, M. Leuther, B. Safai, J. M. Collins, C. E. Myers, and S. Broder. 1988. Phase I studies of 2′,3′-dideoxycytidine in severe human immunodeficiency virus infection as a single agent and alternating with zidovudine (AZT). *Lancet* i:76–81.

4864. Yasukawa, M., A. Hasegawa, I. Sakai, H. Ohminami, J. Arai, S. Kaneko, Y. Yakushijin, K. Maeyama, H. Nakashima, R. Arakaki, and S. Fujita. 1999. Down-regulation of CXCR4 by human herpesvirus 6 (HHV-6) and HHV-7. *J. Immunol.* 162: 5417–5422.

4865. Yasutomi, Y., K. A. Keimann, C. I. Lord, M. D. Miller, and N. L. Letvin. 1993. Simian immunodeficiency virus-specific CD8+ lymphocyte response in acutely infected rhesus monkeys. *J. Virol.* 67:1707–1711.

4866. Yasutomi, Y., S. Koenig, R. M. Woods, J. Madsen, N. M. Wassef, C. R. Alving, H. J. Klein, T. E. Nolan, L. J. Boots, J. A. Kessler, E. A. Emini, A. J. Conley, and N. L. Letvin. 1995. A vaccine-elicited, single viral epitope-specific cytotoxic T lymphocyte response does not protect against intravenous, cell-free simian immunodeficiency virus challenge. *J. Virol.* 69:2279–2284.

4867. Yasutomi, Y., H. L. Robinson, S. Lu, F. Mustafa, C. Lekutis, J. Arthos, J. I. Mullins, G. Voss, K. Manson, M. Wyand, and N. L. Letvin. 1996. Simian immunodeficiency virus-specific cytotoxic T-lymphocyte induction through DNA vaccination of rhesus monkeys. *J. Virol.* 70:678–681.

4868. Ye, P., P. Kazanjian, S. L. Kunkel, and D. E. Kirschner. 2004. Lack of good correlation of serum CC-chemokine levels with human immunodeficiency virus-1 disease stage and response to treatment. *J. Lab. Clin. Med.* 143:310–319.

4869. Yedavalli, V. S., H. M. Shih, Y. P. Chiang, C. Y. Lu, L. Y. Chang, M. Y. Chen, C. Y. Chuang, A. I. Dayton, K. T. Jeang, and L. M. Huang. 2005. Human immunodeficiency virus type 1 Vpr interacts with antiapoptotic mitochondrial protein HAX-1. *J. Virol.* 79:13735–13746.

4870. Yee, C., A. Biondi, X. H. Wang, N. N. Iscove, J. de Sousa, L. A. Aarden, G. G. Wong, S. C. Clark, H. A. Messner, and M. D. Minden. 1989. A possible autocrine role of IL-6 in two lymphoma cell lines. *Blood* 74:789–804.

4871. Yefenof, E., B. Asjo, and E. Klein. 1991. Alternative complement pathway activation by HIV infected cells: C3 fixation does not lead to complement lysis but enhances NK sensitivity. *Int. Immunol.* 3:395–401.

4872. Yeh, M. W., M. Kaul, J. Zheng, H. S. Nottet, M. Thylin, H. E. Gendelman, and S. A. Lipton. 2000. Cytokine-stimulated, but not HIV-infected, human monocyte-derived macrophages produce neurotoxic levels of l-cysteine. *J. Immunol.* 164:4265–4270.

4873. Yeni, P. G., S. M. Hammer, M. S. Hirsh, M. S. Saag, M. Schechter, C. C. J. Carpenter, M. A. Fischl, J. M. Gatell, B. G.

Gazzard, D. M. Jacobsen, D. A. Katzenstein, J. S. G. Montaner, D. D. Richman, R. T. Schooley, M. A. Thompson, S. Vella, and P. A. Volberding. 2004. Treatment for adult HIV infection. 2004 recommendations of the International AIDS Society-USA Panel. *JAMA* 292:251–265.

4874. Yerly, S., S. Jost, M. Monnat, A. Telenti, M. Cavassini, J.-P. Chave, L. Kaiser, P. Burgisser, and L. Perrin. 2004. HIV-1 co/super-infection in intravenous drug users. *AIDS* **18:** 1413–1421.

4875. Yeung, M. C., L. Pulliam, and A. S. Lau. 1995. The HIV envelope protein gp120 is toxic to human brain-cell cultures through the induction of interleukin-6 and tumor necrosis factor-alpha. *AIDS* **9:**137–143.

4876. Yeung, S. C. H., F. Kazazi, C. G. M. Randle, R. C. Howard, N. Rizvi, J. C. Downie, B. J. Donovan, D. A. Cooper, H. Sekine, D. E. Dwyer, and A. L. Cunningham. 1993. Patients infected with human immunodeficiency virus type 1 have low levels of virus in saliva even in the presence of periodontal disease. *J. Infect. Dis.* **163:**803–809.

4877. Yi, Y., S. Rana, J. D. Turner, N. Gaddis, and R. G. Collman. 1998. CXCR-4 is expressed by primary macrophages and supports CCR5-independent infection by dual-tropic but not T-tropic isolates of human immunodeficiency virus type 1. *J. Virol.* **72:**772–777.

4878. Ying, H., X. Ji, M. L. Hart, K. Gupta, M. Saifuddin, M. R. Zariffard, and G. T. Spear. 2004. Interaction of mannose-binding lectin with HIV type 1 is sufficient for virus opsonization but not neutralization. *AIDS Res. Hum. Retrovir.* **20:** 327–335.

4879. Yisastigui, L., J. J. Coull, V. C. Rucker, C. Melandez, R. J. Bosch, S. J. Brodie, L. Corey, D. L. Sodora, P. B. Dervan, and D. M. Margolis. 2004. Polyamides reveal a role for repression in latency within resting T cells of HIV-infected donors. *J. Infect. Dis.* 190:1329–1437.

4880. Ylinen, L. M., Z. Keckesova, S. J. Wilson, S. Ranasinghe, and G. J. Towers. 2005. Differential restriction of human immunodeficiency virus type 2 and simian immunodeficiency virus SIVmac by TRIM5alpha alleles. *J. Virol.* 79:11580–11587.

4881. Yokomaku, Y., H. Miura, H. Tomiyama, A. Kawana-Tachikawa, M. Takiguchi, A. Kojima, Y. Nagai, A. Iwamoto, Z. Matsuda, and K. Ariyoshi. 2004. Impaired processing and presentation of cytotoxic-T-lymphocyte (CTL) epitopes are major escape mechanisms from CTL immune pressure in human immunodeficiency virus type 1 infection. *J. Virol.* 78:1324–1332.

4882. Yolken, R. H., S. Li, J. Perman, and R. Viscidi. 1991. Persistent diarrhea and fecal shedding of retroviral nucleic acids in children infected with human immunodeficiency virus. *J. Infect. Dis.* 164:61–66.

4883. Yonezawa, A., R. Morita, A. Takaori-Kondo, N. Kadowaki, T. Kitawaki, T. Hori, and T. Uchiyama. 2003. Natural alpha interferon-producing cells respond to human immunodeficiency virus type 1 with alpha interferon production and maturation into dendritic cells. *J. Virol.* 77:3777–3784.

4884. Yoo, J., H. Chen, T. Kraus, D. Hirsch, S. Polyak, I. George, and K. Sperber. 1996. Altered cytokine production and accessory cell function after HIV-1 infection. *J. Immunol.* 157:1313–1320.

4885. York-Higgins, D., C. Cheng-Mayer, D. Bauer, J. A. Levy, and D. Dina. 1990. Human immunodeficiency virus type 1 cellular host range, replication, and cytopathicity are linked to the envelope region of the viral genome. *J. Virol.* 64:4016–4020.

4886. Yoshiyama, H., H. Mo, J. P. Moore, and D. D. Ho. 1994. Characterization of mutants of human immunodeficiency virus type 1 that have escaped neutralization by a monoclonal antibody to the gp120 V2 loop. *J. Virol.* 68:974–978.

4887. Youle, R. J., Y. N. Wu, S. M. Mikulski, K. Shogen, R. S. Hamilton, D. Newton, G. D'Alessio, and M. Gravell. 1994. RNase inhibition of human immunodeficiency virus infection of H9 cells. *Proc. Natl. Acad. Sci. USA* 91:6012–6016.

4888. Younes, S. A., B. Yassine-Diab, A. R. Dumont, M. R. Boulassel, Z. Grossman, J. P. Routy, and R. P. Sekaly. 2003. HIV-1 viremia prevents the establishment of interleukin 2-producing HIV-specific memory CD4+ T cells endowed with proliferative capacity. *J. Exp. Med.* 198:1909–1922.

4889. Yu, N., J. N. Billaud, and T. R. Phillips. 1998. Effects of feline immunodeficiency virus on astrocyte glutamate uptake: implications for lentivirus-induced central nervous system diseases. *Proc. Natl. Acad. Sci. USA* 95:2624–2629.

4890. Yu, Q., R. Konig, S. Pillai, K. Chiles, M. Kearney, S. Palmer, D. Richman, J. M. Coffin, and N. R. Landau. 2004. Single-strand specificity of APOBEC3G accounts for minus-strand deamination of the HIV genome. *Nat. Struct. Mol. Biol.*

4891. Yu, X., Z. Matsuda, Q.-C. Yu, T.-H. Lee, and M. Essex. 1993. Vpx of simian immunodeficiency virus is localized primarily outside the virus core in mature virions. *J. Virol.* 67:4386–4390.

4892. Yu, X., M. F. McLane, L. Ratner, W. O'Brien, R. Collman, M. Essex, and T. H. Lee. 1994. Killing of primary CD4+ T cells by non-syncytium-inducing macrophage-tropic human immunodeficiency virus type 1. *Proc. Natl. Acad. Sci. USA* 91: 10237–10241.

4893. Yu, X., Y. Xin, Z. Matsuda, T. H. Lee, and M. Essex. 1992. The matrix protein of human immunodeficiency virus type 1 is required for incorporation of viral envelope protein into mature virions. *J. Virol.* 66:4966–4971.

4894. Yu, X., Y. Yu, B. Liu, K. Luo, W. Kong, P. Mao, and X.-F. Yu. 2003. Induction of APOBEC3G ubiquitination and degradation by an HIV-1 Vif-Cul5-SCF complex. *Science* 302:1056–1060.

4895. Yu, Y., M. Hagihara, K. Ando, B. Gansuvd, H. Matsuzawa, T. Tsuchiya, Y. Ueda, H. Inoue, T. Hotta, and S. Kato. 2001. Enhancement of human cord blood CD34+ cell-derived NK cell cytotoxicity by dendritic cells. *J. Immunol.* 166:1590–1600.

4896. Yu, Z., N. Sanchez-Velar, I. E. Catrina, E. L. Kittler, E. B. Udofia, and M. L. Zapp. 2005. The cellular HIV Rev cofactor hRIP is required for viral replication. *Proc. Natl. Acad. Sci. USA* 102:4027–4032.

4897. Yuen, M. H., M. P. Protti, O. B. Diethelm-Okita, L. Moiola, I. F. Howard, Jr., and B. M. Conti-Fine. 1995. Immunoregulatory CD8+ cells recognize antigen-activated CD4+ cells in myasthenia gravis patients and in healthy controls. *J. Immunol.* 154:1508–1520.

4898. Yuille, M., A. M. Hugunin, P. John, L. Peer, L. V. Sacks, B. Poiesz, R. H. Tomar, and A. E. Silverstone. 1988. HIV-1 infection abolishes CD4 biosynthesis but not CD4 mRNA. *J. Acquir. Immune Defic. Syndr.* 1:131–137.

4899. Yunis, N. A., and V. E. Stone. 1998. Cardiac manifestations of HIV/AIDS. *J. Acquir. Immune Defic. Syndr. Hum. Retrovirol.* 18:145–154.

4900. Yusibov, V., A. Modelska, K. Steplewski, M. Agadjanyan, D. Weiner, D. C. Hooper, and H. Koprowski. 1997. Antigens produced in plants by infection with chimeric plant viruses immunize against rabies virus and HIV-1. *Proc. Natl. Acad. Sci. USA* 94:5784–5788.

4901. Zachar, V., B. Spire, I. Hirsch, J. C. Chermann, and P. Ebbesen. 1991. Human transformed trophoblast-derived cells lacking CD4 receptor exhibit restricted permissiveness for human immunodeficiency virus type 1. *J. Virol.* 65:2102–2107.

4902. Zack, J., A. M. Haislip, P. Krogstad, and I. S. Y. Chen. 1992. Incompletely reverse-transcribed human immunodeficiency virus type 1 genomes in quiescent cells can function as intermediates in the retroviral life cycle. *J. Virol.* 66: 1717–1725.

4903. Zack, J. A., S. J. Arrigo, S. R. Weitsman, A. S. Go, A. Haislip, and I. S. Y. Chen. 1990. HIV-1 entry into quiescent primary lymphocytes: molecular analysis reveals a labile, latent viral structure. *Cell* 61:213–222.

4904. Zack, J. A., A. J. Cann, J. P. Lugo, and I. S. Y. Chen. 1988. HIV-1 production from infected peripheral blood T cells after HTLV-I induced mitogenic stimulation. *Science* 240:1026–1029.

4905. Zagury, D., J. Bernard, R. Cheynier, I. Desportes, R. Leonard, M. Fouchard, B. Reveil, D. Ittele, Z. Lurhuma, K. Mbayo, J. Wane, J.-J. Salaun, B. Goussard, L. Dechazal, A. Burny, P. Nara, and R. C. Gallo. 1988. A group specific anamnestic immune reaction against HIV-1 induced by a candidate vaccine against AIDS. *Nature* 332:728–731.

4906. Zagury, D., J. Bernard, J. Leibowitch, B. Safai, J. E. Groopman, M. Feldman, M. G. Sarngadharan, and R. C. Gallo. 1984. HTLV-III in cells cultured from semen of two patients with AIDS. *Science* 226:449–451.

4907. Zagury, D., J. Bernard, R. Leonard, R. Cheynier, M. Feldman, P. S. Sarin, and R. C. Gallo. 1986. Long-term cultures of HTLV-III-infected T cells: a model of cytopathology of T-cell depletion in AIDS. *Science* 231:850–853.

4908. Zaitseva, M., A. Blauvelt, S. Lee, C. K. Lapham, V. Klaus-Kovtum, H. Mostowski, M. J., and H. Golding. 1997. Expression and function of CCR5 and CXCR4 on human Langerhans cells and macrophages: implications for HIV primary infection. *Nat. Med.* 3:1369–1375.

4909. Zaki, S. R., R. Judd, L. M. Coffield, P. Greer, F. Rolston, and B. L. Evatt. 1992. Human papillomavirus infection and anal carcinoma. Retrospective analysis by in situ hybridization and the polymerase chain reaction. *Am. J. Pathol.* 140:1345–1355.

4910. Zamarchi, R., M. Panozzo, A. Del Mistro, A. Barelli, A. Borri, A. Amadori, and L. Chieco-Bianchi. 1994. B and T cell function parameters during zidovudine treatment of human immunodeficiency virus-infected patients. *J. Infect. Dis.* 170:1148–1156.

4911. Zamore, P. D., T. Tuschl, P. A. Sharp, and D. P. Bartel. 2000. RNAi: double-stranded RNA directs the ATP-dependent cleavage of mRNA at 21 to 23 nucleotide intervals. *Cell* 101:25–33.

4912. Zangerle, R., B. Widner, G. Quirchmair, G. Neurauter, M. Sarcletti, and D. Fuchs. 2002. Effective antiretroviral therapy reduces degradation of tryptophan in patients with HIV-1 infection. *Clin. Immunol.* 104:242–247.

4912a. Zanetti, M., and G. Franchini. 2006. T cell memory and protective immunity by vaccination: is more better? *Trends Immunol.* 27:511–517.

4913. Zanussi, S., M. D'Andrea, C. Simonelli, U. Tirelli, and P. De Paoli. 1996. Serum levels of RANTES and MIP-1α in HIV-

positive long-term survivors and progressor patients. *AIDS* 10:1431–1432.

4914. Zarling, J. M., J. A. Ledbetter, J. Sias, P. Fultz, J. Eichberg, G. Gjerset, and P. A. Moran. 1990. HIV-infected humans, but not chimpanzees, have circulating cytotoxic T lymphocytes that lyse uninfected CD4+ cells. *J. Immunol.* 144:2992–2998.

4915. Zauli, G., D. Gibellini, C. Celeghini, C. Mischiati, A. Bassini, M. La Placa, and S. Capitani. 1996. Pleiotropic effects of immobilized versus soluble recombinant HIV-1 Tat protein on CD3-mediated activation, induction of apoptosis, and HIV-1 long terminal repeat transactivation in purified CD4+ T lymphocytes. *J. Immunol.* 157:2216–2224.

4916. Zauli, G., D. Gibellini, D. Milani, M. Mazzoni, P. Borgatti, M. La Placa, and S. Capitani. 1993. Human immunodeficiency virus type 1 Tat protein protects lymphoid, epithelial, and neuronal cell lines from death by apoptosis. *Cancer Res.* 53:4481–4485.

4917. Zauli, G., M. C. Re, G. Furlini, M. Giovannini, and M. La Placa. 1992. Human immunodeficiency virus type 1 envelope glycoprotein gp120-mediated killing of human haematopoietic progenitors (CD34+ cells). *J. Gen. Virol.* 73:417–421.

4918. Zauli, G., M. C. Re, G. Visani, G. Furlini, and M. La Placa. 1992. Inhibitory effect of HIV-1 envelope glycoproteins gp120 and gp160 on the in vitro growth of enriched (CD34+) hematopoietic progenitor cells. *Arch. Virol.* 122:271–280.

4919. Zaunders, J. J., W. B. Dyer, B. Wang, M. L. Munier, M. Miranda-Saksena, R. Newton, J. Moore, C. R. Mackay, D. A. Cooper, N. K. Saksena, and A. D. Kelleher. 2004. Identification of circulating antigen-specific CD4+ T lymphocytes with a CCR5+, cytotoxic phenotype in an HIV-1 long-term nonprogressor and in CMV infection. *Blood* 103:2238–2247.

4919a. Zaunders, J. J., S. Ip, M. L. Munier, D. E. Kaufmann, K. Suzuki, C. Brereton, S. C. Sasson, N. Seddiki, K. Koelsch, A. Landay, P. Grey, R. Finlayson, J. Kaldor, E. S. Rosenberg, B. D. Walker, B. Fazekas de St. Groth, D. A. Cooper, and A. D. Kelleher. 2006. Infection of CD127+ (interleukin-7 receptor+) CD4+ cells and overexpression of CTLA-4 are linked to loss of antigen-specific CD4 T cells during primary human immunodeficiency virus type 1 infection. *J. Virol.* 80:10162–10172

4920. Zaunders, J. J., M. L. Munier, D. E. Kaufmann, S. Ip, P. Grey, D. Smith, T. Ramacciotti, D. Quan, R. Finlayson, J. Kaldor, E. S. Rosenberg, B. D. Walker, D. A. Cooper, and A. D. Kelleher. 2005. Early proliferation of CCR5(+) CD38(+++) antigen-specific CD4(+) Th1 effector cells during primary HIV-1 infection. *Blood* 106:1660–1667.

4921. Zazopoulos, E., and W. A. Haseltine. 1993. Disulfide bond formation in the human immunodeficiency virus type 1 Nef protein. *J. Virol.* 67:1676–1680.

4922. Zazopoulos, E., and W. A. Haseltine. 1993. Effect of nef alleles on replication of human immunodeficiency virus type 1. *Virology* 194:20–27.

4923. Zeballos, R. S., N. Cavalcante, C. A. Freire, H. J. Hernandez, I. M. Longo, Z. F. Peixinho, N. C. Moura, and N. F. Mendes. 1992. Delayed hypersensitivity skin tests in prognosis of human immunodeficiency virus infection. *J. Clin. Lab. Anal.* 6:119–122.

4924. Zeira, M., R. A. Byrn, and J. E. Groopman. 1990. Inhibition of serum-enhanced HIV-1 infection of U937 monocytoid cells by recombinant soluble CD4 and anti-CD4 monoclonal antibody. *AIDS Res. Hum. Retrovir.* 6:629–639.

4925. Zhang, D., P. Shankar, Z. Xu, B. Harnisch, G. Chen, C. Lange, S. J. Lee, H. Valdez, M. M. Lederman, and J. Lieberman. 2003. Most antiviral CD8 T cells during chronic viral infection do not express high levels of perforin and are not directly cytotoxic. *Blood* 101:226–235.

4926. Zhang, H., G. Dornadula, M. Beumont, L. Livornese, B. Van Uitert, K. Henning, and R. J. Pomerantz. 1998. Human immunodeficiency virus type 1 in the semen of men receiving highly active antiretroviral therapy. *N. Engl. J. Med.* 339: 1803–1809.

4927. Zhang, H., B. Yang, R. L. Pomerantz, C. Zhang, S. C. Arunachalam, and L. Gao. 2003. The cytidine deaminase CEM15 induces hypermutation in newly synthesized HIV-1 DNA. *Nature* 424:94–98.

4928. Zhang, H., Y. Zhang, T. P. Spicer, L. Z. Abbott, M. Abbott, and B. J. Poiesz. 1993. Reverse transcription takes place within extracellular HIV-1 virions: potential biological significance. *AIDS Res. Hum. Retrovir.* 9:1287–1296.

4929. Zhang, L., Y. Huang, H. Yuan, S. Tuttleton, and D. D. Ho. 1997. Genetic characterization of *vif, vpr,* and *vpu* sequences from long-term survivors of human immunodeficiency virus type 1 infection. *Virology* 228:340–349.

4930. Zhang, L., S. R. Lewin, M. Markowitz, H. H. Lin, E. Skulsky, R. Karanicolas, Y. He, X. Jin, S. Tuttleton, M. Vesanen, H. Spiegel, R. Kost, J. van Lunzen, H. J. Stellbrink, S. Wolinsky, W. Borkowsky, P. Palumbo, L. G. Kostrikis, and D. D. Ho. 1999. Measuring recent thymic emigrants in blood of normal and HIV-1-infected individuals before and after effective therapy. *J. Exp. Med.* 190:725–732.

4931. Zhang, L., B. Ramratnam, K. Tenner-Racz, Y. He, M. Vesanen, S. Lewin, A. Talal, P. Racz, A. S. Perelson, B. T. Korber, M. Markowitz, and D. D. Ho. 1999. Quantifying residual HIV-1 replication in patients receiving combination antiretroviral therapy. *N. Engl. J. Med.* 340:1605–1613.

4932. Zhang, L., W. Yu, T. He, J. Yu, R. E. Caffrey, E. A. Dalmasso, S. Fu, T. Pham, J. Mei, J. J. Ho, W. Zhang, P. Lopez, and D. D. Ho. 2002. Contribution of human alpha defensin 1, 2 and 3 to the anti-HIV-1 activity of CD8 antiviral factor. *Science* 298:995–1000.

4933. Zhang, R., J. D. Lifson, and C. Chougnet. 2006. Failure of HIV-exposed CD4+ T cells to activate dendritic cells is reversed by restoration of CD40/CD154 interactions. *Blood* 107:1989–1995.

4934. Zhang, R. D., M. Guan, Y. Park, R. Tawadros, J. Y. Yang, B. Gold, B. Wu, and E. E. Henderson. 1997. Synergy between human immunodeficiency virus type 1 and Epstein-Barr virus in T lymphoblastoid cell lines. *AIDS Res. Hum. Retrovir.* 13:161–171.

4935. Zhang, X., S. Sun, I. Hwang, D. F. Tough, and J. Sprent. 1998. Potent and selective stimulation of memory-phenotype CD8+ T cells in vivo by IL-15. *Immunity* 8:591–599.

4936. Zhang, Y., B. Lou, R. B. Lal, A. Gettie, P. A. Marx, and J. P. Moore. 2000. Use of inhibitors to evaluate coreceptor usage by simian and simian/human immunodeficiency viruses and human immunodeficiency virus type 2 in primary cells. *J. Virol.* 74:6893–6910.

4937. Zhang, Y. M., S. C. Dawson, D. Landsman, H. C. Lane, and N. P. Salzman. 1994. Persistence of four related human immunodeficiency virus subtypes during the course of zidovudine therapy: relationship between virion RNA and proviral DNA. *J. Virol.* 68:425–432.

4938. Zhang, Z., T. Schuler, M. Zupancic, S. Wietgrefe, K. A. Staskus, K. A. Reimann, T. A. Reinhart, M. Rogan, W. Cavert, C. J. Miller, R. S. Veazey, D. Notermans, S. Little, S. A. Danner, D. D. Richman, D. Havlir, J. Wong, H. L. Jordan, T. W. Schacker, P. Racz, K. Tenner-Racz, N. L. Letvin, S. Wolinsky, and A. T. Haase. 1999. Sexual transmission and propagation of SIV and HIV in resting and activated CD4(+) T cells. *Science* 286:1353–1357.

4939. Zhang, Z.-Q., D. W. Notermans, G. Sedgewick, W. Cavert, S. Wietgrefe, M. Zupancic, K. Gebhard, K. Henry, L. Boies, Z. Chen, M. Jenkins, R. Mills, H. McDade, C. Goodwin, C. M. Schuwirth, S. A. Danner, and A. T. Haase. 1998. Kinetics of CD4+ T cell repopulation of lymphoid tissues after treatment of HIV-1 infection. *Proc. Natl. Acad. Sci. USA* 95:1154–1159.

4940. Zhang, Z.-Q., S. W. Wietgrefe, Q. Li, M. D. Shore, L. Duan, C. Reilly, J. D. Lifson, and A. T. Haase. 2004. Roles of substrate availability and infection of resting and activated CD4+ T cells in transmission and acute simian immunodeficiency virus infection. *Proc. Natl. Acad. Sci. USA* 101:5640–5645.

4941. Zhang, Z. Q., T. Schuler, W. Cavert, D. W. Notermans, K. Gebhard, K. Henry, D. V. Havlir, H. F. Gunthard, J. K. Wong, S. Little, M. B. Feinberg, M. A. Polis, L. K. Schrager, T. W. Schacker, D. D. Richman, L. Corey, S. A. Danner, and A. T. Haase. 1999. Reversibility of the pathological changes in the follicular dendritic cell network with treatment of HIV-1 infection. *Proc. Natl. Acad. Sci. USA* 96:5169–5172.

4941a. Zhao, D. M., A. M. Thornton, R. J. DiPaolo, and E. M. Shevach. 2006. Activated CD4+CD25+ T cells selectively kill B lymphocytes. *Blood* 107:3925–3932.

4942. Zhao, Q., L. Ma, S. Jiang, H. Lu, S. Liu, Y. He, N. Strick, N. Neamati, and A. K. Debnath. 2005. Identification of N-phenyl-N'-(2,2,6,6-tetramethyl-piperidin-4-yl)-oxalamides as a new class of HIV-1 entry inhibitors that prevent gp120 binding to CD4. *Virology* 339:213–225.

4943. Zhao, S., W. Li, G. Dornadula, D. Dicker, J. Hoxie, S. C. Peiper, R. J. Pomerantz, and L. Duan. 1998. Chemokine receptors and the molecular basis for human immunodeficiency virus type 1 entry into peripheral hematopoietic stem cells and their progeny. *J. Infect. Dis.* 178:1623–1634.

4944. Zheng, N. N., N. B. Kiviat, P. S. Sow, S. E. Hawes, A. Wilson, H. Diallo-Agne, C. W. Critchlow, G. S. Gottlieb, L. Musey, and M. J. McElrath. 2004. Comparison of human immunodeficiency virus (HIV)-specific-T-cell responses in HIV-1- and HIV-2-infected individuals in Senegal. *J. Virol.* 78:13934–13942.

4945. Zheng, N. N., P. W. McQueen, L. Hurren, L. A. Evans, M. G. Law, S. Forde, S. Barker, D. A. Cooper, and S. F. Delaney. 1996. Changes in biologic phenotype of human immunodeficiency virus during treatment of patients with didanosine. *J. Infect. Dis.* 173:1092–1096.

4946. Zheng, Y., D. Irwin, T. Kurosu, K. Tokunaga, T. Sata, and B. M. Peterlin. 2004. Human APOBEC3F is another host factor that blocks human immunodeficiency virus type 1 replication. *J. Virol.* 78:6073–6076.

4947. Zheng, Y.-H., A. Plemenitas, A. J. Fielding, and B. M. Peterlin. 2003. Nef increases the synthesis of and transports cholesterol to lipid rafts and HIV-1 progeny virions. *Proc. Natl. Acad. Sci. USA* 100:8460–8465.

4948. Zhou, E.-M., K. L. Lohman, and R. C. Kennedy. 1990. Administration of noninternal image monoclonal anti-idiotypic antibodies induces idiotype-restricted responses specific for human immunodeficiency virus envelope glycoprotein epitopes. *Virology* 174:9–17.

4949. Zhou, J. Y., and D. C. Montefiori. 1997. Antibody-mediated neutralization of primary isolates of human immunodeficiency virus type 1 in peripheral blood mononuclear cells is not affected by the initial activation state of the cells. *J. Virol.* 71:2512–2517.

4950. Zhou, N., X. Fan, M. Mukhtar, J. Fang, C. A. Patel, G. C. DuBois, and R. J. Pomerantz. 2003. Cell-cell fusion and internalization of the CNS-based, HIV-1 coreceptor, APJ. *Virology* 307:2003.

4951. Zhou, P., S. Goldstein, K. Devadas, D. Tewart, and A. L. Notkins. 1997. Human CD4+ cells transfected with IL-16 cDNA are resistant to HIV-1 infection: inhibition of mRNA expression. *Nat. Med.* 3:659–664.

4952. Zhou, Y., H. Zhang, J. D. Siliciano, and R. F. Siliciano. 2005. Kinetics of human immunodeficiency virus type 1 decay following entry into resting CD8+ T cells. *J. Virol.* 79:2199–2210.

4953. Zhu, P., E. Chertova, J. Bess, J. D. Lifson, A. O. Arthur, J. Liu, K. A. Taylor, and K. H. Roux. 2003. Electron tomography analysis of envelope glycoprotein trimers on HIV and simian immunodeficiency virus virions. *Proc. Natl. Acad. Sci. USA* 100:15812–15817.

4954. Zhu, P., J. Liu, J. Bess, Jr., E. Chertova, J. D. Lifson, H. Grise, G. A. Ofek, K. A. Taylor, and K. H. Roux. 2006. Distribution and three-dimensional structure of AIDS virus envelope spikes. *Nature* 441:847–852.

4955. Zhu, T., L. Corey, Y. Hwangbo, J. M. Lee, G. H. Learn, J. I. Mullins, and M. J. McElrath. 2003. Persistence of extraordinarily low levels of genetically homogeneous human immunodeficiency virus type 1 in exposed seronegative individuals. *J. Virol.* 77:6108–6116.

4956. Zhu, T., B. T. Korber, A. J. Nahmias, E. Hooper, P. M. Sharp, and D. D. Ho. 1998. An African HIV-1 sequence from 1959 and implications for the origin of the epidemic. *Nature* 391:594–597.

4957. Zhu, T., H. Mo, N. Wang, D. S. Nam, Y. Cao, R. A. Koup, and D. D. Ho. 1993. Genotypic and phenotypic characterization of HIV-1 in patients with primary infection. *Science* 261:1179–1181.

4958. Zhu, T., N. Wang, A. Carr, D. S. Nam, R. Moor-Jankowski, D. A. Cooper, and D. D. Ho. 1996. Genetic characterization of human immunodeficiency virus type 1 in blood and genital secretions: evidence for viral compartmentalization and selection during sexual transmission. *J. Virol.* 70:3098–3107.

4959. Zhu, T., N. Wang, A. Carr, S. Wolinsky, and D. D. Ho. 1995. Evidence for coinfection by multiple strains of human immunodeficiency virus type 1 subtype B in an acute seroconvertor. *J. Virol.* 69:1324–1327.

4960. Zhu, Z. H., S. S. L. Chen, and A. S. Huang. 1990. Phenotypic mixing between human immunodeficiency virus and vesicular stomatitis virus or herpes simplex virus. *J. Acquir. Immune Defic. Syndr.* 3:215–219.

4961. Zhuang, J., A. E. Jetzt, G. Sun, H. Yu, G. Klarmann, Y. Ron, B. D. Preston, and J. P. Dougherty. 2002. Human immunodeficiency virus type 1 recombination: rate, fidelity, and putative hot spots. *J. Virol.* 76:11273–11282.

4962. Ziegler, J. B., D. A. Cooper, R. O. Johnson, and J. Gold. 1985. Postnatal transmission of AIDS-associated retrovirus from mother to infant. *Lancet* i:896–898.

4963. Ziegler, J. L. 1993. Endemic Kaposi's sarcoma in Africa and local volcanic soils. *Lancet* 342:1348–1351.

4964. Ziegler, J. L., J. A. Beckstead, P. A. Volberding, D. I. Abrams, A. M. Levine, R. J. Lukes, P. S. Gill, R. L. Burkes, P. R. Meyer, C. E. Metroka, J. Mouradian, A. Moore, S. A. Riggs, J. J. Butler, F. C. Caranillas, E. Hersh, G. R. Newell, L. J. Laubenstein, D. Knowles, C. Odajnyk, B. Raphael, B. Koziner, C. Urmacher, and B. D. Clarkson. 1984. Non-Hodgkin's lymphoma in 90 homosexual men. Relation to generalized lymphadenopathy and the acquired immunodeficiency syndrome. *N. Engl. J. Med.* 311:565–570.

4965. Ziegler, J. L., W. L. Drew, and R. C. Miner. 1982. Outbreak of Burkitt's-like lymphoma in homosexual men. *Lancet* ii:631–633.

4966. Ziegler, J. L., and D. P. Stites. 1986. Hypothesis: AIDS is an autoimmune disease directed at the immune system and triggered by a lymphotropic retrovirus. *Clin. Immunol. Immunopathol.* 41:305–313.

4967. Ziegler, J. L., A. C. Templeton, and G. L. Voegel. 1984. Kaposi's sarcoma: a comparison of classical, endemic, and epidemic forms. *Semin. Oncol.* 11:47–52.

4968. Zimmerli, S. C., A. Harari, C. Cellerai, F. Vallelian, P. A. Bart, and G. Pantaleo. 2005. HIV-1-specific IFN-gamma/IL-2-secreting CD8 T cells support CD4-independent proliferation of HIV-1-specific CD8 T cells. *Proc. Natl. Acad. Sci. USA* 102:7239–7244.

4969. Zimmerman, E. S., J. Chen, J. L. Andersen, O. Ardon, J. L. Dehart, J. Blackett, S. K. Choudhary, D. Camerini, P. Nghiem, and V. Planelles. 2004. Human immunodeficiency virus type 1 Vpr-mediated G2 arrest requires Rad17 and Hus1 and induces nuclear BRCA1 and gamma-H2AX focus formation. *Mol. Cell. Biol.* 24:9286–9294.

4970. Zimmerman, P. A., A. Buckler-White, G. Alkhatib, T. Spalding, J. Kubofcik, C. Combadiere, D. Weissman, O. Cohen, A. Rubbert, G. Lam, M. Vaccarezza, E. A. Kennedy, A. S. Fauci, T. B. Nutman, and P. M. Murphy. 1997. Inherited resistance to HIV-1 conferred by an inactivating mutation in CC chemokine receptor 5: studies in populations with contrasting clinical phenotypes, defined racial background, and quantified risk. *Mol. Med.* 3:23–36.

4971. Zinkernagel, R. M., and H. Hengartner. 1994. T-cell-mediated immunopathology versus direct cytolysis by virus: implications for HIV and AIDS. *Immunol. Today* 15:262–268.

4972. Ziza, J. M., F. Brun-Vezinet, A. Venet, C. H. Rouzioux, J. Traversat, B. Israel-Biet, F. Barre-Sinoussi, J. C. Chermann, and P. Godeau. 1985. Lymphadenopathy virus isolated from bronchoalveolar lavage fluid in AIDS-related complex with lymphoid interstitial pneumonitis. *N. Engl. J. Med.* 313:183–186.

4973. Zlotnik, A., and O. Yoshie. 2000. Chemokines: a new classification system and their role in immunity. *Immunity* 12:121–127.

4974. Zocchi, M. R., A. Rubartelli, P. Morgavi, and A. Poggi. 1998. HIV-1 Tat inhibits human natural killer cell function by blocking L-type calcium channels. *J. Immunol.* 161:2938–2943.

4975. Zoeteweij, J. P., H. Golding, H. Mostowski, and A. Blauvelt. 1998. Cytokines regulate expression and function of the HIV coreceptor CXCR4 on human mature dendritic cells. *J. Immunol.* 161:3219–3223.

4976. Zolla-Pazner, S., and M. K. Gorny. 1992. Passive immunization for the prevention and treatment of HIV infection. *AIDS* 6:1235–1247.

4977. Zolla-Pazner, S., and S. Sharpe. 1995. A resting cell assay for improved detection of antibody-mediated neutralization of HIV type 1 primary isolates. *AIDS Res. Human Retrovir.* 11:1449–1458.

4978. Zong, J., D. M. Ciufo, R. Viscidi, L. Alagiozoglou, S. Tyring, P. Rady, J. Orenstein, W. Boto, H. Kalumbuja, N. Romano, M. Melbye, G. H. Kang, C. Boshoff, and G. S. Hayward. 2002. Genotypic analysis at multiple loci across Kaposi's sarcoma herpesvirus (KSHV) DNA molecules: clustering patterns, novel variants and chimerism. *J. Clin. Virol.* 23:119–148.

4979. Zou, W., A. Dulioust, R. Fior, I. Durand-Gasselin, F. Boue, P. Galanaud, and D. Emilie. 1997. Increased T-helper-type 2 cytokine production in chronic HIV infection is due to interleukin (IL)-13 rather than IL-4. *AIDS* 11:533–534.

4980. Zou, W., A. Foussat, S. Houhou, I. Durand-Gasselin, A. Dulioust, L. Bouchet, P. Galanaud, Y. Levy, and D. Emilie. 1999. Acute upregulation of CCR-5 expression by CD4+ T lymphocytes in HIV-infected patients treated with interleukin 2. *AIDS* 13:455–463.

4981. Zubiaga, A. M., E. Munoz, and B. T. Huber. 1992. IL-4 and IL-2 selectively rescue Th cell subsets from glucocorticoid-induced apoptosis. *J. Immunol.* 149:107–112.

4982. Zucker-Franklin, D., and Y. Z. Cao. 1989. Megakaryocytes of human immunodeficiency virus-infected individuals express viral RNA. *Proc. Natl. Acad. Sci. USA* 86:5595–5599.

4983. Zuckerman, R. A., W. L. H. Whittington, C. L. Celum, T. K. Collis, A. J. Lucchetti, J. L. Sanchez, J. P. Hughes, J. L. Sanchez, and R. W. Coombs. 2004. Higher concentrations of HIV RNA in rectal mucosa secretions than in blood and seminal plasma, among men who have sex with men, independent of antiretroviral therapy. *J. Infect. Dis.* 190:156–161.

4984. Zufferey, R., D. Nagy, R. J. Mandel, L. Naldini, and D. Trono. 1997. Multiply attenuated lentiviral vector achieves efficient gene delivery in vivo. *Nat. Biotechnol.* 15:871–875.

4985. zur Hausen, H. 1991. Human papillomaviruses in the pathogenesis of anogenital cancer. *Virology* 184:9–13.

4986. zur Hausen, H. 2000. Papillomaviruses causing cancer: evasion from host-cell control in early events in carcinogenesis. *J. Natl. Cancer Inst.* 92:690–698.

4987. zur Megede, J., M. C. Chen, B. Doe, M. Schaefer, C. E. Greer, M. Selby, G. R. Otten, and S. W. Barnett. 2000. Increased expression and immunogenicity of sequence-modified human immunodeficiency virus type 1 *gag* gene. *J. Virol.* 74:2628–2635.

4988. Zwick, M. B. 2005. The membrane-proximal external region of HIV-1 gp41: a vaccine target worth exploring. *AIDS* 19:1725–1737.

4989. Zylberberg, H., and S. Pol. 1996. Reciprocal interactions between human immunodeficiency virus and hepatitis C virus infections. *Clin. Infect. Dis.* 23:1117–1125.

Index

Abacavir, hypersensitivity to, 372
Abrams, Donald I., 213f
Activation, 146–147, 175, 269, 346
Acute HIV infection, 79–87
  antibody production in, 86
  CD4$^+$ cell count in, 433
  CD8$^+$ cell response in, 272–273
  cellular immune response in, 84–86, 84f
  cerebrospinal fluid viral load in, 187
  clinical manifestations of, 80–81, 80t
  definition of, 81
  immunologic findings in, 80t, 82–83
  laboratory findings in, 80t, 81–82, 82t
  natural killer cells in, 229
  postinfection immunization for, 390
  rapid course of, 80
  seroconversion in, 85f, 86
  structured interrupted drug therapy for, 393
  treatment of, 373–375
  viral characteristics and levels in, 83–84, 296
Acute retroviral syndrome, 79–80, 80t; see Acute HIV infection
Adaptive immune system, see also Immune system
  components of, 210t, see also specific components
  vs. innate immune system, 210, 210t, 211f
  in vaccine response, 398–399
Adefovir dipivoxil, 366
Adenovirus, in vaccine development, 409–410, 424
Adhesion molecules
  in neutralizing antibody sensitivity, 244–245
  in viral entry, 71–72, 71t
Adjuvants, for vaccines, 418–420, 418t
Adrenal gland, HIV infection of, 306
Age as a factor, 338–339
Aging, see Telomere
AIDS viruses, discovery of, 1–5, 3t
Alloimmunogens, as vaccine adjuvants, 420
Aluminum phosphate, as vaccine adjuvant, 419
Aluminum sulfate, as vaccine adjuvant, 419
Amman, Arthur J., 252f
Amniotic fluid, viral load in, 28t, 39
Amprenavir, resistance to, 378
Amyloid deposition, 183–184
Anal carcinoma, 310–312, 311f–313f, 311t
Antagonism, T cell receptor, 422
Antibody(ies)
  antilymphocyte, 175
  detune assay, 81
  in autoimmunity, see Autoimmunity HIV, 6, 6f, 8
    in acute infection, 80t, 81–82, 82t, 86
antibody-dependent cell-mediated toxicity and, 227, 251–253
  in breast milk, 38
  vs. clinical stage, 237–238
  complement-fixing, 253
  detection of, 237–238
  enhancing, 247–251, 247f–251f, 421
  isotypes of, 238
  neutralizing, see Neutralizing antibodies
  for passive immunotherapy, 390–391
  HIV type 2, type 2, 6, 6f, 8
  in saliva, 81
  Tat protein, 231
  in vaginal fluids, 42
Antibody-dependent cell-mediated toxicity (ADCC), 227, 251–253
Antibody-dependent cytotoxicity (ADC), 253
Antibody-dependent enhancement (ADE), 247–251, 247f, 421
  clinical relevance of, 250–251
  vs. clinical stage, 247–248, 248f
  mechanisms of, 248–249
  vs. neutralizing antibodies, 248f, 251
  in non-HIV viral infections, 250–251
  in vaccine development, 421
  viral epitope determinants of, 249–250, 249f–251f

Note: Page numbers followed by *f* indicate illustrations; those followed by *t* indicate tables.